Handbook of
ADULT PRIMARY CARE

Handbook of ADULT PRIMARY CARE

Carla Greene, FNP, PA-C, ***Editor***

Ossining Open Door Health Center
Ossining, New York

Robert W. Singer, MD, ***General Consultant***

ILLUSTRATED BY MASAKO HERMAN

A Wiley Medical Publication

JOHN WILEY & SONS

New York / Chichester / Brisbane / Toronto / Singapore

Notice

Medicine is an ever-changing science. As new research and clinical experience broaden our knowledge, changes in treatment and drug therapy are required. The editors and the publisher of this work have made every effort to ensure that the drug dosage schedules herein are accurate and in accord with the standards accepted at the time of publication. Readers are advised, however, to check the product information sheet included in the package of each drug they plan to administer to be certain that changes have not been made in the recommended dose or in the contraindications for administration. This recommendation is of particular importance in regard to new or infrequently used drugs.

Library of Congress Cataloging in Publication Data:

Handbook of adult primary care.

(A Wiley medical publication)
Includes bibliographies.
1. Nursing—Handbooks, manuals, etc. 2. Medicine, Clinical—Handbooks, manuals, etc. 3. Nurse practitioners—Handbooks, manuals, etc. 4. Physicians' assistants—Handbooks, manuals, etc. I. Greene, Carla, 1946– . II. Series. [DNLM: 1. Primary Health Care—nurses' instruction. W 84.6 H236]
RT51.H34 1987 610.73 86–24577
ISBN 0-471-09621-0

Printed in the United States of America

10 9 8 7 6 5 4 3 2 1

To Doug, Craig, and Matt

Contributors and Consultants

CONTRIBUTORS

BARRIGAR–HORNIBROOK, JUDY, BA, *Office Manager, Bruce Heckman, MD, Ossining, New York*

DONIUS, MARY ALICE HIGGINS, RN, BSN, MED, *Director, Undergraduate Program, Columbia University School of Nursing, New York, New York*

FRIEDMAN, BONNIE JONES, RN, ANP, MS, MED, *Assistant Professor, University of North Carolina, Chapel Hill School of Nursing, Adult Nurse Practitioner, Health Maintenance Clinic, North Carolina Memorial Hospital, Chapel Hill, North Carolina*

GREIG, ANN ELIZABETH, MSN, RNC, *Assistant Professor of Nursing, Yale University School of Nursing, Family Nurse Practitioner, Yale–New Haven Hospital, New Haven, Connecticut*

MAIN, CONNIE, BA, *Surgical Assistant, Alan Cohen, DMD, Ossining, New York*

MCTIGUE, MARY, BSN, *Manager of Health Services, Ossining Open Door Health Center, Ossining, New York*

RICH, ELLEN, MS, RNC, FNP, *Clinical Director, Pace University Health Care Unit, Briarcliff, New York*

GENERAL CONSULTANT

ROBERT W. SINGER, MD, *Instructor of Medicine, New York Medical College, Department of Medicine, Attending Physician, Stamford Hospital, Stamford, Connecticut*

CONSULTANTS

Robert P. Bauer, MD, FACS, *Clinical Instructor, Ophthalmology, New York University Medical Center, New York, New York*

Howard Gordon, DDS, *Dental Director, Ossining Open Door Health Center, Ossining, New York*

Katherine Irish, RDH, *Supervisor of Dental Staff, Ossining Open Door Health Center, Ossining, New York*

Weslee Neary McGovern, RN, MA, *Lecturer, Lehman College, City University of New York, New York, New York*

Denise Turnbull, RD, *Manopac, New York*

Preface

The *Handbook of Adult Primary Care* is a clinical reference for primary care providers. It has been written by and is intended for use by nurse practitioners and physician's assistants. Community health nurses will also find this an invaluable reference for everyday practice.

The book is divided into 13 chapters according to body systems. For clinical usefulness, the divisions have been carefully selected to reflect specialty areas for referral. For instance, rather than deal with the mouth (the province of dental specialists and oral surgeons) under the gastrointestinal system (gastroenterologists and general surgeons), separate chapters were developed. The chapters are (1) Eye, (2) Ear, Nose, and Throat, (3) Mouth, (4) Gastrointestinal Tract, (5) Body Nutrients and the Liver, (6) Cardiopulmonary System, (7) Blood and Immunology, (8) Urinary Tract, (9) Reproductive Tract, (10) Skin, (11) Musculoskeletal System, (12) Central Nervous System and Hormone Control, and (13) Psychology.

To emphasize primary care concepts of health, the developmental organization of each chapter is based on normal anatomy and physiology. Clinical problems or considerations are introduced at relevant points in the discussion of anatomy and physiology and are set in boldface italic type for reference. By progressing from normal to abnormal, the etiologic background is naturally established. Information is then provided about how the problem can be recognized and what needs to be done about it. Guidelines for referral are offered and general treatment is outlined. Details of management can be found in a special section at the end of the chapter for any problem marked with an arrowhead symbol in the text.

For each problem in the Details of Management section, four areas are considered: (1) Laboratory tests—those tests advised before initiating therapy. (2) Treatment measures—specific instructions for medications and other therapeutic interventions (heat, cold, exercise, diet, relaxation techniques). Names of medications are used instead of drug classifications in order to be as specific as possible about prescribing instructions. The drug of choice is listed first, and an alternative is given to cover the possibility of allergies. (3) Patient education—any special information that the patient should know about the problem and its treatment, including preventive measures and signs and symptoms that warrant concern. (4) Follow up—guidelines for return visits and referrals.

In addition to normal anatomy and physiology, the text includes information on all problems that may be encountered in primary care settings. An effort has been made to discuss significant conditions, such as dental caries, refractive errors, obesity, and alcoholism, that tend to be ignored by general practitioners. For purposes of patient teaching, relatively benign conditions have been considered as well. Examples are sebaceous cysts, colds, insect bites, and subconjunctival hemorrhage. Changes accompanying aging are also noted.

Preventive health measures are also discussed where relevant. For example, tetanus immunization follows the section on tetanus poisoning and testicular self-exam, the section on testicular cancer. General nutrition is covered in Chapter 6, and special diet requirements are covered for specific problems under each system. Extensive information on family planning appears in Chapter 9.

Problems are introduced at a point of reference that best explains the pathophysiology involved. *This approach must not be confused with any attempt to classify disorders*. Furthermore, it may not always be clear-cut, particularly if the problem affects several systems or is poorly understood.

Readers are referred to other sources for comprehensive information concerning prenatal care and obstetrics. Extremely rare problems have been omitted or mentioned in passing. In order to concentrate on adult primary care, information specific to children and adolescents has also been omitted.

Material has been *deliberately integrated* to preclude a "cookbook" approach to health care. The authors have chosen this format because they believe that knowledge of normal anatomy and physiology is crucial to the recognition and far-sighted management of health problems.

CARLA GREENE

Contents

List of Tables

Iris and Pupil

Albinism
Heterochromia
Miotic pupil
Mydriatic pupil
Anisocoria
Abnormal pupil shape
Anterior uveitis
Cyclitis
Iritis
Iridocyclitis
Posterior uveitis
Chorioretinitis
Panuveitis

Retina and Vitreous

▶ Night blindness as early symptom of Vitamin A deficiency
Color blindness
Tritan (blue)/tetartan (yellow) deficiency
Protan (red)/deutran (green) deficiency
Achromatopsia
Retinal dystrophies and degeneration
Retinitis pigmentosa
▶ Screening far visual acuity
Macular degeneration
Floaters
Retinal detachment
Retinal holes and tears
Photopsia
Metamorphopsia

Optic Nerve

"Asymmetric cupping"
Papilledema
Pseudopapilledema
Papillitis
Ischemic optic neuropathy
Optic neuritis
Retrobulbar neuritis
Uhthoff's syndrome
Optic atrophy
Consecutive optic atrophy
Heterofamilial optic atrophy
Glaucomatous atrophy

Retinal Blood Vessels

Retrolental fibroplasia
Copper and silver wiring
Crossing defects
Macroaneurysms
Hemorrhages and exudates
Microaneurysms
Neovascular fronds
Diabetic retinopathy
Hypertensive retinopathy
Arterial occlusions
Amaurosis fugax
Hollenhorst plaque
Central retinal artery occlusion
Retinal branch vein occlusion
Central retinal venous occlusion
Hemorrhagic retinopathy

VISION

Refraction and Accommodation

Astigmatism
Myopia
▶ Screening far visual acuity
Hyperopia
Presbyopia
▶ Screening near visual acuity
Hard contact lenses
Contact lens overuse syndrome
Contact lens abrasion
Soft contact lenses
Cataract
Nuclear cataract
Posterior subcapsular cataracts
Monocular diplopia
Leukocoria
After cataract
▶ Considerations for post-cataract surgery
Aphakia
Dislocated lens
Hereditary lens dislocation
Traumatic lens dislocation
Iridodonesis

Binocular Vision

Visual field defects
Bitemporal/homonymous defects
Nystagmus
Strabismus
Diplopia
Anisometropia

Amblyopia
Palsy/ophthalmoplegia
Monocular vision
Blindness, near blindness, automobile blindness
▶ Organizations for the blind
▶ Extending courtesies to the visually handicapped

PROTECTIVE FEATURES

Orbits

Exophthalmos
Ophthalmic Graves' disease
Orbital cellulitis
Cavernous sinus thrombosis

Conjunctiva

▶ Nongonococcal bacterial conjunctivitis
Gonococcal conjunctivitis
Viral conjunctivitis
Allergic conjunctivitis
Vernal conjunctivitis
Subconjunctival hemorrhage
Pingueculae
Pterygiums

Eyelids

▶ Contact dermatitis of eyelids
Xanthelasma
Ptosis
Ectropion
Entropion
Trichiasis
Districhiasis
▶ Sty (hordeolum)
▶ Acute blepharitis
▶ Chronic seborrheic blepharitis
▶ Acute meibomianitis
▶ Chalazion

Tears

Dry eye syndrome
Dacryostenosis
Dacryocystitis

Reflexes

Eye injuries
▶ First aid for eye injuries
Chemical burns
Blowout fracture
Black eye
Impaled foreign body
Abrasion
Laceration
Perforation
Superficial foreign body
Rust ring
▶ Eye safety practices

EYEBALL

The eyeball (Fig. 1.1) is a triple-layered sac with an outer coat made up of the sclera and the cornea. A middle coat is formed by the choroid, the ciliary body, the iris, and the pupil opening. To early anatomists, this dark maroon layer attached to the optic nerve looked like a grape skin, or "uvea," hanging from its stalk, hence the term "uveal tract." The innermost coat is the retina, containing the photoreceptors (rods and cones) and a tiny area of specialized cones (the macula). Supported by a gel-like substance (the vitreous fluid), the retina covers the back or "fundus" of the eyeball. Emerging near the center of the fundus are the optic nerve and retinal blood vessels.

Sclera

The sclera is a dense supporting membrane whose posterior portion extends into the bony socket, inaccessible to direct inspection. The anterior portion is readily visible and is referred to as the "white of the eye" even though color variations are common.

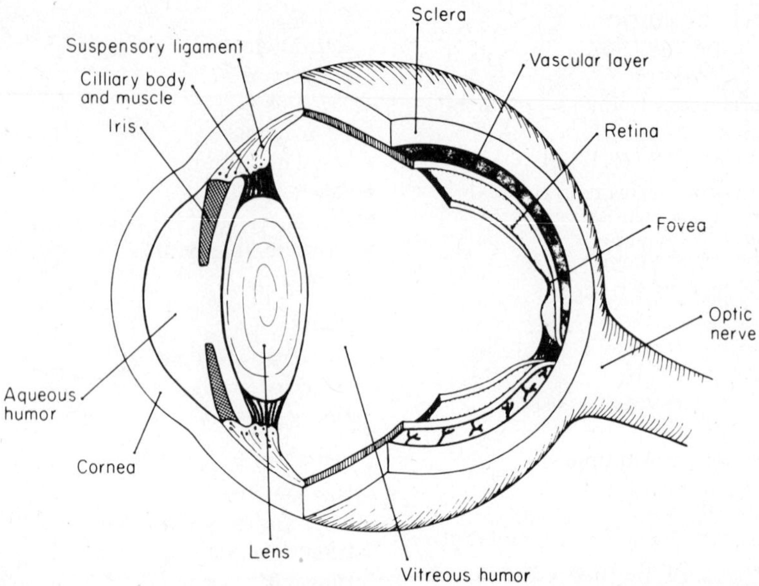

Figure 1.1 Eyeball showing three layers: outermost (sclera and cornea), uveal tract (choroid, ciliary body, iris, pupil), and retina and optic nerve. (From Snyder, M., *A Guide to Neurological and Neurosurgical Nursing,* © 1983, John Wiley and Sons, Inc., New York.)

Small translucent patches of gray develop from ***hyaline degeneration*** with aging. They are both asymptomatic and benign. Pigmented cells in dark-skinned people and fat deposits in older people give the appearance of ***muddy sclera.*** Jaundice leads to yellowing called ***scleral icterus*** (a misnomer in that it is the conjunctiva that stains with bile pigment when the total serum bilirubin exceeds 2.5–3.0 mg%). Icterus occurs with liver, gallbladder, or hemolytic diseases, as discussed in Chapters 5 and 7.

If very thin, the sclera reveals underlying uveal pigment and appears bluish. This is normal in infancy but could signal abnormal thinning of the membrane in adults, called ***scleromalacia.*** Scleromalacia is seen in a number of collagen disorders (osteogenesis imperfecta, Ehlers-Danlos syndrome, pseudoxanthoma elasticum, Marfan's syndrome, pseudohypoparathyroidism) and with congenital anomalies (keratoconus, keratoglobus). It may be associated with scleritis or prolonged use of steroids. Sometimes portions of the underlying uvea pop through the thinning areas and form a painless blue bulge known as ***staphyloma.*** Patients with scleromalacia or staphyloma should be referred to an ophthalmologist for careful observation. Extreme cases could lead to perforation of the globe.

Scleritis may be secondary to granulomatous disease, metabolic disturbances, infections, and irritants, as noted in Table 1.1. However, it usually signals the onset or exacerbation of vasculitis in collagen disease. Inflammation involves the anterior portion of the membrane 95% of the time ***(anterior scleritis),*** being limited to posterior segments ***(posterior scleritis)*** only in extremely rare cases. Anterior scleritis is characterized by multiple, exquisitely tender nodules that sometimes

TABLE 1.1 CONDITIONS ASSOCIATED WITH SCLERITIS

Rheumatoid disorders	Infectious processes
Ankylosing spondylitis	Tuberculosis
Rheumatoid arthritis	Syphilis
Periarteritis nodosa	Leprosy
Relapsing polychondritis	Onchocerciasis (river blindness)
Wegener's granulomatosis	Herpes zoster
Systemic lupus erythematosus	Herpes simplex
Active rheumatic heart disease	Coccidioidomycosis
Psoriatic arthritis	Mumps
Inflammatory bowel disease	Other conditions
Behcet's disease	Gout
Sjögren's syndrome	Thyrotoxicosis
Sarcoidosis	Burns (radiation, thermal, chemical)
Reiter's syndrome	Traumatic injuries

coalesce near the limbus. An area of yellow exudate appears at the center of the nodules and may eventually break down, sloughing necrotic tissue ***(nodular necrotizing scleritis).*** In some cases, focal nodules develop initially, followed by widespread granulation and thickening of the entire sclera as well as the cornea and anterior uveal tract ***(brawny scleritis).*** Rare cases are typified by painless thinning of the membrane and eventual perforation ***(scleromalacia perforans).*** The various types of scleritis are described more fully in Table 1.2. Because the ciliary nerves remain intact, most patients with scleritis have persistent and excruciating eye pain. Depending on the location of the inflammation, they may have uveitis or corneal and fundus changes. Limited movements of the eyelids and extraocular muscles may occur with posterior scleritis. In addition to eye symptoms, flare-up of underlying disease is the rule. In fact, the development of scleritis in patients with rheumatoid arthritis is an ominous sign, concurring with a high rate of fatal cardiopulmonary complications. In one rheumatoid study, patients with ocular involvement had a mortality rate of 46% compared to 18% for other patients. Since successful treatment depends on controlling systemic disease as well as its ocular manifestations, care is best coordinated by rheumatoid and eye specialists. Steroids, as well as immunosuppressive and nonsteroidal antiinflammatory drugs, may be needed. Scleral patch grafting may be undertaken for impending perforation. Intraocular alcohol injections or even enucleation are required in extreme cases of intractable pain.

The sclera is avascular and receives most of its nourishment from a overlying elastic membrane, the episclera. Inflammation of this thin, capillary-rich membrane is known as ***episcleritis.*** Most cases occur as a poorly understood condition in young adults, usually women. The inflammatory reaction causes considerable pain, photophobia, and excessive lacrimation. Diffuse vascular engorgement and edema of the episclera may be noted on examination. Patchy or segmented redness is a telling sign. Patients should be evaluated by an ophthalmologist. Once an underlying scleritis has been ruled out, they can be assured that the problem is self-limiting and rarely lasts longer than 3 weeks. Mild cases require no treatment other than topical decongestants to relieve "red eye" symptoms. More severe cases are treated with topical steroids (e.g., prednisone solution) or antiinflammatory drugs (e.g., Indocin). The problem may be recurrent.

TABLE 1.2 TYPES OF SCLERITIS

Type	Description
Anterior diffuse scleritis	Most common form of scleritis. Usually associated with rheumatoid arthritis, prior herpes zoster opthalmicus, or gout. Causes severe pain, redness, photophobia, and tearing.
Anterior nodular scleritis	Relatively severe form of recurrent scleritis, characterized by nodular formations. Manifesting exacerbation of an underlying vasculitis, it is associated with a high mortality due to cardiopulmonary complications in rheumatoid patients. Most common in women.
Anteror necrotizing scleritis	Most severe type of anterior scleritis, seen as an unremitting complication of an underlying vasculitis (29% of patients die within 5 years). Focal areas of inflammation continually form, with subsequent tissue breakdown. Congestion and necrosis of tissue lead to thinning. Underlying uveal pigment shows through, causing sclera to appear blue (scleromalacia). Elevated intraocular pressure and decreased visual acuity are common.
Scleromalacia perforans	Rare disease that occurs almost exclusively in older women with advanced rheumatoid arthritis. Unlike the others, this variety is quite painless. An initial scleral nodule becomes yellow and necrotic, and sloughs in 6–18 months, thinning or "melting" tissue in the area. The underlying uvea bulges through (staphyloma), and rupture of the globe may follow.
Posteror scleritis	Inflammation is limited to the posterior portions of the sclera, and therefore there are no visible signs. It is associated with severe rheumatoid arthritis. It may be complicated by elevated intraocular pressure, keratitis, uveitis, or cataract formation. Posterior staphyloma or perforation may result from recurrences.
Brawny scleritis	Rare disorder with an initial apearance similar to that of nodular scleritis. However, a widespread granulomatous reaction quickly develops. Thickened tissue gives a brawny appearance to the sclera. It may involve primarily the anterior or posterior segments or both.

Cornea

The sclera continues to the anterior portion of the eyeball, where it meets the clear, slightly bulging structure known as the "cornea" (Fig. 1.1). The cornea consists of five distinct layers of tissue: epithelium, Bowman's layer, stroma, Descemet's membrane, and endothelium. Due to the precise size, shape, and optical clarity of these layers, the cornea acts as the eye's most powerful lens, bending light rays and directing them through the pupil opening onto the retina. Crucial for normal vision, this function may be disrupted by ***congenital disorders*** of the cornea (Table 1.3) or ***corneal degenerations and dystrophies*** (Table 1.4). Some of these conditions are nonprogressive and need no special treatment beyond lenses to correct refractive errors. Others cause severe distortion or opacification, requiring surgical intervention. If an outer layer of the cornea is opacified, its surgical removal ***(superficial keratectomy)*** can sometimes improve vision. An opacity occluding the pupil may be managed by cutting into the iris ***(iridectomy)*** and creating an artificial pupil opening ***(coloboma)*** across from a clear portion of cornea.

When the entire cornea is damaged, the only hope for better vision may be ***corneal transplant*** (keratoplasty). Corneal transplants may involve full-thickness replacements (penetrating keratoplasty) or partial-thickness replacements (lamellar keratoplasty). In full-thickness procedures, success is directly related to the presence of viable endothelial cells, and tissue is preferably obtained from young eye donors within 24 to 48 hours after death. However, with lamellar procedures, donor tissue

TABLE 1.3 CONGENITAL DISORDERS OF THE CORNEA

Anomalies of size, shape, contour
- Megalocornea
- Microcornea
- Cornea plana
- Keratoglobus

Opacities
- Edema resulting from:
  - Hereditary endothelial dystrophy
  - Congenital glaucoma
  - Injury from birth or use of forceps
- Malformations
  - Posterior embryotoxin
  - Axenfeld's anomaly
  - Rieger's anomaly
  - Iridogoniodysgenesis
  - Posterior keratoconus
  - Peter's anomaly
  - Anterior chamber cleavage syndrome
- Tumors
  - Epibulbar
  - Limbal dermoid

Errors of metabolism
- Hurler's syndrome
- Scheie syndrome
- Morquio and Maroteaux-Lamy syndromes
- Cystinosis
- Mucolipidosis
- Gangliosidosis
- Lowe's syndrome
- Riley-Day syndrome
- Von Gierke's disease

Chromosomal defects
- Trisomy 21
- Trisomy 13–15
- Trisomy 18

Postinflammatory diseases
- Maternal rubella
- Luetic interstitial keratitis
- Congenital herpex simplex

can be frozen, dehydrated, or refrigerated for several weeks prior to surgery. In either case, round sections of donor and recipient cornea are removed with a special instrument (trephine) in cookie cutter fashion (trephination). The section of donor tissue is sutured into the trephinated portion of the recipient's eye. The cornea's avascular nature makes healing extremely slow. Patients must stay in the hospital for an average of 5 days, and sutures can remain in place for nearly a year. On the other hand, tissue matching is rarely necessary and rejection rates are low. In fact, the most pressing concern about the procedure is the inability of eye banks to meet transplant requests. Primary care providers may help reduce this shortage by offering important ▶ ***information about organ donations.***

The cornea's optical clarity is partly derived from the avascular, "deturgescent" nature of its five layers. Deturgescence is a state of partial dehydration maintained by the active transport of extracellular fluids by sodium/potassium pumps. ***Corneal edema,*** which would obviously interfere with clarity, is associated with numerous conditions listed in Table 1.5. It usually causes pain and significant visual impairment, particularly colored halos and hazy or blurred sight. On flashlight examination, the edematous cornea may have a "steamy" appearance. Patients should be referred to an ophthalmologist for immediate evaluation. Treatment depends on the underlying cause, for example, steroids for inflammatory conditions, antibiotics for infections, or measures to reduce intraocular pressure with glaucoma. To restore normal deturgescence, hypertonic agents (anhydrous glycerine, 5% sodium chloride, or colloidal osmotic solutions) may be used.

Besides refraction, the epithelial layer of the cornea provides an important protective function. It is richly supplied with sensitive nerve endings, and the slightest irritation elicits a reflex response of pain, lacrimation, and blinking (corneal reflex). Although this helps to ward off or signal injury, the cornea can be damaged by ***abrasions, lacerations, foreign bodies,*** or ***burns.*** These are discussed in a later section on eye trauma.

TABLE 1.4 CORNEAL DEGENERATIVE DISEASES AND DYSTROPHIES

Condition	Description
Degenerative conditions	
Fatty or lipid degeneration	Cause unknown; may begin at any age. Slowly progressive course with generalized (bilateral) stromal deposits of lipid material, macrophageal replacement of Bowman's membrane, and epithelial thickening with some lipid material infiltration. Corneal haziness and thickening (especially in the central zone) produce blurred vision. Poor prognosis (eventual loss of useful vision).
Terrien's marginal deterioration	Rare bilateral noninflammatory disorder, more common in men between 20 and 40 years of age. Slowly progressive course characterized by marginal corneal thinning (especially in the superior peripheral portion), opacity, and vascularization; perforation may occur and lead to iris prolapse. Good prognosis (the central cornea is spared), with mild irritation as the only symptom.
Furrow degeneration	Occurs in older patients in area of arcus senilis. Peripheral corneal thinning with no ulceration, epithelial defect, vascularization, or tendency to perforate.
Furrow degeneration associated with rheumatoid arthritis	Inflammatory thinning of the cornea with epithelial defect and progressive stromal ulceration; potential for perforation, especially with topical steroid treatment.
Calcific band keratopathy	Usually indicates earlier (childhood) uveitis; associated with several inflammatory, metabolic, and degenerative conditions, including rheumatoid arthritis, sarcoidosis, glaucoma, chronic cyclitis, leprosy, hypervitaminosis D, and hyperparathyroidism. Calcified opacity in anterior cornear layers, separated from limbus by a clear zone; disc-shaped holes corresponding to nerve channels may be seen in band. Keratopathy generally limited to interpalpebral area. Symptoms include irritation, injection, and blurring of vision. Treatment for visual and cosmetic purposes involves fairly simple band removal.
Climatic droplet keratopathy (Bietti's or pearl diver's keratopathy, spheroid degeneration)	Recently described acquired keratopathy affecting mainly male adults who work outdoors. Thought to be caused by ultraviolet radiation. Fine yellow (peripheral) subepithelial droplets occur in early stages, which spread centrally as the disease progresses, and eventually cloud cornea and blur vision.
Salzmann's nodular degeneration	Corneal inflammation, particularly phlyctenular keratoconjunctivitis or trachoma, always precedes this disorder. Signs include vascularization and degeneration of superficial corneal layers (stroma, Bowman's membrane, and epithelium); elevated white nodules sometimes appear in chains interspersed among blood vessels. Redness, irritation, and visual blurring are symptoms. In most cases, corneal transplantation greatly improves visual acuity.
Dystrophies	
Meesman's epithelial dystrophy	Dominantly inherited, slowly progressive; changes seen as early as 7 months of age and tend to increase with age. Pathologic changes usually confined to epithelium (small, round intraepithelial cysts). Usually asymptomatic, but may cause mild ocular discomfort and slight decrease in visual acuity (to 20/40 range); treatment not usually necessary, but severe discomfort may be relieved by soft contact lenses; with very severe visual impairment, lamellar keratoplasty may be indicated.
Cogan's microcystic epithelial	Bilateral, more common in women than in men, with no obvious hereditary tendency. Gray-white round or comma-shaped epithelial deposits ("putty marks") at level of basement membrane; may develop into recurrent erosion. Visual acuity and corneal sensation usually unaffected; common complaint of mild foreign body sensation.
Fingerprint dystrophy	Bilateral; no consistent hereditary pattern described. Recognized by fine, wavy, concentric opacites located anterior to Bowman's membrane, best seen by slit lamp retroillumination. Asymptomatic; may be associated with recurrent erosion.
Reis-Buckler's dystrophy	Dominantly inherited condition presenting at about 5 years of age. Recurrent erosion results in diffuse anterior scarring and subsequent opacification; visual acuity and corneal sensation markedly decreased. In mild cases, soft contact lens therapy or corneal scraping suffice, but severe cases may require lamellar keratoplasty.
Vortex dystrophy (cornea verticillata)	May be a manifestation of the asymptomatic carrier state of females with X-linked Fabry's disease; also indicative of chloropromazine, chloroquine, or indomethacin toxicity. Whorls of pigmented lines spread over entire corneal surface (Bowman's membrane, stroma); no significant effect on visual acuity.

TABLE 1.4 *(Continued)*

Condition	Description
Granular dystrophy (Groenouw type I)	Dominantly inherited; may be manifested in first decade of life. Central, dense, whitish, granular-appearing lesions in stroma. Slowly progressive; usually asymptomatic, but slight reduction in visual acuity occurs late in disease. Corneal transplant unnecessary except in very severe or late cases.
Macular dystrophy	Autosomal recessive inheritance; appears between ages of 5 and 9. Diffuse gray clouding in central cornea at level of Bowman's membrane, which gradually spreads peripherally and increases in density with the development of nodular deposits (resulting from local enzyme deficiency). Episodic irritation and photophobia; severe visual impairment often results from recurrent corneal erosion and may require penetrating keratoplasty.
Lattice dystrophy (Biber-Haab-Dimmer)	Dominantly inherited, appearing as early as 2 years of age. Appears as fine, branching, linear opacities in stroma that interlace and overlap at different levels to give appearance of irregular latticework; dots, flakes, and stellate opacities may appear between filaments. Recurrent erosion with progressive central corneal clouding by age 20; severe decrease in visual acuity often necessitates penetrating keratoplasty at about age 40.
Fleck dystrophy (central speckled dystrophy)	Autosomal dominant dystrophy. Oval or round gray-white opacities are well circumscribed and separated from each other by clear cornea; involves all corneal layers. Corneal sensation and visual acuity are usually unaffected.
Central cloudy and parenchymatous dystrophy	Dominantly inherited. Involves deep stromal layers but may extend to Bowman's membrane. Usually no visual impairment occurs; treatment usually not indicated.
Schnyder's crystalline dystrophy	Dominantly inherited condition that may be manifested as early as 18 months. Ring-shaped central corneal opacity (white, yellow, or multicolored crystals in stroma); there may also be peripheral deposits separated from the limbus by a clear line. Normal corneal sensation is typical, but severe decrease in visual acuity may necessitate penetrating keratoplasty.
Congenital hereditary endothelial dystrophy	Dominant thickening due to diffuse milky or ground-glass stromal opacification may be as much as four times normal. Visual acuity varies according to degree of corneal clouding; corneal sensation is normal and vascularization is rare. Asymptomatic relatives may exhibit clear vacuolar lesions surrounded by white haze and irregular mosaic, but have normal corneal thickness and visual acuity. High risk of transmission; poor prognosis for penetrating keratoplasty.
Fuchs' epithelial-endothelial dystrophy	Dominantly inherited condition occurring most often in women 40 to 60 years of age. Slowly progressive condition with central wart-like deposits on Descemet's membrane, thickening of Descemet's membrane, and endothelial thinning and pigmentation, causing epithelial and stromal edema, painful bullous keratopathy, corneal opacification and thickening, and blurring of vision.
Posterior polymorphous dystrophy	Common; autosomal dominant inheritance and early childhood onset. Round, elliptical, or irregular lesions, which often have a vesicular appearance and bulge into the stroma or project into the anterior chamber. Infrequent association with corneal edema may require penetrating keratoplasty to restore vision. Generally benign and nonprogressive.
Ectatic corneal dystrophy (keratoconus)	Uncommon, recessively inherited; typically bilateral. Appears in second decade. Anterior conical ectasia of central cornea with ruptures of Descemet's membrane, and generalized thinning and irregular superficial linear scars at apex of cone that is formed. Signs include conical cornea, Munson's sign (lower lid indentation when patient looks down), irregular retinoscopic shadow, distorted corneal reflection with keratoscope or Placido's disk, reticular scarring, and appearance of a Fleischer ring; stromal corneal nerves become more visible, and there may be fine lines on the internal edge of the Fleischer ring. Corneal distortion prevents clear view of fundi; disruption of endothelium and Descemet's membrane may result in corneal hydrops (severe stromal edema), with pain and sudden decrease in vision. Associated with several ocular anomalies (blue sclera, ectopia lentis, cataract, aniridia, retinitis pigmentosa, optic atrophy) and other conditions (Down's, Ehlers-Danlos, and Marfan's syndromes, Addison's disease, neurofibromatosis, Apert's anomaly, vernal conjunctivitis, atopic dermatitis). Blurred vision is the only symptom (except in cases of painful hydrops); contact lenses may help in early stages, but corneal transplant may be necessary in severe cases.

TABLE 1.5 CAUSES OF CORNEAL EDEMA

Elevated intraocular pressure
From acute angle closure glaucoma
From congenital glaucoma
Endothelial damage
Traumatic: forceps injury (birth trauma), contusion, foreign body penetration, surgical trauma (extraction of cataract, intraocular lens implantation, prolonged or profuse irrigation of anterior chamber)
From dystrophy: Fuchs' dystrophy, congenital hereditary endothelial dystrophy, posterior polymorphous dystrophy, anterior membrane dystrophies, keratoconus
Endothelial dysfunction (secondary to inflammation): uveitis, intraocular inflammation, infectious focal keratitis (bacterial, fungal, viral causes), corneal graft rejection
Epithelial damage
Mechanical, chemical, or radiation injury: contact lens overwear, toxic reaction to medication or anesthetic, etc.

After the resolution of a corneal abrasion, a disturbance called ***corneal erosion*** may appear at the site of an old injury. Suddenly, and for an unknown reason, the regrown epithelium fails to adhere to the basement membrane. After sleep, it is literally pulled off by the opening of the eyelids. Nerve endings are reexposed, causing the typical pattern of morning pain. Ophthalmologists treat an acute erosion with antibiotics and patching until it has healed. They then prescribe nighttime applications of a lubricating ointment, as well as hypertonic saline solutions and the generous use of artificial tears for an additional 6 weeks to help prevent recurrence.

Studded with microvilli, the epithelium provides an adhesive surface for tear film. The bacteriostatic activity of tears is so effective that a break in the epithelial surface is virtually the only way that infection gains entrance to the stroma or inner eye. This may occur in the many types of ***corneal inflammation*** (keratitis) and ***corneal ulceration*** listed in Table 1.6. Development may be favored by the use of drugs (local or systemic corticosteroids, topical anesthetics, antibiotics), local infections (conjunctivitis, blepharitis), and systemic illness (viruses, autoimmune disorders, alcoholism, diabetes). As corneal inflammation develops, irritation of epithelial nerve endings causes tearing, pain, and reflex dilatation of iris vessels. The last symptom produces photophobia, which is quite severe in most cases. Lesions and/or edema may result in blurred vision, particularly with central ulcers ***(hypopyon).*** Patients must be referred to an ophthalmologist for immediate evaluation. The cornea's appearance under slit lamp magnification may provide a clue to the causative organism. For example, *Staphylococcus* remains localized; *Pseudomonas* necrotizes, rapidly giving off a purulent discharge; *Pneumococcus* progresses in a shaggy, undetermined manner; and herpes simplex virus forms distinct "bean-sprout-like" dendrites. Nontheless, lesions should always be scraped for more definitive gram stains and culture. Depending on the result of these tests, hourly administration of steroids, antibiotics, or antifungal or antiviral agents is started. Artificial tears, eye patching, or soft contact lenses may be used to prevent further irritation from lid movements. Silver nitrate cautery, debridement, superficial keratoplasty, or grafts are required in some cases. The goal of such aggressive treatment is to prevent scarring with permanent opacification and/or corneal perforation.

Corneal perforation can result not only from ulceration but from trauma or foreign bodies as well. Threatening to cause partial or complete loss of the anterior chamber, it is an urgent situation requiring immediate attention by an ophthalmolo-

TABLE 1.6 CORNEAL ULCERS AND INFLAMMATIONS

Cause	Type of Corneal Involvement
	Systemic
Allergic (hypersensitivity reaction)	
Immediate/humoral reaction	
Palpebral or limbal vernal keratoconjunctivitis	Possible allergic reaction to pollens; diffuse punctate epithelial keratitis, micropannus, superficial superior oval ulcer, mild corneal scarring.
Atopic keratoconjunctivitis	Superficial peripheral keratitis and vascularization that frequently appears late in patients with atopic dermatitis.
Delayed/cellular reaction	
Phlyctenular keratoconjunctivitis (tubercle bacillus, *Candida albicans, C. aureus, Coccidioides immitis,* staphylococcus, *Chlamydia* lymphogranulomatosis)	Reaction to microbial proteins; corneal phlyctenule (usually bilateral) begins as an amorphous gray infiltrate (severe if induced by tuberculoprotein, mild if induced by staphylococcus protein) that cicatrizes, vascularizes, and eventually scars. Scarring may result in Salzmann's nodular dystrophy.
Gastrointestinal/nutritional disorders	
Avitaminosis A	Bilateral. Includes keratitis sicca (corneal drying, blotchy inferior epithelial keratitis, stromal infiltration, ulceration, thinning, and possible filaments) and xerophthalmia (dry eye). Ulceration is central, gray, indolent; secondary infection and perforation are common.
Avitaminosis B	Drying of cornea can result in keratitis sicca.
Liver disease	Keratitis sicca with associated changes.
Malnutrition	Xerophthalmia.
Inflammatory bowel disease (regional enteritis, ulcerative colitis)	Keratitis
Hypocalcemia (tetany, hypoparathyroidism, etc.)	Bilateral superficial keratitis with corneal vascularization and possible scarring.
Autoimmune diseases	
Rheumatoid arthritis Periarteritis nodosa Scleroderma Midline lethal or Wegener's granulomatosis Ulcerative colitis Relapsing polychondritis Reiter's syndrome Crohn's disease Psoriasis Systemic lupus erythematosus	Keratitis sicca with characteristic peripheral involvement is common. In psoriasis vulgaris, there may be rare marginal corneal ulceration or deep vascularized opacity and possible scarring. Conjunctivitis may lead to obliteration of fornix, lack of precorneal tear film. Long course with poor prognosis (blindness from complete symblepharon and corneal desiccation). Secondary infection and perforation possible.
Disorders of skin and mucous membranes	
Acne rosacea	Corneal infiltrates, keratitis, pannus, ulceration.
Behcet's disease	Keratitis, corneal erosions.
Cicatricial pemphigoid	Corneal drying and perforation.
Epidermolysis bullosa	Subepithelial bullous keratitis, corneal erosion, perforation.
Erythema multiforme	Corneal ulceration, perforation.
Ichthyosis	Corneal drying and associated changes.
Psoriasis	Corneal infiltrates, erosion.

TABLE 1.6 *(Continued)*

Cause	Type of Corneal Involvement
	Systemic
Disorders of skin and mucous membranes *(Continued)*	
Stevens-Johnson syndrome	Corneal drying, secondary infection, and perforation.
Xeroderma pigmentosum	Keratitis.
	Infectious Environmental Causes
Viral	
Adenovirus types 8, 19	Epidemic keratoconjunctivitis (EKC); epithelial keratitis, round subepithelial opacities.
Adenovirus types 3, 4, 7	Pharyngoconjunctival fever, keratitis (PCF, PFK); transient epithelial keratitis, occasional subepithelial opacities.
Rubeola (measles)	Central epithelial keratitis; possible secondary bacterial infection (pneumococcus, *H. influenzae,* etc).
Herpes simplex virus (HSV) Types 1 and 2; primary and recurrent forms	Ulcerative keratitis; dendritic lesions are characteristic, but HSV also causes blotchy, stellate, and filamentary epithelial keratitides.
Varicella-zoster virus (VZV)	Primary form (varicella) causes rare superficial punctate keratitis. Recurrent form (herpes zoster) causes corneal infiltration, vascularization, and edema, limbal or epithelial keratitis, and decreased corneal sensation. Keratitis may be blotchy, disciform, or pseudodendritic.
Mumps (paramyxovirus)	Unilateral interstitial or epithelial keratitis.
Influenza	Mild epithelial keratitis.
Rubella (German measles)	Corneal clouding and edema.
Infectious mononucleosis (Epstein-Barr virus; EBV)	Mild epithelial keratitis.
Molluscum contagiosum virus (pox group)	Unilateral, fine, diffuse, superior or focal keratitis; if chronic and untreated, may lead to subepithelial infiltration, vascularization; corneal involvement thought to be due to toxicity to products released by molluscum nodule (on lid margin) into conjunctival cul-de-sac.
Enterovirus type 70 and coxsackie virus type A 24	Epithelial keratitis follows acute hemorrhagic conjunctivitis.
Bacterial	
Gonorrhea	Keratitis, ulceration, with potential for perforation of intact epithelium.
Brucella (corneal involvement is a complication of brucellosis)	Nummular keratitis (same clinical appearance as EKC), which may occasionally ulcerate and develop into chronic keratitis.
Diphtheria	Corneal ulcer that can penetrate intact epithelium.
Pneumococcus	Corneal ulcer usually appears 24–48 hours after inoculation of abraded cornea. Called "acute serpiginous ulcer" because advancing border is ulcerative and infiltrated, while trailing border heals.
Pseudomonas	Corneal ulcer that often spreads rapidly in all directions; arises from use of contaminated eye solutions and medications.
Moraxella liquefaciens (diplobacillus of Petit)	Corneal ulcer due to pyridoxine (vitamin B_6) depletion in alcoholics; deficiency may also be related to diabetes or other immunosuppressive conditions or to use of isoniazid.
Streptococcus pyogenes, Strep. viridans	Central corneal ulcer, stromal infiltration, and edema; often a hypopyon with *S. pyogenes.*

TABLE 1.6 *(Continued)*

Cause	Type of Corneal Involvement
Klebsiella pneumoniae	Indolent corneal ulcer with occasional stromal edema; no hypopyon.
Staphylococcus epidermis, S. aureus	Central corneal ulcer; usually superficial and indolent, but may be associated with hypopyon and infiltration of surrounding cornea.
Francisella tularensis (ocular tularemia)	Keratitis with potential for perforation.
Mycobacterium fortuitum, Nocardia	Usually associated with eye trauma and contact with soil.
Fungal	Most fungal infections of cornea are opportunistic, following immune system compromise (as in long-term corticosteroid use, use of antibiotics and cytotoxic agents, prolonged use of indwelling intravenous (IV) catheters and hyperalimentation, IV narcotic drug abuse, abdominal surgery, infusion of glucose solutions, malnutrition, diabetes, and debilitating and malignant diseases).
Candidal (*C. albicans*) (See also phlyctenular keratoconjunctivitis)	Exogenously acquired fungal corneal ulcers may have distinct oval outlines and plaque-like surface, and may be associated with relatively indolent stromal infiltration and a large preauricular node. Severe superficial keratitis due to chronic mucocutaneous candidiasis (especially associated with hypoparathyroidism) may result in blindness from corneal scarring.
Filamentous fungi *Fusarium* *Aspergillus* *Coccidioides immitis* *Penicillium* *Cephalosporum* (For *C. immitis,* see also phlyctenular keratoconjunctivitis)	Mild abrasive corneal trauma usually precedes infection of normal eyes, especially if injury was from vegetable matter. Characteristic gray or dirty white keratitis with dry, rough-textured surface and often an elevated margin. Superficial indolent ulcers, gray infiltrate, marked global inflammation, and "satellite lesions." Endothelial plaque formation with deep infections; anterior chamber reaction and hypopyon with large or deep infections.
Nontrue fungi (Actinomycetacea family)	
Actinomyces	May cause superficial nodular keratitis and corneal ulcer.
Nocardia asteroides	May produce chronic, indolent corneal ulcer with gray sloughing base and undermined overhanging edges; possible hypopyon.
Parasitic	
Onchocerciasis (*Onchocerca volvulus*)	Superficial punctate and interstitial sclerosing keratitis; punctate keratitis is due to reaction to individual microfilariae in superficial corneal tissues. Interstitial sclerosing keratitis is reaction to dead microfilariae, with pannus, progressive corneal vascularization, and scarring that begins inferiorly and moves superiorly. May result in blindness.
Loiasis (*Loa loa*)	Keratitis.
Protozoal	
Malaria	Rare ocular involvement includes keratitis.
Chlamydial Trachoma	Epithelial keratitis, corneal infiltrates, superficial vascularization, and micropannus occur in mild cases and heal without causing visual impairment; in more severe cases, trachoma pustules (round subepithelial opacities), Herbert's pits (limbal follicles and their cicatricial remains), gross pannus, and extensive, diffuse subepithelial cicatrization develop and may cause visual damage.
Primary ocular lymphogranuloma venereum	Segmental, highly vascularized interstitial keratitis; diffuse corneal scarring and total pannus may develop and cause blindness.

TABLE 1.6 *(Continued)*

Cause	Type of Corneal Involvement
	Systemic
Protozoal (Continued)	
Feline pneumonitis	Micropannus, central epithelial keratitis, and (rare) subepithelial opacities with little visual significance.
Psittacosis or parakeet keratoconjunctivitis	Corneal involvement is same as that of feline pneumonitis.
Inclusion conjunctivitis (inclusion blennorrhea)	Corneal involvement is same as that of feline pneumonitis.
Others	
Leprosy (mycobacterium)	Typically bilateral, symmetrical; interstitial or punctate epithelial keratitis, deep infiltration, corneal thickening and opacity, pannus, perforation, and scarring. Exposure keratitis may also result from lagophthalmos and corneal anesthesia due to leprotic neuropathy of the seventh and fifth cranial nerves.
Syphilis (spirochete)	Ninety percent of all cases of acute interstitial keratitis are syphilitic. Chronic course involving diffuse interstitial keratitis with widespread, deep stromal infiltration, edema, and diffuse corneal haze; invading vessels remain on corneal stroma after active inflammation has subsided, although devoid of blood ("ghost vessels"). Congenital form is usually bilateral, and acquired form is usually unilateral.
	Noninfectious Environmental Causes
Exposure keratitis	May develop from any condition in which eye is not adequately moistened or covered by eyelid. Corneal desiccation (especially in inferior interpalpebral area) leads to frank epithelial defect and noninfiltrated ulceration. Keratitis is sterile unless secondarily infected.
Radiation injury UV (solar) and infared (laser burns, snow, or eclipse blindness)	Epithelial keratitis, corneal erosion.
Chemical or irritative	Toxic reaction to topical medications, chemicals, or aerosols can produce a diffuse punctate epithelial keratitis.
Drug-induced keratitis	
Use of antiviral medication (idovuridine and vidarabine) and broad- and medium-spectrum antibiotics	Blotchy epithelial keratitis on lower half of cornea and interpalpebral fissure.
Adverse effects of other drugs:	
Antirheumatoid (gold salts and Butazolidin)	Corneal erosion and ulcerative keratitis are rare toxic reactions.
Cardiovascular (hexamethonium, practolol, digitalis/digoxin)	Keratitis sicca and associated changes (corneal thinning, ulceration, opacification, and scarring).
Cholinergic, anticholinergic (isoniazid)	May produce keratitis.

gist. Besides drugs to control infections and inflammation, the specialist may use soft contact badge lenses for splinting and glue-like adhesives for adhesiveness. If these measures prove inadequate, surgical patch grafting or corneal transplant may be necessary. Small perforations sometimes close on their own.

Choroid

Choroid tissue forms the most posterior layer of the uveal tract (Fig. 1.1). It is highly pigmented to prevent internal light reflection and is extremely vascular to nourish the retina. In fact, pigments and vessels in the choroid provide color to the overlying retina. Because of them, the retina often appears pink-yellow in blondes and dark gray in black people.

Examination of the retina may reveal ***degenerative changes*** of the choroid (see also Table 1.11). Breaks in the choroid's lamina (Bruch's membrane) are known as ***angioid streaks.*** Appearing as reddish-brown radiations from the disc, angioid streaks typically develop in middle-aged patients (particularly males) who have a widespread collagen disorder such as pseudoxanthoma elasticum, osteitis deformans, Paget's disease, or senile elastosis of the skin. They are also seen in patients with sickle cell anemia, hypertension, lead poisoning, thrombocytopenic purpura, and familial hyperphosphatemia. Hyperplastic changes of choroid pigments produce translucent yellow deposits known as ***Drusen bodies.*** They represent a senile change and are frequently mistaken for exudates, even though their origin is not vascular. Although isolated Drusen bodies are of no concern, concentrations developing around the macula are associated with macular degeneration. Choroid degeneration may be asymptomatic in the early stages, but as it progresses, serous detachment of the epithelium or neovascularization ***(disciform lesion)*** may develop. Nourishment to the underlying retina is disrupted; if rods are destroyed, night blindness develops, and if the macula is damaged, central and color vision may be lost. Therefore, early ophthalmologic evaluation is always advised. Photocoagulation may prove beneficial in some cases.

Due to its rich pigmentation, the uveal tract is a common site for ***ocular tumors,*** described in Table 1.7. The most worrisome tumor is ***malignant melanoma,*** which affects 0.4% of all eye patients, many of whom are over age 50. Most melanomas occur in the choroid (85%), although some develop in the ciliary body (9%) or the iris (6%). Flashing lights ***(photopsia)*** or blurring may be the only warning before rapid expansion causes retinal damage with visual loss. Earlier stages are usually asymptomatic, but may be discovered as an incidental finding on funduscopic examination. Lesions are typically hyperpigmented, raised, and unilateral. Scattered plaques, orange pigmentation, and large vessels over tumor surfaces indicate rapid growth. Drusen bodies and small, fan-shaped vessels suggest long-standing, less active tumors. Any patient with such findings should be referred to an ophthalmologist immediately. Further information about the location and neoplastic behavior of the tumor may be gained through fluorescein angiography, ultrasonography, or radioactive uptake (^{32}P test). Very small melanomas have an excellent prognosis but may be difficult to differentiate from ***benign nevi.*** If there is any question, lesions are closely monitored for signs of growth with serial photographs and ultrasound studies. Treatment includes photocoagulation, cryotherapy, radiation therapy, or partial resection. Rather than preventing spread, enucleation may actually cause dissemination and is being performed less often. As with other forms of malignancy, pa-

TABLE 1.7 TUMORS OF THE UVEAL TRACT, RETINA, AND OPTIC NERVE

Type	Typical Description
Uveal tract	
Nevus	Flat, pigmented slate gray lesions in the iris ciliary body or choroid. Does not change in size or color. Benign.
Melanoma	Raised, pigmented lesion developing in the uveal tract. Unilateral. Size and appearance change. Highly malignant.
Choroid hemangioma	Solid, elevated lesion with irregular borders near the optic disc. Never pigmented. Associated with Sturge-Weber syndrome. Complicated by serous detachments of the retina and glaucoma.
Medullo-epithelioma (diktyoma)	Rare tumor arising from the ciliary body. May be heteroplastic, containing cartilage, brain, or musculoskeletal tissue. Similar in appearance to retinoblastoma.
Retina	
Retinal angioma	Globular mass in the posterior fundus near engorged retinal vessel. May increase in size. Benign.
Glial hamartoma	Yellow to white mulberry lesion in the posterior fundus (usually near the optic nerve). Associated with tuberous sclerosis (Bourneville's disease).
Retinoblastoma	Yellowish-white nodular growth arising in the posterior retina that may protrude into the vitreous. Often bilateral, seeding numerous satellite lesions. Occurs in all age groups, but 66% of cases appear by age 3. Tumor gradually fills the eye and extends through the optic nerve to the brain.
Optic nerve	
Optic nerve glioma	Abnormal growth of neural connecting tissue leads to enlargement of the optic nerve canal and exophthalmos. Associated with neurofibromatosis and therefore café-au-lait spots.
Meningioma	Originates intracranially or along the optic nerve sheath. Extends along the optic canal or into the orbit.

tients may benefit from the information, services, and support offered by ▶ ***cancer organizations.***

Ciliary Body

The choroid terminates at the serrated margin of a triangle-shaped structure, the ciliary body. Its muscular zone attaches to the zonular fibers, which hold the lens in place. When the ciliary muscles constrict, the zonular fibers decrease tension on the lens. As discussed in a later section, this causes a change in the shape of the lens that allows higher refraction and the ability to focus on nearby objects.

In addition to muscular activity, the ciliary body secretes aqueous humor. This clear fluid circulates in the fixed space between the cornea and the lens. The space is divided by the iris into two compartments: the anterior and posterior chambers (Fig. 1.2). Fluid diffuses from the ciliary processes located in the posterior chamber and circulates through the pupil toward the trabecular meshwork in the anterior chamber. It is then conducted by the canals of Schlemm into the venous system. This constant flow of aqueous humor nourishes the cornea and lens, both structures being avascular.

In some individuals, the angle between the iris and the cornea is very sharp. If the root of the iris pushes the angle closed when the pupil dilates, outflow of aqueous

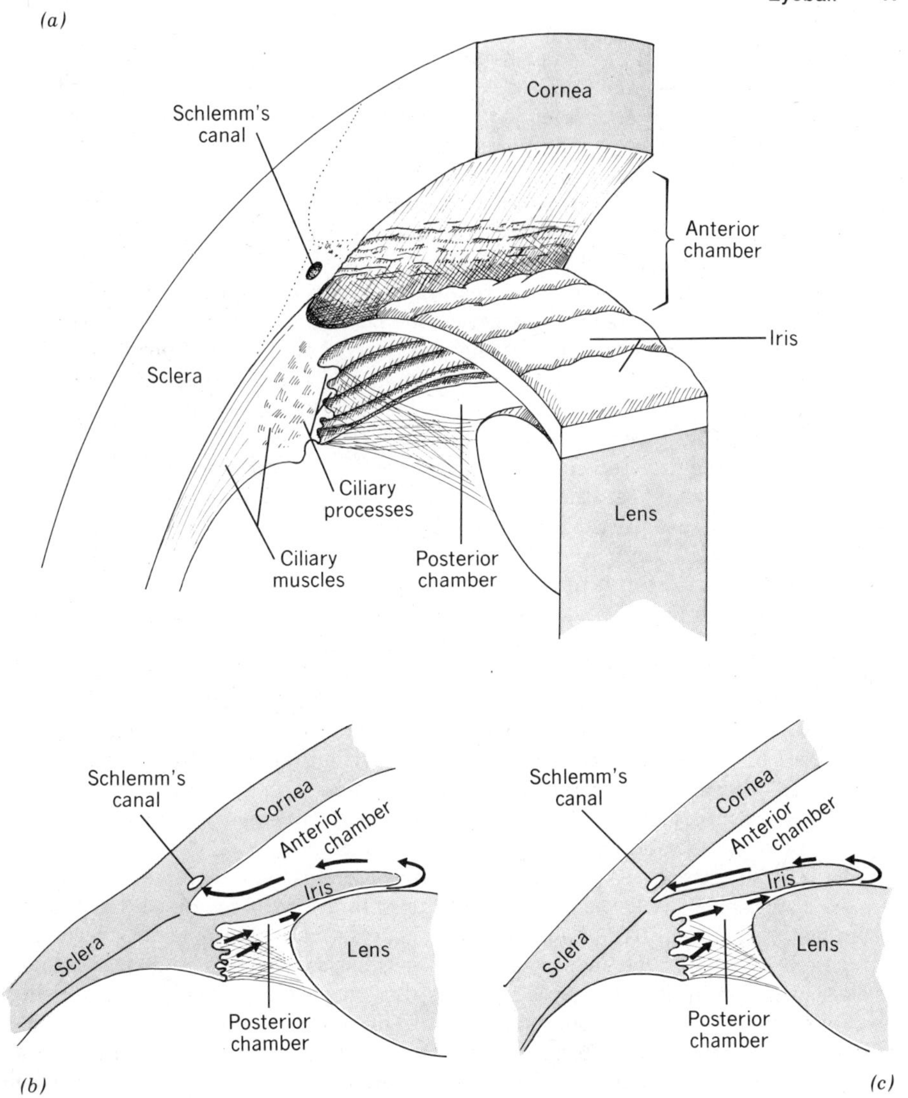

Figure 1.2 Anterior chamber and circulation of aqueous humor in three parts: (*a*) cross section of the anterior and posterior chambers, (*b*) aqueous outflow through the normal anterior angle, and (*c*) aqueous outflow through the narrow anterior angle.

humor becomes blocked. An increase in aqueous fluids raises intraocular pressure. For individuals who have narrow anterior chambers, the mydriatic effects of certain drugs, such as cocaine, atropine, or bronchodilators, or even watching a movie in a darkened theater could dilate the pupils enough to precipitate an attack of ***angle closure glaucoma*** (narrow angle glaucoma). The root of the iris can also be pushed closed by swelling or debris from inflammatory uveitis, intraocular hemorrhage, edematous cataracts, or neoplasms. During an attack, patients experience blurred vision marked by the appearance of colored halos around lights. Pain tends to involve the whole head, rather than being confined to the eyes, and may be severe enough to cause nausea and vomiting. Examination at this time reveals a red eye, with a mid-dilated pupil and a clouded, edematous cornea. Slit lamp evaluation and gonioscopy confirm closure of the angle and flaring of the anterior chamber. With prolonged attacks, the iris stroma develops a gray, atrophied appearance, and the lens may have white anterior opacifications ***(glaukomflecken).*** However, with milder, transient attacks, the examination is sometimes inconclusive and the diagnosis may then depend on provocative tests (dark room, prone position, or mydriatic). Most instances of angle closure glaucoma require emergency hospitalization. Once intraocular pressure is lowered with osmotics, the pupillary block is opened surgically by removing a peripheral portion of the iris ***(peripheral iridectomy).*** However, when elevated pressure has been long-standing, permanent adhesions develop between the peripheral iris and the trabecular meshwork, forming ***peripheral anterior synechiae (PAS).*** They may necessitate surgical deepening of the entire chamber (chamber-deepening technique) or the formation of an opening into the eye (filtration or fistulizing operation). Finally, if angle narrowing is binocular, prophylactic iridectomy is usually performed several days later on the asymptomatic eye.

Open angle glaucoma is quite furtive. Some cases are related to histologic changes that decrease the filtering capacity of the trabecular meshwork (primary open angle), while others follow eye surgery, uveitis, trauma, or systemic diseases (secondary open angle glaucoma). Elevated intraocular pressure cuts off the nutrient supply to the optic nerve, and fibers from the optic nerve are destroyed one after another. Since fibers radiate over the retina in a specific distribution, a predictable pattern of visual field disturbance evolves. Nasal and superior fields are lost relatively early, but "temporal island" and "central" vision remain intact until the end stages of the disease. This condition can be detected with monocular visual field testing (see later section). A current theory holds that vascular insufficiency to the optic nerve may be inherent and not totally related to elevated pressures. It is supported by the strong association of optic atrophy in patients with vascular disorders (diabetes, arteriosclerosis) and by the progressive atrophy that often follows normalization of pressures. Early stages of open angle glaucoma are decidedly asymptomatic but may be suspected by characteristic changes of the optic disc on funduscopic examination. The physiologic cup becomes wider and deeper, increasing the cup-to-disc ratio above normal (0.5). Central areas of the disc turn from a healthy pink color to light gray, and temporal margins appear thinner than normal. Large vessels become nasally displaced. By the time patients become aware of a sensation of eye fatigue, halos around lights, headaches, poor night vision, or blind spots, visual field losses are likely to have occurred. Treatment relies on drugs that decrease the production of aqueous humor or facilitate outflow (Table 1.8).

It is estimated that 1–2% of people over age 35 have glaucoma and that 300,000 cases presently remain undetected. Therefore, ▶***screening for glaucoma*** is extremely important. Schiøtz tonometry requires a relatively inexpensive instrument that can be readily used in primary care settings. It should be routinely done on everyone over age 20 every 3 years and yearly on patients who have a predisposition due to a family history, myopia, or diabetes. There is great variability among individuals in terms of the amount of pressure that can be tolerated before damage occurs. A tonometry reading between 10 and 20 mm is considered normal but does not rule out ocular hypertension, which can have diurnal variations of 3 to 4 mm and

TABLE 1.8 DRUGS USED IN GLAUCOMA TREATMENT

Drug	Usual Dose Ranges	Comment
Direct-acting cholinergic (parasympathetic)		
Pilocarpine hydrochloride 0.5, 1, 2, 3, 4, 6%	1 or 2 drops up to six times a day	In use since 1857; still the most commonly used agent for glaucoma.
Pilocarpine-epinephrine combinations: pilocarpine 1, 2, 3, 4, or 6% to epinephrine 1%	1 or 2 drops up to four times a day	Epinephrine extends action and decreases miosis.
Carbachol 0.75 or 1.5%	1 or 2 drops two to three times a day	Reserved for cases resistant to other drugs, since it has a short duration of action and is poorly absorbed through the cornea. Transient head and eye aching, hyperemia are common.
Reversible indirect-acting anticholinesterase		
Physostigmine salicylate (Eserine) 0.25 or 0.5%	1 or 2 drops three to four times a day	Old, effective drug sometimes combined with pilocarpine. Use limited by short duration of action and allergic reactions.
Neostigmine bromide 2.5 or 5%	1 or 2 drops two to six times a day	Similar to physostigmine.
Irreversible indirect-acting anticholinesterase		
Isofluophate (DFP, Floropryl) 0.1% oil or 0.025% ointment	1 or 2 drops one or two times a day	Causes extreme, long-lasting mitosis and occasional pupillary block. Local irritation common.
Echothiophate iodide (Phospholine) 0.03 or 0.25% solution	1 or 2 drops one or two times a day	Water-soluble and therefore causes less local irritation than physostigmine. However, may cause systemic cholinergic toxicity marked by salivation, nausea, vomiting, and diarrhea. Also thought to be cataractogenic.
Demecarium bromide (Humorsol) 0.12 or 0.25% solution	1 or 2 drops one or two times a day	Similar to echothiophate iodide.
Adrenergic (sympathetic)		
Epinephrine bitartrate (Epitrate) 2%	1 or 2 drops one or two times a day	Epinephrines decrease production of aqueous humor and improve its outflow. They are long-acting (12–72 hours). Since there is no mitosis, they are especially useful in cataract patients. However, local allergies, headaches, and heart palpitations are common.
Epinephrine hydrochloride (Glaucon) 0.5, 1, 2%	1 or 2 drops one or two times a day	
Epinephryl borate (Epinal, Eppy) 0.5, 1%	1 or 2 drops one or two times a day	
Dipivefrin (Propine) 0.1%	1 or 2 drops one or two times a day	
Beta-adrenergic blocking agent		
Timolol maleate (Timoptic) 0.25, 0.5%	1 drop two times a day	Used to treat open angle, aphakic, and certain secondary glaucomas. Does not affect pupillary size or visual acuity. Well tolerated but should be prescribed with caution to patients with asthma and heart failure.
Carbonic anhydrase inhibitors		
Acetozolamide (Diamox) 125, 250 mg	1 or 2 tablets every 24 hours, not to exceed 1 g	By inhibiting carbonic anhydrase production in the ciliary body, drugs reduce the secretion of aqueous humor. They are used when intraocular pressure cannot be controlled with eye drops. Undesirable side effects include dermatitis, hypokalemia, gastric distress, diarrhea, kidney stones, shortness of breath, fatigue, acidosis, and tingling sensations.
500 mg sustained release	1 capsule AM and PM	
Dichlorphenamide (Daranide) 50 mg	25–50 mg three to four times a day after loading	
Ethoxzolamide (Cardase, Ethamide) 125 mg	125 mg two to four times a day	
Methazolamide (Neptazane) 50 mg	50–100 mg two to three times a day	

be quite labile in the early stages. Questionable results or readings above 21 mm should be evaluated by an ophthalmologist.

Iris and Pupil

The last and most visible portion of the uveal tract is the iris. The three posterior layers of the iris are highly pigmented in order to restrict the passage of light through the pupil opening. At birth, the anterior layers have no pigmentation of their own, and the newborn's eyes reflect only the color from posterior pigmentation (blue). By 3 months of age, genetically determined amounts of melanin begin to deposit in the second layers of the iris. If a large quantity is bestowed, eye color turns brown; if little is deposited, it remains blue. Extremely pale iris color occurs in ***albinism*** due to genetic lack of body pigmentation. Patients have white hair and eyelashes, pink skin and eyelids. They appear to have red eyes because the retinal vasculature can be seen through the depigmented iris. Light also shines through the iris unimpeded, explaining the light sensitivity experienced by most albinos and their need for continual protection from sunglasses. Other eye problems include macular hypoplasia, sensory nystagmus, and refractive problems, particularly myopia. Poor vision is the rule.

A defect in iris development may leave the two eyes with different colors (e.g., one blue and one brown). Referred to as ***heterochromia,*** this condition is insignificant unless it is associated with Fuch's iridocyclitis, later described in Table 1.10.

Two types of muscles regulate a central opening of the iris, the pupil. By reflex command of the third cranial nerve, a sphincter muscle contracts the pupil and a radiating muscle dilates it. Construction of the pupil is normally produced with light testing (direct and consensual) and with convergence. Pupils often appear ***miotic*** (less than 3 mm) in the elderly and ***mydriatic*** (more than 7 mm) in blue-eyed or myopic individuals. ***Anisocoria*** (unequal pupils) is a normal variant in 25% of the population. Yet, these findings or any ***abnormality of pupil shape*** (normally, they are perfectly round) might indicate the pathologic effects of drugs, metabolic disease, or neurologic disorders described in Table 1.9. They should always be investigated.

Inflammation occurring anywhere in the uveal tract is referred to by the general term ***uveitis.*** Depending on the location, more specific terms may be used: ***anterior uveitis, cyclitis, iritis,*** or ***iridocyclitis*** for inflammation of the anterior portion; ***posterior uveitis*** or ***chorioretinitis*** for inflammation of the posterior portion; ***panuveitis*** for involvement of the entire tract (extremely rare). The overall annual incidence is 15 per 100,000 people, 12 of which are anterior types. The etiology, signs, symptoms, and outcome vary for each type, as described in Table 1.10. Disorders are most common in whites between the ages of 20 and 50. Women have a higher incidence of anterior uveitis associated with toxoplasmosis or of unknown origin, while men tend to be afflicted by types associated with trauma, ankylosing spondylitis, and Reiter's syndrome. Any suspected case of uveitis should be referred to an ophthalmologist at once. Although eye inflammation can be readily diagnosed by a careful ophthalmologic examination, the underlying cause may be more difficult to establish. Chest or spine x-ray films, or blood, urine, or skin tests, may be used to investigate the possibility of infectious or immunologic processes and therefore determine the best treatment (e.g., antituberculosis or antitoxoplasmic agents). However, in many cases of uveitis, the specific cause and treatment cannot be outlined, and general measures are employed. These include corticosteroids (topical,

TABLE 1.9 PUPIL FINDINGS

Pupil Type	Appearance in Room Light	Light Response	Near Reaction	Comments
Normal	Round, equal size (3–5 diameter).	Equal brisk constriction.	Same as light response. Normal convergence.	Insignificant anisocoria in 25% of population.
Mydriatic	Round, large size (greater than 7 mm).	Constrictive variable.	Normal.	Drug effects. Mid-dilated and fixed types seen in acute glaucoma. Also, ocular contusions, systemic poisoning, neurologic disease. Slight mydriasis normal in blue-eyed people.
Mitotic	Round, small size (smaller than 3 mm).	Already constricted	Normal tracking. Constriction relative.	Common in the aged. Drug effects (antiglaucoma, antiheroin, etc.).
Marcus-Gunn	Normal.	Pupil of affected eye has normal response to consensual light but no response to direct light.	Normal.	Swinging flashlight test. Unilateral damage to sensory retina or optic nerve.
Light-near dissociation	Tend to be mid-sized or enlarged. Often unequal.	Diminished or lost.	Preserved.	Mid-brain lesions. Associated with Parinaud's syndrome, convergence-reaction nystagmus, and limited upgaze.
Argyll Robertson	Small.	Both eyes respond poorly or not at all.	Prompt.	Presumptive evidence of neurosyphilis. Seen also with mid-brain lesions, diabetes mellitus, chronic alcoholism, encephalitis, multiple sclerosis, and central nervous system (CNS) degenerative disease.
Tonic (Adie's) pupil	Enlarged.	Poor response.	Tonic pupil (redilates slowly).	Damage to ciliary ganglion or short ciliary nerves. Usually in combination with lost tendon reflexes (Adie's syndrome). Seen most often in young women.
Pupillodilator (Horner's) dysfunction	Mitotic.	Same as near response.	Same as light response.	Dysfunction of sympathetic chain to pupillodilator fibers (cervical vertebral fractures, tabes dorsalis, syringomyelitis, cervical cord tumor, apical tuberculosis, goiter, enlarged cervical lymph glands m apical bronchogenic carcinoma, mediastinal tumor, aneurysm of the carotid or subclavian artery. Ptosis present. Patients may also have conjunctival erythema, elevation of the lower lid, unilateral facial sweating. Confirmed by cocaine test (if sympathetic damage is present, pupil dilates poorly).

TABLE 1.10 TYPES OF UVEITIS

Description	Treatment	Course
Chronic cyclitis Unknown cause. Affects both sexes equally in young adulthood. Early stages are asymptomatic except for complaints of floaters. However, ophthalmoscopic exam reveals inflammatory cells in aqueous or vitreous fluid and soft, round exudates over the peripheral retina. Vasculitis with perivascular sheathing may also be present. Diagnosis is clinical.	Topical corticosteroids (retrobulbar injections for more severe cases).	Disease remains stationary for 5–10 years and then begins to improve. Some patients develop retinal detachments, glaucoma, or macular scarring. Cataracts are common.
Heterochromic (Fuchs' iridocyclitis) Disease of unknown etiology, accounting for 3% of all cases of uveitis. Beginning in young adulthood, inflammatory cells cause atrophy and depigmentation of the iris and ciliary body. There may be patchy change in eye color (heterochromia), but otherwise no symptoms occur. Cataracts and glaucoma develop in later stages. Diagnosis is clinical.	Treatment not necessary. Glaucoma screening important.	Cataracts and glaucoma develop in 15% of cases.
Histoplasmosis Intracellular fungus (endemic in valleys of Ohio and Mississippi rivers) infects humans via spore-containing dust (inhaled). Causes uveitis characterized by punched-out, depigmented lesions with fine, pigmented borders in the periphery of the retina. These "histo" spots are asymptomatic. However, healed spots are thought to be antigenic to the sensitized choroid, leading to eventual macular changes. Macular lesions may progress to hemorrhagic detachments. Diagnosis is based on systemic findings and positive skin tests.	Advocated treatments include corticosteroids, antihistamines, histoplasmin desensitization, and photocoagulation.	Hemorrhagic detachments of the macula may develop with loss of central vision.
Lens induced Follow leakage of lens material from hypermature or traumatic cataract into the anterior chamber. The lens material causes an inflammatory reaction with painful red eye, mitotic pupil, and markedly reduced vision. The problem also develops after a second cataract procedure if the patient was sensitized to leakage of lens material during the first operation. Glaucoma is a common complication.	Lens extraction.	Both uveitis and secondary glaucoma cured and visual prognosis good if extraction done within 1–2 weeks.
Rheumatoid associated A common development with Marie Strumpell *ankylosing spondylitis, Reiter's syndrome,* and *juvenile arthritis* (the presence of uveitis in an adult with rheumatoid arthritis is considered coincidental). Flares are recurrent, patients presenting with severe pain, photophobia, corneal precipitates, and red eye. Vision may be moderately blurred. Posterior and peripheral anterior synechiae, cataracts, glaucoma, and macular involvement are common complications. Elevated erythrocyte sedimentation rate during active disease.	Control of underlying disease by corticosteroids and mydriatics.	Ocular prognosis is poor.
Sarcoidosis Chronic granulomatous disease of unknown etiology characterized by nodular lesions of the skin, viscera, and bones. Uveal involvement in combination with parotid glands called *Heerfordt's disease;* with lacrimal glands called *Mikulicz's syndrome.* Onset of	Corticosteroids (systemic and topical) and mydriatics during active stages. Potassium supplements.	Recurrence common. Long-term visual prognosis is poor.

TABLE 1.10 (*Continued*)

Description	Treatment	Course
disease occurs in third decade and is more prevalent among blacks than whites. Anterior uveitis (more common) is nodular and may be complicated by development of cataracts and glaucoma. Posterior uveitis is marked by multiple yellowish retinal exudates and perivasculitis. Often bilateral. Patients develop blurred vision, slight photophobia, and ciliary flush. Pain may be minimal or absent. Diagnosis is by rheumatoid work-up.		
Sympathetic ophthalmia Devastating uveitis developing 10 days to several years after penetrating eye injury, retained foreign body, or intraocular surgery involving ciliary area. Thought to be a hypersensitivity reaction to uveal pigments. Inflammatory cells form caseating tubercles in the injured "exciting" eye first and then in the noninjured "sympathetic" eye. Inflammatory process spreads along the optic nerve. Patients present with photophobia, redness, and blurred vision. Diagnosis is based on a history of trauma and bilateral, acute onset.	Enucleation of severely injured eyes within 10 days as prophylactic measure. Enucleation not advised once uveitis is established since injured eye may offer best visual hope. Corticosteroids and atropine in active stages.	Without treatment, disease progresses slowly, ending in complete bilateral blindness.
Toxoplasmosis CNS inflammation with eye involvement caused by the protozoon *Toxoplasma gondii.* Eggs passed to humans in cat feces or infected raw meat. *Congenital form* (fetus affected by maternal infection) results in bilateral, severe chorioretinitis. Cerebral calcifications and mental deficiencies occur in 10% of cases. *Acquired disease* in adulthood is typically unilateral and less severe. Most frequent in white teenage girls, least frequent in blacks. Produces elevated, white, chorioretinal masses obscured by hazy vitreous and (in later stages) punched-out, pigmented lesions revealing the underlying sclera. Vitreous may detach from retina, leaving areas of vitreous precipitates, or the patient may develop a rare reaction with debris formations resembling "grapevines covered with wet snow." Patients have minimal pain but may note blurred vision and slight photophobia. Toxoplasma organisms are recovered from necrotic retinal tissues, and methylene blue dye test is positive.	Pyrimethamine (Daraprim) in combination with trisulfapyrimidines for 4 weeks. Systemic corticosteroids are added if no response occurs in 6 weeks. Subconjunctival/IM injections of clindamycin now under investigation. Cryosurgery photocoagulation may be needed for recurrences.	Lesions remain active for 4 months and then heal, leaving scar tissue. New lesions often develop near old scars, resulting in a chronic course. If macula is involved, loss of central vision is permanent.
Tuberculosis Thought to arise from some tuberculous focus in the body, but rare in patients with active pulmonary disease. Iris nodules and "mutton fat" lesions seen on slit lamp exam if anterior tract is involved; hazy vitreous, yellow chorioretinal masses from caseating tubercles if disease is localized to the posterior tract. Causes moderate infection and blurred vision, but minimal pain.	Atropine drops to dilate pupil. Antituberculous drugs (isoniazid and para-amino-salicylic acid) for 4–6 months. After 6 weeks, corticosteroids added if response is poor.	Resolves after prolonged course, leaving permanently damaged tissue and blurred vision.

systemic, or periocular injections); immunosuppressive therapy (alkylating agents, purine or pyrimidine analogues, or folic acid antagonists); nonsteroidal antiinflammatory agents; and photocoagulation. Mydriatic-cycloplegics are also used to relieve the pain and scarring related to iris sphincter and ciliary muscle spasm.

Retina and Vitreous Fluid

The retina forms the third and innermost coat of the eyeball. It has an outer layer of pigment epithelium (retinal pigment epithelium, RPE) and an inner layer of neural (sensory) tissue that harbors the rods and cones. Rods contain rhodopsin, a chemical extremely sensitive to light and movement, but not to color. As many as 600 rods converge on a single nerve fiber, making vision in dim light possible, but without fine detail. Objects are seen in the dark as colorless masses that have no clear outline.

Rhodopsin is very unstable in bright light and readily breaks down into its component products, retinene and vitamin A. While rhodopsin is in a dissociated state, a temporary but alarming visual loss occurs, such as that caused by the sudden approach of high-beam auto headlights. Once the chemical re-forms, dark adaptation returns. As might be expected, ***night blindness*** (nyctalopia) may develop from ▶ ***vitamin A deficiency.*** Some cases result from a poor diet, but most can be traced to malabsorption of the vitamin (gastrointestinal or pancreatic disorders) or impaired storage (liver disease). Treatment consists of correcting the underlying causes and increasing the intake of foods that are high in vitamin A.

Cones are sensitive to red, blue, and green spectral patterns. Color vision takes place when light waves stimulate one or more of these patterns. The light wave's length (saturation) determines the color, along with its quality of reflection (hue) and its intensity of light (brightness).

When cone sensitivity to a certain spectral pattern is genetically lacking, ***color blindness*** exists. When tested with polychromatic plates such as the Ishihara, Stilling, or Hardy-Rand-Ritler plates, patients are unable to recognize numbers formed by dots of primary colors on background dots of mixed colors. The exact type and severity of color blindness can be defined when patients are tested with a variety of plates. Blue ***(tritan)*** and yellow ***(tetartan)*** deficiencies are very rare. However, red ***(protan)*** and green ***(duetran)*** deficiencies occur in 4% of all males. Since these are X-linked recessive characteristics, only 0.4% of females exhibit any problem. Patients should be counseled to avoid occupations requiring good color vision, but otherwise need no special attention.

Absent or severely abnormal cone function occurs in ***achromatopsia.*** In addition to complete color blindness, patients have nystagmus and poor visual acuity. They naturally avoid bright lights to keep the rods (their only source of vision) in a state of dark adaptation. In fact, the only available treatment consists of providing extra-dark sunglasses with side shields. Since the retina appears normal, the diagnosis of achromatopsia and other problems related to photoreceptor cells may depend on electroretinography (ERG). A contact lens containing electrodes is placed on the eye, and recordings are made of the electrical activity of the retina as various parts are stimulated with external lights. Electro-oculography (EOG) may serve as a supplemental test. By placing electrodes on the skin around the eye and on the cornea, recordings can be made of metabolic changes in the retina, as well as any form of nystagmus.

Retinal dystrophies and degenerations are caused by conditions listed in Table 1.11. Primary disorders are rare. The most commonly encountered of these is ***retinitis pigmentosa.*** As its first symptom in early youth, night blindness signals destruction of rods. Secondary atrophy causes gradual constriction of visual fields ("gun barrel vision") until blindness ensues around age 50 or 60. During this slow process, cells from the damaged RPE migrate along the retinal vessels, giving the fundus a "bone spicule" appearance with scattered clumps of pigmentation. The disk becomes pale and waxy. These changes take place only at later stages of the disease, and early diagnosis may depend on ERG or EOG. As with most retinal dystrophies, there is no treatment.

Over 1 million cones are concentrated in a small oval area in the middle of the retina called the "macula" (Fig. 1.3). Its center (the fovea centralis) contains only cones, each synapsing with its own nerve fiber. This makes the macula the area of highest visual acuity and ►***screening far visual acuity*** a logical test of macular function. As discussed in later sections, screening for visual acuity can also reveal refractive problems.

Although most of the retina receives blood from the central artery as well as the underlying choroid, the macula relies solely on the choriocapillaris for nourishment. For this reason, many cases of ***macular degeneration*** can be traced to disrupted choroid attachment at the RPE or to other changes in the choroid tissues. Others are primary in nature or secondary to systemic diseases and exposure to toxins. Described in Table 1.12, macular degenerations constitute the leading cause of reported blindness. Neither red eye nor pain warns the patient of any problem. Blurred vision made worse by exposure to bright light is the usual presenting symptom. The funduscopic exam may be unremarkable or may reveal angioid streaks, Drusen bodies, an atrophic macular hole, or irregular pigmentation around the macula (poached or scrambled egg appearance). Definitive diagnosis is provided by fluorescein angiography. Some patients may be candidates for photocoagulation, but for many there is no treatment. Preparation for blindness during progressive stages of deterioration facilitates adjustment and continued independence.

The retina is supported by an albuminous substance, the vitreous fluid. As a person ages, the vitreous gel begins to break down, a process that results in the formation of watery cavities. If the shadow of a cavity stimulates the retina, visual awareness of its silhouetted shape occurs. These bits of watery debris that flit in and out of the line of vision are aptly called ***floaters.***

Floaters are common and are usually no cause for concern. However, the sudden development of numerous floaters that seem to descend or swarm over the field of vision could be a warning sign of ***retinal detachment.*** This develops whenever the retina separates from its underlying source of nourishment, the choriocapillaris. Sometimes blood coming from choroidal tumors, or inflammatory or diseased conditions of the retina, causes the two layers to separate. More commonly, the cause is vitreous fluid seeping through a ***retinal hole*** or ***retinal tear.*** Retinal holes represent areas of gradually disintegrated tissue that may be idiopathic or the result of retinal disease. In retinal tears, the tissue rips suddenly during an eye injury or abnormal vitreous traction. The latter is associated with diabetic retinopathy, aging, aphakia, myopia, the use of mitotics with foward displacement of the lens, and scleral ectasia. The retina continues to separate as long as there is seepage of blood or vitreous fluid beneath it. Complete detachment may occur within hours or several years later. It leads to degeneration of rods and cones, with gradual restriction of

TABLE 1.11 POSSIBLE CAUSES OF CHORIORETINAL DETERIORATION

Congenital anomalies
- Morning-glory anomaly of the optic nerve
- Hypoplasia of the optic nerve
- Segmental hypoplasia of the optic nerve
- Optic nerve drusen
- Optic nerve pits
- Macular hypoplasia
- Persistent hyperplastic primary vitreous
- Anterior chamber anomalies
  - Anterior chamber cleavage syndrome
  - Axenfeld's anomaly
  - Iridogonio dysgenesis
  - Peter's anomaly
  - Craniofacial syndromes (Apert's disease, Crouzon's syndrome, craniometaphyseal dysplasia)

Inherited disorders
- Retinitis pigmentosa
- Acanthocytosis (Bassen-Kornzweig syndrome)
- Achromatopia
- Ahlstrom syndrome
- Aicardi's syndrome
- Albinism
- Albipunctuate dystrophy
- Aminoacidurias
  - Homocystinuria
  - Cystinosis
  - Lowe's syndrome
- Apert's syndrome
- Bardet-Biedl syndrome
- Best's vitelliform macular degeneration
- Choroidal sclerosis
- Choroideremia
- Chromosomal abnormalities
  - Trisomy 13 (D trisomy, Patau's syndrome)
  - Trisomy 18 (E trisomy, Edwards' syndrome)
  - Trisomy 21 (Down's syndrome, mongolism)
  - Cri-du-chat (chromosome 5 deletion)
  - Chromosome 13 deletion
  - DeGrouchy syndrome (chromosome 18 deletion)
  - Turner's syndrome (X chromosome deletion)
- Coat's disease (retinal telangiectasia)
- Cockayne's syndrome
- Cone dystrophy
- Ehlers-Danlos syndrome
- Familial hyperphosphatemia
- Friedrich's syndrome
- Goldmann-Favre syndrome
- Gyrate atrophy
- Ichthyosis
- Incontinentia pigmenti
- Juvenile retinoschisis
- Kearnes-Sayre syndrome
- Laurence-Moon-Bardet-Biedl syndrome
- Leber's congenital amaurosis
- Marfan's syndrome
- Mucolipidoses
  - Generalized gangliosidoses
  - Metachromatic leukodystrophy
  - Mucolipidosis type I
  - Farber disease (lipogranulomatosis)
- Mucopolysaccharidosis
  - Type I—Sheie's syndrome
  - Type II—Hunter's syndrome
  - Type III—Sanfilippo's syndrome
  - Type IV—Morquio's syndrome
  - Type VI—Maroteaux-Lamy syndrome
- Myopic choroidal atrophy
- Neuronal lipofuscinosis (Batten-Mayou disease)
- Norrie's disease
- Paget's disease (osteitis deformans)
- Pierre Robin syndrome (clefting syndrome)
- Pseudoinflammatory macular dystrophy of Sorsby
- Pseudoretinitis pigmentosa
- Pseudoxanthoma elasticum (Grönblad-Strandberg syndrome)
- Refsum's disease
- Rendu-Osler-Weber disease (hereditary telangiectasia)
- Ring-D chromosome
- Schmid-Fraccaro syndrome
- Sphingolipidoses
  - Type I—Tay-Sachs disease
  - Type II—Sandhoff's disease
  - Type III
  - Group A—Niemann-Pick disease (infantile)
  - Globoid cell leukodystrophy—Krabbe's disease
- Usher's syndrome
- Wagner's vitreoretinal degeneration

Degenerative changes
- Dry senile degeneration
- Senile retinoschisis
- Paving stone retinal degeneration
- Lattice degeneration
- Retinal holes
- Peripheral cystoid degeneration
- Central serous detachment
- Disciform degeneration
- Pigment epithelial detachment
- Senile degeneration of Bruch's membrane
- Angioid streaks
- Foveal hole

Tumors
- Retinoblastoma
- Malignant melanomas
- Optic glioma
- Hamartomas
- Tuberous sclerosis (Bourneville's disease)
- Neurofibromatosis (von Recklinghausen's disease)
- Von Hippel-Landau disease (angiomatosis retinae)
- Sturge-Weber syndrome (choroidal hemangioma)
- Metastatic (breast, colon, kidney, lung, ovary, cervix, testis, prostate, stomach, pancreas)

Traumatic
- Retinal tears
- Fracture of Bruch's membrane
- Commotio retinae (Berlin's edema)
- Penetrating injury
- Radiation retinopathy (UV, infrared radiation and irradiation of the head and neck)

TABLE 1.11 *(Continued)*

Vascular disorders
- Carotid occlusive disease
- Pulseless disease
- Retinal arterial occlusion
- Retinal venous occlusion (central, branch, and hemorrhagic)
- Hypertension (chronic, malignant, or toxemia of pregnancy)
- Diabetes mellitus
- Arteriosclerosis
- Systemic vasculitis
  - Scleroderma
  - Behcet's disease
  - Epidermolysis bullosa
  - Erythema multiforme
  - Stevens-Johnson syndrome
  - Dermatomyositis
  - Periarteritis nodosa
  - Reiter's syndrome
  - Sarcoidosis
  - Systemic lupus erythematosus
  - Juvenile rheumatoid arthritis
  - Temporal arteritis
  - Wegener's granulomatosis
  - Eales's disease

Hematologic
- Anemia (chronic disease or acute blood loss)
- Sickle cell disease
- Leukemia
- Lymphoma
- Multiple myeloma
- Polycythemia vera
- Thrombocytopenia
- Waldenstrom's macroglobulinemia

Infectious
- Bacterial (brucellosis, septicemia, tularemia, leprosy, tuberculosis)
- Fungal (cryptocossosis, metastatic candidal endophthalmitis, histoplasmosis, actinomycosis)
- Viral (acute posterior multifocal placoid pigment epitheliopathy, cytomegalic inclusion disease, subacute sclerosing panencephalitis from measles virus, fetal exposure to maternal rubella, herpes simplex, chickenpox, herpes zoster, mumps, infectious mononucleosis, influenza)
- Parasitic (tapeworm, toxocariasis, onchocerciasis, toxoplasmosis, echinococcosis, lymphogranuloma venereum)

Toxic
- Neonatal oxygen therapy (retrolental fibroplasia)
- Lead poisoning
- Drugs
  - Antiinflammatory (salicylates, ibuprofen, indomethacin, Butazolidin)
  - CNS drugs (barbiturates, thorazine, ethchlorvynol, monoamine oxidase inhibitors, perphenazine, thioridazine, trimethadione)
  - Cholinergic, anticholinergic (carbachol, atropine)
  - Antiinfective (chloramphenicol, chloroquine, ethambutol, ethionamide, hydroxychloroquine, iodochlorohydroxyquin, diiodohydroxyquin, isoniazid, nalidixic acid, quinine, streptomycin, sulfonamides, tetracycline, triparasimide)
  - Cardiovascular (carbonic anhydrase inhibitors, acetazolamide, chlorothiazides, digitalis, hexamethonium, furosimide, quinadine, reserpine)
  - Hormonal agents (ACTH, corticosteroids, oral contraceptives)
  - Vitamins (vitamin A, nicotinic acid)
  - Other (allopurinol, coumadin, chlorambucil, chloropropamide)

visual fields. If the macula becomes unstuck, there is immediate loss of central vision. Warning symptoms of retinal detachment include the sudden development of vitreous floaters, fiashes of light ***(photopsia),*** and distortions in the contours of objects ***(metamorphopsia).*** They warrant immediate referral to an ophthalmologist. Most detachments begin in the periphery and can be detected only by binocular indirect ophthalmoscopy in the early stages. They appear as translucent bulges with ripples or folds. The first step in treatment is extensive examination of the retina and the construction of a detailed map showing all holes and areas of vitreous traction. After small amounts are removed, vitreous fluid is manipulated until the retina and choroid are reapproximated. All holes and tears are then bonded with cryothermy, diathermy, or photocoagulation. The prognosis is best when seepage of vitreous fluid is still localized.

Optic Nerve

The optic nervehead enters the fundus at a point called the "optic disc" (Fig. 1.3). Magnified 15 times by the ophthalmoscope, this round to oval structure may vary in

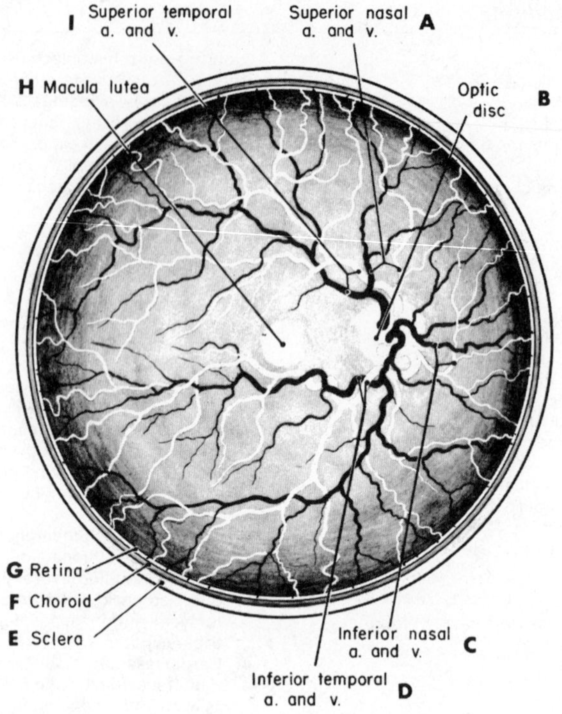

Figure 1.3 Fundus. (From Crafts, *Textbook of Human Anatomy,* © 1985, John Wiley and Sons, Inc., New York.)

size with refractive errors. Thus it appears quite small in farsighted people and excessively large in nearsighted people. For the most part, the disc margin can be clearly delineated from surrounding tissue by differences in pigmentation and texture. The disc itself is generally pink, except for a yellow-tinged depression at its center, the physiologic cup. The cup may normally be absent or occupy up to 80% of the disc space. However, this proportion should be symmetric. ***Asymmetric "cupping"*** suggests the glaucomatous change described earlier.

The optic nerve is a direct extension of the brain, and therefore both unmyelinated and surrounded by fluid-filled meninges. Any increase in intracranial pressure leads to swelling of the optic nerve and congestion of venous outflow known as ***papilledema.*** This may occur in a number of conditions listed in Table 1.13. Once intercranial pressure rises, papilledema develops within 1–5 days (2–8 hours of an acute intracranial bleed). As an early change, thickened nerve fibers and engorged vessels blur the disc margins at the upper and lower poles. At this point, diagnosis may be difficult since hazy disc margins occur as a normal variant ***(pseudopapilledema).*** Pathology is unlikely if pulsations are noted along the central vein or if visual field testing demonstrates a normal blind spot. Later findings in papilledema are unmistakable. The disc becomes elevated and surrounded by flame-shaped, punctate, or splinter hemorrhages. Cotton wool exudates, retinal stress lines, and macular edema with hard exudates (star formation) may occur. Pupil responses are

TABLE 1.12 MACULAR DEGENERATION

Type	Description
Central areolar choroidal sclerosis	Deterioration of the choriocapillaris, inherited as an autosomal recessive or dominant trait. Abnormalities develop early, with slow loss of central vision occurring by middle age. There is no treatment.
Stargardt-Behr disease	Deterioration of the pigment epithelium, transmitted in an autosomal recessive manner. Clinical problems manifest at different ages. Pigment changes develop slowly, the final intensity varying according to family patterns. No treatment available.
Best's vitelliform dystrophy	Autosomal dominant disease marked by diffuse damage to the pigment epithelium. Abnormal deposits of pigment collect around the macula, giving it a poached egg appearance ("sunny side up" in early stages, "scrambled yolk" in advanced stages). Central vision becomes severely reduced. There is no treatment.
Central serous retinochoroidopathy	Problem of unknown etiology, beginning when serous fluid leaks through the RPE into the subretinal space, causing shallow detachment of the sensory macula. Occurring mostly in young men, it causes increased hypermetropia and general decrease of acuity, visual distortion, darkening of visual fields, and poor recovery from glare. These symptoms are usually self-limiting, resolving within 3–6 months, but almost all patients show some ongoing disturbance of the RPE. Cystic edema and lipid deposition may require photocoagulation.
Local detachment of RPE	Similar to central serous retinochoroidopathy in pathophysiology and symptomatology, but involving a greater area and more likely to affect older people. May be associated with Drusen bodies and disciform lesions in the other eye. Entire dome of detachment lights up on fluorescein angiography. Although spontaneous resolution may occur, minor disturbances in visual function often remain. Photocoagulation is of questionable value.
Chorioretinitis	Macular damage following inflammatory (infectious or autoimmune) process of the retina or uveal tract.
Choroid degenerations	Colloid's collections (Drusen bodies), breaks in Bruch's membrane (angioid streaks), or other senile and degenerative changes in the choroid cause serous fluid to collect under the retina, detaching it from the choriocapillaris. Subsequently, the space beneath the RPE becomes occupied by proliferating blood vessels (choriodal neovascular membrane, *CNM*) that can be identified on angiography by a lacy meshwork or "bicycle wheel" distribution of dye. If the CNM hemorrhages, disciform scars form, causing permanent deterioration of central vision. Treatment thus concentrates on early obliteration of the CNM with high-energy contiguous laser lesions.
"Dry" senile changes	Arteriosclerotic changes with chronic ischemia lead to degeneration of the RPE, Bruch's membrane, and choroid. Changes vary from minor atrophy of the RPE to large, punched-out areas of the choroid, overlying RPE, and sensory retina. Visual loss is progressive. Intervention is limited to rehabilitation with low-vision aids and preparation for blindness.
Toxic effects	Degeneration of the RPE results from certain drugs. Daily doses exceeding 150 mg chloroquine base may cause functional changes (scotoma on visual field testing, red-green defect on Ishiahara color tests, abnormal EOG), or horizontal atrophy (bull's-eye appearance on angiography). Doses of thorazine greater than 1 g/day may alter macular pigmentation (central or ring scotomas on visual field testing, altered ERG). Doses of chlorpromazine over 2 g daily for more than 1 year may cause mild pigmentary changes (no significant functional defects).
Gyrate atrophy	Irregular peripheral areas of atrophy develop beneath retinal vessels, beginning in the third decade. Areas enlarge and coalesce, finally involving the macula.

TABLE 1.13 CONDITIONS ASSOCIATED WITH PAPILLEDEMA

Central nervous system Brain tumors (posterior fossa, rarely frontal lobe) Brain abscesses Subdural hematomas (usually traumatic) Hydrocephalis	Hematologic Polycythemia vera Sickle cell disease Waldenström's macroglobulinemia Multiple myeloma
Musculoskeletal Craniofacial syndromes (Apert's disease, craniometaphyseal dysplasia) Crouzon's syndrome	Metabolic Hyperthyroidism Hypoparathyroidism Addison's disease Cushing's disease Hypervitaminosis A and D Avitaminosis A in infants Whipple's disease
Cardiovascular Malignant hypertension Toxemia of pregnancy Aortic arch syndrome (Takayasu) Central retinal vein thrombosis	Toxic Nalidixic acid Tetracycline Chlorambucil Corticosteroids Hormonal agents: ACTH, corticosteroids
Collagen vascular Sarcoidosis Wegener's granulomatosis Systemic lupus erythematosus Periarteritis nodosa	Renal Azotemia (acute and chronic pyelonephritis) Nephrotic syndromes: acute glomerulonephritis, diabetic kidney, systemic lupus erythematosus
Pulmonary Emphysema Tuberculosis Cystic fibrosis of the pancreas	Infectious Toxoplasmosis Cryptococcosis

normal. The blind spot may enlarge, but otherwise visual acuity and visual fields remain unchanged. These findings are usually but not always bilateral. Papilledema is a neuro-ophthalmologic emergency, necessitating immediate hospital admission. Computed tomography (CT) scanning is essential, but lumbar puncture as an initial test is contraindicated due to the risk of brain herniation whenever intracranial pressures are elevated. If underlying causes can be determined and treated quickly, papilledema clears rapidly. However, chronic papilledema may lead to optic atrophy.

Disc swelling in ***papillitis*** evolves from a disorder of the nervehead, either vascular or inflammatory/degenerative in nature (Table 1.14). When the optic nerve and choroid tissues infarct due to a vascular problem, the clinical picture is known as ***ischemic optic neuropathy.*** Most commonly caused by temporal arteritis, it is characterized by pallor and swelling at the disc, dilation of the retinal capillaries, and small hemorrhages or cotton-wool patches of the nerve fiber layers. The affected eye may show a Marcus Gunn pupil, dilation and paralysis of the pupillary sphincter, or a tonic pupil (see Table 1.9). Diplopia is relatively uncommon and pain is unusual. Patients with signs and symptoms of ischemic optic neuropathy should be referred to a neurologist for immediate evaluation. High-dose steroids are given until the results of sedimentation rate and tests and temporal artery biopsy rule out temporal arteritis (see also Chapter 6).

Papillitis evolving from inflammatory/degenerative changes of the optic nerve is referred to as ***optic neuritis.*** Multiple sclerosis is the most common of the many associated conditions noted in Table 1.14. With posterior lesions, papillitis is absent, a variant referred to as ***retrobulbar neuritis.*** The symptoms of optic neuritis are variable. Pain is experienced by the majority of patients but ranges considerably. It

TABLE 1.14 CONDITIONS ASSOCIATED WITH OPTIC NEURITIS AND PAPILLITIS

Degenerative
- Multiple sclerosis
- Late neurosyphilis
- Devic's disease
- Schilder's disease
- Leber's optic atrophy

Toxic
- Abused substances: tobacco, alcohol
- Heavy metals: arsenic, lead, thallium
- Drugs: oral contraceptives, Enterovioform (antidiarrheal sold over the counter abroad), ethambutol, isoniazid, streptomycin, disulfiram, digitalis, chloramphenicol, chloroquine, chlorpropamide, halogenated hydroxyquinones, quinidine, barbiturates, ethchlorvynol, monoamine oxidase inhibitors, perphenazine, ethionamide (antituberculin), sulfonamides, tryparsamide (antisyphilitic, trypanosomiasis), hexamethonium, Butazolidin, salicylates, nicotinic acid

Inflammatory (infectious and autoimmune)
- Temporal (cranial) arteritis
- Behcet's disease
- Reiter's syndrome
- Regional enteritis/ulcerative colitis
- Sarcoidosis
- Erythema multiforme (Stevens-Johnson syndrome)
- Cryptococcosis
- Lens-induced uveitis
- Infective endocarditis
- Bacterial: tuberculosis, brucellosis
- Viral: measles, mumps, chickenpox, influenza, infectious mononucleosis, herpes zoster, Guillain-Barré syndrome
- Protozoal: toxoplasmosis, malaria (may be due to antimalarial drug therapy)
- Fungal: coccidioidomycosis
- Toxocariasis

Other
- Leukemia
- Diabetes mellitus
- Dysthyroidism
- Vitamin deficiencies: beriberi, pellagra
- Hypothyroidism
- Cystic fibrosis of the pancreas

is often described as a dull retro-orbital ache or a sharp discomfort provoked by eye movements and/or pressure on the globe. Visual changes are simultaneous or follow within a few days. They include misty or blurred vision, difficulty in reading, a blind spot, and impaired perception of color, brightness, or depth. In multiple sclerosis or other demyelinating disorders, transient blurring often occurs with physical exertion ***(Uhthoff's syndrome).*** It may also be associated with temperature changes, menstruation, increased illumination, eating, and smoking. On exam, pupils are noted to be equal in size, with normal consensual light reflexes and near responses. A Marcus Gunn pupil is often present. In the early stages, funduscopic abnormalities are limited to blurred disc margins and distention of large veins, whereas fully developed papillitis resembles papilledema with marked disc swelling, obliteration of the physiologic cup, and splinter hemorrhages. Venous sheathing and fine opacities in the vitreous may be observed with a slit lamp. Visual acuity can fall to 20/100 or less, and visual field defects are likely (central scotomas are most common). Patients with signs and symptoms of optic neuritis should be referred to an ophthalmologist. They should also be evaluated for an associated disorder. In most cases, there is no known treatment; systemic corticosteroids have not proved helpful. The natural course is for vision changes to maximize soon after the onset of symptoms and then begin to improve a few days to 3 weeks later. Improvement continues slowly over a period of several months, with vision returning to normal. However, in severe or repeated episodes, secondary optic atrophy may develop.

Optic atrophy is the destruction of nerve bundles located at the optic head. As just noted, this may follow papillitis or chronic papilledema. ***Consecutive optic atrophy*** and ***heterofamilial optic atrophy*** are two other categories described in Table 1.15. ***Glaucomatous atrophy*** was discussed previously. All types of optic atrophy are destructive because nerve bundles send out fibers that radiate over the retina in a specific distribution. When bundles are destroyed at the nervehead,

TABLE 1.16 DIABETIC AND HYPERTENSIVE RETINOPATHY

Type	Description	Course
Diabetic		
Background lesions	Capillary closure due to disease leads to microaneurysms, hemorrhages, cotton wool spots, hard exudates.	Diabetic retinopathy accounts for 12% of all blindness in Western countries. Two-thirds of those with diabetes for 15 years or longer develop retinopathy, the duration of disease being the main factor. The relationship to control of disease has not been established, but it is assumed that normalization of blood sugars delays the onset of retinopathy. *Photocoagulation,* thought to reduce vasoproliferative factors amd delay blindness once neovascularization has occurred, is under widespread clinical trial. Panretinal and focal burns are applied with either an argon laser or a xenon arc photocoagulator. Surgery performed through the pars plana region of the ciliary body (*pars plana victrectomy*) is being used to clear vitreous hemorrhages and reduce the incidence of retinal detachments.
Advanced background lesions (preproliferative)	The ischemic retina elaborates a vasoproliferative factor to stimulate neovascularization in an attempt to establish a better blood supply. This proliferation is heralded by shunt vessels and venous sheathing.	
Proliferative	Fragile new blood vessels develop at interfaces between well-perfused and poorly perfused tissue. They proliferate on the surface of the retina that is attached to the vitreous body. Contraction of the vitreous body results in vitreous hemorrhage. Further traction leads to retinal detachments.	
Hyptertensive[a]		
Group 1 (essential HTN, overall health unchanged)	Moderate arteriole attenuation with focal constriction and copper wire/silver wire light reflexes.	Sustained elevations of blood pressure cause necrosis of smooth muscle in the walls of retinal vessels. Plasma seeps through weakened epithelium into the endothelium, leading to further vessel damage. However, unless there is secondary occlusion of the vessel and retinal ischemia, serious impairment of vision does not usually occur. Retinal changes are important mainly in assessing damage to the heart, brain, and kidneys. Although blood pressure control is mandatory, ocular treatment remains controversial. Photocoagulation is being used in patients who demonstrate funduscopic and fluorescein evidence of deterioration over a period of 6 months. However, even patients with retinal vein occlusions maintain good central vision without treatment.
Group 2 (HTN longstanding, but still no permanent damage)	Pronounced attenuation with diffuse constriction and atrioventricular crossing defects. Hard, shiny deposits and tiny hemorrhages begin to develop.	
Group 3 (malignant HTN; Mean life expectancy 27.6 months)	Focal ischemia leading to retinal edema, hemorrhages, and cotton wool spots.	
Group 4 (end-organ damage; mean life expectancy 10.5 months)	All signs of group 3 plus papilledema.	

[a] Keith-Wagener-Baaker classifications.

TABLE 1.17 CONDITIONS ASSOCIATED WITH TEMPORARY DECREASE OF OCULAR PERFUSION AND AMAUROSIS FUGAX

Mechanical compression of vertebral or carotid arteries	Raised intraocular pressure
Disease of the carotid artery	Papilledema
Dysrhythmia	Migraine
Hypertensive episode	Anemia
Hypotensive episode	Polycythemia
Central artery or vein occlusions	Macroglobulinemia
Retinal emboli	Sickle cell disease
Papillitis	Polycythemia vera

of a gray cloud or the drawing of a window shade. Cholesterol emboli can sometimes be seen on funduscopic exam as a shiny plaque lodged at the bifurcation of retinal arterioles ***(Hollenhorst plaque).*** Patients with any of these signs or symptoms should be referred to a neurologist immediately. The work-up may involve carotid ultrasound or echocardiography (to rule out plaques or thrombi), as well as assessment for conditions known to alter retinal blood flow (Table 1.17). Control of underlying disorders is crucial. High blood pressure should be normalized, but a precipitous fall could compromise blood perfusion to the eye and is to be avoided. If retinal ischemia cannot be halted, optic atrophy with permanent loss of vision quickly develops.

With ***central retinal artery occlusion*** the inner two-thirds of the retina infarcts immediately. Patients experience sudden and complete loss of vision not associated with pain. The fundus takes on a milky white appearance subsequent to reflex constriction of the entire arterial tree and edema. The macula, which receives all of its blood supply from the choriocapillaris, remains perfused and looks like a cherry-red spot in contrast. The direct pupillary response is absent, but the consensual light reaction is normal (Marcus Gunn pupil). While an emergency ophthalmologic referral is being arranged, primary care providers should attempt measures to increase oxygen flow to the retina. They can administer oxygen (100%) or, if this is not available, initiate rebreathing into a paper bag (which produces vasodilatation by altering the CO_2 content). The specialist may massage the globe or remove small amounts of fluid from the anterior chamber, hoping to move the emboli in the central artery to a more peripheral branch. However, this intervention is helpful only within the first two hours, as ischemia that lasts any longer results in tissue death and permanent loss of vision.

Retinal branch vein occlusions (fairly common) and ***central retinal venous occlusion*** (rare) stem from sluggish venous blood flow. Most cases are associated with hypertension, diabetes, sickle cell disease, polycythemia vera, lymphoma, leukemia, macroglobulinemia, or multiple myeloma. Branch occlusions, which usually involve the superior temporal vein, occur at atriovenous crossings, while central occlusions occur at the optic disc. Distal to the obstruction, veins become engorged, tortuous, and hemorrhagic. There is no pain, and loss of vision occurs only when the macula is affected. Patients should be referred to an ophthalmologist for immediate evaluation. Mild bleeding clears with spontaneous return of visual acuity after a few weeks and requires no treatment. However, severe bleeding is often attended by extensive edema, cotton wool spots, and secondary glaucoma. This condition, known as ***hemorrhagic retinopathy,*** leads to cystoid degeneration of fovea, alteration of all retinal layers, and liquefaction of the vitreous. Steroids and photocoagulation have been used with some success. Treatment of underlying blood sludging problems and vascular disorders is also important. Glaucoma, neovascularization, vitreous hemorrhage, and retinal detachment are long-term complications.

VISION

Clear monocular vision occurs as long as light stimulation is kept focused on the macula. This is accomplished by each eye's capacity for refraction and accommodation. Binocular vision, which provides depth perception, is made possible by the fine coordination of the extraocular muscles.

Refraction and Accommodation

Light rays travel fastest in air and are slowed down by transparent media such as water or glass. If light passes through an alternative medium at a nonperpendicular angle, the varying changes in speed cause the light rays to bend. If light enters at a 90 degree angle, all the rays change velocity simultaneously and no bending takes place. This is the principle behind a lens. The curved surface of a lens provides nonperpendicular entry for light while its transparent medium alters the speed of entrance. The shape (convex, concave, or cylindric) determines whether the light rays diverge or converge, and the power of the lens determines the degree of refraction.

Light rays entering the eye are bent by the optically smooth surface of the cornea. An irregularity in the corneal surface causes some of the incoming light to diverge and produces a visual picture that is focused in some planes and blurred in others. This is known as an ***astigmatism.*** Depending on the location and refractive power of the irregularity, either horizontal, vertical, or diagonal lines will appear slanted. Although the brain may correct for out-of-plumb images, it cannot correct for the diminished visual acuity caused by astigmatism. Positive or negative cylindric lenses are usually needed. During the first week of use, or until the brain adjusts to the fact that it is no longer dealing with an image error, patients may experience a tilting sensation while wearing the new lenses.

Light rays entering the eye from a distant object (more than 6 m away) are bent not only by the cornea but also by the aqueous humor, the biconvex lens, and finally the vitreous fluid to converge on a single focal point at the fovea. Because of the optics governing convex lenses, the image formed is inverted, greatly reduced, and reversed from side to side. Luckily, the brain is able to translate such an image correctly.

The distance from the lens to the focal point is normally 16.7 mm. A longer or shorter distance precludes the correct focus of light rays on the retina. In ***myopia,*** the shape of the eyeball is abnormally long, so light from distant objects comes to a focal point in front of the retina (see Fig. 1.4). As the object is brought closer, the image on the retina sharpens. The distance at which it becomes most sharply focused is called the "far point." Because close vision is clearest, the person is said to be "nearsighted." He or she may squint or frown in an effort to delineate distant objects. This is because squinting cuts down on light entering through the pupil and sharpens the image (pinhole effect). The refraction errors is noted on ▶***screening far***

visual acuity and is corrected with concave lenses that bend light rays the extra length to the retina. Understanding that the problem basic to myopia is an elongated globe dispels the popular belief that glasses weaken the eye. Nor is the course of myopia altered by excessive eye strain, inadequate lighting, or eye exercises. There is, however, recent evidence that hard contact lenses may help reduce the degree of nearsightedness by keeping the cornea flattened. Furthermore, a natural tendency exists for myopia to become worse during adolescence and level off at the age of 25. Frequent or drastic changes in refractive status after age 25 suggest a systemic problem, particularly diabetes.

In ***hyperopia*** (farsightedness), the eyeball length is too short and the focal point falls behind the retina (Fig. 1.4). This condition is found in 80% of the general population. Although distant vision is normal, extra effort is needed for accommodation (near vision).

"Accommodation" is a collective term referring to three adjustments undertaken by the eye when an object is viewed from a range of less than 20 ft. Without them, the image falling on the retina would be blurred because light rays from short distances do not enter the eye in parallel lines. First, the ciliary muscles of the iris contract, lessening tension on the zonular fibers. Zonular fibers are attached to the biconvex lens, a transparent, semisolid mass of specialized fibers and proteins enveloped in a thin capsule. As illustrated in Figure 1.4, ligaments are kept taut when the muscles relax (stretch) and slacken when the muscles contract (shorten). When zonular tension decreases, the lens bulges in relief, becoming more convex. Unfortunately, the periphery of the lens in its highly convex state has the ability to scatter light and break it into a prismatic spectrum. To avoid these "spherical" and "chromatic" aberrations, light is prevented from reaching the lens periphery by constriction of the pupil. This constriction is thus the second change that occurs in accommodation. The third change is convergence. This is the tendency of the two eyes to turn toward one another as they track an approaching object into near view.

With severe hyperopia, constant accommodation leads to eye strain, headaches, and even nausea. Patients with these symptoms may need corrective lenses from childhood on. However, people with mild hyperopia make the extra adjustment needed for near vision without too much difficulty. In fact, they enjoy better than average vision until after the age of 40. At that time there is a natural decline in accommodation called ***presbyopia.*** The lens, once soft and pliable, turns stiff and less responsive to changing shape. This results in a blurring of printed material, fatigue from close work, and focal lag when changing from near to distant vision. Symptoms are worse in dim light, early morning, or whenever the patient is fatigued. The problem can be assessed by ▶ ***screening near visual acuity.*** It is corrected with a plus lens (analogous to the close-up lens of a camera), which can be prescribed in several forms. Reading glasses have the correction ground throughout the lens. They are fine for close work but cause a blurring of distant vision and must be constantly taken off. Half-glasses have an open top to mitigate this problem; bifocals and trifocals correct for additional refractive errors as well. When going down stairs, stepping off curbs, or walking on uneven terrain, patients must learn to drop their heads and look through the upper portions of glasses designed for distant vision. By just lowering their eyes, as they were formerly accustomed to doing, they peer through the bottom portion of the glasses, which puts the ground dangerously out of focus.

Besides glasses, contact lenses can be used to correct many refractive errors.

Made from a form of Plexiglas, ***hard contact lenses*** contour the general curvature of the cornea. A continuous flow of tears over and under the lens keeps it in place via surface tension and provides constant oxygen to the cornea. This tear flow also fills in irregularities of the cornea and therefore corrects astigmatism. Hard lenses, if fitting properly, can be worn for 12–14 waking hours at a time. During this period, irritation does not usually occur because blinking slides the lens around the cornea, ensuring tear lubrication and nourishment to all areas. However, sleeping with hard contact lenses in place may lead to the ***contact lens overuse syndrome.*** During sleep, when there is no blinking, the lens remains fixed and tear flow to the area is interrupted. The corneal epithelium decompensates due to lack of oxygen, becoming centrally abrased and edematous. The overuse syndrome may further result in ***contact lens abrasion.*** This problem can also be traced to lenses with defective edges or cracks, a foreign body trapped underneath the lens surface, improper fit, and damage during insertion or removal. Patients note discomfort while wearing the lenses or develop blurred vision, severe pain, and red eye a short time after lens removal. Fluorescein stain may reveal haziness and mild central staining, irregular scratches, or abrasions. Contact lenses should not be worn, and evaluation by an age expert should be arranged. Treatment involves short-acting cycloplegics, pressure dressings for 24 to 48 hours, and prophylactic antibiotics. Contact lens wear can usually be resumed 2 days after all symptoms clear.

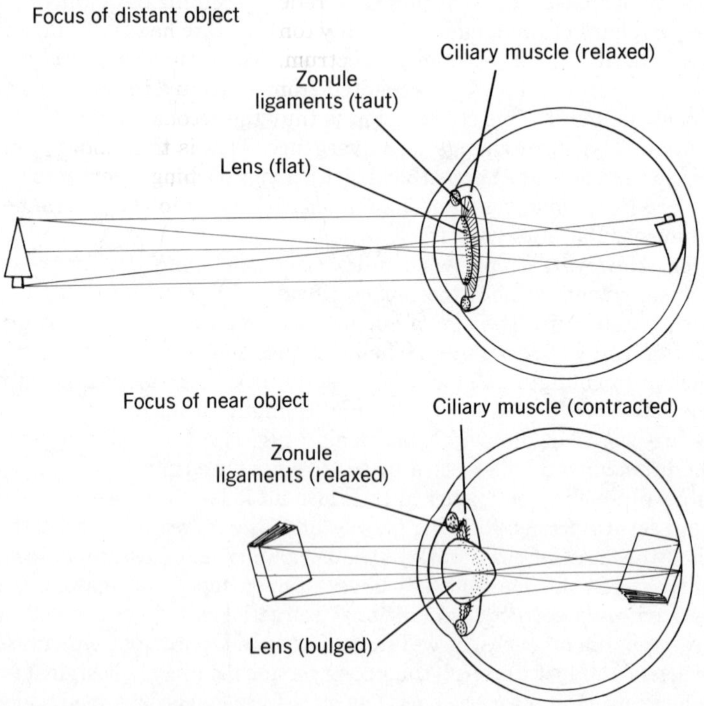

Figure 1.4 Refraction of normal, myopic, hypermetropic, and astigmatic eyes, shown in four parts: (*a*) normal eye focused on a distant object and on a near object, (*b*) myopic eye, (*c*) hypermetropic eye, (*d*) astigmatic eye.

(b) Eyeball abnormally deep: image focuses in front of retina (myopia)

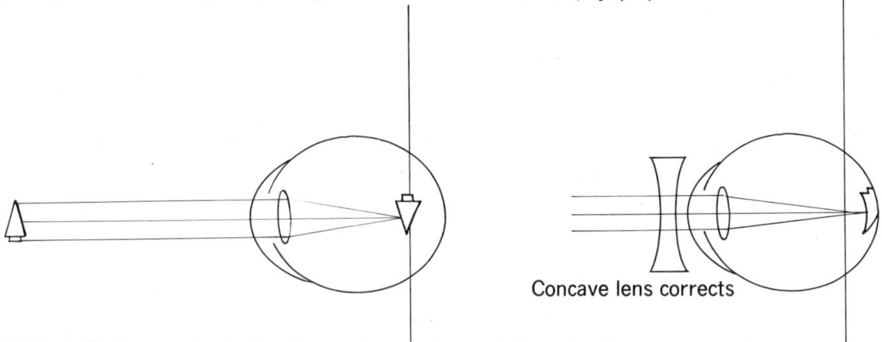

(c) Eyeball abnormally shallow: image focuses beyond the retina (hypermetropia)

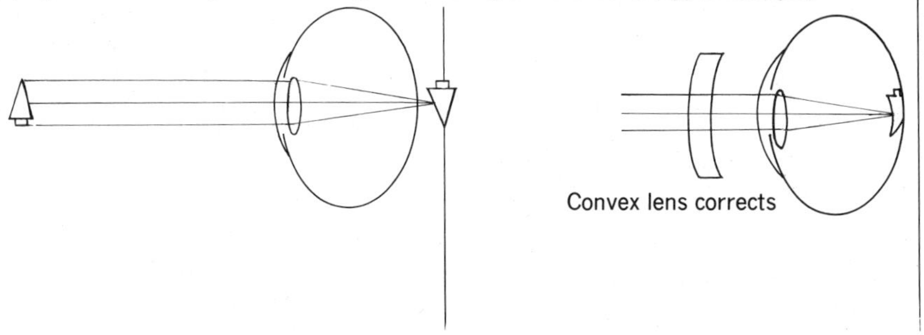

(d) Irregular cornea: image focuses in some planes, not in others (astigmatism)

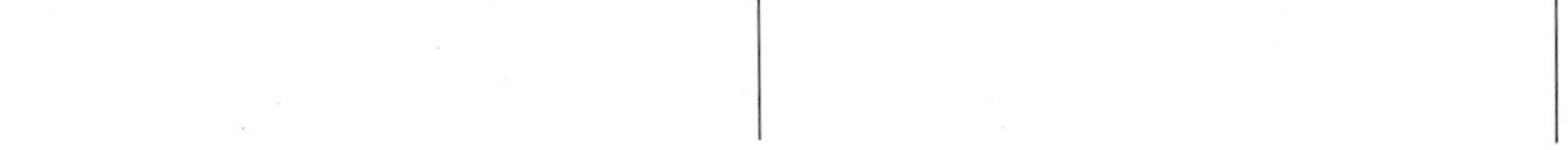

Figure 1.4 *Continued*

Corneal abrasions are less of a problem with ***soft contact lenses.*** For one thing, soft contact lenses are larger than hard lenses. Since they cover the entire cornea, they rarely pop out of place and offer little opportunity for foreign bodies to migrate under the surface. Made out of hydrophilic plastic, they absorb up to 60% of their composition in the form of tears or storing solutions. Thus soft lenses are extremely pliable and permit better oxygenation of the cornea. The wearing time can be several hours longer. Newer gas-permeable lenses can be worn for several days or weeks without removal. On the other hand, traditional soft contact lenses are so flexible that they mold to irregular corneal surfaces and fail to correct astigmatism. Al-

TABLE 1.18 TYPES OF CATARACTS

Congenital	Toxic
Galactosemia	Corticosteroids
Galactokinase deficiency	Mitotics
Neonatal hypoglycemia	Phenothiazines
Neonatal hypocalcemia	Cholinesterase inhibitors
Lowe's syndrome	Infrafred radiation ("glass-blower's")
Myotonic dystrophy	Medical or atomic radiation
Congenital ichthyosis	Microwave radiation (not proven in humans)
Rothmund-Thomson syndrome	Traumatic
Fetal rubella infection	Blunt or penetrating trauma
Werner's syndrome	Foreign bodies containing copper or iron
Hallermann-Streiff syndrome	Electrocution injury
Acquired metabolic	Ocular inflammations
Diabetic (osmotic)	Chronic keratitis
Hypocalcemic (tetanic)	Iritis
Pseudohypoparathyroidism	Posterior uveitis
Aminoaciduria	Neoplasms
Senile	Ocular melanoma
Subcapsular (anterior/posterior)	Retinoblastoma
Cortical (anterior/posterior and equatorial)	Metastatic tumors of the uveal tract
Supranuclear	
Nuclear	

though newer types offer some correction for astigmatism, the vision obtained with soft contact lenses is rarely as good as that with hard lenses. Furthermore, the hydrophilic plastic may absorb bacteria, chemicals, and other impurities, leading to corneal infection or irritation. For this reason, soft contact lenses should always be removed before swimming or applying eye medications. Unlike hard lenses, they cannot be stored dry. Extreme care must be taken to prevent contamination during wet storage by using either of two methods for disinfection (soaking the lens in a chemical solution or heating it in a preservative solution).

Protein, mineral, and fiber alterations of the lens occur with aging. This causes an opacification called ***cataract,*** which is present to some degree in every person older than age 70. However, cataracts are not limited to the aged. They may be congenital or traumatic, as described in Table 1.18. Cataracts are characterized by their location in the lens: anterior, posterior subcapsular, cortical (anterior, equatorial, posterior), supranuclear, or nuclear. The location has a direct bearing on the type of visual disturbance experienced. For example, with ***nuclear cataracts,*** incoming light is blocked centrally. Only angled light reaches the retina, and thus only the periphery is stimulated. Because cones in the periphery are sensitive to yellow/red but not blue/green light, these patients complain of a "yellowing of vision." Although far vision deteriorates, they experience a temporary improvement in near vision because the developing cataract tends to increase the focusing power of the lens. Reading glasses or bifocals are no longer needed, a sign known as "second sight." Unfortunately, once the nuclear zone becomes more opaque, both near and far vision are adversely affected. ***Posterior subcapsular cataracts*** scatter incoming light, causing glare as the principal manifestation. The glare reduces visual acuity, just as sun shining through a dirty windshield impairs a driver's ability to see the immediate road. Glare from headlights of oncoming cars at night is especially bothersome. In fact, difficulty with night driving may be the presenting complaint. Curved distortions of straight edges or overall blurring of images are other symptoms of developing cataracts. Distortions may be significant enough to cause image duplication ***(monocular diplopia).*** Mature cataracts that "white out" the pupil ***(leukocoria),*** and even some immature cataracts that cause whitish, gray, or yellow patches may be noticed on gross inspection. An ophthalmoscope set on +4 diopters held 8 in. from the patient may be needed to assess less developed cataracts. If the opacity appears to move downward with upgaze, it is in the posterior half of the lens. If it moves upward with upgaze, it is in the anterior half. Nuclear cataracts look like a "lens within the lens." Patients with any visual complaint due to the presence of a cataract should be referred to an ophthalmologist. Slit-lamp inspection, refraction testing, retinoscopy, and sonograms help determine the extent, density, type, and location of the deterioration. This knowledge is important in planning the best mode of treatment (see Table 1.19). Formerly, extracapsular surgery had to be delayed until the cataract was "ripe" (consisting of thoroughly decomposed fluid material that could be easily suctioned). This was due to the high incidence of retained debris and secondary inflammation that followed surgery on "immature" cataracts (composed of thick, tenacious material). Patients grew older and their eyesight grew worse while they waited for surgery. Following the procedure, many of them developed an opacifying membrane over the posterior capsule called the ***after cataract.*** For these reasons, the extracapsular method gave way to intracapsular techniques. Today, the ex-

TABLE 1.19 CATARACT TREATMENTS

Type	Description
Surgical	
Intracapsular	Zonule ligaments dissolved with enzymes and entire lens (capsule intact) removed with a forceps or cryophake.
Planned extracapsular	After anterior capsule is opened, the nucleus and residual equatorial cortex are expressed. The posterior capsule is polished and left in place.
Needle aspiration	Anterior capsule opened. Lens cortices and nuclei aspirated, leaving the posterior capsule undisturbed. Not suitable for patients more than 20 years old due to hardness of the adult nucleus.
Phakoemulsification	Nuclear and cortical material emulsified with titanium needle vibrating at ultrasonic frequencies, and then irrigated or aspirated.
Medical	
Mydriatics	Phenylephrine, tropicamide, or cyclopentolate drops may be used in patients with small axial cataracts. Pupil dilation eliminates glare while promoting better light transmission, image formation, and focusing.
Blood sugar control	Careful control of blood sugars can minimize or even reverse early cataract formation in the diabetic. It has no effect on advanced cataracts.
Cataractogenic agent	Ophthalmologic evaluation before, during, and after treatment with corticosteroids, phenothiazines, or other toxic drugs. Eye shielding during radiation therapy to the head. If possible, precipitant should be discontinued early.
Experimental	In animal studies, aldose rectase inhibitors have been shown to block the conversion of glucose to sorbitol, thereby preventing "sugar cataracts." The drugs may prove valuable in patients with diabetes and galactosemia.
Lay treatments	Thiol compounds, oral or injected lens extracts (fish/animal), multivitamins, and fad diets have all been advocated to prevent, delay, or reverse cataracts. None have proven effective.

tracapsular method is back in vogue. In fact, refined by better instruments and combined with intraocular lens insertion, it offers exciting advances in cataract treatment.

The risks of cataract surgery are low, since procedures can be done under local anesthesia and patients are ambulatory almost immediately. Although most normal activities can be readily resumed, those associated with jarring movements or Valsalva maneuvers (contact sports, heavy lifting) should be avoided, since they may weaken or rupture the surgical wound. This also applies to a number of medical conditions (coughing, constipation, etc.). ► ***Considerations for postcataract surgery*** are thus important aspects of primary care. Return to functional vision following cataract surgery depends in part on the optical correction planned for the lensless ***(aphakic)*** eye. Conventionally, cataract glasses are prescribed. These thick convex lenses magnify retinal images by 30%, causing everything to appear deceptively close. At first, patients' proprioception is so disrupted that they may experience severe dizziness. Furthermore, the glasses cover only the central line of vision; peripheral fields remain uncorrected. The blind area that begins at the edge of the spectacles is responsible for a jack-in-the-box phenomenon in which objects pop suddenly into and out of visual existence. If the patient is fitted with contact lenses or an intraocular lens is implanted at the time of surgery, these problems can be avoided because magnification of the retinal image is less than 8% and peripheral vision is maintained.

Cataracts can be associated with a ***dislocated lens*** (ectopia lentis), a problem occurring whenever the lens becomes detached from the zonular ligaments and slips out of place. ***Hereditary lens dislocation*** (associated with colomba homocystinuria, Marfan's syndrome, and Marchesani's syndrome) is usually bilateral, while ***traumatic lens displacement*** (following a blunt blow to he eye) tends to be unilateral. Without the stabilizing effect of the lens, the iris quivers with any kind of eye movement, a classic finding known as ***iridodonesis.*** In partial dislocations, the edge of the lens remains within the pupillary opening and may be observed on flashlight exam. Although the symptoms may be minimal at first, cataract development with reduced vision is a common complication. Complete dislocation into the vitreous space results in immediate blurring of vision and sometimes a red eye. Later on glaucoma may develop, necessitating a pars plana lensectomy. However, surgery involves a high risk of retinal detachment from loss of vitreous fluid, and in most cases, dislocated lenses are best left untreated.

Binocular Vision

The brain receives impulses from two eyes that are set a slight distance apart. Rather than two separate images, a single fused impression is perceived (binocular vision). In order for this to happen, the images must fall on corresponding points of the two retinas at all times. Therefore, each retina is divided into nasal, medial, temporal, and lateral portions.

The visual field from straight ahead to the bridge of the nose is recorded on the temporal half of the retina, while peripheral fields are registered on the nasal half. The optic fibers simply follow the routes that will carry the retinal image to the same part of the brain: at the optic chiasma, fibers from the nasal half of each retina cross and enter the optic tract with the temporal fibers from the opposite eye. For a better explanation, study Figure 1.5. In the figure, note how the light rays from an object at

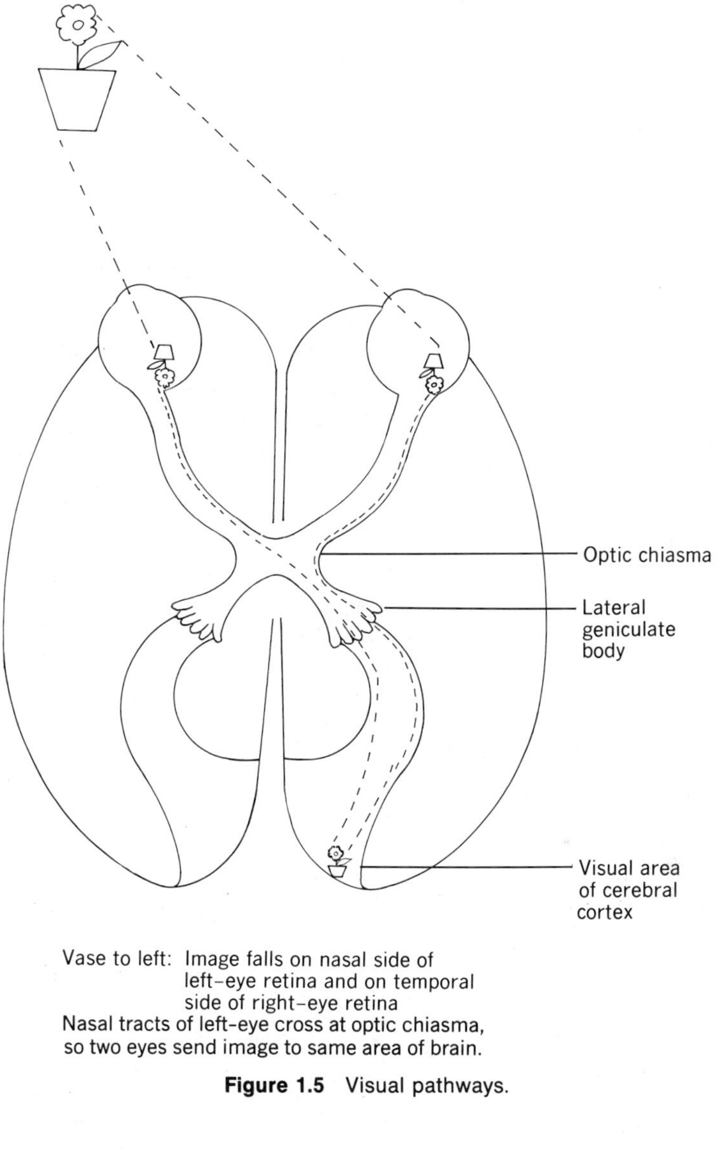
Optic chiasma
Lateral geniculate body
Visual area of cerebral cortex
Vase to left: Image falls on nasal side of left-eye retina and on temporal side of right-eye retina
Nasal tracts of left-eye cross at optic chiasma, so two eyes send image to same area of brain.

Figure 1.5 Visual pathways.

the left, a vase, are recorded on the retina and travel to the right occipital lobes of the cerebral cortex.

The visual pathways are so exact that lesions in the central nervous system can be mapped out by testing the visual fields. When grossly tested with confrontation, fields are considered normal if the patient is able to identify an object at 90 degrees temporally, 50 degrees nasally, 50 degrees upward, and 65 degrees downward. Evaluating the sensitivity within fields requires more refined testing with Amsler charts, the Goldman perimeter, or tangent screens. With the gaze fixed ahead, patients are asked to identify various objects (colored pins, printed grids, white flags) in

TABLE 1.20 VISUAL FIELD DEFECTS

Monocular	Binocular
Superior arcuate scotoma (o.s.) 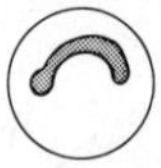	Bitemporal defect. Lesion anterior/inferior to chiasm, compressing the optic nerve. 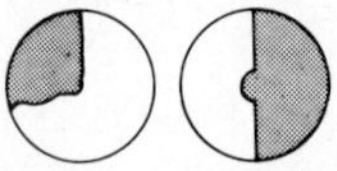
Inferior altitudinal field defect (o.s.) 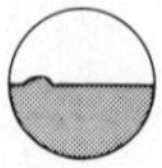	Bitemporal defect. Lesion anterior/superior to chiasm on right side. 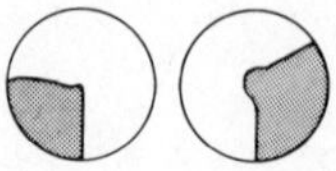
Enlargement of the blind spot (o.s.) 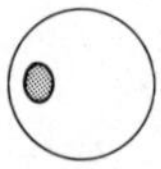	Bitemporal defect. Lesion inferior to chiasm. 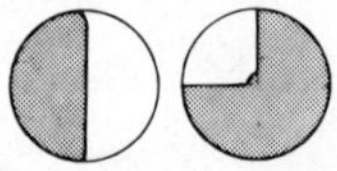
Central scotoma with normal blind spot (o.s.) 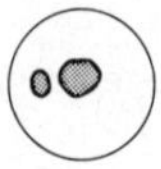	Bitemporal defect: lesion posterior to chiasm. 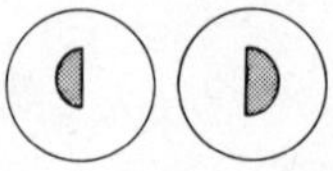
Centrocecal scotoma (o.s.) 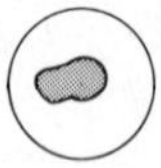	Homonymous "pie in the sky" defect: lesions in left temporal lobe. 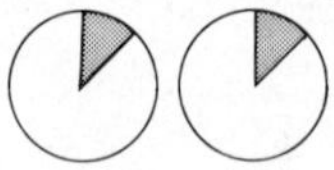
Temporal hemianopia (o.s.) 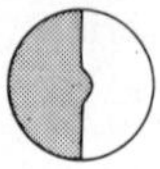	Right superior homonymous quadrantanopsia: lesion in left temporoparietal lobe. 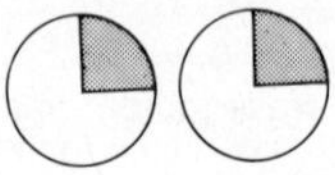
Generalized constriction (o.s.) 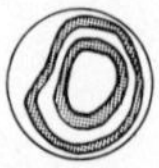	Homonymous "pie on the floor" defect: lesion in parietal lobe. 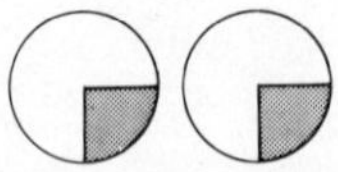
Nonorganic ("corkscrew") (o.s.) 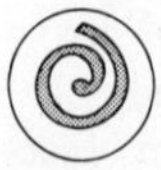	Incongruous right hemianopia: lesion in anterior optic radiations. 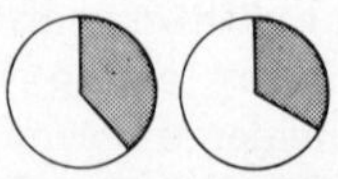
Enlarged blind spot: superonasal Bjerrum scotoma (o.d., early glaucoma) 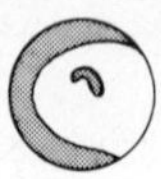	Complete right hemianopia: lesion in left temporoparietal optic radiations or visual cortex. 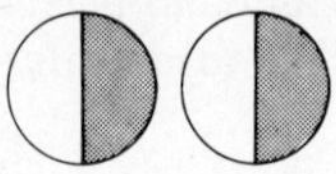

TABLE 1.20 *(Continued)*

Monocular	**Binocular**
Superonasal constriction: advancing Bjerrum scotoma (o.d., middle-stage glaucoma) 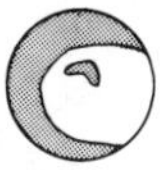	Homonymous congruous scotoma: lesion in right visual cortex. 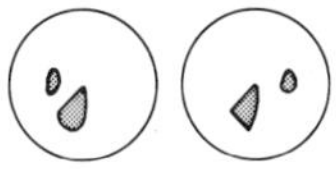
Further superonasal constriction: new inferior defect (o.d., late-stage glaucoma) 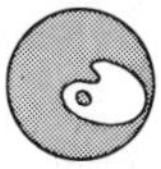	
All fields lost except small area of central vision, temporal island (o.d, end-stage glaucoma) 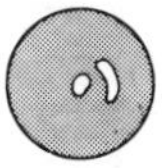	

all fields of vision. The eyes are tested individually to assess the monocular visual fields and together to assess binocular vision. When the responses are mapped out, areas of lost sensitivity, known as ***visual field defects*** (scotomas), may be revealed. More common types are described in Table 1.20. ***Bitemporal*** and ***homonymous*** defects deserve immediate neurologic work-up, since they usually indicate brain lesions in the optic chiasma or higher structures (see also Chapter 12).

Depth perception (stereopsis) is an important advantage of binocular vision. As illustrated in Figure 1.5, it is made possible by the fact that each eye focuses on an object from a slightly different angle (note how the right eye sees a little more of the right side of the flower vase than the left eye, and vice versa). The two retinas, therefore, send images to the brain that are not quite identical. The brain fuses the information into a single image that has depth and solidity.

Binocular vision with fusion and stereopsis is possible only if the two eyes maintain a parallel track for every direction in which they turn. This coordination is undertaken by the six ocular eye muscles: two oblique (superior, inferior) and four rectus (medial, lateral, superior, inferior). Their insertions into the sclera and the complicated movements regulated by the cranial nerves (III, IV, and VI) are described in Figure 1.6.

The parallel action of the two eyes (congruity) can be easily demonstrated by asking the patient to look in the six cardinal positions of gaze. An involuntary jerking motion of the eyes in any or all fields of gaze is called ***nystagmus.*** The mechanism of these downbeat, upbeat, rotary, dissociated, or seesaw movements is unknown. A few of the 38 classifications are described in Table 1.21. They may represent the effects of drugs, vestibular disorders, or brain stem disease. When the cause cannot be readily identified, investigation by a neurologist is indicated.

An imbalance of the extraocular muscles may be present from the time of birth. It causes one or both eyes to wander out of the congruent position ***(strabismus).*** There are many combinations of disjunctive movements. All have the potential to disrupt binocular vision and therefore cause double vision ***(diplopia).*** Young children with

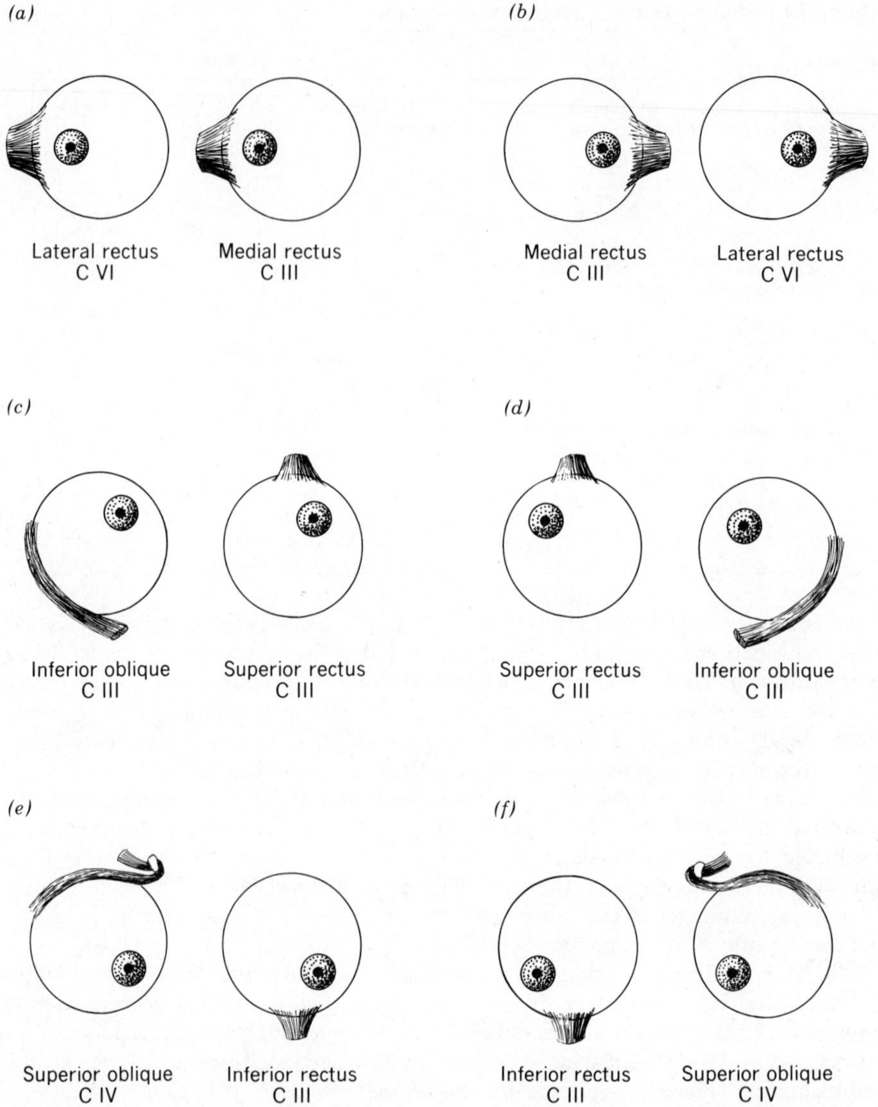

Figure 1.6 Movements in the six cardinal fields (denoting involved muscles and nerves): (*a*) right gaze, (*b*) left gaze, (*c*) up and right, (*d*) up and left, (*e*) down and right, (*f*) down and left.

TABLE 1.21 SOME COMMON TYPES OF NYSTAGMUS

Type	Description
Optokinetic	Physiologic jerking of the eyes as they follow a moving target out of the visual field and then jerk back into position to refix their gaze. Can be elicited by stripes on a moving flag or optikinetic drum in all normal patients or malingerers. Diminished response occurs with parietal occipital disease.
End gaze	Nonsustained horizontal nystagmus of small amplitude elicited in normal patients on far right or left gaze.
Latent	Binocular fixation normal. However, when one eye is occluded, the other eye develops a horizontal jerk that interferes with monocular acuity. Congenital in nature, the problem is poorly understood.
Pendular	Slow pendular movements in primary gaze changing to jerky movements on lateral gaze that decrease with convergence and eye closure. Associated with sensory deprivation due to reduced central vision (macular scarring, macular hypoplasia, achromatopsia, retinal degeneration, or optic nerve hypoplasia).
Jerk	Bidirectional jerking with fast component toward lateral gaze. Patient may keep the head turned to maintain a certain gaze ("null point") at which the nystagmus is decreased or eliminated. The problem is congenital.
Spasmus nutans	Pendular movements (symmetric or asymmetric) combined with head nodding, beginning in infancy and self-resolving by childhood.
Acquired pendular	Pendular movements developing in monocular patients who experience a sudden decrease in acuity of their seeing eye. Also develops in patients with brain stem dysfunction or with sedative or anticonvulsant toxicity.
Gaze paretic	Compression of the brain stem results in slow horizontal movements when gaze is tested toward the side of the lesion and fast, jerky movements when gaze is tested toward the opposite side.
Vestibular	Horizontal or rotary movements associated with vertigo due to malfunction or overstimulation of vestibular apparatus (e.g., Meniere's syndrome, viral labyrinthitis). Normally elicited with cold or warm water irrigation tests: fast component away from side of stimulus with cold water, toward side of stimulus with warm (COWS—cold/opposite, warm/same).
Upbeat	Fast upward jerk elicited on primary gaze. May be congenital, drug induced, or indicative of posterior fossa disease.
Downbeat	Fast downward jerk elicited on primary gaze with posterior fossa disease or on lateral gaze with compression of the foramen magnum.
Rotary	Tortional jerks, usually in combination with horizontal or vertical nystagmus. May be congenital or secondary to brain stem lesions or acute vestibular disease.
Dissociated	Asymmetric horizontal movements that may occur in strabismus (abducting eye) or sixth nerve palsy.
Seesaw	Conjugate pendular motions (one eye rises as the other falls). Associated with lesions in the third ventricle and vascular disease of the upper brain stem.
Nystagmus blockade	Seen in patients with dissociated nystagmus. Since oscillations are increased on abduction and decreased on adduction, patients fix the adducted eye or converge both eyes to obtain clearer vision. Surgical correction of strabismus reduces symptoms.
Ocular monoclonus	Rhythmic pendular movements (usually vertical) associated with synchronous action of the oropharynx and diaphragm. May be secondary to a midbrain lesion.
Ocular bobbling	Rapid downward jerking of both eyes followed by slow return to mid-position. Seen in comatose patients with massive pontine lesions.

strabismus repress central vision in the deviated eye to avoid the confusing effects of diplopia. For the same reason, children who are ***anisometropic*** (myopic in one eye and hyperopic in the other) repress central vision in the hyperopic eye, far vision being less important for most of their activities. The development of central vision takes place from birth to age 6 or 7 and cannot be stimulated at later ages. For this reason, it is important to treat strabismus or anisometropia with patching, corrective lenses, or surgery before permanent dysfunction ***(amblyopia)*** occurs. After age 7, surgical repair may be undertaken for cosmetic purposes, but it will not restore vision and is entirely elective.

Development of dysjunctive ocular movements in previously congruent eyes may be related to ***palsy*** or ***ophthalmoplegia*** (nerve paralysis). Some types are described in Table 1.22. Associated with multiple sclerosis, cerebral aneurysms, encephalitis, neurosyphilis, Parkinson's disease, basilar artery disease, increased intracranial pressure, tumors at the base of the skull, meningitis, diabetic neuropathy, cerebrovascular accidents (CVAs) or trauma, dysjunctive ocular movements always deserve neurologic evaluation.

Obviously, binocular vision ceases whenever sight in one eye is lost. However, people with ***monocular vision*** are completely functional. Though peripheral vision and depth perception are compromised, total visual capacity may remain as high as 90%. The problem rarely interferes with occupational pursuits but must be taken into consideration when engaging in activities that could endanger the remaining eye (e.g., boxing). Monocular vision is not a contraindication for obtaining a driver's license.

Classifications of ***blindness*** and ***near blindness*** have been established by the World Health Organization, although the most widely used standard in the United States is that set by the Internal Revenue Service for tax deduction purposes (Table 1.23). ***Automobile blindness*** is defined as vision too poor to meet standards set by agencies issuing driver's licenses. Requirements vary from state to state and may be less rigid for standard class drivers than for taxi, bus, or truck class drivers. An an example, applicants for a standard class license in New York State must have minimum vision correctable with glasses or contact lenses of 20/40 in one or both eyes. However, people using telescopic lenses can apply for a special license.

Vision classifications are important because rehabilitation programs are most beneficial when geared to the type of visual impairment and the individual's special needs. For example, the child with retrolental fibroplasia may need a number of services to prepare for a lifetime of blindness: schooling for the blind, mobility training, Braille proficiency, job training, psychologic counseling, and financial assistance. On the other hand, the 70-year-old widow who faces slowly diminishing sight from macular degeneration may need (or want) little more than home mobility training, access to special radio stations, and a steady supply of Talking Books. People with residual sight may benefit from large-print newspapers and books, enlarged television screens, or various electronic devices such as the Optacon (which converts visual images of letters into tactile form) or the Apollo electronic visual aid (a camera with a zoom lens, scanning table, and illuminator). ▶ ***Organizations for the blind*** provide important services, information, and support. Individuals can help by ▶ ***extending courtesies to the visually handicapped.***

TABLE 1.22 CRANIAL NERVE PALSIES AND OPHTHALMOPLEGIAS

Type	Description
Palsies	
Congenital third nerve palsy	Ptosis and exotropia with varied limitation of elevation, adduction, and depression. Pupil and ciliary muscles are never involved. Etiology unknown, but a developmental flaw is presumed. Because patients rely on head turning to avoid diplopia, amblyopia may develop. Early surgical treatment is advocated.
Acquired third nerve palsy	Ptosis and exotropia similar to the congenital type. However, intraocular muscles may also be involved, causing paralysis of accommodation with a fixed, dilated pupil. Etiologies include brain stem lesions, meningitis, encephalitis, toxic polyneuritis, intracranial aneurysms, intracranial tumors, multiple sclerosis, and trauma. Diabetes, another cause, is somewhat unusual in that it never affects pupillary muscles and is fairly benign (100% function is usually recovered). The problem requires a search for the underlying cause and aggressive intervention.
Congenital fourth nerve palsy	Developmental abnormality in the cranial nerve's nucleus or motor portion causes paralysis of the superior oblique muscle. Overriding by the inferior oblique muscles leads to eye extortion, with head tilt toward the paretic side (diminishes the disparity resulting from the stronger muscle). Surgery is undertaken to prevent permanent torticollis, facial asymmetry, and scoliosis.
Acquired fourth nerve palsy	Eye extortion and head tilt similar to the congenital type. Usually secondary to head trauma but also associated with intracranial tumors and aneurysms. Once the underlying disease has been controlled, recovery of eye function is usually spontaneous, occurring within 6 months. If not, surgical recession of the antagonistic muscle may limit the extent of deviation.
Congenital sixth nerve palsy	Rare disorder involving trauma or underdevelopment of the cranial nerve's motor nucleus. Causes inward deviation (esotropia) that increases as the eye moves in the direction of the affected muscle. Head tilt away from the paretic eye helps maintain binocular vision. Surgical treatment is usually necessary.
Acquired sixth nerve palsy	Esotropia and head tilt similar to the congenital form. May be secondary to diabetes, heavy metal poisoning, middle ear infection with secondary meningeal irritation or intracranial tumor, aneurysm, or inflammation (particularly viral). After immediate etiologic investigation and treatment of the underlying disorder, ocular manifestations are observed for a period of 3–6 months. If spontaneous recovery from esotropia has not occurred, surgical treatment is advised.
Perinaud's syndrome	Lesions in the subcortical brain centers (particularly tumors of the pineal gland) cause paralysis of upward and downward gaze. May be associated with abnormal pupil reactions to convergence and light. Treatment centers on the underlying disorder.
Ophthalmoplegias	
Thyroid ophthalmoplegia	Hypertrophy of the extraocular muscles from excess mucin deposition in thyrotoxicosis reduces eye motility, particularly elevation. Although correction of the thyroid abnormality may resolve the hypertrophy, patients may be left permanently unable to elevate the eyes due to scar tissue formation around the inferior rectus muscle. They develop a compensatory "chin-up" head tilt to improve vision. Surgical resection of fibrous tissue may be undertaken
Progressive external ophthalmoplegia	Ptosis followed by paralysis of all extraocular muscles (intraocular muscles spared) due to myopathy. Usually beginning with the medial rectus muscle, progression may be asymmetric over years. However, by the time of end-stage disease, both eyes have become permanently frozen in primary gaze. There is no treatment.
Myasthenia gravis	Primary fatigue of all ocular muscle groups due to chronic neuromuscular disease. The problem begins with ptosis (becomes progressively more severe) and later causes weak convergence and upgaze. Alternatively, isolated paralysis of the inferior or lateral rectus muscles may occur. Treatment is medical.

TABLE 1.23 CLASSIFICATIONS OF BLINDNESS

Category	Best Corrected Vision
WHO[a] class 1 (low vision)	Central acuity: 20/70 (6/18, 3/10)
WHO class 2 (low vision)	Central acuity: 20/200 (6/60, 1/10)
WHO class 3 (blindness)	Central acuity: 20/400 (3/60, 1/20) or finger counting at 3 m Visual fields: greater than 5 degrees but less than 10 degrees around central fixation
WHO class 4 (blindness)	Central acuity: 5/300 (1/60, 1/50) or finger counting at 1 m Visual fields: Limited to 5 degrees or less around central fixation
WHO class 5 (blindness)	No light perception
IRS[b] standard	Central vision acuity of 20/200 (6/60) or less in the better eye, with best correction or widest diameter of visual field subtending an angle of no more than 20 degrees.

[a] World Health Organization.
[b] United States Internal Revenue Service.

PROTECTIVE FEATURES

Given the complicated and delicately balanced mechanisms involved in vision, it is little wonder that the eye is so highly protected (Fig. 1.7). Protective features include the bony orbits, conjunctiva, eyelids, tears, and special reflexes.

Orbits

The eyeball is recessed within the bony orbits of the skull. The globe itself occupies one-fifth of the orbital cavity, the remaining space being filled with fat padding. During starvation or illness, the body uses this fat tissue for energy, causing eyes literally to sink into their sockets. "Sunken eyeballs" are also common in very old people.

In addition to fat padding, extraocular muscles and connective tissue encase the back of the eyeball, securing it in place. Swelling or enlargement of these tissues can push the eye forward, resulting in ***exophthalmos*** (proptosis). Caused by tumors (see Table 1.24), vascular abnormalities, or inflammation, exophthalmos is always an indication for prompt ophthalmologic referral. In adults, inflammatory processes account for the majority of cases, particularly ***ophthalmic Graves' disease.*** Besides exophthalmos, hyperthyroidism may lead to lid edema, conjunctival hyperemia, lacrimal gland enlargement, keratitis, and extraocular muscle palsy. Symptoms include tearing, photophobia, foreign body sensation, diplopia, and retrobulbar ache. In severe cases, there may be visual loss secondary to optic nerve involvement. Since some patients with ophthalmic Graves' disease have normal thyroid tests, the diagnosis is established by clinical features alone. Patients are best managed by an ophthalmologist as well as an endocrinologist. In addition to thyroid normalization, a main purpose of treatment is to minimize corneal damage. When there is extensive orbital congestion with optic neuropathy, systemic steroids, surgical decompression, or local radiation may be considered. Extraocular muscle surgery may also be necessary.

A second inflammatory cause of exophthalmos is bacterial invasion of orbital

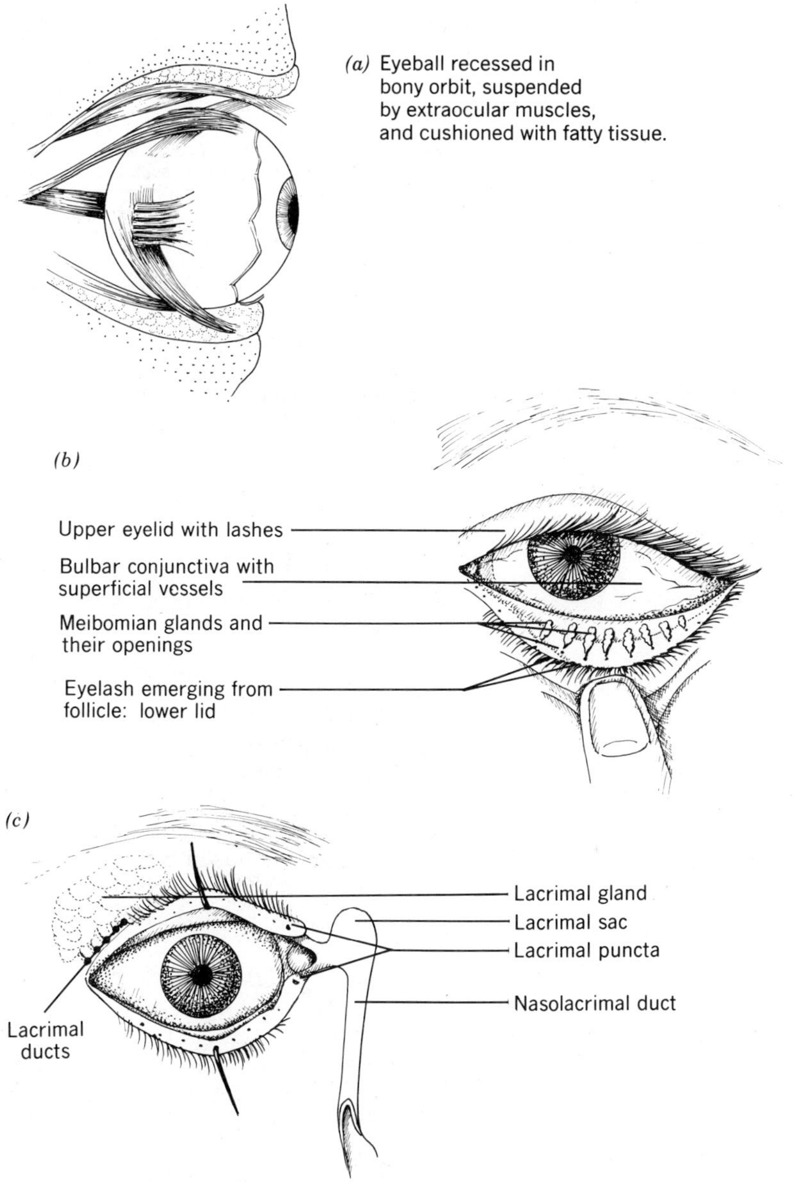

Figure 1.7 Protective structures (in three parts): (*a*) bony orbit and orbit tissues, (*b*) eyelids and lashes, conjunctiva, meibomian glands, (*c*) tear glands and ducts.

TABLE 1.24 SOME TUMORS OF THE EYE ORBITS

Type	Characteristics
Choristomas	Tumors composed of four types of developmental tissue not usually found in the area: *dermoids* (composed of hair follicles and sebaceous material, usually located near the lacrimal glands; *lipodermoids* (solid masses of fat tissue developing beneath the conjunctiva; *epidermoids* (cystic cavities of cholesterol crystals and epithelial debris); *teratomas* (rare tumors arising from multiple germinal layers, containing hair, cartilage, or musculoskeletal tissue). Rupture causes a granulomatous inflammatory reaction, but choristomas are otherwise benign.
Cavernous hemangioma	In adults, the most common benign tumor of the orbit. Causes a retrobulbar mass within the muscle cone.
Lymphangioma	Uncommon tumor. Spontaneous hemorrhage into vascular spaces may cause "chocolate cysts" or sudden enlargement with exophthalmos.
Neurofibromas	Highly vascular tumors usually involving the anterior orbit and upper eyelid, with progressive ptosis and exophthalmos.
Rhabdomyosarcomas	Primary bone lesion causing destruction of orbit walls. Usually occurs in patients under 15 years of age. Early metastases to lymph nodes and lung.
Lymphoproliferative	Benign and malignant tumors of lymphoid origin. Orbit may be primary site, but systemic disease is more likely.
Metastatic	In adults, the primary origin is usually breast or lung cancer. Carcinoids also metastasize to the orbits.

tissues resulting in ***orbital cellulitis.*** The usual source is *Staphylococcus aureus, Streptococcus,* or *Haemophilus influenzae* spread from an infection of nearby sinuses or teeth. Patients present with fever, pain, soft tissue swelling, and restricted eye movements. They should be immediately hospitalized for aggressive antibiotic treatment and close observation. Complications are common and serious, including loss of vision from optic neuritis or panophthalmitis. If the infection spreads along the venous channels draining the orbit to the cavernous sinus in the brain, ***cavernous sinus thrombosis*** may result. Besides exophthalmos, these patients develop septic temperature curves, papilledema, convulsions, severe headaches and other cerebral symptoms. Most of them die.

Conjunctiva

A specialized mucous membrane, the conjunctiva, covers the sclera and underside of the eyelids (Fig. 1-7*b*). The protective nature of the conjunctiva is revealed by its microscopic anatomy. The epithelium, three to seven layers thick, contains goblet cells that secrete the mucoid portion of the tear film. Connective tissue houses numerous blood vessels, nerve endings, and accessory tear glands. Finally, a reticular network enmeshes lymphocytes that collect invading organisms and drain them into the preauricular and submandibular nodes.

These defense mechanisms are so successful that most cases of ***conjunctivitis*** may be considered self-limiting and safely left untreated. Furthermore, although empirical judgment is not always reliable, it is standard practice to diagnose the bacterial, viral, or allergic nature of conjunctivitis by signs and symptoms (Table 1.25). Cultures of discharge to identify bacterial organisms or conjunctival scrapings to check for the presence of eosinophils are often omitted because of the time and expense involved.

TABLE 1.25 DISTINGUISHING FEATURES OF CONJUNCTIVITIS

	Viral	Bacterial	Allergic
Pruritis	Mild	Mild	Severe
Injection	Moderate	Severe	Mild-moderate
Hemorrhage	Occasionally	Occasionally	Not likely
Chemosis	Variable	Common	Common
Exudate	Watery	Purulent	Stringy
Papillae	Not likely	Variable	Common
Follicles	Occasionally	Not likely	Not likely
Preauricular adenopathy	Common	Occasionally	Not likely
Fever/sore throat	Occasionally	Occasionally	Not likely
Neutrophils on stain	Early infection	Yes	No
Monocytes on stain	Yes	No	No
Eosinophils on stain	No	No	Yes

► ***Nongonococcal bacterial conjunctivitis*** is usually caused by *Streptococcus pneumoniae, H. influenzae,* or *S. aureus.* The pathogens typically become established in one eye and are quickly transferred by hand to the other eye. They may also be spread to family members, particularly through shared towels. Bacterial growth with pus formation is most prolific at night. This is due to the slight temperature elevation that occurs in the conjunctival sac when the eyelids are closed during sleep. Some of the accumulating secretions dry along the eyelashes, and in the morning patients may find the lids stubbornly fused shut. They also experience red, watery eyes and a sensation of grittiness. The infection resolves in 1–5 days with antibiotic treatment or in 7–10 days with no intervention.

By contrast, ***gonococcal conjunctivitis*** is aggressively invasive. In adults, the usual etiology is self-inoculation from genital gonorrhea. At first unremarkable, the conjunctivitis quickly evolves into a severe, widespread inflammation. Patients have a copious purulent exudate, marked chemosis, and swollen eyelids. They must be referred to an ophthalmologist for gram stains and cultures and immediate initiation of systemic antibiotic therapy. Without prompt intervention, the infection progresses to corneal ulceration and perforation, sometimes within 24 hours.

Viral conjunctivitis disappears in from 3 days to 3 weeks after the initial symptoms of redness, tearing, and burning. The presence of preauricular nodes is a telling sign. The causes are many, including those viruses known to produce keratitis: varicella, herpes zoster, herpex simplex, pharyngeal conjunctival fever (PCF), and epidemic keratoconjunctivitis (EKC). While antibiotics are of no value, the need for close observation is obvious.

The predominant complaint in ***allergic conjunctivitis*** is itching. Edema of the conjunctiva (chemosis) produces the sensation that the eyes are sinking into the head. Due to constant eye rubbing, the discharge has a ropy texture. In cases of a rare allergic disorder called ***vernal conjunctivitis,*** hypertrophied papillae give a "cobblestone" effect to the palpebra. Treatment is directed toward the allergy (see Chapter 2). It is always tempting to prescribe steroids for any person suffering from allergic conjunctivitis because of the dramatic relief they afford. However, steroids promote fungal invasion or viral proliferation. Corneal perforation, now a recognized complication of herpes simplex virus, rarely occurred prior to the widespread use of topical steroids. Ophthalmic steroid preparations, even those in antibiotic combinations, are prudently left for use by the specialist.

Far more crucial than treatment of nongonococcal forms of conjunctivitis is the determination that no other eye disorder exists. Conjunctival inflammation often accompanies uveitis, keratitis, and glaucoma. The differential key is the history. The conjunctiva may be violently red due to engorged vessels and distinctly uncomfortable from edema, but it never causes pain, photophobia, or blurred vision. The latter symptoms are always an indication for ophthalmologic referral.

Unlike the diffuse inflammation seen with conjunctivitis, a painless red area characterizes ***subconjunctival hemorrhage.*** This disruption of tiny capillaries develops from violent coughing, sneezing, vomiting, or mild trauma. Although the hemorrhage may look very serious, it is quite harmless and usually resorbs within a week, sooner if cold compresses are used for the first 2 days and hot compresses thereafter. Blood pressure should be checked, but hypertension alone is an unlikely cause of spontaneous conjunctival hemorrhage. On the other hand, hemorrhages following severe eye trauma or bilateral hemorrhages suggesting a bleeding disorder require appropriate evaluation.

Two other findings of the conjunctiva are ***pingueculae*** and ***pterygiums.*** Pingueculae are small, yellow fat nodules associated with aging. Pterygiums are clear, triangular wings of thickened membrane that develop in response to constant irritation. Noted in people who work outdoors in hot, dry climates, they usually require no intervention other than protective sunglasses. However, pterygiums that progress over the cornea must be surgically peeled away.

Eyelids

The upper and lower eyelids form a barrier to foreign matter. They also protect the cornea and conjunctiva from excessive exposure and drying. However, eyelid skin lacks extensive stratum corneum and is highly sensitive. ▶ ***Contact dermatitis of eyelids*** results from direct use of eye shadow, eyebrow pencil, eyeliner, mascara, eyedrops, or rubber eyelash curlers. It may also be due to lotions, perfumes, or other substances applied to the hands and inadvertently transferred to the eye area. Furthermore, an acute reaction may develop from the use of nail polish, hair dyes or sprays, or facial cosmetics without any direct eyelid contact. Airborne allergens and irritants, including pollens, dusts, volatile substances, or the burning of poison ivy, may present with or be limited to the eyelids. The clinical picture varies according to the allergen, the intensity and duration of exposure, and the degree of patient sensitivity. It ranges from acute swelling, redness, and vesiculation to chronic lichenified eruptions. Management begins with identifying (through careful questioning or patch testing) and avoiding specific allergens. Boric acid solutions, scale removal, and topical corticosteroids help reduce the symptoms.

Skin changes caused by contact dermatitis should not be confused with ***xanthelasma.*** Representing the most common form of cutaneous xanthomas, these yellowish papules usually appear during middle age and may signal type II or III hyperlipoproteinemia (see Chapter 5). Investigating for the presence of atherosclerosis, diabetes, coronary artery disease, or hyperlipidemia is thus the most important aspect of management. The tumors are otherwise benign. They may be surgically removed for cosmetic purposes.

TABLE 1.26 PTOSIS AND PSEUDOPTOSIS

Type	Description
Congenital ptosis	
Blepharophimosis/ epicanthus	Associated with blepharophimosis–generalized narrowing of the palpebral fissure and epicanthus (semilunar skin fold). The two developmental abnormalities lead to a deficiency of the levator muscle.
Marcus Gunn "jaw winking"	Associated with synkinetic movements of the jaw. As the patient chews or moves the jaw laterally, the ptotic lid elevates. The problem often diminishes as the patient grows older.
Extraocular muscle palsy	Associated with ipsilateral extraocular muscle palsies, particularly of the superior rectus and inferior oblique muscles.
Acquired ptosis	
Myogenic	Secondary to neuromuscular disorders including myasthenia gravis, oculopharyngeal muscular dystrophy, and progressive external ophthalmoplegia.
Neurogenic	Damage to the cranial nerve innervating the levator muscle or decreased sympathetic innervation to Müller's muscle.
Traumatic	Damage to the levator muscle or lid aponeurosis from lacerations or edema.
Mechanical	Movements impeded by scar tissue, tumors, or foreign bodies of the eyelid.
Pseudoptosis	
Normal lid function	Low appearance of the upper eyelid caused by epicanthus, facial asymmetry, excessive upper eyelid skin, palpebral fissure narrowing, contralateral palpebral fissure widening, elongated eyeball, contralateral shortened eyeball, exophthalmos, contralateral exophthalmos.

Eyelids are normally symmetric, the upper and lower margins opening wide enough to allow light to enter the pupil and closing evenly to provide complete protection. Movements are directed by the levator muscle (innervated by cranial nerve III) and the orbicular muscle (innervated by cranial nerve VII), respectively. ***Ptosis*** is an abnormally low position of the upper lid due to one of the congenital or acquired conditions described in Table 1.26. Ophthalmologists evalute the problem by taking palpebral fissure measurements and documenting the abnormalities of eyelid folds or extraocular muscles. Treatment for congenital ptosis is surgical, while that for acquired ptosis centers on the underlying cause.

With ***ectropion,*** the lid margin (usually lower) turns out, leaving a portion of the eye continually exposed. Keratopathy, conjunctival hypertrophy, or (if the lacrimal punctum is everted) excessive tearing may result. Similar problems due to constant irritation develop from ***entropion,*** malposition of the margin inward. Ectropions and entropions can be either congenital or secondary to nerve damage, changes due to aging, scar tissue (from lacerations or burns), and certain diseases (notably trachoma, Stevens-Johnson syndrome, pemphigoid). Patients should be evaluated by an ophthalmologist. Treatment is directed toward the underlying factors and surgical correction of the lid deformity.

The outer margins of the eyelids bear two or three rows of stiff, short eyelashes. These, along with eyebrow hairs, protect the recessed eye from sunlight and small particles of falling debris. Lashes have a normal life span of 5 months and continuously fall out. They regrow within 10 weeks except in old age, when they tend to become sparse. The lashes curl out and back to prevent entanglement with those along the opposing lid. ***Trichiasis*** is abnormal inversion of lashes. ***Districhiasis*** is abnormal growth of extra lashes behind the lid margins. The two conditions can lead to corneal irritation if the surface of the eye is brushed with lid movements. In such cases, the abnormal lashes should be destroyed with cryotherapy, electrolysis, or surgery.

Eyelash follicles harbor sweat and sebaceous glands. Infection of a sebaceous gland in an isolated follicle is called ▶***sty*** (hordeolum). It is usually caused by staphylococcus. The patient experiences lid irritation or foreign body sensation, or notes the sty formation at the base of a lash follicle. If the inflammation is located in the inner canthus, special care must be taken to rule out tear duct infection. Stys resolve with spontaneous drainage, which can be hastened by the use of hot compresses and antibiotics.

Infection of follicles along the entire lid margin is known as ▶***acute blepharitis.*** It, too, is usually caused by staphylococcus. Patients present with widespread swelling and redness of the lid, as well as burning or itching eyes. They typically complain of difficulty in opening their eyes in the morning because purulent secretions dry overnight, gluing the lid margins together. The clinician may note crusted ulcerations that have a bleeding surface when removed. Occasionally, staphylococcus exotoxins produce a hypersensitivity keratitis characterized by pain or photophobia and punctate lesions of the cornea. For this reason, fluorescein staining is advisable whenever there is a purulent lid infection. Treatment of acute blepharitis includes lid hygiene and antibiotics. Care must be taken to avoid spread to family members through poor hygiene or towel sharing. Severe infections can result in loss of eyelashes or thickening of the eyelids.

▶***Chronic seborrheic blepharitis*** is caused by the same seborrheic condition found on the scalp, brows, and ears. Although unsightly, it is neither contagious nor destructive. The patient complains of redness, itching, and flaking around the lid margins without crusting or discharge. The clinician notes an absence of ulceration, intact eyelashes, and easily removable yellow scales. Although the conjunctiva is sometimes mildly irritated, there is never corneal involvement. Treatment includes lid hygiene and control of hair and brow conditions with seborrheic shampoo. Extreme cases may require referral to a dermatologist.

Numerous meibomian glands open behind the eyelash follicles, as illustrated in Figure 1.7*b*. Without the sebum they secrete, tears would continually spill over the bottom rim onto the cheek, and the two lids would be chronically stuck together. Meibomian secretions also leave a film of oil over the cornea, thereby retarding tear evaporation. Occasionally, a plugged duct leads to a secondary staphylococcal infection of the gland known as ▶***acute meibomianitis*** (internal sty). Meibomianitis produces redness, tenderness, swelling of the lid, or a foreign body sensation. By gently everting the lid, the practitioner can readily identify the inflamed gland. In most cases, the infection clears readily with hot compresses and antibiotics. If it does not, the patient should be referred to an ophthalmologist for incision and drainage.

Sometimes acute meibomianitis precedes the development of a ▶***chalazion,*** a painless lesion characterized by the inflammatory granulation of retained meibomian secretions. Chalazia may also arise spontaneously, and while there seems to be an association with rosacea, the precise cause is unknown. Chalazia are quite common and easily recognized as hard, localized nodules beneath the skin surface of the eyelid. The nodules may recede on their own or continue to enlarge. Treatment for chalazia starts with antibiotic eyedrops, lid massage, and warm compresses. Oral tetracycline has been used empirically because of the close association with rosacea. Patients with chalazia unresponsive to medical management should be referred to an ophthalmologist for surgical excision or intralesion steroid injections. Rarely, chalazia are complicated by secondary infections or ulcerations. Very large lesions can exert pressure on the cornea, producing an astigmatism. Recurrence after surgical excision is an indication for a histologic exam to rule out malignancy.

Tears

Each time the eyelids blink, they spread a film of tears over the surface of the eye. Tear fluid is produced by an almond-shaped lacrimal gland located in the upper outer corner of the eyelid (see Fig. 1.7). It consists of three layers: (1) oil to retard evaporation and trap debris, (2) an aqueous solution containing enzymes and gamma globulins to destroy bacteria, and (3) mucin to wet and lubricate the cornea and conjunctiva.

Decreased tear function causes a problem referred to as ***dry eye syndrome.*** It is associated with old age, the inhibiting effects of drugs, systemic disease, and the neurologic abnormalities listed in Table 1.27. Symptoms include grittiness, burning, foreign body sensation, and, paradoxically, excessive tearing. Since "dry eyes" can cause an exposure-type keratitis or leave eye surfaces open to infection, it is extremely important that patients be referred to an ophthalmologist. Tests of quantity (Schirmer I and II), quality (rose bengal staining, conjunctival biopsy, mucous and protein assays), stability (tear film breakup times), and secretion (regurgitation tests, primary/secondary dye tests, canaliculus testing, and dacryocystography) may be needed to pinpoint the problem. Treatment usually begins with specific tear solutions. If this proves inadequate, more complicated measures such as ocular inserts of slowly dissolving polymers, soft contact lenses, tear duct plugs, occlusive shields, or tight-fitting goggles may be employed. Parotid duct transplants and mechanized pump implants have been used experimentally.

Released from the lacrimal gland and spread over the surface of the eye, tears drain through small openings located in the nasal corners of the lids (see Fig. 1.7). These openings empty into the lacrimal sac, which forms the upper end of the nasolacrimal duct. With each blink of the eye, the specialized muscles milk the lacrimal sac and draw excess tears into the duct for drainage into the nose. Obstruction of the nasolacrimal duct is called ***dacrytostenosis.*** Resulting from chronic nasal infection, chronic conjunctivitis, or facial trauma, it requires correction through dilatation, probing, or surgery. Otherwise, a serious infection of the tear duct called ***dacryocystitis*** may develop. Patients who develop dacryocystitis have pain, redness, and swelling around the inner corner of the eye. Excessive tearing, conjunctivitis, or blepharitis may also be noted, along with fever and leukocytosis. Pus can often be expressed from the puctum; if an abscess has formed, it may drain through a fistula. Patients should be referred to an ophthalmologist for immediate evacuation of the infection and aggressive antibiotic therapy. Intramuscular penicillin followed by oral and topical antibiotics are often needed to prevent corneal involvement.

TABLE 1.27 CAUSES OF DRY EYE SYNDROME

- Tear gland hypofunction
  - Congenital causes
    - Riley-Day syndrome (familial dysautonomia)
    - Congenital alacrima (aplasia of the lacrimal gland)
    - Trigeminal nerve aplasia
    - Ectodermal dysplasia
    - Cri-du-chat syndrome
  - Acquired systemic causes
    - Sjögren's syndrome
    - Progressive systemic sclerosis
    - Sarcoidosis
    - Leukemia, lymphoma
    - Amyloidosis
    - Hemochromatosis
  - Infectious
    - Trachoma
    - Mumps
    - Herpes zoster
  - Injuries
    - Traumatic injury
    - Surgical lacrimal gland removal
    - Radiation (UV or infrared)
    - Chemical burn
  - Drug induced
    - Antihistamines
    - Antimuscarinics (atropine, scopolamine)
    - General anesthetics (halothane, nitrous oxide)
    - Beta-adrenergic blockers (timolol, practolol)
  - Neurogenic/neuroparalytic causes (facial nerve palsy, etc.)
- Mucin deficiency associations
  - Avitaminosis A
  - Stevens-Johnson syndrome
  - Ocular pemphigoid
  - Chronic conjunctivitis (rheumatoid arthritis, trachoma, etc.)
  - Chemical burns
  - Drug induced
    - Antihistamines
    - Antimuscarinics
    - Beta-adrenergic blockers
- Lid abnormalities
  - Congenital defects (coloboma, etc.)
  - Ectropion
    - Senile relaxation of orbicularis oculi muscle
    - Seventh nerve palsy (e.g., Bell's palsy)
  - Entropion
    - Senile (spastic)
    - Cicatricial
  - Lid margin keratinization
  - Decreased or absent blink reflex
    - Neurologic (e.g., leprotic neuropathy or other damage to fifth cranial nerve with decreased corneal sensitivity)
    - Hyperthyroidism
    - Riley-Day syndrome
    - Herpes zoster
    - Herpes simplex
    - Contact lenses
    - Drug induced
  - Incomplete eyelid closure (lagophthalmos)
    - Eyelid scar
    - Traumatic loss of part of eyelid
    - Facial nerve injury
    - Atony of orbicularis palpebrarum
    - Exophthalmos (Graves' disease, etc.)
    - Nocturnal lagophthalmos (fatigue, hysteria)
    - Hyperthyroidism
    - Leprotic neuropathy of the seventh cranial nerve
    - Bell's palsy (seventh cranial nerve)
- Conjunctival abnormalities
  - Pterygium
  - Symblepharon

Reflexes

Three special reflexes provide further eye protection. Triggered by exceptionally bright light (dazzle reflex), rapidly approaching objects (menace reflex), or corneal irritation (corneal reflex), they cause flinching, blinking, and/or tearing. In spite of these reflexes and other extensive mechanisms for protection, ***eye injuries*** occur with alarming frequency. Most require emergency room treatment or immediate ophthalmologic referral. However, primary care providers must be prepared to respond to an urgent phone call or initiate ▶ ***first aid for eye injuries.*** The first and most important step is to elicit an exact description of the accident. What was the patient doing when the injury occurred? What was the nature and size of the offending object or substance? Did the object hit the eye socket, or did it blow, fall, or project onto the surface of the eye itself? These questions have a crucial bearing on management. For example, in the event of ***chemical burns*** (from tear gas, mace, sparklers, or flares, as well as household cleaning agents, pesticides, fertilizers, and paints), immediate irrigation is crucial. The victim's eyelids should be held apart and the surface of the eye lavaged for at least 15 minutes with any innocuous liquid available: water from a house or drinking fountain, beer, or even urine. Time spent searching for sterile or neutralizing solutions cannot be spared. The sooner irrigation begins, the better the prognosis, especially for alkali burns. Alkalis are particularly serious because they combine with membrane lipids to penetrate the cornea rapidly. Even mild alkali burns are likely to result in a permanent corneal haze. Acids, on the other hand, activate protein precipitation. This blocks further penetration of the caustic substance and localizes burning to the area of contact. After irrigation, patients should be taken to an emergency room for further evaluation and treatment.

If a blunt object the size of a fist or tennis ball enters the eye socket with enough force, a ***blowout fracture*** may occur from the sudden increase in intraorbital pressure. The fracture frequently traps extraocular muscles, restricting eye motility and causing diplopia (the most common presenting symptom). Sometimes bone fragments and soft tissue herniate into the maxillary sinus, pulling the eyeball down. Other clinical findings include edema, ecchymosis, subconjunctival hemorrhage, and periorbital emphysema (crackling sounds heard with a stethescope placed over the swelling).

Although blowout fractures are relatively rare, the development of a ***black eye*** from facial trauma is a common occurrence. The contusion is often treated at home with cold compresses until the swelling and discoloration resolves. Unfortunately, the injury is sometimes associated with dislocation of the lens and frequently associated with retinal tears. As previously discussed, both conditions can cause complications to develop that threaten eyesight immediately or months later. For this reason, any patient with a black eye should be referred to an ophthalmologist for careful evaluation.

If smaller objects are forcefully projected into the eye (e.g., chips of wood thrown from a chain saw or bits of glass shattered in an auto accident), ***impaled foreign body, abrasion, laceration,*** or ***perforation*** of the globe must be considered. These injuries can also result when the eye is poked (with a fingernail or stick, sharp instrument, paper edge, or leaf blade). They cause intense pain, eyelid spasm, and excessive tearing. Decreased vision, pupil abnormalities, or obvious prolapse of eye fluids usually accompany perforation. Green staining with fluorescein can be noted wherever corneal epithelial cells have been damaged. Immediate evaluation by an eye specialist is imperative. Treatment of an impaled object depends on its toxic or metallic property. Gold, silver, stone, glass, porcelain, and carbon are considered nontoxic and may be left in place if extensive scarring is expected from surgery. Lead, zinc, nickel, aluminum, copper, iron, vegetable matter, cloth, and human or animal tissue are known to cause toxic reactions and must be removed by surgery or magnetic retrieval. Lacerations and abrasions are usually treated with cycloplegics, anesthetics, and pressure dressings to relieve pain. Prophylactic antibiotics may be given for a full week, but steroids and continued anesthetics are ill advised. With prolonged use, anesthetics lose their painkilling effect, interfere with healing, and ultimately lead to epithelial breakdown. Steroids dangerously enhance the opportunity for bacterial, viral, or fungal growth.

Superficial foreign bodies are usually bits of rust, dirt, or plaster that fall into the eye from a ceiling or underside of a car during cleaning/repair. They may also be particles of dirt, vegetation, or animal hairs that blow into the eye. Easily seen, lightly embedded foreign bodies can be removed from the conjunctiva or anesthetized cornea using a moistened sterile cotton swab. However, particles that cannot be dislodged with one or two gentle wipes should be removed by an ophthalmologist under slit lamp magnification, since overzealous swabbing by the nonspecialist will surely cause an abrasion. Cases involving iron particles should also be referred to an ophthalmologist because retained iron leads to opacifying ion deposits known as ***rust rings.*** Once rust rings have developed, they must be removed with a curette or special burr under slip lamp magnification. It must be emphasized that serious eye injuries can exist in the presence of a normal-appearing eye. Regardless of the signs and symptoms, ophthalmologic referred is warranted if there is a history of direct injury. A detailed exam and administration of certain medications by the primary care provider may be ill advised. Eye manipulation, movement, or external pressure intensify the pain and may worsen partial-thickness lacerations or cause prolapse of intraocular fluids. All ointments are contraindicated, since they are irretrievable from the inner eye structures. By pulling away the iris, cycloplegics or mitotics could create a direct opening into the anterior chamber.

Trauma is the main reason for eye-related visits to hospital emergency rooms—288,000 cases annually. According to the National Society to Prevent Blindness, 90% of all accidental eye damage can be avoided by ▶ ***eye safety practices*** such as the use of protective glasses and careful handling of chemicals.

Details of Management

▸ *Eye Bank and Anatomic Donations*

Laborary Tests: None.

Therapeutic Measures: None.

Patient Education: Anyone of legal age can make tissue donations. For children under 18 years of age, parents or legal guardians can arrange the donation. Virtually all tissue is accepted; if not suitable for transplantation, it is used for research or education. All major religions approve and encourage tissue donations. Most organs can be removed without significantly affecting the donor's appearance (eye removal is a simple procedure leaving no visible scars).

In most states, people wishing to donate their body tissue after death can make arrangements at the time of their driver's license renewal. Information and necessary cards can also be obtained from local eye banks (address and phone numbers listed in the telephone directory) or through:

Eye Bank Association of America
6560 Fannin, Level 9
Houston, TX 77030   Phone: (713) 790-6126

The simple process involves filling out a card as follows:

ANATOMIC DONOR CARD

of ______________________________ (printed name of donor)

As indicated below, I hereby make an anatomical gift to take effect upon my death for the purpose of therapy, medical research, or education:

(a) ___ My eyes to the eye bank
(b) ___ Any needed organs or parts
(c) ___ Only the following needed organs or parts: ______________
(d) ___ My body for anatomical study (separate permission for eye disposition required)
(e) ___ Other special donees, limitations, or wishes: ______________

After the card has been filled out and signed by the donor and two witnesses, the eye bank should be notified. Intentions should also be discussed with the donor's family, friends, clergy, and lawyer (their cooperation in notifying hospital personnel, the funeral director, or the eye bank within 6 hours of the time of death is crucial). Donor cards should be carried at all times.

Follow-up: None.

▸ *Cancer Organizations*

Laboratory Tests: None.

Therapeutic Measures: None.

Patient Education: Information about specific types of cancer or problems can be obtained from the following central organizations:

American Cancer Society
777 Third Ave.
New York, NY 10017 Phone: (212) 371-2900
Cancer Connection
H&R Block Building
4410 Main St.
Kansas City, MO 64111 Phone: (816) 932-8543
International Association of Cancer Victims and Friends
7740 W. Manchester Ave.
Playa Del Rey, CA 90291 Phone: (213) 822-5032

Follow-up: Coordinated care as needed.

▸ *Screening for Glaucoma*

Laboratory Tests: On all patients over age 20, do a careful funduscopic exam and obtain a tonometry reading. The Schiøtz tonometer (the most commonly used instrument in ambulatory settings) may be used as follows:

1. Question the patient about an allergy to Novocain. Explain the procedure and have patient remove contact lenses or glasses.
2. With the patient lying comfortably (head flat), place one drop of proparacaine or tetracaine in each eye. *Caution:* Indicator solutions for Hemoccult slides are supplied in similar-looking plastic bottles, and a number of accidental chemical burns have been reported in emergency room settings. Check the label carefully.
3. Have the patient fix his or her gaze on a designated spot straight above. Separate the eyelids and gently place the tonometer (with a 5.5-g weight) in a vertical position directly over the cornea. Allow the plunger to exert its full weight (the pointer should remain fixed except for slight oscillations in either direction reflecting arterial pulse changes) and note the reading. For readings

of less than 3, repeat the procedure using a 7.5-g weight and then a 10-g weight. Note that false readings may result with elongated eyeballs (severe myopia, thyroid exophthalmos) or if the patient squeezes the lids closed.

4. Convert the tonometer reading into millimeters of intraocular pressure using the graph supplied with each instrument.
5. Refer patients with pressures higher than 22 mm Hg to an ophthalmologist. Refer any patient with glaucomatous disc changes (see text) even if the tonometry reading is within the normal range.
6. Sterilize and care for the tonometer according to manufacturer's instructions.

Therapeutic Measures: Per the ophthalmologist.

Patient Education: Explain the disease process. Note that it affects 1.5% of those over age 40 and has resulted in blindness in 50,000 Americans. In many of those cases, blindness could have been prevented by early detection and treatment.

Follow-up: Screen all patients over age 20 every 3 years. Screen patients who have a family history, myopia, or diabetes every year.

▸ *Night Blindness as an Early Symptom of Vitamin A Deficiency*

Laboratory Tests: Serum level of vitamin A.

Therapeutic Measures: Increase vitamin A intake to the Recommended Daily Allowance:

Males (11 years and older)	5,000 IU
Females (11 years and older)	4,000 IU
Pregnant women	5,000 IU
Lactating women	6,000 IU

Adjust for factors that may increase vitamin A requirements:

Increased body weight, cold weather, strenuous physical activity following vitamin A intake

Illnesses such as hepatitis, pneumonia, hyperthyroidism, and diabetes

Use of substances interfering with vitamin A metabolism (notably excess alcohol, mineral oil, tannic acid, nitrates, benzoate, ferrous sulfate, aspirin, and barbiturates)

In order to avoid toxicity, recommended allowances are best obtained through foods: (1) carotene, a substance found in green and yellow vegetables and converted to vitamin A in the body as needed or (2) preformed vitamin A found in fish-liver oil, cream, butter, and certain other animal tissues. However, vitamin A can also be obtained in a number of over-the-counter preparations: (1) synthetic vitamin A (palmitate or acetate) found in multivitamins or as a separate preparation with added oil to ensure multivitamins or as a separate preparation with added oil to ensure absorption, (2) preemulsified vitamin A palmitate, which may be useful in cases of diarrhea, or (3) pure vitamin A obtained from extracts of fish liver oil. Vitamin A_2 is a substance structurally similar to vitamin A but only half as effective in the body. Diabetics need preformed sources of vitamin A since they cannot convert carotene.

Patient education: Provide patients with a list such as the following:

FOOD SOURCES OF VITAMIN A

Food	Vitamin A (IU/100 g)	Food	Vitamin A (IU/100 g)
Winter squash	4,000	Egg yolk	3,400
Cantaloupe	3,400	Endive	3,300
Apricots	2,700	Broccoli	2,500
Pimentos	2,300	Crab	2,200
Swordfish	2,100	Romaine lettuce	2,000
Mangoes	1,800	Nectarines	1,600
Pumpkin	1,600	Peaches	1,300
Cheeses	1,300	Cherries	1,000
Cream	920	Lobster	920
Tomatoes	900	Asparagus	900
Halibut	850	Soybeans	700
Watermelon	590	Mature bean sprouts	550
Okra	520	Mackeral	450
Pink grapefruit	440	Tangerines	420
Green peppers	420	Summer squash	400
Oysters	310	Plums	300
Walnuts	300	Salmon	300

Note that unlike water-soluble vitamins, there is minimal vitamin loss from cooking or processing. Mashing, cutting, or pureeing may actually increase the availability of carotene by releasing the nutrient from cell walls.

Warn patients that although carotene conversion is regulated by the body, preformed vitamin A is fat soluble and excess amounts cannot be eliminated by the kidneys. Doses exceeding the Recommended Daily Allowance may lead to toxicity and liver failure (deaths have been reported).

Inform patients that in addition to night vision, vitamin A is crucial to growth and repair of body tissues, particularly the blood, bones, and teeth, skin, and mucous membranes. It also clears certain toxins and prompts secretion of the gastric juices necessary for the digestion of protein.

Follow-up: As needed.

▸ *Screening Far Visual Acuity*

Laboratory Tests: For routine screening and assessment for medical-legal purposes in *Every* case involving an eye complaint or injury, measure far visual acuity with a

Snellen chart. The chart has several lines marked by descending letter size as pictured below (Fig. 1.8).

Be sure that the chart is at eye level and well lighted. With the patient standing 20 ft away (a distance requiring no focusing effort by the normal eye), have him or her cover the left eye with a card and read the letters line by line using the right eye only. Then test the left eye and both eyes together. Repeat the process using corrective lenses prescribed for general use.

Patients with normal vision are able to read all letters down to the "20" line from 20 ft (recorded as 20/20 vision for that eye). Those with less than average vision are unable to read beyond lines "30" (recorded as 20/30), "40" (recorded as 20/40), and so on. In such cases, *pinhole vision* should be tested by having the patient read the chart

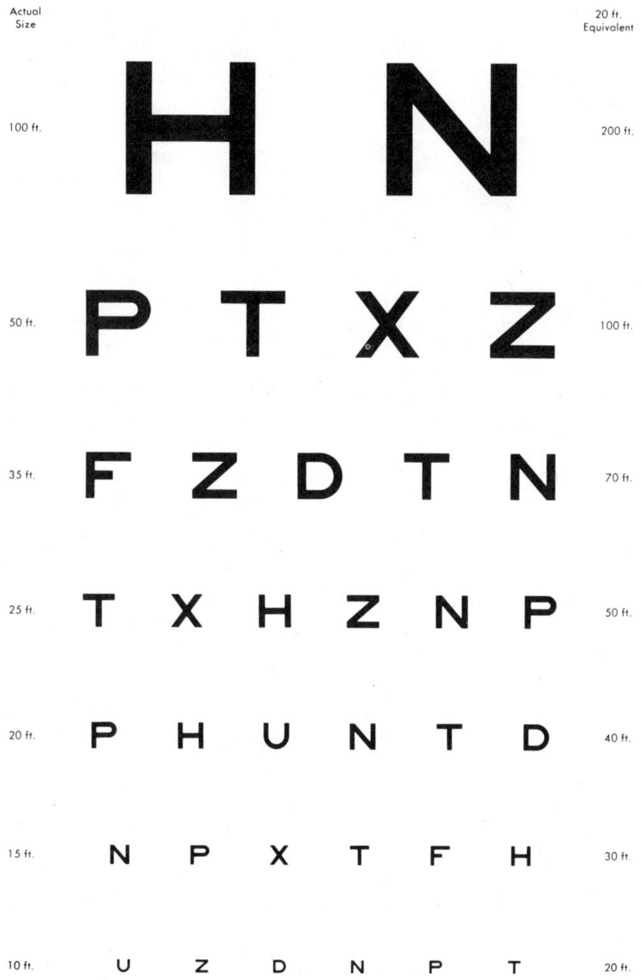

Figure 1.8 Snellen scale. Letter chart for 10 feet. (From National Society to Prevent Blindness, 79 Madison Avenue, New York, NY 10016.)

through a tiny hole punched in a card. This technique improves vision affected by refractive errors but not by macular dysfunction, opacities, or optic nerve disorders.

Patients unable to read letters on the chart at a distance of 20 ft should be tested at 10 ft (10 is recorded as the first number, followed by the number of the line the patient is able to read, e.g., 10/40). Vision progressively lower than this is measured by counting fingers (CF), hand motion (HM), light perception (LP), and finally no light perception (NLP).

It is important to note that opacities such as dense cataracts or severe corneal scarring may cause very low vision even though retinal function remains intact. This is probably the case if patients can differentiate red light from white light or if they see a red area surrounded by retinal blood vessels when the eyeball is gently massaged through a closed lid with a small flashlight.

Therapeutic Measures: Refer patients with previously unnoted or new changes in visual acuity to an ophthalmologist or optometrist. As a convenience to patients renewing driver's licenses, record Snellen chart results on a prescription slip or a special form that can be obtained from state agencies.

Patient Education: Explain the Snellen measurements and various conditions that contribute to reduced visual acuity.

Follow-up: Ideally, screen for visual acuity on a yearly basis.

▸ *Screening Near Visual Acuity*

Laboratory Tests: Measure for close visual acuity with a multipurpose reading card such as the near Vision Screener, which has lines of decreasing print size, similar in principle to the Snellen chart (Fig. 1.9):

Have the patient cover the left eye with a card. Hold the screener 14 in. away and ask the patient to read through the lines with the right eye. Test the left eye in the same manner, and then repeat the process using prescribed reading lenses. For each eye (with and without glasses), record the smallest line patients are able to read as a distance equivalent (e.g., 20/25 or 20/400) or as a Jaegar equivalent (e.g., J-1, J-16).

Suspect presbyopia in patients over age 30 who have difficulty seeing the test card at 14 in. but not at a greater distance.

Therapeutic Measures: Refer patients as needed for further evaluation by an ophthalmologist or optometrist. Corrective reading glasses may be necessary.

Patient Education: Explain the aging process involved in presbyopia and the various lenses used for correction.

Follow-up: Screen patients over age 30 every 2 years.

▸ *Considerations for Postcataract Surgery*

Laboratory Tests: Do not order stressful diagnostic procedures for 6 weeks after cataract surgery or until the eye surgeon has been consulted. Sigmoidoscopy, barium

		DISTANT EQUIVALENT	METER SIZE
5 3		20/800	16M
8 2 6		20/400	8M
4 7 3 9		20/300	6M
2 5 6 8		20/200	4M
7 3 9 4		20/160	3M
2 5 6 8		20/100	2M 18 Pt.
9 3 7	J #10	20/80	1.5M 14 Pt.
6 4 2 8	J #5	20/50	1M 9 Pt.
5 9 3		20/40	.8M 7 Pt.
7 2 4 8	J #1	20/25	.5M 4 Pt.

18 Point Large Type Grades 1 - 3
14 Point Average Book Print Grades 4 - 7
9 Point Magazines, Paper Back Books, Typing
7 Point Newspaper
Distance equivalent calibrated for 40 cm (16 inches)

Figure 1.9 Near vision test. (From the Lighthouse Low Vision Services, 111 East 59th Street, New York, NY 10022.)

enema, pulmonary function studies, and cardiac stress tests are specifically to be avoided.

Therapeutic Measures: Treat respiratory infections, constipation, asthma, vomiting, or any other condition associated with Valsalva maneuvers that may compromise the results of recent eye surgery by elevating intraocular pressure.

Patient Education: Reinforce activity limitations prescribed by the surgeon such as heavy lifting, vigorous exercise, excessive bending from the waist, and avoidance of contact sports.

Follow-up: As needed.

▸ *Organizations for the Blind*

Laboratory Tests: None.

Treatment Measures: None.

Patient Education: For information, services, or support, patients or families may contact the following:

American Foundation for the Blind, Inc. (Offers a "Directory of Agencies Serving Blind Persons in the United States" and a catalogue of "Aids and Appliances" for the blind)
15 W. 16th St.
New York, NY 10011 Phone: (212) 620-2000

Affiliated Leadership League for the Blind of America (ALL)
301 N. Fairfax St., Suite 106
Alexandria, VA 22314 Phone: (701) 548-3804

American Association of Workers for the Blind (AAWB)
206 W. Washington St., Suite 320
Alexandria, VA 22314 Phone: (703) 548-1884

American Council of the Blind (ACB)
1211 Connecticut Ave. N.W., Suite 506
Washington, DC 20016 Phone: (202) 833-1251

Associated Blind
135 W. 23rd St.
New York, NY 10011 Phone: (212) 255-1122

Association for Education of the Visually Handicapped (AEVH)
206 N. Washington St.
Alexandria, VA 22314 Phone: (703) 836-6060

Braille Institute
741 N. Vermont Ave.
Los Angeles, CA 90029 Phone: (213) 663-1111

Library of Congress, Division for the Blind
1291 Taylor St. N.W.
Washington, DC 20016 Phone: (202) 287-5100

Lighthouse Low Vision Services
111 E. 59th St.
New York, NY 10022 Phone: (212) 355-2200

Recordings for the Blind, Inc.
215 E. 58th St.
New York, NY 10022 Phone: (212) 557-5720

Seeing Eye
2130 Maple St.
Baldwin, NY 11510
or
PO Box 1200
San Rafael, CA 94915 Phone: (415) 479-4000

National Society to Prevent Blindness
79 Madison Ave.
New York, NY 10016   Phone: (212) 684-3505

Follow-up: Help patients contact agencies as needed.

▸ *Extending Courtesies to the Visually Handicapped*

Laboratory Tests: None.

Therapeutic Measures: Unless it is clear that a blind person is in distress, do not rush to offer help. However, when intervention seems appropriate, approach the person firmly (on the opposite side of a cane or guide dog). Do not take hold of the person or touch or speak to a guide dog before obtaining permission. Introduce yourself and ask in a friendly voice if help is needed.

Always speak clearly, but quietly and calmly. Use names when talking to people so that the blind person will know who is being addressed. Feel free to discuss the appearance of things and use words such as "see" or "look," but avoid apologetic comments.

Orient sightless persons by guiding them around new surroundings and allowing them to feel furnishings. In order not to interfere with their sense of balance or direction, it is best to offer your arm (not take theirs) and walk slightly ahead. Tell them when approaching stairs, curbs, or inclines, then pause briefly before negotiating the change in terrain. Keep movements smooth and unhurried, since rushing can be very disorienting.

Encourage the use of well-lighted, pleasant surroundings for all blind people. Never rearrange anything without informing them. When joining a sightless person for meals, arrange table settings and food on plates according to familiar patterns. Provide sturdy containers that cannot be easily overturned to serve beverages (not too hot), filling them partway.

Patient Education: For more specific information, contact organizations for the blind.

Follow-up: None.

▸ *Bacterial Conjunctivitis*

Laboratory Tests: Snellen test; fluorescein stain; culture and Gram stain if the discharge is purulent.

Therapeutic Measures: Antibiotics as follows: Sulfacetamide ophthalmic solution 10% (or if the patient is allergic to sulfa drugs, neomycin ophthalmic solution 2.5 mg/mL), 1 or 2 drops four times a day for 7 days. Warm compresses for 10 minutes four times a day at the onset of therapy.

Patient Education: Describe the conjunctival membrane and the bacterial nature of the infection causing the inflammation. Demonstrate the instillation of eye medications. Advise the use of careful hand washing and separate towels to avoid spreading the infection among family members.

Follow-up: As needed.

▸ *Contact Dermatitis of the Eyelids*

Laboratory Tests: Patch test the back or arm in cases of unidentified allergens. Common offenders include eye makeup, eye drops, rubber eyelash curlers, hand creams, nail polishes, hair dyes and sprays, chronic exposure to airborne pollens, dusts, volatile substances, or acute exposure to poison ivy or other *Rhus* species.

Therapeutic Measures: Avoid allergens. Treat acute eruptions with boric acid compresses twice a day. Remove crust formations by gently scrubbing with cotton balls and mineral oil. Apply a low-potency corticosteroid such as Hytone 1% or Kenalog 0.025% twice a day (ophthalmic preparation is not necessary) for up to 10 days.

Patient Education: Eyelids lack thick layers of protective corneum and are therefore highly sensitive. They can develop an allergic dermatitis even though the primary site of contact (e.g., fingers in the case of nail polish sensitivity) remains unaffected. The condition may be unsightly but is relatively benign.

Follow-up: Refer severe or unresponsive cases to a dermatologist.

▸ *Sty (Hordeolum)*

Laboratory Tests: None

Therapeutic Measures: If fluctuant, tweeze the eyelash or lift the head of the sty open with sterile TB syringe to drain the infection. If not fluctuant, use hot compresses for 10 minutes four times a day followed by sulfacetamide ophthalmic solution 10% or neomycin 2.5 mg/mL ophthalmic solution four times a day unil resolution occurs (but not longer than 1 week).

Patient Education: Describe the location of the infection and its benign course. Demonstrate the application of compresses and eye drops. Warn the patient that the problem may be recurrent.

Follow-up: As needed.

▸ *Acute Blepharitis*

Laboratory Tests: Because some lid infections are associated with keratitis, the Snellen test and a fuorescein stain are advised.

Therapeutic Measures: Aggressive treatment three times a day for 7 days as follows: Scrub the lids with cotton balls soaked in a solution of half water, half baby shampoo and apply hot compresses for 10 minutes. Spread a thin layer of erythromycin ophthalmic ointment 1% or neomycin ophthalmic ointment 5 mg/g along the lid and a small amount in the lower fornix.

Patient Education: Discuss the infectious nature of the condition and the possibility of recurrence. Demonstrate the techniques for removing scales and applying compresses and ointments. Advise careful hand washing and the use of separate towels to prevent the spread of infection among family members. Inform the patient that unresolved cases can result in loss of lashes and thickening of lids.

Follow-up: Schedule a return appointment in 1 week. Refer the patient to an ophthalmologist if there is no improvement or if there are any signs of keratitis.

▶ *Chronic Seborrheic Blepharitis*

Laboratory Tests: None

Therapeutic Measures: Treatment twice daily as follows: Remove scales by scrubbing with cotton balls soaked in a solution of half baby shampoo, half warm water. Treat any concurrent condition of the hair and brows with Selsun Blue or any other antiseborrheic shampoo.

Patient Education: Emphasize the nonbacterial nature of the inflammation. Demonstrate the techniques for scale removal. Reassure the patient that unlike acute blepharitis, this condition is not associated with any complications.

Follow-up: As needed. For severe, resistant cases, refer the patient to a dermatologist.

▶ *Acute Meibomianitis*

Laboratory Tests: None.

Therapeutic Measures: Treatment four times a day for 7 days as follows: After applying hot compresses for 10 minutes, instill sulfacetamide ophthalmic solution 10% or neomycin ophthalmic solution 2.5 mg/mL.

Patient Education: Describe the location and bacterial nature of the infection. Demonstrate the use of compresses and eye drops.

Follow-up: If there is no response to medical treatment after 48 hours, refer the patient to an ophthalmologist for I & D.

▸ Chalazion

Laboratory Tests: None.

Therapeutic Measures: Treatment four times a day for 7–10 days as follows: Massage closed eyelids with a hot compress for 10 minutes. Then apply sulfacetamide ophthalmic solution 10% or neomycin ophthalmic solution 2.5 mg/mL (alternatively, oral tetracycline, 250 mg four times a day, has been recommended for chalazia associated with rosacea).

Patient Education: Describe the location and inflammatory nature of the lesion. Demonstrate lid massage and the application of compresses and eye drops.

Follow-up: If the chalazion is unresponsive to medical treatment over a period of 3 months, refer the patient to an ophthalmologist for surgical excision or steroid injections. Recurrence after surgical excision is an indication for a histologic exam to rule out malignancy of the sebaceous gland.

▸ Eye Injuries: First Aid and Prevention

Laboratory Tests: None.

Therapeutic Measures: In the event of an eye injury, initiate first aid as follows:

1. Whenever *any* chemical gets in the eye, *immediately* flood the eye by holding the head under a faucet or pouring water from a clean container. Continue irrigation for *at least 15 minutes,* keeping the lids as wide open as possible. Send the person to an emergency room or ophthalmologist for evaluation and treatment.
2. If a speck blows or falls into the eye, lift the upper eyelid outward and down over the lower lid and let tears wash it out. Do not rub the eye. If the speck does not wash out, bandage the lid lightly closed with a clean piece of gauze or an eye patch held in place with adhesive tape and refer the patient to an emergency room or ophthalmologist for removal.
3. When the surface of the eye is cut, poked, or impaled by a foreign body, bandage the eye lightly and send the patient for immediate ophthalmologic care. Do not wash the eye with water and do not try to remove the foreign body. Never apply ointments or pressure.
4. For direct blows to the eye, advise the patient to apply cold compresses for 15 minutes every hour until the swelling and pain are reduced. For any change in eyesight or the development of a black eye, arrange for immediate ophthalmologic evaluation.

Patient Education: Nearly 1 million Americans have impaired vision as a result of eye injuries, 90% of which could have been avoided by the use of these eye safety measures:

1. Invest in protective eyewear available through ophthalmologists, opticians, or suppliers of safety equipment. Acceptable types are (a) industrial-quality safety glasses with plastic lenses and a specialized frame (no adjustable nose pads, cable-type temples that curve around the ear, or spatula temples with a headband), (b) specially designed sports eye protectors, and (c) protective goggles for general use. Eyewear made with polycarbonate plastic lenses has been shown to provide the greatest impact resistance. Prescription lenses can be incorporated in safety glasses or sports protectors. Sports goggles are also available without lenses, and while they offer some protection, they may still permit objects to strike the surface of the eye. Only industrial-quality lenses meet all the requirements for fire and impact resistance set by the American National Standard Practice for Occupational and Educational Eye and Face Protection (Z 87.1,1979).
2. Wear protective eyewear when:

   Doing yard work: (a) pruning bushes, (b) mowing the lawn, (c) applying pesticides, herbicides, lime, or fertilizers, (d) chopping, sawing, or mulching wood.

   Using household chemicals: (a) oven, drain, or furniture cleaners, (b) lye-containing detergents, ammonia, bleaches, (c) dyes, solvents, paints, inks, varnishes, shellacs, adhesives, and glues, (d) any pressurized spray product.

   Undertaking do-it-yourself projects: (a) plastering, painting, (b) using electric saws, drills, sanders, honing or welding devices, (c) doing ceiling repairs, (d) working on the underside of a car.

   Engaging in sports activities: (a) baseball, volleyball, basketball, hockey, football, soccer, (b) tennis, racquetball, badminton, squash, (c) bicycling, motor biking, (d) archery, riflery
3. Observe general safety practices: (a) read labels and instruction sheets before using a new product, (b) know the composition of chemicals, observing all listed precautions, (c) keep tools in good repair, (d) adhere to all sports rules.

BIBLIOGRAPHY

Abrahamson IA Jr. Cataract update. *American Family Physician,* (Oct.) 1891, 24(4):111–119.

Abramson DH. Retinoblastoma: Diagnosis and management. *Ca-A Cancer Journal for Clinicians,* (May/June) 1982, 32(3):130–143.

Bates B. The head and neck, in *A Guide to Physical Examination,* 3rd ed. Lippincott, Philadelphia, 1983.

Belmont O. Spectacle problems and medical problems that alter the need for glasses. *Medical Clinics of North America,* (Sept.) 1969, 53(5):1131–1144.

Berkow RB (ed.). *The Merck Manual of Diagnosis and Therapy,* 14th ed. Mercke Sharp & Dohme Research Laboratories, Rahway, N.J., 1982.

Boyd-Monk H. (consultant). Taking a closer look at contact lenses. *Nursing 78,* (Oct.) 1978, 39–43.

Boyd-Monk H. Examining the external eye, part 2. *Nursing 80,* (June) 1980, 58–63.

Brown AM, Stubbs DW (eds.). *Medical Physiology.* Wiley, New York, 1983.

Bruce RA Jr, Letson AD. Ocular manifestations of diabetes mellitus. *Postgraduate Medicine,* (Oct.) 1980, 68(4):143–156.

Burkhart CG. How to identify and manage lesions on the eyelids. *Modern Medicine,* (Nov.) 1981, 102–108.

Char DH. The red eye: When can you treat—when should you refer? *Medical Times,* (Dec.) 1979, 107(12):34–40.

Chumbley LC. *Ophthalmology in Internal Medicine.* Saunders, Philadelphia, 1981.

Conn HF, Conn RB Jr (eds.). *Current Diagnosis.* Saunders, Philadelphia, 1980.

Crafts RC. *A Textbook of Human Anatomy,* 3rd ed. Wiley, New York, 1985.

Crouch JE, McClintic JR. *Human Anatomy and Physiology,* 2nd ed. Wiley, New York, 1976.

Elias H, Pauly JE, Burns ER. *Histology and Human Microanatomy,* 4th ed. Wiley, New York, 1978.

Ellis P. *Ocular Therapeutics and Pharmacology.* Mosby, St. Louis, 1977.

Garcia CA, Ruiz RS. Diabetes and the eye. *Clinical Symposia,* 1984, 36(4):2–32.

Gordon DM. Diseases of the eye. *Clinical Symposia,* 1962, 14(4):115–142.

Goroll AH, May LA, Mulley AG. *Primary Care Medicine: Office Evaluation and Management of the Adult Patient.* Lippincott, Philadelphia, 1981.

Gray H, Goss C (eds.). *Gray's Anatomy,* 29th American ed. Lea & Febiger, Philadelphia, 1973.

Greenberg D. Evaluation of dry eye, in: Goroll AH, May LA, Mulley AG (eds.): *Primary Care Medicine: Office Evaluation and Management of the Adult Patient.* Lippincott, Philadelphia, 1981, 735–739.

Greene J. The ABC's of contact lenses. *FDA Consumer,* U.S. Dept. of Health and Human Services, Rockville, Md., February 1980.

Guyton AC. *Textbook of Medical Physiology,* 6th ed. Saunders, Philadelphia, 1981.

Hoole AJ, Greenberg RA, Pickard CG Jr. *Patient Care Guidelines for Nurse Practitioners.* Little, Brown, Boston, 1982.

Isselbacher KJ, et al. (eds.) *Harrison's Principles of Internal Medicine,* 9th ed. McGraw-Hill, New York, 1980.

Kelley WN, et al. *Textbook of Rheumatology,* Vols. I and II. Saunders, Philadelphia, 1981.

Kingham JD. Retrolental fibroplasia. *American Family Physician,* (Nov.) 1979, 20(5):119–125.

Krupp MA, Chatton MJ, Werdegar D (eds.). *Current Medical Diagnosis and Treatment 1985.* Lange, Los Altos, Calif., 1985.

Kupper C, Kaiser-Kupper M. *Differential Diagnosis: Disorders of the Eye and Visual System.* Arco, New York, 1978.

Langley L, Telford I, Christensen J. The special senses, in *Dynamic Anatomy and Physiology,* 4th ed. McGraw-Hill, New York, 1974, 304–329.

Lawyer T Jr. Diagnosis: External neurological examination of the eye. *Hospital Medicine,* (June) 1980, 35–43.

Leibowitz H, Pratt M, Flagstad I, et al. Human conjunctivitis: Diagnostic evaluation. *Archives of Ophthalmology* 1976, 94:1747.

Leitch CJ, Tinker RV. *Primary Care.* Davis, Philadelphia, 1978.

Luckmann J, Sorensen KC. *Medical Surgical Nursing: A Psychophysiologic Approach,* 2nd ed. Saunders, Philadelphia, 1980.

Mandell GL, Douglas RG Jr, Bennett JE. *Principles and Practice of Infectious Diseases.* Wiley, New York, 1979.

Mehalas TJ, Kollarits CR. Pupillary clues to neuroophthalmic diagnoses. *Postgraduate Medicine,* (Mar.) 1982, 71(3):199–210.

Miller RW. Keeping an eye on glaucoma. *FDA Consumer,* U.S. Dept. of Health and Human Services, Rockville, Md., June 1980.

Monk C. Primary care for ocular emergencies, part II. *Physician Assistant and Health Practitioner,* (Aug.) 1979, 16–20.

National Society to Prevent Blindness. *Eye Safety Is No Accident.* New York, 1980.

National Society to Prevent Blindness. *Facts and Figures.* New York, February 1980.

Newell F, Ernest J. *Ophthalmology Principles and Concepts,* 3rd ed. Mosby, St. Louis, 1974.

Newton D. Eye disorders, in Leitch CJ, Tinker RV (eds.): *Primary Care.* Davis, Philadelphia, 1978, 109–133.

Ophthalmology Newsletter. Glaucomatous cupping. (June) 1982, 2(3):

Paton D, Craig JA. Glaucomas: Diagnosis and management. *Clinical Symposia,* 1976, 28(2):3–47.

Pavon-Langston D (ed.). *Manual of Ocular Diagnosis and Therapy.* Little, Brown, Boston, 1980.

Purcell J, Spaeth G. Ocular trauma, in *Principles and Practice of Emergency Medicine.* Saunders, Philadelphia, 1978.

Rapp DA. Primary glaucoma. *Physician Assistant and Health Practitioner,* (Apr.) 1982, 14–30.

Records RE. Diabetic retinopathy: Current concepts of management. *Continuing Education,* (Oct.) 1981, 103–112.

Richter C. Evaluation of impaired vision, in Goroll AH, May LA, Mulley AG (eds.): *Primary Care Medicine: Office Evaluation and Management of the Adult Patient.* Lippincott, Philadelphia, 1981, 728–732.

Scheie H, Albert D. *Adler's Textbook of Ophthalmology,* 10th ed. Saunders, Philadelphia, 1981.

Schwartz GR, (eds.). *Principles and Practice of Emergency Medicine,* Vols. 1 and 2. Saunders, Philadelphia, 1978.

Silverstein A. The sense organs: Sight, in *Human Anatomy and Physiology.* Wiley, New York, 1980.

Simon RP. The pupillary exam: Easy and essential. *Diagnosis,* (May) 1980, 62–65.

Spector RH. Ocular clues to neurologic disease. *Emergency Medicine,* (Oct.) 1981, 66–99.

Squillacote D, Osborn HH. Corneal abrasions. *Physician Assistant and Health Practitioner,* (Oct.) 1982, 16–32.

Steinert R. Evaluation of the red eye, in Goroll AH, May LA, Mulley AG (eds.): *Primary Care Medicine: Office Evaluation and Management of the Adult Patient.* Lippincott, Philadelphia, 1981, 723–728.

Trevar-Roper P. *The Eye and Its Disorders.* Blackwell, Oxford, 1974.

Vaughan D. Asbury T. *General Ophthalmology.* Lange, Los Altos, Calif., 1980.

Victor M, Adams R. Common disturbances of vision, ocular movement, and hearing, in: Isselbacher KJ, *Harrison's Principles of Internal Medicine,* 9th ed. McGraw-Hill, New York, 1980, 101–108.

Wolff E. *Anatomy of the Eye and Orbit.* Saunders, Philadelphia, 1968.

Wyngaarden JB, Smith LH Jr (eds). *Cecil Textbook of Medicine,* 16th ed., Vols. 1 and 2. Saunders, Philadelphia, 1982.

Zinn KM. Pars plana vitrectomy: Current techniques. *New York State Journal of Medicine,* (Oct.) 1979, 1734–1743.

2

Ear, Nose, Throat

Carla Greene and Mary McTigue

Outline

EAR

External Ear

Congenital anomalies
Perichondritis
Lacerations
Hematoma
Cauliflower ear
Ear piercing
▶ Furuncles
Trapped insects
Foreign bodies
▶ Impacted cerumen
▶ Otitis externa
Malignant otitis externa

Middle Ear

▶ Traumatic perforations
▶ Bullous myringitis
Otosclerosis
▶ Eustachian tube dysfunction
▶ Serous otitis media
▶ Acute otits media
Mastoiditis
Chronic otitis media
Cholesteatoma
Conductive hearing loss

Inner Ear

Sensorineural hearing loss
Noise-induced hearing loss
Acoustic neurofibroma
Drug-induced hearing loss
Presbycusis
▶ Proper use and care of hearing aids
▶ Courtesies and commonsense measures for people with hearing loss
▶ Organizations for the deaf
▶ Labyrinthitis
▶ Motion sickness
Meniere's disease

NOSE AND THROAT

Nasal Structure

▶ Folliculitis
Fissures

▶ Nasal furuncles
Squamous papilloma
Septal deviation
Nasal fractures
Septal hematoma
Septal abscess
Septal perforation
Rhinoplasty

Nasal Mucosa

Viral infections
▶ Common cold
▶ Vitamin C intake
▶ Allergic rhinitis
Nonallergic vasomotor rhinitis
Sampter's syndrome
Rhinitis medicamentosa
Nasal polyps
Tumors of the nasal cavity
▶ Nosebleed

Olfactory Cells

Disturbances of smell

Paranasal Sinuses

▶ Acute sinusitis
Sinus headache
Chronic sinusitis
Sinus tumors

Pharynx

Chronic adenoid infection
▶ Acute viral pharyngitis/tonsillitis
▶ Acute streptococcal pharyngitis/tonsillitis
Peritonsillar infection
Peritonsillar abscess
Chronic tonsillitis
Infectious mononucleosis
▶ Gonococcal pharyngitis
Diphtheria
▶ Primary diphtheria immunization for adults
Pharyngitis medicamentosa

Larynx

▶ Acute laryngitis
Chronic laryngitis
Intrinsic carcinoma of the true vocal cords
Extrinsic carcinoma of the larynx
Acute epiglottitis

EAR

The ear (Fig. 2.1) is divided into external, middle, and internal compartments.

External Ear

The external ear consists of the auricle and the ear canal. Supported by cartilage and covered by skin, the auricles have a number of specially shaped areas diagrammed in Figure 2.2. Although many normal variations in size and shape exist, ***congenital anomalies*** may indicate malformations of other organs, particularly those that developed during the same embryonic stage as the ear. For instance, small or absent ear lobes have been associated with kidney problems; a deep diagonal groove in the lobe with heart attacks; and low-set ears with mental retardation.

Ear cartilage is avascular. It is nourished only by diffusion of materials from the blood vessels of an outer membrane, the perichondrium. For this reason, ***perichondritis,*** an infection that spreads from overlying skin, can be extremely destructive. Pus gathering behind the membrane cuts off the blood supply to the inner cartilage and causes necrosis. Because perichondritis is an indolent process, patients may have few if any systemic signs. However, there may be local adenopathy and the auricle is usually red, swollen, and tender. Patients should be sent to a surgeon or

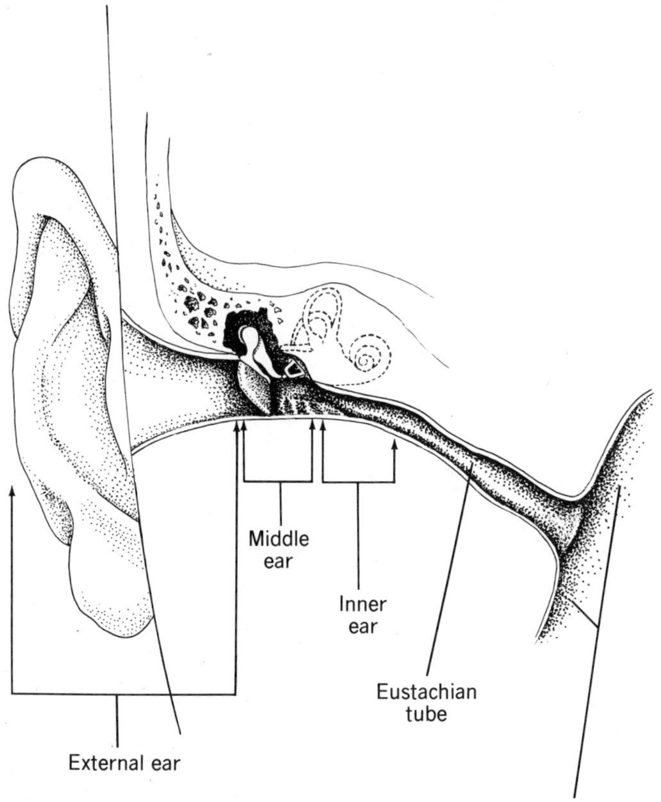

Figure 2.1 Divisions of the ear: external canal, middle canal, inner canal, eustachian tube.

ear, nose, and throat (ENT) specialist for immediate drainage. In order to reinstate contact of the perichondrium with the underlying cartilage, pressure bandages are usually applied. Antibiotics guided by culture and sensitivity tests are also required. The usual pathogens are gram-negative rods.

To prevent perichondritis, all cases of trauma to the outer ear should be promptly treated. ***Lacerations*** that penetrate the cartilage need to be skin sutured and splinted. Sutures should not extend into the cartilage because the tissue has such poor reparative ability that it may become infected.

Hematoma, a blood collection between the perichondrium and the cartilage, causes the outer ear to become a shapeless purple mass; it must be evacuated. Patients should be sent to a surgeon for incision and drainage. Following this procedure, the skin and perichondrium must be molded onto the cartilage and a pressure bandage applied to ensure adequate circulation. Without these measures, the hematoma may calcify into hard bulbous masses called ***cauliflower ear.*** Cauliflower ear is fairly common among boxers and wrestlers, and may be seen in battered adults.

The common practice of ***ear piercing*** may also lead to complications. Unsterile conditions during piercing may cause local infection or perichondritis. Even clean, newly pierced ears may become infected if the grade of gold of the first earrings

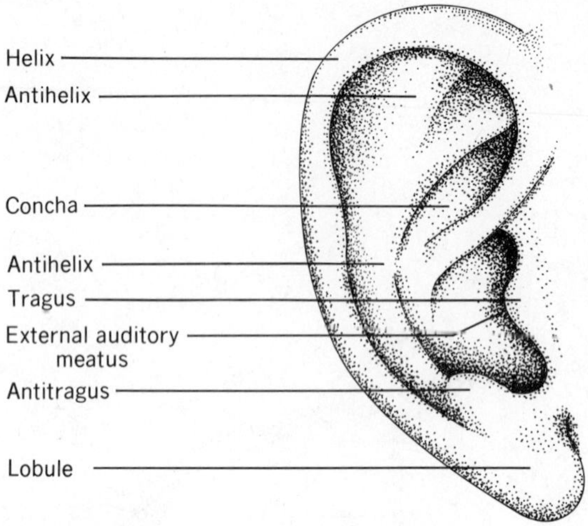

Figure 2.2 Details of the external ear (lateral view): auricle, ear canal.

inserted is not 14 carat or greater. This is due to the high incidence of allergic responses to other metals, especially nickel (gold allergies also occur but are less common). The metals cause contact dermatitis marked by inflamed, weeping skin that often becomes secondarily infected, particularly around the metal post behind the lobe. Topical steroid creams or antibiotics may be needed if the area is infected. Gold hoops, which allow maximum air circulation, or hypoallergenic earrings help alleviate chronic problems.

Behind the tragus (Fig. 2.2) opens the ear canal. The narrow outer portion contains numerous sebaceous glands and hair follicles. These may become infected and form ▶ ***furuncles*** (boils). Even small boils in the ear canal cause severe pain, which is exacerbated by chewing or movement of the auricle. Patients may also note a sensation of fullness in the ear or decreased hearing. The involved area is often red and severely swollen. Fever, adenopathy, and adjacent cellulitis are not uncommon. The treatment consists of hastening fluctuation and drainage. This can be accomplished by placing a gauze wick into the canal and instructing the patient to wet it every few hours with half-strength Burrow's solution. Along with intermittent heat applications, this measure usually brings the boil to a head within 48 hours. The apex can then be opened. In the meantime, codeine may be needed to relieve pain, and systemic antibiotics are given if there is fever or cellulitis.

The ear canal is lubricated and protected by secretions of the ceruminous glands. Although the brown, bitter-tasting "ear wax" is thought to discourage insects from entering the canal, ***trapped insects*** occur with some frequency. The wriggling, buzzing, or wing beating of an insect inside the canal is both uncomfortable and frightening, and patients are likely to seek immediate attention. Luckily, the problem is easily managed. The insect sometimes exits on its own when attracted to a light held at the meatus. If this does not work, it must be killed by filling the canal with mineral oil. The dead insect is then removed with gentle irrigation, using tepid water and a soft rubber syringe.

A number of ***foreign bodies*** other than insects may become embedded in the ear canal. Children often stuff jelly beans, pills, or bits of crayon in their ears. Adults may forget cotton wicks or ear plugs, or may break off matchsticks trying to clean the canal. Such objects can usually be removed with a curette or small pair of tweezers. Irrigation may also be used unless the foreign body is hydrophilic (e.g., a dried bean or wood particle). Hydrophilic foreign bodies may absorb water and swell, thus complicating removal. Patients should be referred to an ENT specialist if there is any chance that removal of the foreign body may be difficult or may jeopardize the ear drum.

Through actions of the jaw, cerumen is continually worked out of the ear canal, and carries with it particles of dust and dirt. Attempts to clean the ears with cotton swabs or bobby pins interrupt this self-cleaning mechanism. Paradoxically, they promote accumulation of debris and may lead to ▶***impacted cerumen.*** When the ear canals becomes occluded by wax, patients complain of pain, itching, ringing, or decreased hearing. The wax is clearly visible on otoscopic exam, and unless there is a concurrent infection in the canal or middle ear, fever and adenopathy are absent. Soft brownish wax can usually be removed by gentle flushing with tepid water alone. However, it is better to soften white, hardened wax with Ceruminex drops 15 minutes before attempting to irrigate. Irrigation is contraindicated if the patient has any signs of an active middle ear infection, a history of recurrent ear infections, or any possibility of a perforated drum. For chronic problems, ear-softening agents can be prescribed for intermittent use at home.

Although usually protective, ear wax can absorb water during swimming or bathing and form an ideal medium for an infection of the ear canal. Because of this connection, ▶***otitis externa*** is often called "swimmer's ear." However, the problem also follows trauma from attempts to clean or scratch the ear canal; allergic responses to hair dyes or sprays; and chronic seborrhea, eczema, or psoriasis that becomes secondarily infected. The organisms involved are most frequently *Pseudomonas aeurginosa,* occasionally *Staphylococcus aureus,* and rarely fungi. Patients with otitis externa describe pain, itching, a clogged sensation, and decreased hearing. Fever and adenopathy may be present, and traction on the auricle exacerbates the pain. On otoscopic exam, the underlying skin in the canal appears red and swollen with a weepy crust. It bleeds easily and is exquisitely sensitive. There may be a liquid, solid, or "cottage cheese" exudate, which is either white or yellowish and often foul-smelling. The eardrum, if it can be visualized, may have the same appearance as the canal, but it moves with the pneumatic otoscope and shows no signs of bulging. For treatment, topical ear solutions containing antibiotics and corticosteroids are given for several days. To ensure that medication reaches the infected skin, exudate should be removed frequently. This can be accomplished with gentle use of a cotton stylet or hydrogen peroxide drops. Cool or warm compresses and analgesics may relieve some of the discomfort. Recurrences can be prevented by using drops of a vinegar and water solution after swimming and avoiding other predisposing factors.

Elderly diabetics with ear canal infections should be watched closely, since they are at risk for developing a lethal variety of the infection called ***malignant otitis externa.*** Invariably due to *P. aeruginosa,* this infection can progress rapidly to invade soft tissue cartilage, nerve, and skull bone. Osteomyelitis, cranial nerve impairment, and even death can result. Mortality rates are as high as 50–75%, and early hospitalization is imperative.

Middle Ear

The middle ear is illustrated in Figure 2.1. The tympanic membrane, which lies at the end of the ear canal (Figure 2.3*a*) forms the lateral wall. Shiny and pearly gray in appearance, it is positioned obliquely and pulled in at the center by the malleus (Fig. 2.3*b*). The relatively thin membrane can be accidentally torn if Q-tips, bobby pins, or small tree branches protrude into the canal. ▶ ***Traumatic perforations*** can also follow sudden increases in atmospheric pressure (airplane descent, diving, or a forceful open-handed slap over the ear). The patient experiences sudden, severe pain and hearing change; occasionally, blood is discharged from the canal. Small tears heal spontaneously within a few days to several weeks. Patients are given penicillin

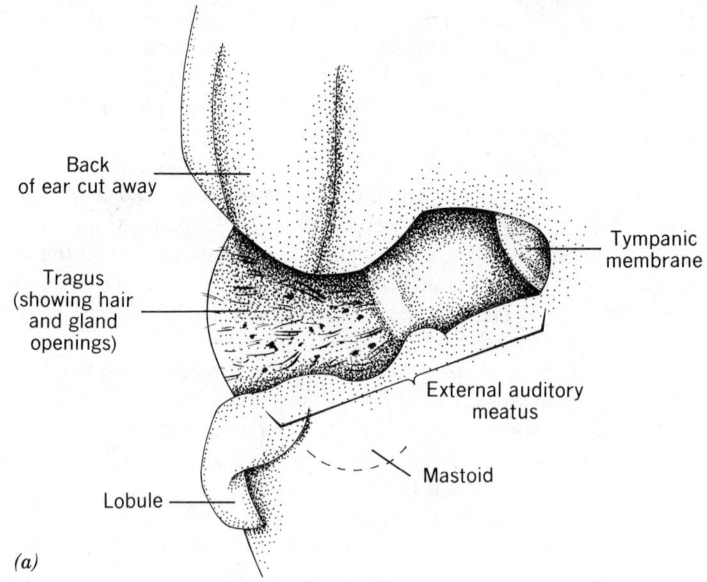

(*a*)

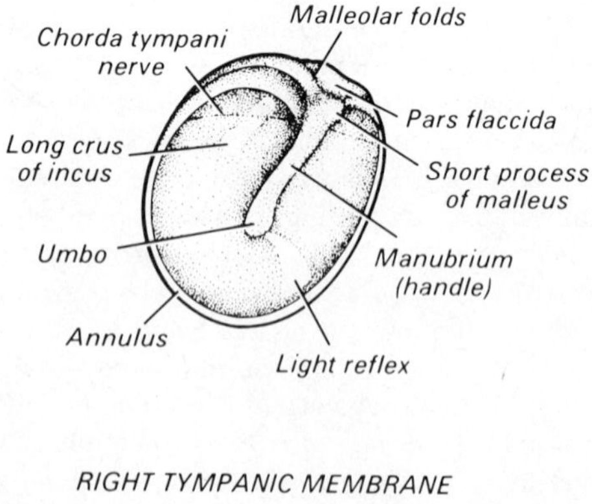

(*b*)

Figure 2.3 Tympanic membrane: (*a*) at end of ear canal (posterior view) (*b*) as seen through an otoscope.

for 7 days to prevent middle ear infection. They should also be advised to keep water or any other fluids from entering the canal (no swimming and ear plug protection during bathing or hair washing). Patients with large tears, persistent pain, or tears that do not heal within 3 weeks should be referred to an ENT specialist. Displaced flaps may need to be realigned, the edges of ragged wounds cauterized, or the opening of large perforations grafted. Furthermore, patients with persistent conductive hearing loss may need middle ear exploration to rule out damage to the ossicles.

An infection of the eardrum, ▶ ***bullous myringitis,*** can be exceedingly painful. It is probably the extension of a middle ear infection, since studies show that the same organisms (see Table 2.1) are usually involved. Contrary to a well-accepted notion, mycoplasma is probably an unusual cause. With infection, the membrane becomes inflamed and develops herpetic-like vesicles that can reach blister size or fill with blood. Since a clinical distinction between viral and bacterial etiologies cannot be made, antibiotic therapy is always called for. To relieve pain, most patients need strong analgesics, and a few require ENT referral for rupture of the vesicles.

On the other side of the middle ear cavity is a bony partition separating the middle from the inner ear. Through the bone is a membrane-covered opening called the "oval window." The middle ear cavity contains three tiny bones (ossicles). The first ossicle (malleus) protrudes into the tympanic membrane. It connects through the second ossicle (incus) to the third (stapes), which sits on the oval window. Set into motion by a vibrating eardrum, the ossicles act as a series of levers to increase pressure in the oval window and thus stimulate the fluid-filled chambers of the inner ear. Sometimes diseased bone in the middle ear is replaced by sclerotic tissue, and the oval window becomes covered. The stapes becomes immobilized, a condition called ***otosclerosis.*** Occurring in 4% of the population, otosclerosis has a familial tendency and affects mainly women in their twenties or thirties. Fixation of the stapes may advance rapidly during pregnancy and sometimes causes damage to the eighth cranial nerve. All patients who notice tinnitus and progressive loss of hearing should be referred to an otolaryngologist. Complete audiology testing and surgical evaluation are needed. Usually the damaged stapes can be replaced with a plastic prosthesis and a new eardrum formed out of grafted material. A hearing aid may also be necessary.

The middle ear is connected to the nasopharynx by the eustachian tube (refer to

TABLE 2.1 CULTURE FINDINGS IN ACUTE OTITIS MEDIA

No growth (indicating viruses or anaerobes)
Streptococcus pneumoniae
Hemophilus species
Streptococcus pyogenes (group A)
Staphylococcus aureus
Branhamella (formerly *Neisseria*) *catarrhalis*
Miscellaneous or mixed infections

Source: Based on David Fairbanks, *Antimicrobial Therapy in Otolaryngology.* Washington, D.C., American Academy of Otolaryngology, 1983.

Fig. 2.1). For the most part, its slit-like opening in the throat remains closed. However, a sneeze, yawn, or swallow flips the slit open, exposing the middle ear to atmospheric pressure. Without the pressurization provided by the eustachian tube, the ear drum would rupture. Blockage of the tube from allergies or respiratory infections (measles, mumps, influenza, scarlet fever, pneumonia, or the common cold) creates enough negative pressure in the middle ear to cause considerable discomfort. This is known as ▶***eustachian tube dysfunction.*** The tympanic membrane retracts, producing a popping or clogged sensation and pain that is sharpened by jaw movements. If the eustachian tube remains dysfunctional, a sterile transudate, drawn from the blood vessels in the mucous lining, collects behind the drum. This condition, called ***serous otitis media,*** is responsible for conductive hearing loss and symptoms of pain and tinnitus (ringing, buzzing, or roaring in nature). On otoscopic exam, the eardrum has an amber-gray appearance and may reveal an air-fluid level or bubbles in the middle ear cavity. The presence of fluid is further confirmed with pneumatic or impedance testing. Treatment of eustachian tube dysfunction centers on the underlying cause. For example, some patients may need desensitization for allergies. Gum chewing (to equalize atmospheric pressure in the tube) and decongestants help facilitate drainage. Intervention by an ENT specialist (blowing open the tube or evacuating fluid through a myringotomy) is indicated for persistent problems that do not respond to medical management.

Whenever there is negative pressure from eustachian tube dysfunction, pathogens from the nose and throat can be sucked up into the middle ear. This is the major cause of ▶***acute otitis media,*** although pathogens also gain entrance from forceful nose blowing and backlogged water during swimming or diving. As suggested by culture studies, the most common organisms are listed in Table 2.1. As septic fluid accumulates in the closed space, patients with acute otitis media experience pain, fever, adenopathy, and decreased hearing. The eardrum is usually bulging, red, and unresponsive to pneumatic testing. There may be purulent fluid or blood in the canal if spontaneous perforation has occurred. Treatment includes a 10-day course of antibiotics and decongestants to help restore eustachian tube function. Heat applications, codeine, or aspirin may be helpful in relieving the pain. Patients who do not respond readily to this treatment, noting decreased fever and pain within 48 hours, should be referred to an ENT specialist. This is extremely important, since a number of complications could arise: mastoiditis, meningitis, brain abscess, deafness, facial paralysis, cavernous sinus thrombosis, and labyrinthitis.

Mastoiditis is the extension of a middle ear infection to the air-filled cells of the mastoid bone (see Fig. 2.3). It becomes clinically evident 2 or more weeks after the onset of otitis media, causing increased fever and earache, and sometimes a profuse discharge from the ear canal. With bone destruction, a red, swollen, painful mass develops over the mastoid process, and changes can be seen on x-ray films. Intramuscular (IM) or intravenous (IV) antibiotics guided by culture and sensitivity tests are given for at least 2 weeks. If the infection does not respond, mastoidectomy is performed. Fortunately, mastoid infections are now rare.

Recurrent cases of acute ear infections are a major factor in the development of ***chronic otitis media.*** This condition is characterized by a persistent effusion or, more often, by a painless discharge from the ear canal. The discharge may be odorless or foul-smelling, and typically increases with upper respiratory infections. Most often caused by the pathogens listed in Table 2.2, the ongoing infection leads to changes in the ear mucosa and eventually destroys the ossicles, with inevitable loss

TABLE 2.2 CULTURE FINDINGS IN CHRONIC OTITIS MEDIA

Infections characterized by effusions	Infections characterized by discharge
Hemophilus influenza	Mixed aerobes/anaerobes
Diphtheroids	*Pseudomonas* species
Streptococcus pneumoniae	Staph. *aureus*
Branhamella catarrahalis	Staph. *epidermidis*
Staphylococcus aureus	*Escherichia coli*
Streptococcus pyogenes	*Proteus* species
Variable anaerobes	*Diphtheroides*
	Streptococcus species
	Variable anaerobes

Source: Based on David Fairbanks, *Antimicrobial Therapy in Otolaryngology.* Washington, D.C.: American Academy of Otolaryngology, 1983.

of hearing. Patients with symptoms of chronic otitis should be referred to an ENT specialist. Sometimes the problem is improved by a medical program that includes (1) regular debridement of the discharge, (2) systemic antibiotics or antibiotic powders blown into the middle ear, and (3) ear drops containing corticosteroids or drying agents. However, surgical procedures such as mastoidectomy, myringoplasty (eardrum repair), or tympanoplasty (middle ear reconstruction) may also be necessary.

As a result of an acute or chronic process in the middle ear, squamous epithelium could become trapped in the tympanic membrane and/or mastoid cells. The epithelim sheds keratin and forms a retention cyst called ***cholesteatoma.*** It can be identified on otoscopic exam as a white lesion lying in the middle ear cavity. Becoming quite extensive, the lesion can perforate the periphery of the eardrum and erode bone tissue. The painful perforations are filled with a cheesy, seborrheic debris that causes a sterile brownish discharge. Occasionally, cholesteatomas invade the inner ear, resulting in vertigo. Patients with suspected cholesteatomas need ENT evaluation. Surgical debridement and tympanoplasty are the usual treatments.

Problems in the ear canal or middle ear interfere with the mechanical reception or amplification of sound and therefore produce ***conductive hearing loss*** (Table 2.3). Patients with conductive hearing loss are unable to distinguish low tones and vowels. The Weber test shows a better response in the affected ear, and the Rinne test shows greater bone conduction than air conduction. In many cases, the underlying cause (impacted wax, furuncle, middle ear effusion) can be easily identified and treated. If not, the patient should be sent for audiology evaluation to help pinpoint

TABLE 2.3 CAUSES OF CONDUCTIVE HEARING LOSS

Disorders of the external canal	Disorders of the middle ear
Impacted cerumen	Perforation of the tympanic membrane
Foreign body	Scarring of the tympanic membrane
Otitis externa	Acute otitis media
Furuncle	Chronic otitis media
	Serous otitis media
	Congenital malformation of the ossicles
	Trauma to the temporal bone with disruption of the ossicles
	Otosclerosis
	Cholesteatoma

the area of dysfunction (see Table 2.7). Problems such as a scarred tympanic membrane, otosclerosis, or cholesteatoma need further care by an ENT surgeon.

Inner Ear

The inner ear (cochlea) is a coiled, fluid-filled structure in the temporal bone (Fig. 2.4). Whenever the ossicles transmit sound waves across the oval window, the fluid in the cochlea is set in motion. This motion is translated into nerve impulses by the hair cells of the organ of Corti. Picked up by the acoustic branch of cranial nerve VIII, the impulses travel via complicated pathways to the brain; these paths are diagrammed in Figure 2.4*b*. Discrimination of pitch, intensity, and timber takes place in the auditory cortex. The cortex aids in localization of sound and is necessary for comprehension of the spoken word.

Any abnormality of the cochlea, acoustic nerve, or central pathways may result in ***sensorineural hearing loss.*** Abnormalities can be congenital or acquired, as described in Table 2.4.

Prolonged exposure to sound levels in excess of 95 dB may lead to ***noise-induced hearing loss.*** Workers in factories, construction sites, mills, and airports are at particularly high risk. Thirty percent of all discotheque disc jockeys suffer hearing damage, along with many members of rock bands and avid fans of loud music. Recently, Walkman-type radios and tape recorders with earphones have been implicated in an alarming increase in hearing damage. When turned up enough to drown out noise from a lawn mower or city traffic, the volume of these instruments may reach 120 dB (the equivalent of an unmuffled jackhammer). Many otologists believe that the standard of 95 dB set by the Occupational Safety and Health Administration (OSHA) is too lenient and that any noise greater that 85 dB is damaging. This is a disturbing thought in view of the high decibel ratings of many commonly encountered sounds (Table 2.5). The onset of noise-induced hearing loss is characterized by a decrease in sensitivity to sound with a rise in the threshold for sound perception. If noise exposure is reduced during this stage, the damage is reversible and hearing returns to previous levels. The problem is that patients remain unaware of the change because speech frequencies (500, 1,000, and 2,000 cycles/sec) are initially unaffected. By the time hearing loss is noted, nerve damage is usually irreversible. To protect susceptible individuals, OSHA has established regulations for acceptable noise levels in work environments. In addition, many industries require preemployment audiometric screening, along with periodic retesting, and encourage their workers to wear protective apparatus. Rubber or plastic ear plugs come in standard sizes or can be custom made from molded impressions of the ear canal. Ear plugs, acoustic ear muffs, and head shields should be used by workers directly exposed to jet engines or explosions.

Another cause of sensorineural hearing loss is ***acoustic neurofibroma*** (neurinoma), a rare, benign tumor of the eighth cranial nerve. It develops at the point where the nerve is transformed from brain to peripheral tissue, usually within the internal auditory meatus. Tinnitus, vertigo, and hearing loss progress over several years. Reaching sizes of 4 to 6 cm, some tumors eventually cause eye or ear pain, weakness, numbness, and/or twitching of facial muscles, difficulty in talking or swallowing, and disturbances of gait and balance. Mental changes, along with papilledema with headache, visual disturbance, and vomiting, are late changes. Patients should be sent to a neurologist for evaluation. The diagnosis is revealed by

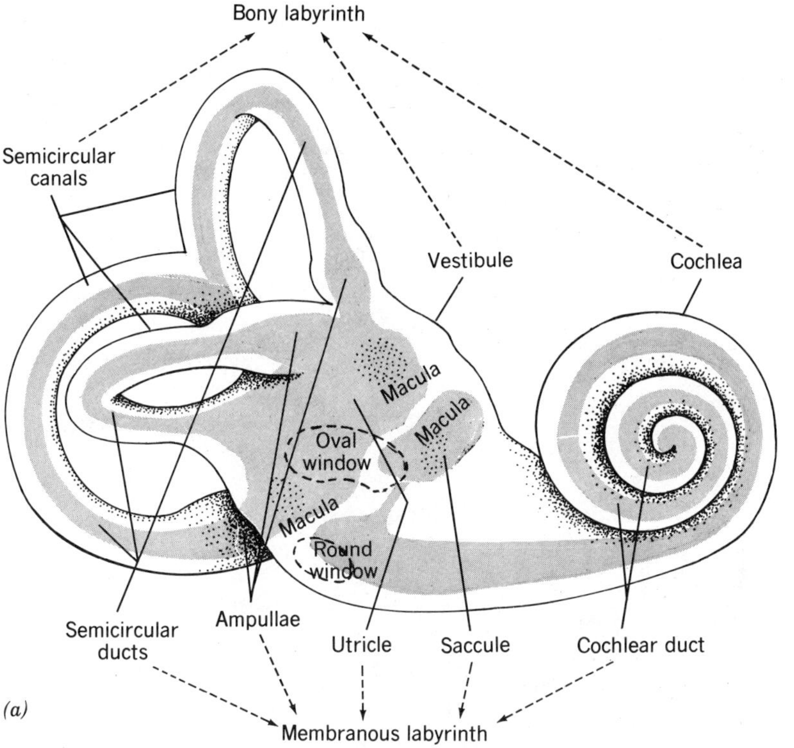

(a)

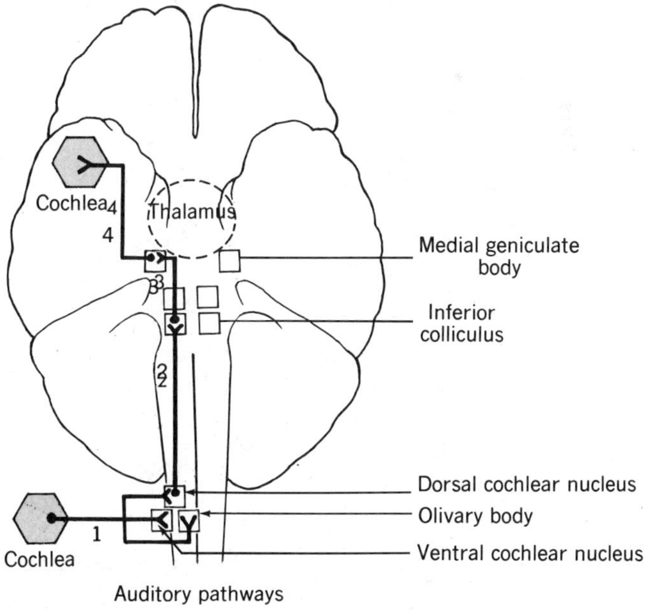

(b)

Figure 2.4 Details of the inner ear: (*a*) labyrinths and (*b*) auditory pathways.

TABLE 2.4 CAUSES OF SENSORINEURAL HEARING LOSS

Congenital
- Maternal rubella infections
- Maternal exposure to ototoxic drugs
- Anoxia at birth
- Birth trauma causing bleeding into the inner ear
- Erythroblastosis fetalis
- Hereditary syndromes including albinism, Hurler's disease, and Waardenburg's syndrome

Acquired
- CNS embolism, thrombosis, or hemorrhage
- Vasculitis
- Viral infections affecting the inner ear, specifically mumps, measles, influenza, chickenpox, mononucleosis, and adenoviruses (complete or partial recovery is the rule)
- Meningitis
- High fevers in childhood
- Prolonged exposure to loud noise
- Degenerative changes associated with aging
- Ototoxic drugs
- Fractures of the temporal bono
- Bleeding into the inner ear following trauma
- CNS tumors, notably acoustic neurinoma
- Meniere's disease

the following findings: elevated protein levels on spinal fluid analysis; an enlarged internal auditory meatus visible on x-ray films; and deformities of the ventricles on computed tomography (CT) scan. Surgery is the only treatment. Complete tumor removal is possible in more than 60% of the cases, using combined approaches through the labyrinth and cranium.

A number of drugs have toxic effects on the auditory nerve (Table 2.6). ***Drug-induced hearing loss*** is a distinct complication of the aminoglycoside antibiotics. Ethacrynic acid, furosemide, and quinidine are other common but less potent offenders. Marked by tinnitus, salicylate poisoning causes mild nerve irritation that is completely reversible. Since damage caused by other drugs may be permanent, drug levels should be carefully monitored and the drug withdrawn at the first signs of hearing impairment.

Of all the causes of sensorineural hearing loss, ***presbycusis,*** the degeneration of the nerve cells in the cochlea associated with aging, is the most common. Since the degenerative decline starts at age 20, almost all people experience some hearing loss by age 60. Men are affected more often and more severely than women. It is typical that these patients can hear people talking but have difficulty deciphering the words, and find that shouting by others only exacerbates the problem. They may initially notice decreased sensitivity to doorbell or telephone rings, since sensorineu-

TABLE 2.5 DECIBEL RATINGS OF SOME COMMONLY ENCOUNTERED SOUNDS

Sound	Decibel Rating	Sound	Decibel Rating
Whisper	10	Motorcycle	90
Rustle of leaves	20	Power lawn mower	100
Light traffic	50	Amplified rock music	115
Normal conversation	60	Pneumatic jackhammer	120
Air conditioner	60	Jet takeoff	120
Freeway traffic	65	Walkman-type radio	Up to 130
Television	70	High-power siren	130
Dishwasher	75	New York City subway	135
Crowded restaurant	80	Shotgun blast	140

TABLE 2.6 DRUGS THAT ARE OTOTOXIC

Aminoglycosides	Other antibiotics	Loop diuretics
Amikacin	Chloramphenicol	Ethacrynic acid
Gentamicin	Colistin	Furosemide
Kanamycin	Erythromycin	Other drugs
Neomycin	Minocycline	Quinine
Netilmicin	Polymyxin	Quinidine
Streptomycin	Vancomycin	Salicylates
Tobramycin	Viomycin	Cisplatin

ral problems are characterized by lost acuity for high-frequency sound waves. Sometimes there are complaints of heightened sounds, but more often there is a failure to notice or an attempt to conceal hearing changes. Problems should be suspected in any patient who displays certain manners: speaking with an unusually loud or soft voice; tilting the head or straining facial muscles while listening; requesting frequent clarification; or appearing inattentive or failing to respond when spoken to.

Examination of patients with sensorineural hearing loss reveals no obstruction in the canal or abnormality of the tympanic membrane. The Weber test shows lateralization to the good ear, and the Rinne test shows reduced bone and air conduction with a normal ratio. However, to locate the exact area of dysfunction, extensive audiology tests described in Table 2.7 are needed. Depending on the results, an audiologist can estimate the effects of any hearing loss and prescribe the best means of rehabilitation. Lip reading, sign language, speech therapy, auditory training, or specially trained dogs may be suggested in certain instances of severe impairment. In many cases, hearing aids will improve communication ability. They work by amplifying sound and are particularly useful in patients with conductive hearing loss. However, hearing aids may compound the problem for those people who have nerve damage and are unable to tolerate loud sounds. Amplification of background noise can also be disturbing but may be alleviated to some extent by binaural aids (hearing aids for both ears). Binaural aids can be built into the earpieces of eyeglasses. The other basic types are bone conduction receivers worn behind the ear or air conduction receivers worn as a mold in the canal. ▶ ***Proper use and care of hearing aids*** maximizes their benefit. A number of ▶ ***courtesies and common sense measures*** may also improve communication for people with hearing loss. ▶ ***Organizations for the deaf*** offer important services, information, and support systems.

In addition to hearing, the inner ear provides senses of posture and equilibrium. Housed within the bony labyrinth is the vestibular apparatus. As illustrated in Figure 2.4, it is a membranous sac consisting of two parts, the semicircular canals and the maculae (utricle and sacculi). The semicircular canals are three fluid-filled channels placed in perpendicular planes to one another. Receptors in the channels are sensitive to head movements and provide information that controls extraocular muscles. In spite of changes in head position, the eyes remain fixed on the same point.

The maculae provide information about the position of the head relative to the force of gravity. They play a role that is helpful in, but not essential to, maintaining an upright position. In fact, people with destroyed vestibular systems have postural

TABLE 2.7 AUDIOLOGY TESTING

Test	Description	Implications of Findings
Pure tone reception threshold	Test tones at various frequencies (250–8,000 cps) are first conducted through ear phones and then via the mastoid bone. Decibel ratings (dB, volume) at which the patient is able to identify the tones are plotted on a graph.	Patients with perfect hearing can detect all sounds without any increase in volume (O dB). They detect tones better through the ear phones than via the mastoid bone (air conduction is greater than bone conduction). Patients who need volume increases of up to 20 db to detect tones are considered to have normal hearing. Those who need increases above 30 dB have a clinically significant hearing loss. A better score via the mastoid bone than through ear phones indicates a conductive hearing loss. If the underlying cause is uncorrectable, these patients do extremely well with hearing aids. Equal loss by air and bone conduction indicates an inner ear problem. With damage to the eighth cranial nerve or central pathways, air and bone conduction thresholds coincide; hearing ranges from normal to severe loss. Loss of acuity to high-frequency sounds is characteristic of noise-induced damage.
Speech reception threshold	Same testing procedure as for pure tones, except that words instead of sounds are used. The point at which the patient just barely hears words is noted as the threshold.	Measurements normally coincide with pure tone reception.
Speech discrimination	Patients are given a series of 50 one-syllable, high-pitched words (e.g., "thin"). A score for the total number of correctly recognized words is assigned (each word represents 2%).	Patients with conductive hearing loss have normal speech discrimination. With sensorineural damage, patients may need a decibel increase above 40 dB to discriminate words. The benefit from hearing aids is variable. Very poor speech discrimination is a red flag for acoustic neurinoma.
Recruitment or short-increment sensitivity test (SISI) or loudness balancing	Patients are subjected to a continuous tone with 1-db increases at 5-second intervals. This process is repeated at the various frequencies (one type of test).	The normal response to the increase is: (1) unable to hear, (2) barely able to hear, (3) hears easily, (4) sound too loud, (5) sound uncomfortable. Patients with conductive or neural hearing loss have no recruitment abnormality. In patients with cochlear damage, the response is: (1) unable to hear, (2) barely able to hear, (3) barely able to hear, (4), barely able to hear, (5) sound uncomfortable (positive recruitment). Hearing aid prescription is difficult but not impossible with these patients. Positive recruitment is evidence against acoustic neurinoma.
Tone decay test	With the opposite ear masked, the patient is given a continuous tone for a total of 60 minutes. Whenever he or she indicates that the tone is heard for a longer period, the intensity is increased by 5 dB. The procedure is repeated at various frequencies (one type of test).	In normal cases, the tone is perceived unchanged for the full 60 seconds. With middle ear problems, there is little or no tone decay. Patients with inner ear problems may need up to 30-dB increases. Rapid fatique with more than 30-dB increases occurs with eighth cranial nerve damage. No tone decay occurs in disorders of central pathways.

TABLE 2.7 (*Continued*)

Test	Description	Implications of Findings
Bekesy test	Combines both SISI and Tone decay tests. Given tones that become louder and louder, then weaker and weaker, the patient presses a switch at the point where the sound is first heard and releases it when the sound is no longer heard. This process is repeated at progressively higher frequencies, first using a tone that is interrupted every 2.5 seconds and then using a sustained tone. Results are recorded on the same graph, showing one of four types of curves.	Patients with normal hearing show the type I curve (continuous and interrupted tones superimposed on one another). The type I curve is also seen in patients with conductive hearng loss who have intact sensorineural functions. Patients with cochlear disease have the type II curve (the tracing remains normal until frequencies rise above 1,000 cps. Continuous tones then fall below the interrupted tones, and swings become smaller). Patients with eighth cranial nerve disorder have the type III curve (as frequencies increase, the continuous tone tracing shows diminished and then absent hearing). Patients with severe cochlear damage or Meniere's disease have the type IV curve (similar to type II except that the continuous tone falls below the interrupted tone at all frequencies).

instability only in instances in which visual reference is lacking, such as while walking in darkness, on uneven ground, or down stairs. By contrast, an acute disturbance of the vestibular system, ▶ ***labyrinthitis,*** can be severely disabling. There are several types, including benign positional, acute purulent, and toxic. These are described in Table 2.8. Symptoms of labyrinthitis include dizziness, nausea, and vomiting. Patients also describe nonspecific feelings such as whirling, confusion, pulsating blankness, or giddiness. They either have the sensation that they themselves are turning or that their environment is turning around them. ▶ ***Motion sickness*** is a form of labyrinthitis. In response to movement, they experience cyclic episodes of nausea and vomiting preceded by hyperventilation, profuse cold sweating, and pallor. Dizziness, headache, and fatigue may be the prevalent symptoms. Labyrinthine nystagmus, slow rhythmic movements of the eyes in one direction followed by rapid compensatory movement in the opposite direction, may be noted. The most important aspect of managing motion sickness or labyrinthitis is to rule out other, more urgent causes of dizziness listed in Table 2.9. Functional labyrinthitis responds to meclazine and avoidance of precipitating movements or positions. In cases of motion sickness, a semireclining position is preferred. Flat positions, alcohol, large meals, cigarette smoking, or reading during travel should be avoided. Prophylactic antihistamines, sedatives, or transdermal scopolamine may be necessary.

An overproduction of fluid in the inner-ear organs causes a vestibular disturbance known as ***Meniere's disease.*** The etiology and pathophysiology are poorly understood, but a symptom triad of vertigo, tinnitus, and gradual hearing loss is well known. Occurring with greatest frequency among men between the ages of 40 and 60, the problem causes attacks of vertigo, nausea, and vomiting that may last for periods ranging from a few minutes to several hours. Impairment of hearing and equilibrium is usually unilateral, both ears being involved in only 10–15% of cases. Other serious disorders may mimic symptoms of Meniere's disease (see Table 2.9), and these should be ruled out before referring patients for ENT evaluation. Although there is no cure, symptomatic relief is sometimes obtained from atropine,

TABLE 2.8 TYPES OF LABYRINTHITIS

Type	Description	Etiology	Course
Benign positional (most common type; accounts for 25% of all cases of dizziness)	Spinning sensation (lasting for less than 5 minutes) brought on *only* by sudden head movement, sometimes accompanied by nausea, vomiting, ataxia; often provoked by lying on the side or rolling over in bed. Nystagmus elicited by the Barany maneuver (changing the patient's position from sitting to lying, with the head resting at a 45-degree angle below the horizontal plane and turned to the side). Fifty percent of patients have depressed labyrinthine function in one ear. Hearing is uninvolved.	Sometimes follows head trauma or ear surgery; granulation masses have been demonstrated in the posterior semicircular canal. May occur in association with a wide variety of lesions of central or peripheral origin, including tumors, degenerative neurologic diseases, labyrinthine vascular insufficiency, and drug intoxications. Abnormalities of the neck, particularly those involving the cervical vertebrae (and arteries), may also cause this condition.	Disappears in several weeks. Sometimes recurrent over the course of years.
Acute (vestibular neuronitis)	Spontaneous bout of severe vertigo, accompanied by nausea, vomiting, diaphoresis, ataxia, and nystagmus. Symptoms intensified by rapid positional changes of the head and alleviated by lying quietly in a darkened room. No associated hearing loss or tinnitus. Most common in adolescents and young adults.	Thought to be neuronitis involving the vestibular portion of the eighth cranial nerve. May be viral or bacterial in origin, since in a high proportion of cases, onset of symptoms is associated with illness involving fever, particularly an upper respiratory infection.	Self-limited condition that may occur as a single episode or as a series of frequent attacks, becoming less frequent and less severe and disappearing after 18 months. Acute symptoms last for 48 hours to 14 days; a residual off-balance sensation may persist for months.
Purulent (suppurative)	Symptoms are severe vertigo and nystagmus, nausea, and vomiting, which are increased if the patient lies on the affected side. Possibly accompanied by signs of meningeal irritation, including nuchal rigidity, opisthotonus (dorsal arched position of the body in which the feet and head touch the floor or bed), and Kernig's sign (reflex contraction and pain in hamstring muscles when attempting to extend the leg after flexing the thigh upon the body). Followed by facial paralysis if associated with chronic otitis media and cholesteatoma. Invariably results in total hearing loss.	Secondary to acute bacterial infection of the middle ear, which may or may not involve the mastoid; labyrinthine involvement may be due to toxins, or to actual bacterial invasion via the emissary veins, or to bony necrosis and erosion into the semicircular canals.	Labyrinthectomy is necessary for drainage of the inner ear; treatment also involves radical mastoidectomy and massive antibiotic therapy. Actual purulent meningitis may occur from bacterial invasion of the meninges. Brain abscess may result from chronic mastoiditis.

TABLE 2.8 *(Continued)*

Type	Description	Etiology	Course
Toxic or allergic	Acute episode of vertigo with associated nausea and vomiting.	Direct toxic effect of certain drugs or allergic manifestation of the ingestion of foods. Drugs with known ototoxic potential include aminoglycoside antibiotics, salicylates, quinine and its synthetic substitutes, ethacrynic acid, and furosemide. Tobacco and alcohol commonly produce vertigo in sensitive individuals, as well as allergic food reactions (particularly to shellfish).	Permanence or potential reversibility of hearing or vestibular symptoms is dependent on the drug that is involved; oxotoxic effect of certain drugs increased by the presence of renal insufficiency.

antihistamines, barbiturates, or antianxiety medications. A number of procedures, including shunts, irradiation, and cryosurgery, may relieve the vertigo but invariably destroy hearing. These measures are advocated in cases in which attacks are frequent and disabling.

NOSE AND THROAT

Nasal Structure

Bone and cartilage form the anatomic chambers of the nose, as illustrated in Figure 2.5. These chambers are specially designed to filter, warm, and humidify air en route to the lungs. Air first enters the vestibule. Vibrissae, short stiff hairs, project from the skin and screen out insects and large dust particles. The follicles of these numerous hairs may be the site of a localized infection called ▶ ***folliculitis.*** Inflammation, tenderness, and recurrent crusting just inside the vestibule are the usual signs. The infection tends to spread from one follicle, particularly if the patient picks at crust formations. Treatment consists of topical ointments containing antibiotics and sometimes cortisone.

Facial skin joins the mucous membrane just inside the vestibule. At this junction, ***fissures*** often develop, and the crusts that form over broken skin prove painful when removed. Usually of little consequence, fissures may be treated with an antibiotic ointment or ammoniated mercury, or cauterized with silver nitrate.

When breakages in the skin are invaded by staphylococcal or streptococcal organisms, ▶ ***nasal furuncles*** (boils) develop. The area becomes extremely sensitive. Swelling and redness develop around the tip and sides of the nose, as well as on the upper lip. Fever may be present. The infection is potentially dangerous, since the venous supply of the nose drains into the brain's cavernous sinus. Aggressive treatment is indicated. Antibiotics should be started and hot wet packs used to bring the boil to an early head. No attempt at drainage should be made prior to fluctuation due to the danger of spreading the infection to the cavernous sinus.

The vestibule is also a site of ***squamous papilloma,*** small wartlike growths

TABLE 2.9 CAUSES OF DIZZINESS

Central nervous system	Cardiovascular
Subdural hematomas	Orthostatic hypotension
Tumors (particularly of the cerebellopontine angle)	Cardiac arrhythmias
Normal pressure hydrocephalis	Carotid sinus hypersensitivity
Cerebrovascular disease involving the basilar or vertebral arteries	Vasovagal response
Pathology of vestibular nuclei or their connections	Cough/micturition syncope
Parkinson's disease	Other
CNS degenerative disease (syphilis, multiple sclerosis, Cogan's syndrome, tuberculosis)	Hypoglycemia
Encephalitis	Severe anemia
Migraine	Hyperventilation
Seizure disorders	Hypoxia
Herpes zoster involving the eighth cranial nerve	Hypercapnia
Labyrinthine	Postcataract surgery
Benign positional (precipitated by sudden head movement)	Anxiety states
Acute or recurrent labyrinthitis following upper respiratory tract or other infection	Psychosis
Meniere's disease	Hypothyroidism
Toxic labyrinthitis following drug or alcohol ingestion	Dysproteinemia
Head trauma	Diabetes
Disorders of the cervical spine	Pregnancy
Otitis media	Menopause
Hypoactive or asymmetric labyrinthine function	

thought to be of viral origin. These growths are not premalignant, but they may be unsightly and annoying. A small incisional removal, rather than simple excision, by an ENT specialist prevents recurrence.

Cartilage divides the nose into two lateral halves (refer to Fig. 2.5). Obstruction to the normal passage of air may be caused by structural irregularity of this septum. ***Septal deviation*** often results from birth trauma. The infant's twisted nose ("greenstick" injury) usually rights itself after a few days, but deviation of the septum may persist. There is also a tendency for the septum to become deviated to one side or the other as part of normal aging. By adulthood it is uncommon to see a perfectly midline septum. For the most part, this causes no problem unless the passage of air through the nasal cavity is disrupted. Obstructive deviation may cause headache and sinusitis as a result of impingement on sinus openings. Resection (nasal septal reconstruction) is indicated when the airway is greatly reduced and is causing discomfort to the patient.

Septal deviation may also result from ***nasal fractures.*** Fractures follow several types of facial trauma, as described in Table 2.10. Common causes include blows from blunt objects (fists, bats, balls) or from direct impact (automobile or diving accidents, falls). In most cases, the diagnosis is obvious from swelling and bone displacement, and can be readily confirmed using x-ray films. By reducing the fracture, an ENT specialist can usually restore a satisfactory airway and the original appearance of the nose and face. However, it is essential to rule out brain or cervical damage prior to performing reduction procedures.

After injury to the nose, ***septal hematoma*** may develop. Blood collects between the septum and the perichondrium (a membrane covering the septum). Cut off from

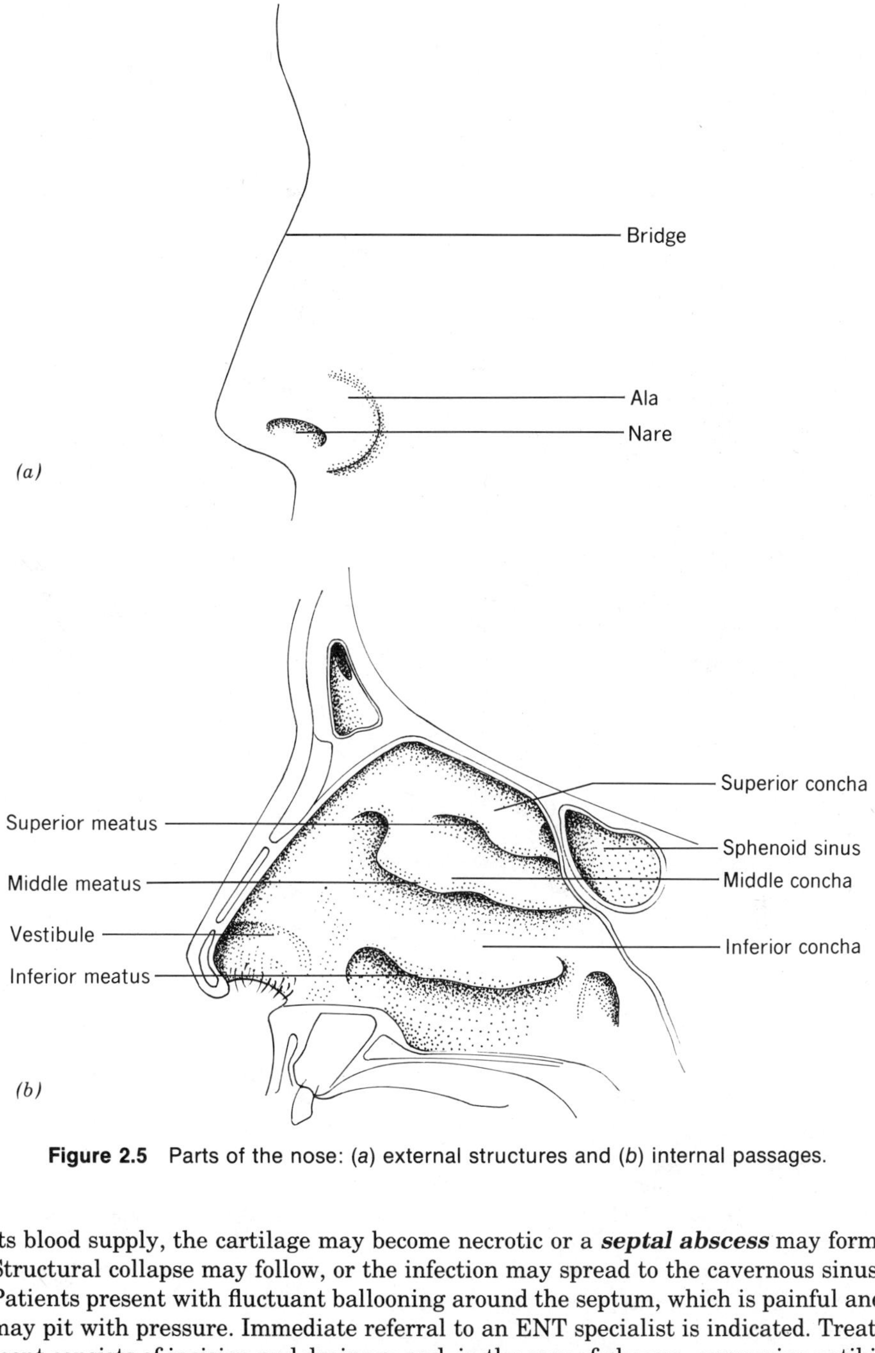

Figure 2.5 Parts of the nose: (*a*) external structures and (*b*) internal passages.

its blood supply, the cartilage may become necrotic or a ***septal abscess*** may form. Structural collapse may follow, or the infection may spread to the cavernous sinus. Patients present with fluctuant ballooning around the septum, which is painful and may pit with pressure. Immediate referral to an ENT specialist is indicated. Treatment consists of incision and drainage and, in the case of abscess, aggressive antibiotic therapy. During drainage procedures, care is taken to avoid a through-and-through incision of the septum (septal perforation).

Surgical complication is only one cause of ***septal perforation.*** Others include

TABLE 2.10 CAUSES AND DESCRIPTIONS OF COMMON FACIAL FRACTURES

Type of Fracture	Most Common Cause	Description
Maxillary	Severe direct trauma due to blow with fist, fall, auto accident	Flat face. Protrusion of mandibular teeth. Rocking maxilla.
Blowout	Blunt trauma to orbit	Double vision. Orbital fat and muscles may press through the fracture into the maxillary sinus; extraocular muscles may be incarcerated.
Zygomatic	Direct blows. Often accompanies maxillary fractures.	Zygomatic arch is depressed, losing normal convexity.
Mandibular	Direct or blunt trauma	Abnormal occlusion. Mobility and irregularity of dental arch; pain when jaw is clenched.
Nasal	Birth trauma Direct blow ("right cross")	Nasal bones may be smashed to one side or inward. Septum may be twisted.

chronic infections exacerbated by repeated trauma (e.g., nose picking), cocaine sniffing, syphilis, and tuberculosis. Symptoms are not always apparent, but recurrent nosebleeds, nasal crusting, and whistling on breathing may be clues. Nor is the perforation always obvious on exam, particularly since there is a tendency to mistake normal mucosa in the opposite cavity for continuation of cartilage. Although surgical closure is possible, management aims at controlling symptoms with the use of bland ointments to minimize crusting, packing or cautery to control bleeding, and patient education.

Deformities of nasal appearance or function can be corrected through ***rhinoplasty.*** Techniques and procedures vary and are subject to constant revision. The typical rhinoplasty operation is done under local anesthesia and involves several incisions and manipulations of the nasal cartilages and bones. Silicone implants may be employed. Patients seeking rhinoplasty should be referred to an ENT or plastic surgeon specialist.

Nasal Mucosa

The inferior, middle, and superior turbinates protrude from the lateral walls of the nasal cavity. Along with the septum, they provide surface area for the mucosal lining. Entering air ricochets off these structures, leaving particles trapped in the sticky secretions manufactured by the mucosa's goblet cells. Some of the particles are destroyed by leukocytes. The remainder are swept by cilia toward the pharynx, where they are either expectorated or swallowed. Swallowed debris is destroyed by the high acid content of gastric juices.

Ciliary and leukocyte activity of the nasal mucosa is so successful that the environment of the lower respiratory tract is kept practically sterile. However, the upper respiratory tract is quite susceptible to a variety of ***viral infections*** (see Table 2.11). Viruses have the pathogenic ability to damage ciliary action and inhibit leukocyte emigration, and thus facilitate bacterial invasion.

The most typical of the mild viral infections that attack the upper respiratory

TABLE 2.11 COMMON ORGANISMS IN UPPER RESPIRATORY INFECTIONS

Site	Organism
Nose	*Staphylococcus* *Streptococcus*
Paranasal sinuses	*S. pneumoniae* *Hemophilus influenzae* Group A streptococcus *Staph. aureus* Anaerobes
Nasopharynx	Enteroviruses Influenza viruses Adenoviruses Parainfluenza viruses Respiratory syncytial virus Rhinoviruses *H. influenzae* *Neisseria meningitidis* *Corynebacterium diphtheriae*
Pharynx	Group A streptococcus (also groups C and G) *Staph.* aureus *H. influenzae* *C. diphtheriae* Adenoviruses Infectious mononucleosis Enteroviruses Influenza and parainfluenza viruses Herpes simplex virus Other viruses: measles, rubella, rhinoviruses, cytomegalovirus, reoviruses, respiratory syncytial virus *M. pneumoniae* *Candida* species
Tonsils	Group A streptococcus (See also Pharynx)
Larynx	Group A streptococcus *C. diphtheriae* *H. influenzae* Infectious mononucleosis (See also Pharynx)
Epiglottis	*H. influenzae* Group A streptococcus

tract is the ▶ ***common cold.*** Large numbers of cold viruses have been isolated, the usual incubation period being 48 to 72 hours. Modes of transmission include inhalation of airborne droplets and direct contact with infectious secretions on skin and environmental surfaces. Close physical contact is probably necessary for efficient spread. Patients with a cold present with nasal stuffiness, discharge, sneezing, cough, and general malaise. They may also note a "scratchy" or mildly sore throat, watery eyes, and a feeling of pressure in the ears. Decreased appetite accompanies decreased ability to smell and taste. Low-grade fever may be present. On exam, redness and swelling of the nasal mucosa is obvious and the membranes may have a glossy appearance. A clear, thin nasal discharge becomes mucoid or purulent as the illness resolves and often leads to local skin irritation. Mild inflammation of the pharynx or serous otitis may also be noted. Most colds resolve spontaneously in 4–7 days, and only symptomatic treatment is necessary. Fluids, aspirin or Tylenol, decongestants, and rest can be advised. Although no cure has been discovered for cold viruses a preventative measure may soon be available. Trials have shown that use of interferon nasal spray by household members of a cold sufferer greatly reduced their chances of contracting illness. Unfortunately, the spray is only effective against rhinoviruses (responsible for 30–50% of colds) and seems to offer little if any protection against influenza or other respiratory viruses.

The therapeutic value of ▶ ***vitamin C intake*** for the treatment or prevention of colds remains unclear. Some studies indicate that large doses of vitamin C can stimulate defense mechanisms (increased interferon production, immunoglobulin production and T-lymphocyte activity). The recommended daily allowance of vitamin C is 600 mg. While doses in excess of 1 g/day fail to decrease the number of colds, they appear to lessen cold symptoms. Linus Pauling, in a widely followed and controversial book, *Vitamin C and the Common Cold,* recommends 1–5 g daily and up to 15 g/day with cold symptoms. However, such large doses of vitamin C are potentially toxic. They may cause increased absorption of lead and mercury from the gut, depressed leukocyte function, mobilization of calcium from bone and resultant formation of urinary tract calculi, and increased intestinal contractions that cause nausea, diarrhea, and abdominal cramps. Megadoses of vitamin C have been linked to abortion, stillbirth, and abnormal bleeding during pregnancy. They can interfere with drug action, particularly that of anticoagulants, and result in false interpretations of diabetic urine and stool hemoccult tests.

The nasal mucosa is highly vascularized and is thus sensitive to allergens and irritants. In cases of ▶ ***allergic rhinitis,*** nasal congestion develops in response to inhalation of an allergen that forms antigen–IgE complexes on receptors in the nasal mucosa (see Chapter 7). The condition has a familial tendency. It is referred to as "acute" and "seasonal" when the antigen is a pollen from trees, grasses, or flowers, or "chronic" and "perennial" when the allergens are dusts, molds, foods, or animal dander. Seasonal conditions are more common than perennial ones. Patients with allergic rhinitis have an itching sensation of the nose, throat, and eyes that is most severe in the morning. Persistent postnasal drainage and stuffiness typify the perennial form of the disorder, while sneezing, rhinorrhea, and stuffiness mark the seasonal form. Both contribute to the incidence of upper respiratory infections and sinusitis. The symptoms of perennial allergic rhinitis are usually less severe than those of the seasonal variety, but present more of a treatment challenge since the associated allergen may be difficult to isolate. Boggy, pale turbinates are most commonly noted on exam; however, not infrequently, they appear bluish or a dull red. An allergic facies (dark circles and edema beneath the eyes) is also evident. Microscopic exam of nasal secretions is useful for diagnostic confirmation. In allergic rhinitis, the number of eosinophils may run as high as 90% (normal secretions contain few if any). Allergy testing and recommendations for allergen removal or desensitization is the preferred treatment. When this is not possible, antihistamines, corticosteroid nasal sprays, and general measures to reduce the allergen load are helpful.

Nonallergic vasomotor rhinitis is characterized by symptoms similar to those seen in allergic rhinitis. Two variations are ***Sampter's syndrome*** (submucosal edema and polyp formation correlated with aspirin hypersensitivity, particularly in asthmatics) and ***rhinitis medicamentosa*** (rebound edema from habitual use of decongestant nasal drops or sprays). In addition, vasomotor rhinitis can be related to psychologic stress or endocrine disturbances, particularly hypothyroidism. Occasionally, it develops during pregnancy and resolves only after delivery. Although nasal secretions may contain high eosinophil counts, there is no IgE mediation or sensitivity to inhaled allergens. An ENT consultation is indicated to rule out nasal pathology. Otherwise, treatment depends on the underlying cause. Thyroid supplements are given for documented cases of hypothyroidism. Aspirin is avoided in cases of Sampter's syndrome, and nasal sprays are discontinued in rhinitis medicamentosa. Symptoms usually resolve within 2–3 weeks.

Patients with rhinitis (notably allergic rhinitis) are prone to develop ***nasal polyps.*** These soft, pale gray, nontender, mobile tumors are frequently the result of recurrent localized swelling of the sinus or nasal mucosa with submucosal edema.

Partial or complete nasal occlusion is the presenting symptom. If the condition has been present for a long period of time, changes in nasal bone and bridge structure may be seen; the nasal bone spreads and the bridge widens. When polyps arise from the paranasal sinuses, the sinuses show changes on x-ray films. Surgical removal is the required treatment; however, polyps tend to recur if the underlying allergy cannot be well controlled. In severe cases, more extensive procedures such as ethmoidectomy and sphenoidectomy may be indicated.

Other than polyps, ***tumors of the nasal cavity*** are unusual. Significant symptoms are unilateral nasal obstruction and a blood-tinged discharge. The most common malignant lesions are squamous cell carcinoma, adenocarcinoma, and melanoma. Referral for biopsy and removal is in order.

The nasal mucosa plays an important role in air humidification as well as filtration. It is covered by a mucous and serum blanket that transfers varying amounts of water to inspired air as needed. The moisturized air is warmed by the mucosa's dense network of blood vessels. If any aspects of this process are disrupted, ▶***nosebleed*** (epistaxis) may occur. Aging is a contributing factor in nosebleeds, since atrophy of the mucosa and sclerotic changes in vessels commonly occur after the age of 50. Excessively dry environments cause crusting of the mucosal blanket. Picking of the crusts may open small blood vessels. Mucosal damage with bleeding also results from trauma, cocaine use, and exposure to chemicals. Respiratory infections, rheumatic fever, hypertension, leukemia, disturbances in blood-clotting mechanisms (particularly from aspirin overuse) may also be the underlying cause of epistaxis. The most frequent site of bleeding is the anterior aspect of the nasal septum (Kiesselbach's venous plexus), in which a moderate amount of blood drains from the front of the nose when the patient is in the upright position. If there is posterior involvement, bleeding is more rigorous since the source is more likely arterial. Arterial bleeds usually occur as the result of trauma or sclerotic vessel rupture. Most nosebleeds are self-limited. However, profuse, uncontrolled bleeding can be life-threatening. Proper management depends on identifying the cause and location of the bleeding. The patient should remain in an upright position, applying firm, continuous pressure against the side of the nose for 10–15 minutes. Ice and/or epinephrine can act as vasoconstrictors. If bleeding does not stop readily, patients should be referred to an ENT specialist for cauterization or packing. Persons prone to repeated nosebleeds should apply petroleum jelly or mineral oil to maintain mucosal moisture and relieve crusting. They should also be warned against picking the nasal mucosa or forceful nose blowing.

Olfactory Cells

The olfactory sense organ is limited to a small, irregular area in the upper part of the nasal cavity (Fig. 2.6). Hair-like projections of neurons respond to odoriferous substances that have entered the nostrils and dissolved in the mucosa. Impulses are sent upward through the cribriform plate of the ethmoid bone to a second set of neurons residing in the olfactory bulb. Perception of the smell results as the impulses continue through the olfactory nerve in the cortex of the temporal lobe. Olfactory receptors are sensitive to seven primary odors: camphor, musk, floral, peppermint, ether-like, pungent, and putrid. Two or more primary odors combine to form other fragrances. Although olfactory cells are stimulated by even very slight odors, they

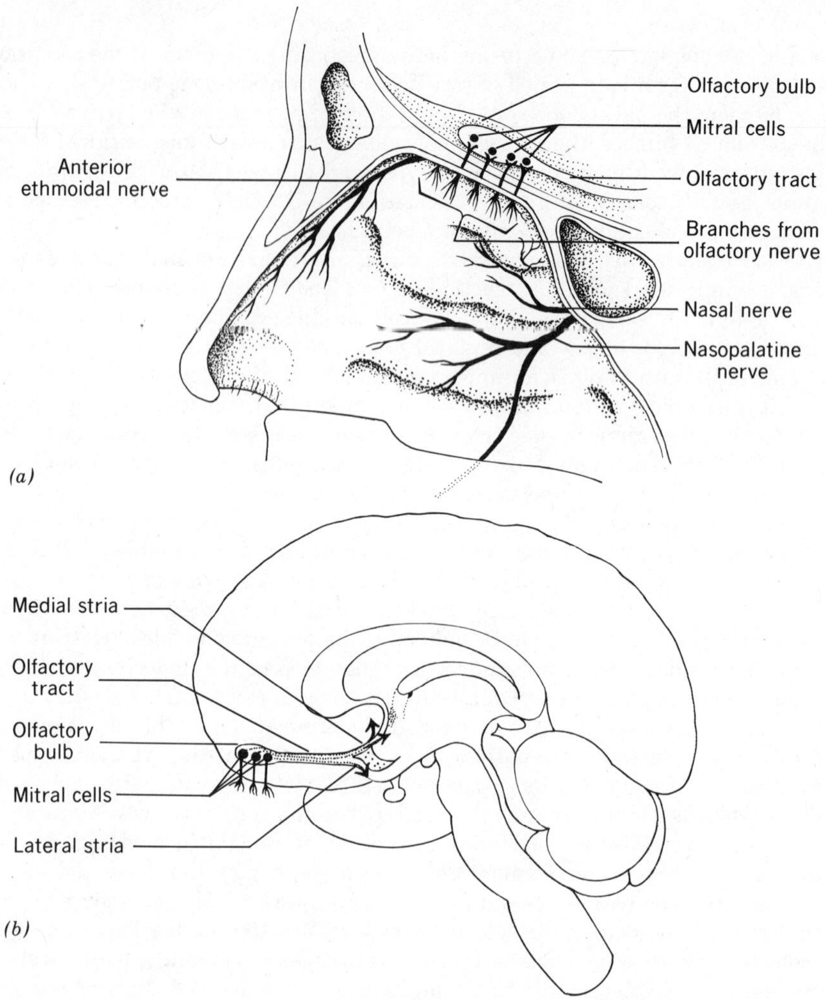

Figure 2.6 Olfactory structures: (*a*) CNS pathways and (*b*) local sense organs.

are also easily fatigued. Thus, odors that are very noticeable at first are not sensed at all after a short time.

Disturbances of smell (anosmia) may indicate the existence of underlying disease, as outlined in Table 2.12. They frequently develop in the aftermath of nasal surgery, particularly correction of a deviated septum. From 5 to 10% of all cases of head trauma lead to some impairment. Aging and numerous drugs have been implicated, and familial syndromes have been described. Clinicians may detect a disturbance of smell by testing sensitivity to the primary odors. No specific treatment for anosmia is available unless the underlying cause can be corrected. Zinc sulfate therapy is now under investigation, since low serum zinc levels have been found in various disorders associated with anosmia. However, anosmia is often irreversible.

Olfactory receptors also play an essential role in taste distinction. They enhance stimulation of the specialized taste receptors (taste buds) concentrated in the surface

TABLE 2.12 FACTORS ASSOCIATED WITH DISTURBANCE OF SMELL

ENT pathology	Drugs
Rhinitis (acute and chronic)	Vasoconstrictive nose drops
Sinusitis	Antithyroid agents
Polyps	Antibiotics (tetracycline, streptomycin)
Tumors	Morphine
Sarcoidosis	
Radiation therapy	Metabolic disorders
	Turner's syndrome
Neurologic	Hypothyroidism
Head trauma	Pseudohypoparathyroidism
Tumors (bilateral gliomas or meningiomas)	Hypo- and hypergonadotropic hypogonadism
Meningitis	Diabetes mellitus
Brain abscess	Viral hepatitis
Parkinson's disease and levodopa therapy	Renal failure
Multiple sclerosis	
Korsakoff's syndrome	
Hydrocephalus	
Minor strokes	
Aneurysm of the internal carotid artery or circle of Willis	

of the tongue. Disorders of taste (hypogeusia and dysgeusia) are considered in the next chapter.

Paranasal Sinuses

Four groups of paranasal sinuses are found in the maxillary, ethmoid, sphenoid, and frontal bones of the skull and are named accordingly (Fig. 2.7a). These sinuses lighten the bones of the skull, contribute mucus to the nasal cavity, and act as resonating chambers for production of sound. They are connected with the nasal cavities to allow ventilation and drainage.

Under normal conditions, cilia remove mucous secretions from the sinuses to help maintain their sterility. As noted in Figure 2.7b, these secretions continually drain through the sinus openings (ostia). When this cleaning mechanism fails to prevent bacteria from gaining access, ▶***acute sinusitis*** results. Failure is usually due to inflammation of the mucous membrane and/or blocked drainage. This may be triggered by an upper respiratory infection or a chronic condition of the nose (polyps, rhinitis, deviated septum). Once the mucosa becomes infected, there may be rapid accumulation of purulent fluid in the sinus cavity. The most common pathogens involved are streptococci, staphylococci, and pneumococci. Acute sinusitis begins with a feeling of stuffiness and pressure over the involved sinus that becomes more defined within 48–72 hours. The alteration of pressure leads to ***sinus headache.*** These headaches tend to be worse in the morning and subside after the patient is up and about. They are intensified by bending over, jostling, straining, coughing, or any factor contributing to mucosal engorgement (cold air, sexual excitement, pregnancy, menstruation, alcohol ingestion). Rather than headache, some patients with acute sinusitis experience severe facial pain and tenderness. The location of the pain may not correspond to the sinuses that are involved. Patients with maxillary sinusitis may experience a dull ache in the cheek or upper teeth. Ethmoid and sphenoid pain may be referred to the occipital region, while frontal sinus infection causes pain in

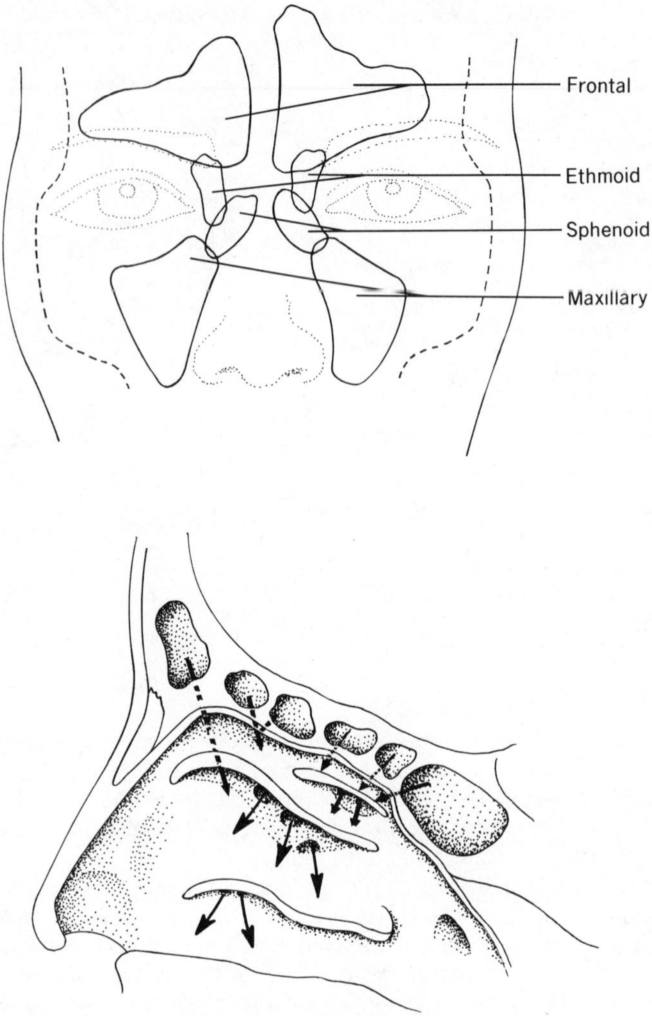

(a)

Openings of sinuses for drainage

(b)

Figure 2.7 Paranasal sinuses: (*a*) frontal, ethmoid, sphenoid, and maxillary cavities; (*b*) drainage openings.

the forehead above the eyebrow. The nasal discharge may be blood-tinged in the first 24–48 hours but rapidly becomes purulent and copious. Postnasal drip causes irritation and inflammation of the throat. Fever and elevated white blood cell counts are not characteristic. If present, they may indicate a concomitant infection. Disruption of smell can also occur. Physical exam finds the nasal mucosa red and swollen and the turbinates enlarged. Pus that has drained through the ostia is present in the nasal cavity unless the ostia is completely blocked. There may be tenderness to percussion of an affected sinus. Transillumination of the maxillary and frontal sinuses may be reduced (due to their position, the sphenoid and ethmoid sinuses cannot be tested for light transmission). Radiologic exam can confirm the diagnosis; however, an absence of pathology on x-ray films does not rule out an infection. Treatment of acute sinusitis aims at relieving pain, shrinking the nasal mucosa, and controlling the infection. Hot wet packs applied continuously or at 2-hour intervals relieve symptoms and facilitate inflammation reduction. Limited use of nose drops or sprays is also useful. Analgesics are prescribed for pain and antibiotics to eliminate infection. In cases where pain is excessive or pus fails to drain, patients should be referred for surgical intervention. If the nasal discharge persists after the resolution of acute symptoms, ENT referral is indicated. Failure to resolve the infection may lead to more severe complications such as meningitis, epidural abscess, or abscess of the frontal lobe.

Repeated bacterial invasion and chronic inflammation of the sinus mucosa cause the irreversible tissue changes characteristic of ***chronic sinusitis.*** A purulent nasal discharge is the constant and often the only symptom. Recurrent headache or persistent pain is uncommon and may indicate impending complications or a malignancy. Although a small percentage of patients respond to antibiotics, antihistamines, or repeated irrigation, the primary treatment is surgery.

The maxillary sinus is the most common site of ***sinus tumors.*** Early symptoms may include a unilateral, foul-smelling, purulent discharge or bleeding. Advanced growth is marked by nasal obstruction, pain, hyperesthesia over the cheek and upper lip, displacement of the eye upward, tearing, unilateral stuffiness of the ear, and serous otitis media. Ethmoidal neoplasms may present with unilateral nasal obstruction, discharge, and bleeding. Later symptoms are orbital pain and frontal headaches. Sphenoid tumors are characterized by discharge and bleeding, as well as bizarre headaches, ocular palsies, and proptosis. Signs and symptoms of panhypopituitarism may also be present. Metastatic tumors of all of the sinuses are most commonly identified by severe epistaxis and local swelling. Any suspected growth should be referred for biopsy and removal, since most neoplasms of this area are malignant.

Pharynx

The pharynx extends from the base of the skull to the esophagus and is divided into three parts: the nasopharynx, the oropharynx, and the laryngopharynx, as illustrated in Figure 2.8. The latter two serve both the respiratory and digestive systems. Their specialized musculature maintains the structure of the passageway and permits swallowing. The mucosal membrane extends from the nasal and sinus cavities to line the pharynx. As respiratory tissue, it contains ciliated goblet cells. These cells produce a mucous blanket that continuously traps and moves foreign particles toward the back of the throat, where they can be swallowed or expectorated.

Four concentrations of lymph tissue (Waldeyer's ring) surround and protect the entrance of the lower air and food passages, as shown in Figure 2.8. The adenoids lie in the nasopharynx and are present in all infants and children. They regress just before puberty and are usually absent in adults. In children, obstruction of the nasal passages and eustachian tubes are the result of ***chronic adenoid infection*** and inflammation. When adenoid hypertrophy is present without chronic infection of the tonsils, adenoidectomy is often recommended. The tonsils also undergo atrophy during aging.

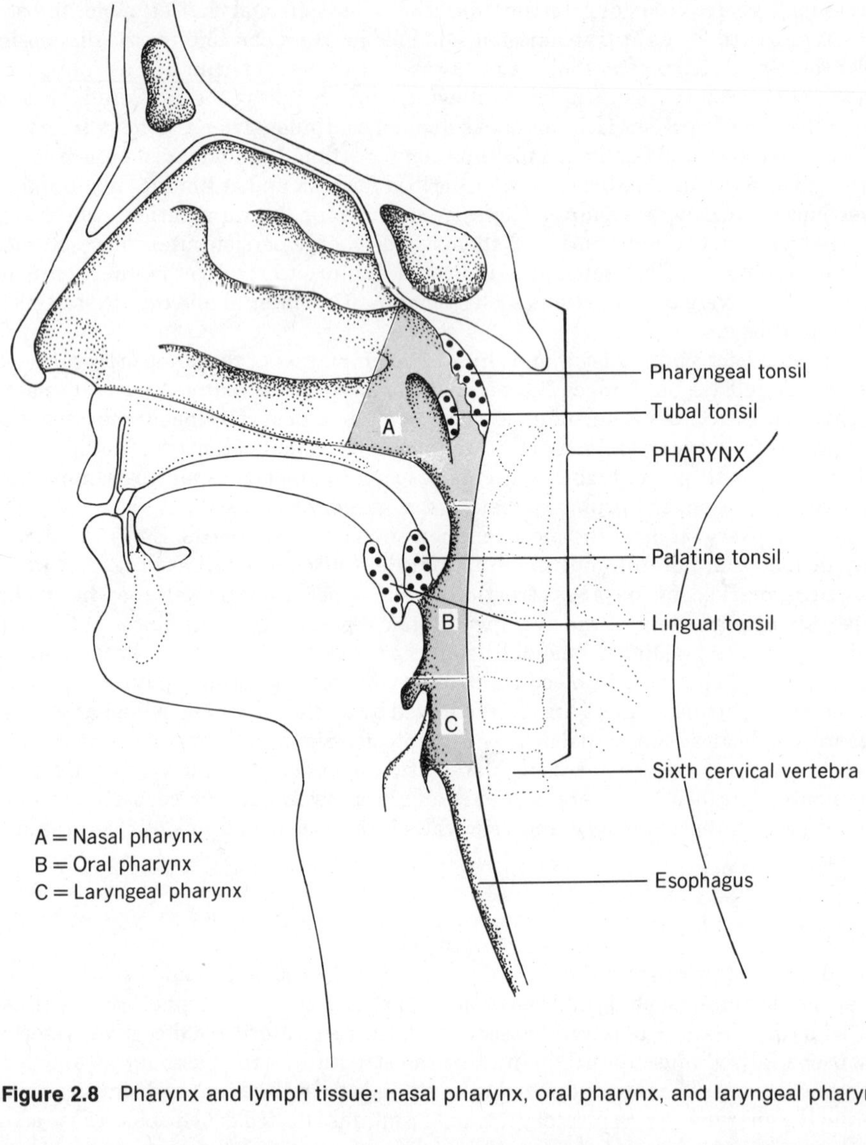

Figure 2.8 Pharynx and lymph tissue: nasal pharynx, oral pharynx, and laryngeal pharynx.

The nasopharyngeal mucosa and lymph tissue can be affected by a number of infectious organisms. ***Acute viral pharyngitis/tonsillitis*** produces a burning pain or scratchiness of the throat and/or nasal symptoms often associated with conjunctivitis and cough. Viewed with a postnasal mirror, the nasopharynx may show petechial hemorrhages, a white exudate, and swelling. Fever may be present along with pharyngeal erythema, cervical adenopathy, and tonsillar enlargement. A throat culture should be taken to rule out bacterial infection (specifically streptococcus). The practice of obtaining overnight throat cultures on all sore throats was questioned in the past. Newer antibody tests may prove more practical; in addition to being more accurate, the results are readily available. If the test is negative, the patient is treated with rest, warm saline gargles, decongestants, and analgesics. Symptoms typically resolve in 10 days. Antibiotics may be started before culture results are available in patients with very severe symptoms or prolonged illness.

► ***Acute Streptococcal pharyngitis/tonsillitis*** is more serious than a viral infection since group A streptococcus may be complicated by an immunologic reaction responsible for rheumatic fever or glomerulonephritis (see Chapters 6 and 8). Most prevalent in the winter months (November to May), streptococcal infections account for 10–15% of sore throats in adults. Sometimes they are mild and mimic viral pharyngitis. Usually, however, patients have sudden onset of chills and temperature elevation that may reach over 101°F (38.3°C). They complain of pain in the throat on swallowing, headache, and generalized malaise. Unlike viral infections, coughing is not present. Pharyngeal erythema, edema of the uvula, and tender cervical adenopathy may be noted on exam. If the pallatine tonsils are infected, the tissue is readily noted to be swollen, red, and often covered with exudate. Infection limited to the lingual tonsils is more difficult to diagnose due to the location of these tonsils at the extreme back of the tongue (see Fig. 2.8). In such cases, the patient's history is the key. Patients complain of low throat pain, a feeling of a lump in the throat, and difficulty in swallowing. Leukocytosis frequently exists. Throat cultures or streptococcus antibody testing is necessary to distinguish the cause of the infection. When the test is positive, antibiotics are required. Bed rest, gargling, and analgesics help relieve symptoms. Treatment of affected household members is important in cases of streptococcal infection.

Acute streptococcal tonsillitis may lead to ***peritonsillar infection.*** The symptoms of tonsillitis seemingly improve prior to an increase in one-sided throat pain and swallowing difficulty. Drooling, a muffled voice ("hot potato voice"), and referred pain in the ear are present. Examination finds tonsil displacement and swelling of the soft palate and anterior pillar. Antibiotic therapy may be sufficient to resolve the infection. Hot saline irrigations are helpful to relieve symptoms. Incision and drainage can become necessary if ***peritonsillar abscess*** develops and does not drain on its own. Since peritonsillar abscess is recurrent, tonsillectomy is frequently recommended following subsidence of the infection.

Frequent infections of tonsils is called ***chronic tonsillitis.*** In addition to antibiotics for acute symptoms, patients should be referred to an ENT specialist. Tonsillectomy may be advised if there is hypertrophy of the tonsils and adenoids to the point of obstruction. It is also indicated for diphtheria carriers, recurrent purulent otitis media with hearing loss, or a definite relationship between tonsillitis and exacerbation of other conditions such as arthritis, iritis, rheumatic fever, or asthma.

Caused by the Epstein-Barr virus (EBV), ***infectious mononucleosis*** can markedly affect lymph tissue in the pharynx. Not only do patients experience painful inflammation of the tonsils, but as many as 15–30% develop secondary streptococcal infections. A systemic disease marked by diffuse hyperplasia of lymphatic tissue throughout the body and increased production of lymphocytes, infectious mononucleosis is discussed in Chapter 7.

► ***Gonococcal pharyngitis*** must be considered in patients who engage in oral-genital sexual activity. The patient may be asymptomatic or have a sore throat. A pharyngeal exudate and lymphadenopathy are observed by the practitioner. The diagnosis is confirmed by a pharyngeal Gram stain and culture. Antibiotic treatment is necessary.

The gram-positive organism *Corynebacterium diphtheriae* is the cause of ***diphtheria.*** Transmitted by secretions of infected humans, diphtheria is most prevalent in winter months and in crowded living conditions. It is characterized by a gray or white ulcerative membrane that forms over the mucosal tissue of the pharynx. The onset is gradual, occurring over 1–2 days, and is accompanied by a low-grade fever, throat soreness, and a weak but rapid pulse. Patients are severely ill and require hospitalization. Once the diagnosis is confirmed by cultures taken from beneath the membrane, antitoxins and penicillin can be initiated. Aggressive treatment continues for 14 days, and eradication should be documented by three consecutive negative cultures. If the advancing membrane extends into the trachea, it may obstruct airflow, necessitating tracheotomy.

Although outbreaks of diphtheria still occur in fully or partially vaccinated populations, primary diphtheria immunization has greatly reduced the occurrence of the disease. Three shots are given in combination with tetanus and pertussis vaccines (DPT) before the age of 6. After age 6, vaccine containing increased tetanus but reduced diphtheria toxoids (Td) must be used. It contains no pertussis toxoid due to its association with CNS complications in older age groups. ▶ ***Primary diphtheria immunization for adults*** involves three shots of Td given over the course of a year. In addition, boosters are recommended every 10 years.

Pharyngitis medicamentosa results from prolonged use of irritating solutions and medications. Inflammation or even ulceration can be attributed to over-the-counter gargles (medicinal or breath-cleansing), antibiotic lozenges, or ammoniated tooth powders. Long-term use of saline solutions has also been implicated. Recognition and withdrawal of the irritant is curative.

Larynx

The larynx (voice box) connects the pharynx with the trachea and is divided into three portions (see Fig. 2.9). Sound is produced as air passes against its bands of elastic cartilage. The larynx also participates in coughing, swallowing, expectorating, breathing, and protecting the lower regions of the respiratory tract from foreign objects.

▶ ***Acute laryngitis*** is an inflammation of the larynx that is usually associated with generalized upper respiratory tract infection, the common cold, and influenza. However, isolated inflammation and infection of the vocal cords can occur. Acute laryngitis may be precipitated by voice abuse and occasionally by foreign bodies, excessive smoking, and inhalation of irritant gases. Hoarseness and/or aphonia is the chief symptom. Fever, a nonproductive cough, throat scratchiness, and pain aggravated by talking are common. The disease has a rapid onset. Vocal cords viewed with a laryngeal mirror are red rather than white and have rounded rather than sharp edges. An obstructive membrane may indicate streptococcal infection, laryngeal diphtheria, aspiration of a caustic substance, or trauma from hot gases. No specific treatment is required in most cases of acute laryngitis. Symptoms subside with the resolution of associated disorders. Antibiotics, steam or aerosol therapy, and voice rest are indicated for fever, persistent cough, and/or air obstruction. Relief of pain is facilitated by the use of throat lozenges.

Smoking, constant use (or misuse) of the voice, and related chronic respiratory conditions are causes of ***chronic laryngitis.*** Hoarseness, persistent, nonproductive cough, and throat tiredness or achiness are common symptoms. Voice use is greatly limited. Both the true and false vocal cords are red and thickened or edematous and

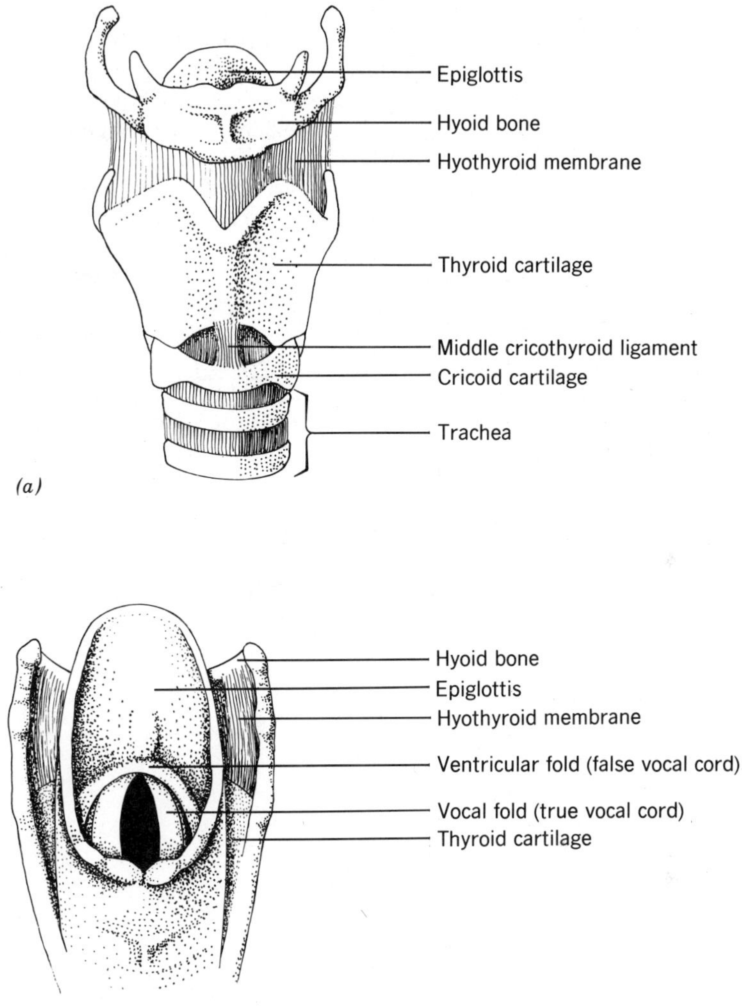

(b)

Figure 2.9 Larynx: (*a*) anterior view and (*b*) posterior-superior view.

polypoid. Tissue changes may be irreversible. Removal of the cause is the best treatment. Symptoms, however, are alleviated by inhalation of unmedicated steam and voice rest. Referral is indicated to rule out malignancy if symptoms persist, if vocal cord paralysis occurs, or if visible laryngeal disease is noted on physical exam.

Persistent hoarseness is an early symptom of ***intrinsic carcinoma of the true vocal cords.*** Pain is not a usual symptom, but difficulty in breathing may occur in later stages. Patients with intrinsic malignancies have an excellent prognosis if treatment is begun early. Metastasis occurs at a much later stage than with other laryngeal malignancies since lymphathics are scarce in the area of the true vocal cords.

The earliest symptom of ***extrinsic carcinoma of the larynx*** is frequently pain from ulceration. Hoarseness occurs later in the disease process, as does dysphagia, breathing difficulty, weight loss, foul breath, and general debility. A muffled hot potato voice may be present. Due to the large number of lymph vessels in the larynx, metastasis is common. Patients should be referred to an ENT specialist for evaluation. Using a laryngeal mirror, true vocal cord lesions can be seen on one or both of the cords. Extrinsic malignancy greatly distorts the normal appearance of the larynx. Bleeding is often common, though not profuse. The diagnosis is confirmed with laryngoscopy and biopsy. Surgery and radiation are necessary treatment interventions.

The epiglottis, a small flap of skin that prevents foreign objects from entering the trachea, may become involved in any bacterial infection (primarily *Hemophilus influenzae*) of the throat. Occurring almost exclusively in children aged 1 to 6 years but occasionally seen in adults, ***acute epiglottitis*** produces abrupt-onset severe sore throat, drooling, croupy cough, and difficulty in breathing. Patients typically have temperature elevations of 101 to 105°F and significantly elevated white blood cell counts (18,000–24,000). Due to the high potential for respiratory obstruction, the problem is a medical emergency requiring immediate hospitalization and ENT consultation. The swollen epiglottis may be seen on a lateral x-ray film of the neck or with direct laryngoscopy. The latter procedure should be done only by the specialist in a setting well equipped for emergency tracheotomy. Treatment consists of airway maintenance and aggressive antibiotic therapy (ampicillin and/or chloramphenicol).

Details of Management

▸ *Ear Furuncles*

Laboratory Tests: None.

Therapeutic Measures: Insert a cotton wick into the affected canal. Have the patient wet the wick, using an eye dropper filled with half-strength Burrows solution every few hours, and apply heat to the outer ear for 10 minutes four times a day. When the boil is fluctuant (usually in 24–48 hours with soaks), lift the head with a sterile tuberculosis syringe to drain. Continue soaks for another 24 hours. Advise the use of aminosalicylic acid (ASA) or Tylenol, 2 tablets every four hours, for pain. If cellulitis develops, prescribe an antistaphylococcal penicillin such as dicloxacillin 250 mg qid or a cephalosporin such as Keflex 250 mg qid for 5–10 days. As a less expensive alternative, erythromycin 250 mg qid for 5–10 days may also be used.

Patient Education: Demonstrate application for ear wick soaks. Instruct patient to report fever, chills, or extension of infection. Review antibiotic use. Advise the following prophylactic measures: (1) keep ear canals reasonably clean, using a wet wash cloth over the fingertip (never use Q-tips or bobby pins); (2) protect canals with ear plugs during swimming.

Follow-up: As needed.

▸ *Impacted Cerumen*

Laboratory Tests: None.

Therapeutic Measures: Irrigate ears using a rubber bulb syringe or Water Pik (on a low setting) with tepid solution of one-half tap water and one-half hydrogen peroxide (irrigation is contraindicated in patients who have perforated eardrums or a history of recurrent otitis media). Soften dry, hard wax by filling the ear canal with Ceruminex drops 15 minutes before irrigation. As an alternative to irrigation, prescribe Debrox otic solution, 3 drops in the affected ear, nightly for 7 days.

Patient Education: Explain that production of ear wax is normal, and attempts should never be made to remove it with Q-tips or other instruments (this practice actually pushes wax into the canal or may cause perforation of the eardrum). Ear canals are properly cleaned with a damp wash cloth wrapped around a fingertip. Debrox ear solution, 3 drops in each ear at night for several days on an intermittent basis, can be prescribed for prophylactic use.

Follow-up: As needed.

▸ *Otitis Externa*

Laboratory Tests: None.

Therapeutic Measures: Gently remove debris from the ear canal, using suction or a cotton stylet. Prescribe cortisporin otic solution, 4 drops three times daily for the affected ear. An hour before using the drops, have the patient debride the canal by filling it with hydrogen peroxide warmed to room temperature and removing residual fluids with a cotton wick. Suggest ASA or Tylenol, 2 tablets every 4 hours, for pain and itching. Treat concurrent dandruff infections of the scalp or eyebrows with a dandruff control shampoo. Advise prophylactic use of a one-third white vinegar, two-thirds rubbing alcohol solution, 4 drops, after swimming (dries the canal and alters the pH). Ointments should not be used.

Patient Education: Point out the site of infection on a diagram of the ear. Discuss predisposing factors such as trapped moisture in the canal, allergic responses to hair dyes and sprays, and seborrhea. Demonstrate debridement and instillation of ear drops.

Follow-up: As needed.

▸ *Traumatic Perforations*

Laboratory Tests: None.

Therapeutic Measures: Large, unclean tears of the eardrum should be referred to an ENT specialist. For small, uncomplicated perforations, instruct the patient to protect the canal from moisture; a shower cap or ear plugs should be used for showering and hair washing; swimming should be avoided. Prescribe penicillin, 250 mg, or erythromycin, 250 mg qid, for 5 days to prevent middle ear infection. ASA or Tylenol can be used for pain. Ear drops should not be used.

Patient Education: Reassure the patient that small perforations usually heal spontaneously within days and that hearing is not permanently impaired. Emphasize the importance of preventing middle ear infections by taking oral antibiotics and keeping the ear canal dry.

Follow-up: Weekly visits are needed until the perforation has closed. If spontaneous healing does not take place within 3 weeks, refer the patient to an ENT specialist.

▸ *Bullous Myringitis*

Laboratory Tests: None.

Therapeutic Measures: Since there is no way to distinguish a viral from a bacterial process, prescribe erythromycin, 250 mg plus sulfonamide (e.g., Gantrisin) 500 mg qid or amoxicillin 250 mg tid for 10 days. Apply heat, using compresses or a hot water bottle, for 15 minutes several times a day. Prescribe anesthetic ear drops such as Auralganotic solution, enough to fill canal every 1 to 2 hrs until pain relieved.

Patient Education: Point out the eardrum on a diagram of the ear as the site of infection. Review medication use.

Follow-up: Reevaluate the patient in 24–48 hours and refer him or her to ENT specialist for I&D of blebs if there is no improvement.

▸ *Eustachian Tube Dysfunction and Serous Otitis Media*

Laboratory Tests: None.

Therapeutic Measures: Prescribe a decongestant or a combination decongestant/antihistamine for 3 weeks as follows: Sudafed 60 mg tid, Dimetapp Extentabs bid, or Actifed tid. Prescribe Otrivin 0.1% nasal spray bid for 3 days. In cases of allergic rhinitis, also give Beconase or Vanceril inhaler, 1 spray tid for 14 days. Have the patient chew gum.

Patient Education: Point out the relationship of the eustachian tube to ear symptoms. Instruct patients to use Otrivin nasal spray as follows: (1) spray the right nostril; (2) tip the head toward the right and back for 30 seconds; (3) spray the left nostril; (4) tip the head toward the left and back for 30 seconds; (5) wait 5 minutes and repeat the entire process. Warn against overuse of nasal sprays.

Follow-up: Evaluate the patient in 3 weeks. If the condition has not resolved, continue the therapy along with a second course of Otrivin for 2 more weeks. Then refer the patient to an ENT specialist.

▸ *Acute Otitis Media*

Laboratory Tests: Have a throat culture taken to rule out concurrent pharyngeal infection (the identity of the otitis pathogen cannot be assumed from results of throat culture).

Therapeutic Measures

For infection: Start amoxicillin 250 mg tid, erythromycin 250 mg plus sulfonamide (e.g., Gantrisin) 500 mg qid, or cefaclor (Ceclor) 250 mg tid for 10 days.

Local heat in the form of a hot water bottle or heating pad applied to the outer ear for 10 minutes several times a day may hasten resolution.

To improve eustachian tube function: Prescribe a decongestant or a combination of decongestant/antihistamine for 3 weeks as follows: Sudafed 60 mg tid, Dimetapp Extentabs bid, or Actifed tid. Prescribe Otrivin 0.1% nasal spray bid for 3 days. Have the patient chew gum.

For pain: Prescribe Auralgan otic drops, enough to fill the ear canal, every 1–2 hours until the pain is relieved (contraindicated in cases of perforated tympanic membrane). Depending on the degree of discomfort, ASA, Tylenol, or Tylenol with codeine every 4 hours may also be needed.

Patient Education: Point out the middle ear canal as the area of infection and the part played by the eustachian tube in the development and resolution of infection. Emphasize the importance of antibiotics. Instruct patients to use Otrivin nasal spray as follows: (1) spray the right nostril; (2) tip the head toward the right and back for 30 seconds; (3) spray the left nostril; (4) tip the head toward the left and back for 30 seconds; (5) wait 5 minutes and repeat the entire process. Warn against overuse of nasal sprays.

Follow-up: Evaluate the patient in 3 days. If the condition has not improved, refer the patient to an ENT specialist. Myringotomy should be promptly performed in cases marked by continued pain, fever, bulging ear drum, increasing hearing loss, or vertigo.

▸ *Proper Use and Care of Hearing Aids*

Laboratory Tests: None.

Therapeutic Measures: Cerumen removal as needed.

Patient Education: Assess the patient's knowledge about the parts, use, and maintenance of the prescribed type of hearing aid. For general measures of care, offer the following advice:

1. Handle and store the hearing aid carefully.
2. Turn off the instrument when it is not in use.
3. Wash ear molds with soap and water daily (reinsert only when dry).
4. Clean the cannula with a small pipe cleaner periodically.
5. Open the battery compartment at night to avoid accidental power drainage.

For malfunction, offer the following advice:

1. Check the on/off switch.
2. Make sure that the ear mold and cannula are clean.

3. Check battery power and insertion (dead or improperly placed batteries are the most common reasons for malfunction).
4. Keep extra batteries on hand at all times (usual life, 2 days to 2 weeks).
5. Check the cord for breaks and improper insertion (keep an extra cord on hand).
6. If whistling is the problem, check ear mold insertion.
7. Have handy the name, address, and phone number of a local service center and do not hesitate to call if any problems occur.

Follow-up: As needed.

▸ *Courtesies and Commonsense Measures for People with Hearing Loss*

Laboratory Tests: None.

Therapeutic Measures: Avoid startling patients by approaching them from behind. Allow time for patients to adjust hearing aids. Whenever possible, minimize background noise (e.g., close the door). Face the patient and make sure that the lighting is adequate. Speak slowly and distinctly. Do not shout or lower your voice at the end of sentences. Avoid eating, smoking, or gum chewing while talking, as these movements interfere with lip reading. Open the conversation by stating the main topic to be discussed (e.g., "Back. Tell me how you hurt your back"). To help convey messages, use facial expressions, hand gestures, pointing, or restatements. Pronounce new or unfamiliar words carefully and then write them down (always keep paper and pen or a slate board readily available). In some cases, it may help to speak to the patient through a stethoscope or rolled-up magazine. Patients should be politely informed if they are speaking too loudly. Encourage those who have associated speech disorders to use their verbal communication skills. However, if the listener is unable to understand a message, he or she should ask for clarification in writing. Share the above suggestions with friends and family members.

Patient Education: Suggest to patients with hearing impairment that they:

1. Have an audiology evaluation if they have not already done so.
2. Position themselves in a corner or near a wall for better sound reflection.
3. Sit or stand with the better ear toward speakers.
4. Arrange good lighting.
5. Have a spouse or friend keep them informed of any changes in conversation topics.
6. Arrange buzzers and amplifiers for telephones and plug-in earphones for televisions and radios.

Follow-up: As needed.

▸ *Organizations for the Deaf*

Laboratory Tests: None.

Therapeutic Measures: None.

Patient Education

National Association of the Deaf (NAD)
814 Thayer Ave.
Silver Springs, MD 20910 Phone: (301) 587-1788
Serves as a clearinghouse for information on deafness.

Better Hearing Institute
1430 K St. N.W., Suite 600
Washington, DC 20005 Phone: (202) 638-2848
Consumer-oriented "Hearing Helpline."

Self Help for Hard-of-Hearing People
P.O. Box 34889
Bethesda, MD 20033 Phone: (301) 365-3548
Educating members and the public about hearing problems.

National Association for Hearing and Speech Action
10801 Rockville Pike
Rockville, MD 20852 Phone: (301) 897-8682
Concentrates on prevention, preservation, and rehabilitation of hearing problems.

National Captioning Institute
5203 Leesburg Pike, Suite 1500
Falls Church, VA 22041 Phone: (703) 998-2400
Provides captioning for public events and television.

National Hearing Aid Society
20361 Middlebelt Rd.
Livonia, MI 48152 Phone: (313) 478-2610
Specialists test for hearing aid selection and instruct on the care and use of devices.

Follow-up: None.

▸ *Labyrinthitis and Motion Sickness*

Laboratory Tests: None.

Therapeutic Measures

Positional labyrinthitis: Teach the patient to avoid provocative positions.

Acute or recurrent labyrinthitis: Prescribe Antivert, 12.5 or 25 mg qid.

Motion sickness: Advise Dramamine, 50 mg, one-half before travel or a Transderm-Scóp (formerly Transderm-V) patch containing 1.5 mg scopolamine behind one ear several hours before the effect is needed. The patch provides 3 days of continuous therapy before replacement is necessary (contraindicated for patients with glaucoma; use with caution in the elderly, in cases of gastric/intestinal/bladder obstruction, in the presence of metabolic/renal/hepatic disease; pregnancy category C).

Patient Education

Labyrinthitis: Explain the etiology of the problem. Review medication use.

Motion sickness: For ocean cruises, suggest cabin arrangements amidship; for plane travel, suggest seating over airplane wings; for automobile rides, advise sitting in the front seat. Semireclining positions should be used whenever possible. Reading should be avoided. For extended periods of travel, patients should take frequent small amounts of food and fluids. Alcohol consumption and exposure to cigarette smoke should be limited.

Follow-up: As needed.

▸ *Nasal Folliculitis*

Laboratory Tests: None.

Therapeutic Measures: Prescribe bacitracin or neomycin ointment rubbed into the nasal vestibule three times a day until symptoms disappear and for 2 weeks thereafter to prevent recurrence.

Patient Education: Explain that the infection occurs in the hair follicles and that spread can be limited by avoiding nose picking.

Follow-up: As needed.

▸ *Nasal Furuncles*

Laboratory Tests: None.

Therapeutic Measures: Arrange an appointment with an ENT specialist for incision and drainage. In the meantime, start an antistaphylococcal penicillin such as dicloxacillin 250 mg qid or a cephalosporin such as Keflex 250 mg qid for 5–10 days. As a less expensive alternative, erythromycin 250 mg qid may also be used for 10 days, along with applications of wet packs for 15 minutes as often as possible to hasten fluctuation. Advise the use of ASA or Tylenol every 4 hours for pain.

Patient Education: Emphasize the importance of leaving the furuncle alone. Explain the serious consequences of nose picking or premature squeezing (venous drainage from this part of the nose can spread infection to the brain).

Follow-up: Per ENT specialist.

▸ *Common Cold*

Laboratory Tests: None.

Therapeutic Measures: Advise rest and adequate fluid intake. Prescribe ASA or Tylenol, two tablets every 2 hours as needed for body aches; pseudoephedrine, 60 mg three or four times daily, and/or phenylephrine 0.25% or 0.5% nasal spray every 4 hours for nasal stuffiness; Robitussin DM or Pherergan DM 1 tsp every 4 hours for cough. Suggest the use of a cold vaporizer at night, along with petroleum jelly to minimize nasal irritation and warm saline or baking soda gargles to alleviate sore throat.

Patient Education: Explain why antibiotics are not indicated for viral infections. Review the proper use of decongestant nasal sprays. Inform patients that transmission of the cold can be minimized if they avoid close contact with others and practice careful hand washing when symptoms are most pronounced.

Follow-up: Instruct patients to return if symptoms persist or worsen, since secondary bacterial infections can develop when resistance is lowered by a virus.

▸ *Vitamin C Intake*

Laboratory Tests: None.

Therapeutic Measures

Diet: Increase as follows:

RECOMMENDED DAILY REQUIREMENTS FOR VITAMIN C

Males (15+ years)	60 mg
Females (15+ years)	60 mg
Pregnant women	80 mg
Lactating women	100 mg

Supplements: Since most people fail to meet the Recommended Daily Allowance through diet alone, daily supplements (vitamin C liquids, powders, crystals, or pills) may be beneficial. The usual dose is 250 mg, one to four times a day with meals. To reduce cold symptoms, advise the use of 1,500–2,000 mg in divided doses at the onset of illness.

Patient Education: Inform patients about natural sources of vitamin C such as fresh fruits and vegetables. Advise them that smoking and heavy drinking decrease the level of vitamin C in the blood. Provide a list such as the following:

VITAMIN C (mg/100 g OF FOOD)

Parsley	170	Strawberries	57
Green peppers	110	Spinach	51
Chives	70	Oranges	50

Cabbage	47	Nectarines	13.0
Grapefruit	38	Cucumbers	11.0
Lemons	35	Onions	10.0
Cantaloupe	33	Bananas	10.0
Green onions	32	Cranberries	10.0
Radishes	24	Apricots	10.0
Tangerines	23	Cherries	8.7
Tomatoes	23	Carrots	8.0
Squash	22	Peaches	6.1
Raspberries	18	Pears	4.0
Romaine lettuce	18	Apples	4.0
Pineapple	17	Grapes	3.6
Honeydew melon	15.0	Watermelon	3.2
Avocadoes	14.0	Lettuce	2.4
Blueberries	14.0	Plums	1.9

Warn that megadoses of vitamin C supplements on a long-term basis can lead to stomach irritation (discomfort, indigestion, ulcers) and urinary tract problems.

Follow-up: None.

▸ *Allergic Rhinitis*

Laboratory Tests: Wright's smear for eosinophils.

Therapeutic Measures: Suggest referral to an allergist for allergen testing and desensitization. Prescribe Beconase or Vanceril nasal spray tid for 14 days. Prescribe Chlor-Trimeton 8 mg bid or Teldrin 12 mg bid prn.

Patient Education

General: Review medication use. Note high association with aspirin use and development of nasal polyps and asthma in allergic patients.

Seasonal: Instruct patients to avoid wooded or grassy areas during periods of pollination and to remain indoors when symptoms are severe and pollen counts are high (hot, windy, sunny days). Note that air conditioners provide relief from heat but that filters do not remove airborne pollens.

Perennial: Review measures of controlling allergens in the home such as (1) damp mopping two or three times a week, especially in the bedroom, to remove dust, (2) removing feather pillows and covering pillows and mattresses with plastic, (3) eliminating areas where mold can collect, such as piles of old newspapers and magazines or old furniture left in damp areas, (4) limiting contact with or removing domestic animals, (5) using nonallergic cosmetics, and (6) eliminating or limiting the intake of chocolate, nuts, soy products, rice, corn oil, oranges, oats, milk, and eggs as the most common food allergens.

Follow-up: As needed.

▸ Nosebleeds (Epistaxis)

Laboratory Tests: Hematocrit in cases of substantial blood loss. If bleeding dysfunction is suspected, the prothrombin time, partial thromboplastin time, bleeding time, and platelet count should be obtained.

Therapeutic Measures: Have the patient sit upright to reduce venous pressure. Encourage expectoration of accumulated blood. Apply firm, continuous pressure for 10–15 minutes to both sides of the nose above the nasal alar cartilage. The use of ice may facilitate vasoconstriction. If bleeding persists, insert cotton balls that have been soaked in 1:1,000 epinephrine and apply pressure for several minutes. If bleeding still persists, refer the patient to an ENT specialist or emergency room for packing or cauterization. After bleeding stops, insert daily (for the next 7–10 days) cotton balls covered with an antibiotic ointment (neosporin or bacitracin) to aid healing and prevent crusting. Thereafter apply petroleum jelly to the rims of the nostrils to prevent crusting.

Patient Education: Instruct patients to sit upright for the remainder of the day and elevate the head to 30 degrees while sleeping. Suggest humidifier use. Warn against nose picking or forceful nose blowing.

Follow-up: As needed or per ENT specialist.

▸ Acute Sinusitis

Laboratory Tests: Curettage and suction of the discharge from the ostia. Consider sinus x-ray films.

Therapeutic Measures

For infection: Pending culture results, start ampicillin or erythromycin (250–500 mg) four times a day for 10 days.

For drainage: Prescribe Actifed tid, or Chlor-Trimeton 8 mg bid, or Ornade bid for 10–14 days. Suggest short-term use (3 days only) of Afrin or Dristan nasal spray. Cold or hot compresses (whichever provides more relief) can be used for 15 minutes three times a day.

For headaches and sinus discomfort: Aspirin or Tylenol, 2 tablets every 4 hours prn.

Patient Education: Point out areas of infection on a diagram of the sinuses. Review the medication schedule. Instruct patients on proper use of nasal sprays to shrink swollen tissue around the ostia as follows: (1) spray the right nostril; (2) tip the head toward the right and back for 30 seconds; (3) spray the left nostril; (4) tip the head toward the left and back for 30 seconds; (5) wait 5 minutes and repeat the entire process. Have patients report persistent, generalized headache, high fever, and eye symptoms such as blurred vision or pain.

Follow-up: If symptoms persist or worsen.

▸ *Acute Viral Pharyngitis/Tonsillitis*

Laboratory Tests: Throat culture or streptococcal antibody test.

Therapeutic Measures: Suggest rest and high fluid intake. Advise the use of warm saline gargles and lozenges, ASA or Tylenol, 2 tablets every 4 hours for pain and fever.

Patient Education: Explain why antibiotics are not indicated for treatment. Instruct patients to report signs of superimposed bacterial infection.

Follow-up: As needed.

▸ *Streptococcal Pharyngitis/Tonsillitis*

Laboratory Tests: Throat culture or streptococcal antibody test.

Therapeutic Measures: Prescribe penicillin V-K, 250 mg, or erythromycin, 250 mg, four times a day for 10 days. For patients who are unlikely to finish the full course of oral antibiotics, consider benzathine penicillin, 1.2 million units IM. ASA or Tylenol, 2 tablets every 4 hours, rest, extra liquids, and warm saline gargles are also helpful.

Patient Education: Explain the possible complications of streptococcal infections. Emphasize the importance of completing the full 10-day course of the antibiotic. Advise throat cultures for family members.

Follow-up: As needed.

▸ *Gonococcal Pharyngitis*

Laboratory Tests: Pharyngeal Gram stain and gonorrhea culture. Serologic tests for syphilis.

Therapeutic Measures: One of the following regimens is effective:

1. Procaine penicillin G, 4.8 million units divided into two IM injections, combined with probenecid, 1 g orally.
2. Tetracycline, 500 mg four times daily for 7 days.
3. Trimethoprim 80 mg-sulfamethoxazole 400 mg (e.g., Bactrim regular strength) 9 tablets daily for 5 days.

Report cases to the local health department.

Patient Education: Discuss the necessity of treating contacts.

Follow-up: Repeat the pharyngeal gonorrhea culture in 1 week. Patients receiving ampicillin or tetracycline should have follow-up serologic tests in 3 months (only procaine penicillin is effective for incubating syphilis).

▸ *Adult Primary Diphtheria Immunization*

Laboratory Tests: None.

Treatment Measures: After age 6, give adult-type tetanus/diphtheria toxoids (Td) adsorbed as follows:

Starting dose—0.5 ml IM.
Second dose—0.5 ml IM 4 weeks after the starting dose.
Third dose—0.5 ml IM 1 year after the starting dose

Patient Education: Explain that complete immunization requires all three doses and stress the importance of returning 1 year later for the third dose.

Follow-up: Td boosters at 10-year intervals.

▸ *Acute Laryngitis*

Laboratory Tests: Throat culture.

Treatment Measures: If the throat culture is positive, prescribe penicillin V-K or erythromycin, 250 mg four times a day for 10 days. Advise voice rest, adequate liquid intake, throat lozenges (particularly those containing benzocaine), and aspirin or Tylenol, 2 tablets every 4 hours, to help alleviate symptoms.

Patient Education: Point out the area of inflammation on a diagram of the throat. Review medication use. Stress the importance of resting the voice.

Follow-up: If symptoms persist or worsen.

BIBLIOGRAPHY

A more casual approach to strep throat. *Emergency Medicine,* (May) 1983, 139–142.

Abramowicz M. *Handbook of Antimicrobial Therapy,* rev. ed. The Medical Letter, New Rochelle, N.Y., 1980.

Bates B. *A Guide to Physical Examination,* 3rd ed. Lippincott, Philadelphia, 1983.

Berkow RB (ed.). *The Merck Manual of Diagnosis and Therapy,* 14th ed. Merck Sharp & Dohme Research Laboratories, Rahway, N.J., 1982.

Bertz JE. Maxillofacial injuries. *Clinical Symposia,* 1981, 33(4):2–32.

Black FO, Correia MJ, Stucker FJ. Easing proneness to motion sickness. *Patient Care,* (Mar. 30) 1980, 114–128.

Bozian RC (consultant). Therapeutic controversy: Talking vitamin C with your patients. *Patient Care,* (May 15) 1983, 18–74.

Brown AM, Stubbs DW (eds.). *Medical Physiology.* Wiley, New York, 1983.

Caplan LR. A logical approach to dizziness. *PA Drug Update,* (Mar.) 1984, 27–42.

Conn HF, Conn RB Jr (eds.). *Current Diagnosis.* Saunders, Philadelphia, 1980.

Crafts RC. *A Textbook of Human Anatomy,* 3rd ed. Wiley, New York, 1985.

Crouch JE, McClintic JR. *Human Anatomy and Physiology,* 2nd ed. Wiley, New York, 1976.

Dewing LR, Humble JO. Sinusitis. *Physician Assistant and Health Practitioner,* (Mar.) 1982, 18–25.

Duval AJ III, Lowel SH. The "chronic" ear: How to manage mild to severe otitis. *Postgraduate Medicine,* (Aug.) 1979, 66(2):94–101.

Elias H. Pauly JE, Burns ER. *Histology and Human Microanatomy,* 4th ed. Wiley, New York, 1978.

Fahey DJ. Tonsillectomy, adenoidectomy, and otitis: The real world. *New York State Journal of Medicine,* (Dec.) 1979, 2019–2022.

Fairbanks DNF. *Pocket Guide to Antimicrobial Therapy in Otolaryngology,* 2nd ed. American Academy of Otolaryngology—Head and Neck Surgery Foundation, Inc., Washington, D.C., 1983.

Farmer HS. A guide for the treatment of external otitis. *American Family Physician,* (June) 1980, 21(6):96–101.

Glasscock ME III. Meniere's disease. *Hospital Medicine,* (Dec.) 1979, 48–58.

Goodhill V. Of age and hearing. *Transition,* (June) 1983, 19–36.

Gordon CB. Practical approach to the loss of smell. *American Family Physician,* (Sept.) 1982, 26(3):191–193.

Goroll AH, May LA, Mulley AG (eds.) *Primary Care Medicine: Office Evaluation and Management of the Adult Patient.* Lippincott, Philadelphia, 1981.

Gray H. *Anatomy of the Human Body,* 29th American ed. (CM Goss, ed.). Lea & Febiger, Philadelphia, 1973.

Guyton AC. *Textbook of Medical Physiology,* 6th ed. Saunders, Philadelphia, 1981.

Harner SG. Evaluating the patient with a hearing loss. *Continuing Education for the Family Physician,* (May) 1981, 14(5):22–30.

Holliday MJ. Some common ear problems. *Hospital Medicine,* (May) 1981, 13–32.

Hoole AJ, Greenberg RA, Pickard CG Jr. *Patient Care Guidelines for Nurse Practitioners.* Little, Brown, Boston, 1982.

Isselbacher KJ, et al. *Harrison's Principles of Internal Medicine,* 9th ed. McGraw-Hill, New York, 1980.

Kasanof DM (staff ed.). Current care for otitis media. *Patient Care,* (Dec. 15) 1980, 31–49.

Krupp MA, Chatton MJ, Werdegar D (eds.). *Current Medical Diagnosis and Treatment 1985.* Lange, Los Altos, Calif., 1985.

Lipman AG. Which drugs may induce deafness? *Modern Medicine,* (Dec.–Jan.) 1981, 147–148.

Luckmann J, Sorensen KC. *Medical Surgical Nursing: A Psychophysiologic Approach,* 2nd ed. Saunders, Philadelphia, 1980.

Mandell GL, Douglas RG Jr, Bennett JE. *Principles and Practice of Infectious Diseases.* Wiley, New York, 1979.

Middleton DB. A logical approach to managing sore throats. *Modern Medicine,* (Nov.–Dec.) 1980, 40–48.

Pfizer Laboratories Division. Sinusitis: What You Should Know. Pamphlet No. X011X83B. Pfizer, Inc., New York, August 1983.

Rhea JT, Deluca SA. Acute sinusitis. *American Family Physician,* (Apr.) 1982, 25(4):121–122.

Rice DH, et al. Cranial complications of frontal sinusitis. *American Family Physician,* (Nov.) 1980, 22(5):145–149.

Richardson MA, Donaldson JA. Middle ear fluid. *American Family Physician,* (June) 1981, 23(6):159–163.

Ruben RJ. Otolaryngologic problems of the old. *Hospital Practice,* (Aug.) 1977, 73–87.

Rudick J, Bimonte R. *Tuning in On Hearing Aids.* FDA Consumer, Dept. of Health and Human Services, Rockville, Md, May 1980.

Sasaki ER. Epistaxis: A step-by-step approach to treating nosebleeds. *PA Practice,* 1983, 3–7.

Silverstein A. *Human Anatomy and Physiology.* Wiley, New York, 1980.

Wyngaarden JB, Smith LH Jr (eds.). *Cecil Textbook of Medicine,* 16th ed., Vols. 1 and 2. Saunders, Philadelphia, 1982.

Wyre HW Jr. The diagonal earlobe crease: A cutaneous manifestation of coronary artery disease. *Cutis,* (Mar.) 1979, 23:328–331.

3

Mouth

Mary McTigue
Howard A. Gordon, DDS, and Katherine Irish, RDH,
Special Consultants

Outline

Pulpitis
Dead tooth
Root canal
Tooth abscess
Gum boil
Apiectomy

Gums

Lead line
Gingival hypertrophy
► Acute necrotizing ulcerative gingivitis
Chronic gingivitis
Periodontal disease
Periodontitis
Marginal periodontitis (pyorrhea)
Gingivectomy
Periodontosis
► Prevention and control of periodontal disease
Keyes method
Mouth trauma
Emergency procedures for mouth trauma
Dentures
► Proper denture care

TONGUE AND SALIVARY GLANDS

Tongue

Macroglossia
Halitosis
Hairy tongue
Glossitis
Geographic tongue
Hypoguesia
Tongue-tied

Salivary Glands

Sjögren's syndrome
Mikulicz's syndrome
Sialolithiasis
► Sialandenitis
Mumps
Childhood mumps immunization
Adult mumps immunization
Tumors of the salivary glands

LIPS AND ORAL MUCOSA

Lips

The lips are formed from a mucosal membrane that converges with facial skin at a line of demarcation known as the "vermillion zone." Structured by striated muscle and connective tissue, they are reddened by a rich subcutaneous network of capillaries. Inflammation of the lips, ***cheilitis,*** occurs in response to infectious or systemic disease, allergens, irritants, and vitamin deficiencies, as described in Table 3.1. ***Angular cheilitis*** refers to the development of fissures at the corner of the mouth, ***perleche*** to the development of a secondary bacterial or fungal infection. Underlying problems, upon which diagnosis and treatment are based, are discussed in other chapters of this book.

Lacking keratin, the lips are readily affected by sun exposure. An acute sunburn results in an extremely painful inflammation called ***actinic cheilitis.*** The lips become blistered, red, shiny, and swollen. If damage from sunburn is severe, tissue necrosis causes a yellow exudative membrane to form. Treatment consists of Burrow's solution compresses, corticosteroid ointments, and surgical debridement of necrotic tissue to prevent infection. Sun protection (minimized exposure, hats or visors, and sunscreens) is an important preventive measure.

Individuals who spend a lot of time outdoors (particularly redheads with fair skin) develop excessively dry lips and brown areas of erosion known as ***actinic cheilosis.*** The latter is a premalignant change that may lead to ***lip cancer.*** In addition to sun exposure, risk factors for lip cancer include heavy alcohol and tobacco use. The most

TABLE 3.1 TYPES OF CHEILITIS

Type	Description	Treatment
Actinic cheilitis	Acute sunburn of lip tissue with swelling and necrosis.	Burrows solution compresses; debridement of necrotic tissue; sun protection.
Allergic cheilitis	Sensitivity reaction to food, chemicals, or cosmetics. Causes shiny erythema with slight swelling, itching, dryness, burning, and desquamation.	Remove irritant; use topical corticosteroids.
Nutritional chelitis	Caused by deficiency of vitamin B_{12}, riboflavin, pyridoxine, folate. Fissuring and scaling at vermillion surfaces and angles of mouth.	Correct deficiency.
Perleche	Secondary bacterial or fungal infection. Causes white or purulent exudate to form over preexisting cheilitis.	Topical fungal or bacterial ointment.

common type, squamous cell carcinoma, usually appears as a nonhealing, indurated ulcer (less commonly as a keratotic patch) fixed to the lower lip border. Other types of ***neoplastic lip changes*** are described in Table 3.2. If there is any question about malignancy, patients should be referred to a dermatologist for biopsy and removal. If lip cancer is treated early, the prognosis is excellent.

Sun irritation is also a triggering factor in ▶ ***cold sores*** (fever blisters). This common problem is caused by herpes simplex type 1 virus. After the primary infection, the virus remains dormant in nerve ganglia. Activated by stress, sunlight, fever, allergy, pregnancy, menses, systemic infection, local irritation, and certain foods or drugs, it produces skin lesions that classically appear as grouped vesicles on an erythematous base. The lesions usually occur on the outer edges of the lips but sometimes develop around the cheeks, oral and nasal cavities, genitalia, and/or cornea. Eruption is preceded by swelling and an itching, burning, or tingling sensation; it is followed, in a few days, by drying of serous fluids and yellow crust formation. Healing begins in 7–10 days and is complete by 21 days without scar formation (except in cases of recurrent lesions at the same site, which may cause atrophy and scarring). For the most part, treatment is symptomatic. Intermittent cleansing with soap and water is recommended. However, it is best to keep lesions dry, since continuous moistness aggravates the inflammation and delays healing. Acyclovir (Zovirax) may alleviate discomfort and shorten the course of the disease. Since herpes virus is shed from skin lesions, patients with an active eruption should be advised to avoid direct contact with others, particularly newborns and immunocompromised persons who are at risk for developing a systemic herpes infection. Sunscreens and avoidance of triggering factors help prevent recurrences.

Oral Mucosa

The mucous membrane that forms the lips extends into the mouth, where it becomes the oral mucosa (Fig. 3.1). The portion covering the inside of the cheeks is called the "buccal mucosa." Inflammatory lesions within the mouth are referred to as ***stomati-***

TABLE 3.2 NEOPLASTIC CHANGES OF THE LIPS

Type	Description
Actinic chelosis (premalignant)	Lips are dry, with erosive areas. Most common in redheads with fair skin and persons who spend a lot of time outdoors. Patients should be seen every 3–6 months for follow-up. Prolonged exposure to sun should be avoided.
Mucocele (benign)	Obstruction of the duct that carries mucoid secretion to the mucosal surface results in cyst formation (obstruction is usually the result of trauma or infection). Cryosurgery is the treatment of choice.
Smoker's patch (premalignant)	Firm, brownish, keratotic plaque on vermillion border of lower lip. Most common in smokers who hold pipe or cigarette in one location. Cessation of smoking and careful observation are necessary.
Squamous cell carcinoma (malignant)	Usually seen on vermillion border of lower lip as a nonhealing ulcer with a convex, indurated margin or, less commonly, as a keratotic patch. Excellent prognosis if treated early.
Warts (usually benign; in rare cases, premalignant or malignant)	Most often of viral origin. Usually found on vermillion border. Treatment of choice is simple excision. Multiple warts may indicate Cowdin's syndrome. Pathology studies needed to rule out verrucous carcinoma.

tis. They occur in response to infectious or systemic disease, allergens and irritants, and vitamin deficiencies, as described in Table 3.3. The underlying problems are the main concern; they are discussed in other chapters of this book.

▶ ***Thrush*** (monilia, candidiasis) is caused by the yeast-like organism *Candida albicans.* Although most common in infants and small children, thrush occurs in adults with diabetes mellitus, severe debilitation, or immunodeficiency. It may also develop in patients receiving long-term antibiotic therapy (antibiotics eliminate normal bacteria in the mouth that prevent yeast overgrowth). The chief complaint is painful swallowing. Exam reveals creamy white, raised patches resembling milk curds in the mouth and throat. These patches can be scraped away, leaving a raw, bleeding surface. The diagnosis is confirmed by fungal smears or culture. The treatment is an antifungal medication.

▶ ***Canker sores*** (apthous ulcers) commonly affect the oral mucosa. Often they develop in response to trauma, such as accidental raking of the gum line with a toothbrush or scraping of the buccal mucosa from jagged braces. However, canker sores may also indicate viruses, stress, allergies, anemia, or gastrointestinal disease. Recurrences in women have been associated with menses. The lesions begin as small, reddened macules that develop into small ulcers with gray-white necrotic centers. Appearing singly or in small groups, the ulcers are extremely painful, particularly when talking, swallowing, or eating (especially salty, spicy, or acidic foods or alcoholic beverages). Burning, itching, or a tingling sensation may be present in the area 24–48 hours before the lesions appear. Lymphadenopathy is not present unless secondary infection supervenes. Canker sores usually heal spontaneously in 8–12 days. Topical pain medications, debridement, and tetracycline suspension relieve discomfort and hasten the healing process.

Recurrent clusters of canker sores affecting the oral mucosa and/or the mucocutaneous membranes of the eye and genital tract (scrotum, penis, vulva, vagina) are a presenting manifestation of ***Behçet's disease.*** An immune disorder of unknown etiology, Behçet's disease generally appears in the third decade, striking

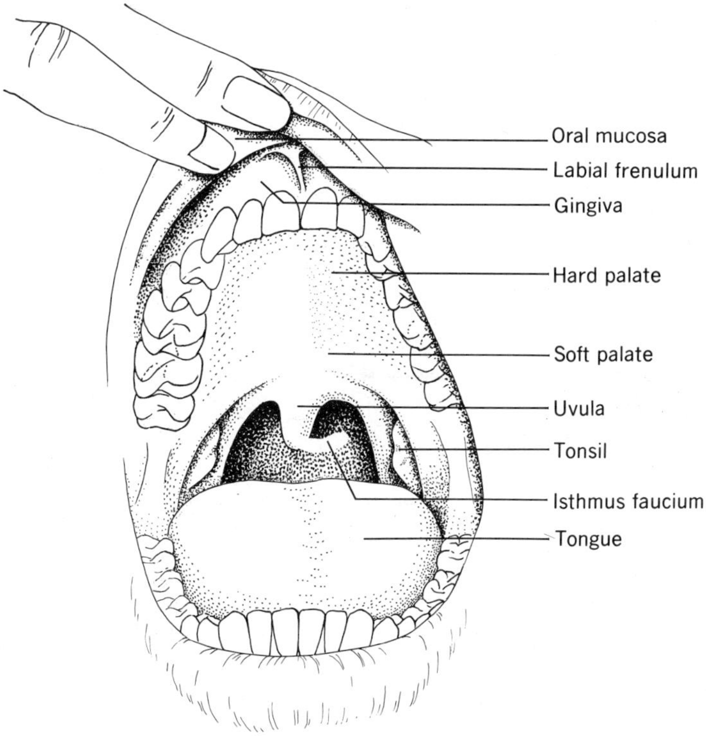

Figure 3.1 Oral cavity: lips and buccal mucosa, upper and lower teeth, tongue, tonsils, and uvula.

men twice as often as women. Following an outbreak of aphthous ulcers, patients develop vasculitis in one or several organs. As a consequence, they may experience uveitis, vascuar skin lesions, nondestructive arthritis, colitis, or CNS damage. Laboratory tests are nonspecific. Diagnosis is based on the presence of a rheumatoid process with a history of recurrent aphthous ulcers. The disease is characterized by periods of remission and relapse extending over several decades. Mild cases can be managed by primary care providers (see canker sores). Cases marked by serious vasculitis should be referred to a rheumatologist and/or ophthalmologist. High doses of systemic prednisone (60–80 mg/day) and immunosuppressive drugs (cyclophosphamide and azathioprine) have been used with some success.

Neoplastic changes affecting the oral mucosa are described in Table 3.4. The ***benign tumors*** (fibromas, lipomas, neurofibromas, and hemangiomas) represent overgrowth of normal tissue. They cause few problems and can be easily excised. By contrast, ***leukoplakia*** represents abnormal keratosis of the oral mucosa. It is caused by chronic irritation from cheek biting, ill-fitting dentures, malocclusion, habitual lozenge use, malnutrition, diets of highly seasoned foods, and heavy use of alcohol or tobacco. Leukoplakia can develop anywhere in the mouth, but the buccal mucosa is the most common site. A number of variations are observed, all potentially malignant. The typical lesion appears as a clearly delineated area having a coarse, wrinkled surface. Usually gray-white or yellow, its surface may be brown in smokers.

TABLE 3.3 CAUSES OF STOMATITIS

Disease	Oral Manifestations
Anthrax	Ragged ulcers and edema.
Diphtheria	Oral pseudomembrane associated with paralysis of the soft palate.
Erythema multiforme	Hemorrhagic ulcerations of the oral mucosa developing in response to viral infections, drug sensitivities, and systemic disease.
Gonorrhea	Yellowish-white patches, inflamed, swollen gingiva (similar to Vincent's infection).
Leprosy	Granulomatous nodules (lepromas) of mucosal membranes, tongue, and soft palate.
Leishmaniasis	Chronic mucocutaneous ulcerations.
Lymphogranuloma venereum	Papules, vesicles, and ulcers (lymphogranulomatous chancres) in oral mucosa. Fibrotic, blister-like lesions. Enlargement, scarring, and retraction of the tongue.
Measles	Enanthema characterized by white spots on the buccal mucosa (Koplik's spots).
Nutritional deficiencies	Beefy red changes in oral mucosa and tongue caused by vitamin B_{12}, folate, pyridoxine, and iron deficiencies, which are associated with abnormal epithelial cell turnover.
Sjögren's syndrome	"Burning mouth" syndrome and chronic changes in oral mucosa caused by decrease in salivary flow.
Stevens-Johnson syndrome	Severe variation of erythema multiforme.
Streptococcal infections	Stomatitis scarlatina, strawberry tongue, raspberry tongue.
Syphilis	Chancres, recurrent mucous patches, gummas, syphilids, congenital lesions.
Tularemia	Ulcers resembling syphilitic chancres, grayish-white oral mucosal lesions, generalized stomatitis.

Lesions involving the tongue are characterized by loss of taste buds, those on the palate by nodular or ring-like elevations around palatal glands. Velvety red lesions with white speckling ***(erythroplakia)*** are particularly premalignant. Unfortunately, leukoplakic lesions are painless. By the time there is any discomfort from fissures or erosions, malignant change is likely.

Patients with any suspicious lesion should be referred to an oral surgeon or ENT specialist for evaluation. Tissue exam by exfoliative cytology or biopsy is essential. The most informative specimens are taken from areas with white flecks characteristic of granulation tissue. If the lesion is small enough, excisional biopsy is recommended. Patients with premalignant changes (inflammation or hyperkeratosis) must be taught to maintain careful oral hygiene and eliminate chronic irritants such as tobacco, alcohol, and highly seasoned foods. Although ill-fitting dentures are known to cause hyperkeratosis, properly fitting ones may actually prevent tissue changes. Supplements of the vitamin B complex and vitamin C help to improve the general condition of the oral mucosa. Even more important may be the topical application of vitamin A for a period of 4–6 months. Local absorption of vitamin A has been found to interfere with keratinization and reduce the lesions. Follow-up tissue exams are done every 6–12 months. Evidence of early malignant change ***(dyskeratosis)*** is an indication for surgical removal of lesions. "Stripping" of an entire area of the mouth may be required in cases of widespread involvement. Fol-

TABLE 3.4 NEOPLASTIC CHANGES OF THE ORAL MUCOSA

Change	Description
Melanocytic nevi	Benign. Pigmented nevi (lentigos, blue, junction, compound, and dermal). Excision indicated.
Macules (amalgam tattoos)	Benign. Traumatic inoculation of amalgam particles from dental work causes bluish-brown lesions on the posterior gingivae and adjacent buccal mucosa.
Oral pigmentation	Benign. Accompanies heavy metal exposure, antimalaria drugs, phenothiazine therapy, Addison's disease, hemochromatosis, neurofibromatosis, and Peutz-Jegher's syndrome.
Fibromas and papillomas	Benign. Pedunculated, fibrous epithelial masses found anywhere in the oral mucosa. Simple excision is indicated.
Leukoplakia ("speckled" type of erythroplakia)	Premalignant or malignant. White keratotic patch on erythematous base. Biopsy imperative.
Squamous cell carcinoma	Malignant. Follows chronic glossitis or leukoplakic change. Deep ulcer with smooth, indurated, rolled margin. Common in heavy users of alcohol and tobacco. Syphilis is another predisposing factor.
Rhabdomyoma	Malignant. Commonly found on tongue as a palpable interior mass. Excision and/or chemotherapy indicated.

lowing surgery, patients are managed in the same manner as those with hyperkeratosis. Smoking must be discontinued forever. Early diagnosis and intervention, along with a commitment to therapy, may prevent invasive cancer and be truly lifesaving. ▶ ***Oral self-examination*** plays an important part in this process.

PALATE, TEETH, AND GUMS

Palate

The oral cavity (Fig. 3.1) is roofed by the bony hard palate and the anterior portion of the soft palate. The hard palate, formed by the maxillae and palatine bones, is covered with a thick mucoperiosteum. Excess bone growth in the midline of the hard palate is referred to as ***torus palatinus*** and is a problem only when dentures are necessary.

Striated muscle fibers covered with mucous membrane form the soft palate, which attaches to the posterior margin of the hard palate and ends at the uvula. Through the action of the nasopharyngeal muscles, the soft palate draws up, preventing food or liquids from entering the nasopharynx during swallowing. This closing mechanism may not function if a person talks or laughs while swallowing, causing liquids to back up into the nose. Saying a prolonged "ah" elevates the soft palate, providing visualization of the posterior pharyngeal wall.

Teeth

Twenty primary (deciduous) teeth erupt gradually between the ages of 4 months and 3 years. They hold space in the jaw for the permanent teeth and are shed in early childhood. Normally, there are 32 permanent teeth, which erupt gradually from age 6 years through young adulthood. Additional ***(supernumerary) teeth*** or ***absent***

teeth are congenital variations that occur with some frequency. They are a chief cause of malocclusion, a problem discussed subsequently.

The last teeth to erupt are the four ***wisdom teeth*** (third molars). One or more of the wisdom teeth may be congenitally missing. If present, they usually, but not always, emerge between the ages of 17 and 21. Failure to appear is nothing to worry about and may actually be an advantage. Wisdom teeth are difficult to clean and highly prone to decay. This is particularly true of those that emerge at an angle, creating a stagnation area for food particles. ***Impacted wisdom tooth*** occurs if growth is impeded by gum, bone, or another tooth. A 1971 study of 5,600 persons between 17 and 24 years of age found that 65.6% of those radiographically surveyed had at least one impacted tooth. Prophylactic removal ***(exodontia)*** at this age, before root formation is complete, is often recommended because the problem can lead to a number of complications. For one thing, an impacted wisdom tooth can push nearby teeth out of position once it starts to grow. Furthermore, it creates a pocket in the gum. The pocket becomes an area of cyst formation, which some studies have linked to malignant change. Alternatively, it traps food and bacteria, causing infection to develop around the embedded tooth ▶***(pericoronitis).*** Patients with pericoronitis develop swelling and redness of the overlying gum, pain when chewing, and an unpleasant taste. They should be started on antibiotics and referred to an oral surgeon. Once the active infection has cleared, the impacted tooth is removed.

Full-grown teeth are arranged in two opposing arches. The maxillary arch (upper jaw) is fixed, and the mandibular arch (lower jaw) is movable (see Fig. 3.1). The relationship of the upper and lower teeth when the mouth is closed is referred to as "occlusion." With normal occlusion, the upper teeth slightly overlap the lower ones and the points of the molars alternate. The teeth are straight, regularly spaced, and neither too big nor too small for the jaws. Because teeth and jaw patterns are a combination of characteristics inherited from each parent, few persons have perfect teeth.

When the teeth of the maxillary and mandibular arches fail to come in proper contact, ***malocclusion*** exists. In addition to heredity, malocclusion may result from premature loss of baby teeth, extra or missing permanent teeth, tongue thrusting, and/or thumb sucking. Dental evaluation is important because malocclusion can interfere with proper chewing and teeth cleaning, both of which lead to caries and gum disease. Furthermore, severe malocclusion can contribute to ENT problems and seriously affect the self-image. Treatment ***(orthodontics)*** depends on the type and severity of the condition. Removal of teeth (exodontia), jaw surgery, crownwork, bridgework, and/or braces may be advised. Braces are usually most effective during childhood and early adolescence, when the teeth and jaws are still developing and the texture of the bone facilitates tooth movement. However, they are also being used successfully and much more frequently in adults. Hypertrophied gums, gingivitis, caries, facial pain, bone damage, and trauma to the oral mucosa may occur during treatment. Thus, close attention by the orthodontist is mandatory.

Malocclusion is a major cause of ***bruxism*** (gnashing of teeth). This automatic reflex of the neuromuscular system during sleep may be exacerbated by stress and anxiety. Thousands of pounds of pressure per square inch can be exerted on teeth, gums, alveolar bone, and jaws. To prevent damage to these structures, patients should be referred to an orthodontist.

The temporomadibular joint serves as a hinge for the lower jaw. If ligaments attaching the condyles of the jaw into the base of the skull become overstretched,

► ***temporomadibular joint (TMJ) syndrome*** may develop. Contributing factors include aging, arthritis, trauma to the jaw or head, malocclusion, having the mouth open too wide for prolonged periods, or biting down on hard food. Once the ligaments are damaged, even normal chewing and biting result in further stretching and spasm of the masseter muscles. Muscle spasm produces erratic jaw movements, clicking noises, and pain below the ear. The TMJ syndrome affects as many as 60 million people, or 20% of the population, annually. Women between the ages of 20 and 40 are particularly susceptible. Because it contributes to head and neck pain, clogged ears, dizziness, sinusitis, tic doloureux, migraine, and tinnitus, TMJ syndrome has been referred to as "one of medicine's great impostors" (Goldberg et al., 1983). Primary treatment aims at reducing pain and muscle tension. This is accomplished in part by the use of heat, massage, and pharmacologic agents. Attention to the underlying disorder is important. Referral to a dental specialist to correct the occlusion or to be fitted with a mouthpiece is often necessary. Bite plates reposition and redistribute stress on the jaw and teeth. Patients should also be instructed to avoid aggravating jaw movements and to modify their diet.

An individual tooth is basically composed of pulp, dentin, cementum, and enamel, as shown in Figure 3.2*a*. The living portion, pulp, contains tissue, blood vessels, and nerves. It is responsible for tooth sensitivity to heat, cold, pressure, and pain. The bulk of the tooth consists of nonliving, calcified tissue, dentin, which contains millions of tiny canals leading to the pulp. Dentin in the root (the portion of the tooth anchored in the alveolar bone) is covered and held in place by cementum; dentin in the crown (the portion of the tooth above the gum) is covered by enamel.

Dentin reflects through the clear enamel covering to give teeth their color. Although usually light yellow, normal tooth color can vary among individuals and among teeth in the same individual. ***Tooth discoloration*** results from bacteria, food debris, aging, chemicals, or disease, as outlined in Table 3.5. ***Fluorosis,*** that is, overexposure to fluoride, is responsible for permanent color changes: excessively white patches in mild cases, gray patches in moderate cases, and brown eroded areas in more severe cases.

After eating, a sticky substance called ***plaque*** forms in the mouth. Consisting of mucus, food particle, and bacteria, it collects between the teeth and along the lines where teeth and gums meet. Certain bacteria in the plaque (acidogenic streptococci, lactobacilli, actinomyces, and others) react with carbohydrates, particularly sucrose, to form an acid. If plaque remains in contact with tooth surfaces, the acid can erode tooth enamel, resulting in ***dental caries*** (cavities).

Prevention is one of the most important aspects of the problem. It has three aspects, the first being to maximize the density of enamel. Related to calcification during years of tooth formation, density of enamel depends on ingesting adequate amounts of vitamins A, C, and D, calcium, phosphorus, and fluorine. Most of these nutritional substances are readily obtained in a diet containing well-balanced servings from the Four Basic Food Groups. Fluorine is not. For this reason, ***fluoride supplementation*** (through public water systems, applications by dentists, tablets, or school rinse programs) is recommended from infancy through age 18. Fluorinated toothpastes should be used by all age groups. Reducing bacteria/plaque contact with tooth surfaces is the second aspect of prevention of dental caries. The most recent advance toward this end is the development of a vaccine that, successful in rats and monkeys, is now under investigation for use in humans. Future developments in plaque control may depend on some interesting findings about enzyme deficiencies in

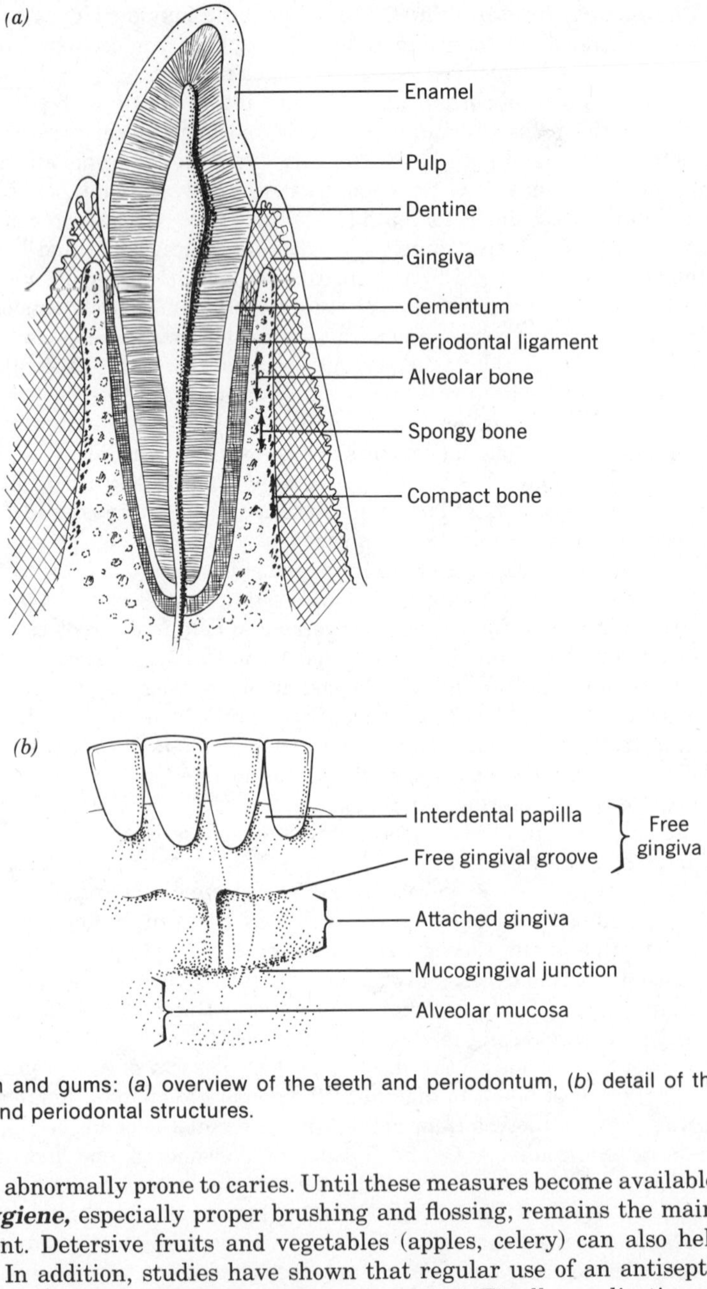

Figure 3.2 Teeth and gums: (*a*) overview of the teeth and periodontum, (*b*) detail of the individual tooth and periodontal structures.

groups of people abnormally prone to caries. Until these measures become available, ▶***good oral hygiene,*** especially proper brushing and flossing, remains the mainstay of treatment. Detersive fruits and vegetables (apples, celery) can also help remove plaque. In addition, studies have shown that regular use of an antiseptic mouthwash lowers the amount of damaging bacteria by 50%. Finally, applications of ***dental sealants*** to fill in deep pits and fissures of occlusal surfaces help prevent plaque buildup in hard-to-brush areas (first and second molars and second bicuspids). Widely used in younger age groups, dental sealants are now being advocated for adults as well. The third aspect of prevention of dental caries is reduction of

TABLE 3.5 CAUSES OF TOOTH DISCOLORATION

Physiologic Aging Pulp stones Inadequate fluid exchange between dentin and pulp Idiopathic internal dentin resorption (pink to reddish-brown discoloration) Fibrosis, degeneration, and aseptic necrosis of pulp (progressive grayness or black) Dental caries (yellow or green/brown discoloration) Foods and beverages Dark berries, beets Spices, licorice Coffee, tea, cola drinks Tobacco	Drugs and chemicals Excess fluorine (diffuse cloudiness, white flecks, yellow-brown lines, brownish-black patches) Tetracycline (yellow to brownish-gray discoloration in adults only after prolonged use) Iron compounds, manganese silver (black-brown discoloration) Mercury, lead (gray discoloration) Iodide, bromide (brown discoloration) Copper, antimony, nickel (green-blue discoloration) Mercury, nitrate acid (green discoloration) Chromic acid (deep orange discoloration) Cadmium (yellow discoloration) Potassium permanganate (deep violet discoloration) Mercurial salts in local antiseptics (green, orange, or red discoloration) Blood and bacterial pigments High bilirubin (green discoloration) Heme (blue-black discoloration) Methemoglobin (red-brown discoloration) Hematoidin (orange discoloration) Sulfmelhemoglobin (green discoloration)

sucrose in the diet. Forms of sucrose that stick to enamel (e.g., carmel candy, raisins) or remain in contact with enamel for long periods (hard candies, gum) are particularly destructive. They are most damaging between meals when brushing is unlikely.

► ***Prevention and control of dental caries*** is important because enamel is acellular; once a cavity develops, the body cannot repair it. A small cavity may not cause any symptoms, but can be noted by the dentist with explorer instruments or x-ray studies. To treat it, the dentist drills away all traces of decay and shapes the hole to retain a secure filling. The hole is filled with a mixture of silver/tin/mercury or quartz/plastic resin.

When asymptomatic caries are left untreated, acid eats thorugh the enamel and exposes the underlying dentin. Bacteria travels through the minute dentin canals that lead to the pulp. If bacteria reaches the pulp, an inflammatory response, called ***pulpitis,*** develops. Patients experience pain in the tooth, which is exacerbated by eating something hot, cold, or sweet. They may also note sharp stabbing pains in the surrounding jaw. Immediate dental attention is crucial. The large area of decay must be drilled away and the cavity filled. Severely decayed, broken, cracked, or brittle teeth may require special treatment whereby the dentist shapes a portion of the natural tooth into a peg and takes molds of the area. Special laboratories use the molds to create a hollow shell of white porcelain or gold alloy (*crown*). The crown is cemented in place, using the portion of natural tooth as an anchor.

A ***dead tooth*** is the invariable result of untreated pulpitis. It may also follow trauma and sometimes occurs for no apparent reason. A cavity may cease to be painful, and eventually the tooth turns slightly gray. Otherwise, the death is accompanied by no explicit symptoms and is noted only on routine x-ray films. Once detected, it should be specially treated with a ***root canal.*** The procedure (endodontics) begins with measures to remove all debris from the pulp chamber and root canal. Both areas are then disinfected and sealed.

If a dead tooth is not prepared with endodontic procedures, the nonviable pulp decomposes. Bacteria from the decaying matter can seep into the root canal, setting up an infection in the tissue around the tip of the tooth's root (apex). Pus collects in the area and ***tooth abscess*** develops. This may also occur from bacteria associated with deep decay. Patients note fever and general malaise. Swelling of the lips and cheeks accompanies abscess of an upper tooth, while the jaw is found to be swollen with abscess of a lower tooth. Gnawing, continuous pain in these areas may be aggravated by heat or cold. Patients often attribute such symptoms to a sinus or ear problem. Examination, however, confirms the existence of tooth pathology. The tissue surrounding the affected tooth is edematous, inflamed, and tender. The tooth itself is tender to percussion, mobile, or discolored. Lymphadenopathy, leukocytosis, dehydration, and facial cellulitis may be present in the acute stage. Advanced abscesses may be accompanied by the formation of the fistulous tract through the bone. In such cases, a fluctuant mass develops along the gum ***(gum boil).*** If the gum boil bursts, foul-tasting pus drains into the mouth and the pain is suddenly relieved. As in the case of pericoronitis, patients with a tooth abscess should be started on antibiotics, hot saline mouth rinses to encourage fluctuation, and strong analgesics. Immediate dental referral should be arranged. The dentist drills open the pulp cavity to relieve pressure and promote drainage of the infection. Once the acute inflammation is under control, root canal is performed (see above). If the infection cannot be cleared through the root canal, the tip of the tooth is removed and the area debrided in a surgical procedure ***(apiectomy).*** In some cases, extraction is necessary.

Gums (Periodontum)

The periodontum (Figure 3.2*b*) surrounds and supports the teeth. It consists of complex structures that are divided into two units (gingiva and attachment), as described in Table 3.6. The gingivae (gums) are made of fibrous tissue covered with a mucous membrane that surrounds and attaches the teeth to the alveolar bone. Its color varies from light coral to dark pink, depending on the person's complexion and skin color. While a dark gray coloration along gum margins is normal in black people, it may also represent abnormal pigmentation ***(lead line)*** that is characteristic of lead poisoning (see Chapter 7). Many of the nerves around the teeth are found in the gingivae. Thus, patients reporting toothaches may actually be experiencing referred pain from the periodontal tissues and surrounding bone.

Gingival hypertrophy is overgrowth of gum tissue. It may be evidence of periapical abscess or the result of a local irritating factor, poor oral hygiene, or systemic disease. Dilantin therapy may lead to generalized enlargement of the gums, particularly in combination with poor dental hygiene. Dental prophylaxis, surgical excision, and a mouth guard may reduce regrowth in such cases. Patients with leukemia may experience gingival hypertrophy with hemorrhaging. In such cases, careful oral cleansing is recommended, but surgery is contraindicated. Another condition leading to enlargement of the gingiva is mouth breathing (runners are prone to the condition for this reason). These patients should be advised to breathe through the nose.

▶***Acute necrotizing ulcerative gingivitis*** (ANUG, trench mouth, Vincent's disease) is an acute destructive inflammation of the gingiva. Caused by a mixed infection of spirochetes and fusiform bacilli, the condition is associated with poor

TABLE 3.6 STRUCTURES OF THE PERIODONTUM

Free gingiva	Extends from the gingival margin to the base of the gingival sulcus (the crevice between the free gingiva and the tooth, normally no deeper than 2.5 mm); closely adapted around each tooth in a collar-like manner.
Junctional epithelium	Encircles the tooth and provides the actual attachment on the cementum at full eruption. The attachment recedes along the root of the tooth with disease and wear.
Interdental gingiva (papilla)	Occupies the space between the teeth and is continuous with the free gingiva at the top and lateral borders. The shape varies from flat to tapered according to the spacing of the teeth. Most periodontal disease begins in the center of this area because the tissue here is not keratinized.
Attached gingiva	Firmly bound to the underlying cementum and alveolar bone. Follows the depression between the eminences of the roots of the teeth.
Alveolar mucosa	Loosely attached to the underlying bone. Joins the attached gingiva at the mucogingival junction and continues to the vestibule of the mouth. Is composed of lining mucosa and has a deeper red color than the gingiva.

oral hygiene, malnutrition, lowered host resistance, and stress. Gingival margins, particularly between the teeth, become necrotic and painful. There is invariably a fetid odor and usually a low-grade fever. Systemic antibiotics followed by removal of necrotic tissue by a dental specialist is the treatment.

Though mild, ***chronic gingivitis*** is significant as the initial stage in the development of ***periodontal disease.*** The inflammation results from irritation caused by tartar (calculus), which is mineralized plaque. Tartar builds up along the gum line in the presence of poor oral hygiene, or structural or tissue changes of the teeth and gums due to malocclusion, aging, trauma, or disuse (e.g., in persons on soft or liquid diets). The first signs of gingivitis are slight swelling and redness of the gums not associated with pain. Bleeding from even minor trauma such as tooth brushing is common. Inflammation is furthered by bacteria trapped under the tartar. If the tartar and inflammatory debris are not removed with special instruments (scaling), the process extends to the periodonal ligaments, causing ***periodontitis.*** The most common type of periodontitis in adults is ***marginal periodontitis (pyorrhea).*** The bacteria trapped beneath the tartar forms subgingival pockets. In addition to bleeding, gums recede. Reaching depths of 5–9 mm (normal depth is 2–3 mm), the pockets create sites for deep-seated infections that cannot be reached unless the gums are surgically trimmed ***(gingivectomy).*** If uncontrolled, periodontitis causes ligament structures to break down ***(periodontosis).*** Teeth separate from the alveolar bone and loosen in their sockets. Tapping produces a dull sound rather than the sharp sound of a firmly set tooth. Furthermore, when the erosive process reaches the cementum (sensitive tissue covering the root), teeth begin to ache on exposure to anything hot, cold, or sweet. Splinting may be attempted but is rarely successful. Eventually teeth simply fall out or must be removed. Therefore, ▶***prevention and control of periodontal disease*** is the most viable approach to care. If treated early and aggressively, gingivitis can usually be reversed. With the first warning signs, patients should be referred to the dentist for scaling and a possible course of antibiotics. Good oral hygiene must be practiced faithfully. This may be modified with special techniques for brushing and flossing using baking soda and peroxide solutions ***(Keyes method).***

Periodontal disease and caries are the two most significant causes of tooth loss. ***Mouth trauma*** is a third cause. Although most cases necessitate immediate referral to a dentist or oral surgeon, primary care providers may need to initiate or advise ▶ ***emergency procedures for mouth trauma.*** Reinforcing the use of mouth guards during contact sports and seat belts in cars is a sensible preventive measure.

Following significant tooth loss, patients should be fitted for partial or complete ***dentures.*** Dentures are important not only for the self-image and nutrition but also for maintaining the integrity of the oral mucosa, gums, and facial features. Patients should be warned to expect certain changes with dentures. They may be sensitive to alterations in appearance and may experience some awkwardness when chewing or speaking. These problems, however, can be minimized by ▶ ***proper denture care*** and a positive mental attitude. Regular adjustment of dentures is of great importance in long-term management. As the patient ages the bone and gum ridges recede and shrink, causing dentures to become loose and unstable. Improper alignment leads to more rapid shrinkage of the jaw and irritation of the soft tissues of the mouth. Open sores, which have the potential for malignant change, may result. Thus, any patient with signs of ill-fitting or damaged dentures should be referred to the dentist.

TONGUE AND SALIVARY GLANDS

Tongue

The tongue is illustrated in Figure 3.3. ***Macroglossia,*** enlargement of the entire tongue, can develop in response to tumors, infections, and metabolic disorders (especially hypothyroidism and acromegaly). It also accompanies amyloidosis, angioneurotic edema, superior vena cava syndrome, and sarcoidosis. Macroglossia is reversed with treatment of the underlying disorder.

The upper side of the tongue is covered with a specialized gray-colored mucosa. It has a roughened surface from numerous minute projections, the papillae. Trapping of food particles and plaque by the papillae is one of the most common causes of ***halitosis*** (bad breath). The problem can also result from periodontal disease, dental caries, sinusitis, pharyngitis, and/or fermentation of food particles in the mouth. Occasionally it can be traced to systemic conditions, notably hepatic encephalopathy, diabetic ketoacidosis, respiratory disease, or neoplasms. Treatment consists of maintaining good oral hygiene and correcting any underlying disorder.

In response to antibiotics or mouthwash, smoking or radiation therapy, the epithelium on the papillae can grow very long and dark. This benign condition, referred to as ***hairy tongue,*** is easily treated by discontinuing the use of the offending substance, brushing the tongue with a soft-bristle toothbrush, and applying hydrogen peroxide solution. In more severe cases, the abnormally long papillae must be snipped away and the area covered with 15% tricholoroacetic acid. Several treatments are usually required.

Inflammation of the tongue results in epithelial loss, causing the surface to become very smooth, red, and beefy-looking, a condition referred to as ***glossitis.*** The problem is associated with nutritional deficiencies (of vitamin B_{12}, folic acid, niacin, iron), infections, and allergic responses. The initial complaint is a burning, tingling sensation, which continues after the changes in color and topography appear. Treatment of the underlying disorder is indicated. Symptomatic relief may be obtained from antiseptic mouthwashes and avoidance of hot, spicy food, alcohol, and tobacco.

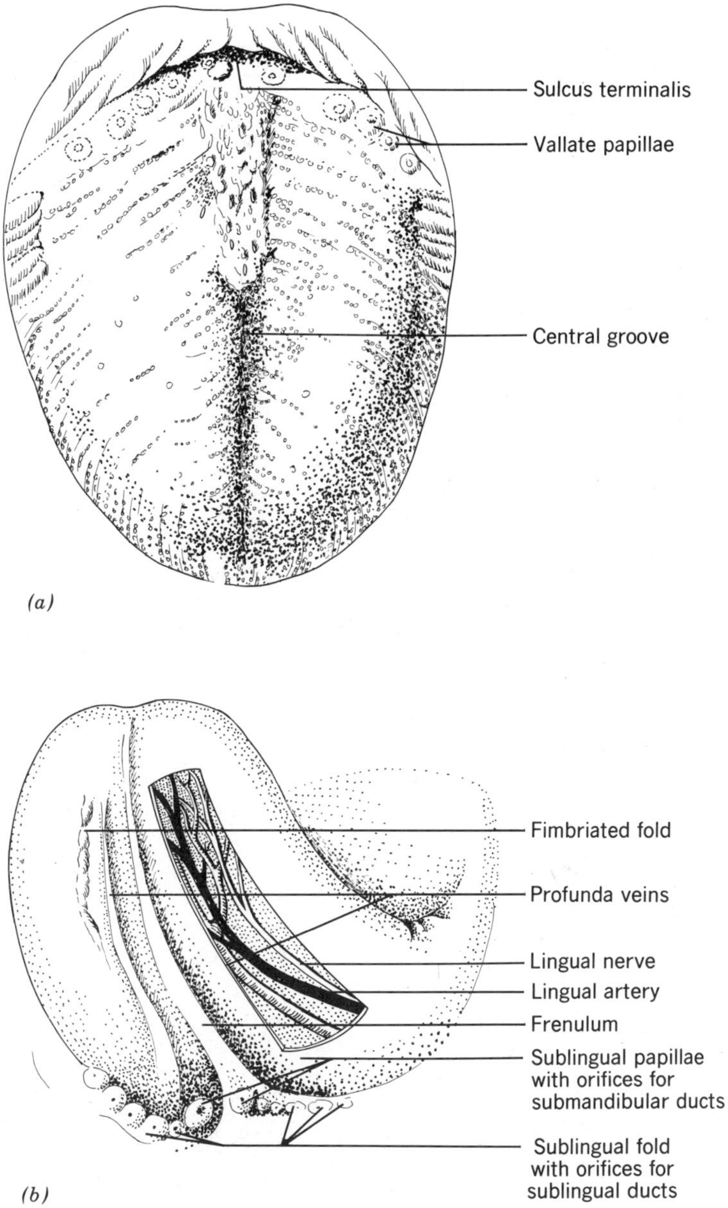

Figure 3.3 Tongue: (*a*) dorsum and (*b*) inferior surface.

Geographic tongue results from patchy areas of denuded epithelium that come and go. Since the cause is unknown, there is no curative treatment. As in the case of glossitis, avoidance of hot, spicy foods, alcohol, and tobacco, and the use of antiseptic mouthwashes, may provide some relief.

Taste receptors (taste buds) in the papillae respond to chemical substances dissolved in saliva. They are sensitive to four primary tastes: bitter, sweet, sour, and salt. The sense of taste is greatly enhanced by the sense of smell. Its loss, ***(hypoguesia),*** occurs with diseases of the tongue, injury to the seventh or ninth cranial nerve, or damage to the brain's sensory area for taste. Treatment is aimed at correcting the underlying disorder.

The sublingus (underside of the tongue) is visualized when the tongue is raised. It has a smooth, glistening appearance free of papillae. Extremely vascular and covered by only a thin layer of mucosa, the sublingual area can be used for the absorption of soluble drugs such as nitrites. The posterior lateral portion of the sublingus is a common site for squamous cell carcinoma of the oral cavity (see Table 3.4). Careful examination is therefore important. This is best accomplished by wrapping a folded gauze pad around the anterior tongue and gently pulling it outward and to the side.

The tongue attaches to the floor of the mouth via a fold of oral mucosa called the "frenulum." Congenital shortening of the frenulum reduces mobility of the tongue and interferes with normal speech. This ***tongue-tied*** condition is easily corrected by cutting the binding membrane.

Salivary Glands

There are three major pairs of salivary glands, as illustrated in Figure 3.4. The parotid glands are located near the angle of the jaw. They open into the oral cavity through Stenson's ducts opposite the two upper second molars. The submaxillary glands lie on the inner surface of the mandible and open through Wharton's ducts behind the lower incisors. Located beneath the mucous membranes of the floor of the mouth, the sublingual glands have several small ducts. A number of minor salivary glands also exist.

Each salivary gland produces a unique chemical substance. The composite of these various watery substances constitutes saliva. Salivary flow is affected by the type of gland, as well as by the season, time of day, and degree of stimulation. Averaging a liter a day in healthy adults, it cleanses the mouth and plays an important role in digestion. Saliva contains the enzyme ptyalin (which initiates the chemical breakdown of complex carbohydrates), as well as mucus (which lubricates food and helps prevent abrasion of the esophagus during swallowing).

Decreased salivary flow is one component of ***Sjögren's syndrome.*** Two other components are keratoconjunctivitis sicca and collagen disease (rheumatoid arthritis, scleroderma, systemic lupus erythematosus, or polymyositis). Involvement of the salivary and lacrimal glands without connective tissue association is called ***Mikulicz's syndrome*** (a benign lymphoepithelial lesion). It is unclear whether Sjögren's and Mikulicz's syndromes are different disorders or variations of the same process. They are thought to be autoimmune in origin. In addition to antibodies directed against the salivary gland, many patients have a number of other immunologic abnormalities. These include hypergammaglobulinemia, rheumatoid factor, antinuclear antibody, anti-DNA antibodies, and an elevated erythrocyte sedimentation rate. The disease presents between the ages of 40 and 60. Nearly 9 out of 10 patients are women. Symptoms of Sjögren's syndrome tend to develop gradu-

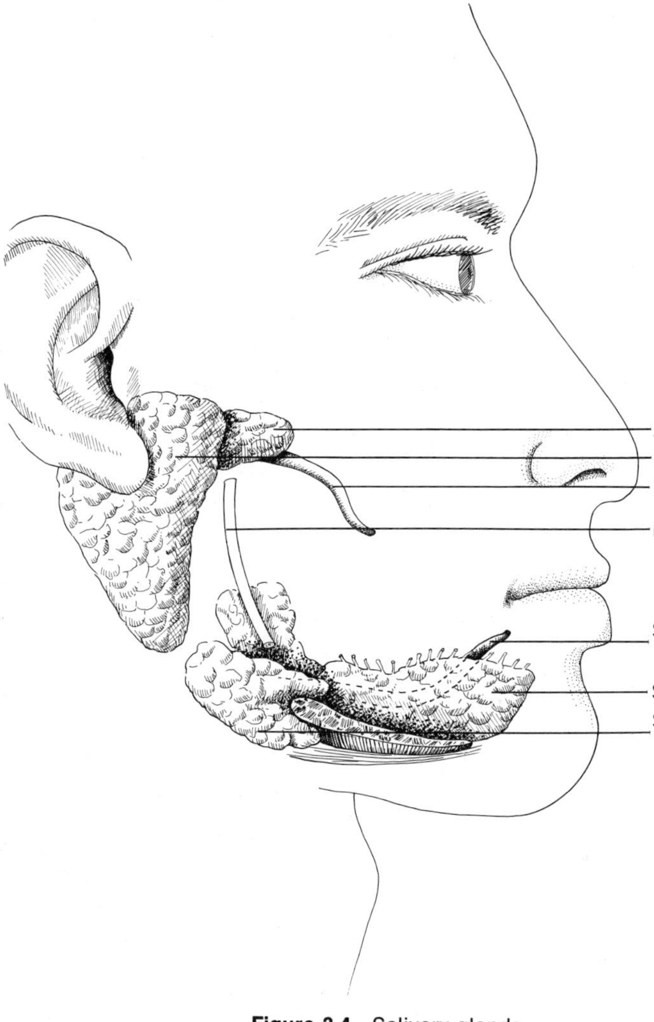

Figure 3.4 Salivary glands.

ally. Lack of saliva leads to a dried-out oral mucosa, which in turn results in dental caries, denture problems, or secondary infections of the mouth. Eventually, patients have difficulty in eating and find that they need sips of water in order to swallow food. Enlargement of the salivary glands (usually parotid or submandibular) is a variable finding. It may be unilateral or bilateral, intermittent or chronic, slight or severe.

Lacrimal gland involvement may lead to conjunctivitis or, more seriously, to corneal ulceration. Some patients experience dryness of the upper respiratory tract and/or genital mucosa as well. Problems related to collagen disease tend to develop later. Lymph node enlargement, most marked along the cervical chain, also occurs and is associated with the subsequent development of lymphoma. Several laboratory tests help to confirm the diagnosis of Sjögren's syndrome. In addition to a collagen work-up, the Schirmer test can be used to measure decreased tear production.

Parotid flow rate, minor salivary gland biopsy, or x-ray scans are used to evaluate salivary gland function. Sialography shows changes only in very advanced cases. Since the disorder is irreversible, little treatment may be offered. Instructing the patient to suck on sugarless candy may stimulate residual functioning of saliva glands. Topical methylcellulose of glycerin is often helpful in more advanced cases. Complications such as thrush, dental caries, and gingivitis should be cared for promptly. Their occurrence may be minimized by good oral hygiene.

Stone formation within a salivary gland or ductal system is called ***sialolithiasis.*** If the stones are small, the patient may be asymptomatic. Larger stones cause swelling and localized pain, especially at mealtime. The obstruction can be palpated or evaluated with special x-ray films called "sialograms." Sometimes giving plenty of liquids and stimulating salivary flow with warm compresses and sour candy clears the problem. If not, patients need to be referred to an oral surgeon for duct dilation or removal of the stone.

▶ ***Sialadenitis*** (bacterial parotitis) is a bacterial infection of the glands. Associated with decreased salivary flow, the condition is seen most often in the elderly, debilitated, or postoperative patient. It causes acute painful swelling, usually unilateral. There may be localized signs of heat and redness, along with generalized signs of fever and leukocytosis. Purulent drainage from the duct orifice confirms the diagnosis. After the drainage is cultured, patients should be started immediately on antibiotics and increased fluid intake. They should also be referred to an oral surgeon for possible surgical drainage. Aggressive treatment is important, since a number of deaths have been attributed to sialadenitis.

Mumps (viral parotitis) is an acute viral infection manifested by swelling of the salivary glands. The virus is transmitted by droplet infection of saliva for approximately 9 days before and 9 days after the onset of symptoms. The patient complains of fever, headache, and anorexia. Muscle pain may exist 24–48 hours prior to pain around the ear and jaw. Swollen parotid glands (unilateral or bilateral) are observed, and the ear lobe is distorted upward. Unilateral orchitis may occur within the first 2 weeks of infection, but sterility is a rare outcome. Other complications include meningoencephalitis, nerve deafness, and pancreatitis. For the most part, however, mumps is generally self-limited and no treatment is necessary. Patients should be isolated until gland swelling and other symptoms subside. Mumps immune globulin, once thought to protect exposed persons against the disease, is no longer manufactured.

Due to mandatory programs for ***childhood mumps immunization,*** mumps is

TABLE 3.7 NEOPLASTIC CHANGES OF THE SALIVARY GLANDS

Change	Description
Hypertrophy	Benign. Usually secondary to chronic alcoholism.
Pleomorphic adenoma (mixed tumor)	Malignant. Both major and accessory glands are affected; 60% are found in the parotid. Swelling in the parotid is very painful. Facial paralysis results if there is spread or if a facial nerve is compressed. In submandibular involvement, pain is encountered when the lingual branches or the trigeminal nerve are compressed.
Mucoepidermoid carcinoma	Malignant. As above.

now a rare disease. Mumps vaccine is usually given in combination with measles and rubella (MMR) at 12 months of age or older. Although 15% of reported cases occur in older patients, who suffer more severe illness (up to 20% of postpubescent men develop orchitis), ***adult mumps immunization*** is not recommended. For one thing, over 90% of older persons have natural immunity. Identifying the small number of persons who may still be susceptible remains the problem. Due to subclinical or forgotten cases of childhood disease, the history is unreliable. For screening purposes, skin tests are of no use, and immune titers are too expensive.

As described in Table 3.7, ***tumors of the salivary glands*** are usually benign. Adenocarcinoma, the most frequent malignant tumor, occurs primarily in the submaxillary and parotid glands. Both benign and malignant tumors cause gland enlargement, malignant enlargement occurring at a faster rate than benign enlargement. Pain develops when pressure is exerted on sensory nerves. Treatment is based on the type and extent of growth or spread.

Details of Management

▸ *Cold Sores (Herpes Simplex Type 1 Lesions)*

Laboratory Tests: None.

Therapeutic Measures: Although not specifically approved by the Food and Drug Administration (FDA) for oral lesions, acyclovir (Zovirax) ointment 5% applied topically q3h at the first signs of an outbreak may greatly alleviate the symptoms and shorten the course. Ascorbic acid, 400 mg tid, and/or lysine tablets, 500 mg tid for 3 days, beginning with the first signs may also prove helpful.

Patient Education: Explain the viral nature of herpes, the difference between oral and genital types, and the triggering factors. Note that the virus can be spread by kissing or by sharing cosmetics when lesions are present. Emphasize the importance of sun protection and good eating and sleeping habits, and stress reduction to minimize recurrences. Discourage the use of drying agents (alcohol, ether, chloroform) that may facilitate the invasion of resistant and mutagenic strains and corticosteroids, which can cause spread of the virus.

Follow-up: None.

▸ *Thrush*

Laboratory Tests: Smears or culture to isolate *C. albicans*.

Therapeutic Measures: Prescribe nystatin oral rinse (Mycostatin oral suspension) 100,000 U held in the mouth for 2 minutes and then swallowed qid for 10 days; or nystatin vaginal tablets (Mycostatin vaginal tablets) used as oral lozenges qid for 10 days; or Mycolex Troche, one lozenge five times daily for 14 days. To keep the mouth clean, advise the patient to rinse with $\frac{1}{2}$ tsp of sodium bicarbonate in 250 ml (8 oz) warm water.

Patient Education: Explain the fungal nature of thrush and its relationship to systemic disease, immunosuppression, or antibiotic therapy.

Follow-up: Patients should return for a general physical exam if the condition has not improved within 2 weeks. If no underlying disorder can be found, refer patients to an oral surgeon or ENT specialist for biopsy.

▸ *Canker Sore*

Laboratory Tests: Usually none. For recurrent or prolonged cases, check serum ferritin, vitamin B_{12}, and folic acid assays.

Therapeutic Measures: After applying topical lidocaine, debride individual ulcers by rubbing the surface with dry cotton gauze until light bleeding results. Prescribe tetracycline oral suspension (250 mg/15 ml); hold 1 tsp in the mouth for 2–5 minutes and then swallow, qid for 10 days. For pain, prescribe 2% viscous lidocaine; swish 1 tsp in the mouth and then expectorate q3h as needed. Treat underlying nutritional deficiencies as needed.

Patient Education: Note the possible causes. Reassure the patient that the ulcers are self-limiting. Warn the patient that recurrences are common and that thrush may result from tetracycline therapy.

Follow-up: If lesions do not heal.

▸ *Oral Self-Examination*

Laboratory Tests: None.

Therapeutic Measures: None.

Patient Education: Give patients a handout with the following instructions:

1. Neck and jaw: Using the right hand, check for lumps in the left neck and the area under the left jaw. Reverse the process and check the right side.
2. Lips: Look for color changes and feel for lumps on the outside. Pull the bottom lip down, using the thumb and forefinger. Check for color changes and feel the inside for lumps. Pull the top lip up and repeat the process.
3. Gums: With the lips pulled away, examine gums for color changes. Using the forefinger, feel for lumps.
4. Cheeks: Draw the right cheek away from the teeth by pulling on the corner of the mouth with the right thumb and forefinger. Using a good source of light, examine the inside for color changes. Close the mouth slightly and use the left fingers to feel for lumps. Reverse the process to examine the left cheek.
5. Tongue: Look at and touch the top surface of the extended tongue. Feel both sides of the tongue. Examine the underside by touching the tip of the tongue to the back roof of the mouth. Feel for lumps with the forefingers.
6. Palate: Tilting the head slightly backward and, using a good source of light, examine the roof of the mouth for color changes. Use the forefinger to check for scaling or lumps.

Follow-up: Yearly oral exams as part of a health physical or dental checkup.

▸ *Pericoronitis/Tooth Abscess*

Laboratory Tests: None.

Therapeutic Measures: Care is often initiated by the primary care giver. Prescribe penicillin V-K, 250–500 mg q6h; erythromycin, 250 mg q6h; or tetracycline, 250 mg q6h for 5 days. Give Tylenol with codeine, 30–60 mg q3–4h for pain relief. Advise the use of warm saline mouth rinses every 2–4 hours to induce fluctuation. Arrange a dental referral as soon as possible.

Patient Education: Stress the importance of following through on the dental referral, since abscesses can led to more serious infections (sinusitis, mastoiditis, meningitis).

Follow-up: Per specialist.

▸ *TMJ Syndrome*

Laboratory Tests: None.

Therapeutic Measures: Emphasize that resting jaw ligaments and avoiding further stretching is the main treatment. To relieve the pain caused by the associated muscle spasm, suggest the application of moist heat to the area for 5 minutes every half hour until acute symptoms subside.

Patient Education: Explain the etiology of the problem. Instruct patients on the following:

1. Avoid hard-to-chew foods such as nuts, crusts of bread, caramel, and gum.
2. Never bite off pieces of hard or brittle food with the front teeth. Instead, cut or tear food by hand into into bite-size pieces and chew the pieces slowly with the back teeth.
3. Limit the degree of mouth opening to less than 1 in. when laughing, yawning, or eating.
4. Avoid making protruding gestures of the jaw while talking, smoking, or applying lipstick.
5. Do not sleep with weight on the jaw.
6. Minimize jaw-clenching or teeth-grinding habits by keeping the lips together and the teeth apart.

Follow-up: If the above measures fail to reduce the symptoms, refer the patient to an orthodontist.

▸ *Good Oral Hygiene*

Laboratory Tests: None.

Therapeutic Measures: Advise brushing and flossing after every meal and regular use of mouthwashes. If this is not possible, suggest rinsing after food intake and/or eating detersive fruits and vegetables.

Patient Education: For the above procedures, provide specific information as follows:

Toothpaste: Use a fluoride toothpaste, since fluoride combines with tooth enamel, making it more resistant to decay. Not all fluoride toothpastes have been proven effective, so use only those that carry the seal of the American Dental Association Council on Dental Therapeutics. Some approved brands are Crest, Aim, Colgate MFP, Macleans Fluoride, and Aquafresh. Be sure that the toothpaste you choose is not too abrasive (it should be mildly abrasive), since use of very abrasive pastes wears away tooth enamel.

Toothbrush: Choose a brush with a straight handle; a flat, multitufted brushing surface and soft, rounded, polished bristles is best (electric toothbrushes are helpful for patients with poor manual dexterity). Avoid hard-bristle brushes, since their use can cause gum irritation and recession. Replace toothbrushes every 3–4 months.

Correct brushing: Place the head of the brush along the side of the teeth with the bristle tips angled against the gum line. Using short strokes and a gentle scrubbing motion, move the brush back and forth. With the bristles angled against the gum line, brush the outer surface of all teeth. Scrub the biting surfaces of all teeth. Tilting the brush vertically and using its "toe" (front tip), clean the inside surfaces of all the teeth and gum tissue with several gentle up-and-down strokes. Gently brush the tongue to give the mouth a fresher feeling. Refrain from compulsive brushing, since it can wear away tooth enamel.

Correct flossing: Break off about 18 in. of floss. Wind some of it around the middle finger of one hand and the rest around the finger of the opposite hand (the source of fresh floss for each tooth). Using the thumb and forefinger with an in. of taut floss between them, gently guide the floss between the two teeth to the gum line (never "snap" it). Once at the gum line, curve the floss into a C shape against one tooth and gently slide it into the space between the gum and the tooth until there is resistance. Move the floss up and down away from the gum against the side of the tooth. Repeat this procedure on the rest of the teeth. Establish a pattern that ensures flossing of all gum surfaces.

Rinsing and detersive foods: When brushing and flossing is not possible after eating, rinse the mouth to remove excess food debris. Eating raw cauliflower, celery, carrots, or an apple at the end of a meal also helps control plaque.

Water Pik and interdental devices: As an additional option (never as a substitute for brushing and flossing), use oral water irrigating devices (Water Pik) and interdental devices (rubber-tipped toothbrushes or toothpicks) to remove loose food debris and/or to clean around fixed bridgework or orthodontic appliances.

Mouthwash: Consider the regular use of Listerine, Scope, and another approved antiseptic mouthwash to reduce harmful mouth bacteria. After brushing, rinse the oral cavity with $\frac{1}{2}$ oz of mouthwash for 20 seconds and then expectorate. Discontinue this practice if irritation develops.

Disclosing substances: To evaluate the effectiveness of brushing and flossing techniques, staining (disclosing) solutions or tablets can be used to reveal plaque.

Follow-up: Review good oral hygiene with patients during health maintenance exams or during visits for other medical problems.

▸ *Prevention and Control of Dental Caries in Adults*

Laboratory Tests: None.

Therapeutic Measures: Institute measures for good oral hygiene. Reduce the amount of sticky, retentive sucrose in the diet and foods that can erode enamel directly. Encourage regular dental checkups and prompt evaluation for symptoms of caries.

Patient Education: For the above procedures, provide specific information as follows:

Oral hygiene: See above.

Diet: Limit candy, cake, cookies, pastry, ice cream, candied popcorn/apples, gum, honey, peanut butter and jelly sandwiches, graham crackers, dried fruits, raisins, hard candies, lollipops, breath mints, and cough drops, particularly between meals. Have milk, cheese, luncheon meats, raw fruits/vegetables, unsweetened fruit juice, vegetable juice, crackers, toast, pretzels, corn chips, or popcorn for between-meal snacks instead. Do not eat raw lemons, limes, or citrus fruit peelings. Limit carbonated beverages.

Regular dental checkups: See your dentist once or twice a year for routine checkups and dental cleaning.

Signs and symptoms of caries: See your dentist immediately if a tooth develops sensitivity to heat, cold, or sweets or becomes painful when chewing.

Follow-up: Per dentist.

▸ *Acute Necrotizing Ulcerative Gingivitis*

Laboratory Tests: None.

Therapeutic Measures: Prescribe Pen VK, 250 mg qid, or tetracycline, 250 mg qid, for 7 days. Start patients on mouth rinses of 3 oz hydrogen peroxide mixed with 3 oz warm water swished and expectorated bid. Arrange a dental referral for scaling by day 5 of antibiotic treatment.

Patient Education: Explain the bacterial nature of the infection and the relationship to poor oral hygiene. Stress the importance of dental follow-up to prevent periodontal disease. Reassure the patient that with proper treatment, the problem will resolve.

Follow-up: Per dentist.

▸ *Prevention and Control of Periodontal Disease*

Laboratory Tests: None.

Therapeutic Measures: Stress the importance of good oral hygiene to prevent plaque buildup and routine dental cleanings to remove tartar (tartar cannot be removed by brushing and flossing alone). Evaluate patients for signs and symptoms of gum disease and urge prompt dental attention. Reinforce the Keyes method if advised by the dentist.

Patient Education: For the above measures, provide specific directions as follows:

Good oral hygiene: See the previous section.

Routine dental cleanings: Have dental cleanings with scaling at least once a year (persons with malocclusions, smokers, or others who are prone to tartar formation should be seen every 6 months).

Signs and symptoms of periodontal disease requiring immediate dental attention.

1. Bleeding of gums when the teeth are brushed.
2. Redness, swelling, or tenderness or recession of gums.
3. Bad breath.
4. Expression of pus along gum lines.
5. Loosened or separating teeth.
6. Change in bit or the fit of bridges.

Keyes method:

Weekly

1. Mix 1 tsp baking soda and a capful of 3% peroxide in 2 oz of water.
2. Smear the mixture across the necks of the teeth with a finger or rubber tip.
3. Work the mixture into the gum crevice with the tip.
4. Do this throughout the entire mouth on both the cheek and the tongue side.
5. Floss.
6. Brush with the mixture that is left after completing steps 1–3.

Daily

1. Using only baking soda, complete the procedures described above.

Patient Education: Describe the causes and progressive nature of peridontal disease to emphasize the importance of the above measures. Note that gum disease is the number one cause of tooth loss in adults.

Follow-up: Evaluate patients for signs of gum disease as part of routine health maintenance.

▸ *First Aid for Mouth Trauma*

Laboratory Tests: None.

Therapeutic Measures

Knocked-out tooth: Place the tooth in water or wrap it in a piece of gauze (do not clean the tooth). Arrange emergency referral to a dentist.

Broken tooth: Clean dirt and debris from the injured area with warm water. Apply cold compresses on the face next to the injured area to reduce swelling. Arrange a dental referral as soon as possible.

Irritation from braces: If a wire or piece of jagged metal is irritating the cheek or gums, cover the end with cotton or gauze and advise immediate orthodontic evaluation. Have the patient save and bring any broken parts to the orthodontist. Do not attempt to remove wires or embedded metal.

Bitten tongue or lip: Place direct pressure on the bleeding area with a clean cloth. Apply cold compresses to reduce swelling. Send patients with severe injuries to the emergency room for further treatment.

Object wedged between teeth: Try to remove the object with dental floss, never with a sharp or pointed instrument. If removal is unsuccessful, arrange a dental referral as soon as possible.

Possible fractured jaw: Immobilize the jaw with a handkerchief, tie, or towel and send the patient to the emergency room.

Patient Education: Reinforce appropriate use of seat belts and mouth guards as preventive measures.

Follow-up: Per specialist.

▸ *Denture Care*

Laboratory Tests: None.

Therapeutic Measures: None.

Patient Education: Reinforce information provided by the dentist, such as the following:

General adjustments: Expect new dentures to feel bulky, cause the tongue to feel crowded, or cause a slight gagging sensation. Until the muscles of the cheeks and tongue develop, dentures may loosen and tip when chewing or talking.

Eating: In the beginning, select soft foods. Gradually progress to coarser foods. Since the mouth is less sensitive with dentures in place, be sure to remove all bones when preparing foods and allow hot foods and liquids to cool. Cut food into small pieces. Avoid very hard or sticky foods. Always chew slowly and at the back of the mouth to avoid tipping dentures.

Speaking: In the beginning, read aloud to hasten adjustment to new dentures. Speak slowly to prevent clicking (if clicking persists, consult a dentist).

Denture care: At least once a day, remove dentures and brush them thoroughly with a special dentrifrice and denture brush (available at most drugstores). Remove persistent stains and calculus with nonabrasive household cleansers (e.g., Clorox if dentures contain no metal parts) or white vinegar. Thoroughly rinse dentures after cleaning and before inserting in mouth. Whenever dentures are not in the mouth, store them in water or a cleansing solution (dry dentures lose their shape). Never place dentures in hot solutions or water, since heat can warp plastic fittings. Always handle dentures with care; if dropped, porcelain teeth can break. Never attempt do-it-yourself adjustments. Ill-fitting dentures can cause a premalignant change due to chronic irritation and should always be evaluated by the dentist.

Oral care: Rinse the mouth thoroughly with a warm saline solution after each meal and before retiring. Brush the tongue, palate, and gums gently with a soft-bristled brush daily to remove plaque and stimulate circulation.

Follow-up: Careful oral exams with dentures in place and removed as part of routine health examinations.

▸ *Sialadenitis*

Laboratory Tests: Culture and sensitivity of duct drainage.

Therapeutic Measures: Start an antistaphylococcal penicillin such as dicloxacillin 250 mg qid or a cephalosporin such as Keflex 250 mg qid for 5–10 days. As a less expensive alternative, erythromycin 250 mg qid may also be used. Increase fluid intake to 6–8 full glasses daily. Arrange immediate ENT referral for possible surgical excision and drainage.

Patient Education: Stress the importance of following through on the ENT referral. Review good oral hygiene measures, since they are important in preventing the disease.

Follow-up: Per specialist.

BIBLIOGRAPHY

American Dental Association. *Dentures: What You Don't Know Can Hurt You.* Pamphlet G-35. Chicago, 1978.

American Dental Association. *What to Do After the Extraction of a Tooth.* Pamphlet G-20. Chicago, 1980.

American Dental Association. *Your New Dentures.* Pamphlet G-4. Chicago, 1980.

American Dental Association. *Como Limpiar los Dientes y las Encilas.* Pamphlet W-136 (Spanish). Chicago, 1981.

American Dental Association. Keyes technique. *ADA News,* Dec. 14, 1981.

Bates B. *A Guide to Physical Examination,* 3rd ed. Lippincott, Philadelphia, 1983.

Berkow RB (ed.). *The Merck Manual of Diagnosis and Therapy,* 14th ed. Merck, Sharp & Dohme Research Laboratories, Rahway, N.J., 1982.

Brand R, Isselhard D. *Anatomy of Orofacial Structures.* Mosby, St. Louis, 1977.

Brown AM, Stubbs DW (eds.). *Medical Physiology.* Wiley, New York, 1983.

Brown R, Clinton D. Vesicular and ulcerative infections of the mouth and oropharynx. *Postgraduate Medicine,* (Feb.) 1980, 67(2):107–116.

Burket L (Lynch M, ed.). *Burket's Oral Medicine,* 7th ed. Lippincott, Philadelphia, 1977, 2–24.

Colwell Systems, Inc. *Information on Periodontal Diseases.* Pamphlet 4946, Champaign, Ill.

Conn HF, Conn RB Jr (eds.). *Current Diagnosis.* Saunders, Philadelphia, 1980.

Conn R (ed.). *Current Therapy.* Saunders, Philadelphia, 1983.

Crafts RC. *A Textbook of Human Anatomy.* 3rd ed. Wiley, New York, 1985.

Crouch JE, McClintic JR. *Human Anatomy and Physiology,* 2nd ed. Wiley, New York, 1976.

Dreizen S. Aphthous ulcers. *Postgraduate Medicine,* (June) 1981, 69(6):158.

Elias H, Pauly JE, Burns ER. *Histology and Human Microanatomy,* 4th ed. Wiley, New York, 1978.

Friedman MH, Weisberg J. Screening procedures for temporomandibular joint dysfunction. *American Family Physician,* (June) 1982, 25(6):157–160.

Goldberg MH, Nemarich AN, Marco WP. The impacted third molar: Referral patterns, patient compliance, and surgical requirements. *Journal of the American Dental Association,* (Sept.) 1983, 107:439–441.

Gorlin RJ, Goldman HM (eds.). *Thomas's Oral Pathology,* Vols. 1 and 2. Mosby, St. Louis, 1970.

Gray H. *Anatomy of the Human Body,* 29th American ed. (CM Goss, ed.). Lea & Febiger, Philadelphia, 1973.

Guichet NF. The night grind. *Family Health,* (June) 1970.

Guyton AC. *Textbook of Medical Physiology,* 6th ed. Saunders, Philadelphia, 1981.

Hefley DC, et al. Periodontal disease. *Physician Assistant and Health Practitioner,* (Oct.) 1982, 99–104.

Hess JW, Margolis FJ. The physician's role in caries prevention. *American Family Physician,* (Oct.) 1981, 24(4):171–173.

Hoole AJ, Greenberg RA, Pickard CG Jr. *Patient Care Guidelines for Nurse Practitioners.* Little, Brown, Boston, 1982.

Isselbacher KJ, et al. *Harrison's Principles of Internal Medicine,* 9th ed. McGraw-Hill, New York, 1980.

Johnson J, Edwards P. The asymptomatic smooth palatal mass. *Postgraduate Medicine,* (Sept.) 1980, 68(3):96–104.

Johnson J, Newman R, Olson J. Persistent hoarseness. *Postgraduate Medicine,* (May) 1980, 67(5):122–126.

Kamen S, Tideiksaar R. Dental care for geriatric patients. *Physician Assistant and Health Practitioner,* (Dec.) 1982, 31–46.

Kasanof D (staff ed.). Current care for pharyngitis. *Patient Care,* (Dec. 15) 1980, 50–91.

Krupp MA, Chatton MJ, Werdegar D (eds.). *Current Medical Diagnosis and Treatment 1985.* Lange, Los Altos, Calif., 1985.

Last JM (ed.). *Maxcy-Rosenau Public Health and Preventive Medicine,* 11th ed. Appleton-Century-Crofts, New York, 1980.

Luckmann J, Sorensen KC. *Medical Surgical Nursing: A Psychophysiologic Approach,* 2nd ed. Saunders, Philadelphia, 1980.

Mandell GL, Douglas RG Jr, Bennett JE. *Principles and Practice of Infectious Diseases,* 2nd ed. Wiley, New York, 1985.

Maxey K, Rosenau M (Last J, ed.). *Public Health and Preventive Medicine,* 11th ed. Appleton-Century-Crofts, New York, 1980.

Meyers BR, Lawson W. Infections of the oral cavity, in Mandell GL, Douglas RG Jr, Bennett JE (eds.): *Principles and Practice of Infectious Diseases.* Wiley, New York, 1979, 466–480.

Miller AJ, Brunelle JA. A summary of the NIDR community caries prevention demonstration program. *Journal of the American Dental Association.* (Aug.) 1983, 107:265–269.

National Institute of Dental Research. *Tooth Decay.* NIDR pamphlet 81-1146. April 1981.

National Institute of Dental Research. New directions for improving oral health. *Journal of the American Dental Association,* (Mar.) 1983, 106:304–313.

Newland JR, Fasser CE, Smith QW, et al. Clinical diagnosis of localized intraoral swellings. *Physician Assistant and Health Practitioner,* (Jan.) 1983, 88–99.

Schwartz R, Quinnell R. Throat cultures in the office. *American Family Physician,* (June) 1980, 21(6):72–78.

Silverstein A. Anatomy of the digestive system, in *Human Anatomy and Physiology.* Wiley, New York, 1980.

Smith QW, et al. Dental caries. *Physician Assistant and Health Practitioner,* (Sept.) 1982, 32–36.

Topazian RG, Goldberg MH. *Management of Infections of the Oral and Maxillofacial Regions.* Saunders, Philadelphia, 1981.

Van Sickels JE, Dolwick MF. The patient with temporomandibular joint pain. *Physician Assistant.* (Aug.) 1983, 63–69.

Wyngaarden JB, Smith LH Jr (eds.). *Cecil Textbook of Medicine,* 16th ed., Vols. 1 and 2. Saunders, Philadelphia, 1982.

Zegarelli E, Kutscher A, Hyman G. *Diagnosis of Diseases of the Mouth and Jaws.* Lea and Febiger, Philadelphia, 1980.

4

Gastrointestinal Tract

Bonnie Friedman

Outline

The gastrointestinal tract is a long, muscular tube that propels and mixes gastrointestinal contents, secretes digestive juices, digests food, and absorbs nutrients. It is divided into the esophagus, stomach, small intestine, colon, and rectum (Fig. 4.1).

ESOPHAGUS

The esophagus extends from the cricopharyngeus muscle, or upper esophageal sphincter (UES), down to and including the lower esophageal sphincter (LES). About 25 cm long and 2 cm in diameter, it lies posterior to the heart and trachea and passes through a hiatus in the diaphragm, as illustrated in Figure 4.2.

Across the lumen of the upper esophagus, a thin membrane known as an ***esophageal web*** may form. Composed of squamous epithelium, it is occasionally congenital but more commonly is the result of ulceration, local infection, hemorrhage or mechanical trauma, or exostoses of cervical vertebrae. In premenopausal women with severe iron deficiency, a diaphanous web can develop along with splenomegaly, glossitis, and spooning of the nails ***(Plummer-Vinson syndrome).*** Most esophageal webs cause significant dysphagia for solid foods. Often missed on routine barium swallow, they are best diagnosed by cinefilms. Esophagoscopy is mandatory to rule out carcinoma and may be curative by disrupting the membrane. In some cases, bougienage is necessary.

The walls of the esophagus contain layers of smooth muscle. During swallowing, muscular action creates peristaltic waves that carry food from the pharynx to the

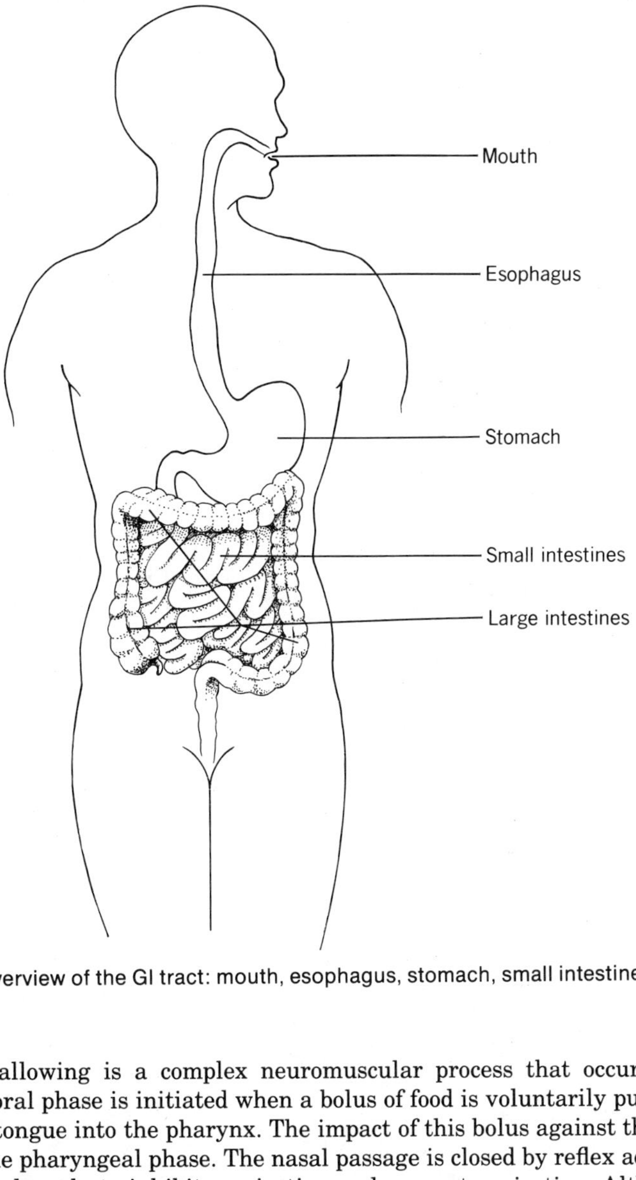

Figure 4.1 Overview of the GI tract: mouth, esophagus, stomach, small intestines, and large intestines.

stomach. Swallowing is a complex neuromuscular process that occurs in three phases. The oral phase is initiated when a bolus of food is voluntarily pushed backward by the tongue into the pharynx. The impact of this bolus against the pharynx stimulates the pharyngeal phase. The nasal passage is closed by reflex action of the soft palate and uvula to inhibit respiration and prevent aspiration. Although it is impossible to inhale and swallow at the same time, it is possible to swallow significant amounts of air. Caused by habitual mouth breathing, ill-fitting dentures, nasal obstruction, or postnasal drip, ***air swallowing*** may lead to the development of gastrointestinal gas. This problem is discussed further in a later section.

While the nasal passage is closed, the third phase of swallowing, the esophageal phase, incorporates peristaltic waves that propel food down to the LES. Motor function of the upper esophagus is controlled by the glossopharyngeal nerve, and the remainder of the esophagus is controlled by the vagus nerve.

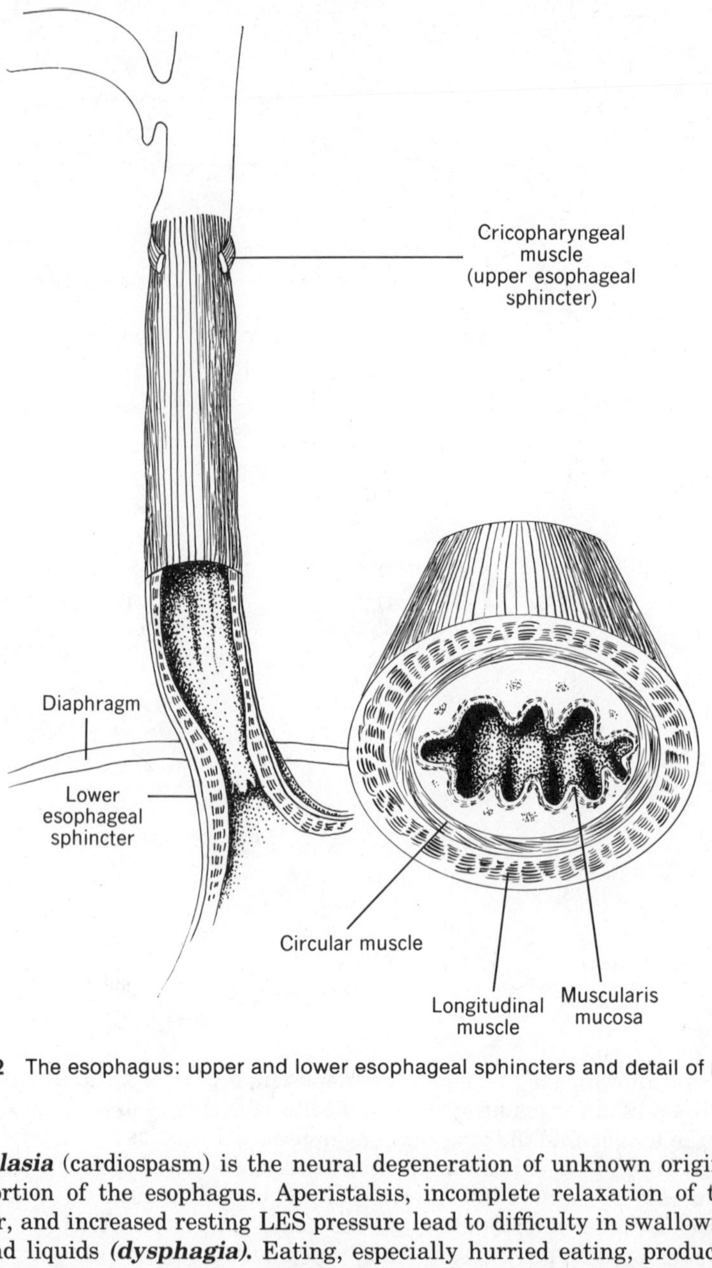

Figure 4.2 The esophagus: upper and lower esophageal sphincters and detail of muscular walls.

Achalasia (cardiospasm) is the neural degeneration of unknown origin in the lower portion of the esophagus. Aperistalsis, incomplete relaxation of the LES sphincter, and increased resting LES pressure lead to difficulty in swallowing both solids and liquids ***(dysphagia).*** Eating, especially hurried eating, produces spasmodic substernal pain. Initial symptoms usually begin in middle age and gradually worsen over months or years. Weight loss is common. As the disease progresses, dilatation of the esophagus results in regurgitation of food. Patients with this history should be referred to a gastroenterologist for manometry and endoscopy. A barium x-ray film shows a classic beak-like narrowing of the lower esophagus. The treatment is surgical correction.

TABLE 4.1 CAUSES OF DYSPHAGIA

Nonesophageal	Esophageal
Cerebral vascular accident	Obstructive
Myasthenia gravis	Tumor
Muscular dystrophy	Esophageal stricture (acid or alkali ingestion, chronic stomach acid reflux, prolonged herpes or monilial infection, nasogastric intubation)
Amyotrophic lateral sclerosis	Motor
Parkinson's disease	Achalasia
Bulbar polio	Scleroderma
Enlarged thyroid	Diffuse esophageal spasm
Aortic aneurysm	Presbyesophagus
Mediastinal tumor	Schatzki's ring
	Esophageal web

Ineffective peristaltic contractions and prolonged esophageal emptying time also develop as a result of aging. Failure of the LES to relax, with progressive difficulty in swallowing, is then known as ***presbyesophagus.***

Abnormal deposits of connective tissue cause esophageal dysfunction in 80% of patients with ***scleroderma*** (see Chapter 11). Other causes of dysphagia are listed in Table 4.1. Unless the underlying problem can be corrected, treatment of dysphagia centers on measures to ease swallowing and minimize the possibility of aspiration. Eating soft foods, eating slowly, and drinking only small amounts of fluids at a time may be helpful. Good posture and upright positions while eating are also important.

Disorders of esophageal motility are often associated with ▶ ***diffuse esophageal spasm.*** This is not a specific disease but a sensation of pain caused by spastic contractions that irritate sensory nerve fibers in esophageal tissue. The sharp substernal pain may be confused with angina, particularly since it is described as being "squeezing" or "pressing." Symptoms frequently occur at night and may be triggered by eating, by tension, or by drinking very hot or very cold liquids. The condition is suspected by the patient's history and confirmed by barium swallow. In mild cases of esophageal spasm, reassurance is frequently all that is necessary. Antacid therapy, eating small meals, and elevating the head of the bed provide symptomatic relief. When prescribing antacids (for esophageal spasm or various other gastrointestinal disturbances), the buffering capacity and sodium content of the various brands should always be considered. These are noted in Table 4.2.

Once the bolus of food has been milked down the esophagus, the LES relaxes briefly so that it can enter the stomach. Sphincter tone is quickly restored and the area is maintained under high pressure (12–30 mm Hg) to prevent any backwash of gastric fluids. The esophageal mucosa is normally alkaline and unable to tolerate the highly acidic contents of the stomach. An incompetent LES leads to ▶ ***esophageal reflux,*** with symptoms of heartburn and indigestion. Heartburn is a burning sensation that starts behind the sternum and rises toward the throat. It usually develops after large meals containing fatty, spicy, high-acid foods, alcohol, and caffeine, and is aggravated by lying down, bending, or stooping. Some patients experience an upwash of acid liquid or bile into the mouth (pyrosis). Persons with symptomatic esophageal reflux have an LES pressure of less than 10 mm Hg. Pregnancy, obesity, and ***hiatus hernia,*** a benign condition whereby a portion of the stomach slips up through the diaphragm, may be contributing factors. It should be noted that

TABLE 4.2 BUFFERING CAPACITIES AND SODIUM CONTENT OF COMMON LIQUID ANTACIDS

Antacid	Contents	mEq of Buffer per 30 ml	Number of Milliliters Needed for a 140-mEq Dose	Sodium Content per 30 ml
Mylanta II[a]	Mg-Al[b] hydroxides	124	34	8
Maalox	Mg-Al hydroxide gel	78	54	15
DiGel	Mg-Al hydroxides	76	58	5
Riopan[c]	Mg-Al hydroxides	66	64	4
Amphojel	Al hydroxide gel	58	74	23
Gelusil	Mg-trisilicate Al hydroxide gel	40	108	5

[a] Mylanta II has best buffering dose per milliliter and a low sodium content.
[b] Mg-Al, magnesium-aluminum.
[c] Riopan has the lowest sodium content.

hiatus hernia can be present without causing esophageal reflux. On the other hand, a number of hormones, foods, drugs, and positions raise or lower LES pressures, as described in Table 4.3. This information can be helpful in managing the problem. Antacid therapy is the other mainstay of treatment.

Chronic esophageal reflux can cause ►***esophagitis,*** an inflammation of the esophageal mucosa with changes in epithelial architecture. Esophagitis leads to bleeding and stricture formation. Patients have symptoms of reflux that are not improved by medical therapy. The diagnosis is suspected by the results of barium swallow and endoscopy and confirmed by a biopsy demonstrating inflammatory changes. Management includes all antireflux measures as well as agents to block gastric secretion (e.g., cimetidine). If this does not help, surgery may be necessary.

When normal squamous epithelium is completely destroyed and replaced by columnar epithelium similar to that found in gastric mucosal lining, the complication is called ***Barrett's esophagitis.*** This change in cell structure is one of the main risk factors in the development of ***esophageal cancer.*** Others are heavy smoking or alcohol use or previous severe corrosive burns of the esophagus. The victims are usually over 60, and 80% are men. One of the first signs of esophageal cancer is progressive difficulty in swallowing solids. Substernal burning may occur when hot liquids are swallowed. Pain under the sternum, in the back, or in the neck may be caused by spasm, esophagitis, or spread of the tumor through the wall of the esophagus. With severe stenosis, regurgitation of esophageal contents is common. Diagnosis is by barium x-ray substantiated by esophagoscopy, biopsy, and brushings of the lesion for cytological examination. Patients should be referred to a specialist for treatment, which may include surgery, radiation, or a combination of these modes. Palliative measures include dilatation or placement of a silastic tube through the affected area. Metastasis to the liver or lung occurs frequently, and to bone, the kidneys, or the adrenal glands occasionally. There may be dramatic invasion of adjoining structures, such as aortic perforation.

Zenker's diverticulum is a pouch that occurs in the posterior portion of the upper esophagus. It is seen mostly in men over age 60. Symptoms include dysphagia, regurgitation of stagnant food, and nocturnal coughing. There may be fullness or a

TABLE 4.3 COMMON FACTORS THAT AFFECT LES PRESSURE

Factor	Increase	Decrease	Mechanism of Action	Comments
Foods				
Protein	Yes		Gastrin release.	Gastrin is a gastric secreted hormone known to increase LES pressure.
Carbohydrate	Yes, slight		Gastrin release probable.	
Fat		Yes	Cholecystokinin.	Cholecystokinin is a hormone secreted by the duodenum that induces gallbladder contraction.
Orange/tomato products		Yes	Uncertain; probable local effect.	
Chocolate		Yes	Increased cyclic adenosine monophosphate (cAMP), which has a direct effect on muscles.	Intracellular cAMP promotes specific function of organs.
Drugs				
Ethanol				
Low dose	Yes		Gastrin release.	
High dose		Yes	Direct smooth muscle relaxation.	
Nicotine (smoking)		Yes	Unknown; probable smooth muscle relaxation.	
Nitrates/nitrites		Yes	Smooth muscle relaxation.	Nitrites can be helpful in treatment of diffuse esophageal spasm.
Atropine		Yes	Decreases tone of LES through inhibition of vagal impulses.	
Xanthines (caffeine, theophylline)		Yes	Smooth muscle relaxation.	
Isoproterenol		Yes	Relaxes smooth muscle.	
Bethanecol (Urecholine)	Yes		LES stimulation.	
Hormones				
Progesterone (oral contraceptives)		Yes	Not known; possible smooth muscle relaxation.	Lower LES pressures also seen during all phases of pregnancy.
Position				
Recumbent, bending		Yes	Antigravity; increase in intra-abdominal pressure with poor LES response.	

visible bulge in the neck. X-ray films with contrast material are diagnostic. Patients should be referred to a surgeon for myotomy or diverticulectomy. Small diverticulae in the middle and distal esophagus are usually not symptomatic.

In the distal portion of the esophagus, a congenital abnormality of the submucosa known as ***Schatzki's ring*** may cause narrowing of the lumen. Persons with small ring formations and lumen diameters that remain greater than 2 cm are usually asymptomatic. However, larger rings may result in dysphagia for solid foods or even obstruction. The problem is diagnosed by barium swallow and corrected with endoscopic rupture, pneumatic dilatation, or surgical resection. Milder cases may be managed by diet modifications alone. These include soft or blenderized foods, slow thorough chewing, and upright eating positions.

The cardioesophageal junction is the site of ***esophageal varices.*** These are collateral channels of thin-walled, dilated veins that are subject to massive, life-threatening bleeds. They develop as a consequence of portal hypertension and as a major complication of liver disease (see Chapter 5).

STOMACH

The stomach is divided into the fundus, body (forming the greater and lesser curvatures), and pyloric antrum. It lies somewhat obliquely, from left to right, across the left upper quadrant and epigastrium of the abdomen. The diaphragm is above it and the transverse colon below it (Fig. 4.3). Its shape, size, and position depend a great deal on body build, age, posture, and degree of gastric distention.

The inner mucosal layer of the stomach is arranged in longitudinal folds called "rugae," which allow for distention. The relaxed stomach can adapt to an increase in volume (up to a normal capacity of 1,000–2,000 cc) with no increase in pressure. Three types of glands are found in the mucosal layer and are named "cardiac," "gastric," and "pyloric" according to their location. As described in Table 4.4, these glands contain a variety of cells that produce mucus for protection, as well as hydrochloric acid (HCl), enzymes, and gastrin for digestion. In addition, parietal cells secrete intrinsic factor, a transporting agent essential for vitamin B_{12} absorption. Damage to the parietal cells from gastric surgery or disease leads to ***pernicious anemia*** (see Chapter 7).

Gastric secretion takes place in phases before, during, and after the time food is in the stomach. Initiated by the vagus nerve, the cephalic phase stimulates gastric glands to produce HCl, pepsinogen, and mucus at the first thought, sight, or taste of food. Vagal stimulation, which can result in up to 500 ml of gastric secretions per hour, continues throughout the gastric phase. As food enters the stomach, it sets off vagal nerve endings found in the mucosa. In addition, both the bulk of food stretching the antrum and local stimulation by substances such as digested proteins, alcohol, and caffeine cause the release of gastrin. Gastrin is absorbed by the blood and carried to the gastric glands, where it stimulates low rates of secretion (200 ml/h) for the several hours during which food remains in the stomach. Together, vagal and gastrin stimulation cause gastric secretions to peak after meals.

Food is continuously mixed by peristaltic waves of the stomach walls and then propelled by stronger contractions into the duodenum. Gastric emptying is controlled by the pyloric sphincter, which is influenced by volume, viscosity, acidity, physiological or emotional state, and exercise. External heat retards gastric empty-

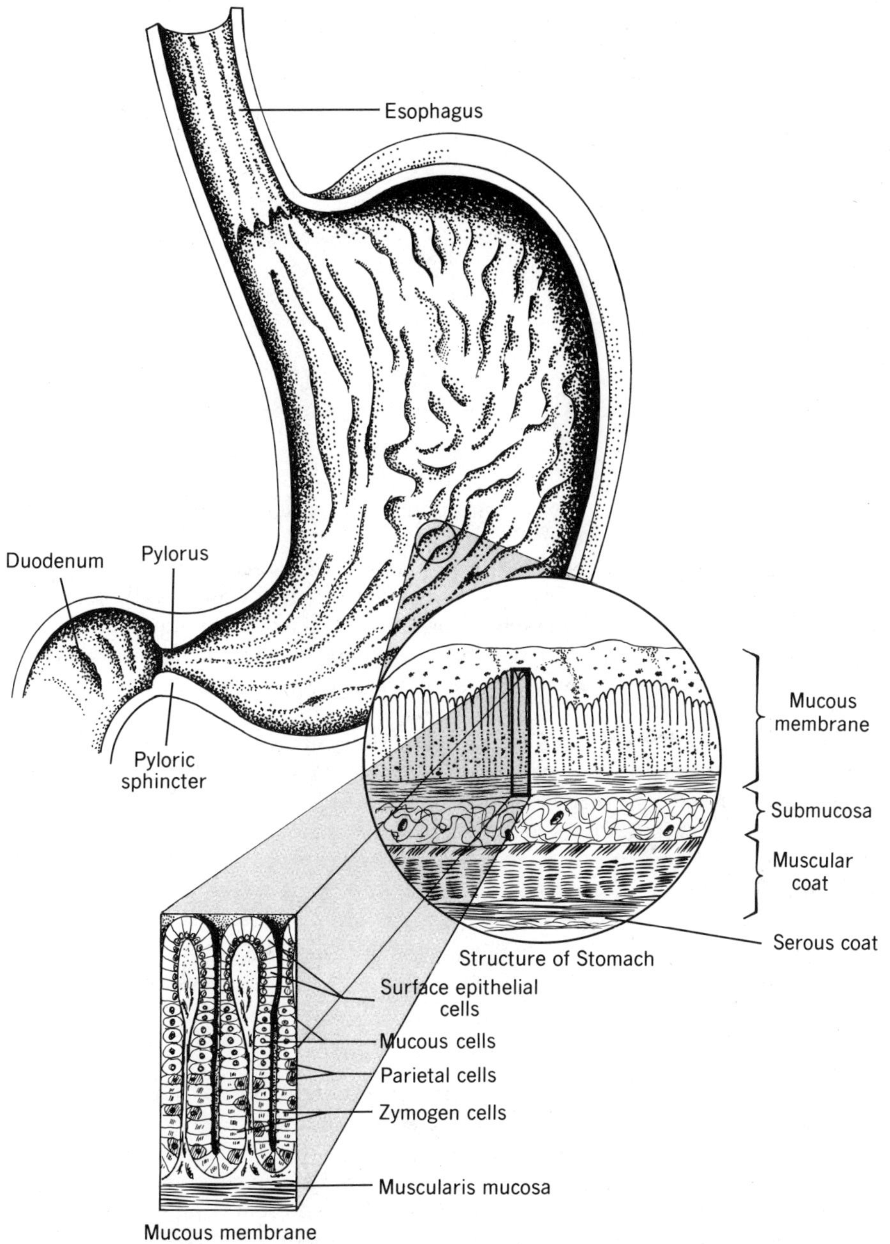

Figure 4.3 The stomach: relationship to esophagus and duodenum, pyloric sphincter, and detail of mucosal layers.

TABLE 4.4 STOMACH GLANDS

Gland	Cells/Secretion	Action
Cardiac	Mucous	Protective lubrication.
Gastric	Chief cells: pepsinogen, HCl, pepsin	Protein digestion.
	Parietal cells:	
	HCl	Protein digestion.
	Intrinsic factor	Absorption of vitamin B_{12} in distal small bowel.
	Neck cells: mucus	Protective lubrication.
Pyloric	Gastrin	Stimulates secretion of HCl, pepsin, intrinsic factor; stimulates gastric and intestinal motility; promotes receptive relaxation of stomach.

ing and cold accelerates it. The pyloric sphincter also helps to prevent backflow of duodenal contents into the stomach.

If the stomach (or any part of the gastroinestinal tract) becomes excessively irritated or distended, impulses are transmitted to the vomiting center of the medulla, which initiates contractions of the diaphragm and abdominal muscles. The stomach and its contents are squeezed between them, and ***vomiting*** results. Vomiting is a symptom, the circumstances of which often provide valuable diagnostic information (Table 4.5).

Although pepsin has profound proteolytic activity and gastric acid has a pH of 0.8 (4 million times the hydrogen ion concentration of arterial blood), the stomach mucosa is able to resist their corrosive effects. Mucus secretions coat and neutralize the surfaces to some extent. However, most of the protection comes from the gastric mucosal barrier. This tight junction formed between the epithelial cell surfaces prevents a back fusion of hydrogen ions into underlying tissue. When the mucosal barrier is interrupted because of disease, irradiation, extreme stress, or irritants, ***gastritis*** can develop. The stomach mucosa becomes edematous and hyperemic, with diffuse surface erosions. Epigastric pain, anorexia, nausea, and vomiting result. Diagnosis is based on the patient's history, radiography, or endoscopy. Irritants should be discontinued and antacids and a clear liquid diet prescribed. Hospitalization may be necessary.

Gastritis can contribute to the formation of ▶***gastric ulcers.*** Appearing usually at the lesser curvature or the junction of the antrum, these acid-induced injuries to the mucosa occur most frequently in men of ages 55–64. Pain, precipitated by food intake and relieved by antacids, may radiate from the epigastrium to the back or substernum. Anorexia, nausea, and vomiting may be present. Diagnosis is based on barium x-ray films, gastroscopy, and gastric analysis. Antacids, H2-receptor antagonists (cimetidine, ranitidine), and diet modifications (small, frequent meals, slow eating, avoiding known irritants) are the mainstays of treatment. As an alternative to H2-receptor antagonists, sucralfate (Carafate) is also being employed with excellent results and may prove to be particularly useful for treatment of alcohol-induced necrosis. Offering the advantage of nonsystemic action, this drug results in the formation of a proteinaceous complex at the ulcer site, protecting injured tissue from

TABLE 4.5 CHARACTERISTICS OF VOMITING AND ASSOCIATED CONDITIONS

Characteristics	Associated Conditions
Epidemic affecting any number of people. Accompanied by diarrhea, abdominal pain, fever, malaise. Malodorous if bacterial.	Acute gastroenteritis: nonbacterial (viral) or bacterial (staphylococcus enterotoxin).
Occurs during or within 1 hour after a meal.	Psychoneurotic, pregnancy.
Delayed; occurs more than 1 hour after eating; undigested contents.	Gastric outlet obstruction, diabetic gastric atony.
Occurs in the morning.	Pregnancy, uremia, alcoholism, postnasal drip.
Acute onset without nausea.	Drug induced, e.g., cardiac glycosides (direct effect on vomiting center in medulla).
Projectile, unexpected, not related to ingested food; occurs with or without nausea.	Increase in intracranial pressure.
Relieves epigastric or abdominal pain.	Peptic ulcer, obstruction due to peptic ulcer.
Does not relieve abdominal pain.	Pancreatitis, biliary tract disease.
Situational.	Motion sickness.
Accompanied by vertigo with or without tinnitus, hearing loss.	Inner ear disease.
Antabuse-type reaction (flushing, throbbing in head or neck, respiratory difficulty, nausea, copious vomiting, sweating, thirst, chest pain, palpitations, dyspnea, hyperventilation, syncope, uneasiness, blurred vision, confusion precipitated by ETOH intake)	Aminopyrine (in some combination analgesics), chloramphenicol (Choloromycetin, Mychel), chlorpropamide (Diabinese), cyclothiazide (Anhydron), dimercaprol (British anti-lewisite in oil), Ethacrynic acid, metroniazide (Flagyl).
With or without chest pain, explosive diarrhea, burping, and hiccups	Myocardial infarction of posterior wall.

the damaging effects of acid, pepsin, and bile salts. Since acid must be present for therapeutic effect, the drug should be taken on an empty stomach (30–60 minutes before meals). While neither cimetidine nor ranitidine should be used concomitantly, antacids may still be employed for pain if taken at least 1 hour before or after sucralfate administration.

Biopsy of any suspicious or nonhealing ulcer is indicated to rule out ***gastric cancer.*** Gastric carcinoma is declining in the United States but still affects some 20,000 persons annually. Men older than 65 are at highest risk. Nonwhite and low socioeconomic groups are also significantly affected, as are persons with gastric pathology, pernicious anemia, and atrophic gastritis. Studies have linked high rates of gastric cancer to ingestion of smoked and salted foods among the Japanese, Finns, and Icelanders. Nitrosamines (primarily from meats cured with nitrates and nitrites) are associated with a high incidence of disease in Chile and the United States. The presentation of gastric cancer may be subtle. Some patients have epigastric discomfort and anorexia accompanied by nausea. Weight loss, dyspepsia, and early satiety are later symptoms, the presence of which always warrants referral to a gastroenterologist for a complete work-up. Barium x-ray films, endoscopy, and cytologic studies help confirm the diagnosis. Surgery followed by chemotherapy is the usual treatment. Long-term care includes dietary adjustment as well as analgesic and antiemetic medications. Unfortunately, over 80% of these patients die within 5 years.

SMALL INTESTINE AND PANCREAS

Approximately 12 ft long, the small intestine is divided into the duodenum, jejunum, and ileum (Fig. 4.4). Food entering through the pyloric sphincter stretches the duodenum and stimulates a complex feedback system of nerves and hormones (enterogastric reflex) that slows the rate of gastric secretions. In this way, gastric secretions in the empty stomach are curtailed.

The small intestine has a higher pH than the stomach, and the mucosal barrier of the duodenum often breaks down due to the acid effects of gasric emptying. This may result in ▶ ***duodenal ulcers.*** Duodenal and gastric ulcers are classified together as peptic ulcers. However, there are fundamental differences between them, as noted in Table 4.6. Duodenal ulcers are more common, with 10% of the population developing symptoms and up to 70% having evidence of disease on autopsy. Clinical manifestations are most prevalent among men between the ages of 45 and 55. Seasonal trends (spring and fall), familial tendencies, blood type O, and aspirin intake have also been associated with duodenal ulcers. The classic symptom is pain that begins 2–3 hours after a meal or awakens the patient at night. Unlike the symptoms of gastric ulcer, those of duodenal ulcer tend to be relieved by food. Approximately 15% of patients have at least one episode of acute GI bleeding. The diagnostic procedures are similar to those for gastric ulcers, except that biopsies are not indicated. Duodenal ulcers are not associated with malignancy. Treatment measures are the same as those for gastric ulcers.

The pancreas (Fig. 4.5) is both an endocrine and an exocrine gland. The endocrine portion produces insulin, which is necessary for the metabolism of carbohydrates and fats (see Chapter 5). The exocrine portion produces a number of enzymes, which are described in Table 4.7. These enzymes continue digestive processes that are initiated in the stomach. They help break down carbohydrates into mono- and disaccharides; proteins into amino acids and peptides; and fats into monoglycerides and fatty acids. Bicarbonate in the pancreatic secretion neutralizes the acid chyme from the stomach and provides a conducive pH environment for these enzymatic actions. Its production is stimulated by secretin, a hormone manufactured by the duodenal mucosa in response to HCl. Secretin also stimulates the liver to produce bile, which aids the digestive process by emulsifying fats. Bile salts act as detergents by breaking fats into smaller globules and creating more surface area on which enzymes can act. Simultaneously, breakdown products of fats (and proteins) stimulate the duodenal mucosa to release another hormone, cholecystokinin (pancreozymin), which causes the pancreas to produce its enzyme-rich juice and the gallbladder to contract.

Many people have a deficiency of the enzyme lactase, which is needed to break down milk sugar (lactose). Undigested lactose fails to be absorbed, leading to an osmotic shift of fluids into the intestinal tract with symptoms of ▶ ***lactose intolerance.*** Primary lactase deficiency seems to be hereditary and is discovered soon after birth. However, lactose intolerance may not become evident until adolescence or later as the enzyme decreases with age. Lactase activity is further decreased by alcohol abuse. It has been estimated that up to 55% of the general U.S. population and 70% of U.S. blacks have lactose intolerance. There is also a high prevalence among Japanese and Middle Eastern people. The problem may be suspected from a history of nausea, bloating, and abdominal cramps occurring 30 minutes to a few hours after the ingestion of 5–12 g of lactose (the amount contained in less than 8 oz

(a)

(b)

(c)

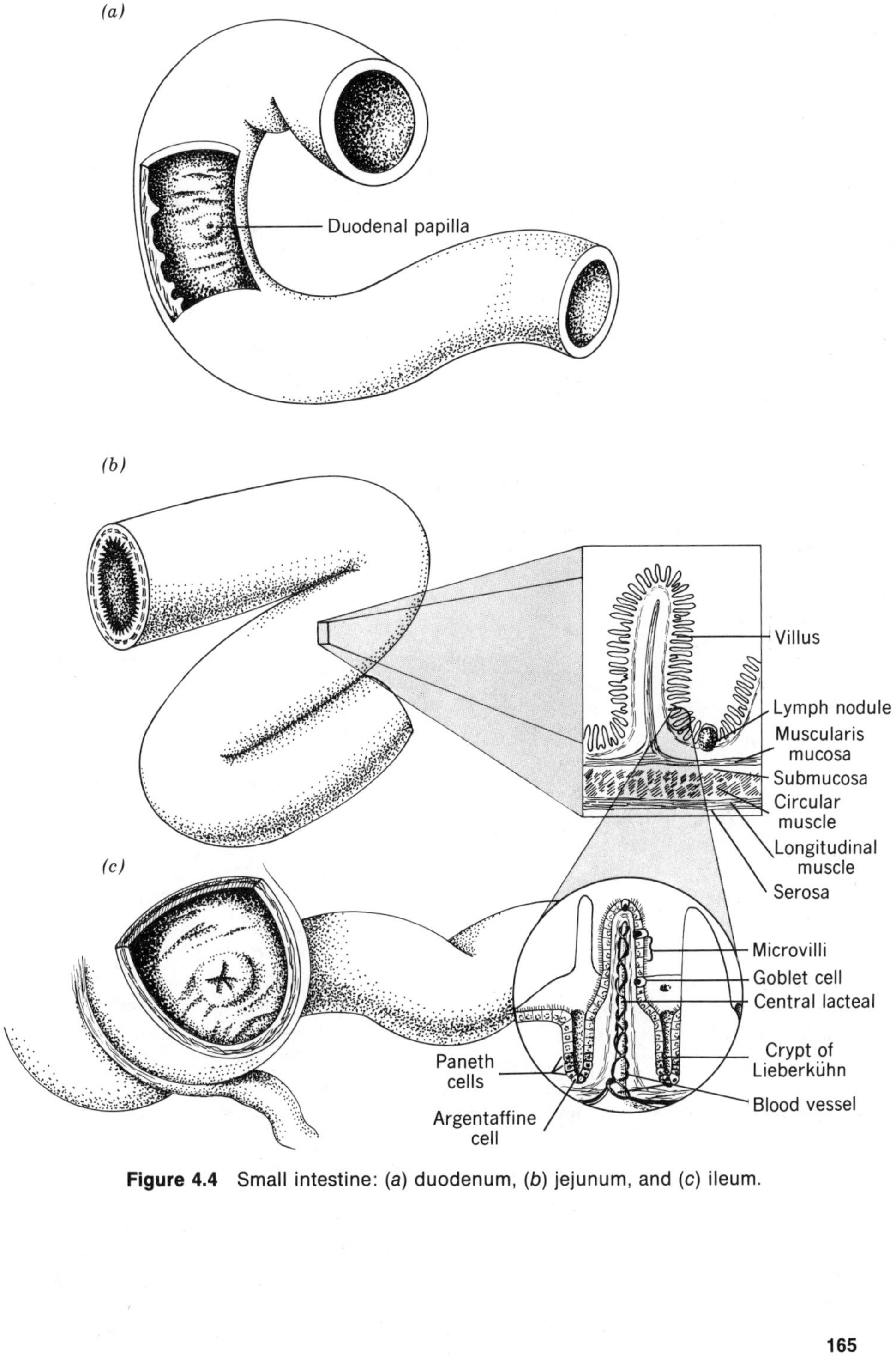

Figure 4.4 Small intestine: (*a*) duodenum, (*b*) jejunum, and (*c*) ileum.

TABLE 4.6 DIFFERENTIAL FEATURES OF DUODENAL AND GASTRIC ULCERS

	Duodenal	Gastric
Incidence	Peak age: 50+ years; male:female = 2.2:1	Peak age: 40+ years; male:female = 1.1:1
Pathophysiology		
Parietal cell secretion	Normal to increased.	Normal to decreased.
Gastric acid secretion	Normal to increased.	Normal to decreased (no achlorhydria).
Gastrin		
Circulating	Normal to mildly elevated.	Normal to elevated.
Response to meals	Excessive and prolonged.	
Mucosal barrier	Not affected.	Abnormal.
Pyloric function	Not affected.	Abnormal with bile reflux.
Course	Chronic pain pattern with remissions and exacerbations.	Less of a remission/exacerbation pattern; high recurrence rate.
Associations	Seasonal trend (spring, fall); familial tendency; blood group O nonsecretor; also associated with chronic obstruction, pulmonary disease, hepatic cirrhosis, pancreatic insufficiency, hyperparathyroidism.	Ulcerogenic drugs: steroids, aspirin, indomethacin, alcohol, nicotine (from smoking).

of milk). Greater milk intake is likely to initiate diarrhea, along with the other symptoms. Diagnosis is based on such a history and is confirmed by lactose challenge tests or breath tests that measure the amount of radioactive labeled CO2 or hydrogen (more specific). Most people with lactose intolerance are aware that their symptoms are associated with milk and tend to avoid it. However, they may not realize the connection with a number of milk products. A carefully explained lactose-free or -controlled diet may be all that is needed to prevent further problems. Suitable alternatives to milk include most cheese, yogurt, and other fermented dairy products. Lactose-hydrolyzed milk can also be given.

Pancreatitis is usually associated with alcoholism or chronic gallbladder disease. It is characterized by the sudden onset of sharp, steady epigastric pain frequently radiating to the midback. The pain, often precipitated by alcohol ingestion, is more intense when the patient is lying flat and is somewhat relieved by sitting with the knees drawn up. Nausea, vomiting, and/or dry heaves and fever may be noted. Appearing acutely ill, patients are restless and have cold, clammy skin. Jaundice may be present along with tachycardia, hypotension, and hypoactive bowel sounds. The abdomen is tender, rigid, and distended, with guarding over the area of the pancreas and rebound tenderness. After 2 or 3 days, bruising may appear around the upper thigh (Turner's sign) or around the navel (Cullen's sign). No laboratory test will specifically and unequivocally identify acute pancreatitis, but serum amylase is elevated in approximately 70% of cases. Hospitalization for fluid replacement, nasogastric suction, and pain relief may be necessary.

▸ ***Chronic pancreatitis*** develops as a consequence of repeated attacks of acute inflammation. When it is caused by gallstones, surgery is curative. However, when it is secondary to alcoholism (80–90% of all cases), the disease progresses slowly and irreversibly. Hypercalcemia and hyperlipidemia may be associated with chronic

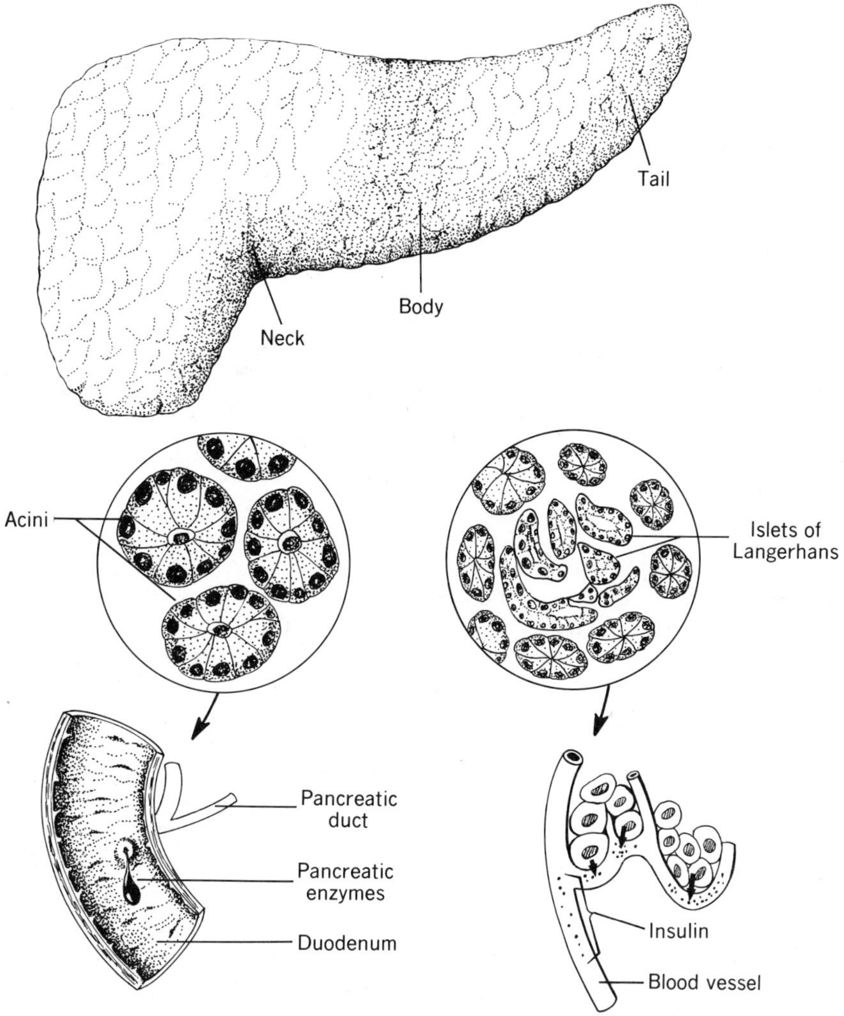

Figure 4.5 Pancreas: pancreatic acini and enzyme flow; islets of Langerhans and insulin secretion.

pancreatitis. Typically, the patient is a thin, emaciated man in his late thirties. Intermittent abdominal pain of varying intensity, vomiting, and nausea are common symptoms. Attacks, which are brought on by drinking alcohol or eating, become less intense but more frequent and lead to serious malabsorption problems. Diabetes is a late complication of advanced disease. Diagnosis is based on the history, abdominal x-ray films, ultrasound, and pancreatic function tests. Unlike acute pancreatitis, there may be no elevation of serum amylase and lipase. Treatment consists of alcohol withdrawal and a diet limited in fats and proteins. Since narcotics may be addictive, chronic pain is often managed with aspirin or Tylenol.

Pancreatic carcinoma is a devastating disease that afflicts men much more

TABLE 4.7 PANCREATIC ENZYMES

Enzyme	Action
Lipase	Breaks down some fats to fatty acids and glycerides.
Amylase	Breaks down starch to maltose.
Sucrase	Splits sucrose into glucose.
Maltase	Splits maltose into glucose.
Lactase	Splits lactose into glucose.
Trypsin and chymotrypsinogen	Split proteins into peptides and amino acids.
Chymotrypsin and renin	Splits proteins into peptides and amino acids (coagulates milk).
Carboxypeptidase	Degrades peptides to amino acids.
Nucleases	Break down nucleic acid to release simple nucleotides.

commonly than women. Most patients are more than 40 years old (the peak incidence is between 60 and 70), and many are smokers or diabetics. The tumor usually arises from ductal epithelium and causes weight loss, abdominal pain, and anorexia. Other symptoms include nausea, weakness, fatigue, vomiting, diarrhea, and dyspepsia. On exam, jaundice may be noted if the tumor has involved the head of the pancreas. The liver is often enlarged, and an abdominal bruit can sometimes be heard in the right upper quadrant. Patients with symptoms of pancreatic carcinoma should be referred to a gastroenterologist as early as possible for diagnostic work-up. This may involve exocrine pancreatic function tests, ultrasound, a computed tomography scan, arteriography, percutaneous biopsy, and endoscopic retrograde cholangiopancreatography (ERCP). Pancreatectomy (Whipple procedure), radiation therapy, and chemotherapy are possible treatments. However, since the tumor has already metastasized in 60% of patients by the time of diagnosis, the prognosis is poor.

The mucosal layers of the small intestine are arranged in circular folds that extend into the lumen. The folds are covered with villi, surface projections just visible to the naked eye. They contain absorptive cells with outer surfaces of microvilli that form a brush-like border (Fig. 4.4). The end products of digested carbohydrates, fats, and proteins are absorbed (transferred) across the brush border to the vascular and lymphatic circulations for use by body cells. Although many substances are absorbed throughout the entire length of the small bowel, there are principal sites of absorption for specific nutrients: iron, calcium, fats, sugars, amino acids, and fat-soluble vitamins from the duodenum; sugars and amino acids from the jejunum; bile salts and vitamin B_{12} from the ileum. Knowledge of these sites is important for identifying some of the actual or potential ***malabsorption syndromes*** described in Table 4.8.

Water, electrolytes, all intestinal secretions including saliva, gastric, and pancreatic juices, and bile are reabsorbed in the small intestine. Any loss through vomiting or diarrhea is actually a loss of extracellular fluid, which can cause significant electrolyte imbalance (dehydration). This is a concern in the common presentation of ▶ ***viral gastroenteritis.*** It usually occurs in epidemics during the fall and winter. Patients experience an abrupt onset of nausea, vomiting, diarrhea, and abdominal cramps. Headache, low-grade fever, and general malaise may accompany the intestinal symptoms. On exam, patients appear ill and have diffuse abdominal tenderness with hyperactive bowel sounds. However, guarding and rebound tenderness should be absent. Treatment is symptomatic, and the infection is self-limiting.

TABLE 4.8 SOME CAUSES OF MALABSORPTION SYNDROME

Stomach disorders Following gastric surgery	Small intestinal disorders Inflammatory bowel disease (ulcerative colitis, regional ileitis) Bowel resection Infectious acute enteritis Giardiasis/parasitic infestation Lactase deficiency
Pancreatic disorders Chronic pancreatitis Pancreatic cancer Cystic fibrosis	Chronic oral drug use Neomycin Dilantin (can inhibit intestinal absorption of calcium)
Liver disorders Cirrhosis Chronic hepatitis	

Bacterial gastroenteritis is caused by a large number of organisms described in Table 4.9. As noted, these organisms fall into three categories depending on their predominant mode of action: enterotoxins acting on the small intestine, systemic invasion with gastroenteritis as a main feature (enteric fever), or local invasion of superficial bowel mucosa. For the most part, enterotoxins produce a watery "plasma-like" diarrhea, and organisms that invade the bowel mucosa produce bloody diarrhea. The confusing aspect of the disease is that some strains of the same species work in different ways. For example, *Salmonella typhi* (which causes typhoid fever) and *S. enteritidis* (which causes paratyphoid) are systemic in action, while other *Salmonella* strains are more local. There are enterotoxigenic strains of *Escherichia coli* (ETEC) causing mild, self-limiting diarrhea and enteroinvasive (EIEC) strains causing severe dysentery. To add to the confusion, some organisms have the capacity for more than one mechanism of action. *Vibrio parahaemolyticus,* for example, may cause a mild form of food poisoning from enterotoxins or a severe form from intestinal invasion. Although anyone may become infected by the organisms listed in Table 4.9, travelers who have never built up immunity through exposure are particularly susceptible. People with hypochlorhydria (the elderly, gastrectomy patients, patients taking cimetidine, and possibly marijuana users) are also at higher risk, since gastric acid secretions normally help destroy ingested bacteria.

Cholera serves as the model for understanding bacteria-induced diarrhea caused

TABLE 4.9 BACTERIAL ENTEROPATHOGENS CLASSIFIED BY MODE OF ACTION

Bowel irritation from high bacterial load and/or enterotoxins
- *Vibrio cholerae, V. Eltor, V. metchnikovii, V. proteus, V. parahaemolyticus*
- Enterotoxigenic *Escherichia coli* (ETEC), varied serotypes
- *Staphylococcus aureus*
- *Bacillus cereus*
- *Clostridium perfringens*

Systemic disease with enteritis as a main component (enteric fever)
- *Salmonelli typhi, S. enteritidis* (paratyphi A, B, and C), *S. arizonae, S. cholerasuis, S. schottmuelleri, S. sendai, S. typhimurium* (rare)
- *Yersinia enterocolitica, Y. pseudotuberculosis*

Invasion of bowel mucosa with inflammatory response
- *Salmonella arizonae, S. derby, S. enteritidis, S. gallinarum, S. typhimurium*
- *Shigella flexneri, S. sonnei, S. boydii, S. dysenteriae*
- *Campylobacter fetus* (*Vibrio coli, V. fetus, V. jejuni*)
- Enteroinvasive *E. coli* (EIEC)

by enterotoxins. The aerobic rod (*Vibrio cholerae*) is passed through food or water that has been contaminated by the feces of infected persons, humans being its only host. From 1 to 3 days after entering the body, the organism quickly colonizes the gut and produces a toxin that stimulates massive secretions from the small intestine. Similar to plasma except for a higher bicarbonate level and the absence of proteins, these secretions overwhelm the absorptive capacity of the colon and pass through the rectum as stool. Painless diarrhea may exeed 1 L/h. Diagnosis is confirmed by cultures (rectal swabs or fresh stool samples) and agglutination by specific antisera. As water, potassium, salt, bicarbonate, and glucose continue to be lost, patients develop signs of dehydration and metabolic acidosis: intense thirst, fever, sunken eyes, oliguria, muscle cramps, weakness, and marked loss of tissue turgor. Unless hydration is maintained, patients soon die. Fortunately, although the colon's reabsorptive capacity is overwhelmed, its reabsorptive ability remains normal. This explains the effectiveness of ▶ ***oral fluid and electrolyte replacement in gastroenteritis.***

Patients with cholera should be hospitalized, the health department notified by phone, and ▶ ***enteric precautions*** observed. With prompt and aggressive treatment, sensitive antibiotics eradicate the *Vibrio,* terminating diarrhea within 48 hours; 99% of patients recover. Untreated disease is self-limiting within 3–5 days, but mortality ranges from 20 to 80%.

Primary care providers are unlikely to see active cases of cholera in the United States (there have been occurrences on the Gulf Coast). However, they may be called on to give ▶ ***cholera vaccinations*** to patients traveling to portions of Asia, the Middle East, and Africa where cholera is still endemic or to any area undergoing an outbreak. Natives of these areas are likely to have lifetime immunity from past disease; for this reason, U.S. Public Health Service does not require cholera vaccination for incoming visitors. While the vaccine may boost immunity for them, it has little value for most Americans who are "immunologic virgins." It is not recommended for U.S. citizens, no matter what their destination, unless they are at high risk for hypochlorhydria. However, the vaccine is still given to travelers entering countries that require proof of vaccination for entry.

▶ ***Enterotoxigenic E. coli*** (ETEC, "turista") causes more than half of all cases of diarrhea suffered by travelers. Several strains (other than those commonly residing in the large bowel) may be spread by infected persons or carriers through food or water. Within hours, their endotoxins produce a sudden onset of abdominal cramps, borborygmi, nausea, and sometimes vomiting. Loose and then watery stools follow with great urgency. All symptoms are most severe during the first 24 hours, with a gradual abatement and complete recovery in 3–7 days. Stool tests are nonspecific, with the absence of leukocytes or red blood cells on fecal smears and negative culture. However, ETEC strains can be identified with more complicated tests: agglutination or immunofluorescence with antisera or a demonstration of heat-labile toxins. Such tests, which are generally unavailable, are not indicated for routine cases. Fluid replacement is the main treatment.

Toxin-producing bacteria growing in food may cause short-lived bouts of "food poisoning." ***Staphylococcal food poisoning*** is relatively common, since *S. aureus* inhabits the human nose and skin and exists in cuts, acne pimples, boils, and sores. The organism is transferred by hand or via the respiratory tract (from a sneeze or cough) to food. There it multiplies and produces a toxin that causes nausea, vomiting, urgent diarrhea, and abdominal cramps 3–8 hours after ingestion.

Reheated fried rice is the usual source of ***Bacillus cereus* food poisoning.** After the contaminated rice is eaten, enterotoxins form in the gut, causing vomiting 1–6 hours later and diarrhea 8–16 later. Recovery in 24 hours is the rule. By contrast, ***Vibrio parahaemolyticus* food poisoning** develops from infected crabmeat or other types of shellfish. It causes abrupt onset of diarrhea and sometimes vomiting that lasts for 1 to 3 days.

In ***Clostridium perfringens* food poisoning,** the organism multiplies on food that has been inadequately cooked. Most infections can be traced to meats, poultry, and gravies originally cooked in large quantities and reheated by catering services, restaurants, or cafeterias. When large amounts of bacteria are ingested, they produce an enterotoxin in vivo that results in moderate to severe midepigastric cramps and watery diarrhea 8–24 hours later. Fever is absent and vomiting unusual. (Another species, *Clostridium botulinum,* is responsible for a life-threatening neuromuscular toxin known as "botulism," discussed in Chapter 12).

A comparison of the four types of food poisoning is presented in Table 4.10. In all cases, symptoms are usually self-limiting and no specific treatment is required. However, the control measures should be emphasized to prevent future outbreaks.

Several ***Salmonella*** strains (there are over 2,200) cause systemic illnesses with gastroenteritis as a major component (Table 4.9). **Typhoid** (*S. typhi*) and its mimic, **paratyphoid** (*S. paratyphi* or *S. enteritides*), are still prevalent in much of the world, excluding North America, Scandinavia, and most of Western Europe. The typhoid organism is shed by healthy carriers (in stool) or patients with active disease (in urine and stool), and is transmitted through contaminated water, milk, and food. Flies may serve as vectors, but infection through direct contact probably does not occur.

After its entrance via the GI tract, the organism invades the lymphatic channels and finally enters the bloodstream. Three days to 3 weeks later, the patient shows the first signs of disease: chills, malaise, headache, backache, anorexia, and consti-

TABLE 4.10 COMMON TYPES OF BACTERIAL FOOD POISONING

	Staphylococcus aureus	*Bacillus cereus*	*Clostridium perfringens*	*Vibrio parahemolyticus*
Description of organism	Gram + cocci found in air, respiratory tract of asymptomatic carriers, common skin infections (pimples, boils, abscesses, impetigo).	Gram + spore-forming rod. Naturally distributed in dusts and soil and on plants.	Anaerobic spore-forming gram + rod. Isolated from soil, milk, female genital tract. Produces five toxin types (A–E) in vivo.	Gram—motile rod. Natural inhabitant of sea water.
Foods affected	Meats and dairy products left unrefrigerated.	Meats, vegetables, refried rice.	Meat/gravy dishes inadequately cooked and reheated.	Shellfish, particularly crabs and oysters.
Incubation period	1–18 hours.	1–16 hours.	8–24 hours.	5–92 hours.
Fever	None.	None.	None.	One-half of cases.
Vomiting	All cases.	Variable.	All cases.	One-third of cases.
Diarrhea	One-third of cases.	Variable.	Unusual.	All cases.
Recovery	24–48 hours.	24 hours or less.	1–4 days.	1–3 days.
Control	Thoroughly cook and properly refrigerate all foods including shellfish. Divide large quantities of food into small portions for storage and reheating. Keep foods covered. Screen food handlers for staphylococcal carriage and active skin lesions.			

pation. Although temperature rises daily, bradycardia may be present. Diagnostic crops of "rose spots" (which blanch with pressure) erupt over the abdomen, and hepatosplenomegaly may be present. Florid diarrhea develops in later stages. Severe dehydration, delirium, leukopenia, and anemia are the rule. Complications include intestinal hemorrhage and perforation from ulcer formation.

Diagnosis of typhoid fever is confirmed by positive culture yields from stool, blood, urine, or bone marrow. Serologic tests (febrile agglutinins or a Widal test) have a high rate of both false-positive and false-negative results and are somewhat limited in value. Without prompt hospitalization for fluid and electrolyte replacement and antibiotic therapy, the mortality is 30%. A 2-week course of chloramphenicol is given, along with corticosteroids in severe cases. Antipyretics have been known to cause drastic falls in body temperature and are avoided. As a preventive measure, parenteral ampicillin or cholecystectomy is recommended for chronic carriers. To increase resistance to infections, ▶***typhoid immunization*** is recommended for travelers to areas of endemic disease, household contacts of chronic carriers, and laboratory workers who have frequent contact with the organism. The vaccine is not recommended in instances of disease outbreaks. A better oral vaccine is being produced in Switzerland but is not yet available in this country.

Nontyphoidal strains (Table 4.9) are responsible for ▶***acute salmonella enterocolitis.*** The epidemiology is more complicated than that of typhoid fever, since infection is spread by direct contact through animals and animal products as well as the human oral-fecal route. Contaminated meats, poultry, and eggs have led to a steady increase in the incidence of active infections and healthy carriers. Their preparation on wooden butcher blocks, which may harbor organisms, further compounds the problem. Pet turtles and wild birds are other important sources of infection. After a short incubation period of 12–48 hours, patients experience transient fever followed by mild abdominal discomfort and diarrhea. The loose, pasty stools may contain blood and mucus, although this is rare. Ocassionally the diarrhea is more severe and cholera-like. Septicemia is a possible complication. Diagnosis of salmonella enterocolitis depends on positive stool culures (neutrophils and red blood cells may be noted on a smear but are inconclusive).

The treatment in noncomplicated cases is symptomatic. Antibiotics do not shorten the course of disease and have been found to prolong the carrier state. However, they are warranted in high-risk groups (infants or patients with cancer, hemoglobinopathy, chronic gastrointestinal disease, or immune deficiency). Enteric precautions should be maintained until stool cultures are negative. Control measures include pasteurization of milk, sanitation or sterilization of contaminated water, careful processing of all possible food sources (particularly poultry), and proper sewage disposal. It may also be sensible to screen food handlers and prohibit the sale of pet turtles (which are common carriers).

▶***Shigellosis,*** caused by a gram-negative rod belonging to the *Shigella* family, is seen more frequently in children than in adults. Having no animal reservoirs, the organism is spread solely through human feces containing contaminated food, water supplies, or inanimate objects. Houseflies serve as vectors. Outbreaks, which are associated with poor sanitation systems and crowded living conditions, often occur in institutional settings (e.g., Indian reservations, day-care centers, and residential homes for the retarded). In most cases, shigellosis causes a mild infection marked by loose, watery stools that last for several days and are of little consequence. Some patients, however, encounter more serious infections, as forewarned by the abrupt onset of fever and headache. Soon afterward they develop vomiting, abdominal cramps, and tenderness, along with frequent diarrhea—20 small-volume stools per day (which may contain blood and mucus). The diagnosis may be suspected by stool smears revealing neutrophils and red blood cells. It is confirmed by culture.

Treatment includes antibiotics, Pepto Bismol, and fluid replacement. Enteric precautions should be maintained until cultures are negative. The disease offers no immunity, but some prophylactic protection may be obtained from a recently developed live oral vaccine. Although it is not yet available for public use, field trials have shown considerable success.

Also caused by a gram-negative rod, ▶ ***Campylobacter enteritis*** affects people of all ages and produces a clinical picture similar to that of shigellosis. Animals may become infected and are an additional source of disease (particularly puppies and kittens). Diagnosis is based on stool cultures achieved by special laboratory techniques. Mild cases require only fluid replacement, but more serious infections are treated with antibiotics. Enteric precautions are advised until stool cultures turn negative.

Unlike the mild, self-limiting bout of diarrhea caused by enterotoxigenic *E. coli*, ▶ ***enteroinvasive E. coli*** (EIEC) passed in contaminated food or water produces a picture of severe dysentery. Patients have fever, vomiting, and profuse diarrhea (frequently bloody) accompanied by tenesmus and abdominal pain. The disease is diagnosed by the Sereny test (guinea pig conjunctival sac inoculation) or special tissue cultures. Antibiotics and Pepto Bismol may avoid prostration and help shorten the course. Fluid replacement is crucial.

For ▶ ***prevention of bacterial gastroenteritis,*** travelers to endemic regions should have recommended typhoid and cholera vaccinations. If there is any question about the purity of the water supplies, they should boil drinking water or treat it with chlorine or iodine. Although ice or bottled water should be avoided, carbonated beverages may be safely used, since carbonzation lowers the pH and thereby kills or inhibits bacteria. In addition, travelers should eat only thoroughly cooked or properly preserved food, avoiding salads and unpeeled fruits and vegetables. They should also be wary of food and water contamination through insect and bird droppings. Doxycycline may be effective against tetracycline-sensitive *E. coli* and shigellae but has the potential for causing photosensitivity reactions, tooth discoloration in children, and the development of drug-resistant organisms. Therefore its use should be carefully determined by the patient's age, as well as the type and length of travel.

The ***parasites*** described in Table 4.11 also cause gastroenteritis but, until recently, were considered exotic findings in the United States. However, the influx of Asian, Central American, and Caribbean refugees in the 1970s has caused a steady increase in related diseases. Because most laboratory workers and clinicians may be facing a problem never before encountered, the Center for Disease Control has established the Parasitic Disease and Drug Service. Primary care providers should rely on this service or on experts from state health departments and universities to answer questions about diagnosis and treatment. General guidelines are offered in Table 4.11, and further discussion of parasitic disease can be found in Chapter 7.

Unlike most parasites, ▶ ***Giardia*** is endemic in the United States, particularly the Rocky Mountain and Northern Cascade regions. It is prevalent in the Soviet Union and other foreign countries. Cysts of this protozoon contaminate water sources and remain viable in cold temperatures for as long as 2 months. In addition to drinking water, fecal-oral, food-borne, and venereal spread have been implicated.

TABLE 4.11 PARASITIC DISORDERS CAUSING GI SYMPTOMS

Disorder	Causative Organism	Where Acquired	Source of Human Infection
Amebiasis	*Entamoeba histolytica*	Worldwide distribution.	Feces-contamined food or water. Person-to-person spread.
Anisakiasis (herring worm disease)	Anisakis, Phocanema	California, Holland, Japan.	Eating raw infected saltwater fish.
Ascariasis (giant roundworm)	*Ascaris lumbricoides*	Rural areas throughout the world, especially warm, moist climates.	Eating vegetables grown in soil with human fertilizer.
Balantidiasis	*Balantidium coli*	Hog-raising locales.	Food or water contaminated by hog manure.
Beef tapeworm	*Taenia saginata*	Worldwide. Common in Kenya, Ethiopia, Yugoslavia, Moslem countries, Latin America.	Eating raw or poorly cooked beef infected with larvae.
Dwarf tapeworm	*Hymenolepis nana*	Institutions in the United States. Africa, South America, Eastern Europe.	Eggs in soil to mouth.
Echinococcosis	*Echinococcus granulosus*	Greece, Lebanon, Australia, New Zealand, South America, parts of Africa.	Eggs in canine feces to mouth.
Enterobiasis (pinworms, seatworms)	*Enterobius vermicularis*	Fifteen percent of U.S. population mostly institutionalized persons and children.	Eggs passed from anus to mouth.
Eosinophilic gastroenteritis	*Angiostrongylus costaricensis*	Central and South America.	Eating infected snails or vegetation contaminated by them.
Fish tapeworm	*Diphyllobothrium latum*	Finland, Sweden, Japan, Baltic countries, Canada, United States.	Eating raw freshwater fish infected with larvae.
Giardiasis	*Giardia lamblia*	Worldwide. Endemic in Rocky Mountains, Northern Cascades, parts of New York State.	Drinking water containing cysts. Oral/fecal spread.
Intestinal capillariasis	*Capillaria philippinensis*	Central Luzon region of Northern Philippines. U.S. infections imported from the Orient and tropics.	Ingestion of raw infected fish.
(Intestinal fluke)	a. *Fasciolopsis* b. *Heterophyes, Metagonimus* c. *Echinostoma*		a. Vegetation b. Freshwater fish. c. Snails.
Pork tapeworm	*Taenia solium*	Latin America, Asia, USSR, Eastern Europe, Africa, India. Rare in United States.	Undercooked pork infected with larvae.
Schistosomiasis (blood fluke)	a. *Schistosoma japonicum* b. *S. mansoni* c. *S. haematobium*	a. Orient. b. Latin America, Africa. c. Near East, Africa.	Larvae in water enter body through skin or mucous membranes.
Strongyloidiasis (threadworm)	*Strongyloides stercoralis*	Southern United States, tropics.	Larva in dirt enter skin through feet.
Trichuriasis (whipworm)	*Trichuris trichiura*	Warm, moist climates. Rare in United States.	Eggs in contaminated soil to mouth.

Signs and Symptoms	Diagnosis	Treatment
Usually mild intestinal symptoms or asymptomatic. Sometimes feverish dysentery with ulceration of the colon. Abscesses may form in the liver, lungs, brain and skin.	Identification of trophozoites or cysts in stool.	Metronidazole or diiodohydroxyquin.
Acute gastrointestinal symptoms mimicking diverticulosis. Peritonitis or obstruction may develop. Modest eosinophilia.	Isolation of larva in tissues.	None.
Colicky abdominal pains from worms. Larval stage produces bronchial symptoms and eosinophilia.	Eggs found in stool; worms in stool or vomitus.	Pyrantel pamoate, mebendazole.
Nausea, vomiting, bloody diarrhea in acute form. Intermittent diarrhea with chronic disease.	Examination of fresh stool or sigmoid scrapings.	Tetracycline or diiodohydroxyquin.
Usually asymptomatic, but sometimes causes abdominal distress similar to that of acute appendicitis.	Eggs found around anus; proglottids in stool.	Niclosamide, paromomycin.
Abdominal discomfort and diarrhea.	Eggs in stool.	Niclosamide, paromomycin.
Abdominal pain and mass. Pulmonary symptoms and "coin" lesions.	Positive serology; cysts on lung/liver scans.	Surgical excision of cysts.
Perineal irritation and pruritis ani worse at night.	Eggs on "scotch tape test," anal swabs. Adult worms per anum.	Pyrantel pamoate or mebendazole.
Fever, anorexia, vomiting, and pain mimicking acute appendicitis. Rarely, intestinal obstruction.	Recovery of eggs from intestinal wall. Precipitin test.	Surgical excision of granulomatous tissue and bowel resection.
Mild gastrointestinal symptoms. Pernicious anemia.	Eggs in stool.	Niclosamide or paromomycin.
Asymptomatic or abdominal pain and mucous diarrhea.	Cysts in stool, stomach, or duodenal aspirate.	Metronidazole or quinacrine.
Severe protein-losing enteropathy. High mortality rate.	Eggs and parasites in stool.	Thiabendazole, acute support.
Usually asymptomatic. At times, abdominal pain, diarrhea, intestinal obstruction, toxemia.	Eggs in stool.	Tetrachloroethylene.
Asymptomatic or acute gastrointestinal distress that may be mistaken for appendicitis.	Eggs and worms in stool. Eggs near anus.	Niclosamide or paromomycin.
Dysentery. Fibrotic changes of bladder, intestine, liver (a, b). Hematuria (c).	Eggs in stool (a, b). Eggs in urine (c).	Antimony potassium tartrate (a). Niridazole (b, c).
Diarrhea and radiating stomach pain.	Larvae in stool or duodenal aspirate.	Thiabendazole.
Diarrhea, abdominal pain, weight loss, and anemia.	Eggs in stool.	Mebendazole.

After entering the body, the cysts release trophozoites that infest the duodenum and the upper small bowel and/or biliary tree. Seventy-five percent of patients remain asymptomatic. However, with heavy infestations, abdominal cramps and high-volume, explosive diarrhea occur. Since the diarrhea is persistent, dehydration, malabsorption, and weight loss are common. Stool analysis is often the only test undertaken for diagnostic purposes, although it has been shown to be nonproductive 50% of the time. A duodenal aspirate is more dependable (85% yield) and small bowel biopsy is most accurate (100% correlation). Treatment with antiparasite drugs is quite effective.

Outbreaks of diarrhea caused by *E. coli, Shigella,* or *Giardia* may appear with no history of travel in homosexual populations. This condition is called the ***gay bowel syndrome.*** The symptoms and treatment are specific for the types of diarrheal disease just discussed.

While gastroenteritis and the common parasite infections are relatively benign, some serious inflammatory changes occur in ***Crohn's disease.*** The changes, which develop for unknown reasons, involve all layers of the intestinal wall but are most marked in the submucosa. Mucosal edema and lymphocytic infiltration appear first, followed by extensive fibrosis. Patchy ulcerations surrounded by edematous tissue create the characteristic "cobblestone" or "thumbprint" picture on x-ray films. Portions of the bowel remain untouched by this process (skip areas) and contrast sharply to diseased segments, hence the term "regional" enteritis. The ileum is involved in 50% of Crohn's cases, the ileum and colon in 40%, and the colon alone in only 10%. Arthritis, uveitis, canker sores, and leg ulcers are associated manifestations. The disease has ethnic (more common in Jews than other groups) and familial tendencies but affects men and women equally. The peak incidence is the second decade, with most cases occurring before age 40. Among the initial symptoms are cramping, abdominal pain, and intermittent constipation alternating with diarrhea, anorexia, and weight loss. Obstruction, fistula formation, and abscesses are the inevitable complications of progressing disease or, in some cases, the presenting features. Dysuria may be the first complaint if a fistula tract forms between the diseased ileum and the bladder. Fever may be expected, along with laboratory findings of anemia, leukocytosis, elevated erythrocyte sedimentation rate, and hypoalbuminemia. Inflammation and thickening of the anus on rectal exam is an important finding.

Crohn's disease can usually be diagnosed by radiographic changes. A barium enema shows reflux into the terminal ileum along with thick, stiff, nodular intestinal walls. A small bowel series demonstrates the nature and extent of the lesions. Sometimes complete recovery follows a single attack (acute ileitis). More often, there are lifelong exacerbations and progressive structural changes. Surgical interventions are necessary for obstructions, abscesses, or fistulas, but resection of diseased portions of bowel ameliorates symptoms only temporarily. Anticholinergics, narcotics, steroids, antibacterials, and bulk preparations are among the medical treatments. Given its chronic and serious nature, Crohn's disease is best managed by a gastroenterologist.

Peristalsis occurs throughout the gastrointestinal tract and is most typically demonstrated in the small intestine. It is a circular constrictive movement much like that produced by circling fingers tightly around a soft tube of paste and pulling along the tube. Any material in front of the fingers will be squeezed forward. Peristaltic movement can go in any direction, but it normally moves toward the anus ("law of the gut"). ***Intestinal obstruction*** (ileus) halts this movement. Common causes include duodenal ulcer, inflammatory processes (Crohn's disease, diverticulitis, enteritis), abscesses or tumors, fecal impaction, and adhesions. Patients with intestinal obstruction have intense, spasmodic pain that starts suddenly. They may be restless and move about frequently in an attempt to find a comfortable position. Intervals between painful episodes last for 4–5 minutes with upper bowel obstructions and for 10–15 minutes with lower bowel obstructions. Steady pain can indicate strangulation or perforation. Depending upon the location of the obstruction, patients may vomit clear gastric juices or recently ingested food, bile, or fecal matter. There may be abrupt cessation of bowel movements or alternating constipation and diarrhea. Feces below the obstruction may continue to be expelled for some time. Hospital evaluation and treatment are necessary in all cases.

COLON

The colon is illustrated in Figure 4.6. The cecum, located in the right lower quadrant, comprises the first 2 or 3 in. It is separated from the small intestine by the ileocecal valve, through which liquid fecal material advances. The flow of liquid from the smaller lumen of the ileum to the larger lumen of the cecum causes bowel sounds to be heightened in this area. It is a good place to begin auscultation of the abdomen.

The appendix hangs from the cecum. If its point of attachment becomes obstructed by hardened stool, seeds, overgrown tissue, or strictures, ***acute appendicitis,*** a surgical emergency, develops. Most commonly seen in adolescents or young adults, it presents with the gradual onset of steady, generalized abdominal pain. One or two episodes of nausea or vomiting follow the onset of pain. If they precede the pain, appendicitis is unlikely. After several hours, the pain shifts to the right lower quadrant and localizes at the appendix. Low-grade fever may occur, with the temperature rising to 38.3°C, and the pulse rate increases after several hours. Patients prefer to lie quietly, frequently with the right leg flexed. Peristalsis is decreased and may stop altogether in the later stages. Because of guarding, abdominal palpation for rebound tenderness may be easier during the pelvic or rectal exam. The white blood cell count may be elevated or normal. As many as 20% of patients present with ***atypical appendicitis.*** These include the elderly, the acutely ill, and patients receiving steroids, as well as those with an atypically positioned appendix (persons with congenital retrocecal appendix, pregnant women, and the obese). The gangrenous appendix may not be recognized before rupture. Since almost all morbidity and mortality associated with appendicitis occur in patients with an atypical presentation, any abdominal pain in those known to be at risk should be carefully monitored in the hospital. In most cases, surgery is more readily tolerated than complications of the disease.

Ruptured appendix or other intra-abdominal infections are common causes of ***peritonitis,*** or inflammation of the lining of the peritoneal cavity. Chemical irritation from leakage of gastric acid, bile, blood, or urine may cause peritonitis secondary to perforated peptic ulcer or rupture of the gallbladder or bladder. Primary peritonitis rarely occurs. The presenting symptoms depend on the underlying pathology (see the discussion of pancreatitis, tubo-ovarian abscess, etc.). A temperature elevation up to 40°C, a board-hard abdomen, a high white blood cell count and

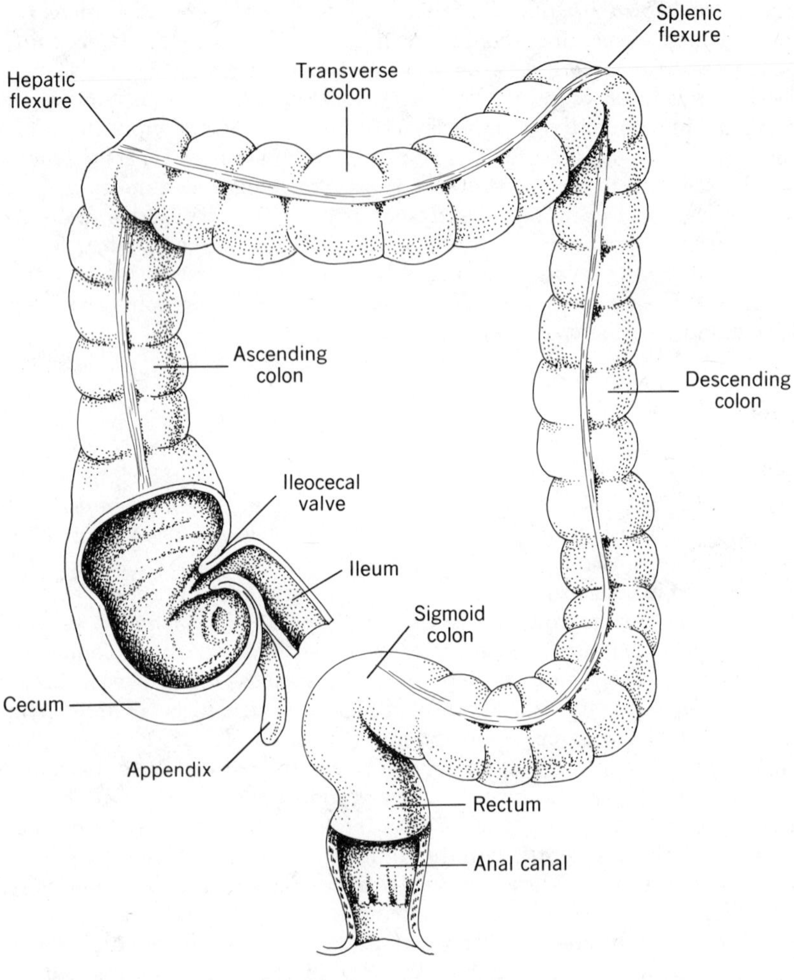

Figure 4.6 Colon: ileocecal valve, cecum, appendix; ascending colon; transverse colon; descending colon; sigmoid colon; rectum and anal canal.

signs of shock may be present. Since the anterior rectal wall lies adjacent to the peritoneum, tenderness will be present on rectal exam. Immediate surgical consultation is required.

Following the cecum are the ascending, transverse, and descending loops of the colon. They are divided by the hepatic and splenic flexures (see Fig. 4.6). The sharp turn of the splenic flexure is anatomically significant because trapped gas can cause acute abdominal pain in some individuals. This benign but distressing condition is called ***splenic flexure syndrome.***

The mucosal layer of the large intestine is thicker than that of the small intestine. Fibrous bands cause the intestinal walls to pucker and form small sacs called "haustra," the size and shape of which are determined by the state of colonic contraction. On a plain x-ray film of the abdomen, haustra make up the irregular outline of the colon. The intestinal glands are found deep in the mucosa and have numerous goblet cells. These cells produce mucus to lubricate the passage of stool and protect the mucosa. However, no enzymes are secreted in the large intestine.

Bacteria in the colon synthesize vitamin K and several vitamins of the B group. These bacteria also act on undigested materials from the small intestine and form a number of gases including ammonia, hydrogen, carbon dioxide, and methane. Some of these gases are given off in the feces, while others are absorbed, detoxified by the liver, and excreted in the urine. Excessive ▶***gastrointestinal gas*** is marked by repeated belching, abdominal bloating, mild abdominal pain, and excessive flatus. Carbohydrates such as those found in legumes and the flour in some pastas pass into the colon partially undigested and ferment, releasing gas. Although annoying, the condition is benign and can be treated symptomatically with antiflatulent agents. Correcting any factors that contribute to air swallowing and prescribing diets of highly digestible foods are other important measures.

The most important function of the large intestine is the absorption of water and electrolytes, which is largely completed in the right side of the colon. Every day, approximately 2,000 ml of fluid are reabsorbed and routed back into the extracellular spaces. However, the fecal mass must maintain a certain amount of fluid, or it hardens and resists peristalsis. This leads to bowel spasm and mucosal irritation, both of which have been implicated in a number of intestinal problems ranging from constipation to cancer of the colon. Plant fibers, which pass through the intestine undigested, are necessary to maintain optimal bulk and hydration of stool. Because of their beneficial effects (Table 4.12), a ▶***high-fiber diet*** is an important preventive health measure. It may also be used in the treatment of constipation and anal disorders.

To allow increased time for absorption, the bowel employs slow churning and kneading contractions as well as mass peristalsis to move the fecal mass forward. This normal motility is disturbed by a number of drugs (Table 4.13) that decrease transit time as well as interfere with the secretory and osmotic mechanisms of the bowel. Caused by food additives, antibiotics, magnesium-containing antacids, laxatives, or alcohol, ***drug-induced diarrhea*** can be chronic or recurrent. Elimination of the causative factors is usually curative (refer to Tables 4.2 and 4.13).

An exception is ***Pseudomembranous colitis,*** a serious inflammatory bowel disorder. An opportunistic organism, *Clostridium difficile,* becomes established when an imbalance of normal gut flora develops from the use of broad-spectrum antibiotics

TABLE 4.12 EFFECTS OF DIETARY FIBER

Actions	Benefits
Absorbs water in colon.	Stool bulk and frequency increased: decreased intraluminal pressure; decreased straining at stool.
Normalizes intestinal passage time.	Decreased intestinal exposure to potential carcinogens in stools.
Decreases reabsorption of bile salts in intestine, thereby increasing fecal excretion of cholesterol.	Decreased serum cholesterol; decreased incidence of cholesterol gallstones.
Facilitates slower absorption of glucose from food.	Reduction of postprandial blood sugars and glycosuria.
Demands longer chewing and eating times.	Early satiety with decreased food intake.

TABLE 4.13 SOME DRUGS KNOWN TO CAUSE DIARRHEA

Antacids (magnesium hydroxide)	Laxatives
Antibiotics, including tetracyclines	Ponstel (mefenamic acid)
Alcohol	Guanethidine
Caffeine	Quinidine
Colchicine	Reserpine
Digitalis	Clindamycin
Ergot (breast milk)	

in the presence of a disrupted vascular supply as a result of GI surgery, shock, mercury poisoning, or uremia. *Clostridium* toxins cause histologic changes of the bowel mucosa including necrosis, edema, inflammatory infiltration, and vascular thrombosis. Usually developing 2–7 days after GI surgery, symptoms include colicky pain, nausea, abdominal distention, and fever. A profuse, offensive diarrhea that is yellowish-green and often bloody occurs in less than half of these patients. Because barium enema is contraindicated, diagnosis rests on sigmoidoscopy and plain films of the abdomen. Fluid and electrolyte replacement, albumin infusions, and other measures of supportive care are initiated. The offending antibiotic should be stopped and severe cases of colitis treated with cholestyramine or oral vancomycin. Intravenous corticosteroids or colectomy may be lifesaving in fulminant cases.

Bowel motility is also interrupted in ▶ ***irritable bowel syndrome*** (mucous colitis, spastic colitis, nervous diarrhea, functional bowel syndrome). For inapparent reasons, motility is either increased or decreased significantly and may involve both the small and large intestines. Neither anatomical abnormality nor inflammation has been identified. However, three clinical patterns exist: spastic colon with constipation, painless diarrhea with mucus, and alternating diarrhea and constipation. These disturbances usually begin in early adult life and rarely present after age 50. Infectious diarrhea and laxative abuse seem to contribute to the occurrence of irritable bowel syndrome. Also, there is a well-substantiated correlation with stress. This is not to say that irritable bowel syndrome reflects a psychologic disorder, but rather that patients have an exaggerated, heightened bowel response to internal or external stress. They may also have a lower threshold to intestinal pain. The most common symptom in irritable bowel syndrome is a crampy pain in the lower abdomen that is relieved with the passage of flatus or stool. There may be constipation characterized by hard, pellet-like stool formations or diarrhea accompanied by a sense of urgency and the painful sensation of incomplete rectal emptying (tenesmus). The diarrhea is low in volume and semiliquid, and may contain mucus. Dyspepsia, postpradial fullness, anorexia, belching, nausea, and bloating are other commonly reported symptoms.

The physical exam in irritable bowel syndrome may be completely within normal limits. Often, however, localized abdominal tenderness is noted on deep palpation that abates with continuous pressure. The rectal area may be excoriated and tender, with evidence of inflamed hemorrhoids or sphincter spasm. The stool guaiac test is negative. For the most part, the diagnosis is based on the history and physical exam. Sigmoidoscopy reveals a normal or dilated, engorged bowel with increased mucus. Treatment measures include diet modifications (high-bulk foods, xanthine elimination), heat, exercise/rest programs, and anticholinergic or sedative drugs.

While irritable bowel syndrome is a functional problem, severe inflammatory changes take place in ***ulcerative colitis.*** This disease of unknown etiology occurs at all ages but most commonly presents between ages 15 and 40. It usually begins in the rectosigmoid area and extends backward, eventually involving the entire large intestine. A more benign form of the disease, ***ulcerative proctitis,*** remains limited to the rectum. Pathologic changes evolve from inflammation of the mucosa, perhaps as a result of localized vasculitis. The mucosa becomes hyperemic and infiltrated with neutrophils and eosinophils. Goblet cells are destroyed and their housing crypts drop out or become abscessed. Mucus production decreases. Epithelial necrosis, mucosal ulceration, and fibrosis ultimately develop. With repeated bouts of inflammation, the bowel shortens, not so much from fibrosis but from a peculiar retraction of the longitudinal muscles. Other than retraction, the muscular layer remains untouched by the disease. The mucosa, however, may be completely denuded and replaced by hyperplastic tissue known as "inflammatory polyps" (pseudopolyps).

Episodic attacks of bloody diarrhea, marked by extreme urgency to defecate and lower abdominal cramps, is the usual presentation of ulcerative colitis. However, a number of patients have a fulminant onset of disease with violent diarrhea, high fever, and signs of peritonitis, and nearly 10% die from hemorrhage, perforation, sepsis, and/or toxemia. Another 10% not only recover completely from the first attack but have no further problems. Unfortunately, the majority suffer from repeated exacerbations of increasing severity. Stools, 10–15 per day, become looser and frequently consist entirely of blood, mucus, and pus. Abdominal cramps and tenesmus awaken the patient at night. A number of extracolonic manifestations may also be associated with ulcerative colitis, including arthritis, uveitis, ankylosing spondylitis, aphthous ulcers, erythema nodosum, and pyoderma gangrenosum (foot ulcers). On exam, patients have diffuse abdominal tenderness but no masses. Weight loss, fever, and anemia are common, along with an elevated white blood cell count, an increased erythrocyte sedimentation rate, and hypoalbuminemia.

Patients thought to have ulcerative colitis should be referred at once to a gastroenterologist. The disease is confirmed by proctoscopy, and the patient may be started on corticosteroids and sulfa drugs. Once controlled, the disease should be staged by more extensive tests. Ongoing care includes a milk-free diet (milk products seem to aggravate symptoms), maintenance doses of sulfa, retention enemas containing steroid preparations, or, in more severe cases, surgery. Because there is an increased risk of colon cancer, screening biopsies and prophylactic protocolectomy have been advocated.

The descending colon takes an S-shaped turn at the left iliac crest and forms a short segment called the "sigmoid colon" (Figure 4.6), which stores fecal matter until it is expelled. Because the sigmoid colon is narrower and has higher pressures than other portions of the large intestine, it is the most common location for the development of ▶ ***diverticulae.*** Raised further by spasm or irregular contractions of the musculature, pressures force thin layers of mucosa to herniate through weakened areas of bowel wall, usually around blood vessels. Diverticulae also form in the cecum or ascending colon; although far less numerous than those in the sigmoid colon, they are more likely to ulcerate and bleed. Associated with bowel spasm and irregular pressures, inadequate dietary bulk and overuse of laxatives are thought to be responsible for the formation of diverticulae in 30–40% of the population over age 50.

Most patients with diverticulae are asymptomatic, but some experience lower abdominal pain and distention. These symptoms are typically intermittent and may be relieved by defecation. Constipation and constipation alternating with diarrhea are also common. On exam, loops of colon filled with stool can often be palpated in the left lower quadrant. The area may also be tender, but without signs of peritoneal irritation. Diverticulae are diagnosed by barium enema. The concurrent presence of polyps or carcinoma should be ruled out with proctoscopy and/or biopsy, particularly if there is evidence of rectal bleeding. Measures to reduce bowel spasm and intraluminal pressures are the basis of treatment. They include high-fiber diets, adequate fluids, exercise, and weight reduction. Caffeine, alcohol, and laxatives should be avoided.

Diverticulae can become filled with fecal matter and particles of undigested food. If the thin wall of the mucosa becomes inflamed or infected, ***diverticulitis,*** a potentially fatal condition, develops. Abscesses form that may be absorbed, drain into the bowel lumen, or create fistulous tracts. Inflamed segments of bowel often adhere to walls of the bladder or nearby pelvic organs and may become obstructed. In an extremely serious complication, the abscesses may perforate and contaminate the peritoneal cavity with purulent fecal material. The presenting sign of diverticulitis is pain, usually in the left lower quadrant. Crampy pain is associated with small bowel adhesions, while pain aggravated by urination suggests bladder adhesions. Severe pain accompanies peritonitis. Patients are usually febrile and have elevated leukocyte counts. A mass may be palpated in the left lower quadrant, and there may be signs of peritonitis. Patients with acute diverticulitis require hospitalization for administration of intravenous (IV) fluids and antibiotics. Emergency resection may be needed in cases of perforation. Prophylactic resection is advocated for patients with recurrent diverticulitis. Performed when the bowel is quiescent, elective surgery prevents recurrence and is associated with few complications.

RECTUM

The rectum (Figure 4.7) makes up the last portion of the large intestine. The terminal inch of the rectum, the anal canal, contains internal and external layers of sphincter muscles. Slips from some of these muscles attach to skin around the anus, giving it a puckered appearance. Inside, veins project into the lumen, forming anal columns. The depressions between these columns are called the "anal sinuses," into which empty the anal glands (crypts of Morgani). A continuous blanket of mucous membrane covers the irregular sinus contours and, by bridging their bases, forms the pectinate line.

The anus is supplied with somatic sensory nerves and is extremely sensitive. For this reason, lesions, infections, or dermatologic conditions of the perianal area can cause great discomfort (Table 4.14). Probably the most painful is ***rectal abscess.*** Rectal abscesses can develop below the levator ani muscle (perianal and ischiorectal) or, less commonly, above it (supralevator). They form from fecal matter that has collected in deep folds of the anal sinuses or from bacterial invasion of preexisting lesions such as hidradenitis, cryptitis, hematomas, sclerosed hemorrhoids, or anal fissures. Rectal abscess is more likely to occur in patients with diabetes, alcoholism, neurologic disease, and leukemia. General malaise and fever precede by days the development of localized tenderness and swelling with lower abscesses or by weeks with supralevator abscesses. There may be vague pelvic discomfort. In men, inflammation near the base of the bladder may cause misleading urinary symptoms. The abscess may eventually drain through the skin of the peritoneum, the groin, or the

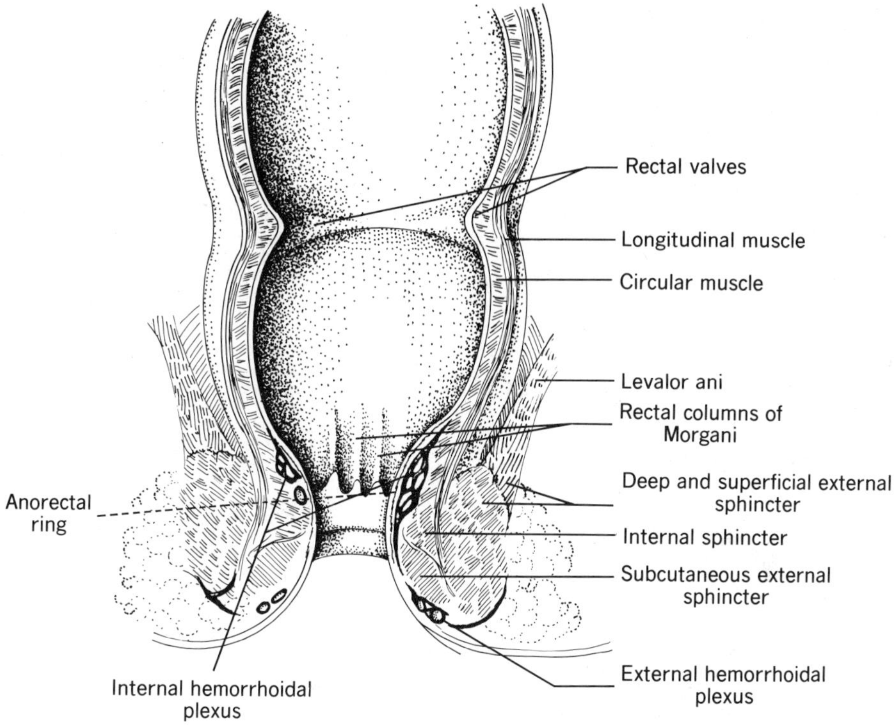

Figure 4.7 Rectum.

buttocks. Treatment consists of pustular drainage and surgical excision of fistulas. Antibiotics should be guided by culture and sensitivity. Analgesics are prescribed for pain. Since rectal abscesses are the forerunners of inflammatory bowel disease, a complete GI work-up is indicated for nonhealing or recurring lesions.

Pilonidal cysts are the result of abnormal embryologic development. The residual cysts are located at the base of the sacrum and are prone to abscess formation from embedded hairs. Infection causes inflammation, acute pain, and swelling. Fistular tracts may drain into the rectal region. Surgical excision is the necessary treatment, and the healing process is lengthy. Recurrence can be prevented by complete drainage of the infection and removal of hairs in the area.

Superior, middle, and inferior hemorrhoidal veins drain the rectum and anal canal. These veins anastomose with the portal system. Dilatation of hemorrhoidal veins results from portal hypertension, straining at stool, upright posture, obesity, pregnancy, or familial weakness of vascular walls and leads to ▶***hemorrhoids.*** Dilated veins above the pectinate line (see Fig. 4.7) are called ***internal hemorrhoids.*** Covered by recal mucosa that lacks sensory fibers, internal hemorrhoids are painless. However, they can become substantially enlarged, protrude through the anal canal, and bleed. ***External hemorrhoids*** (dilated veins below the pectinate line) are covered by squamous epithelium containing numerous nerve fibers. They can be extremely painful, particularly if their blood supply is cut off. This may lead to sudden swelling, inflammation, and sometimes profuse bleeding known as a

TABLE 4.14 ANORECTAL LESIONS

Cancer	May resemble a polyp or lipoma with or without ulceration.
Cryptitis	Inflammation of a crypt or follicle that drains an anal gland. Stasis due to obstruction or trauma precedes the inflammation.
Fissure (ulcer)	Crack in the lining of the anus with severe burning pain after defecation. Most fissures are posterior midline, but chronic fissures can also be found anteriorly. A hemorrhoidal tag may signal the presence of a fissure.
Gonorrheal proctitis	Inflammatory reaction of the rectum with soreness, burning, and purulent anal discharge.
Hemorrhoids	
Internal	Range from no detectable prolapse or prolapse that can be reduced to permanent prolapse outside the anus.
External	Bluish, rounded, swollen, dilated inferior hemorrhoidal veins with pain and itching.
Tag	Sequel to an acute hemorrhoid consisting of two or more folds of anal skin.
Herpes genitalis	Painful single or clustered blisters (vesicular lesion) that may also involve the penis or vulva. May be accompanied by fever.
Hidradenitis (apocrinitis)	Inflammation of the perianal sweat glands.
Infection	
Abscess	Acute phase. Localized to anal glands and obvious as a red, painful swelling close to the anal verge. Pain on sitting or coughing.
Fistula	Chronic phase. Tract that connects and drains abscess or anal canal out to the perianal region.
Pilonidal cyst	Swelling or draining sinus midline in area of natal cleft above anus. Multiple sinuses may be present. Most common in men aged 16–30.
Viral warts (condylomata)	Soft, filiform, multiple growths that may also involve the penis and vulva. Single lesions may enlarge and become confluent.

▶ ***thrombosed hemorrhoid.*** Thrombosed hemorrhoids reduce spontaneously, but because the condition is so painful, surgical excision may be elected. Without surgery the clot absorbs within 5 days, leaving a protruding tag of hypertrophied tissue. These ***skin tags*** are usually asymptomatic but sometimes annoy the patient with continual itching. ▶ ***Inflamed hemorrhoids*** can also cause extreme discomfort and are the most common cause of rectal bleeding. Treatment includes suppositories, stool softeners, sitz baths, and careful hygiene. Surgery is indicated in the following cases: bleeding sufficient to cause anemia; prolapse of hemorrhoidal tissue, especially if associated with bowel movements; and intolerable discomfort.

Defecation is a reflex involving volunary and involuntary muscles of the rectum and anal canal. When feces distend the wall of the rectum, it stimulates the mass peristaltic movement. As the distended rectum contracts, the levator ani muscle relaxes and the anal canal straightens out. The internal and external sphincters then relax and defecation occurs. Increased intra-abdominal pressure (Valsalva's maneuver or straining) substantially facilitate this process. Parasympathetic nerve fibers are responsible for the contraction of the rectum and the relaxation of the internal sphincter. Conscious inhibition of the defecation reflex can be accomplished by the contraction of the levator ani and external sphincter muscles. In general, there is a decrease in the tone of the anal sphincter with aging.

▶ ***Constipation*** is defined as fewer than three stools per week or as a decrease from the patient's usual routine. Stools are hard and difficult to pass. Constipation is

TABLE 4.15 CAUSES OF CONSTIPATION

Impaired motility
  Inadequate dietary fiber
  Sedentary lifestyle/inactivity
  Pregnancy
  Aging
  Dehydration
  Laxative abuse
  Irritable bowel syndrome
  Inflammatory bowel disease
  Cancer/tumor
  Diverticulosis/diverticulitis
  Hypothyroidism
  Hypokalemia
  Scleroderma
  Drugs
    Antacids (calcium and aluminum hydroxides)
    Anticholinergics
    Antihistamines
    Tricyclic antidepressants
    Opiates
	Obstruction
	  Cancer/tumor
	  Stricture
	  Volvulus
	Neurologic problems
	  Multiple sclerosis
	Anorectal problems
	  Hemorrhoids
	  Fissures
	  Abscesses
	Emotional disorders
	  Depression
	  Bowel function fixation

associated with inadequate dietary fiber, dehydration, a number of drugs, and weight reduction diets. It may also result from hectic lifestyles and inadequate exercise. On the other hand, constipation may be the presenting symptom of serious underlying pathology (Table 4.15). This latter possibility should be considered before treatment with increased fiber and fluid, exercise programs, and bowel habit retraining. Laxatives, described in Table 4.16, should be used sparingly, if at all.

Chronic constipation often leads to ▶ ***anal fissures,*** longitudinal tears in rectal skin (see Table 4.14). A burning or tearing sensation is felt with passage of stool, along with slight bleeding. Severe muscle spasm of the sphincter usually accompanies chronic fissures. Patients may avoid defecation, thus exacerbating the condition. Most fissures heal spontaneously and respond well to sitz baths, local analgesics, stool softeners, and anal hygiene. Occasionally, surgical excision of damaged tissue is required.

Perianal itching can be caused by fissures, hemorrhoids, venereal infections, and parasites. ▶ ***Idiopathic pruritis ani*** is diagnosed when these conditions have been excluded. It is a form of dermatitis that develops when urine or stool is wiped into cracks in the skin, excessively alkaline stool, or in reaction to perfumes and feminine sprays. Diet exacerbates the symptoms, especially the intake of caffeine and spicy foods. Scratching leads to severe excoriation and hyperpigmentation. Soft stools, perianal hygiene, and cortisone ointments are the cornerstones of treatment.

Cancer of the colon and rectum is the second most common malignancy and accounts for 20% of all deaths due to neoplastic disease. Polyps, ulcerative colitis, diet, and heredity have been associated with this disease, but the cause is unknown. Disease occurs at all ages, with the highest incidence after the age of 50. Women are more likely to develop colonic cancer, while men are more prone to rectal malignancies. Although there are several types of tumors, all tend to invade the lymphatic system, and metastasis is common. Carcinoma affecting the left side of the colon tends to produce a change in bowel habits (diarrhea, constipation, and/or tenesmus). Since rectal bleeding occurs in 70% of cases, malignancy should be ruled out before

TABLE 4.16 COMMONLY USED LAXATIVES

Laxative	Dosage	Side Effects
Bulk-forming		
Psylluim hydrophilic mucilloid (Metamucil)	1 tsp dissolved in 1–2 glasses of water one to three times a day. Onset of action occurs within 24 hours; full effect is apparent in 3 days.	Flatulence; rare risk of obstruction. Binding of digitalis, nitrofurantoin, salicylate. Decreases the effect of these drugs.
Saline		
Magnesium hydroxide (milk of magnesia)	15–30 mL at bedtime; results occur in 3–8 hours.	Prolonged diarrhea may lead to water loss and electrolyte disturbances. Contraindicated in renal insufficiency because of possibility of magnesium toxicity.
Sodium biphosphate and sodium phosphate (Fleet enema)	4 oz (rectal only); results occur in 30 minutes.	Repeated use contraindicated in cardiac disease.
Lubricant		
Mineral oil	15–45 mL at bedtime; results occur in 8–24 hours.	Malabsorption of fats and fat-soluble vitamins. Lipoid pneumonia occurs if aspirated. Decreases prothrombin levels.
Dioctyl sodium sulfosuccinate (Colace)	100–600 mg daily for 1 week; full effect achieved in about 3 days.	Possible hepatoxicity. Enhances absorption of mineral oil to cause granuloma formation if given concomitantly.
Glycerin/Dulcolax	One suppository; results occur in 30 minutes. Also available in enema form.	Rectal irritation.
Stimulant		
Bisacodyl (Dulcolax)	10–20 mg orally; results occur in 3–12 hours. Or give 10-mg rectal suppository; results occur in 15–60 minutes.	Gastric irritation (oral); rectal irritation (suppository).
Castor oil	15–60 ml; results occur in 2–6 hours.	Prolonged diarrhea and crampy abdominal pain.

attributing the presence of blood to hemorrhoids or rectal fissures. Occasionally, patients develop severe anemia and present with symptoms of failure. Pain is a variable finding. Anorexia, weight loss, and malaise develop at any time.

Cancer of the large bowel is curable if discovered early. Approximately one-half of rectal cancers are within reach of digital examination. For this reason, rectal examinations are important aspects of routine health care. Stool tests for occult blood provide the most efficient and economical screening measure. False-positive tests are reduced by testing six stool samples while the patient is on a meat-free diet. Patients with any signs or symptoms of malignancy should undergo sigmoidoscopy and barium enema. Suspicious lesions noted during these procedures must be biopsied. The primary treatment for cancer of the colon and rectum is surgical resection of the bowel. Chemotherapy may follow if there is evidence of metastasis to lymph nodes or the liver.

Details of Management

▸ *Diffuse Esophageal Spasm*

Laboratory Tests: EKG. Barium swallow and manometry may be helpful for diagnosis.

Therapeutic Measures: Reassurance (particularly that the problem is not cardiac) and stress reduction are the most important aspects of treatment. Low-dose sublingual nitroglycerin such as Nitrostat, 0.15–0.3 mg, may give occasional relief, but anticholinergics and smooth muscle relaxants have not been found to be successful. Calcium channel blockers are a future possibility. Prescribe H2-receptor antagonists and antacids if esophagitis is present (see the following section).

Patient Education: Explain the relationship between stress and symptoms. Teach stress reduction techniques (see Chapter 13).

Follow-up: Periodic weight checks and symptom review. Refer progressive or unresponsive cases to a gastroenterologist.

▸ *Esophageal Reflux and Esophagitis*

Laboratory Tests: EKG. Barium swallow or endoscopy may be necessary.

Therapeutic Measures: Prescribe liquid antacids, 30 ml 1 and 3 hours after meals and at bedtime, to neutralize residual gastric contents. Use magnesium-containing antacids (e.g., Maalox), since calcium-containing antacids (e.g., Tums) cause rebound hyperacidity (see Table 4.2). If no improvement occurs, start cimetidine, 400 mg HS, to suppress gastric secretions and limit nocturnal reflux, or prescribe Reglan, 1 tablet 30 minutes before each meal and at bedtime for 2–4 weeks, to speed gastric emptying and reduce reflux following food intake. All medications should be taken with ample amounts of water. Advise the use of small meals and the limitation of foods that cause symptoms such as spices, citrus juices, coffee, excess carbohydrates, fats, and chocolate. Eliminate alcohol, smoking, and, whenever possible, anticholinergic drugs. Instruct patients to elevate the head of the bed by placing 6-in. blocks under the head posts. Have them refrain from lying down immediately after eating and advise them to avoid eating 4 hours before bedtime. Start overweight patients on weight loss programs and advise all patients not to wear tight clothing around the waist.

Patient Education: Discuss the nature of the condition and the rationale for therapeutic measures. Emphasize that when all measures are undertaken together, symptoms usually subside. Warn patients that diarrhea may result from magnesium-containing antacids.

Follow-up: If no improvement occurs in 4 weeks, refer the patient to a gastroenterologist.

▸ *Gastric and Duodenal Ulcers*

Laboratory Tests: Stool guaiac test, upper gastrointestinal series, endoscopy and biopsy of suspicious or nonhealing lesions.

Therapeutic Measures: Start antacids (see Table 4.2), 2 tbsp 1 hour and 3 hours after meals and at bedtime. Keep in mind that antacids enhance the effect of dicumarol and L-dopa and decrease the effect of phenothiazines, sulfa, isoniazid, penicillin, and tetracyclines. Although most patients do well on antacid therapy alone, recent studies show that cimetidine (Tagemet), 300 mg with meals and at bedtime, or ranitidine (Zantac), 150 mg bid for up to 4 weeks, is effective in the treatment of uncomplicated gastric and duodenal ulcers. As an alternative to H2-receptor antagonists (particularly in alcohol-induced cases), prescribe sucralfate (Carafate) 1 gm qid for 4–8 weeks. Since acid must be present for therapeutic effect, sucralfate should be taken on an empty stomach (30–60 minutes before meals). While neither cimetidine nor ranitidine should be used concomitantly, antacids may still be employed for pain if taken at least 1 hour before or after sucralfate administration. Advise a regular diet of three meals a day, limiting substances that are known to increase acid secretion (caffeine, alcohol, etc.). Have patients avoid bedtime eating to reduce postprandial acid stimulation. Discourage smoking and discontinue drugs that are gastric irritants.

Patient Education: Explain the relationship of ulcer disease and acid secretion. Educate patients to read labels of foods and over-the-counter drugs for caffeine (in soft drinks and chocolate) and salicylates (in many cold preparations and Alka Seltzer). Discuss the role of stress and the production of stomach acid. Prescribe simple relaxation techniques (see Chapter 13). Educate patients about signs and symptoms that need immediate evaluation (increased pain, vomiting, rectal bleeding, anorexia, or weight loss).

Follow-up: Arrange an appointment in 6 weeks (sooner if symptoms do not improve). If the patient is asymptomatic, antacids can be discontinued. Endoscopy with biopsy should be performed if the ulcer does not heal 8–12 weeks after initiation of therapy or if it recurs soon after healing. Perform periodic stool guaiac tests.

▸ *Lactose Intolerance*

Laboratory Tests: Diagnosis is usually based on the patient's history. It may be confirmed by breath tests that measure the amount of radioactive labeled CO_2 or hydrogen. Oral lactose tolerance tests are also performed but are less specific.

Therapeutic Measures: Since tolerance varies in adults, begin by removing all sources of lactose for 3 weeks:

All milks	Ice cream	Cottage cheese
American cheese	Milk chocolate	Party dips
Sherbets	Puddings	Pie fillings
Cream soups	Medications (some tablets and vitamins)	
White bread or other bakery products made with milk		

Gradually reintroduce these foods. Limit dietary intake of lactose to the point of tolerance (established by the development of symptoms). As an alternative to milk elimination, patients can buy fresh lowfat milk in which the lactose has been hydrolyzed (converted into galactose and glucose). This can be found under the brand LactAid but is not available in all areas of the country. Patients may also hydrolyze their own milk by adding 4–10 drops of prescription LactAid to 1 quart of milk, depending on the degree of lactose conversion desired (4–5 drops yields 70%, while extra drops and/or time yields up to 100%). LactAid products are contraindicated in patients with galactosemia. Women on strict lactose-free diets should start taking calcium supplements (see Chapter 11).

Patient Education: Explain the etiology of the disease and the fact that the enzyme lactase decreases naturally with age. Alcohol abuse can also cause decreased lactase activity. Teach patients to check labels on food packages for lactose content or the presence of milk solids. Diabetics using LactAid should note that hydrolysis converts the milk sugar in each quart into readily available glucose (25 g) and galactose (25 g). Diet adjustments should be made accordingly.

Follow-up: If a strict lactose-free diet is followed, monitor the patient's weight and calcium intake. If there is no abatement of symptoms with lactose control, consider other causes of symptoms.

▸ *Chronic Pancreatitis*

Laboratory Tests: Serum amylase, lipase, and creatinine clearance ratios may or may not be helpful. Other tests are a flat film of the abdomen, an oral cholecystogram, serum calcium, and fasting triglyceride levels.

Therapeutic Measures: Prescribe a low-fat diet (see Chapter 5) and start daily multivitamin supplements. Discontinue all alcohol. For steatorrhea, give a pancreatic supplement such as Cotazyme or Pancreatin, 1 or 2 capsules during meals and 1 capsule with snacks. Prescribe Librax, 1 or 2 capsules tid with meals and at bedtime, or other sedative/anticholinergic combinations to alleviate pain symptoms. Aspirin and Tylenol may also be used but, whenever possible, avoid narcotics to prevent addiction. In extreme cases, methadone may be necessary. Arrange for surgical treatment of correctable biliary tract disease.

Patient Education: If the disease is associated with alcohol abuse, discuss the patient's drinking habit frankly and explore its treatment options with the patient and family. Use diet teaching as needed. Plan an exercise program for improved fitness and sense of control. Advocate relaxation techniques or alternative methods for dealing with pain.

Follow-up: See the patient every 3–4 months for medication review and continued support regarding alcohol control and diet. Periodic evaluation is needed for early symptoms of carcinoma, pancreatic pseudocyst, pancreatic insufficiency (diarrhea and weight loss), biliary tract disease, and abnormal glucose tolerance.

▸ *Viral Gastroenteritis*

Laboratory Tests: None.

Therapeutic Measures: Replace fluids and electrolytes with clear juices, cola drinks, tea with sugar, Gatorade, or popsicles (solutions with sugar facilitate absorption of water and give needed energy). Avoid milk products and excessive caffeine. Progress to easily digested foods such as crackers and bananas. Advise rest until the acute symptoms have resolved and then suggest progressive activity. Give Tylenol or aspirin, 2 tablets every 4–6 hours, for fever and myalgia.

Patient Education: Explain that the infection is caused by a virus and will resolve spontaneously in 24–48 hours. Emphasize that antidiarrheal, antiemetic, and antibiotic medications are not effective and may prolong the illness. Stress the importance of fluid replacement. Have the patient report increasing or persistent symptoms.

Follow-up: As needed.

▸ *Oral Fluid and Electrolyte Replacement in Gastroenteritis*

Laboratory Tests: Only for signs of depletion. Specific gravity of urine, hematocrit, serum electrolytes.

Therapeutic Measures: Prepare in the office or have patients prepare at home an oral rehydration solution (ORS) recommended by the World Health Organization. All necessary salt, potassium, bicarbonate, glucose, and fluid are provided as follows:

Formula 1	Formula 2
1 L (qt) pure water	1 glass fruit juice
½ tsp table salt	½ tsp honey or corn syrup
½ tsp baking soda	1 pinch of table salt
4 tbsp sugar	
¼ tsp Kcl	

Other well-balanced sources are Pedialyte, Gatorade, and, in the tropics, green coconut milk. Prescribe an amount of solution intake equal to the amount of body fluids lost (approximately an 8-oz glass per diarrheal stool). Bananas and citrus fruits provide potassium; popsicles provide sugar and small amounts of fluid.

Patient Education: Stress the fact that in all cases of gastroenteritis, replacement of fluids and electrolytes is crucial to recovery. Instruct patients to keep a record of fever, amount and frequency of stool, and fluid intake. Have patients report any worsening of signs immediately.

Follow-up: As dictated by the specific nature of the disease.

▸ *Enteric Precautions*

Laboratory Tests: Stool cultures as dictated by the specific organism.

Therapeutic Measures: Advise separate sleeping and bathroom arrangements for patients in nursing homes or other institutional settings or for incontinent patients being treated at home (otherwise, special arrangements are not needed). Have clothes, bedding, towels, bathroom fixtures, and other objects that become contaminated by the patient's stool and urine carefully disinfected or discarded. Cleaning products such as chlorine bleach may be used for this purpose. Clothes should be washed separately in extra hot water and then thoroughly sun or machine dried. To cut down on the amount of soiled clothing and the inconvenience of changing, advise any person attending incontinent patients to wear an apron. Attendants or visitors *must* wash hands carefully after any direct contact with the patient or contaminated objects even if gloves are worn. It is also crucial that the patient practice careful hand washing after urination and defecation.

Patient Education: Emphasize that infection is spread only through fecal material, not by any type of direct contact. It cannot be spread by an ill patient who merely touches or breathes on someone. Furthermore, the fecal material must somehow be ingested by a noninfected individual before causing disease. This happens most commonly when unnoticed fecal matter passes from the hands or an inanimate object to the mouth (thus the necessity of careful hand washing). Alternatively, fecal material can filter into water systems where sanitary conditions are inadequate or passed by dirty hands to food. People then contract a disease by eating contaminated food or water.

Follow-up: Give job clearance for patients only after signs of infection have resolved. With some organisms (notably *Salmonella typhi, Shigella,* and *Campylobacter*), three negative cultures obtained at 24-hour intervals are advised.

▸ *Cholera Vaccination*

Laboratory Tests: None.

Therapeutic Measures: At present, the U.S. Public Health Service recommends that cholera vaccine (which offers little if any protection) be given only to U.S. citizens traveling to endemic areas of the world who are at high risk for developing disease (hypo- or achlorhydric patients). Such patients should be given a full series as follows:

Series	Adult Dose	Schedule
First	0.5 ml IM or SQ	To start
Second	Same	1–4 weeks after the starting dose and
Booster	Same	every 6 months thereafter as needed

Give low-risk patients who must have evidence of cholera immunization for entry into certain areas (e.g., Asia, the Middle East, and Africa) a single 0.5-ml primary or booster dose within 6 months of expected arrival. Do not give cholera vaccine at the same time or within 3 months of yellow fever vaccine. Safety of vaccination during pregnancy has not been established.

Patient Education: Warn patients that pain, redness, and swelling may occur at the site of injection, along with fever, malaise, and headache lasting for 1–2 days. Advise patients not to have future vaccinations if they experience more serious symptoms.

Follow-up: Usually none. For high-risk patients, every 6 months for boosters as needed.

▸ *Enterotoxigenic* **E. coli** *(ETEC, "Turista")*

Laboratory Tests: Usually none are indicated. Stool smears are reassuring in that neutrophils and red blood cells should be absent. Agglutination or immunofluorescence with antisera or demonstration of heat-labile toxins may be specially ordered tests.

Therapeutic Measures: Replace fluids as previously described. Prescribe Peptol Bismol, 30 ml every 30 minutes, to reduce symptoms. Antibiotics are not indicated, and Lomotil or opiates may prolong the course of the disease. Advise the use of enteric precautions (see the previous section) until symptoms resolve.

Patient Education: Reassure the patient that the problem is self-limiting and should resolve in 3–7 days. Explain that antibiotics may compromise the problem by further upsetting bowel flora and that antidiarrheal agents may favor bacterial growth by slowing gastric motility. Warn against the use of Entero-Vioform, an antidiarrheal agent associated with optic neuritis, which is available over the counter in some countries.

Follow-up: As needed for work clearance.

▸ *Typhoid Immunization*

Laboratory Tests: None.

Therapeutic Measures: Vaccinate patients traveling to areas with poor food and water sanitation (check with the U.S. Public Health Service for specific information) as follows:

Series	Adult Dose	Preferred Schedule
First	0.5 ml SQ	To start
Second	Same	4 or more weeks after first dose
Booster	Same	Every 3 years as needed

or

Series	Adult Dose	Alternative Schedule (Less Effective)
First	0.5 ml SQ	To start
Second	Same	1 week after the first dose
Third	Same	1 week after the second dose
Booster	Same	Every 3 years as needed

Give only a booster even if more than 3 years have elapsed since the primary series. Do not give the vaccine during pregnancy.

Patient Education: Note that the vaccine protects 70–90% of recipients depending on the amount of exposure. Emphasize that even vaccinated individuals should be cautious with food and water when traveling (see the next section). Warn that vaccination may cause a local reaction (erythema, induration, and tenderness), as well as fever, malaise, and headache within 24 hours.

Follow-up: Every 3 years for boosters as needed.

▸ *Acute Salmonella Enterocolitis*

Laboratory Tests: Stool guaiac test. Methylene blue or Gram stain. If fecal leukocytes and/or red blood cells found, a stool culture is needed. If symptoms of diarrhea are accompanied by systemic illness, obtain blood cultures and serotype them to rule out *S. typhi.*

Therapeutic Measures: Advise enteric precautions and fluid replacement as previously described. Prescribe Pepto Bismol, 3 tbsp every 30 minutes, in six doses. Antibiotics may prolong carriage in the GI tract and are warranted only in high-risk cases where cancer, hemoglobinopathy, chronic GI disease, or immune deficiency coexist. Drugs of choice are ampicillin (100 mg/kg intravenously or orally) or chloramphenicol (50–100 mg/kg orally) until signs of improvement appear.

Patient Education: Explain that even though the infection is caused by a bacterial agent, the disease is self-limiting within 3–5 days and that antibiotics do not shorten the course of symptoms. Emphasize the importance of fluid replacement. For future precautions, advise patients to wash hands after manipulating uncooked meats (especially poultry); to eat only thoroughly cooked meats (particularly following defrosting); and to be wary of picnic tables under trees (bird droppings can contain salmonella). Have pet turtles checked for disease.

Follow-up: Arrange daily phone contact to monitor the patient's hydration status. Severely ill patients may need hospitalization for intravenous fluid replacement and antibiotics. Reevaluate the patient as soon as symptoms have subsided. Continue isolation until three consecutive stool cultures 24 hours apart prove negative.

▸ *Shigellosis,* Campylobacter *Enteritis, and Enteroinvasive* E. coli *(EIEC)*

Laboratory Tests: Fecal stain for leukocytes and red blood cells. Stool cultures with sensitivity tests for *Shigella* and *Campylobacter* (there is a high incidence of resistant strains). *Shigella* is heat labile, so multiple samples may be needed. EIEC is identified only by special tissue cultures such as guinea pig conjunctival sac inoculation.

Therapeutic Measures: Start fluid replacement and enteric precautions as previously described. Prescribe trimethoprim/sulfamethoxazole (Bactrim or Septra) DS bid; ampicillin or erythromycin 250 qid for 3–5 days. Stop the use of antibiotics at the earliest signs of improvement. Advise the use of aspirin or Tylenol, two tablets every 4–6 hours, for general discomfort. Do not give opiates or anticholinergics, since they decrease bowel motility (which is conducive to bacterial growth).

Patient Education: Emphasize the importance of fluid intake. Advise patients to respond to the body's need for more rest by reducing travel activities. Warn travelers not to take Entero-Vioform, an antidiarrheal drug (associated with optic neuritis), available over the counter in many foreign countries.

Follow-up: If symptoms persist beyond 7–10 days, evaluate the patient for parasites or other causes of diarrhea. The patient should observe enteric precautions until symptoms subside and three cultures are negative.

▸ *Prevention of Bacterial Gastroenteritis*

Laboratory Tests: None.

Therapeutic Measures: Give cholera and typhoid vaccinations for travelers as recommended by the U.S. Public Health Service. Give doxycycline, 200 mg on day 1 followed by 100 mg daily, or trimethoprim/sulfamethoxazole, DS daily, as effective prophylaxis against sensitive *E. coli* and shigellae. Since these drugs may lead to adverse reactions and resistant organisms, reserve their use for patients taking short nonrecreational trips (lasting for fewer than 2–3 weeks) during which symptoms would impose a serious hardship. Medication should be continued for 2–3 days after returning from travel to prevent a delayed attack. Peptol Bismol in large doses (2 oz four times a day) has also been found to reduce the incidence of diarrhea.

Patient Education: Note that disease can be spread through homosexual practices, and a high incidence occurs in homosexual populations. Since patterns of disease are ever-changing, advise patients to check with the U.S. Center of Disease Control for current guidelines when planning trips outside the country. The yearly publication *Health Information for International Travel,* published by the U.S. Department of Health and Human Resources, Public Health Service (CDC), Atlanta, Georgia, 30333, can be obtained for a small charge. Give patients a handout containing the following advice:

Never drink from streams, lakes, or untested wells. If there is any question about local supplies, drink only water that has been boiled for 15 minutes or treated as follows:

	Clear Water	Cloudy Water
(Chlorine/L)		
1%	10 gtt	20 gtt
4–6%	2 gtt	4 gtt
7–10%	1 gtt	2 gtt
Iodine (not effective against giardia cysts)		
2%	5 gtt	10 gtt

Refrain from using ice or bottled water. Carbonated beverages and beer may be safely used, since carbonation lowers the pH and thereby kills or inhibits bacteria. Eat only thoroughly cooked or properly preserved food, avoiding salads and unpeeled fruits and vegetables. Be wary of food and water contaminated by insect and bird droppings (e.g., on picnic tables under trees).

▸ Giardia

Laboratory Tests: Stools for cysts or trophozoites. If stool tests are negative and disease is strongly suspected, an exam of a duodenal aspirate or intestinal mucosal biopsy is warranted for evidence of protozoa.

Therapeutic Measures: Prescribe metronidazole (Flagyl), 250 mg tid for 10 days, or quinacrine (Atabrine), 100 mg tid for 7 days. Start fluid replacement as previously described for significant diarrhea. Monitor the patient's weight.

Patient Education: Instruct patients to avoid alcohol intake while taking Flagyl. Explain that no isolation procedures are required but that exposed persons may want to have stools examined for evidence of disease. Warn about venereal spread of disease. Review preventive measures (especially avoidance of drinking stream water unless it is properly treated with chlorine; iodine does not kill *Giardia* cysts).

Follow-up: None necessary unless symptoms persist.

▸ *Gastrointestinal Gas*

Laboratory Tests: None.

Therapeutic Measures: If possible, correct conditions that contribute to air swallowing: arrange a dental visit for denture adjustment; ear, nose, and throat (ENT) evaluation for nasal obstruction or polyps; and treatment of rhinitis, postnasal drips, and so on. Identify and eliminate air-swallowing habits such as gum chewing, sucking on hard candies, drinking with a straw, gulping drinks, and smoking. Point out that air swallowing is often related to stress and discuss various approaches to stress reduction (see Chapter 13). Give patients a diet sheet listing foods to avoid (broccoli, cabbage, beans, peas, turnips, radishes, onions, bran, and large amounts of fruit). Note that fatty or fried foods and foods with air whipped into them (souffles, milkshakes, carbonated beverages including beer) cause belching. Have patients modify certain eating practices as follows: eat slowly (spend 30–60 minutes per meal), chew food thoroughly, and limit liquids while eating (they tend to wash down unchewed food and distend the stomach). Avoid large meals and eating when tense or upset. Instruct patients not to wear tight clothing. Prescribe a sensible exercise program. For abdominal distention with discomfort, advise placing a heating pad on the area and/or antacid therapy (Mylanta, 2 tbsp after meals and at bedtime). Simethicone (Mylicon), 1–2 chewable tablets after meals and at bedtime, can also be tried, but its efficacy has been questioned.

Patient Education: Explain the relationship of gas symptoms to air swallowing and diet. Reassure the patient that there is no serious organic disease.

Follow-up: As needed.

▸ *High-Fiber Diet*

Laboratory Tests: None.

Therapeutic measures: Review the recommended daily allowance for fiber (10–30 g). Some experts advise the ingestion of up to 50 g/day. Give patients a list of foods with high fiber contents such as the following:

Food	Grams of Crude Fiber/100 g
Miller's bran	10.0
Bran cereals (100% bran)	7.8
Sunflower seeds (kernels)	3.8
Bran flakes (40% bran)	3.6
Raisin Bran	3.0
Peanuts with skins	2.7
Almonds with skins	2.6
Shredded wheat, Wheaties	2.3
English walnuts	2.1
Puffed wheat	2.0
Peanut butter (2 tbsp)	1.9
Bran muffin	1.8
Fresh fruit with skin (1 average)	1.5
Whole wheat bread (1 slice)	1.3
Oats (Cheerios, granola)	1.2
Raw vegetables (1 serving)	1.1
Cooked vegetables	1.1
Fresh fruit without skin	1.0
Whole-grain bread (1 slice)	0.9
Mixed cereals (Special K, Quaker Natural Cereal)	0.8

Gradually increase the amount of fiber in the diet to prevent or minimize flatulence, abdominal distension, bloating, or diarrhea, which may occur from overzealous introduction of fiber. A hydrophylic psyllium seed preparation (Metamucil) may be given (1 tsp [7 g] one to three times a day) if the patient is unable to conform to a high-fiber diet.

Patient Education: Note the association of a high-fiber diet with reduced colon cancer and better glucose tolerance. Advise patients to ingest small amounts of bran throughout the day initially. Explain that if flatulence does occur, it will diminish within 1–3 weeks of continued use. If cereals are used as a source of fiber, a practical rule of thumb is that the cereal's name must include "bran" to be of sufficient benefit. Care should be taken to continue eating a well-balanced diet in addition to the supplemental fiber. The pure bran taste is bland, so it is helpful to add fruits, honey, or other foods to make it more palatable.

Follow-up: None needed.

▸ *Irritable Bowel Syndrome*

Laboratory Tests: None.

Therapeutic Measures: Instruct the patient to keep a diary of food intake and exacerbation of symptoms in order to identify lactose intolerance or other bowel irritants. Eliminate foods known to cause symptoms, as well as xanthine derivatives (foods or medications containing theophylline or caffeine), which produce smooth muscle relaxation. With those exceptions in mind, prescribe a well-balanced, high-fiber diet (see the previous section). Offer information on stress reduction (see Chapter 13). Initiate a good exercise program. Avoid the use of laxatives, enemas, and opiates.

Patient education: Discuss the nature of the problem and the contributing factors. Emphasize that irritable bowel is not to be confused with inflammatory bowel disease or gastroenteritis (i.e., it has no ominous prognosis and is not contagious). Reinforce diet instructions with written handouts.

Follow-up: Until symptoms are under control, schedule brief visits every 2 weeks to emphasize practitioner interest and the medical nature of the problem (it is a common misconception that irritable bowel syndrome is a psychiatric illness). Refer patients with persistent or increasingly severe symptoms to a gastroenterologist.

▸ *Diverticulae*

Laboratory Tests: Stool guaiac test. Barium enema.

Therapeutic Measures: Initiate a high-fiber diet (see the previous section) and adequate fluid intake. Decrease or eliminate milk products (if the patient is lactose intolerant), coffee, and alcohol (which cause bowel hypertonicity). Start a weight reduction program if indicated. Since stress can affect bowel motility and increase intraluminal pressure, stress reduction may be an important aspect of therapy (see Chapter 13). Avoid laxatives, enemas, and opiates.

Patient Education: Using a diagram, discuss the pathology involved and the contributing factors. Reinforce diet instructions with written handouts. Explain that diverticulitis is a possible complication and that the patient should report persistent abdominal pain, fever, or rectal bleeding.

Follow-up: As needed. Stools for a yearly guaiac test.

▸ *Thrombosed Hemorrhoid*

Laboratory Tests: None.

Therapeutic Measures: Instruct the patient to apply ice packs or iced witch hazel to the anal area for 5 minutes every half hour as often as possible. Prescribe a topical anesthetic (Xylocaine) or an oral pain medication (Tylenol with codeine, 30–60 mg q4h, or Dolobid, 500 mgq12h) as needed for pain. For comfort, suggest a prone position with the buttocks elevated by a pillow placed under the pelvis. Discuss the option of surgical intervention.

Patient Education: Explain the etiology of a thrombosed hemorrhoid and the self-limiting nature of the problem (an acute process that resolves in 3–5 days). Warn patients that a painless skin tag of connective tissue will remain permanently. Have patients report increased pain or bleeding.

Follow-up: Refer patients who have too much discomfort to undergo spontaneous resolution to a general surgeon.

▸ *Inflamed Hemorrhoid*

Laboratory Tests: Stool guaiac test. Anoscopy.

Therapeutic Measures: Prescribe rectal suppositories containing a hydrocortisone preparation such as Anusol-HC 1 am, 1 hs, for 3–6 days. Advise hot sitz baths for 15–20 minutes four times a day (before insertion of suppositories). Give dioctyl sodium sulfosuccinate (Colace), 100 mg three times a day, until symptoms resolve. Discuss prophylactic measures for constipation (see the following section). Advise patients not to use irritant laxatives and to refrain from straining at stool, lingering on the toilet, or vigorous wiping after bowel movements. Warn against long periods of standing or irritating activities (e.g., horseback or bike riding, bumpy car rides).

Patient Education: Explain the etiology of the condition and the association with factors that raise venous pressure. Tell patients that symptoms normally subside in 3–5 days and that they should report persistent pain or bleeding. Review proper use of suppositories. Discuss surgical alternatives.

Follow-up: As needed.

▸ *Constipation*

Laboratory Tests: As needed to rule out pathology (see Table 4.15). Stool guaiac test.

Therapeutic Measures: Prescribe a high-fiber diet (see the previous section). If it is not tolerated, prescribe Metamucil, 1–2 tsp in 8 oz of liquid three times a day. If possible, have patients avoid constipating foods (eggs, cheese, white bread) and medications (codeine, calcium- or aluminum-based antacids, vitamins with iron). Warn against the use of unprescribed enemas or laxatives (for extreme discomfort, prescribe glycerin suppositories). Advise the use of 7–12 daily glasses (1,000–2,500 cc) of water unless the patient is on fluid restriction for renal or cardiac problems. Initiate a sensible exercise program. Initiate a bowel-retraining program.

Patient Education: Explore with the patient factors that have contributed to the condition. Explain that bowel retraining requires patience and attention to details which may seem overly simple, such as the following: Since the gastrocolic reflex is greatest after the first meal of the day, eat a fairly large breakfast that includes fruit, a bran cereal or whole wheat bread, and coffee or another hot fluid. Go to the toilet at the same time each day, 15–45 minutes after a meal. Allow 10–15 minutes on the toilet without interruption and tension; a book, magazine, or music may provide relaxation. Sit with the feet on a footstool, since the squatting position is more natural and enhances muscle control. Do not strain or push forcefully. Applying petroleum jelly around the anus before defecation and using a sitz bath afterward eases rectal discomfort from the passage of hard stool. Explain that a bowel movement may not occur for 2–4 days and that it may take 4–6 weeks for normal function to return. Emphasize that most cases of constipation are functional, but that those that represent a significant change in bowel pattern may be the sign of a serious problem and should be medically evaluated.

Follow-up: Keep in touch with the patient weekly, since a supportive role is important. Phone consultations may be all that is needed.

▸ *Anal Fissures*

Laboratory Tests: None.

Therapeutic Measures: Initiate warm sitz baths two to three times a day or hot, wet towels or compresses to the fissured area for 15–20 minutes three to four times a day until it is healed. Prescribe an anesthetic ointment or hydrocortisone 0.25% (ointment or spray) to be applied after compresses. Institute measures for constipation if needed (see the previous section) and careful perianal hygiene.

Patient Education: Explain that fissures are generally caused or worsened by local trauma and/or abrasive, hard stool. Instruct patients to maintain careful perianal hygiene as follows: Use a soft wet wash cloth or wet cotton balls to clean the area after each bowel movement; pat the area dry with a soft material (don't wipe with dry, scratchy toilet paper); avoid tight undergarments, perfumed sprays, and powders. Anal sexual practices can cause or worsen anal fissures; liberal lubrication is very important. Reassure patients that most fissures will heal in a few days to a week with treatment.

Follow-up: As needed. If the condition becomes chronic, surgical stretching of the anal canal under anesthesia may be necessary.

▸ *Idiopathic Pruritis Ani*

Laboratory Tests: None.

Therapeutic Measures: Initiate a program for careful perianal hygiene. Prescribe witch hazel compresses or Tucks, to be applied to the irritated area for 15–20 minutes three to four times a day for several weeks, and topical hydrocortisone ointment 0.25% after compress use. Have patients maintain soft, regular stools (see the previous section on constipation).

Patient Education: Explain that the itching developed from the irritating effects of stool being wiped into the skin. Reassure the patient that most cases resolve within 3–4 weeks of therapy and will not recur if the patient maintains careful hygiene. Instruct patients to modify hygiene as follows: Use a soft wet wash cloth or wet cotton balls to clean the area after each bowel movement; pat the area dry with a soft material (don't wipe with dry, scratchy toilet paper); avoid tight undergarments, perfumed sprays, and powders.

Follow-up: As needed.

BIBLIOGRAPHY

Abramowicz M (ed.). Drugs for parasitic infections. *The Medical Letter on Drugs and Therapeutics,* (Dec.) 1979, 21(26):105–112.

American Cancer Society. Guidelines for the cancer-related checkup . . . Recommendations and rationale. *Ca—A Cancer Journal for Clinicians,* (July/Aug.), 1980.

Anderson P. When and how to use hemocult slides. *Consultant,* (Oct.) 1979.

Bates B. *A Guide to Physical Examination,* 3rd ed. Lippincott, Philadelphia, 1983.

Berkow RB (ed.). *The Merck Manual of Diagnosis and Therapy,* 14th ed. Merck Sharp & Dohme Research Laboratories, Rahway, N.J., 1982.

Blankenhorn DH. Lipoproteins and the progression and regression of atherosclerosis. *Cardiovascular Reviews and Reports,* 1982, 30–32.

Brown AM, Stubbs DW (eds.). *Medical Physiology.* Wiley, New York, 1983.

Capell P. *Ambulatory Care Manual for Nurse Practitioners.* Lippincott, Philadelphia, 1976.

Chlebowski RT. Cancer of the colon. *Hospital Medicine,* (Mar.) 1982, 71–78.

Conn HF, Conn RB Jr. (eds.). *Current Diagnosis.* Saunders, Philadelphia, 1980.

Cooper H. Irritable bowel syndrome: Diagnosis by exclusion. *Geriatrics,* (Jan.) 1980.

Crafts RC. *A Textbook of Human Anatomy,* 3rd ed. Wiley, New York, 1985.

Crouch JE, McClintic JR. *Human Anatomy and Physiology,* 2nd ed. Wiley, New York, 1976.

DeLuca SA, Rhea JT. Colonic volvulus. *American Family Physician,* (June) 1982, 25(6):135–136.

Dembert ML. Giardiasis: Aids to diagnosis and treatment. *Modern Medicine,* (July) 1981, 131–134.

Drossman D. The irritable bowel syndrome. *Gastroenterology,* (Oct.) 1977.

Drossman D. Diagnosis of the irritable bowel syndrome. *Annals of Internal Medicine,* (Mar.) 1979.

DuPont HL. Using OTC drugs for acute diarrhea. *PA Drug Update,* (May) 1983, 39–49.

Elias H, Pauly JE, Burns ER. *Histology and Human Microanatomy,* 4th ed. Wiley, New York, 1978.

Ellis FH, Jr. Carcinoma of the esophagus. *Ca—A Cancer Journal for Clinicians,* (Sept./Oct.) 1983, 33(5):264–278.

Farmer RG. Diarrhea. *Consultant,* (May) 1981.

Farmer RG, Ferguson DR, Sivak MV. *Primary Care: Clinics in Office Practice,* Vol. 8, No. 2, Saunders, Philadelphia, 1981.

Farthing MJG, Keusch GT. Giardiasis: The wilderness disease. *PA Drug Update,* (June) 1982, 34–43.

Fry RD, Kodner IJ. Anorectal disorders (M Erdelyi-Brown, ed.). *Clinical Symposia,* 1985, 37(6):2–32.

Gillin JS, Shike M. Nutritional aspects of common GI diseases. *Physician Assistant,* (Nov.) 1983, 21–36.

Goroll AH, May LA, Mulley AG. *Primary Care Medicine: Office Evaluation and Management of the Adult Patient.* Lippincott, Philadelphia, 1981.

Gray H. Anatomy of the Human Body, 29th American ed. (CM Goss, ed.). Lea & Febiger, Philadelphia, 1973.

Greenberger N. *Gastrointestinal Disorders: A Pathophysiologic Approach.* Year Book Medical Publishers, Chicago, 1981.

Guyton AC. *Textbook of Medical Physiology,* 6th ed. Saunders, Philadelphia, 1981.

Hoole AJ, Greenberg RA, Pickard CG Jr. *Patient Care Guidelines for Nurse Practitioners.* Little, Brown, Boston, 1982.

Isenberg J. Cimetidine versus low dose antacid for benign gastric ulcer. *New England Journal of Medicine* (June), 1983.

Isselbacher KJ, et al. *Harrison's Principles of Internal Medicine,* 9th ed. McGraw-Hill, New York, 1980.

Kaplan WM, Fisher RS. Diffuse esophageal spasm. *Chest Pain: Problems in Differential Diagnosis,* 1980, 6(3):1–7.

Kaye MD. Recognizing and managing esophageal spasm. *Drug Therapy,* (Mar.) 1982, 137–147.

Kaye MD. Extraintestinal manifestations of gastrointestinal disease. *Continuing Education,* (Dec.) 1982, 41–50.

Keusch GT. Advice to travelers 1983. *PA Drug Update,* (Aug.) 1983, 47–54.

Kodner IJ, Fry RD (B Bekiesz, ed.). Inflammatory bowel disease. *Clinical Symposia,* 1982, 34(1):2–32.

Krupp MA, Chatton MJ, Werdegar D (eds.). *Current Medical Diagnosis and Treatment 1985.* Lange Medical Publishers, Los Altos, Calif., 1985.

Lamb C (ed.). Simplifying diagnosis of malabsorption. *Patient Care,* (Oct.) 1981, 128–178.

Levitt MD, et al. Flatulence. *Annual Review of Medicine,* 1980, 31:

Luckmann J, Sorensen KC. *Medical Surgical Nursing: A Psychophysiologic Approach,* 2nd ed. Saunders, Philadelphia, 1980.

McGuigan MA. Treatment of poisoning. (AH Trench, ed.). *Clinical Symposia,* 1984, 36(5):3–32.

Mellow MH. Treating primary esophageal motility disorders. *PA Drug Update,* (Mar.) 1984, 47–50.

Mendeloff A. Dietary fiber and gastrointestinal disease: Some facts and fancies. *Medical Clinics of North America,* 1987.

Nuccio MA, Sparks C (LB Pearson, ed.). Intestinal parasites: Diagnostic and treatment guidelines. *Nurse Practitioner,* (Jan.) 1983, 47–50.

Ouyang A, Cohen S. Achalasia. *Chest Pain: Problems in Differential Diagnosis,* 1981, 7(1):1–8.

Palmer E. Idiopathic gastritis. *American Family Physician,* (June) 1981.

Patten R. Salmonellosis. *American Family Physician,* (Jan.) 1981.

Price S, et al. *Pathophysiology.* McGraw-Hill, New York, 1978.

Rogers AI. Answers to questions on the irritable bowel syndrome. *Hospital Medicine,* (May) 1981, 36A–36J.

Sachar D. Differentiating types of diarrhea. Consultant, (Mar.) 1980.

Schroeder S, Conte JE Jr. How to tell what's causing acute bacterial gastroenteritis. *Modern Medicine,* (Dec./Jan.) 1981, 135–136.

Silverstein A. *Human Anatomy and Physiology.* Wiley, New York, 1980.

Sleisenger M. *Gastrointestinal Disease.* Saunders, Philadelphia, 1978.

Spiro H. *Clinical Gastroenterology,* 3rd ed. Macmillan, New York, 1983.

Stratton JW, Mackeigan JM. Treating constipation. *American Family Physician* (June), 1982, 25(6):139–142.

Tedesco FJ. Cimetidine or antacids for peptic ulcer: Where we stand now. *Modern Medicine,* (July) 1981, 52–65.

Tollison J. High fiber diet and colorectal disease. *American Family Physician,* (July) 1980.

Verm RA. Gastrointestinal parasites, part I: Protozoal infections. *American Family Physician,* (Apr.) 1982, 25(4):170–175.

Verm RA. Gastrointestinal parasites, part II: Helminthic infections. *American Family Physician,* (May) 1982, 25(5):216–225.

Villeneuve J. Clinicopharmacologic perspective of duodenal ulcer therapy. *Southern Medical Journal,* (Sept.) 1978.

Weissmair J. Infectious diarrhea: When should you start to worry? *Medical Times,* (Sept.) 1977.

Wilkins R. *Medicine.* Little, Brown, Boston, 1978.

Wintrobe M, et al. *Harrison's Principles of Internal Medicine,* 7th ed. McGraw-Hill, New York, 1975.

Wolf JL (consultant). Infectious diarrhea: What's the cause? (prepared by Joanne Hornick) *Patient Care,* (May) 1983, 79–115.

Wolfe MS (Trench AH, ed). Diseases of travelers. *Clinical Symposia,* 1984, 36(2):2–32.

Wyngaarden JB, Smith LH Jr (eds). Cecil Textbook of Medicine, 16th ed., Vols. 1 and 2. Saunders, Philadelphia, 1982.

5

Body Nutrients and the Liver

Ellen Rich and *Carla Greene*
Denise Turnbull, RD, Special Consultant

Outline

Hyperosmolor nonketoic diabetic coma
Vascular changes in diabetes
Silent heart attack
Diabetic retinopathy
Diabetic nephropathy
Diabetic neuropathy
Somatic neuropathy
Visceral neuropathy
Gastroparesis diabeticorum
Diabetic enteropathy
Diabetic male sexual dysfunction
▶ Diabetic foot
▶ Diabetes organizations
Inborn errors of carbohydrate metabolism
Glycogen storage disease

FATS

▶ Screening for hyperlipidemia
▶ Type I hyperlipidemia
▶ Type IIa hyperlipidemia
Secondary hypercholesterolemia
▶ Type IIb or Type III hyperlipidemia
▶ Type IV hyperlipidemia
▶ Type V hyperlipidemia
Familial lecithin cholesterol acyltransferase (LCAT) deficiency
Secondary hypertriglyceridemia
Rare lipid disorders
Gaucher's disease

FAT STORAGE

Obesity
Juvenile-onset obesity
Adult-onset obesity
Night eating syndrome
Binge eating
Bulimia
Anorexia nervosa
Medical causes of obesity
▶ Weight reduction diet
▶ Support groups for weight loss

CLEARING INFECTIOUS AGENTS

Viral hepatitis
▶ Hepatitis A virus (HAV)
Prophylaxis for HAV
▶ Immune serum globulin
▶ Hepatitis B virus (HBV)
▶ Chronic HBV carrier state
Delta hepatitis (HDV)
HBV prophylaxis
▶ Hepatitis B immune globulin (HBIG)
▶ Hepatitis B vaccine
▶ Non-A, non-B (NANB) hepatitis
Prophylaxis for NANB hepatitis
Fulminant hepatitis
Chronic persistent hepatitis
Chronic active hepatitis (CAH)
Autoimmune CAH
Pyogenic abscesses
Amebic abscesses
Entamoeba histolytica

REGULATING HORMONE AND DRUG ACTIVITY

Toxic hepatitis
Methyldopa hepatitis
Halothane exposure
Thorazine-related hepatitis
INH hepatitis
Acetaminophen overdose
Alcoholic hypoglycemia
Steatosis (fatty liver)
▶ Alcoholic hepatitis
▶ Laennec's cirrhosis
Macronodular cirrhosis
Micronodular cirrhosis
Noncirrhotic fibrosis
Banti's syndrome

PORTAL CIRCULATION

Budd-Chiari syndrome
Portal hypertension
Caput medusae
Hemorrhoids
Varices (esophageal, gastric)
Portal systemic encephalopathy (PSE)
Fetor hepaticus
Asterixis
▶ Early stages of PSE
Shunts
▶ Ascites

Metastatic liver cancer
Primary hepatic carcinoma
Hepatic adenoma

BILE

Unconjugated hyperbilirubinemia
Nonobstructive jaundice
► Gilbert's syndrome
Crigler-Najjar syndrome
Bleeding problems
Wilson's disease

BILE FLOW

Conjugated hyperbilirubinemia
Obstructive jaundice
Dubin-Johnson syndrome
Rotor syndrome
Chronic progressive nonsuppurative cholangitis
Malignancy of the bile ducts
Benign tumors of the bile ducts

BILE STORAGE

Gallstones
Cholesterol gallstones
Pigment gallstones
Cholelithiasis
Chronic cholecystitis
Acute cholecystitis
Choledocholithiasis
Chronic choledocholithiasis
Secondary biliary cirrhosis
Cholangitis
Suppurative cholangitis
Gallbladder cancer

The liver is one of the body's most versatile organs. It receives freshly absorbed nutrients from venous blood draining the gastrointestinal (GI) tract and uses them for processing proteins, carbohydrates, and fats for body use. The liver clears infectious organisms and influences the activity of many hormones and drugs. Such functions are made possible by a unique portal circulation. The liver also produces bile, a crucial digestive substance, which is stored in the gallbladder.

NUTRIENT SUPPLY

Fifty or more nutrients are needed to maintain body functions. They are divided into five major classes, which are described in Table 5.1. Although some of the body's exact requirements for all of these nutrients remain unknown, important standards have been set (recommended dietary allowances or RDAs) for many. They may differ with age, medical condition, and sex. The standards are reviewed every 5 years by the Food and Nutrition Board of the National Research Council.

The ► ***Four Food Group System,*** developed over 25 years ago, remains one of the best tools for educating patients about good nutrition. It translates the body's complicated chemical requirements into four practical groups known as (1) milk (2) meat (3) fruits and vegetables, and (4) breads and cereals. Serving sizes, listed for each group, reflect the varying amounts of the foods needed to provide comparable nutrients. It should be stressed that these are nutritional, not caloric, equivalents. Four scoops of ice cream (1,200 calories) are needed to supply the same amount of calcium found in an 8-oz glass of skim milk (90 calories). By learning to place foods within the appropriate group and eating a variety of the recommended servings from all four groups each day, patients can be assured of obtaining 80–100% of the RDA for most nutrients. A variety of foods is essential, no single food provides adequate

TABLE 5.1 PRINCIPAL BODY NUTRIENTS

Nutrient	Function	Main Sources
Water	Main constituent of blood, lymph, all tissues, secretions/excretions (three-fourths of body weight). Basic to electrolyte/PH balance, blood volume, urine output, metabolic activity.	All beverages, fruits, vegetables, meats, dairy products.
Protein	Formation and repair of body tissues, disease resistance.	Animal products such as egg white, milk, meat, poultry, and fish. Combinations of cereals, grains, nuts, seeds, and legumes.
Carbohydrate	Blood sugar for quick cellular energy.	Honey, cereal grains, fruit, vegetables.
Fat	Stored energy, vitamins A D, E, K depot, skin oils, cell membrane function.	Dairy products, flaxseed, beef, cold-water fish, nuts, vegetable oils, soybeans, arachidonic acid.
Vitamins		
B_1 (thiamine)	Nerve cell function, carbohydrate metabolism.	Yeast, whole grains, enriched cereals, nuts, legumes, potatoes, pork, liver.
B_2 (riboflavin)	Protein metabolism, integrity of mucous membranes, cellular energy.	Eggs, cheese, meat, liver, milk, enriched cereals, whole grains.
B_6 (pyridoxine)	Porphyrin/heme synthesis, transamination, tryptophan and linoleic acid conversion.	Fish, organ meats, dried yeast, whole-grain cereals, legumes.
B_{12} (cobalamin)	DNA synthesis (folate coenzyme), neural activity, red blood cell maturation, acetate and methionine synthesis.	Beef, pork, organ meats, eggs, milk, fish.
Niacin (nicotinic acid)	Carbohydrate metabolism, oxidation/reduction reactions.	Whole grains, enriched cereals, legumes, dried yeast, organ meats.
Biotin	Amino and fatty acid metabolism, carboxylase activity (carbon dioxide formation).	Nuts, legumes, yeast, egg yolk, liver, kidney, cauliflower.
Folic acid	Purine and pyrimidine synthesis, maturation of red blood cells.	Fresh leafy green vegetables, organ meats, fruits, dried yeast.
C (ascorbic acid)	Formation of collagen/bone tissue, integrity of blood vessels, wound healing, cell respiration.	Citrus fruits, tomatoes, potatoes, cabbage, parsley, green peppers.
A	Rod photoreception, epithelial integrity, lysosome stability, glycoprotein synthesis.	Fish oil, liver, green leafy vegetables, yellow vegetables, egg yolk, butter, cream, fortified foods.
D	Calcium and phosphorus absorption, bone mineralization.	Fortified milk, sunshine, fish oil, butter, egg yolk.
E	Cell membrane stability, intracellular antioxidant.	Wheat germ, leafy vegetables, vegetable oils, legumes, egg yolk.
K	Prothrombin formation.	Leafy vegetables, vegetable oils, pork, liver, intestinal bacteria.
Pantothenic acid	Component of C.A. Involved in metabolism of fats, carbohydrates, proteins, enzyme activity.	Present in all types of food.

RDA*	Effects of Excess	Effects of Deficiency
Replacement of loss (insensible loss, urine output, sweating). Normally 2,000 mL, but increased for lactation, hot weather, exercise, fever, vomiting, etc.	Fluid overload.	Dehydration.
14% of total calorie intake.	Obesity.	Infections, edema, abnormal growth, body wasting.
51% of daily calorie intake.	Obesity.	Muscle wasting.
30–35% of daily calories.	Obesity, atherosclerosis.	Poor skin turgor, temperature regulation.
M: 1.4 mg, F: 1.0 mg (decreases with age), P: 1.4, L: 1.5 mg	Not described.	Peripheral neuropathy, cardiac failure, beriberi, Wernicke-Korsakoff syndrome.
M: 1.6 mg, F: 1.2 mg (decreases with age), P: 1.5, L: 1.8 mg	Not described.	Cheilosis, stomatitis, corneal vascularization, amblyopia.
M: 2.2 mg, F: 2.0, P: 2.6, L: 2.5	Peripheral neuropathy.	Anemia, neuropathy, seborrhea-like dermatitis.
M: 0.003 mg, F: 0.003, P: 0.004, L: 0.004	Not described.	Pernicious anemia, neuropathy, mental status change, amblyopia, abnormal epithelial turnover.
M: 18 mg, F: 13 (decreases with age), P: 15, L: 18	Flushing, hypotension, lipid function tests, abnormal GTT	Glossitis, dermatosis pellagra, GI problems, central nervous system changes.
100–200 μg/day	Not described.	Glossitis, dermatitis from excessive intake of egg whites (contains a biotin antagonist, avidin)
M: 400 μg, F: 400, P: 800, L: 500	Not described.	Megaloblastic anemia, GI disturbances, fertility problems, skin disorders.
M: 50 mg, F: 50, P: 60, L: 80	Stomach irritation, diarrhea, kidney stones.	Scurvy, infections, poor wound healing, easy bleeding.
M: 5,000 IU, F: 4,000, P: 5,000, L: 6,000	Hair and skin dryness, symptoms of increased intracranial pressure, joint pain, hepatosplenomegaly.	Night blindness, keratinization of the cornea, conjunctiva, GI and UT epithelia. Susceptibility to infection.
M: 5 μg, F: 5, P: 10, L: 10	Elevated calcium level with impaired renal function, weakness, irritability.	Osteomalacia hypocalcemia, renal failure.
M: 10 mg, F: 8, P: 10, L: 11	Not described.	Hemolysis, creatinurea, flaky dermatitis, edema.
70–140 μg	Hemolysis, especially in glucose 6-phosphate deficiency.	Prolonged prothrombin time.
4–7 mg. Diet intake much more than needed (5–20 mg).	Not known.	Not described.

TABLE 5.1 (*Continued*)

Nutrient	Function	Main Sources
Fatty acids (linoleic, linolenic, arachidonic)	Prostaglandin synthesis, cell membrane structure.	Corn and safflower oils, sunflower seeds, shellfish, dairy products, red meat, linseed oil, cold-water fish, soy oil, walnuts.
Minerals		
Sodium	Acid-base balance, nerve transmission, muscle concontraction, cellular pumps, osmotic pressure.	Present in all goods. Highest in snack foods, cheese, beef, pork, pickles, and olives.
Chloride	Acid-base balance, bicarb shift in red blood cells, component of gastric acid.	Sodium chloride, potassium chloride.
Potassium	Nerve transmission, muscle contraction, intracellular acid-base balance.	Bananas, prunes, raisins, citrus fruits, sunflower seeds, milk.
Calcium	Neuromuscular activity, myocardial contraction, blood coagulation, bone formation/preservation.	Milk, eggs, cereals, fruits, vegetables, fish, meat.
Phosphorus	Component of nucleic acid, acid-base balance, cell energy.	Poultry, fish, meat, milk, cheese, cereals, nuts, legumes.
Magnesium	Nerve conduction, muscle contracton, enzyme activity, bone formation.	Nuts, grains, seafood, green leafy vegetables.
Iron	Enzyme activity, formation of hemoglobin and myoglobin.	Found in most foods except for dairy products. High in red meat, clams, raisins, peaches.
Iodine	T3 and T4 formation.	Seafood, iodized salt, dairy products, some water sources.
Fluoride	Bone mineralization.	Fluorinated water, supplements, coffee, tea.
Zinc	Enzyme and insulin component. Growth, wound healing.	Most foods and water. High in vegetables.
Copper	Component of enzymes.	Nuts, dried legumes, whole grains, oysters, organ meats.
Cobalt	Component of vitamin B_{12} molecules.	Green leafy vegetables.
Chromium	Component of glucose tolerance factor.	Most foods. High in brewer's yeast.
Selenium	Key component of antioxidant enzyme, glutathione peroxidase.	Seafood, meat, grains, garlic, mushrooms, asparagus.
Molybdenum	Component of several enzyme systems. Active in reduction of ferritin and purine metabolism.	Legumes, whole grains, milk, eggs, organ meats.
Sulfur	Active in detoxification reactions; constituent of connective tissue, insulin, CoA, and sulfur bonds.	Eggs, meat, fish, poultry, milk, cheese, nuts.

RDA*	Effects of Excess	Effects of Deficiency
?	Not known.	Dermatosis.
Not to exceed 7.5 g.	Linked with hypertension and fluid retention.	Nausea, diarrhea, abdominal pain, muscle cramps. Rarely due to dietary deficiency alone.
1,700–5,100 mg. Normal diet more than adequate.	Primary hyperchloremia not described.	Fluid-electrolyte imbalance due to sodium-restricted diet or vomiting.
Diet normally supplies adequate amount.	Cardiac disturbances, paralysis.	Weakness, muscle cramps, cardiac disturbance.
M: 800 mg, F: 800, P: 1,200, L: 1,200	Renal failure, psychosis, GI disturbance. Rarely occurs from dietary excess alone.	Tetany, neuromuscular irritability.
M: 800 mg, F: 800, P: 1,200, L: 1,200	GI disturbance, renal damage, convulsions.	Poor bone mineralization; irritability, weakness; blood cell, GI, and renal disorders.
M: 350 mg, F: 300, P: 450, L: 450	Hypotension, respiratory failure, cardiac disturbance.	Neuromuscular irritability.
M: 10 mg, F: 18, P: 18+, L: 18, 30–60 supplements.	Hemochromatosis, DM cirrhosis.	Anemia, nail changes, esophageal web, GI disturbance.
M: 150 μg, F: 150, P: 175, L: 200	Possible myxedema.	Goiter, cretinism, deaf/mutism.
1.5–4.0 mg	Mottling and pitting of teeth, exostosis of spine.	Predisposition to dental caries, possible connection with osteoporosis.
M: 15 mg, F: 15, P: 20, L: 25	Not described.	Retarded growth, poor wound healing, hypogeusia.
2–3 mg/day. Diet more than adequate (2.5–5 mg).	Liver disturbance.	No primary deficiency.
See vitamin B_{12}		
0.05–0.20 mg daily.	Not known.	May play a part in diabetes, and cardiovascular disease.
0.05–0.20 mg (diet furnishes about 0.15 mg).	Nausea, sour milk taste, loss of hair and nails.	Premature aging due to decreased tissue elasticity.
0.15–0.50 mg (found in most diets).	Not known.	Not known.
Not established. Provided in high-protein diet.	Not known.	Not known.

amounts of the major nutrients within a group, and some nutrients work only in combination with others.

The Four Food Group System not only helps patients assess the quality of their diet and monitor their food choices on a daily basis but also provides the basis for a number of therapeutic diets. For example, it can be easily modified to teach a hypertensive patient to restrict salt intake, the patient taking lithium to replace salt, or a breast-feeding mother to meet her need for increased calcium. Intake of calories, potassium, fiber, lactose, carbohydrates, fats, proteins, and other substances can be altered while overall nutrition is maintained. Such dietary considerations are discussed, along with specific clinical conditions discussed throughout this book.

PROTEINS

Body proteins are made from organic compounds called "amino acids." Of the 80 or more amino acids found in nature, only 20 are used by the body for metabolism and growth (Table 5.2). Eleven of them can be synthesized by the body and are thus called "nonessential," while the remaining nine must be supplied by the diet and are referred to as "essential." Complete proteins (milk, cheese, eggs, and meat) contain all of the essential amino acids, while incomplete proteins (vegetables, legumes, and grains) contain only some of them. Incomplete proteins can be combined to provide a full complement of essential amino acids.

After they are broken down from protein foods by the GI tract, the amino acids pass through the intestinal wall and the portal vein into the blood to form a circulating pool. The tissue cells draw from the circulating pool whatever amino acids they need to make their own proteins (tissue proteins). Hepatocytes use the rest of the amino acids to manufacture the proteins that circulate in plasma (plasma proteins). These may be globular, fibrous, or compound in structure, as outlined in Table 5.3.

The ratio of tissue proteins to plasma proteins is maintained at 33:1 even during starvation or debilitating diseases. This is because production of the plasma proteins is suppressed whenever the availability of amino acids is low. However, when plasma proteins become relatively depleted, enzymes known as "cathepsins" decompose tissue proteins into amino acids. The acids are transported out of cells and back into the blood for use by hepatocytes. Conversely, when tissue proteins need replacement, the plasma proteins are broken down. In addition to the part they play in maintaining tissue proteins, the plasma proteins perform other important functions. Albumin maintains oncotic pressure, preventing plasma loss from capillaries. Many globulins perform enzyme functions, and gamma globulins are responsible for antibodies and immunity. Fibrinogen polymerizes into long threads whenever a blood vessel is damaged, helping to clot blood and repair leaks in the circulatory system.

Proteins are continually broken down and re-formed, but very few escape from the body under normal conditions. Acute losses may occur with severe burns or shock. Chronic wasting may take place in certain GI and kidney disorders: both large and small molecular weight proteins pass through the gut walls, but only smaller proteins (mostly albumin) pass through glomerular membranes. Macroglobulins pass into urine only when kidney damage is extreme. To compensate for such losses, the liver can double its activity rate and synthesize up to 100 g of protein a day.

When protein losses exceed replacement, ***hypoproteinemia*** develops. As might

TABLE 5.2 AMINO ACIDS

Essential	Nonessential
Histadine	Alanine
Isoleucine	Aspartic acid
Leucine	Arginine
Lysine	Citrulline
Methionine	Glutamic acid
Phenylalanine	Glycine
Threonine	Hydroxyglutamic acid
Tryptophan	Hydroxyproline
Valine	Norleucine
	Proline
	Serine

be expected, hypoproteinemia results from malnutrition or liver disease, as well as from nephrotic syndromes. It may follow any kind of lymphatic obstruction from constrictive pericarditis, congestive heart failure, and so on in that high venous pressures force proteins through the intestinal walls. A complete list of conditions associated with hypoproteinemia appears in Table 5.4. Although the signs and symptoms vary with the underlying cause, edema is fairly universal. With lowered albumin levels, oncotic pressures fall and circulating blood neither holds nor draws water from body tissues. This leads to dependent edema and contributes to ascites formation. Treatment of hypoproteinemia centers on the treatment of the underlying disease. Protein levels can be raised by nutritional improvements or, if necessary, by intravenous hyperalimentation.

Unused amino acids are metabolized in the liver or by the action of bacteria in the gut. In cases of ***amino acid anomalies*** described in Table 5.5, faulty metabolism leads to a buildup of toxic waste products. ***Phenylketonuria*** is prototypic. Normally, phenylalanine is reduced to tyrosine by the enzyme phenylalanine hydroxylase and thus is eliminated by the body. In patients with phenylketonuria, the

TABLE 5.3 TYPES OF BODY PROTEIN

Globular Proteins (named for their elliptical shape). Consist of three relatively simple types:
- *Albumin.* Constitutes a major part of the plasma proteins and is found to some degree inside cells.
- *Globulin.* Distributed widely in plasma as well as inside cells. Globulin products make up most of the cellular enzymes.
- *Histone and protamine.* Protein component of nucleoproteins. Contain large quantities of basic amino acids.

Fibrous Proteins. Consist of three types:
- *Collagen.* Foundation of ligaments, cartilage, and bone.
- *Elastin.* Make up flexible fibers found in tendons and arterial walls.
- *Keratin.* Building material of hair and nails.

Conjugated Proteins. Combined with nucleic acids, mucopolysaccharides, lipids, or other nonprotein substances. There are several types:
- *Nucleoprotein.* DNA, principal constituent of genes, and RNA, director of protein synthesis.
- *Mucoprotein.* A compound highly resistant to acid destruction found in gastric lining.
- *Lipoprotein.* HDL and LDL, lipid transporters.
- *Chromoprotein.* Contains special pigments (e.g., hemoglobin and cytochromes).
- *Phosphoprotein.* Contains phosphorus.
- *Metalloprotein.* Contains magnesium, copper, iron, zinc, or other metallic ions, all of which are important enzymes.

TABLE 5.4 CONDITIONS ASSOCIATED WITH HYPOPROTEINEMIA

Idiopathic	Hepatic
Intestinal lymphangiectasia	Toxic hepatitis
Gastrointestinal	Infectious hepatitis
Whipple's disease	Cancer
Crohn's disease	Portal hypertension
Ulcerative colitis	Cirrhosis
Pseudomembranous enterocolitis	Renal
Gastric carcinoma	Infectious glomerulonephritis
Lymphoma	Rapidly progressive glomerulonephritis
Gastric rugal hypertrophy	Chronic glomerulonephritis
Tropical sprue	Other
Celiac sprue	Starvation
Infectious diarrhea	Severe burns

enzyme is absent and, as a consequence, phenylalanine accumulates in the blood. The end products of the amino acid, even though they are eventually excreted in urine, produce a number of changes. Children often develop light-colored skin, hair, and eyes, as well as a "mousy" body odor caused by phenylacetic acid in their urine and sweat. Neurologic complications are manifested as petit and grand mal seizures, abnormal reflexes, hyperactivity, psychosis, and/or severe mental retardation. Electroencephalograms (EEGs) are abnormal in 75–90% of patients. Early diagnosis and treatment can prevent most of these problems. Therefore, screening programs are mandatory in a number of states. The Guthrie inhibition test is performed on capillary blood 48 hours after birth, just long enough for the infant to consume moderate amounts of phenylalanine in milk. Other tests are done at 4–6 weeks of age when abnormal levels of phenylalanine end products appear in the urine. Treatment of phenylketonuria is simple, but must begin during the first few days of life in order to prevent mental retardation. It consists of limiting phenylalanine intake. Milk is replaced by a product such as Lofenalac or Phenyl-free, which has been treated with casein hydrolysates to remove the phenylalanine, and other foods are limited to those with low phenylalanine contents (fruits, vegetables, and certain cereals). Treatment must last until age 10, when myelinization of the brain is complete.

CARBOHYDRATES

Carbohydrates constitute the body's major source of energy. Readily available in foods, they are subdivided into monosaccharides, disaccharides, and polysaccharides, as described in Table 5.6. To be absorbed, dietary carbohydrates must be in the form of monosaccharides. Polysaccharides are broken down to disaccharides by the action of ptyalin (salivary amylase) in the mouth and pancreatic amylase in the small intestine. In the intestinal mucosa, disaccharides are broken down into monosaccharides (glucose, galactose, and fructose) by three enzymes (sucrase, lactase, and maltase). Glucose, galactose, and fructose are then absorbed and sent to the hepatic portal system. The liver immediately converts galactose and fructose to glucose.

Of the total glucose provided by the diet, three-fourths remains in the liver, where most of it is broken down through glycolysis. As noted in Figure 5.1, glycolysis yields adenosine triphosphate (ATP), pyruvic acid, and other substances needed for cellu-

TABLE 5.5 AMINO ACID ANOMALIES

Disorder	Abnormality of (Amino Acid)	From Defective (Enzyme)	Clinical Features	Treatment
Albinism	Tyrosine	Tyrosinase	Absent skin, hair, eye pigment	Sun protection
Alkaptonuria	Tyrosine	Homogentisic oxidase	Arthritis, dark urine	None
Alpha-methyl-acetoacetate	Isoleucine	Acetyl-CoA thialase	Acidosis, retardation	Controlled-isoleucine diet
Argininemia	Arginine	Arginase	Retardation, spasticity, seizures	Essential amino acids; low- protein diet
Argininosuccinic acidemia	Argininosuccinic acid	Argininosuccinase	Retardation, seizures	Arginine; essential amino acid mixture; low-protein diet
Beta-alaninemia	Beta-alanine	Beta-alanine and alpha-ketoglutarate amino transferase	Seizures, death	? Pyridoxine
Beta-hydroxyisovaleric aciduria	Leucine	Beta-methylcrotonyl-CoA carboxylase	Retardation, muscle wasting, malodorous urine	Controlled-leucine intake
Branched chain ketoaciduria (maple syrup urine disease)	Leucine, isoleucine, valine, alloisoleucine	Branched chain keto acid decarboxylase	Malodorous urine, sweat; hypertonicity, convulsions, coma, death	Controlled intake of affected amino acids; transformations and dialysis during acute periods
Citrullinemia	Citrulline	Argininosuccinic acid synthetase	Vomiting, seizures, coma	Essential amino acids; keto acid analogs; arginine
Cystathioninemia	Methionine	Cystathionase	Mostly asymptomatic; possible retardation	Large doses of pyridoxine
Cystinosis	Cystine	Not known	Cystine accumulation in reticuloendothelial system; white blood cell and corneal abnormalities; Fanconi's syndrome; renal failure	Treatment of Fanconi's syndrome; kidney transplant for failure
Glutamicacidemia	Glutamic acid	Not known	Physical and mental retardation; seizures	Not known
Glycinemia (ketotic)	Isoleucine, valine, threonine, methionine	Methylmalonul-CoA mutase	Mental and physical retardation; acidosis, lethargy, coma	Controlled intake of affected amino acids; massive doses of vitamin B_{12}
Glycinemia (non-ketotic)	Glycine	Glycine cleavage enzymes	Retardation; seizures	Low-protein diet; strychnine
Histidinemia	Histidine	l-Histidine ammonia lysase	Retardation, neurologic symptoms; may be benign	Controlled histadine intake; low-protein diet
Homocitrullinemia	Homocitrulline	Mitochondrial transport defect	Retardation; seizures	Low-protein diet
Homocystinemia	Methionine	Cystathionine synthetase	Retardation; skeletal anomalies	Massive doses of pyridoxine; controlled methionine intake; folic acid and cystine supplements
Hydroxyprolinemia	Hydroxyproline	Hydroxyproline oxidase	Retardation; central nervous system manifestations; sometimes benign	Low-protein diet

TABLE 5.5 (*Continued*)

Disorder	Abnormality of (Amino Acid)	From Defective (Enzyme)	Clinical Features	Treatment
Hyperammonemia (type I)	Ammonia	Carbamylphosphate synthetase	Acidosis, vomiting, lethargy, death	Arginine; essential amino acids; keto acid analogs; low-protein diet
Hyperammonemia (type II)	Ammonia	Ornithine transcarbamylase	Acidosis, vomiting, irritability seizures, coma; fatal in males.	Same as type I
Isovaleric acidemia	Leucine	Isovaleryl CoA carboxylase	Retardation; acidosis, vomiting, lethargy; sweaty foot odor; neonatal death	Glycine; controlled leucine intake
Lysinemea	Lysine	Lysine-ketoglutarate reductase	Retardation; weakness; sometimes benign	Controlled lysine intake
Lysine intolerance	Lysine; arginine	Lysine NAD oxidoreductase	Vomiting; coma	Controlled lysine intake; low-protein diet
Ornithinemia	Ornithine	Ornithine keto acid transaminase	Gyrate atrophy of choroid and retina	Low-protein diet
Phenylketonuria	Phenylalanine	Phenylalanine hydroxylase	Retardation; neurologic symptoms	Controlled phenylalanine intake
Pipecolicacidemia	Lysine	Pipecolate oxidase	Retardation	Controlled lysine intake
Prolinemia (type I)	Proline	Proline oxidase	Nephritis; deafness; sometimes benign	None
Prolinemia (type II)	Proline	Delta-pyrroline-5 carboxylate dehydrogenase	Mental retardation; seizures	Controlled lysine and glutamic acid intake; low-protein diet
Pyroglutamic acidemia	Pyroglutamic acid	Not known	Retardation; episodic vomiting	Not known
Saccharopinuria	Lysine	Pipecolate oxidase	Retardation	Controlled lysine intake
Sarcosinemia	Sarcosine	Sarcosine dehydrogenase	Retardation; sometimes benign	None
Tyrosinemia	Tyrosine	Tyrosine aminotransferase	Retardation; liver disease; Fanconi's syndrome; keratitis; dermatitis	Controlled phenylalanine, tyrosine, methionine intake
Valinemia	Valine	Valine aminotransferase	Retardation	Controlled valine intake

lar energy. Pyruvic acid is oxidized to acetyl coenzyme A (CoA), which provides fuel for the Krebs cycle and acts as a substrate for many important reactions, particularly the synthesis of hepatic fatty acids (see the next section). The other one-fourth of dietary glucose enters the general circulation, causing a transitory rise in blood sugar for a few hours after feeding. The rise in blood sugar normally results in the release of insulin, a hormone produced by the beta cells in the islets of Langerhans tissue of the pancreas (see Fig. 4.5). Insulin combines chemically with receptor sites located on the surface of many body cells to initiate a series of reactions. It enhances the transport of glucose into the cells and stimulates glycolysis. It promotes the conversion of excess glucose into glycogen for storage through a process called "gly-

TABLE 5.6 TYPES OF CARBOHYDRATES

Classifications	Comments
Monosaccharides Glucose Fructose Galactose Mannose Xylose Arabinose	Simple sugars.
Disaccharides Maltose Maltotriose Sucrose Lactose	Composed of two or more sugars bonded together; split by the disaccharidases maltase, sucrase, lactase, and isomaltase into monosaccharides and oligosaccharides.
Oligosaccharides G4 G5 Limit dextrins	Glucose molecules joined by alpha-1,4 bonds; split by the disaccharidases maltase and isomaltase into maltose, maltotriose, and glucose.
Polysaccharides Amylose Amylopectin Glycogen Cellulose Pectin Pentosans	Complex carbohydrates; amylose and amylopectin are the principal nutritional starches; small amounts of glycogen are ingested from meat and liver; cellulose pectins and pentosans are nondigestible fibers.

cogenesis." Glycogenesis takes place in many body tissues, most notably liver and muscle.

A few hours after feeding, blood sugar and insulin levels drop. This stimulates secretion of glucagon, a hormone produced by the alpha cells in the islets of Langerhans tissue of the pancreas (see Fig. 4.5). Secretion of glucagon and insulin is influenced by the factors listed in Table 5.7. The fall of insulin and the rise of glucagon bring about a shift from anabolic to catabolic processes. Glycogenolysis, the process whereby stored glycogen is broken down, is particularly important. In most body cells, glycogenolysis yields glucose 6-phosphate, which can be used as energy within the cell, but nowhere else. However, liver and kidney cells contain phosphatase, an enzyme that cleaves phosphate from glucose 6-phosphate, resulting in the release of free glucose. This process maintains blood sugar levels during short periods of fasting or increased exercise (exercise normally lowers blood glucose levels because of the added requirement for glucose by muscle tissue). As might be expected, the fuel reserves provided by glycogenolysis run out when glycogen stores become depleted. When this happens, hepatocytes must turn to noncarbohydrate sources (fatty acids from the breakdown of adipose tissue and amino acids from the breakdown of skeletal muscle) to create glycogen. Referred to as "glyconeogenesis" or "gluconeogenesis," this process maintains blood sugar levels during periods of prolonged fasting and/or exercise (e.g., marathon running). In addition to glucose, sustained gluconeogenesis results in the release of free fatty acids and ketone bodies, both of which can be used by certain body cells for energy.

Glycolysis, glycogenesis, glycogenolysis, and gluconeogenesis maintain blood sugar levels within relatively narrow ranges through periods of feeding as well as fasting. The controlled rise, fall, and maintenance of blood sugar levels is referred to

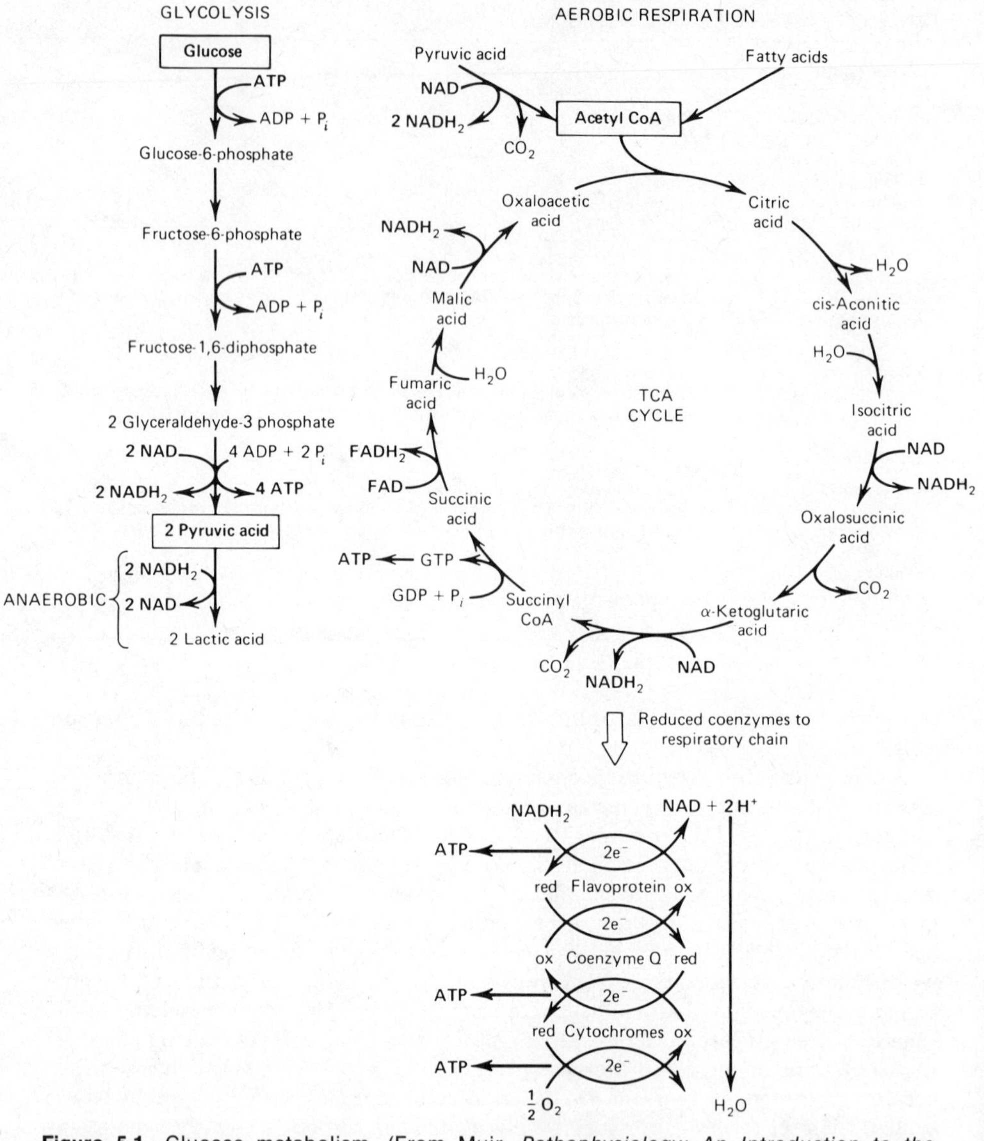

Figure 5.1 Glucose metabolism. (From Muir, *Pathophysiology: An Introduction to the Mechanisms of Disease,* © 1980, John Wiley & Sons, Inc., New York.)

TABLE 5.7 FACTORS AFFECTING INSULIN AND GLUCAGON SECRETION

	Insulin	Glucagon
Stimulating effect	Acetylcholine Beta stimulation[a] D-Glucose (strongest single stimulant) D-Glucosamine Fatty acids (weak stimulant) Glucagon Intracellular cyclic AMP Intracellular calcium Isoproterenol Ketones L-Amino acids[a] Sulfonylureas	Beta stimulation Cholecystokinin Hypoglycemia L-Amino acids Prostaglandins Starvation Strenuous exercise
Inhibiting effect	Alpha stimulation (epinephrine, norepinephrine) 2-Desoxyglucose Somatostatin[a,b] Starvation Strenuous exercise	Fatty acids Hyperglycemia Insulin Ketones Somatostatin

[a]Affects insulin and glucagon in the same manner.
[b]Hormone produced by D cells of the pancreatic islets.

as ***glucose tolerance.*** It is extremely important since blood, peripheral nerve, and renal medulla cells are primarily dependent on glucose and since, under normal circumstances, brain cells are totally dependent. Normal and altered patterns of glucose tolerance are presented in Table 5.8.

Hypoglycemia is defined as a fall in blood sugar below 45–50%. It is of clinical concern only if symptoms occur, since 23% of the normal population, particularly women, can demonstrate blood sugar levels below 50 mg%. Symptoms, in turn, are related to both central nervous system changes (inadequate glucose supply to brain cells) and/or stimulation of the autonomic nervous system (catecholamine release). The earliest symptoms include hunger, sweating, restlessness, and palpitations. Rapid, severe falls in blood sugar may be attended by altered mental status, stupor, or seizures. The diagnosis is confirmed with an oral glucose tolerance test (OGTT). Treatment depends on the underlying cause; the more common causes are covered in the following paragraphs. ***Alcoholic hypoglycemia*** is discussed in a later section.

▶ ***Functional postprandial hypoglycemia*** results from an abnormal response to food intake. In some cases this is due to excessive secretion of insulin following high carbohydrate intake, but in many cases the cause remains unknown. The

TABLE 5.8 GLUCOSE TOLERANCE PATTERNS[a]

Subject	Fasting	½–1½ hours	2 hours
Normal	Less than 115	Less than 200	Less than 140
IGT[b]	Less than 140	200 or more[c]	140–199
Diabetic	140 or more[d]	More than 200[c]	200 or more

[a]Measured as plasma glucose (milligrams per deciliter), which is normally 15% higher than blood glucose.
[b]Impaired glucose tolerance.
[c]One or more occasions.
[d]At least two occasions.

OGTT reveals a normal glucose response within the first 2 hours but the development of symptomatic hypoglycemia during hours 2–5. Dietary modifications are the mainstay of treatment: frequent, small meals composed of high-protein foods. Reassurance is also important, since it is a common misconception that the problem causes the future development of diabetes.

Insulinoma is a rare but important cause of hypoglycemia resulting from tumors of pancreatic islet cells. Single or multiple tumors develop at the head or tail of the pancreas, near the surface or deep within. Ectopy, within or near the duodenum, may also occur. Because the tumors (85% of which are benign) produce insulin inappropriately and at uncontrolled rates, clinical presentations are extremely variable. Combinations of confusion, abnormal behavior, diplopia, blurred vision, sweating, palpitations, and weakness may occur, along with amnesia and seizures. Although such manifestations have been documented in the early morning, late afternoon, or several hours after a meal, they are typically precipitated by fasting and exercise. The problem is suggested by blood tests showing high insulin levels coexisting with hypoglycemia. Hyperinsulinemia following the tolbutamide test is also characteristic of insulinoma. The diagnosis is confirmed by arteriography. Small, confined tumors are removed. Large, multiple, or malignant tumors may necessitate partial or total pancreatectomy.

► ***Insulin/sulfonylurea reactions*** are a common complication of diabetic drug therapy. Medication overdose, omitted meals, and increased physical activity are the usual precipitating events. Use of the drugs listed in Tables 5.13 and 5.16 may also contribute to the problem. Patients should be taught to recognize early symptoms (e.g., headache, irritability, shaking, sweating) and to eat something immediately. Severe reactions may necessitate administration of glucagon or intravenous glucose.

Hyperglycemia is defined as a rise in blood sugar above normal levels of glucose tolerance. ***Secondary hyperglycemia*** may develop in the presence of pancreatic disease, hemochromatosis, endocrine disorders, genetic syndromes, and drug use, as noted in Table 5.9. Treatment is aimed at correcting the underlying disorder. Patients require diabetic intervention only if the fasting plasma glucose level rises above 140 mg/dL.

Diabetes mellitus accounts for most cases of hyperglycemia. It is characterized by lack of insulin or resistance to its action. The various types of diabetes are listed in Table 5.10.

TABLE 5.9 SECONDARY CAUSES OF HYPERGLYCEMIA

Drugs	Genetic disorders
Alcohol	Cystic fibrosis
Diazoxide	Inborn errors of carbohydrate metabolism
Epinephrine	Leprechaunism
Estrogens (including oral contraceptives)	
Furosemide	Insulin receptor abnormalities
Glucocorticoids	Acanthosis nigricans
Hydantoins	Muscular dystrophy
Thiazide diuretics	
	Pancreatic disease
Endocrine disease	Glucagonoma
Acromegaly	Pancreatectomy
Aldosteronism	Pancreatitis
Cushing's disease	Pancreatic carcinoma
Hyperthyroidism	
Pheochromocytoma	

TABLE 5.10 CLASSIFICATIONS OF DIABETES MELLITUS

Impaired glucose tolerance (IGT)
Gestational diabetes mellitus (GDM)
Previous abnormality of glucose tolerance (PrevAGT)
Potential abnormality of glucose tolerance (PotAGT)
Diabetes type I
Diabetes type II
Nonobese subset
Obese subset

Impaired glucose tolerance (IGT) is defined as fasting plasma glucose levels below 140 mg/dL and a 2-hour postprandial level between 140 and 200 mg/dL. Previously referred to as "chemical," "subclinical," "asymptomatic," "borderline," or "latent diabetes," the problem is accompanied by no overt signs of hyperglycemia. It is usually discovered as an incidental finding on blood and urine tests. Patients have accelerated atherosclerosis, but rarely develop other complications of diabetes. For the obese patient, weight loss via a calorie-restricted diet is essential. Otherwise, no specific treatment is recommended. Plasma glucose levels should be checked once or twice a year.

Gestational diabetes mellitus (GDM) is a condition of a small group of women who develop abnormal glucose tolerance during pregnancy. It is diagnosed by a 3-hour modified OGTT. Following a standard glucose load of 100 g, at least two plasma glucose levels must exceed the established upper limits of normal (105 mg/dL fasting, 190 mg/dL at 1 hour, 165 mg/dL at 2 hours, and 145 mg/dL at 3 hours). If such elevations are demonstrated, patients are treated meticulously with insulin throughout the prenatal period, since high rates of fetal death are associated with uncontrolled hyperglycemia. As sulfur derivatives, oral hypoglycemic agents are contraindicated during pregnancy.

Previous abnormality of glucose tolerance (PrevAGT) applies to patients who at one time developed and then recovered from hyperglycemia secondary to obesity, pregnancy, or stress (infection, myocardial infarction, surgery). ***Potential abnormality of glucose tolerance (PotAGT)*** refers to patients who have close relatives with diabetes and women who have given birth to babies weighing more than 4.5 kg. Because both groups of patients are at higher risk for decreased glucose tolerance in later life, fasting plasma glucose levels should be checked at least yearly. Except for ideal weight maintenance, no treatment is necessary.

Type I diabetes is caused by an absolute deficiency of insulin that follows damage to pancreatic beta cells. Developing prior to adulthood, it accounts for less than 15% of all cases of diabetes. Genetic predisposition undoubt plays a role, since most patients are human leukocyte antigen (HLA) types DW3, DW4, B8, or B15. However, type I diabetes is not inherited. The precipitating event is thought to be coxsackie B, mumps, rubella, cytomegalovirus, or another virus that invades pancreatic beta cells and then induces their humoral and cell-mediated destruction. Breast feeding, perhaps by providing passive immunity to many viruses, may be protective. A recent study in Scandinavia found that children who had been breast fed for 3 months or more were much less prone to develop the disease later in life.

The presentation of type I diabetes is usually dramatic. Falling insulin levels render body cells (except for liver and brain cells) incapable of utilizing glucose. The resultant hyperglycemia and cellular starvation lead to the four cardinal symptoms

TABLE 5.11 SIGNS AND SYMPTOMS OF DIABETES: PATHOLOGIC PROGRESSION

Hyperglycemia

Falling insulin levels render body cells (except for liver and brain cells) incapable of utilizing glucose. As unused glucose accumulates in the blood, hyperosmolarity develops. An osmotic shift in fluids results in general cellular dehydration and, if significant amounts of fluid are drawn from the lens, sudden changes in vision. The kidneys attempt to normalize osmolarity by eliminating excess glucose in the urine. Patients then demonstrate *glycosuria*. They also develop *polyuria* because the high osmolar load created by the glucose in tubular fluids causes fluid to be drawn into the urine (*osmotic diuresis*). With fluid loss, patients become plagued by excessive thirst and *polydipsia*. If fluids are not replaced at the same rate as they are lost, general dehydration develops.

Cellular Starvation

As glucose remains unusable and glycogen becomes depleted, body cells become desperate for fuel. The rate of gluconeogenesis in hepatocytes is increased. Because raising blood glucose levels, even further, this action results in the mobilization of fat and the breakdown of muscle tissue. Patients lose weight, experience excessive hunger (*polyphagia*), and feel generally unwell. Fatigue can be significant. Nonetheless, tissue breakdown is an important compensatory mechanism. It releases fatty acids and amino acids, both of which can be used by many body cells for fuel. Furthermore, free fatty acids supply a substrate used by hepatocytes to manufacture ketones (*ketogenesis*). Ketone bodies (acetoacetate, beta-hydroxybutyrate, and acetone) are picked up from the liver by the blood (*ketosis*). Although some are eliminated in the urine (*ketonuria*), most are transported to peripheral tissues. The acids acetoacetate and beta-hydroxybutyrate serve as sources of fuel, particularly for cardiac muscle, renal cortex, and skeletal muscle. Unfortunately, they also lower the pH of blood and may lead to *ketoacidosis*.

of polyuria, polydipsia, polyphagia, and weight loss, as described in Table 5.11. Strongly suggested by these symptoms, the diagnosis of type I diabetes is readily confirmed by the presence of glycosuria, with or without ketonuria, and a significantly elevated blood sugar level (usually well over 300 mg/dL). By the time patients reach adulthood, they have invariably been under treatment for many years. However, ▶***supervision of type I diabetes*** is a lifelong concern. Primary care-givers play an important role in enforcing the diet, prescribing exercise, and adjusting insulin levels. ▶***High-carbohydrate, high-fiber diet*** of sufficient caloric content to maintain ideal body weight has been found to lower blood sugar levels and insulin requirements. ▶***Exercise for the diabetic*** improves glucose tolerance, minimizes atherosclerotic changes (see the later section on this topic), and enhances feelings of health and well-being. However, strenuous programs should be undertaken only when blood sugar levels are under good, constant control and should be avoided or modified by patients who have retinopathy, diabetic foot, and cardiovascular disease. Diet and/or insulin adjustments may also be needed.

▶***Insulin therapy*** involves careful titration with one or a combination of the preparations listed in Table 5.12. ***Complications of insulin therapy*** include ***rebound hyperglycemia (Somogyi effect), insulin allergy, insulin immunoresistance, lipodystrophy, insulin edema,*** and ***insulin presbyopia.*** Each is described in Table 5.13, along with management approaches (insulin reactions were previously discussed). Properly choosing and rotating injection sites, as illustrated in Figure 5.2, minimizes lipodystrophy and uneven insulin uptake. Human insulin (derived from genetically coded bacteria) is associated with the fewest complications but may be prohibitive in cost. Drugs that interfere with insulin action (Table 5.14) should be used with extreme care. The overall goal is to balance insulin intake with diet and exercise in order to keep fasting blood sugar levels below 140 mg/dL without instigating episodes of hypoglycemia. Toward this end, ▶***home glucose moni-***

TABLE 5.12 INSULIN PREPARATIONS

Type	Brand Name (Source)[a]
Regular, rapid-acting Onset: ½–1 hour Peak action: 2–4 hours Duration: 5–7 hours	Actrapid (PP) Actripid Human (H) Humulin R (H) Regular[b] (P) Regular Iletin I[b] (B/P) Regular Iletin II (PB or PP) Regular Concentrated[b] (PP)
Zinc suspension, prompt-acting Onset: 1–3 hours Peak action: 2–8 hours Duration: 12–16 hours	Semilente Iletin I[b] (B/P) Semilente (B) Semitard (PP)
Zinc suspension, intermediate-acting Onset: 1–3 hours Peak action: 8–12 hours Duration: 24–48 hours	Lente @ (B) Lentard (PP/PB) Lente Iletin I[b] (B/P) Lente Iletin II (PB or PP) Monotard (PP) Montard Human
Isophane Insulin Suspension (NPH), intermediate-acting Onset: 3–4 hours Peak action: 6–12 hours Duration: 24–28 hours	NPH (B) NPH Iletin I (B/P) NPH Iletin II (PB or PP) Insulatard NPH (PP) Protaphane NPH (PP) Humulin N (H)
NPH and regular mixture, prompt/intermediate-acting Onset: ½ hour Peak action: 4–8 hours Duration: 24 hours	Mixtard (PP)
Protamine Zinc Insulin (PZI), long-acting Onset: 4–6 hours Peak action: 14–24 hours Duration: 36 hours	PZI I[b] (B/P) PZI II (PB or PP)
Zinc suspension, extended-action Onset: 4–6 hours Peak action: 18–24 hours Duration: 36 hours	Ultralente (B) Ultralente Iletin I[b] (B/P) Ultratard (PB)

[a] Source notations as follows: B = beef, P = pork, PP = purified pork, PB = purified beef, B/P = 70% beef/30% pork combination, H = human (synthesized by a strain of *E. coli* genetically altered by the addition of a human gene for insulin production).
[b] Comes in U-40 as well as U-100 forms.
[c] U-500.

toring is imperative (most specialists agree that urine testing should be reserved for ketone detection). Periodic measurements of glycosylated hemoglobin (HbAlc) are also helpful in determining long-term control. The test is based on the concept that glucose and other sugars become attached to hemoglobin and hemoglobin fractions during the 120-day life span of the red blood cell. The higher the average blood glucose level during this period, the higher the assay.

▶ ***Type II diabetes (obese*** and ***nonobese subsets)*** is a milder form of the disease caused by antagonism to the action of insulin. Target cells demonstrate a reduction in (1) insulin receptor-binding capacity, (2) glucose transport across the cell membrane (prereceptor defects), and (3) utilization of glucose within the cell

TABLE 5.13 COMPLICATIONS OF INSULIN THERAPY

Complication	Description
Rebound hyperglycemia (Somogyi effect)	Insulin-induced hypoglycemia stimulates release of epinephrine, glucagon, cortisol, and growth hormone. This leads to hyperglycemia by stimulating hunger and gluconeogenesis, as well as inhibiting the peripheral actions of glucose. The infrequent problem is managed by using lower split-dose combined insulin regimens.
Insulin allergy	A systemic allergy to insulin related to the production of IgE insulin antibodies. Manifested as a local reaction at injection sites. Develops infrequently with purified insulin preparations. Desensitization using purified regular insulin (Lilly Desensitization Kit) is highly effective.
Insulin resistance	IgG insulin-binding antibodies develop that prevent insulin from gaining access to receptor sites. Insulin requirements rise steadily while diabetic control declines. The problem is most common among allergy-prone patients who are obese. It is also associated with the use of low-purity insulin preparations, infection, cirrhosis, and hyperendocrinopathies. Patients should be shifted to a highly purified pork or human insulin. Steroids are sometimes given as well.
Lipohypertrophy	Fibrofatty masses develop at overused sites of insulin injection. Treatment consists of avoiding affected sites. When this is done, the masses slowly regress.
Lipoatrophy	Subcutaneous fat disappears at injection sites. Patients should be shifted to a highly purified pork or human insulin and instructed to give subsequent injections into the perimeter of atrophic areas. These measures result in a gradual replacement of subcutaneous fat.
Insulin edema	Rapid correction of hyperglycemia leads to temporary salt imbalance with fluid retention. The condition disappears gradually on its own, sooner with salt restriction and diuretics.
Insulin presbyopia	Dehydration and/or glycosylation of the eye lens occurs with severe or long-standing hyperglycemia. Refraction changes result. They are reversed with normalization of blood sugar. Since the prescription for glasses can change several times during the period of adjustment, refraction studies should be postponed until 6 weeks after blood sugar levels are controlled.

(postreceptor defects). The etiology of these changes is not fully known, though a strong genetic determinant is clear. The disease is usually expressed in autosomal dominant patterns of inheritance. Neither HLA types nor islet cell antibodies are associated with it. However, diet plays an important part, a large subset of patients (at least 60–80%) being obese. Obesity contributes to the disease in that adipose cells with large stores of fat are particularly prone to problems with insulin binding, glucose transport, and glucose utilization. Unlike diabetes type I, insulin remains available. In fact, insulin levels are usually high in the obese patient and normal or reduced in the nonobese one. Nonetheless, insulin antagonism reduces cellular uptake of glucose. Unused glucose accumulates in the blood, and hyperosmolarity develops. As described in Table 5.11, this leads to polyuria and polydipsia, along with possible changes in vision. Some utilization of glucose, though lessened, remains. Gluconeogenesis and ketosis are therefore unusual except during periods of stress, trauma, or infection. Consequently, weight loss and polyphagia are uncommon markers.

Diagnosis of diabetes type II is made on the basis of an elevated fasting plasma glucose (FPG) level greater than or equal to 140 mg/dL and a glucosylated hemoglobin (HbAlC) level greater than or equal to 8% measured simultaneously. Random plasma glucose or 2-hour postprandial concentrations above 200 mg/dL associated with abnormal elevations of plasma glucose are also indicative. In the event of

Setting Up An Easy Rotation Cycle

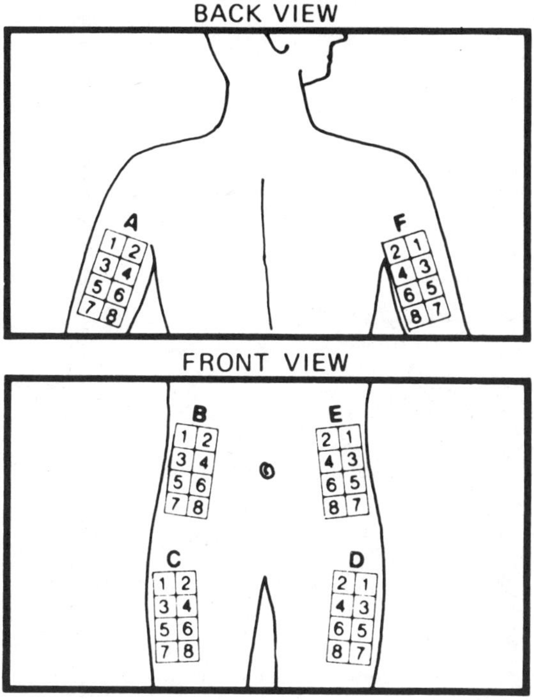

Injection Log

SITE		1	2	3	4	5	6	7	8
right arm	A								
right abdomen	B								
right thigh	C								
left thigh	D								
left abdomen	E								
left arm	F								

Figure 5.2 Insulin rotation sites. (From Loebl et al., The *Nurse's Drug Handbook,* 4th ed., © 1986, John Wiley & Sons, Inc., New York.)

TABLE 5.14 DRUGS NOTED TO INTERFERE WITH INSULIN ACTION

Increases Risk of Hypoglycemia	Increases Risk of Hyperglycemia
Alcohol	Corticosteroids
Anabolic steroids	Dextrothyroxine
Disopyramide	Estrogens
Guanethidine	Ethacrynic acid
Monoamine oxidase inhibitors	Furosemide
Sulfonylureas	Thiazide diuretics
Salicylates (large doses)	Phenytoin
Ethylenediaminetetraacetic acid (EDTA)	Thyroid hormones
Oxytetracycline	
Propranolol[a]	

[a]Does not contribute to hypoglycemia, but may mask warning signs.

borderline elevations on either test, a 2-hour glucose tolerance test is advised. Otherwise, it is considered unnecessary. The use of HbAlc alone for diagnosis is presently not recommended. The treatment of type II diabetes depends on the subset. Nonobese patients are usually given insulin preparations (Table 5.12) or an oral hypoglycemic agent (Table 5.15). Oral hypoglycemic agents work by stimulating insulin secretion from the pancreas and by increasing the number and affinity of the insulin receptor sites on target cells. Their action may be adversely affected by the drugs listed in Table 5.16. Obese type II diabetics are given hypocaloric diets for weight reduction. If the response is poor, semistarvation diets of 800 calories for short periods (7–10 days) has been advocated. Adherence to a hypocaloric diet usually improves plasma glucose concentrations even before substantial amounts of weight are lost. In contrast, oral hypoglycemic agents or insulin seem to compound the problem. By stimulating appetite, either may contribute to weight gain and exacerbate the factors involved in insulin antagonism. Furthermore, insulin requirements tend to rise steadily in patients who are already insulinophethoric. Nonetheless, for many type II obese patients who fail to adhere to their diet, drug therapy remains the only recourse.

Complications of diabetes affect virtually every system of the body. One of the most life-threatening is ***diabetic ketoacidosis (DKA)***. As previously mentioned, ketogenesis develops as a compensatory mechanism in type I diabetes. The acids acetoacetate and β-hydroxybutyrate serve as sources of fuel, particularly for cardiac muscle, renal cortex, and skeletal muscle. Unfortunately, large amounts of keto acids accompanying more severe states of cellular starvation can significantly lower the pH of blood. Patients may then develop metabolic, respiratory, cardiovascular, and neurologic changes. Early symptoms of DKA include abdominal pain, nausea, and vomiting. The patient who has had severe vomiting with loss of hydrogen, potassium, and chloride ions or who has taken alkalis for abdominal symptoms may present with ***diabetic ketoalkalosis.*** A fruity breath odor (like that of decaying apples) indicates high concentrations of plasma acetone. It may not be prominent in patients whose ketone production is shifted toward β-hydroxybutyrate. Kussmaul breathing, preceded by tachypnea, signals the fall of serum bicarbonate to around 10 mEq. These respiratory changes help to lower the carbon dioxide pressure (P_{CO_2}) and thus serve as important buffering mechanisms. However, if acidosis becomes more severe, respiratory drive is lost and Kussmaul breathing cannot be sustained. The

TABLE 5.15 ORAL HYPOGLYCEMIC AGENTS

Generic Name	Brand Name	Tablet Dose (mg)	Usual Dosage (mg)	Duration of Action	Excretion
Acetohexamide	Dymelor	250 and 500	250–1,500, once or divided bid	10–20 hours	Renal
Chlorpropamide	Diabinese	100 and 250	50–750, once a day	24–36 hours	Renal
Glipizide	Glucatrol	5 and 10	5–15, single dose or up to 40 divided bid	6–12 hours	Hepatic, renal, and biliary
Glyburide	Micronase	1.25, 2.5, and 5	1.25–10 single dose, 10–20 divided bid	10–20 hours	Hepatic, renal, and biliary
Tolbutamide	Orinase	500	1,000–3,000 divided bid or tid	6–8 hours	Hepatic and renal
Tolazamide	Tolinase	100, 250, and 500	100–1,500 once or divided bid	12–24 hours	Renal

mental status in DKA varies from full alertness to drowsiness or deep coma. Any of these clinical findings in the presence of glucosuria, ketonuria, and low arterial pH is diagnostic. Usually the progression of unattended disease in a new diabetic, ketoacidosis developing in long-standing patients under established treatment is more likely to be precipitated by one of the factors listed in Table 5.17. Particularly with elderly patients, ruling out infection, abdominal problems, silent myocardial infarction, or other underlying conditions becomes an important consideration.

Treatment for all cases of DKA requires hospitalization. Over a period of 12–24 hours, water and salt are replaced at the respective rates of 75 mL and 8 mEq per kilogram of body weight. For this purpose, half-strength saline is used if serum sodium is above 155 mEq/kg, normal saline if serum sodium is under 155 mEq/kg. Insulin is given in a continuous low-dose intravenous infusion of 4–8 U/h or as small intramuscular (deltoid) doses of 5–10 U/h. Continuous low-dose regimens of insulin decrease blood glucose levels at predictable rates of 80–100 mg%/h. This, in turn, seems to lower the incidence of cerebral edema. It also minimizes problems related to shifts and/or precipitous falls of potassium, phosphate, lactate, and magnesium. All

TABLE 5.16 DRUGS KNOWN TO INTERFERE WITH THE ACTION OF ORAL HYPOGLYCEMICS

Increases the Risk of Hypoglycemia	Increases the Risk of Hyperglycemia
Alcohol	Corticosteroids
Anabolic steroids	Epinephrine
Chloramphenicol	Estrogens
Clofibrate	Nicotinic acid
Monoamine oxidase inhibitors	Phenytoin
Sulfonamides	Thiazide diuretics
Cyclophosphamide	Dextrothyroxine
Salicylates (large doses)	Ethacrynic acid
Phenylbutazone and derivatives	Glucagon
Probenecid	Phenothiazines
Beta blockers[a]	Thyroid preparations
Oxytetracycline	Triampterene (Dyrenium)
Coumarins	Calcium channel blockers

[a]May mask warning signs of hypoglycemia.

TABLE 5.17 FACTORS PRECIPITATING DIABETIC KETOACIDOSIS

- Decreased secretion or antagonism of endogenous insulin
  - Acromegaly
  - Cushing's syndrome
  - Pancreatitis
  - Pheochromocytoma
  - Previously undiagnosed diabetes (notably type I)
  - Thyrotoxicosis
  - Viral infections of the pancreas
- Failure of exogenous insulin
  - Change in diet or exercise
  - Insulin resistance
  - Patient error in calibration/injection
    - Inadequate education
    - Mental or physical incapability (particularly poor vision)
  - Prescription error (inadequate dose or type of insulin)
- Stress
  - Acute psychiatric illness
  - Infection (particularly of the teeth or gums, pneumoia, UTI, gangrene)
  - Myocardial Infarction
  - Pregnancy
  - Surgery
  - Trauma

four of these substances tend to be depleted in DKA and may require replacement even though serum levels remain within normal ranges. Alkali therapy has been adversely associated with (1) accentuation of intracellular shifts of potassium and phosphate, (2) development of cellular hypoxia, (3) paradoxical acidosis of cerebrospinal fluid with coma, (4) induction of metabolic alkalosis, (5) hypocalcemia and/or hypomagnesemia, and (6) sodium overload. It is thus reserved for patients with a pH of 7.0 or less and/or patients with cardiopulmonary compromise (e.g., cardiac arrhythmia, abnormal elevation of P_{CO_2}).

Whereas DKA is associated with severe type I diabetes, ***hyperosmolar nonketotic diabetic coma*** typically afflicts elderly patients with mild or previously unknown disease. Responsible for a steady increase in the number of hospital admissions (DKA admissions are declining), this problem can usually be traced to the use of a drug that inhibits endogenous insulin release or alters glucose metabolism (Table 5.18). Patients present with central nervous system changes ranging from depressed sensorium to frank coma. The picture mimics cerebrovascular accident, an unfortunate happenstance, since early and correct diagnosis is the most crucial factor in recovery. More distinguishing features include glucose levels in excess of 600 mg/dL, absence of ketosis or ketoacidosis, and serum osmolality greater than or equal to 350 mosm per kilogram of water. Management in an intensive care unit is essential. Treatment consists of administering large amounts of hypotonic fluid and continuous low doses of insulin. Mortality rates have approached 40–70%.

Vascular changes in diabetes affect both large vessels (macroangiopathy) and small vessels (microangiopathy). Histologically, arteriosclerotic changes resemble those occurring in nondiabetic patients. However, arteriosclerosis in the diabetic is earlier in onset, more extensive, and more progressive. As a result, hypertension is common. Diabetics suffer three-fourths of all strokes and more than one-half of all myocardial infarctions in the United States. They have a fivefold increase in coronary occlusive disease compared to the nondiabetic population. An extraordinary

TABLE 5.18 DRUGS KNOWN TO PRECIPITATE NONKETOTIC DIABETIC COMA

Asparaginase	Diuretics Chlorthalidone Ethacrynic acid Furosemide Hydrochlorothiazide
Beta blockers	Glucocorticoids
Chlorpromazine	Phenytoin
Cimetidine	
Diazoxide	

proportion of these patients are premenopausal women and patients with no history of hypertension or significant hyperlipidemia. The risk of a ***silent heart attack*** is also high. Furthermore, diabetic victims of heart attacks are younger and have a shorter life expectancy than the population at large. Microangiopathy is characterized by distinct lesions that affect small vessels in the eye ***(diabetic retinopathy)*** and kidney ***(diabetic nephropathy),*** problems discussed in Chapters 1 and 8, respectively.

Diabetic neuropathy, which can involve virtually every system in the body, may be divided into somatic and visceral types. ***Somatic neuropathy*** usually affects nerves of the lower extremities in a bilateral, symmetric pattern. Outstanding symptoms are pain and paresthesia. The pain may be dull, cramp-like, aching, stabbing, or crushing. Paresthesia produces sensations of coldness, numbness, tingling, or burning and sometimes foot drop. Worsening in the middle of the night, it causes skin to become so sensitive that the touch of clothing or sheets cannot be tolerated. Pacing the floor may offer some relief. The upper extremities are commonly affected as well. In such cases, patients present with amyotrophy, asthenia, sensory impairment, and/or radiculitis. Other manifestations include depression, irritability, and anorexia. ***Visceral neuropathy*** results in symptoms that simulate many other diseases. It can cause a number of GI changes including (1) impaired esophageal motility, (2) delayed gastric emptying with marked gastric distention ***(gastroparesis diabeticorum),*** and (3) current nocturnal or postprandial diarrhea with associated incontinence ***(diabetic enteropathy).*** Visceral neuropathy may be associated with bladder dysfunction or ***diabetic male sexual dysfunction.*** In the latter case, there is involvement of the nerves erigentes (which is responsible for dilating arteries to the penis). An erection cannot be sustained, though libido, sensation, orgasm, and ejaculation are unaffected. In new diabetics, sexual dysfunction may be transient, developing only during periods of poor blood sugar control. However, in long-term patients, it tends to be chronic, whether blood sugar levels are well controlled or not. General involvement of the autonomic nervous system leads to vasomotor instability (postural hypotension, tachycardia, dependent edema) and a number of skin changes (anhidrosis, trophic disturbances, and reversal of skin temperature). These symptoms, in turn, may contribute to stroke, myocardial infarction (particularly the silent variety), and gangrene.

Diagnosis of diabetic neuropathy is clinical, since there are no specific pathognomonic markers. Absent or reduced knee/ankle jerk and modest elevation of cerebrospinal fluid protein levels may be the only objective findings. Some of the lesions, particularly external ocular palsies, resolve spontaneously. Though neuritis also resolves, Dilantin or Tegretol may be required for pain control. Enteropathies frequently respond to broad-spectrum antibiotics. Resection of the internal vesical sphincter is advocated for neurogenic bladder that fails to respond to more conservative measures such as drug therapy. In cases of erectile impotence, surgical implantation of a silicone rod or prosthesis into the penis may be considered.

▶ ***Diabetic foot*** is a particularly common problem. Diabetics characteristically develop multiple arterial occlusions in the major distal vessels, particularly the tibial and popliteal ones. Due to the diffuse nature of these occlusions, collateral circulation fails to develop. Consequently, arterial runoff below the lesions to the feet remains negligible. Peripheral neuropathy often coexists. Impairment of the autonomic nervous response, pain conduction, and temperature perception predispose the extremity to unperceived trauma and lowered tissue resistance. In conjunction with vascular insufficiency and hyperglycemia, infection becomes a major threat, particularly since it may quickly develop into osteomyelitis or gangrene. Five out of every six amputations for gangrene are related to diabetes. These complications are described more fully in Table 5.19, along with the symptoms and interventions. They may be minimized by a number of preventive measures. Control of blood sugar and avoidance of tobacco are foremost. Special attention to foot care is also mandatory. Properly fitting shoes, warm woolen socks, avoidance of heat applications (hot water, heat lamps), and daily inspection of the feet are extremely important. Trimming of nails, corns, and calluses should be done by a podiatrist. Signs of infection should be promptly treated with antibiotics as determined by culture and sensitivity tests. As with other aspects of the disease, ▶ ***diabetes organizations*** can provide important information about care and referral.

In contrast to diabetes, which is an acquired disease, are the ***inborn errors of carbohydrate metabolism.*** As described in Table 5.20, many of them result from the genetic absence of a particular enzyme needed for the formation and breakdown of glycogen ***(glycogen storage disease).*** All forms are quite rare. Diagnosis is made on the basis of clinical findings, as well as biopsy of affected tissue to demonstrate an enzyme deficiency. For most types of glycogen storage disease, no effective treatment is known. Sometimes ketosis and hypoglycemia can be controlled in types 0, I, and III patients by continuous intragastric infusions of dextrin at night and small, frequent feelings of carbohydrates and proteins during the day. Limiting muscle use is advocated in type V to cut down on muscle cramps.

FATS

Fats are chemical compounds classified as triglycerides (neutral fats), phospholipids, or cholesterol (Table 5.21). Both triglycerides and phospholipids contain fatty acids, the most common being stearic acid, oleic acid, and palmitic acid. Cholesterol contains a sterol nucleus synthesized from products of fatty acid degradation. Therefore, although cholesterol molecules contain no fatty acids, they have many of the physical and chemical properties of the two other lipids. All three types of fats are obtained from food or synthesized in the body.

Fats from foods are digested in the small intestine. Bile salts emulsify small particles of cholesterol and phospholipids, while pancreatic enzymes break down triglycerides into fatty acids and glycerol. Small amounts of short chain fatty acids enter the portal blood directly. All other fats pass into the lymph in the form of dispersed droplets called "chylomicrons." They travel to the thoracic duct and empty into the venous blood. After a meal, chylomicrons in the blood rise from 2%, giving

TABLE 5.19 Diabetic Foot Complications

Complication	Description	Diagnosis	Treatment
Arterial insufficiency	Atherosclerotic lesions develop in large vessels as well as small arteries, arterioles, and capillaries. Lesions tend to be multisegmental rather than isolated. As a result, collateral ("runoff") circulation does not develop, as it may in nondiabetic disease. Patients present with intermittent claudication, pain on resting, ischemic ulcers, and secondary infection.	Arterial blood pressure measurements of thigh, calf, and ankle using ultrasound; arterial pulse contour studies; arteriography.	Conservative measures include control of hyperglycemia, weight reduction, cessation of smoking, analgesics for pain. Patients should be instructed to elevate head of bed 6 in. and started on a program of passive foot exercises (Buerger's exercises). Bed rest for 1–2 weeks may improve mild rest pain. Arterial reconstruction is a possibility if the patient does not have small vessel disease.
Neuropathy	Almost universal after 15 years of diabetes. May affect the motor nerve supply of muscles, diminish sensory acuity, or damage the sympathetic nerve supply. Muscular weakness leads to deformities such as hammer toes and medial deviations of small toes. It also results in damage to ankle ligaments and joint capsules. Painless but severe osteoarthritic changes (Charcot's joint) may occur. Calluses form over abnormal prominences. Due to diminished sensation, there may be continuous unknown trauma to these areas. Pressure necrosis (neuropathic ulcers) develop, with inflammation and swelling. If the sympathetic nerve supply is involved, the feet become anhydrotic (dry and nonsweating) and vasodilated.	For neuropathic ulcers, x-ray films to rule out osteomyelitis, cultures to rule out skin infection. X-ray films reveal Charcot's joint.	Neuropathic ulcers require that the foot be kept at rest with a short-leg walking cast until inflammation subsides. The cast is then removed and replaced with a molded polypropylene orthosis to provide continuing support for the foot.
Infection	Easily established in the presence of hyperglycemia, vascular insufficiency, and/or neuropathy. There are three types, each of which may progress readily to gangrene. *Mal perforans ulcers* develop in patients who have neuropathy but no evidence of ischemia. Usual site is plantar surface of toes or feet. If untreated, infection spreads to underlying fascia, tendons, bones, and joints. A spreading cellulitis, *nonsuppurative phlegmon,* develops on the dorsum of the foot. Associated with necrosis of overlying skin. Penetration by a foreign body, spread of local toe infection, or ulceration of a bunion may lead to *deep abscess.* The sole of the foot becomes edematous, with obliteration of the arch.	Cultures and sensitivity tests	Bed rest and large doses of sensitive antibiotics. Surgical debridement and drainage as necessary. Toe, toe and metatarsal head, transmetatarsal, below-knee, or above-knee amputation when infection cannot be arrested and involves underlying bone, joints, or connective tissue.

plasma a turbid, yellow appearance. However, most chylomicrons are cleared within 1–8 hours as they circulate through heart, muscle, and adipose capillaries, where significant amounts of the enzyme lipoprotein lipase (LPL) are stored. These capillary enzymes hydrolyze about 80% of meal-generated chylomicrons into fatty acids. The acids diffuse through the membranes of local cells, becoming fuel for intracellular energy.

The remaining chylomicrons travel to the liver, where most of them are processed into special types of body fats. These "synthesized" fats are bound to albumin (also

TABLE 5.20 ERRORS OF CARBOHYDRATE METABOLISM

Disorder	Abnormality	Clinical Features	Treatment
Galactosemia	Inherited absence of galactose-1-phosphate uridyl transferase prevents the conversion of galactose to glucose.	Infant appears normal at birth but after several days of breast feeding becomes severely ill with GI symptoms, liver failure, proteinuria, and aminoaciduria.	Milk elimination even by mother during pregnancy. Diet substitutes of synthetic galactose and lactose-free milk until age 6.
Galactokinase deficiency	Galactose fails to be metabolized due to inherited deficiency of galactokinase; blood and urine levels rise.	Cataract development but no GI or central nervous system disturbance.	Same as galactosemia.
Glycogen storage	Impaired synthesis or breakdown of glycogen due to missing:	Abnormal deposition of galactose in:	
Type O	UDPG-glycogen transferase	Liver, muscle.	Frequent, small carbohydrate feedings and high protein intake during the day; high dextrin infusions overnight.
Type I	Glucose 6-phosphatase.	Liver, kidney, bowel	Same as type O.
Type II	Lysosomal glucosidase.	All organs.	No effective treatment.
Type III	Debrancher system.	Liver, muscle, heart.	Same as type O.
Type IV	Brancher enzyme.	Liver (amylopectin).	No effective treatment.
Type V	Muscle phosphorylase	Skeletal muscle.	Exercise limitation to reduce muscle cramps.
Type VI	Liver phosphorylase.	Liver.	No effective treatment.
Type VII	Phosphofructokinase.	Skeletal muscle.	No effective treatment.
Types VIII, IX, X	Phosphorylase control mechanisms.	Mild liver changes.	No effective treatment.
Hereditary fructose intolerance	Inability to utilize fructose due to absence of 1-phosphofructoaldolase.	Severe hypoglycemia, even seizures or coma, with high fructose intake. Smaller amounts cause renal tubular acidosis, cirrhosis, and mental deterioration.	Exclusion of fructose, sucrose, and sorbital from diet. Glucose for hypoglycemic episodes.
Fructosuria	Absence of fructokinase prevents normal utilization of ingested fructose.	Harmless elevations of fructose in blood and excretion in urine (may lead to false diagnosis of diabetes mellitus).	No treatment necessary.
Pentosuria	Absence of L-xylulose dehydrogenase prevents normal utilization of ingested fructose.	Harmless excretion of L-xylose in urine (may lead to false diagnosis of diabetes mellitus).	No treatment necessary.
Disaccharidase deficiencies Lactose intolerance	Lack of lactase prevents splitting of the disaccharide lactose into monosaccharides glucose and galactose.	Intestinal pain, gas, diarrhea, or constipation with ingestion of milk products.	Diet with controlled lactose intake or lactose conversion with LactAid.
Glucose-galactose intolerance	Transport system for monosaccharides lacking in small bowel. Sugars fail to be absorbed.	Watery diarrhea with intake of galactose, glucose, sucrose, or lactose.	Fructose, carbohydrate-free formulas in infancy. Controlled diet throughout life.
Sucrose-isomaltose intolerance	Absence of sucrase or isomaltase prevents splitting of these disaccharides into monosaccharides.	Intestinal irritation with ingestion of sucrose and maltose. Often asymptomatic.	Diet controlled in sucrose and maltose.

TABLE 5.21 IMPORTANT TERMS IN FAT METABOLISM

Type	Description
Cholesterol	Organic compounds containing no fatty acids, but similar properties due to a sterol nucleus made from degradation products of fatty acids. Dietary cholesterol is absorbed in chylomicron particles.
Fatty acids	Water-insoluble organic acids of two types: (a) *saturated* (acetic, butyric, caprylic, capric, lauric, formic, myristic, palmitic, and stearic acids), containing single bonds; (2) *unsaturated* (oleic, tiglic, hypogeic, palmitoleic, physetoleic, linoleic, linolenic, clupanodonic, arachidonic, hydrocarpic, and chaulmoogric acids), containing double or triple bonds.
Triglycerides	Animal and vegetable fats consisting of glycerol and three fatty acids (usually stearic, oleic, and palmitic). Dietary triglycerides absorbed in chylomicrons and broken down by LPL.
Short chain fatty acids	Small fraction of dietary fat that can be absorbed directly into the bloodstream. All others must first enter lymph in chylomicrons.
Essential fatty acids	Fatty acids (linoleic, linolenic, and arachidonic) that cannot be made by the body and must be provided in the diet.
Free fatty acids	Variable amounts of fatty acids (3–30 molecules) combined with albumin in the liver for transport to other parts of the body.
Lipoproteins	Complexes consisting of an inner core of cholesterol ester and triglyceride and an outer surface of protein, phospholipids, and unesterified cholesterol. They function to transport fats in a stable and soluble form throughout the body. The complexes become progressively smaller in size but greater in protein density. Five stages are described.
Chylomicrons	Largest complexes formed from dietary fat. They normally clear within 1–8 hours after a meal.
VLDL (prebeta lipoproteins)	Very-low-density complexes from hydrolysis of chylomicrons by LPL.
LDL (beta-lipoproteins)	Low-density complexes formed from the remnants of intermediate-density lipoprotein (IDL). They deliver cholesterol to peripheral tissues or to the liver.
HDL (alpha-lipoproteins)	High-density complexes of lighter (HDL2) and heavier (HDL3) types. Action of LCAT causes its structural cholesterol to move to the core, leaving the surface free to pick up excess cholesterol from tissues. Thus it is thought to protect vessels from atherosclerotic changes.
Apoproteins	Protein portion of the complexes that play crucial roles in their structural maintenance and metabolic function. There are live major groups and subgroups. The principal ones are as follows:
ApoA-I	Found in chylomicrons and HDL. Activates LCAT.
ApoA-II	Found in chylomicrons and HDL. Activates LPL.
ApoA-IV	Found in chylomicrons.
ApoB-48	Minor component of chylomicrons. Manufactured in the intestine.
ApoB-100	Major protein of LDL. Produced in the chylomicrons and broken down by LPL.

made in the liver), forming transporting complexes called "lipoproteins." The complexes contain (1) a core of nonpolar lipids (triglycerides and cholesterol esters), (2) an outer layer of polar lipids (phospholipids and free cholesterol), and (3) specialized surface proteins (apoproteins). The apoprotein C-II activates LPL. Other apoproteins ensure uptake of the lipoproteins by particular body cells. For example, E is recognized by receptors on hepatocytes, and B is recognized by both hepatic and extrahepatic cells.

Lipoproteins are separated into groups according to the density of protein—low or high (see Table 5.21). Lipoproteins with low concentrations of protein have high concentrations of lipids, and those with high concentrations of proteins have low concentrations of lipids. Very-low-density lipoproteins (VLDL) transport nearly all endogenous triglycerides. Such triglycerides are generated from carbohydrates, while those found in chylomicrons are derived from fats.

Up to 150 g of triglycerides enter and leave plasma each day, compared to 1–2 g of cholesterol. Seventy-five percent of this cholesterol is transported by low-density lipoproteins (LDL). LDL is created by the removal (via lipase-like enzymes) of glyceride and surface porteins from VLDL. LDL has an unknown fate. It is probably directed by apoproteins to receptor sites on fibroblasts or other cells and removed from circulation. High-density lipoprotein (HDL) binds the remaining 25% of cholesterol. Plasma concentrations of the various lipoproteins can be determined by electrophoresis (phenotyping). Beta lipoproteins correspond to LDL and alpha lipoproteins to HDL.

► ***Screening for hyperlipidemia*** is clinically important because of the condition's high association with atherosclerosis. However, the mechanisms by which hyperlipidemia contributes to atherosclerosis are not known, and the studies have two seeming contradictions. First, treatment to lower abnormally high lipid levels results in a regression of plaque formation but not in a significant reduction of the major sequela, namely, myocardial infarction. Second, atherosclerotic acceleration is related less to triglycerides than to cholesterol. Heart disease rises in linear fashion with cholesterol levels, a fact consistent with the higher cholesterol levels found in men and postmenopausal women. However, the cholesterol in HDL has an inverse effect: high HDL levels actually lower the risk of cardiovascular disease (possibly by removing cholesterol from peripheral tissues and preventing its accumulation in arteries).

Once hyperlipidemia has been diagnosed, the lipoprotein pattern should be established in order to select the best therapy. Five types have been defined, as outlined in Table 5.22. A deficiency of LPL with impaired clearance of chylomicrons is called ► ***type I hyperlipidemia.*** This rare disorder is almost always genetic, but occasionally develops as a consequence of systemic lupus erythematosus, dysgammaglobulinemia, or insulinopenic diabetes mellitus. By young adulthood, patients have usually developed cutaneous deposits of fat (xanthomas) over pressure points and

TABLE 5.22 COMPARISON OF THE HYPERLIPIDEMIAS

	Prevalence	Involved Lipoprotein	Cholesterol Level	Triglyceride Level
Type I	Very rare	Chylomicrons	Normal to high	High
Type IIA	Common	LDL	High	Normal
Type IIB	Most common	VLDL and LDL	High	High
Type III	Rare	LDL	Variably high	Variably high
Type IV	Common	VLDL	Normal to high	High
Type V	Rare	Chylomicrons	High	High

extensor surfaces of joints. Lipemia retinalis and hepatosplenomegaly are also common. Pancreatitis-like abdominal pain may be the presenting symptom. Overindulgence in fats not only exacerbates the pain but has been known to cause severe, even fatal, hemorrhagic pancreatitis. Interestingly enough, there is no evidence that this form of lipidemia leads to atherosclerosis. Type I hyperlipidemia should be suspected when any patient with the above presentation is found to have extremely high triglyceride levels but relatively normal cholesterol levels. Triglycerides may be higher than 5,000 mg/dl and typically are eightfold higher than cholesterol.

The diagnosis can be confirmed by demonstrating chylomicrons in a fasting specimen. This is done by placing a tube of serum upright in a refrigerator overnight. If chylomicrons are present, they form a "cream" layer on the top of an otherwise clear plasma (positive chylomicron test). Failure of LPL activity to increase after injection of intravenous heparin is also diagnostic. This is called postheparin lipolytic activity (PHLA) test. In treating patients with type I hyperlipidemia, the goal is to reduce circulating chylomicrons, thereby minimizing abdominal problems. This is accomplished by a diet markedly reduced in all fats except medium chain triglycerides, which do not require chylomicron formation for absorption.

▶ ***Type II hyperlipidemia*** (hypercholesterolemia) is characterized by elevated serum cholesterol levels resulting from delayed LDL clearance. In most cases, the problem is traced to a genetic defect in LDL receptors. However, ***secondary hypercholesterolemia*** results from biliary cirrhosis, hypothyroidism, hypopituitarism, diabetes mellitus, nephrotic syndrome, acute porphyria, or dietary excess. A benign form of hypercholesterolemia may be related to increased levels of HDL, as commonly seen in postmenopausal women or women taking oral contraceptives. Patients with hypercholesterolemia may be asymptomatic or develop xanthomas, usually over extensor tendons of the fingers, patella, or Achilles tendon. Achilles tendinitis is not uncommon. Atherosclerosis advances at much faster rates than normal, particularly among men. Most accelerated in the coronary arteries, it is responsible for a high incidence of myocardial infarction. In fact, two out of three afflicted men have heart attacks by age 60.

Refrigerated Plasma	CAD Risk Factor	Diet Modifications	Drug Choices
Top layer creamy, rest clear	0	Low fat	None
Clear	2+	Low cholesterol; high polyunsaturated fat	Cholestyramine, Probucol, choloxin, gemfibrozil, niacin
Turbid	2+ to 3+	Low cholesterol; controlled fat; weight control; limited (ETOH)	Same as type IIA
Turbid	4+	Same as type IIB	Nicotinic acid, clofibrate
Turbid	1+	Controlled weight; moderate cholesterol; limited ETOH	Gemfibrozil, niacin, clofibrate
Top layer creamy, rest turbid	1+ to 3+	Low fat; moderate cholesterol; weight control	None

TABLE 5.23 LIPID-LOWERING DRUGS

Drug	Action	Dose
Cholestyramine (Questran, Cuemid (Colestipol)	Increases formation of bile acids from cholesterol	8–12 g bid
Clofibrate (Atromid-S)	Decreases synthesis/release of VLDL and fatty acids	500 mg tid
Nicotinic acid (Niacin)	Inhibits lipolysis and activates LPL	100 mg tid, increased to 1 g tid
Sodium *d*-thyroxine (Choloxin)	Increases bile excretion of cholesterol	1 mg daily, increased to 6 mg
Probucol	Unknown; thought to inhibit LDL formation	500 mg bid
Gemfibrozil	Unknown; thought to inhibit lipolysis and decrease VLDL production	600 mg bid

The diagnosis is confirmed by elevated serum cholesterol levels shown to be from increased LDL on phenotyping. The plasma is translucent (LDL does not refract light regardless of its concentration), and triglycerides are normal. The most effective way to lower serum LDL is to avoid foods containing cholesterol and saturated fats. As described in Table 5.23, several drugs are known to increase LDL removal but are associated with a number of side effects. Clofibrate has no effect on serum cholesterol. Since it contributes to gallstone formation and other metabolic problems, it should not be used in type II hyperlipidemia.

▶ ***Type III hyperlipidemia*** (broad beta disease) is an uncommon familial disorder resulting from the failure of triglyceride-rich VLDL to convert to LDL. As a consequence, both triglycerides and cholesterol become elevated, predisposing the patient to severe premature atherosclerosis. Xanthomas appear over the extensor surfaces of the fingers, patella, or Achilles tendon, as they might in other hyperlipidemias. Palmar xanthomas, however, are pathognomonic for type III hyperlipidemia. Claudication or angina may signal vascular disease. In addition to equally high cholesterol and triglyceride levels, cloudy serum with a slight chylomicron layer helps to make the diagnosis. Electrophoresis that traces these abnormalities to VLDL confirms it. Treatment for type III hyperlipidemia centers on a low-cholesterol, low-carbohydrate diet. Since lipid levels tend to normalize at ideal body weight, weight reduction and maintenance may be important considerations for many patients. Drug therapy with clofibrate or niacin may also be needed.

In ▶ ***type IV hyperlipidemia,*** triglyceride levels fluctuate in response to stress, alcoholism, or dietary indiscretion (high intake of refined carbohydrates, including large amounts of fruit juices). The problem is common, particularly among American men. Whether or not it leads to premature coronary artery disease is still a question. The condition should be suspected when triglyceride levels are intermittently elevated while cholesterol levels remain relatively normal. Serum is turbid and electrophoresis indicates that the source is VLDL. Weight reduction alone is

Uses	Contraindications	Main Side Effects	Comments
Type II only	Malabsorption syndromes	GI discomforts	No triglyceride effect; may interfere with drug and vitamin absorption
Types III, IV	Heart disease	GI problems, gallstones	Prudent use, since many problems are being revealed.
All but type I	Peptic ulcer, liver disease, DM, uricemia	Flushing, rare GI discomfort, hypotension	Potentiation of antihypertensives
Type IIa	Heart disease	Angina, arrhythmias	Reserve for special cases; no effect on triglycerides
Cholesterol only	Hypersensitivity	GI upset, changes in complete blood count	Variable effect on triglycerides
Triglycerides	Hepatobiliary and renal diseases	Changes in liver enzymes and complete blood count; GI upset	No effect on cholesterol

often enough to bring lipid levels under control. Weight should be maintained at normal levels, with ongoing restriction of carbohydrates and alcohol. Niacin and clofibrate also reduce triglycerides in these patients, but have many bothersome side effects and should be considered as a last resort.

Defective clearance of triglycerides leads to ► ***type V hyperlipidemia.*** The problem can be genetic, as in the case of ***familial lecithin cholesterol acyltransferase (LCAT) deficiency.*** The LCAT enzyme normally esterifies cholesterol in plasma. Its absence causes not only hypertriglyceridemia but also hypercholesterolemia and hyperphospholipidemia with renal damage. LCAT deficiency and other familial forms of type V hyperlipidemia are quite rare. Unfortunately, ***secondary hypertriglyceridemia*** from acute alcoholism, long-term uncontrolled diabetes (diabetic lipemia), nephrosis, or drugs (estrogens, thiazides, or corticosteroids) is more common. Neither familial nor secondary hypertriglyceridemia predisposes to atherosclerosis. However, both are associated with peripheral neuropathy and pancreatitis. Tending to be severe and recurrent, the pancreatitis can lead to cyst formation or hemorrhage. Other developments include xanthomas, lipemia retinalis, and hepatosplenomegaly. Abdominal pain, exacerbated by ingestion of dietary fats, is a common complaint. The diagnosis is based on markedly elevated triglyceride levels with only modest elevations of cholesterol. The serum is cloudy and the chylomicron test is positive, but LPL tests are usually normal. The latter finding helps to distinguish the disorder from type I hyperlipidemia. Attention should focus on the underlying causes and on maintaining patients at ideal body weight. Fat and alcohol intake must be restricted. Niacin and clofibrate may also be necessary.

Other than hyperlipidemia, there are several ***rare lipid disorders.*** As described in Table 5.24, most of them result from rare genetic defects for which there is no treatment. Many patients die in early childhood. One notable exception is ***Gaucher's disease.*** Presenting at any age, this disorder is characterized by the deposition of fatty substances (glucocerebrosides) in reticuloendothelial cells found

TABLE 5.24 RARE LIPID DISORDERS

Disorder	Description
Hypolipidemia	Abnormally low lipoproteins either as a familial disorder (rare) or secondary to hyperthyroidism, anemia, malabsorption, malnutrition.
Hypobetalipoproteinemia	Reduced levels of LDL without symptoms.
Abetalipoproteinemia (Bassen-Kornzweig syndrome)	Impaired fat absorption due to congenital absence of beta lipoproteins. Leads to mental retardation, retinitis pigmentosa, acanthocytosis, and steatorrhea. Vitamins E and A used to delay neurologic sequelae.
Alpha-lipoproteinemia (Tangier disease)	Decreased serum cholesterol and HDL associated with hepatosplenomegaly, lymphadenopathy, and polyneuropathy. No known treatment.
Gaucher's disease	Failure of glucocerebrosides to be broken down (lack of glucocerebrosidase), with abnormal deposition in tissues.
Neimann-Pick disease	Failure of sphingomyelin to be broken down (lack of sphingomyelinase), with accumulation in reticuloendothelial cells and myelination. Patients develop mental retardation, hepatosplenomegaly with pancytopenia, lymphadenopathy, skin pigmentation, and xanthomas. No known treatment.
Fabry's disease	Abnormal catabolism of glycolipids in men due to sex-linked deficiency of alpha-galactosidase. Ceremide accumulates in skin (producing angiokeratomas), eyes, and blood vessels. Heart, central nervous system, and kidney problems result. Heterozygous women exhibit attenuated symptoms. No effective treatment.
Wolman's disease	Accumulation of neutral lipids in body tissue, leading to hepatosplenomegaly, adrenal calcification, steatorrhea, and death within the first year of life.
Cholesterol ester storage disease	Deficiency of cholesteryl ester hydrolase leads to lipid accumulation in lysosomes of the liver, spleen, and lymph nodes.
Beta-sitosterolemia	Increased absorption of plant sterols with accumulation in tendons, blood, and other tissues. Clinical course poorly defined. Treatment consists of a diet low in plant sterols.
Refsum's syndrome	Deficiency of phytanic acid hydrolase leads to accumulation of phytanic acid in plasma and tissues. Patients develop peripheral neuropathy, retinitis pigmentosa, and bone and skin changes. Treatment consists of a diet low in phytanic acid.
Tay-Sachs disease	Deficiency of hexosaminidase A leads to accumulation of sphingolipids in the brain. Progressive retardation, paralysis, and blindness occur, and death follows by age 4.
Generalized gangliosidosis	Accumulation of the ganglioside GM1 in the nervous system, causing progressive deterioration and death by age 2.
Metachromic disease	Deficiency of cerebroside sulfatase results in accumulation of metachromic lipids in myelin, kidney, spleen, and other tissues. Deterioration begins by age 2 and progresses relentlessly.

in the liver, spleen, lymph nodes, and bone marrow. These cells become distorted and enlarged, leading to varying degrees of hepatosplenomegaly, lymphadenopathy, bone pain, and joint swelling. Spleen and marrow involvement may cause blood dyscrasias. Brown pigmentation of the sclera (pingueculae) and skin are commonly noted. The diagnosis is made by finding abnormal reticuloendothelial cells on marrow, spleen, or liver biopsy and by demonstrating the absence of glucocerebrosidase activity in cell cultures. Patients who survive into adolescence may live for many years. Longevity may be favored by splenectomy, blood transfusions, and replacement of glucocerebrosidase (still experimental).

FAT STORAGE

As mentioned previously, the liver absorbs about 20% of the chylomicrons generated from a meal (the proportion normally left after tissue cells have met their requirement for immediate energy). It uses whatever is needed for hepatocellular energy and converts any excess back to triglycerides for reserve storage by adipose tissue. The latter process requires carbohydrate, protein, or fatty acid substrates, which are measured in calories. A calorie is the unit of heat required to raise the temperature of 1 pint of water 4°F. Fat supplies 9 calories/gram, while carbohydrates and proteins each supply 4 calories/gram.

The number of calories needed to maintain body weight depends on the person's activity level. Someone who is moderately active must eat the equivalent of 15 calories per body pound to maintain weight. In other words, if this person weighed 150 pounds, he or she needs 2,250 calories/day (daily caloric maintenance allowance). The calories should be proportionately derived from proteins, fats, and carbohydrates to ensure proper nutritional intake. The recommended balance is no less than 12–14% of protein and no more than 35% of fat, with the rest in carbohydrates. The Four Food Group System takes these food proportions into account.

Whenever the caloric content of the diet exceeds the energy requirements of the body, ***obesity*** may result. Patients with ***juvenile-onset obesity*** are typically normal in weight at birth but become overweight during childhood. They also experience excessive weight gain during puberty. This is particularly true of girls, who then tend to become permanently heavier with each successive pregnancy. These patients develop increased numbers of fat cells (hence the term "hyperplastic obesity"). Normally, the number of fat cells increases during the first 2 years of life and then stabilizes. Another period of proliferation occurs just before puberty. In the patient with juvenile-onset obesity, fat cells are added as long as there is caloric excess. Hypertrophy (enlargement of the cells) may also occur. In the normal child, once growth ceases, so does the formation of fat cells. From this point on, the fat cells can increase in size, but not number. However, those that have developed remain for life, and persons with juvenile-onset obesity have up to five times the number found in persons with normal weight or in those who develop obesity later. For this reason, the odds against an obese adolescent becoming a normal-weight adult are 28:1. Weight, which can be lost only by reducing the size of excess cells, is particularly difficult to lose. When lost, it tends to return to prereduction levels almost as if preset.

Bottle feeding may predispose the infant to hyperplasia of fat cells. This is because the mother can see how much formula is left and often forces the remaining amount on the infant. In contrast, the breast-feeding mother produces milk only in accordance with the child's demand. Early introduction of solid foods is another cause of excessive caloric intake. Parental attitudes toward eating also contribute to the problem. For example, fatness in a baby is considered a sign of health, while in older children it becomes the object of derogatory concern. In many families, food is served rather than offered on a help-yourself basis. In such cases, equal portions of food may be given to all family members, regardless of age or degree of hunger. Adults often pressure children to clean their plates. Food may be used as a reward and withdrawn as punishment. Snacking while watching television and eating junk foods are not discouraged. Such eating patterns affect weight gain in childhood and throughout life. They are associated with the socioeconomic background, with lower-class individuals having much higher obesity rates (women, six times; men, two times) than individuals from the upper classes.

Inactivity contributes to weight gain, sometimes to a greater degree than excessive caloric intake. This is especially true for the adolescent. Studies show that overweight teenage girls eat less than control subjects but also exercise less (up to 67% of their activities are sedentary). Decreased activity with age is the basis of ***adult-onset obesity.*** Caloric intake begins to exceed energy requirements beginning at age 20 and, unless adjustments are made, leads to weight gain (mostly in girth). One-third of American men and one-half of American women exceed by 20% the desirable weight noted in Table 5.25. This "middle-age spread" is unlike the general obesity seen in juvenile types. Since fat cells increase only in size, not in number, weight is easier to control. Obesity affects well-being in a number of ways. For example, hypertrophied fat cells are resistant to insulin. To compensate, beta cells of the pancreas become stimulated and a feedback hyperinsulinism develops. Weight reduction at this point reduces hyperinsulinism. Without it, beta cells become exhausted and patients develop diabetes. Obesity complicates and is a risk

TABLE 5.25 IDEAL WEIGHTS FOR HEIGHT AND BODY FRAME

	Men			Women		
Height	Small Frame	Medium Frame	Large Frame	Small Frame	Medium Frame	Large Frame
4′10″				102–111	109–121	118–131
4′11″				103–113	111–123	120–134
5′0″				104–115	113–126	122–137
5′1″				106–118	115–129	125–140
5′2″	128–134	131–141	138–150	108–121	118–132	128–143
5′3″	130–136	133–143	140–153	111–124	121–135	131–147
5′4″	132–138	135–145	142–156	114–127	124–138	134–151
5′5″	134–140	137–148	144–160	117–130	127–141	137–155
5′6″	136–142	139–151	146–164	120–133	130–144	140–159
5′7″	138–145	142–154	149–168	123–136	133–147	143–163
5′8″	140–148	145–157	152–172	126–139	136–150	146–167
5′9″	142–151	148–160	155–176	129–142	139–153	149–170
5′10″	144–154	151–163	158–180	132–145	142–156	152–173
5′11″	146–157	154–166	161–184	135–148	145–159	155–176
6′0″	149–160	157–170	164–188	138–151	148–162	158–179
6′1″	152–164	160–174	168–192			
6′2″	155–168	164–178	172–197			
6′3″	158–172	167–182	176–202			
6′4″	162–176	171–187	181–207			
			Or Calculate			
		106 lb for first 5 ft 6 lb for each additional inch.			100 lb for first 5 ft 5 lb for each additional inch.	

Source: Metropolitan Life Insurance Company, 1983.

factor for the development of hypertension, heart disease, osteoarthritis, and some pulmonary conditions; it also affects surgical outcomes. It may also be a social disadvantage. Studies have shown that school admission and job placement are more likely to be awarded to individuals of normal weight.

Although obesity may affect body image, it is not associated with more serious psychological problems. In fact, very few obese individuals suffer marked psychologic impairment (psychoses). On the other hand, stress and emotional disturbance may lead to deviant eating habits. For example, 10% of obese individuals exhibit ***night eating syndrome,*** a pattern characterized by morning anorexia, evening hyperphagia, and insomnia. ***Binge eaters*** comprise 5% of the obese. They suddenly and compulsively consume large amounts of food in a very short period of time. These binges are typically followed by agitation, self-condemnation, and sometimes ***bulimia*** (cycles of binging and self-induced purging with laxatives or vomiting). ***Anorexia nervosa*** may be an outcome of binge eating and bulimia. Patients with these conditions may benefit from psychiatric intervention (see Chapter 13 for a detailed discussion and specifics of treatment). In addition to psychologic problems, there are certain ***medical causes of obesity*** (Table 5.26). These conditions account for less than 1% of all weight problems. It should be noted that a number of diagnoses of hypothyroidism were based on false interpretations of tests. Using basal metabolic rates (BMR) to indicate thyroid function, these earlier studies failed to account for the effects of increased body mass on oxygen consumption. With the development of T3 and T4 tests, it became evident that most obese persons have normal levels of thyroid hormone. Whatever the contributing factors, the main treatment for obesity is a ▶ ***weight reduction diet.*** The most successful programs are based on a well-balanced, reduced-calorie diet tailored to the patient. Exercise programs (see Chapter 11) and ▶ ***support groups for weight loss*** are important adjuncts.

CLEARING INFECTIOUS AGENTS

As shown in Figure 5.3, hepatocytes are assembled in plates, one cell thick, that form central spaces known as "lacunae." These lacunae contain sinusoids, cylindric arrangements of porous capillaries filled with extra amounts of blood. In the event of blood loss, the sinusoids drain into the peripheral circulation to provide an emergency blood supply. The internal surfaces of the sinusoids are lined with Kupffer

TABLE 5.26 MEDICAL CAUSES OF OBESITY

Neurologic	Hypothalamic injury from craniopharyngiomas, encephalitis, trauma; Klein-Levin syndrome (hypersomnia and hyperphagia); a rare seizure syndrome characterized by EEG changes and preoccupation with food (responds to Dilantin).
Endocrine	Hypothyroidism; Cushing's syndrome; Stein-Leventhal syndrome; pregnancy; eunuchism; hyperinsulin states.
Drugs	Appetite stimulation with many psychiatric drugs (amitriptyline, tricyclic antidepressants, chlorpromazine, thioridazine, trifluoperazine, haloperidol). Cyproheptadine, corticosteroids.
Genetic	Laurence-Moon-Bardet-Biedl syndrome; Alstrom's syndrome; Prader-Willi syndrome; hyperostosis frontalis interna.

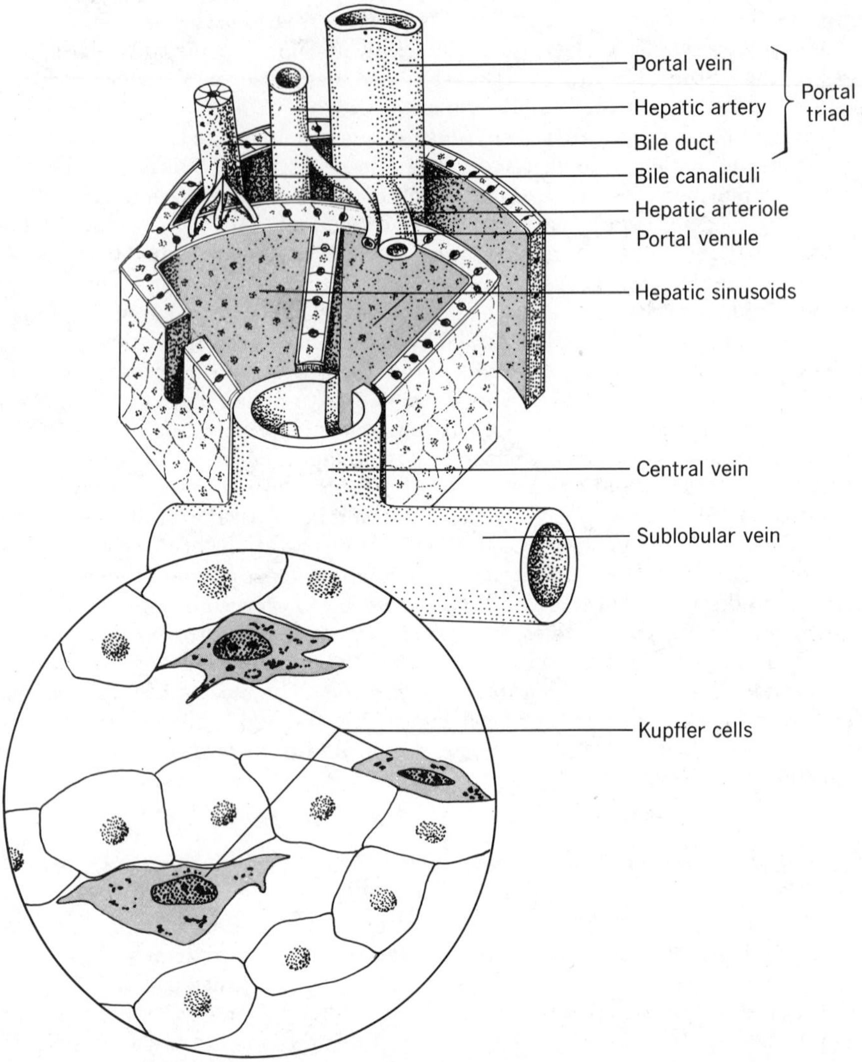

Figure 5.3 Hepatocellular architecture: sinusoids showing the central vein and portal triad; details of hepatocytes and Kupffer cells.

cells, macrophagic cells that kill 99% of the bacteria entering portal blood from the colon.

Despite Kupffer cell activity, infectious organisms sometimes invade the liver. The viruses listed in Table 5.27 can be particularly devastating because they replicate in hepatocyte nuclei. ***Viral hepatitis*** may lead to parenchymal cell degeneration and necrosis, with accumulation of inflammatory cells and proliferation of Kupffer cells.

▶***Hepatitis A*** (formerly known as "infectious or short-incubation hepatitis") tends to be the most benign but also the most contagious form. Hepatitis A virus

TABLE 5.27 VIRUSES CAUSING HEPATITIS

Hepatitis A	Yellow fever	Herpes simplex	Rubeola
Hepatitis B	Epstein-Barr	ECHO	Rubella
NANB (retrovirus)	Cytomegalovirus	Coxsackie	Varicella

(HAV) appears in the blood and stool during the incubation period (15–45 days) and during early illness. Transmission occurs mainly through oral-fecal routes and is thus favored by crowded living conditions, oral-anal or oral-genital sexual practices, and poor hygiene related to defecation. Food and water contaminated by human feces are other sources. Public swimming pools are not a concern, since the virus is readily inactivated by chlorine. Found in neither saliva, urine, tears, semen, nor cervical secretions, HAV presents little threat to fellow workers, classmates, or casual contacts. Theoretically, one is highly unlikely to contract the infection by kissing, sharing cigarettes, or drinking from a common glass, although oropharyngeal secretions have been implicated in a number of cases. On the other hand, since the virus is found in blood during the early stages of disease, it would seem quite possible to develop disease from blood product transfusions; however, this has never been documented. Disease in childhood is usually mild or even subclinical; it tends to be more severe in adults.

The many clinical and laboratory findings described in Table 5.28 establish the diagnosis of hepatitis A. Determining that HAV is the specific agent can be done by serologic measurements of anti-HAV antibodies, either IgM or IgG. IgM antibodies appear only in the initial phase of the immune response. They begin to rise 2 weeks after inoculation, peak along with clinical symptoms 4–6 weeks later, and then disappear within the next 6 months. Thus, measurement of anti-HAV IgM anti-

TABLE 5.28 CLINICAL FINDINGS IN VIRAL HEPATITIS

Stage	Complaints	Laboratory Findings
Incubation	None	Positive HBsAg in late period.
Prodrome	Nonspecific—malaise, headache, fatigue, anorexia; distaste for cigarettes. Right upper quadrant discomfort low-grade fever. Extrahepatic (thought to be related to immune complex deposition in other body tissues)—arthralgias, symmetric distal arthritis, urticarial skin rash. Rare extrahepatic (HBV only)—polyarteritis nodosa, glomerulonephritis, myopericarditis, Guillain-Barré–like neuropathy.	Positive HBsAg.
Acute	Dark urine or jaundice; clay-colored stools; pruritis; continuation of above symptoms.	Tenfold or more increase in SGPT, SGOT; mild increase in alkaline phosphatase, lactic acid dehydrogenase; elevated serum bilirubin, urine bilirubin; increased prothrombin time in severe cases. HBsAg turns negative.
Convalescent	Disappearance of jaundice and major symptoms; malaise/fatigue may persist for weeks.	Falling enzyme and bilirubin levels; anti-HAV, anti-HBsAg eventually turn positive.

bodies is used to diagnose the acute infection. Anti-HAV IgG antibodies also begin to rise 2 weeks after inoculation. They peak when IgM antibodies disappear and persist for a lifetime. Since 45% of U.S. adults are positive for anti-HAV IgG, repeated tests documenting a rise in titers are needed to diagnose current disease. Management of hepatitis A patients centers on reassurance, counseling, and observation. Guidelines for fluid replacement, diet alterations, activity levels, enteric precautions, and reportable symptoms must be given. In general, patients can expect complete recovery in 3–16 weeks. Fulminant courses are extremely rare, and neither carrier states nor chronic hepatitis follows. The disease confers lifetime immunity.

Prophylaxis for HAV is complicated by the fact that peak shedding of the virus tends to occur 1 week before the clinical illness. Once symptoms or laboratory changes confirm the disease, excretion of the virus is usually minimal. For this reason, ▶***immune serum globulin*** (ISG, IG, gamma globulin) is recommended only in high-risk persons (such as household members or sexual contacts) and only if exposure occurred 2 weeks before to 1 week after the illness began. The serum is consistently advised for travelers to endemic areas. It is also given for exposure to hepatitis B and non-A, non-B hepatitis when hepatitis B immune globulin is unavailable.

▶***Hepatitis B*** (serum hepatitis, long-incubation hepatitis) is potentially a more dangerous disease, although cases range greatly in severity. Hepatitis B virus (HBV) is present in the saliva, blood, breast milk, and semen of infected individuals and is transmitted via skin abrasions, needle punctures, insect vectors, across mucosal surfaces, and through the placenta. Although the fecal-oral route plays a considerably less important part than in hepatitis A, it must be considered. Furthermore, a ▶***chronic HBV carrier state*** occurs in up to 10% of patients, perpetuating a sizable infectious reservoir. The incubation period for HBV ranges from 45 to 160 days, and illness presents with the symptoms and laboratory findings described in Table 5.28. The onset is characteristically more insidious than that of hepatitis A. A prodromal period (attributed to the deposition of immune complexes) may be marked by arthralgia, urticaria, and a serum- sickness–like syndrome.

HBV changes in size and shape during its life span. The various pleomorphic stages provide three distinct antigen–antibody systems to help measure viral replication and infectivity. The largest form, the Dane particle, is believed to be the complete infectious virus. It is composed of (1) a core, (2) a double-shelled surface, and (3) an outer coating of spherical and tubular substances that lack nucleic acid. Surface particles provide the first antigen (HBsAg, hepatitis surface antigen, formally Australia antigen) that can be measured in the blood. Appearing 4 weeks after initial exposure to the disease, HBsAg precedes clinical symptoms by 4–8 weeks. A second distinct antigen (HBeAg) becomes detectable almost simultaneously. HBeAg is clinically important because it is associated with high infectivity. DNA polymerase activity is another marker of increased infectivity. Becoming detectable when titers of HBsAg peak, these enzymes reflect viral replication and remain elevated in chronic carriers. HBsAg, on the other hand, can persist with or without infectivity. Its persistence is usually associated with asymptomatic carrier states or chronic hepatitis. In most cases, HBsAg clears from the blood once the patient begins to recover from illness. Some time later, anti-HBs begins to rise, eventually providing immunity to future disease and signaling noninfectivity. However, patients may still be infectious after the HBsAg disappears and before anti-HBs titers become sufficiently elevated. This gap (serologic window) may be detected by the presence of antibodies to the virus's inner core (anti-HBc). When the Dane particle breaks up early in the infection, its inner core lodges in the nucleus of the infected hepatocytes and the patient remains infectious until it is completely cleared. Although blood cannot be used to measure core antigens (which are found only in hepatocyte nuclei), it can be used to measure core antibodies. Anti-HBc corresponds to the onset of clinical illness and may persist after most symptoms and HbsAg have cleared. Thus it is particularly useful for screening donated blood.

Management of acute illness attributed to HBV involves counseling and close observation. Patients must be given specific guidelines for fluid replacement, diet alterations, activity levels, infection control, and reportable symptoms. Liver function tests should be followed until they return to normal (typically in 3–16 weeks). Persistent elevations of these tests beyond 6 months require biopsy evaluation, since hepatitis B has been associated with both chronic active and chronic persistent inflammation. Fulminant hepatitis, membranous glomerulonephritis, and polyarteritis nodosa are other complications.

Delta hepatitis is caused by a defective virus labeled hepatitis D virus (HDV). Dependent on hepatitis B virus for replication, HDV causes clinical disease only in patients with a history of hepatitis B. Perinatal, sexual, and percutaneous transmission is probable, making IV drug users and homosexuals high risk groups. HDV causes a coinfection in patients with active hepatitis B that usually resolves. It causes a superinfection in hepatitis B carriers that typically leads to chronic active hepatitis. Furthermore, both coinfection and superinfection have been associated with fulminant hepatitis (see later section). HDV is diagnosed by detection of serum markers (delta-antigen, IgM anti-delta during acute infection and delta-antibody after infection), but many of these tests are available only in research laboratories. Treatment is the same as for hepatitis B. Prevention is particularly important; toward this end, hepatitis B carriers should be warned that engaging in homosexual activities and abusing IV drugs greatly increases the risk of developing HDV.

There are several choices available for ***HBV prophylaxis.*** ISG contains HBV antibodies and offers some protection in cases of known exposure. However, its titers of 1:100 are probably too low to prevent disease. With titers greater than 1:100,000, ►***hepatitis B immune globulin (HBIG)*** is preferable. If given within 1 week of exposure and then 1 month later, HBIG can prevent disease in 75% of cases. Hesitation to use the serum may be related to its high cost ($150 per dose). High-risk persons (health care professionals, dialysis patients, male homosexuals, families of HBsAG carriers) should be advised about ►***hepatitis B vaccine.*** Vaccination, which requires three doses given over a period of 6 months, has been shown to produce antibodies in 90% of healthy persons and causes minimal side effects. Although it is known that antibodies persist for at least 3 years, the exact duration of protection and indications for boosters have not yet been established.

►***Non-A non-B (NANB) hepatitis*** is a third major form of viral hepatitis and the most frequent form in the United States today. It accounts for 90% of transfusion-associated hepatitis (TAH) as well as 25–50% of hepatitis cases in the general population. NANB hepatitis virus is transmitted by both oral-fecal and systemic routes. Accidental needlesticks, transfusions of blood products, and intravenous drug use are the most common and clearly documented forms of transmission. Two forms of retrovirus, and perhaps more, are thought to be involved in NANB hepatitis. This theory helps to explain incubation periods ranging from 42 to 103 days. Acute phases tend to be relatively mild, with minimal elevations of hepatic enzymes and serum bilirubin. In fact, 50% of these patients are asymptomatic, and the rest demonstrate a wide range of the clinical findings noted in Table 5.28. Jaundice is infrequent. Because serologic markers have not been identified, the diagnosis of NANB is made by excluding HAV, HBV, or the other viruses listed in Table 5.27. As with all types of viral hepatitis, treatment includes rest, a nutritious diet, and avoidance of alcohol and hepatotoxins. The prognosis, however, is somewhat more guarded. One study found 27% of fulminant hepatitis to be NANB in origin. Furthermore, 20–40% of these patients develop chronic persistent or chronic active disease, with sequelae not predicted by the severity of the acute illness.

Prophylaxis for NANB hepatitis is also more complicated. Carrier states and asymptomatic illness are common, and the absence of serologic markers prevents screening of donor blood. Since the probability of developing NANB with nonpercutaneous exposure is 20% and with percutaneous exposure 80%, ISG is strongly advised, although its effectiveness is uncertain. The serum is given according to the same guidelines used for hepatitis A.

Fulminant hepatitis occurs in less than 1% of patients with viral hepatitis, although it may be precipitated by Reyes syndrome or by exposure to halothane or other hepatotoxins. It is characterized by a rapidly progressive course of jaundice, clotting abnormalities, hepatic encephalopathy, and finally coma. Massive necrosis occurs and the liver shrinks. In-hospital supportive therapy is all that can be offered. The mortality is high.

In some patients infected with HBV and NANB, liver function fails to return to normal within the usual period of 3–6 months. This long-lasting inflammation, known as ***chronic persistent hepatitis,*** can also be related to drug-induced hepatitis or inflammatory bowel syndrome. Abnormalities are usually confined to serum glutamic oxaloacetic transaminase (SGOT) and serum glutamic pyruvic transaminase (SGPT) and rarely involve bilirubin, alkaline phosphatase, total protein, albumin, or prothrombin concentrations. Patients have no other signs and are asymptomatic, with the possible exception of fatigue and vague right upper quadrant discomfort. Nonetheless, they should be referred for liver biopsy for a definitive diagnosis, since more serious causes of inflammation such as cirrhosis, malignancy, or chronic active hepatitis must be ruled out. Although problems with reliability have been noted, postprandial serum cholyglycine tests (used in the identification of chronic active hepatitis) may also be performed. Pathologic findings in chronic persistent hepatitis are characterized by mixed inflammatory infiltrates in portal tracts. The architecture of the hepatic lobules remains undisturbed, and there is little evidence of hepatocellular necrosis. Once the diagnosis is firmly established, patients can be reassured of an excellent prognosis. Since the condition eventually resolves on its own, treatment is unnecessary.

Chronic active hepatitis (CAH) is a second, far more serious cause of prolonged inflammation of the liver. It may follow infection with HBV, HDV, or NANB. It is also related to autoimmune disorders associated with positive antinuclear antibody and lupus erythematosus preparations ***(autoimmune CAH,*** formerly called "lupoid CAH"). Abnormal liver functions lasting for more than 6 months may be the first indication of the disease. These may be limited to SGOT and SGPT or may also involve bilirubin, alkaline phosphatase, total protein, albumin, and prothrombin concentrations. Although patients may initially be asymptomatic, they eventually manifest signs of chronic liver disease including jaundice, weakness, anorexia, splenomegaly, ascites, and a firm liver. They should be referred to a gastroenterologist for diagnosis and ongoing care. The specialist can confirm the disorder by testing serum cholyglycine levels, smooth muscle antibodies, and antinuclear antibodies (positive in autoimmune CAH) and by performing a liver biopsy. Since lesions in CAH develop in a spotty fashion, laparoscopy may sometimes offer the best route for biopsy. It allows general inspection of the liver and procurement of several specimens from the most suspicious areas. Pathologic findings are characterized by hepatocellular necrosis, often piecemeal, and monocytic infiltration. Fibrosis may be present in advanced disease.

Once the diagnosis of CAH is firmly established, patients are usually started on prednisone, sometimes in combination with azathioprine. Although such treatment has been credited with remission or improvement (particularly in autoimmune CAH), recent studies suggest that steroid therapy may be associated with increased mortality. Improvement (demonstrated by the histologic picture becoming similar to that of chronic persistent hepatitis) may also occur spontaneously. Unfortunately, relapses occur in 50% of all cases, usually within 1 year. Progression is the rule, and the prognosis is poor.

Viral infections of the liver are common and can affect healthy persons. By contrast, ***pyogenic abscesses*** are rare and develop only in compromised individuals. The bacteria (commonly an anaerobe, *Escherichia coli,* or *Staphylococcus aureus*) usually originate from an obstructed and/or inflamed biliary tree, appendix, or pancreas. They can also be implanted through the abdominal wall by gunshots, stab wounds, or portal blood flow in cases of septicemia. Fever is the initial, sometimes the sole, symptom of abscess formation in the liver. Characteristically high and spiking, it is often attended by sweats and chills. Other presenting complaints include anorexia, nausea, vomiting, weight loss, and pain over the epigastrium or right hypochondrium. On exam, patients appear sick and may be icteric. The liver is usually enlarged and quite tender. Its surface may be smooth or interrupted by localized bulges. Blood tests often reveal anemia, a very high white blood cell count with a prominent left shift, and elevated bilirubin and liver enzymes. Elevation of the diaphragm may be noted on chest x-ray films if the abscess is large and occupies the right portion of the liver. Multiple hepatic defects demonstrated by radioisotope scanning are most consistent with disease. Patients should be given antibiotics effective against coliform organisms. Those who do not show immediate improvement should be hospitalized for culture samples from surgical drainage of the abscess. The mortality rate for unrecognized, untreated cases is 60% for small multiple abscesses and 90% for large solitary ones.

Worldwide, but not in the United States, ***amebic abscesses*** are more common than pyogenic abscesses of the liver. In 95% of cases, the causative organism is ***Entamoeba histolytica,*** a protozoan parasite present throughout the world, particularly in tropical areas. Contaminated food or water, person-to-person contact, and flies or other vectors are all possible sources of transmission via cysts. Once ingested, *Entamoeba* cysts lodge near the ileocecal valve, where they release trophozoites. These usually multiply in colonic fecal matter and are shed with little disturbance. In some cases, however, trophozoites invade bowel mucosa and/or the liver, producing microabscesses that enlarge and coalesce. Intestinal disease is marked by high fever, colicky abdominal pain, vomiting, and diarrhea. Stools (5–20 per day) first contain fetid, pasty fecal matter, but later only blood, mucus, and necrotic tissue. Liver manifestations are characterized by steady high fever, anorexia, nausea, severe upper abdominal pain, and prostration. They may develop with or without concurrent or antecedent intestinal disease. On exam, the liver is usually enlarged, extending below the costal margin or sometimes pushing the rib cage forward. Enlargement may produce dullness, rales, or diminished diaphragm movement at the right lung base. The liver is extremely tender, and its surface is smooth or interrupted by localized bulges. Blood tests often reveal anemia, mild elevation of the white blood cell count with no eosinophilia, and normal or mildly elevated liver functions. A high diaphragm may be noted on chest x-ray films. Hepatic defects (often multiple, sometimes massive) can be demonstrated with ultrasound, radioisotope, or computed tomography (CT) scanning.

Since trophozoites are difficult to detect in stool samples, diagnosis may depend on specific antibody tests (hemagglutination, agar-gel methods, or the enzyme-linked immunosorbent assay). Patients invariably require hospitalization, with care coordinated by infectious disease specialists and gastroenterologists. Treatment involves fluid and electrolyte correction, antiamebic drugs (e.g., metronidazole or chloroquine), and careful aspiration of abscesses. With early, aggressive intervention, the prognosis for complete recovery is good. Without it, abscesses may rupture and death may follow.

REGULATING HORMONE AND DRUG ACTIVITY

Many hormones and drugs are regulated by the liver and thus are affected by liver disease. For one thing, levels of drugs and hormones that are transported by proteins manufactured by the liver may rise in the blood with protein depletion. Furthermore, a number of drugs and hormones are metabolized and excreted by the liver. They may be shunted away from the liver in portal hypertension, remain unmetabolized by damaged hepatocytes, or fail to be secreted via bile in the event of cholestasis.

Because so many drugs and chemicals are metabolized or cleared by the liver, ***toxic hepatitis*** occurs with some frequency. Liver injury may be due to either a hypersensitivity reaction or direct toxicity. Common hepatotoxins and their effects are enumerated in Table 5.29.

Methyldopa hepatitis occurs as a hypersensitivity response in a few patients, especially women. Hepatic damage (to the parenchymal cells) usually begins within the first month of therapy. A prodrome of malaise, fatigue, fever, anorexia, nausea, and vomiting usually precedes jaundice by 1–2 weeks. Liver injury (with possible progression to chronic active hepatitis) is reversible if the drug is withheld before jaundice occurs. Continued use or rechallenge with methyldopa can cause massive hepatic necrosis. Thus, careful monitoring of patients during the months following initiation of Aldomet therapy is crucial. They must be advised to report any of the above symptoms promptly.

Repeated exposure to fluorinated anesthetic agents such as ***halothane*** may cause a hypersensitivity response. Postoperatively, patients develop symptoms mimicking those of acute viral hepatitis. Tracing the problem to its toxic source may be difficult. However, mortality is high (15–50%), and if hypersensitivity to fluorinated anesthetics is suspected, further exposure must be avoided.

Thorazine-related hepatitis occurs in a small percentage of patients. It is characterized by bile stasis and obstruction. Predominant complaints include nausea, vomiting, skin eruptions, and arthralgias. Jaundice, lymphadenopathy, and

TABLE 5.29 DRUGS AND CHEMICALS ASSOCIATED WITH HEPATOTOXICITY

	Hypersensitivity	
Direct Toxic Effect	**Hepatitis**	**Cholestasis**
Acetaminophen	Aspirin	Anabolic steroids
Antimony	Amitriptyline	Erythromycin stearate
Arsenic	Chloramphenicol	Haloperidol
Berryllium	Diphenylhydantoin	Nitrofurantoin
Ethanol	Gold	Oral contraceptives
Carbon tetrachloride	Halothane	Phenothiazines
Chlorates	Indomethacin	
Chlorinated hydrocarbons	Isoniazid	
Copper	Methyldopa	
Dinitro-0-cresol (herbicides)	Nitrofurantoin	
Halogenated hydrocarbons (DDT)	Oxacillin	
Mushrooms (phalloidine species)	Quinidine	
Nitrosamines	Rifampin	
Phosphorus	Sulfonamide	
Vinyl chloride		

hepatomegaly are usually present on exam. Complete recovery is common with discontinuance of the drug, but chronic cholestasis may develop.

Almost everyone receiving isoniazid (INH) demonstrates a mild subclinical rise in liver function tests of no lasting consequence. However, approximately 10% of patients being treated with the drug develop a hypersensitivity reaction referred to as ***INH hepatitis.*** The incidence of this complication is low in patients under age 35 but rises sharply thereafter. Resembling viral hepatitis, most cases develop within the first 3 months of therapy. They range in severity from patchy inflammation to massive hepatic necrosis; from mild symptoms to a fulminant course ending in death. Therefore, all patients taking INH must be followed carefully. They should be evaluated periodically. Most importantly, they must be instructed to report any symptoms of hepatitis immediately. If the drug is discontinued at once, the clinical and histologic changes can be reversed.

Acetaminophen is metabolized to an intermediate compound that is quite toxic to hepatocytes. Thus ***acetaminophen overdose,*** either as a suicide attempt or an accidental ingestion, may lead to acute liver damage. In fact, a single dose of 10 g by an adult causes centrilobular necrosis within the first 12 hours and a dose of 15 g or more is usually fatal. Although signs and symptoms of liver failure may not appear for 1 or 2 days after the overdose, emergency treatment must be started at once. The best chance for recovery occurs if the drug is removed from the body by emesis or gastric lavage within the first 30 minutes of ingestion, followed by the antidote *N*-acetylcysteine (Mucomyst, Respaire) administered every 4 hours for 4 days. If the patient survives, minimal cirrhosis persists.

Alcohol is detoxified almost exclusively by the liver. Persistent, intensified detoxification with high alcohol intake may interfere with other hepatocellular processes. One effect is inhibition of glyconeogenesis. Alcoholics, who are likely to have depleted glycogen stores due to poor nutrition, are prone to ***alcoholic hypoglycemia***. Dangerous decreases in blood sugar are manifested by weakness, shakiness, sweating, hunger, blurred vision, abnormal behavior, or loss of consciousness. Treatment consists of abstinence and frequent nutritious meals.

TABLE 5.30 CONDITIONS ASSOCIATED WITH FATTY LIVER

Condition	Mechanism
Alcoholism	Decreased fatty oxidation due to increased reducing environment, which occurs during the detoxification of ETOH.
Caloric infusion from hyperalimentation	Fatty acid synthesis outstrips the liver's ability to secrete lipids.
Early starvation	Fatty acids mobilized from adipose tissue and partly converted to triglycerides in the liver.
Protein malnutrition	Impaired lipoprotein synthesis due to choline deficiency.
Obesity	Excess adipose tissue allows for increased release of free fatty acids.
Jejunoileal bypass surgery	Possibly similar to protein starvation.
Juvenile-onset diabetes mellitus	Increased lipolysis and decreased clearance.
Adult-onset diabetes mellitus	Possibly increased CHO ingestion
Pregnancy	Unknown. Can progress to fulminant hepatitis.
IV tetracycline (>2 g/day)	Unknown
Corticosteroid prescriptions and Cushing's disease	Increased lipolysis, mobilization of fatty acids.
Hepatotoxins	Direct toxicity to cells prevents triglyceride metabolism.
Reye's syndrome	Membrane and mitochondrial damage to cells.

Overuse of alcohol may also lead to abnormal deposition of lipids in liver tissue. Known as ***steatosis (fatty liver),*** this condition may also be caused by a number of factors described in Table 5.30. The signs and symptoms vary depending on the degree of fat infiltration. Most patients are asymptomatic, although most develop tender hepatomegaly. In cases of massive infiltration, right upper quadrant pain (caused by stretching of Glisson's capsule) may be present. A liver biopsy will confirm the diagnosis. Fatty liver is often reversible after removal of the primary cause; in fact, in the alcoholic, significant amounts of hepatic fat disappear within 6 weeks of initiation of a program that combines alcohol abstinence with adequate nutritional intake. In patients who continue to drink, fatty liver may progress to cirrhosis, but this does not always occur.

Overconsumption of alcohol may cause an inflammatory reaction known as ▶ ***alcoholic hepatitis.*** Polymorphonucleocytes and lymphocytes infiltrate centrilobular regions, destroying tissue. The damaged liver cells typically contain clumps of eosinophils and hyaline material known as Mallory bodies. The process can be virtually asymptomatic or severe and life-threatening. Manifestations include anorexia, nausea, vomiting, malaise, weight loss, and jaundice. Fever is fairly common, affecting more than half of these patients. An enlarged, possibly tender liver is frequently palpated, and splenomegaly is present in one-third of the patients. If the case is severe, signs of extreme hepatic decompensation such as ascites and hepatic encephalopathy appear. Laboratory findings include an elevated white blood cell count, moderately elevated bilirubin and alkaline phosphatase, and a possibly elevated prothrombin time. SGOT and SGPT are mildly increased, usually in a ratio that exceeds 1:2. Sepsis must be considered in the febrile patient and treated if present. Otherwise, management of alcoholic hepatitis begins with alcohol abstention. A high-calorie, high-protein diet (unless signs of encephalopathy are present) with moderate salt restriction is an important measure. Since many alcoholics have concurrent nutritional deficiencies, vitamin supplementation will help counteract symptoms. For example, folic acid and pyridoxine often help correct related anemia, and parenteral thiamine (vitamin B_1) may improve Wernicke-Korsakoff's disease. However, it must be stressed that adequate nutrition and vitamin supplementation will not protect the liver from further insult due to alcohol ingestion.

Bouts of alcoholic hepatitis tend not only to recur but to increase in severity. In many cases, there is progression to ▶ ***Laennec's cirrhosis,*** in which bands of fibrous scar tissue form around the areas of inflammatory necrosis. These bands, which become infiltrated by monocytes, are inelastic. By constricting blood and lymph vessels, they may eventually produce portal hypertension (see the section on "Portal Circulation"). Between the fibrotic bands appear nodules of regenerated hepatocytes as the liver attempts to replace lost cells. These alterations in the hepatic parenchyma typify biopsy changes. Presentation of Laennec's cirrhosis may range from a gradual progression of symptoms to the sudden onset of ascites or an acute GI bleed. In early disease, patients often experience malaise, anorexia, nausea, vomiting, a dull abdominal ache, constipation or diarrhea. On exam, the liver is usually firm, possibly tender, and sometimes nodular in consistency. It may be either enlarged or shrunken. Splenomegaly or other sequelae of portal hypertension (see the section on "Portal Hypertension") may be concurrent. Local vasodilation often produces a distinct redness on the fingertips and the base of the palm (palmar erythema), and an increased estrogen effect may lead to the development of spider angiomas over the face, neck, shoulder, back of the hands, or umbilicus. The presence of jaundice suggests active necrosis. There is a strong association with parotid gland enlargement, macrocytic anemia, and Wernicke-Korsakoff's syndrome, all related to malnutrition from alcoholism. Dupuytren's contractures of the hands, testicular atrophy, gynecomastia, and amenorrhea, as well as hyperaldosteronism, Cushing's syndrome, and hyperthyroidism, may develop secondary to altered hormone activity. All of the manifestations of chronic liver disease, including typical laboratory abnormalities, are summarized in Table 5.31. Glucose intolerance (as opposed to hypoglycemia due to acute alcohol overconsumption) is common in the cirrhotic and is associated with increased plasma glycogen levels and insulin resistance.

Alcohol withdrawal is mandatory. Because success usually depends on strong psychologic support, this difficult problem is covered in Chapter 13. In addition to withdrawal, adequate nutritional and vitamin intake and palliation of disease are the mainstays of treatment in milder cases. Interventions for the complications of portal hypertension (esophageal bleeds, ascites, encephalopathy, etc.) are discussed in a later section. Cirrhotic changes cannot be reversed, but progression can be arrested.

Although chronic alcohol use is the prime cause, cirrhosis can be induced by other conditions described in Table 5.32. The pathology is variable. ***Macronodular cirrhosis*** is characterized by irregular, large regeneration nodules and broad bands of fibrous tissue. Small, uniform regeneration nodules typify ***micronodular cirrhosis.*** Sometimes occurring in the same liver, both conditions lead to loss of functional hepatocytes and liver failure. Because the underlying causes are often untreatable, management may be limited to relieving symptoms and maintaining nutrition as described for Laennec's cirrhosis.

Rarely, fibrotic changes take place in liver tissue without any necrosis. Called

TABLE 5.31 SIGNS OF CHRONIC LIVER DISEASE

Sign	Secondary to:
Jaundice	Impaired bilirubin metabolism/excretion; hemolysis
Palmar erythema	Local vasodilation
Spider angiomas	Increased estrogen
Firm, nontender liver with irregular edge	Fibrosis, regenerative nodules
Hepatomegaly	Acute inflammation
Splenomegaly	Portal hypertension
Esophageal varices	Portal hypertension with formation of collateral circulation
Hemorrhoids	Same as above
Dilated abdominal veins	Same as above
Bleeding tendency	Deficiency of clotting factors V, VII, IX, X, and prothrombin
Ascites	Hypoalbuminemia; obstruction of blood flow through liver with transudation of fluid
Hyperaldosteronism	Transudation of fluid decreases circulatory volume, stimulating aldosterone secretion
Dyspnea	Pressure against diaphragm from severe ascites
Deterioration of memory, handwriting, cognitive function	PSE
Wernicke-Korsakoff syndrome	Nutritional deficiency
Macrocytic anemia	Same as above
Testicular atrophy	Decreased androgen and/or increased estrogen
Amenorrhea	Same as above
Gynecomastia	Same as above
Anovulatory cycle	Same as above
Hyperthyroidism	Poorly understood
Cushing's syndrome	Altered excretion of hormone

noncirrhotic fibrosis, this condition can be congenital or secondary to schistosomiasis. It can also be idiopathic ***(Banti's syndrome).*** Since hepatocytes suffer no direct injury, they usually remain functional. For this reason, patients who require a portacaval shunt tend to do well.

PORTAL CIRCULATION

The key functions just discussed (processing nutrients, clearing infectious organisms, influencing the activity of hormones and drugs) are made possible by a unique circulation of blood and lymph (Fig. 5.4). Major vessels enter the liver via the porta hepatis, a fissure above the quadrate lobe. The hepatic artery brings oxygenated blood from the heart, and the portal vein drains venous blood containing nutrients and colonic bacteria from the stomach, pancreas, and spleen. Subdividing into smaller and smaller branches, hepatic arterioles and portal venules flow toward the

TABLE 5.32 CAUSES OF CIRRHOSIS

Chronic alcoholism (typically 1 + pints of whiskey or several quarts of wine, or equivalent amount of beer daily for at least 10 years)	Exact mechanism unknown. Fatty liver from alcohol detoxification or malnutrition may contribute.
Sequelae of viral hepatitis	Not known.
Primary biliary cirrhosis	Not known. Possibly a disease of the small bile ducts or immune system.
Idiopathic cirrhosis	Possibly from asymptomatic undiagnosed cases of viral hepatitis.
Secondary biliary cirrhosis	Extrahepatic biliary tract obstruction with bile stasis.
Cardiac cirrhosis	Long-standing congestive heart failure leads to congestion of poorly oxygenated blood in the liver. Hepatocytes become hypoxic and necrose.
Hemochromatosis	Iron deposition in the liver.
Wilson's disease	Copper deposition in the liver.
Drug-induced	Hepatocellular necrosis from direct toxicity or hypersensitivity.

hepatocytes. As noted in Figure 5.3, hepatocytes are arranged like single-layered brick walls around central spaces called "sinusoids." Several sinusoids converge on a central vein to form a lobule. The central vein from each lobule (50,000–100,000 of them) empties into vessels of increasing caliber: sublobular veins, the large hepatic vein, and finally the inferior vena cava.

Arterioles and portal venules run through canals whose walls are supported by tough fibrous tissue (Glisson's capsule). If cirrhosis, tumor, thrombosis of the hepatic vein ***(Budd-Chiari syndrome),*** or other disease interrupts this flow, hydrostatic pressure within the portal vein or one of its tributaries increases, creating ***portal hypertension.*** To bypass the congested liver, collateral vesels form in several areas. A network of subcutaneous veins, known as ***caput medusae,*** may radiate from the umbilicus, producing a venous hum heard with a stethoscope. Visually, it is most prominent when the patient is standing. Another network may form between the inferior mesenteric and internal iliac veins, resulting in extensive ***hemorrhoids.*** Finally, ***esophageal varices*** and ***gastric varices*** may develop in submucosal layers of the upper GI tract. Thin-walled, dilated, and tortuous, they are prone to rupture and hemorrhage. Thus, hematemesis, melena, or, less commonly, chronic anemia are the presenting symptoms. Patients with bleeding varices require immediate hospitalization. Iced saline lavage and intravenous or splanchnic infusions of vasopressin are initiated. If they fail to control the bleeding, tamponade is attempted with the use of an inflated balloon. A Sengstaken-Blakemore tube is employed for esophageal bleeds and a Linto-Nachlas tube for gastric bleeds. Another second-line treatment is injection sclerotherapy (injecting varices with a sclerosing agent). Unfortunately, no matter what interventions are used, up to 50% of patients die during the first episode. Those who survive are prone to more serious rebleeds.

The altered circulation in portal hypertension may cause splenomegaly with resultant thrombocytopenia. It may also lead to a dangerous rise in blood levels of ammonia as blood containing ammonia from the gut is shunted away from the liver. Normally, hepatocytes convert this ammonia, a by-product of amino acid degrada-

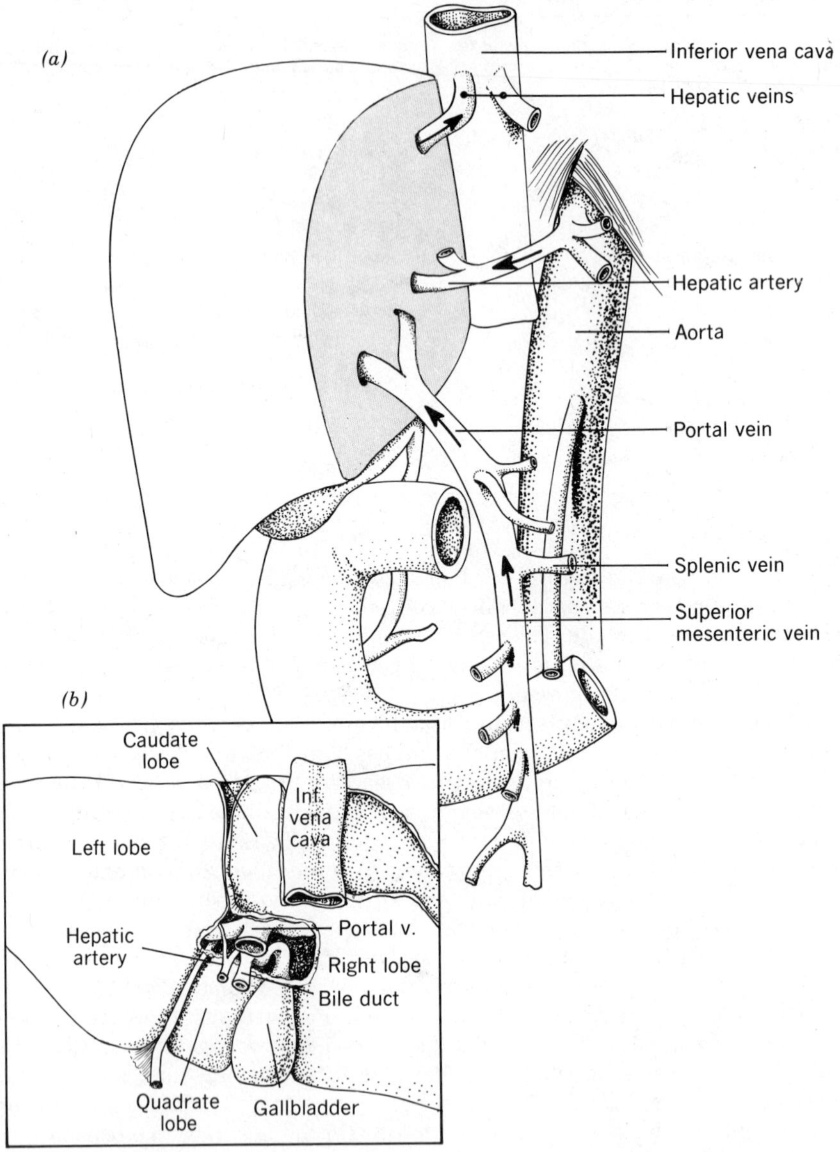

Figure 5.4 Portal circulation: (*a*) anterior view; (*b*) posterior view.

tion, into glutamine and urea, a water-soluble substance that can be excreted in urine. When conversion fails, ammonia blood levels rise. The toxin is taken up by gray matter in the brain, especially by astrocytes (positioned near the capillary membrane of the blood–brain barrier). Either by reducing the chemical transport of oxygen and glucose across neuron membranes or by interfering with neurosynaptic transmission, ammonia causes an altered state of consciousness known as ***portal systemic encephalopathy*** (PSE, hepatic encephalopathy, portosystemic encephalopathy). Mercaptains and short chain fatty acids and other substances usually metabolized in the liver may also be involved in the process. Patients with a history of alcoholism, surgical creation of a portal systemic shunt, acute viral hepatitis, drug abuse, sclerosing cholangitis, pericholangitis, or biliary cirrhosis are at high risk for developing PSE.

The symptoms and signs of PSE may be subtle and gradual or may fluctuate rapidly. Deterioration of handwriting is one of the earliest and most reliable clues. Memory, attention span, and concentration may become slow and speech slurred. Decreased problem-solving ability and sluggish tracting of extraocular muscles can be revealed by simple tests of mental function such as number connection tests. Personality changes include depression, euphoria, anxiety, irritability, paranoia, and lack of concern for other people and property. Mild lethargy can progress to deep coma. ***Fetor hepaticus*** may be noted. This characteristic musty odor of the breath is probably caused by unmetabolized mercaptans. Another classic sign, ***asterixis,*** may be elicited by having the patient stretch out both arms and then dorsiflex the hands for 30 seconds. Unlike twisting-type tremors, true asterixis is manifested by spasms at the wrist joint that range from an occasional irregular flap to continuous, exaggerated flapping. Hyperreflexia with clonus and ataxia may be revealed during the neurologic exam. Abnormal electroencephalogram waves are the rule.

Early detection of encephalopathy may favorably influence the prognosis. However, the diagnosis is mainly clinical and may be difficult to establish. It is based on the history, the physical exam, and exclusion of other conditions known to alter mental status (notably electrolyte imbalances, hypoglycemia, drug effects, head trauma, psychosis, or organic brain disorders). Treatment is aimed at the primary disease as well as reducing systemic ammonia. Dietary proteins are restricted to reduce bacterial action on amino acids in the intestine. For the same reason, GI bleeding (a source of protein in the bowel) must be controlled. Constipation results in stasis of wastes in the colon, and bowel cleansing may be employed to prevent ammonia buildup. For patients with late prehepatic coma and actual coma, administration of neomycin in large oral doses often relieves symptoms by destroying colonic bacteria. Diarrhea secondary to depletion of intestinal flora and impaired vitamin K absorption are adverse effects of this therapy. Lactulose has been shown to decrease ammonia production by lowering the intestinal pH and may be useful on a long-term basis in the patient with chronic liver disease who tends to develop hepatic coma. Finally, blood pH must be carefully controlled, since alkalosis favors ammonia diffusion across the blood–brain barrier. ▶ ***Early stages of PSE*** can often be managed with diet or even lactulose and neomycin on an outpatient basis. More advanced disease requires hospitalization.

Shunts can be formed surgically to alleviate some of the problems associated with with portal hypertension. However, the patient with chronic liver disease frequently is a poor operative candidate. Portacaval shunting is accomplished by anastomosing the portal vein or one of its tributaries to the vena cava, thus bypassing the congested liver. This rerouting does not allow the blood to be detoxified by the liver and hepatic encephalopathy may occur. It was assumed that splenorenal shunts that divert some but not all portal blood from the liver would relieve pressure while ensuring better detoxification. However, initial enthusiasm for this procedure has diminished due to the higher incidence of rebleeding.

One-third to one-half of the body's lymph is produced in the liver. Lymph vessels empty, along with intestinal lymphatics, into the thoracic duct. Small increments in hepatic venous pressure (as little as 3–5 mm Hg), as seen in portal hypertension, cause a marked increase in lymph production and linkage of fluid through the liver's outer surface. As the pressure builds to 10–15 mm Hg, lymph flow may increase 20-fold, and the "sweating" from the liver's surface causes an accumulation of fluid in the peritoneal cavity. This collection of free fluid in the abdomen is referred to as ► ***ascites.*** Sodium retention by the kidney tubules is an important factor in ascites formation, although the exact etiology is unclear. Secondary hyperaldosteronism may be implicated. Systemically, a lowered colloidal osmotic pressure due to hypoalbuminemia (the hypofunctioning liver cannot synthesize sufficient plasma proteins) is a contributing factor. Blocked lymphatic drainage is another cause. Clinically, ascites is manifested by abdominal distention and may be evaluated by serial measurements of abdominal girth. Weight gain is noted. Free fluid in the abdominal cavity seeks the lowest point to settle. Therefore, percussion of the abdomen with the patient first supine, then in a lateral position, will reveal areas of shifting dullness. A fluid wave may be observed crossing the abdomen when one side of the belly is firmly tapped. In massive ascites, urinary output may decrease and fluid collection will cause elevation of the diaphragm and subsequent respiratory compromise. Umbilical and/or inguinal hernias may appear. Sheer fluid overload can cause impairment of cardiac function. In patients with concurrent bacteremia, bacterial seeding of ascitic fluid can cause spontaneous bacterial peritonitis, a very dangerous condition. It has been postulated that the increased pressure exerted by ascites can cause gastroesophageal reflux. If esophageal varices are present, this acid reflux would favor erosion and possible eruption of the vessels.

Fluid accumulation limits physical activity and may cause significant discomfort. Management of ascites is somewhat dependent upon the underlying cause. To mobilize the fluid, general principles include bed rest, along with careful adjustment and restriction of fluid and sodium intake. Frequent monitoring of weight, intake and output, hematocrit, electrolytes, serum BUN, or creatinine is imperative. If these measures do not induce mobilization of ascitic fluid, cautious use of diuretics, including an aldosterone inhibitor, may be indicated. However, diuretic therapy is merely a symptomatic approach and may lead to serious electrolyte imbalances. Paracentesis may be indicated for temporary relief of respiratory compromise in patients with massive ascites. Refractory cases require peritoneovenous (LeVeen) shunts.

The extensive blood and lymph flow through the liver makes this organ a prime target for cancer metastases. ***Metastatic liver cancer*** is 20 times more common than primary liver cancer and is the second leading cause of fatal liver disease (cirrhosis is the first). The diagnosis is usually made during evaluation of a primary tumor, liver metastases being common in cancers of the breast, lung, GI tract, or skin (malignant melanoma). In many cases, patients are asymptomatic or may exhibit nonspecific symptoms including weakness, fever, weight loss, and diaphoresis. Less frequently, the patient may present with signs of active liver disease such as ascites, jaundice, abdominal pain, and hepatomegaly. With extensive involvement, one may observe signs of portal hypertension, a friction rub, and a large, tender, and/or indurated liver. Initially, the only laboratory abnormality may be an increased alkaline phosphatase level. Later, serum albumin may drop as liver enzymes rise. Ultrasound or a CT scan will readily identify abnormal masses. Radioisotope scans are less reliable, and liver biopsy is diagnostic in only 60–80% of cases. Treatment is palliative. Chemotherapy, usually with 5-fluorouracil and methotrexate, may slow cancer growth and alleviate some symptoms but has a doubtful effect on the prognosis. Intrahepatic chemotherapy via an inflatable infusion pump delivers a higher concentration of drugs to the liver. It has proved more effective and is attended by fewer systemic side effects.

Whereas metastatic liver cancer is common, ***primary hepatic carcinoma*** (hepatoma) is responsible for only 2% of the malignancies in the United States. The incidence is highest in patients over age 60 and among men. A history of chronic HBsAg-positive blood, hemochromatosis, exposure to aflatoxins (metabolites of food contaminated with fungus), androgen use, and infection with liver flukes are associated factors. There is also a strong association with cirrhosis of the liver (40 times the normal risk). In fact, sudden clinical deterioration of the cirrhotic patient may signify tumor growth. Palpation of the right upper quadrant of the liver may show tenderness, an enlarged and/or nodular liver, or a discrete mass. Auscultation in the same area may reveal a bruit, hum, or friction rub. Laboratory analysis (including alpha fetoprotein levels, which tend to be increased with hepatoma), liver scan, and liver biopsy help confirm this diagnosis. Unfortunately, early detection of hepatoma is not the rule and surgical resection is rarely possible. Chemotherapy, with infusions directly into the hepatic artery, is the usual approach. The mortality is high.

Hepatic adenoma is a benign growth associated with long-term use of oral contraceptives and Laennec's cirrhosis (5–10% risk). Although nonmalignant, it may result in a sudden fatal hemorrhage. Tumors associated with oral contraceptives are known to regress spontaneously after withdrawal of the drug.

BILE

Hepatocytes constantly form small amounts of bile, a mixture of water, bile salts, cholesterol, bilirubin, lecithin, and electrolytes. Many of these components play a part in emulsifying dietary fats for digestion by pancreatic lipase. Like all nutrients, fats must be in a water-soluble form in order to be broken down by enzymes and assimilated. Bile salts, synthesized from cholesterol by the hepatocytes, possess a detergent action that breaks down fat globules into tiny particles (emulsification). They also aid in the absorption of lipids from the intestinal tract. Lecithin emulsifies fats and keeps the cholesterol component of bile soluble in water. Electrolytes keep bile alkaline and thus compatible with the environment of the small intestine.

Bilirubin has no digestive function. It is a pigmented organic ion that comes from the breakdown of hemoglobin. As an insoluble waste product, bilirubin must be converted (conjugated) to a water-soluble form of excretion. This is the overall purpose of bilirubin metabolism, as diagrammed in Figure 5.5.

As noted in Table 5.33, problems with bilirubin clearance may occur before conjugation. If this happens, ***unconjugated hyperbilirubinemia*** and ***nonobstructive jaundice*** may result. Yellow pigmentation of the skin develops, most notable in the

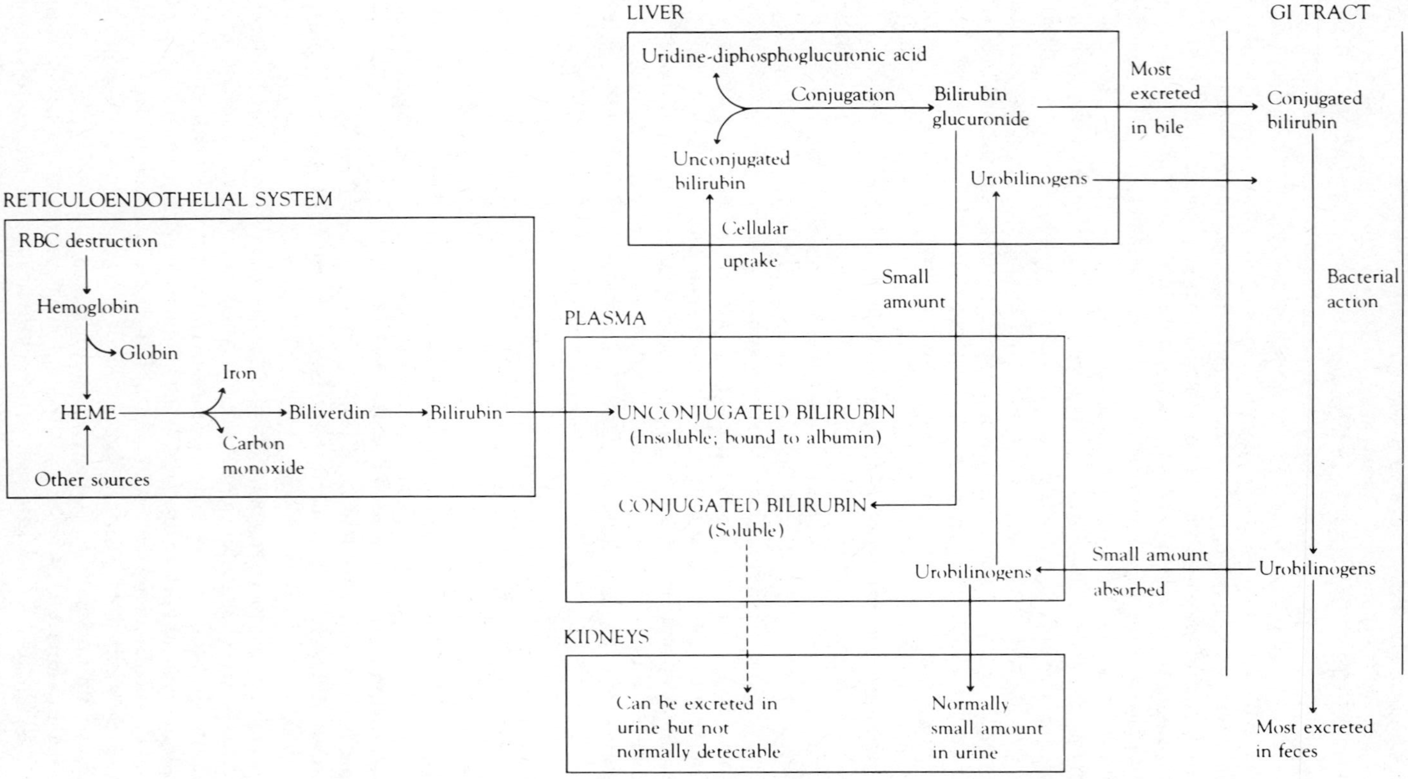

Figure 5.5 Bilirubin metabolism. (From Muir, *Pathophysiology: An Introduction to the Mechanisms of Disease,* © 1980, John Wiley & Sons, Inc., New York.)

TABLE 5.33 CAUSES OF HYPERBILIRUBINEMIA AND JAUNDICE

Increased production of bilirubin from hemolysis (unconjugated)
- Congenital red blood cell abnormalities (membrane defects, enzyme deficiencies, hemoglobinopathies)
- Antibody response (transfusion, autoimmune reaction, drugs)
- Mechanical damage (microangiopathic hemolytic anemia, cardiac valve hemolysis)
- Infections (malaria, *Bartonella,* clostridia)
- Toxins (snake and spider venoms, mushroom and plant poisons, copper, arsenic)
- Splenomegaly

Reduced hepatic uptake of bilirubin (unconjugated)
- Gilbert's syndrome
- Acute viral hepatitis after recovery
- Congestive heart failure
- Portacaval shunt surgery

Reduced bilirubin conjugation (unconjugated)
- Neonatal jaundice (immaturity of the hepatic excretory system)
- Crigler-Najjar syndrome (congenital absence of glucoronyl transferase)

Reduced excretion of conjugated bilirubin (conjugated)
- Dubin-Johnson syndrome
- Rotor syndrome
- Hepatocellular injury
- Drug interference with bilirubin metabolism or bile ducts (e.g., estrogens, testosterone, thorazine)
- Hepatic infiltration (neoplasm, granuloma, infection)
- Extrahepatic bile duct obstruction

sclera and oral palate. Urine remains normal in color because unconjugated bilirubin is not soluble in water. The most common cause of unconjugated hyperbilirubinemia is hemolysis (see Chapter 7). Normally, the liver is capable of clearing excess amounts of bilirubin generated from abnormal breakdown of red blood cells. Even in cases of brisk hemolysis, serum levels rarely exceed 3–5 mg/dL, which is slightly above the normal range of 1–2 mg/dL. However, when hemolysis occurs in the presence of liver disease, severe hyperbilirubinemia may result.

Unconjugated hyperbilirubinemia also occurs in ▶ ***Gilbert's syndrome*** (idiopathic, unconjugated hyperbilirubinemia). The cause is twofold: defective uptake of bilirubin by hepatocytes and low glucuronyl transferase activity. Many patients also have a reduced red blood cell survival rate. Once considered rare, Gilbert's syndrome is now known to affect 3–5% of the population. The defect is thought to be genetic. Hyperbilirubinemia is mild, and liver function tests are normal. Jaundice may occur intermittently; fasting, intercurrent illness, or hemolysis can cause exacerbations.

Gilbert's syndrome may represent a benign form of ***Crigler-Najjar syndrome.*** Characterized by serious deficiencies of glucuronyl transferase, two types of Crigler-Najjar syndrome have been described. Type I is inherited as an autosomal recessive trait. Extreme elevations of unconjugated bilirubin usually cause fatal kernicterus and central nervous system damage within the first year of life. Type II, inherited as a dominant trait, is less severe. Most patients reach adulthood without suffering damage from kernicterus. By inducing the deficient glucuronyl transferase, phenobarbital may diminish jaundice.

Bile plays a key role in the absorption of vitamin K because the vitamin is fat soluble. Since vitamin K is necessary for the production of fibrinogen, prothrombin, and factors V, VII, IX, and X, these blood-clotting factors may become dangerously low in liver disease as an indirect consequence of decreased bile production by hepatocytes. Patients have ***bleeding problems,*** marked by prolonged prothrombin and bleeding times. They note easy bruising, fresh blood from gums or hemorrhoids, or excessive bleeding from superficial cuts. Urine or stool testing may reveal occult blood. In most cases, parenteral administration of vitamin K corrects the serum prothrombin time. Sometimes, however, diseased hepatocytes are unable to synthesize the clotting factors regardless of vitamin K availability. In such cases, treatment must center on preventive measures. Patients should be advised to use an electric razor and a soft toothbrush. They should avoid aspirin, straining at stool, and vigorous nose blowing.

Copper, an important trace element stored by hepatocytes, is excreted in bile. A rare autosomal recessive inherited illness, ***Wilson's disease,*** is characterized by a disturbance in biliary excretion of copper. Copper accumulates in the liver, eventually causing cirrhosis. When the hepatocytes have become damaged, they release copper into the system, which then collects in other tissues, including the brain, kidneys, and corneas. Symptoms may begin in childhood or young adulthood and include tremors, incoordination, ataxia, and possibly an atypical, prolonged case of hepatitis. Wilson's disease is diagnosed by decreased serum ceruloplasmin, increased urine copper, and golden-brown pigment deposits that form a ring just inside the iris (Kayser-Fleischer rings). If improperly diagnosed or untreated, Wilson's disease can be fatal. A low-copper diet combined with long-term use of a chelating agent such as D-penicillamine can avoid overloading of copper.

BILE FLOW

Once formed, bile is secreted into canaliculi, tiny grooves running between hepatocytes (see Fig. 5.3). Completely sealed off from the lacunae and sinusoids, the canaliculi form an independent, gradually enlarging ductal system. From them, bile empties into the terminal bile ducts and then flows peripherally through progressively larger bile ducts, eventually reaching the hepatic duct and the common bile duct (Fig. 5.6). Although separate, bile ductules share canal space with blood and lymph vessels. As blood flows to the hepatocytes, bile and lymph flow away from sinusoids in the opposite direction, a traffic arrangement known as the "portal triad" (see Fig. 5.3).

Conjugated hyperbilirubinemia and ***obstructive jaundice*** may result when passage of conjugated bilirubin through the ductal system into the GI tract is blocked. This may be caused by the conditions noted in Table 5.33. Lack of bilirubin and its pigmented breakdown products is indicated by clay-colored stools. The kidneys excrete some excess serum bilirubin (only conjugated bilirubin will pass through the glomerulus), and the urine may become darkened or tea-colored. Bile salts, which may also be blocked from excretion, may accumulate in the skin, causing pruritis. Prolonged obstructive jaundice can also lead to elevations of serum cholesterol, with xanthoma formation of the eyelids, neck, or palm creases. Treatment is directed to the underlying cause. Cholestyramine resins that bind bile salts for excretion and antihistamines may provide some relief from symptoms.

In the case of ***Dubin-Johnson*** and ***rotor syndromes,*** defects of bilirubin metabolism interfere with bile transport across membranes. Although conjugated successfully, bilirubin is selectively retained, along with BSP and cholecystographic dyes. Other bile substances are secreted normally. These benign conditions are both inherited as autosomal recessive traits. More common in women than in men, Dubin-Johnson syndrome should be suspected when jaundice from conjugated hyper-

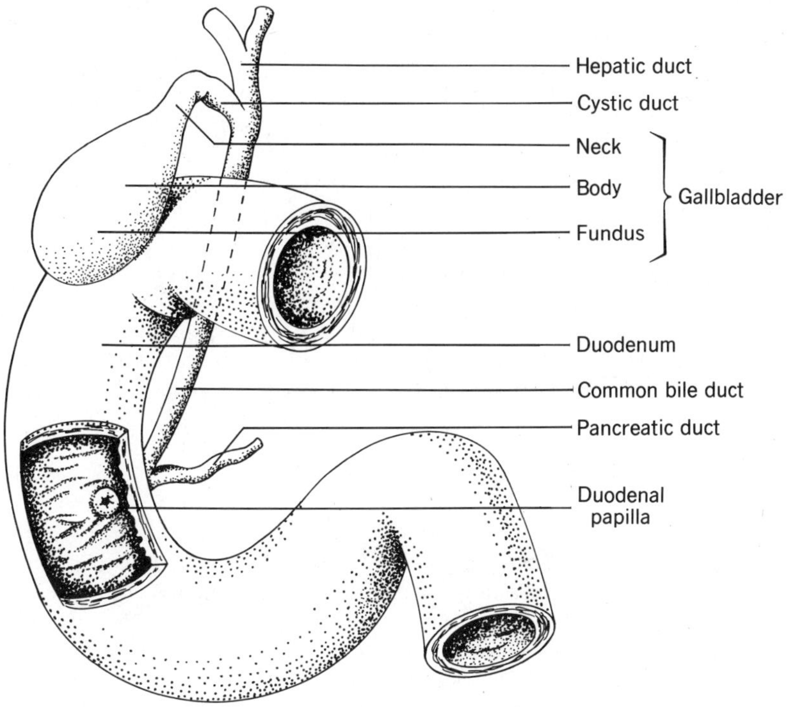

Figure 5.6 Bile ducts and gallbladder.

bilirubinemia develops during pregnancy. It also causes a curious dark pigmentation of the liver. Rotor syndrome is not associated with any liver changes, and its clinical significance is limited to a mild jaundice. No treatment is needed for either disorder.

Injury of unknown etiology to the bile duct system causes ***chronic progressive nonsuppurative cholangitis*** (primary biliary cirrhosis, PBC). Perhaps due to better recognition, PBC is no longer considered extremely rare. Ninety percent of cases occur in women. The problem is believed to be autoimmune, since it is associated with increased IgM, positive antimitochondrial antibodies, and a history of autoimmune disease (notably Sjögren's syndrome, thyroiditis, and scleroderma). Duct damage from an inflammatory exudate leads to chronic intrahepatic cholestasis with eventual fibrosis and cirrhosis. Pruritis is usually the presenting symptom, since significant elevation of alkaline phosphatase appears early. Diagnosis is often delayed, since patients initially seek the aid of a dermatologist and may then be referred to a psychiatrist when no apparent cause can be found for the itching. Only symptomatic treatment can presently be offered. A low-fat diet decreases steatorrhea, replacement of vitamins D and K should be given, and cholestyramine resin may be used to manage pruritis. The prognosis varies with the degree of symptomatology.

Malignancy of the bile ducts may also occur, but usually not until later in life. Seventy is the average age of diagnosis, although tumors have been found in younger patients, particularly those with a history of ulcerative colitis or exposure to the carcinogens benzidine and toluene. Groups at higher risk are Japanese, Mexican-

Americans, and women. As bile flow becomes blocked by the malignant growth, intrahepatic biliary stasis causes gradual hepatocellular damage and/or secondary hepatobiliary infection. Symptoms include deep jaundice, mild upper abdominal pain, weight loss, and possibly pruritis. On abdominal exam, hepatomegaly without splenomegaly is present. Although a distended, nontender gallbladder may be felt, a bile duct tumor is rarely palpable. Very high serum bilirubin levels (mean, around 18 mg/ml) with smaller increases in alkaline phosphatase and SGOT are observed. Transhepatic cholangiography will demonstrate the site of the mass. Malignant bile duct tumors are often inoperable, since important contiguous structures are usually involved. In these cases, biliary enteric anastomoses to bypass the mass and allow bile drainage are palliative measures. The prognosis is poor, with less than a 1-year survival being common. Cure rates remain below 10%. ***Benign tumors of the bile ducts*** also exist, but these are quite rare.

BILE STORAGE

From the common bile duct, bile is released into the duodenum for immediate digestive purposes or diverted to the gallbladder for storage. The gallbladder is a hollow, pear-shaped organ nestled in a fossa on the underside of the liver. It is divided into four sections: the fundus, body, infundibulum, and neck (see Fig. 5.6). Able to hold only 40–70 ml of bile, the gallbladder must concentrate much of the 800–1,000 ml of bile produced daily by the liver. This is accomplished by a lining of specialized columnar epithelial cells tipped by many microvilli. When tight junctions between these cells are allowed to open, water and electrolytes are resorbed into intercellular spaces, then into capillaries, and finally into the cystic vein. The remaining bile salts, cholesterol, bilirubin, and lecithin are thus concentrated from 5- to 10-fold.

Beneath the epithelial lining of the gallbladder is a thick muscular layer. Adequate quantities of fat, amino acids, and acid in food entering the small intestine stimulate the release of cholecystokinin from the intestinal mucosa. This hormone is absorbed into the bloodstream; when it reaches the gallbladder, it stimulates the muscular layer to contract. This contraction raises the pressure in the gallbladder above that in the common bile duct, lifts the fundus, and thus forces the concentrated bile out through the cystic duct. The gallbladder's contractions and/or direct action by cholecystokinin cause inhibition of the sphincter of Oddi (which under fasting conditions is tonically contracted), and the bile passes into the duodenum. Peristaltic waves in the duodenum also cause intermittent relaxation of the sphincter of Oddi, allowing bile in the common bile duct to squirt into the small intestine. Bile salts are later recycled by resorption through the intestinal wall. They are then bound to albumin in the portal blood and delivered to the liver, to be used again in the formation of bile.

Alteration of the composition of bile can cause precipitation of bile constituents, with the formation of ***gallstones***. Reduced water content and increased alkalinity of bile are predisposing factors. Sluggish bile flow in the gallbladder (as in pregnancy, oral contraceptive use, diabetes, cirrhosis, pancreatitis, and celiac disease) and inflammation of the gallbladder epithelium are also implicated. Excessive hepatic secretion of cholesterol (with obesity and a high-fat diet) causes an imbalance of bile components; bile salts become saturated and excess cholesterol precipitates out of solution, forming insoluble crystals. Too much absorption or inadequate production of bile salts has the same effect. More debris and cholesterol tend to accumulate, and

TABLE 5.34 FACTORS PREDISPOSING TO GALLSTONE FORMATION

Cholesterol stones (increased cholesterol and/or decreased bile acid)
- Obesity
- Oral contraceptives
- Clofibrate

Ileal
- Genetic

Pigment stones (increased unconjugated bilirubin)
- Cirrhosis
- Chronic hemolytic anemia
- Biliary infections

the stone enlarges. ***Cholesterol gallstones*** constitute 75% of gallstones in Western cultures. They affect three times as many women as men, with the highest incidence occurring in female American Indians. ***Pigment gallstones*** account for the other 25% and occur mostly in the elderly. They are composed of calcium bilirubinate and other inorganic and organic solids. Factors predisposing to the two types of gallstones are noted in Table 5.34. When stones form in the gallbladder, the condition is called ***cholelithiasis.*** Many persons have cholelithiasis without being aware of any problem, since total obstruction has not occurred. The asymptomatic gallstones, which are often discovered by chance on flat plate abdominal x-ray films (see Table 5.35 for other diagnostic tests for biliary tract disease), require no intervention. However, careful observation is in order.

If a stone occludes the cystic duct, it causes increased pressure, dilation, and inflammation of the gallbladder. The resultant pain is called "biliary colic," which is a symptom of ***chronic cholecystitis.*** The onset of biliary colic is often triggered by ingestion of a large or fatty meal. Cramp-like pain escalates rapidly and remains severe for 1 or more hours before gradually subsiding into a long-lasting soreness. It may be referred to the back (scapula level), but more typically begins in the epigastrium or left upper quadrant and later localizes to the right subcostal area. Vomiting, flatulence, heartburn, and belching may be associated. Attacks may occur rarely or daily. The diagnosis may be confirmed by the tests described in Table 5.35.

TABLE 5.35 DIAGNOSTIC TESTS FOR BILIARY TRACT DISEASE

Test	Use
Flat plate of abdomen	Reveals calcified stones only.
Oral cholecystogram (radiopaque tablets swallowed)	Nonacute cases. Dependent on good intestinal absorption, hepatic secretion, and gallbladder uptake.
Ultrasonography	Demonstrates dilated biliary tree. Can visualize small stones. False-positive results rare, but false-negative ones common. Good for screening.
CT scan	Same as ultrasonography, but more costly.
Percutaneous transhepatic cholangiography (PTC) (needle inserted into hepatic duct and dye injected)	Very effective for visualizing dilated biliary tree. Helps differentiate between obstructive and hepatocellular jaundice. Not indicated if patient has prolonged prothrombin time.
Endoscopic retrograde cholangiography (ERC) (endoscope passed via duodenum into common duct)	Depends on skill of endoscopist. Good for visualization of undilated biliary tree. Helps R/O biliary tract obstruction.
(HIDA) scan (IV injection of radionuclide)	Shows functional patency of ducts. Used to R/O acute cholecystitis. Radiation exposure equivalent to lung scan.

It is important to note that only 15% of gallstones are radiopaque, two-thirds of which are more uncommon pigment types. Decreasing the intake of fat may alleviate symptoms. For those whose symptoms are not severe, oral therapy with chenodeoxycholic acid (CDCA) may help dissolve radiolucent cholesterol stones within 1–2 years. CDCA causes increased bile salt secretion and a lowered output of cholesterol from the liver. It may cause reversible hepatotoxicity and increased levels of LDL cholesterol. Cholecystectomy is a more definitive treatment. It is advised for all patients who are a good operative risk as well as those who may have future complications. The latter category includes diabetics (who have an exceptionally high mortality from acute cholecystitis) and persons with nonfunctional gallbladders, calcified gallbladders (associated with malignant changes), and large (greater than 2 cm in diameter) or radiopaque stones.

Whenever the cystic duct is blocked by a stone, concentrated bile trapped within the gallbladder may cause an inflammation of the mucosa called ***acute cholecystitis.*** As the blockage continues, gallbaldder inflammation worsens and secondary bacterial infection develops. Two-thirds of patients with acute cholecystitis have previously experienced biliary colic. The pain is similar in quality but does not subside. Nausea, vomiting, anorexia, and moderate fever are common. On physical exam, the right subcostal region is typically tender, with guarding and a positive Murphy's sign (while the subhepatic area is being palpated, the patient is instructed to take a deep breath; a sudden increase in tenderness with inspiratory arrest is a positive finding). Palpation of the distended gallbladder is diagnostic. Mild jaundice and leukocytosis may be present. When the surgical risk is high, the physician may attempt to manage the patient with nasogastric suction, replacement of lost fluids and electrolytes, and possibly intravenous antibiotics. However, if empyema (a pus-filled gallbladder), gangrene, perforation, or septicemia threaten, emergency cholecystectomy or cholecystostomy (opening and drainage of the gallbladder) may still be necessary.

Besides the gallbladder, stones can lodge in the small liver bile ducts, the hepatic duct, the cystic duct, the pancreatic duct, or the terminal ileum. When they form in the common bile duct, the condition is known as ***choledocholithiasis.*** Blockage may be intermittent, causing episodes of biliary colic, or, if the blockage is below the pancreatic duct, pancreatitis. Levels of conjugated bilirubin and alkaline phosphatase may rise and fall. ***Chronic choledocholithiasis*** often leads to obstructive jaundice with cirrhotic changes. The latter condition, known as ***secondary biliary cirrhosis,*** also results from strictures, cancer, or pancreatitis. Relief of the blockage, if possible, is the primary treatment goal. Supportive care is indicated for the patient exhibiting the complications of cirrhosis.

Obstruction in the area may also cause ***cholangitis***, an inflammation and infection of the common duct. Symptoms mimic those of biliary colic, with varying degrees of systemic sepsis. The patient appears to be toxic, and hospital management is required to prevent progression to ***suppurative cholangitis.*** In this severe disease, the infection is purulent and the mortality is about 50%.

Gallbladder cancer also seems related to gallstones. Over 50% of these cancer victims have had gallstone symptoms for several years, and 10% of patients over 70 with gallbladder symptoms have carcinoma of the gallbladder. With a penchant for early metastasis to the liver and hilar lymph nodes, this disease accounts for 1% of cancer deaths and affects women three times as often as men. Early diagnosis offers the best hope for survival and is often made incidentally at the time of cholecystectomy. By the time the tumor has reached palpable size, the prognosis is poor.

Details of Management

▸ *Four Food Group System (Basic Diet)*

Laboratory Tests: None.

Therapeutic Measures: None.

Patient Education: To teach patients about the Four Food Group System, provide them with the following sample sheet:

Group	Major Nutrients	Foods/Serving Sizes
Milk	Calcium; vitamin B_2 (riboflavin); protein; vitamin D	8 oz milk; 1½ oz cheese; 1 c yogurt; 2 c cottage cheese; 1 c custard or pudding; 4 scoops of ice cream
Meat (or meat substitute)	Protein; niacin; iron; vitamins B_1 (thiamine) and B_{12}	2 oz cooked meat or fish; 2 eggs; 1 c dried beans or peas; 2 oz cheese; 4 tbsp peanut butter; ½ c nuts or seeds
Fruits and vegetables	Vitamins A and C; folic acid; complex carbohydrates;	½ c cooked fruits or vegetables; ½ c juice; 1 c raw fruit;
Bread and cereal (whole grains)	Vitamin B_1 (thiamine); iron; niacin	1 slice bread; 1 c ready-to-eat cereal; ½ cooked cereal, rice, pasta, grits, barley, millet, or oats

Use the sheet to identify the Four Food Groups, the nutrients supplied by each group, and sample foods. Note that varying amounts of the different foods may be required to provide equivalent amounts of nutrients, and this has been accounted for in the nutritional servings. Emphasize that nutritional servings do not imply calorie equivalents; 4 scoops of ice cream (1,200 calories) are required to provide the same amount of calcium as 8 oz of milk (165 calories).

Teach patients how to place common and/or customary foods into the Four Food Groups. Most foods are readily categorized. However, mixed foods such as pizza or casseroles need to be broken into their components (cheese, tomatoes, bread, etc.) and then classified separately.

Assure healthy patients that they can meet 80–100% of all of their nutrient requirements by eating a variety of foods from each group daily. Note that the number of servings should vary according to the life stages, the recommendations being as follows:

Group	Adolescents (Servings)	Adults (Servings)	Pregnancy/Lactation (Servings)
Milk	4	2	4
Meat /protein	2	2	3
Fruit/vegetable	4	4	4
Bread/cereal	4	4	4

In addition to specific instructions on the Four Food Groups, provide patients with general dietary guidelines for good health as follows:

Eat a variety of foods
Maintain ideal weight
Eat foods with adequate starch and fiber
Avoid too much total fat, saturated fat, and cholesterol
Avoid too much sugar
Avoid too much sodium
Avoid processed foods and chemical additives
If you drink alcohol, do so in moderation.

Follow-up: Refer patients who need in-depth counseling to a registered dietitian.

▸ *Functional Postprandial Hypoglycemia*

Laboratory Tests: 5-h OGTT.

Therapeutic Measures: Start patients on a balanced diet (see the Four Food Group System) with an appropriate caloric intake to achieve and maintain ideal weight (see "Weight Reduction Diet"). Divide the total caloric intake into six or more feedings per day. Restrict carbohydrate intake to 50 g per feeding. Limit simple carbohydrates and high-calorie, complex carbohydrates.

Patient Education: Explain that a high intake of carbohydrates (particularly refined sugars) contributes to symptoms of spontaneous hypoglycemia by stimulating oversecretion of insulin. Stress the functional nature of the problem. Note that hypoglycemia is not considered a preliminary stage of diabetes. Provide a handout such as the following:

FOOD GUIDELINES FOR FUNCTIONAL HYPOGLYCEMIA. Avoid foods in list A as much as possible. Choose a variety of foods from lists B and C for breakfast, midmorning snack, lunch, midafternoon snack, dinner, and bedtime snack. Limit foods in list B to one or possibly two servings per feeding. Limit foods in list C as needed for calorie restriction.

A (to be avoided)	B (permitted in limited amounts)	C (permitted)
Condensed milk	Whole, nonfat milk	Cheese (except whey)
Candy	Cottage cheese	Eggs
Flavored yogurt	Plain yogurt	All meats
Apple juice	Unsweetened canned fruit	All fish
Grape juice		All poultry
Pineapple juice	Strawberries	Bean sprouts
Dried fruits	Grapefruit	Green beans
Corn	Cantaloupe	Wax beans
Dried peas	Oranges	Broccoli
Lima beans	Papayas	Brussel sprouts
Navy beans	Raspberries	Cabbage
Kidney beans	Honeydew melon	Cauliflower
Blackeyed beans	Watermelon	Celery
Split peas	Tangerines	Chicory
Lentils	Bread	Cucumber
Barley	Bagels	Escarole
Baked beans	Biscuits	Eggplant
Hominy	Muffins	Beet greens
Parsnips	Sandwich rolls	Swiss chard
White potatoes	Cornbread	Collard greens
Sweet potatoes	Graham crackers	Dandelion greens
Yams	Melba toast	Kale
Creamed vegetable soup	Oyster crackers	Mustard
	Saltines	Spinach
Sugar-coated cereal	Ry-Crisp	Turnips
Instant breakfasts	Tortillas	Lettuce
Pancakes	Hot cereal	Mushrooms
Waffles	Unsweetened cereals	Okra
Sweet rolls	Cooked rice cereal	Green and red peppers
Coffee cake	Spaghetti	Radishes
Doughnuts	Macaroni	Sauerkraut
Sweetened gelatin	Noodles	Summer squash
Puddings	Popcorn	Tomatoes
Custards	Dietetic desserts	Watercress
Ice cream	Dietetic syrups	Broth
Sherbet	Gravy	Bouillon
Pies	Cream sauces	Consomme
Pastries	Cheese sauces	Plain gelatin
Candy	Nuts	Artificially sweetened jellies, jams
Regular chewing gum	Catsup	
Cakes		Sugar substitutes
Cookies		Butter
Jelly and jam		Margarine

A (to be avoided)	B (permitted in limited amounts)	C (permitted)
White sugar		Mayonnaise
Brown sugar		Heavy cream
Confectioner's sugar		Bacon
Molasses		Salad dressings
Honey		Oil
All syrups		Shortening
Coconut		Diet soft drinks
Alcohol		Coffee substitute
Nondiet soft drinks		Tomato juice
Sweetened fruit punch		Dill pickles
Sweet pickles		Olives
		Hollandaise sauce
		Sauce bearnaise
		Herbs, spices, lemon, mustard, horseradish, vinegar au jus

Tear-out sheets with similar information can be obtained by requesting *Hypoglycemia Diet* from the Carnation Company, P.O. Box 610, Dept. 99, Pico Rivera, California 90665.

Follow-up: As needed.

▸ *Insulin/Sulfonylurea Reactions*

Laboratory Tests: Stat blood sugar determination whenever possible.

Therapeutic Measures: Early, mild reactions. Have patients immediately take one of the following as soon as symptoms of hypoglycemia appear and repeat it in 5 minutes as needed:

½ glass fruit juice or nondiet soda
1 glass milk
2 large sugar cubes
2 tsp honey, syrup, sugar
6–7 Lifesavers
½ candy bar
2 pieces of hard candy
Any available food

More severe reactions: If the patient is having difficulty swallowing, give glucagon 0.5–1 mg IM or SC (use with caution in undernourished patients or those with renal or hepatic disease). If this is not available or if the patient fails to respond within 5–20 minutes, arrange emergency transportation to a hospital for IV glucose, 10- to 20-g push.

Postreaction: Have patients eat a serving of a slowly digested food such as bread, cottage cheese, or crackers and milk or a scheduled meal to prevent a second drop in blood sugar.

Recurrent and/or nighttime reactions: Review the use of any drugs that may stimulate the hypoglycemic effect of insulin or sulfonylurea (Tables 5.14 and 5.16). Adjust diet, exercise, and medication (see the next sections).

At all times: Make sure patients have diabetic identification.

Patient Education: Explain the cause and effects of hypoglycemia. Teach patients to recognize the following signs and symptoms:

1. Early mild reactions
   Hunger
   Mood change (irritability, tearfulness, dullness)
   Headache, lightheadedness, numbness of the lips or tongue
   Paleness or moistness of the skin
   Tremulousness
2. More severe reactions
   Dizziness, confusion
   Loss of coordination
   Difficulty swallowing
   Unconsciousness
3. Nighttime reactions
   Excessive dreaming
   Night sweats
   Morning headache

As preventive measures, advise patients to:

1. Take insulin as prescribed.
2. Adhere to the planned diet, eating at regular intervals.
3. Eat extra food before prolonged or strenuous exercise.
4. Eat something before driving if more than 2 hours have elapsed since the time of the last meal.

Stress the importance of carrying some form of candy at all times and of treating symptoms promptly. Teach relatives or care-givers how to administer glucagon.

Follow-up: As needed.

▸ *Supervision of Type I Diabetes*

Laboratory Tests: Home glucose monitoring (see the subsequent section on "Home Glucose Monitoring"). Test glycosylated hemoglobin (hemoglobin Alc) levels every 4–6 months (this should be done while the patient is fasting).

Therapeutic Measures: HCF diet, exercise, insulin therapy, and home glucose monitoring as described below. Measures for insulin reaction (see the previous section).

Patient Education: Review the etiology of the disease. Constantly reinforce the fact that balancing diet, exercise, and insulin is crucial to controlling the disease. Teach preventive measures for diabetic foot care and encourage patients to contact diabetic organizations (see below). Provide educational material such as "Understanding Your Diabetes," available from Pfizer Laboratories, Professional Service Department, 235 E. 42 Street, New York, New York 10017 or "Managing Your Diabetes," obtained from Eli Lilly and Company, 307 E. McCarty Street, Indianapolis, Indiana 46285.

Follow-up: Schedule visits every 4–6 months. Perform careful screening for hypertension, hyperlipidemia, coronary heart disease, neuropathy, nephropathy, and retinopathy.

▶ High-Carbohydrate, High-Fiber (HCF) Diet

Laboratory Tests: None.

Therapeutic Measures: Begin by estimating the patient's ideal body weight (IBW) from Table 5.25. Convert IBW to kilograms (divide by 2.2). Depending on the patient's stature and activity level, multiply the kilograms of IBW by the appropriate number below to arrive at the daily caloric requirement:

	Activity Level		
Stature	Inactive	Moderately active	Very active
Obese	25	30	35
Normal weight	30	35	40
Underweight	35	40	45

For example, a very active normal-weight woman weighing 110 lb (50 kg) requires a 2,000-calorie/day diet.

Divide the daily caloric requirement into proteins, carbohydrates, and fats by multiplying by 20, 50, and 30%, respectively. Convert calories into grams of protein, carbohydrates, and fats by dividing by 4, 4, and 9, respectively. Thus, a 2,000-calorie diet would be balanced as follows:

20% protein (4 calories for every gram of protein)
  2,000 calories multiplied by 20% = 400 calories.
  400 calories divided by 4 = 100 g.
50% carbohydrates (4 calories for every gram of carbohydrate)
  2,000 calories multiplied by 50% = 1,000 calories.
  1,000 calories divided by 4 = 250 g.
30% fat (9 calories for every gram of fat)
  2,000 calories multiplied by 30% = 600 calories.
  600 calories divided by 9 = 67 g.

Thus, the complete diet description for a very active, normal-weight woman weighing 50 kg is 2,000 calories, 100 g protein, 250 g carbohydrates, and 67 g fat.

Use the diet prescription to compile exchange lists by which the patient can plan six feedings a day (breakfast, midmorning snack, lunch, afternoon snack, dinner, and evening snack). Exchanges should specifically include complex carbohydrates and high-fiber foods. Some experts advocate 35–45 g of plant fiber per 1,000 calories. Twenty percent of the total caloric intake should be allotted to each regular meal and the remaining 40% divided among snacks. Detailed information about diet planning can be obtained from *HCF Diets: A Professional Guide,* University of Kentucky Diabetes Research and Education Fund. In addition to the prescribed exchanges, patients must avoid refined sugars.

Patient Education: Stress the key role of diet in diabetes. Explain the beneficial effects of complex carbohydrates and fibers and the deleterious effects of refined sugars and simple starches in controlling blood sugar. Provide general information about the various exchanges such as the following:

Fruit exchanges (e.g., apples, oranges, peaches, berries, cherries, bananas): Natural desserts high in vitamins, minerals, and fiber (if eaten whole). Can be eaten raw, canned in their own juice, unsweetened, or artificially sweetened. Portion sizes are important because some fruits have more calories than others even though their size is comparable.

Meat exchanges (e.g., meats, poultry, fish, cheese, and egg whites). Provide high-quality protein. Very small servings (3–5 oz) should be used to complement vegetable proteins for well-balanced intake of amino acids. Because diabetics are prone to accelerated atherosclerosis, proteins from animal sources (high in fat and cholesterol) should be limited.

A and B vegetable exchanges (e.g., green beans, yellow beans, tomatoes, sprouts, carrots, cauliflower, celery, cucumbers, peppers, lettuce, mushrooms, summer squash, cabbage, brussel sprouts, broccoli): Divided into A or B groups depending on the calorie difference due to the method of preparation (raw, cooked, canned). Both types are low in calories but high in vitamins and minerals. A vegetables are high in fiber and slightly lower in calories than B vegetables.

C vegetables (e.g., barley, corn, parsnips, sweet potatoes, white potatoes, spaghetti, macaroni, rice, winter squash): of all the vegetable groups, this one is highest in calories. However, these vegetables are excellent sources of complex carbohydrates.

Milk exchanges (e.g., skim milk, yogurt, buttermilk): Provides protein, calcium, and several vitamins. Low-fat forms should be used exclusively.

Fat exchanges (e.g., margarine, mayonnaise, corn oil, safflower oil, olive oil, soybean oil, nuts): As fats and concentrated sources of calories, should be carefully limited.

Cereal exchanges (e.g., oatmeal, grits, All-Bran, shredded wheat, Grape-Nuts, Bran Buds): Can be used as good sources of bran and as snacks. Avoid cereals containing refined sugars. Use artificial sweeteners or a fruit exchange as a sweetener.

Bread exchanges (e.g., rye, whole wheat, graham crackers, rye crackers, muffins): Good sources of B vitamins and complex carbohydrates. Should be prepared with whole-grain flour and liquid oil, and should be free of sucrose, honey, molasses, or butter.

Provide specific exchange lists based on the patient's calorie requirement. These lists can be obtained by writing for the *Diabetic Diet Plan* (a basic plan for 1,500 calories adjusted for 1,000, 1,200, and 1,800 calories), Carnation Company, P.O. Box 610, Dept. 99, Pico Rivera, California 90665 or the *American Diabetic Association,* 2 Park Ave., New York, New York 10016. In addition, give patients a handout such as the following:

SELECTION OF SWEETS

Avoid	Use Instead
All sugars	Artificial sweeteners
Regular soft drinks	Diet soft drinks containing fewer than 5 calories
Regular chewing gum	Sugarless gum
Sweetened cereals	Natural cereals
Pies, pastries, rich desserts	Artificially sweetened or natural gelatin, fresh fruit
Syrups, honey, molasses, jams, jellies	Artificially sweetened products

Follow-up: Diet review and weight checks on each follow-up visit.

▸ *Exercise for the Diabetic*

Laboratory Tests: See the section on prescribing exercise in Chapter 11.

Therapeutic Measures: Advise exercise training as described in Chapter 11, with the following modifications:

1. Vigorous activities should never be undertaken when blood sugar is poorly controlled.
2. Patients with peripheral sensory neuropathy and/or vascular insufficiency should avoid jogging, rope jumping, soccer, or other forms of exercise that may cause trauma to the feet.
3. Patients with diabetic retinopathy should avoid weight lifting, jogging, rope jumping, or any exercise that may induce hemorrhage.
4. Patients taking hypoglycemic agents should be instructed to eat about 15 additional grams of carbohydrates for every 30 minutes of strenuous exercise, to carry a source of glucose, and to wear medical identification.
5. Patients taking insulin may have to decrease the dose by 10–20 U prior to planned exercise if hypoglycemia becomes a problem. They should also inject insulin at a nonexercise site (e.g., the stomach rather than the thigh before jogging).

Patient Education: See the section on prescribing exercise in Chapter 11.

Follow-up: As needed.

▶ *Insulin Therapy*

Laboratory Tests: Home glucose monitoring (see the next section). Test glycosylated hemoglobin (hemoglobin Alc) levels every 4–6 months (should be done while the patient is fasting).

Therapeutic Measures: Individualize therapy carefully. No single prescription can be offered to all patients, but the following guidelines may prove helpful.

Preparations: Any of the preparations listed in Table 5.12 may be used initially, except for regular concentrated Iletin and possibly fixed combinations. Human and purified pork preparations seem to be associated with fewer complications but are more expensive. A change from one insulin preparation to another (refinement, purity, strength, brand, type, or source) should be made with extreme caution. Either hypoglycemia or hyperglycemia may result with the first dose or over a period of several weeks. To prevent hypoglycemia (the more common reaction), it may be wise to reduce the dose of a new preparation by 10–20% initially and titrate upward as needed. Regular crystalline insulin may be mixed with NPH or lente insulins in any proportion. If mixed with PZI, it combines with protamine and becomes long-acting. Lente, Semilente, or Ultralente may be mixed with regular insulin and with one another, but not with any other type of modified insulin.

Single-dose regimen (use is usually limited to new onset of type II disease): Start with 10–20 U of an intermediate- or long-acting preparation (NPH, Lente, Ultralente). Give one-half hour before breakfast (before dinner for patients who work nights). Increase the dose by 4–5 U every other day until fasting blood sugar levels are controlled (less than 140 mg/dL). If control requires more than 50 U, consider switching to a split-dose regimen.

Split-dose regimen (improves glucose control during the night): An intermediate-acting preparation (NPH or Lente) is best for this purpose, since a dose taken before breakfast gradually influences glucose absorption during the day, has its maximal effect at dinnertime, when it is needed most, and lasts throughout most of the night. By contrast, long-acting preparations taken in sufficient amounts to control glucose throughout the day create the risk of hypoglycemia during the night. Split the total daily dose by giving two-thirds in the morning and one-third at night. The usual starting dose is 15 U NPH or Lente, 10 U before breakfast and 5 U before dinner. Test the effect of the morning dose by checking blood sugar before dinner; check the effect of the evening dose by checking blood sugar before breakfast. Increase the total dose in increments of 5 U every other day (adding 3 U before breakfast and 2 U before dinner) until morning and evening blood sugar levels are controlled.

Split-dose combinations (improves postprandial control): Titrate the split dose of intermediate-acting insulins as above. Do not use PZI, since protamine combines with regular insulin, rendering it long-acting and defeating its purpose. Convert established morning and evening doses into combinations as follows: 40% intermediate-acting, 60% regular in the morning, 60% intermediate-acting, 40% regular in the late afternoon, or 40% lente, 60% regular in the morning, 40% lente, 20% ultralente, 40% regular in the late afternoon. Test the combined morning dose by checking blood sugar before lunch and the combined evening dose by checking blood sugar at bedtime.

Physiologic coverage (closest to natural control and provides flexibility in mealtime/exercise scheduling): Prescribe regular insulin before each meal and NPH before sleep or regular insulin before each meal and Ultralente before breakfast and/or dinner. Withhold or adjust regular insulin for missed meals or for deviations in work or exercise patterns.

Special control: Refer hard-to-control patients to a special center for multidisciplinary focus and evaluation for an insulin delivery device. For short-term use, a butterfly needle may be implanted subcutaneously and left in place for several days. The patient injects insulin into the butterfly instead of the skin. The pen pump is kept in the patient's pocket. When it is time for an injection, a plunger is pushed to inject a predetermined amount of insulin (the ratio of long-acting and regular insulin cannot be altered). Continuous pumps (a device worn on a belt) achieve tight glucose control and normalize other metabolites such as lactate, 3-hydroxybutyrate, triglycerides, free fatty acids, and branched chain amino acids. Immunosuppressive therapy is being used in the early stages of type I diabetes. Transplantation of beta cells is being done successfully in animals and may be ready for use in humans within the next 2 years.

Patient Education: Explain the various insulin preparations, duration of action, sources, purities, and concentrations. Emphasize that U-40 insulin must be used with U-40 syringes, U-100 insulin with U-100 syringes, and U-500 insulin with U-500 syringes. Note that different brands of syringes have variable amounts of space between the needle and the first marking. For these reasons, teach patients to check for and question any change in the brand of insulin and/or syringes by the physician or pharmacist (which could result in dosage error). Instruct the patient on the general use of insulin, as well as specific techniques for injections. In addition to demonstrations, give written information such as the following:

GENERAL INSTRUCTIONS FOR INSULIN USE

1. Buy the specific syringes and insulin prescribed. Check for any changes each time you pick up a new prescription. Do not use a different brand/calibration of syringes or a different brand/type/source/strength of insulin without checking with the physician. To do so may result in a dosage error.
2. Check the dates on new bottles of insulin to make sure that they have not expired.
3. Store insulin in a refrigerator, but warm it to room temperature before using it. Avoid exposing it to direct sunlight, warm temperatures (above 80°F), or freezing temperatures.
4. Read the drug insert for information about the normal appearance of your preparation. Basically, all preparations except regular and globin insulin are cloudy. Discard any vial with clumped, granular, or solidified particles of precipitate.
5. Take your insulin as directed every day. Do not omit it when you are ill.
6. Change the insulin dose only according to instructions.
7. Always carry candy to take when the first symptoms of hypoglycemia appear. Keep glucagon at home, work, or school (see the previous section).

HOW TO PREPARE AN INJECTION WITH ONE INSULIN

1. Assemble the insulin, syringe, and alcohol wipe in a clean, uncluttered area with good lighting.
2. Use only a new disposable or sterile reusable syringe. Sterilize the latter by boiling all parts (syringe, plunger, needle) in water for 5 minutes or by immersing the parts in 70% ethyl alcohol (bathing, rubbing, or medicated alcohol is not suitable) for 5 minutes. Remove all liquid from the syringe by pushing the plunger in and out several times and allow it to dry
3. Wash your hands.
4. Check the expiration date on the insulin. Make sure that the syringe size matches the insulin concentration and that there has been no change in the prescription.
5. Gently roll the insulin bottle several times to mix the preparation. Do not shake the bottle.
6. Look for any change in the usual appearance of the insulin.
7. Wipe the rubber stopper on top of the bottle with an alcohol swab. Never remove the rubber cap.
8. Remove the protection cap from the needle. Draw air into the syringe by pulling back on the plunger until it reaches the marking of the insulin dose you need.
9. Push the needle straight through the rubber top of the insulin bottle and push in the plunger.
10. Turn the bottle and syringe upside down. Tipping the bottle so that the insulin covers the needle, slowly draw back on the plunger. Pass the marking for the desired dose and then return to it to force out any air bubbles. Though harmless if injected, air bubbles can invalidate the measurement.
11. Pull the bottle off the needle, taking care not to change the position of the plunger.
12. Double check the dose.
13. If you are visually impaired, obtain help from family members, a visiting nurse, or via special devices. Information about the latter can be obtained by writing for "Devices for Visually Impaired Diabetics," New York Diabetes Association, 104 East 40th Street, New York, New York 10016, or "An Evaluation for Insulin Dependent Visually Handicapped Diabetics," The New York Association for the Blind, 111 East 59th Street, New York, New York 10022.

PREPARING AN INJECTION WITH TWO INSULINS

1. Following steps 1 through 9 above, prepare short-acting insulin and inject air into the bottle. Remove the empty syringe.
2. Following steps 1 through 9 above, prepare the longer-acting preparation. Draw up the correct dose, following steps 10 through 12.
3. Take the syringe containing the correct dose of long-acting insulin and insert the needle into the vial of short-acting insulin. Do not push down on the plunger.
4. Turn the bottle and syringe upside down. Tipping the bottle as needed so that

insulin covers the needle, slowly draw back on the plunger until the marking for the desired dose is reached. Arrive at this marking by adding the doses of long-acting insulin and short-acting insulin together, that is, 40 U for a prescription of NPH U-24 and Regular U-16. Do not inject any preparation back into the vial.

5. Pull the bottle off the needle, taking care not to change the position of the plunger.
6. Double check your dose.
7. Although it does not matter initially, never change the established order in which the two insulins are drawn up.

CHOOSING AN INJECTION SITE

1. Inject insulin into areas that have a layer of fat under the skin and are free of large blood vessels and nerves.
2. Avoid injections around joints (danger of infection), and around the groin, the navel (highly vascularized), and the midline of the abdomen (very sensitive nerve supply).
3. To minimize tissue damage (mild dimpling to deep pits in the skin), allow 3–4 cm between injection sites and use insulin warmed to room temperature.
4. Do not inject the same site for at least 1 month.
5. Set up a rotation cycle, using the sites and injection log noted in Figure 5.2.
6. Because absorption may be accelerated, avoid arms and legs as injection sites prior to strenuous exercise.

INJECTING INSULIN

1. Wipe the injection site with an alcohol swab.
2. Using your nondominant hand, pinch up a large area of skin between the thumb and forefinger.
3. Using your dominant hand, pick up the syringe as you would a pencil.
4. Insert the needle at a straight angle to the hub (a quick stab proves to be the most comfortable method for most people).
5. Once the needle is fully inserted, push the plunger in all the way. The practice of pulling back on the plunger is not advocated by many experts (it adds to patient anxiety, may result in dislodgement of the needle, and may contribute to tissue damage). If correct sites are used, there is very little danger of injecting insulin into blood vessels.
6. Hold the alcohol swab near the needle and pull the needle straight out.
7. Press the swab over the injection site for several seconds, but do not massage, since this may interfere with the rate of absorption.
8. After putting the cap back on the needle, destroy disposable syringe by quickly snapping the syringe and the needle together like breaking a stick. Throw away the parts. Sterilize reusable syringes as previously described.
9. Store insulin in the refrigerator and all other equipment in a safe place away from small children.
10. Record the injection on the site chart.

Follow-up: Arrange daily sessions until the patient demonstrates a good understanding of insulin therapy and feels comfortable giving injections.

▸ *Home Glucose Monitoring*

Laboratory Tests: Blood sugar testing at home two to four items a day.

Therapeutic Measures: Patients will need finger lancets, reagent strips, and a photometer (optional in some cases). Sterile disposable finger lancets can be used alone or with a spring-loaded holder (closed, open arc, or pen design). Reagent strips can be used directly (color chart interpretation) or with a reflectance photometer. Color charts provide only a range, while the photometer provides an actual reading. While less precise, reagent strips for color chart interpretation are readily portable and relatively inexpensive ($0.40 to 0.90 per strip; some strips are wide enough to cut in half). Photometers are extremely accurate and require no color interpretation but are quite expensive—$100 to $400 for the initial cost of the machine plus reagent strips (which cannot be cut in half). With either method, reagent strips must be carefully prepared. Furthermore, most photometers must be calibrated according to the manufacturer's instructions. Some of the products available are as follows:

Device	Manufacturer	Comment
Automatic lancets		
Autoclix	Bio-Dynamics	Closed design
Autolet	Ulster Scientific and Ames	Open arc
Hemalet	Med Probe	Closed design
Monojector	Sherwood Medical	Closed design
Penlet	Life Scan, Inc.	Pen-shaped
Test strips (for direct color chart interpretations)		
Chemstrip	Bio-Dynamics	Dry wipe; 20- to 800-mg/dL range
Dextrostix	Ames	Only up to 250 mg/dL on color chart; cannot be cut
Visidex	Ames	Wet wash; 20- to 800-mg/dL range
Test strips (for use with photometer)		
Dextrostix	Ames	For use with Glucometer
Glucoscan	Life Scan, Inc.	For Glucoscan II meter
Star-Tek	Bio-Dynamics	For Stat-Tek meter only
Photometers		
Dextrometer	Ames	For use with Dextrostix
Glucometer	Ames	For use with Dextrostrix; battery; built-in timer
Glucoscan	Life Scan, Inc.	Needs no calibration; requires battery
Stat-Tek	Bio-Dynamics	Not portable
Accu-Chek	Bio-Dynamics	Has calibration strips; requires battery

Help patients gather information about systems, and base the choice on the cost, availability of supplies, and portability. Be sure to fill out insurance forms and/or press for third-party payment (most broad-coverage insurance plans reimburse up to 80% of the cost). Once patients have obtained their equipment, demonstrate its use and set up a schedule for testing. Have patients take readings before breakfast and before dinner each day (patients on split doses/regular coverage should take additional readings at noon and at bedtime). Teach them to record each day's readings, along with the insulin dosage, on a graph such as the following:

	AM	N	PM	HS
More than 250	______	______	______	______
200	______	______	______	______
150	______	______	______	______
100	______	______	______	______
50	______	______	______	______
Long-acting	______		______	
Regular	______	______	______	______

Patient Education: Point out the advantages of home monitoring, particularly direct and immediate feedback about the effects of diet, exercise, and medication. Fasting levels of 70–120 mg/dL, 1-hour postprandial levels of less than 180 mg/dL, 2-hour postprandial levels of less than 150 mg/dL, and preprandial bedtime readings of 80–120 mg/dL demonstrate excellent control. Stress the importance of following the manufacturer's instructions for all testing procedures. Work to correct some common causes of error such as the following.

1. Failing to obtain sufficient blood to cover the reagent strip. Advise patients to stick the finger from the side of the fingertip, where there is a smaller concentration of nerves, and to strip the finger distally to create a thick drop of blood.
2. Timing the steps incorrectly. A clock with a sweep second hand or a digital display must be available (some systems have built-in timers), and equipment must be well organized.

Follow-up: Have patients bring daily recordings to each follow-up visit (Chemstrips and Visidex have a fixed endpoint, so patients can save the strips and bring them for review). Adjust insulin levels if fasting readings are persistently above 140 mg/dL or below 50 mg/dL (see the previous section). Arrange for patients to bring in their monitoring equipment and redemonstrate their technique every 4–6 months.

▸ *Type II Diabetes, Obese Subset*

Laboratory Tests: Fasting blood glucose level. Insulin level is optional.

Therapeutic Measures: Attain and maintain ideal body weight by adopting a hypocaloric, high-carbohydrate, high-fiber diet (see the section "High-Carbohydrate, High-Fiber (HCF) Diet"). Avoid using hypoglycemic agents or insulin if at all possible. When blood sugar levels are under control, start a regular exercise program (see Chapter 11).

Patient Education: Explain the effects of obesity on glucose tolerance. Note that diet and exercise are crucial to the control of blood sugar and that medications often compound the problem. Review diabetic foot care (see the section "Diabetic Foot").

Follow-up: Schedule visits every 4–6 months to support the diet and check the glucose with glycosylated hemoglobin. Careful screening is needed for hypertension, hyperlipidemia, coronary heart disease, neuropathy, nephropathy, and retinopathy.

▸ *Type II Diabetes, Nonobese Subset*

Laboratory Tests: Fasting blood glucose levels. Insulin levels suggested.

Therapeutic Measures: Maintain ideal body weight by adopting a high-carbohydrate, high-fiber diet with the correct caloric requirement (see the section "High-Carbohydrate, High-Fiber (HCF) Diet"). If this diet does not readily improve the blood sugar level, start to use one of the hypoglycemic agents listed in Table 5.15. Titrate the drug according to the manufacturer's directions. For example, if you are using Glucotrol (one of the newer agents), start with 5 mg once daily before breakfast and adjust upward or downward in increments of 2.5–5 mg every several days according to the patient's blood sugar readings. Dose increases beyond 15 mg must be divided bid, the total daily dose not to exceed 40 mg. If the response remains inadequate with maximum doses, switch to another agent or insulin. Use the medications listed in Table 5.15 with care. When blood sugar levels, are under control, start a regular exercise program (see Chapter 11).

Patient Education: Explain the etiology of the disease and the beneficial effects of diet and exercise on glucose tolerance. For patients who are starting oral hypoglycemic agents, describe the hypoglycemic reactions and home glucose monitoring (see the previous sections). Start measures for diabetic foot care (see the following section).

Follow-up: Schedule visits every 4–6 months. Review diet, exercise programs, medication, and the results of glucose monitoring. Check long-term blood sugar control with glycosylated hemoglobin. Screen for hypertension, hyperlipidemia, coronary heart disease, neuropathy, nephropathy, and retinopathy.

▸ *Diabetic Foot*

Laboratory Tests: Depending on the complication, may include culture and sensitivity tests, x-ray films, or vascular testing (e.g., arterial blood pressure measurements of the ankle, calf, and thigh using ultrasound, arterial pulse contour studies, arteriography).

Therapeutic Measures: For any complication, early recognition and treatment referral are essential, as noted in Table 5.19. Elevation of extremities is contraindicated in patients with vascular insufficiency, even though signs of edema and inflammation may be present.

Patient Education: Explain the various types of foot complications associated with diabetes. Provide information such as the following:

MEASURES TO PREVENT DIABETIC FOOT PROBLEMS

General measures: Keep blood sugar and lipid levels under control with the prescribed diet, medication, and exercise. Do not smoke.

Foot inspection: Check every portion of your feet in the morning and at night for sores, drainage, color change, temperature change, dryness, cracking, fissures, or callus formation (use a mirror for hard-to-observe areas). Report any changes to the physician.

Foot hygiene: Gently wash your feet every day, using a soft washcloth, lukewarm water, and mild soap. Dry them thoroughly, especially between the toes, with a soft absorbent towel. Apply a bland lubricating cream (lanolin or petroleum jelly) to the top and bottom of the feet (but not between the toes) to prevent the development of cracks or fissures. Apply mild talcum powder between the toes to discourage fungal infections.

Toenails: If possible, have a podiatrist provide care. Cut nails straight across, leaving them long at the corners. Use emery boards with extreme care.

Corns or calluses: See a podiatrist. Do not cut or rub these growths or use chemical agents.

Shoes: Wear only comfortable shoes made of soft leather that fit snugly (neither too loose nor too tight). If you have hammer toes or bunions, make sure that the toe box is high and wide enough to prevent rubbing. Extra-depth shoes or shoes with molded insoles may be specially ordered. If you have a narrow heel, buy a double last shoe. Generally, a heel height of less than 1.5 in. is best for everyday shoes. When breaking in new shoes, walk with shorter strides for the first day or so. Before wearing shoes, always check them for any defects or foreign objects that may irritate the skin. Never wear wet shoes.

Socks and stockings: Buy socks or stockings that fit snugly but not tightly over the foot, calf, and upper thigh. For most seasons and everyday activity, thin socks of 33% wool, 32% cotton, and 35% nylon keep feet driest and coolest. For extremely cold weather and/or strenuous athletic activity, thicker socks of 65% orlon, 25% cotton, and 10% nylon are warmer and less likely to wrinkle. Wear only clean, dry socks or stockings.

Exposure: Avoid heating pads, hot water bottles, hot baths, and excessive cold. Never walk barefooted, either indoors or outdoors.

Foot exercises (Buerger's exercises): Hold the feet elevated for 1 minute, dependent for 3 minutes, and horizontal for 6 minutes. Wiggle them gently for the entire 10 minutes. Repeat this cycle three to six times a day.

Follow-up: Carefully inspect the feet at each follow-up visit.

▸ *Diabetes Organizations*

Laboratory Tests: None.

Therapeutic Measures: None.

Patient Education: American Diabetes Association
2 Park Avenue
New York, New York 10016 Tel.: (212) 683-7444

Follow-up: Help patients make contact as needed.

▸ *Screening for Hyperlipidemia*

Laboratory Tests: Screen healthy persons once during adolescence and once during middle adulthood. Take blood samples following a 12- to 14-hour overnight fast. Since lipid concentrations may be affected by weight change or illness, baseline values should be established before dieting and at least 8 weeks after an MI, trauma, or severe illness. If feasible, estrogens, steroids, contraceptive pills, and other lipid-altering drugs should be discontinued 3–4 weeks before testing.

Therapeutic Measures: None unless an abnormality is found.

Patient Education: Hyperlipidemia should be recognized and treated because it contributes to the development of atherosclerosis. Generally, any fasting triglyceride level greater than 150–175 mg/dL is considered abnormal. The risk of CAD is associated with age-adjusted levels of cholesterol as follows:

Patient's Age	Mild Risk	Moderate Risk	High Risk
20–29 years	172–199	200–220	>220
30–39	194–219	220–240	>240
40+	206–239	240–260	>260

Follow-up: If lipid concentrations are found to be high, at least two confirmatory samples should be taken. If they are high on three occasions, do phenotyping and begin appropriate treatment.

▸ *Type I Hyperlipidemia*

Laboratory Tests: Hyperlipidemia screening (see above). Overnight refrigeration of plasma (creamy top layer). Phenotyping showing type I hyperlipidemia (uncleared chylomicrons).

Therapeutic Measures: To reduce symptoms of abdominal pain and other complications, restrict fat intake to 25–35 g/day. Since this level is very low, the fat content of all types of food must be considered. There is no need to limit cholesterol, carbohydrates, or protein, but alcohol is not recommended. Suggest the use of medium chain triglycerides for cooking or as an added ingredient to make the diet more palatable.

Patient Education: Give general instructions such as the following: eliminate all separated fats (butter, margarine, shortening, oils) and nuts. Use only lean, well-trimmed meat. Exclude dairy products and baked goods containing fat. Eat enough calories to maintain ideal weight (carbohydrates may have to be increased).

Provide the specific instructions and sample menus found in "Diet 1 for Hyperchylomicronemia." Booklets containing 50 tear-out sheets can be ordered free of charge from:

Hyperlipoproteinemia Diets
National Heart, Lung, and Blood Institute
National Institutes of Health
Bethesda, Maryland 20014

Follow-up: Diet reinforcement every 4–6 months.

▸ *Type IIa Hyperlipidemia*

Laboratory Tests: See the section "Screening for Hyperlipidemia." Phenotyping showing the type IIa pattern (high cholesterol, normal triglycerides). Evaluation of family members, since the problem is often familial.

Therapeutic Measures: To reduce the risk of atherosclerosis, restrict cholesterol to less than 300 mg/day. Reduce the intake of saturated fats and increase that of polyunsaturated fats. Carbohydrates and protein need not be limited, and alcohol can be used in moderation. If diet measures fail to lower cholesterol levels, prescribe niacin (e.g., Nicolar, 500 mg, 2–4 tablets daily) until cholesterol is controlled or until its use is limited by side effects (maximum dose, 8 g). Niacin is contraindicated in patients with hepatic dysfunction or active peptic ulcer. As an alternative, start cholestyramine (e.g., Questran, 4 g or 9 g/packet mixed with 2–6 oz water, soup, milk, fruit juice, or another noncarbonated fluid; it should not be taken dry).

Patient Education: Explain that cholesterol is contained in foods of animal origin, particularly egg yolk, organ meats (e.g., sweetbreads, kidney, heart, liver), meat, meat fat, and shrimp. These foods should be omitted or limited. Fats of animal origin such as butter, cream, whole milk, and whole milk products are saturated (their molecular structure is not completely filled, and they are therefore unable to dissolve or combine). Vegetable fats are usually unsaturated (their molecular structure is not completely filled, and therefore they are capable of combining or dissolving). Exceptions include coconut oil, palm oil, and cocoa butter (a fat contained in chocolate), as well as unsaturated oils that are saturated by a special process (hydrogenation). In the case of hydrogenated oils, the degree of hardness offers some guide to the degree of saturation (a stick of margarine being more saturated than a tub of margarine). Saturated fats increase cholesterol levels and should be limited in the diet. Unsaturated fats lower cholesterol levels and should be increased.

Provide the specific instructions and sample menus in "Diet 2 for Hypercholesterolemia." Booklets containing 50 tear-out sheets can be ordered free of charge from the National Heart, Lung, and Blood Institute (address previously given).

Follow-up: Every 4–6 months.

▸ *Type 11b or Type III Hyperlipidemia*

Laboratory Tests: See the section "Screening for Hyperlipidemia." Refrigerated serum (turbid appearance). Phenotyping.

Therapeutic Measures: For overweight patients, institute a reduction diet to obtain the ideal body weight (see the section "Weight Reduction Diet"). For patients of ideal weight, prescribe a diet based on a daily caloric maintenance allowance balanced in fat and carbohydrates and increased in protein as follows:

Caloric Allowance:	1,500	1,800	2,000	2,200	2,400	2,600	2,800	
As 20% protein	75	80	90	115	120	120	125	(g)
40% fat	70	80	95	100	110	120	130	(g)
40% carbohydrate	135	180	195	210	225	255	285	(g)

The ratio of unsaturated to saturated fats should be increased. Cholesterol should be limited to less than 300 mg/day. Two servings of alcohol may be substituted for part of the daily carbohydrate intake. Consider iron supplementation, since the diet will not meet the iron requirements. If diet measures do not lower lipid levels, prescribe gemfibrozil (e.g., Lopid, 600 mg bid taken 30 minutes before the morning and evening meals). This medication is contraindicated in liver or gallbladder disease.

Patient Education: Give general guidelines on cholesterol and fat modification described in the previous section. Provide the specific instructions and sample menus in "Diet 3 for Hypercholesterolemia and Endogenous Hypertriglyceridemia." Booklets containing 50 tear-out sheets can be ordered free of charge from the National Heart and Lung Institute (address previously given).

Follow-up: Every 4–6 months. Watch for biliary changes.

▸ *Type IV Hyperlipidemia*

Laboratory Tests: See the section "Screening for Hyperlipidemia." Phenotyping.

Therapeutic Measures: For overweight patients, prescribe a reduction diet to obtain ideal body weight (see the section "Weight Reduction Diet"). For ideal-weight patients, prescribe a diet based on a daily caloric maintenance allowance controlled in carbohydrates as follows:

Calorie Allowance:	1,500	1,800	2,000	2,200	2,400	2,600	2,800	
45% as carbohydrate	165	210	225	240	270	285	315	(g)

Protein and fat intake is not limited, but the ratio of unsaturated to saturated fats should be increased. Cholesterol should be moderately restricted. Two servings of alcohol may be substituted for part of the daily carbohydrate intake. Consider iron supplementation, since the diet will not meet the iron requirements. If diet measures do not lower lipid levels, prescribe gemfibrozil (e.g., Lopid, 600 mg bid taken 30 minutes before the morning and evening meals). This medicated is contraindicated in liver or gallbladder disease.

Patient Education: Give general guidelines on cholesterol and fat modification described for type II hyperlipidemia. Provide the specific instructions and sample means in "Diet 4 for Endogenous Hyperglyceridemia." Booklets containing 50 tear-out sheets can be ordered free of charge from the National Heart and Lung Institute (address previously given).

Follow-up: Every 4–6 months.

▸ Type V Hyperlipidemia

Laboratory Tests: See the section "Screening for Hyperlipidemia." Phenotyping. Consider screening for abnormal GTT and hyperuricemia (often associated).

Therapeutic Measures: For overweight patients, prescribe a reduction diet to obtain ideal body weight (see the next section). Weight reduction alone usually results in normal concentrations of lipids and greater tolerance for minor excesses of dietary fat and carbohydrates. For ideal-weight patients, prescribe a diet based on a daily caloric maintenance allowance high in protein and moderately controlled in fats and carbohydrates as follows:

Caloric Allowance:	1,500	1,800	2,000	2,200	2,400	2,600	2,800	
As 20% protein	90	100	105	130	135	140	145	(g)
30% fat	50	50	65	70	70	85	85	(g)
50% carbohydrate	180	235	250	265	310	325	370	(g)

The ratio of unsaturated to saturated fats should be increased and cholesterol should be moderately restricted. Alcohol is not recommended, since it may increase triglyceride levels and exacerbate abdominal pain. Consider iron supplementation, since the diet will not meet iron requirements. Drugs are usually not indicated, though niacin (e.g., Nicolar, 500 mg, 2–4 tablets daily) until cholesterol is controlled or until niacin is limited by side effects (maximum dose, 8 g) has been used. It is contraindicated in patients with hepatic dysfunction or active peptic ulcer.

Patient Education: Give general guidelines on cholesterol and fat modification described under type IIa hyperlipidemia. Provide the specific instructions and sample menus in "Diet 5 for Mixed Hyperglyceridemia." Booklets containing 50 tear-out sheets can be ordered free of charge from the National Heart and Lung Institute (address previously given).

Follow-up: For patients on medication, review every 4–6 months. Otherwise, perform yearly lipid level tests and weight checks to monitor the success of the diet.

▸ Weight Reduction Diet

Laboratory Tests: None.

Therapeutic Measures: Before planning the diet, have patients conduct a personal review of present eating habits. Have them:

1. List their favorite foods.
2. Keep a record of everything they ate or drank for at least a 24-hour period (include snacks, side dishes, alcohol, and condiments).
3. Use the record to indicate the type of food preparations they use (fried, boiled, baked, etc).
4. Note whether breakfast, lunch, dinner, and between-meal snacks are eaten on a regular basis and which are considered most important.
5. Indicate meals eaten at restaurants and how often.
6. Determine whether food intake is more or less on weekends.
7. Specify (a) daily amounts of bread, water, milk, tea, coffee, soft drinks, beer, whiskey, cereal, desserts, and sweets; (b) use of mayonnaise, catsup, and mustard on food; (d) addition of cream, milk, and sugar to coffee or tea.
8. Note any eating changes (more or less) in response to nervousness, depression, or excitement.
9. Describe eating habits: (a) taking second helpings, (b) leaving food on the plate, (c) helping oneself to food, (d) being served, and (e) the size of served portions.

Use the personal review to evaluate the patient's knowledge of the Four Food Group System. Identify imbalanced eating habits. Plan a reduced calorie intake for the patient. Calculate the patient's daily caloric maintenance allowance (present weight × 15 for a moderately active person) and subtract 1,000 calories/day for a 2-lb/week weight loss. Teach patients to eat the recommended number of servings from each group every day, but to select low-calorie foods. Give them a list of foods comparing calories per serving such as the following:

Have a Serving of:	No. of Calories	Rather Than a Serving of:	No. of Calories
		Milk Group	
Skim milk/buttermilk	80	Whole milk	165
Cottage cheese	25	Blue/cheddar/cream/swiss	105
Yogurt	60	Ice cream	150
Nonfat pudding	60	Regular pudding	140
Cocoa/milk and water	105	Cocoa/milk	140
Margarine	70	Butter	100
Coffee-Mate	10	Cream	94
		Meat Group	
Boiled/poached egg	78	Scrambled egg	120
Canned crabmeat	80	Canned tuna	165
Swordfish	140	Fish sticks	200
Chicken	160	Duck	310
Pot roast	160	Loin roast	290
Fried liver	210	Swiss steak	300
Lean hamburger	145	Regular hamburger	240
Veal chop	185	Pork chop	340
Boiled ham	200	Sausage	405

Have a Serving of:	No. of Calories	Rather Than a Serving of:	No. of Calories
	Fruit and Vegetable Group		
Asparagus	30	Lima beans	160
Cauliflower	30	Corn	185
Summer squash	30	Winter squash	75
Spinach	40	Succotash	260
Cantaloupe	40	Banana	85
Fresh peas	115	Canned peas	145
Peach	35	Grapes	65
Boiled potatoes	100	Mashed potatoes	245
Baked potatoes	100	Fried potatoes	480
	Bread and Cereal Group		
Rice	100	Spaghetti	210
Rice-a-Roni	130	Elbow macaroni	210
Frozen waffle	120	Pancakes	240
Thomas' Protein Bread	45	Rye bread	70
Puffed rice	50	Rice flakes	110
Puffed wheat	50	Cream of wheat	100

Use this list to point out that the preparation can change the calorie content. Boiling, baking, steaming, and broiling are preferable, since frying, breading, and the use of gravies, sauces, and creams add calories. This fact is a major influence on the high calorie content of many fast foods. Patients who eat a lot of these foods should be provided with a list such as the following:

Popular Food	No. of Calories
Meat	
Burger King Whopper	606
McDonald's Big Mac	541
Burger Chef hamburger	285
Dairy Queen Brazier Dog	273
Chicken	
Kentucky Fried Original Dinner	830
Kentucky Fried Crispy Dinner	950
Fish	
Arthur Treacher's fish sandwich	440
Burger King Whaler	486
McDonald's Filet-O-Fish	402
Long John Silver's fish	318
Other entrees	
Pizza Hut thin pizza ($\frac{1}{2}$ pie)	450
Pizza Hut thick pepperoni ($\frac{1}{2}$ pie)	560
McDonald's Egg McMuffin	352

Popular Food	No. of Calories
Other entrees *(Continued)*	
Taco Bell taco	186
Taco Bell tostada	179
Taco Bell beef burrito	446
Side dishes	
Burger King french fries	214
Arthur Treacher's cole slaw	123
Dairy Queen onion rings	300
Beverages	
Burger King vanilla shake	332
McDonald's chocolate shake	364
Small cola drink	95
Small orange drink	117
Small root beer	103
Small Sprite	95
Desserts	
McDonald's apple pie	300

Source: Senate Committee on Nutrition and Human Needs.

Although fast foods are high in calories, they do have substantial nutritional value (particularly since salad bars are now offered by many chains). This distinguishes them from "junk foods" such as candy, cookies, and soda. Having little nutritional value, the latter merely add "empty calories," which must be eliminated from any weight reduction diet.

Stress that portions must be watched in order for low-calorie substitution to work. Eating larger-than-recommended portions defeats the purpose of the diet. For this reason, teach patients how to weigh, measure, and read the labels of all foods they eat. A measuring cup, food scale, and comprehensive calorie chart are needed. Calorie charts can be found in paperback or reference books on food values. Two good sources are:

Composition of Foods—Raw, Processed, Prepared. United States Department of Agriculture Handbook No. 8. Available from the Superintendent of Documents, U.S. Government Printing Office, Washington, D.C. 20402.

Nutrition: A Preventive Medicine Institute/Strang Clinic Health Action Plan by Cheryl Corbin. New York: Holt, Rinehart and Winston, 1980.

Explain that exercise is an important adjunct to diet in weight reduction. Calories expended in increased activity can be credited to the weekly food allowance. For example, 240 calories are burned up by the person who bicycles to work at a moderate pace for 30 minutes. These calories cancel out two scrambled eggs or a club steak added to the day's food plan. If not replaced by food, these calories will contribute to faster weight loss. Therefore, provide patients with a chart showing the number of calories expended in various activities such as the following:

Activity	Calories/ Minute	Activity	Calories/ Minute
Sedentary		Active	
Sleeping	1.2	Sawing wood	6.9
Sitting	1.4	Tennis	7.0
Reading	1.4	Shoveling	7.1
Kneeling	1.4	Rowing	8.0
Typing	1.5	Slow cycling	8.0
Sewing	1.5	Bowling	8.0
Eating	1.6	Basketball	8.6
Standing	1.6	Skiing	10.0
Sweeping floors	1.7	Squash	10.0
Playing cards	1.7	Handball	10.0
Driving a car	2.0	Fast cycling	11.0
Moderate		Swimming	12.1
Sailing	2.6	Running	17.0
Washing clothes	2.9	Stair climbing	20.0
Cooking	3.0		
Horseback riding	3.0		
Playing pool	3.0		
Walking indoors	3.4		
Showering	3.7		
Dancing	4.0		
Ironing	4.2		
Ping pong	4.8		
Chopping wood	4.9		
Making beds	5.3		
Mopping floors	5.3		
Stacking wood	6.1		
Walking outdoors	6.1		

Patients will need a well-planned program to start strenuous exercising (see Chapter 11).

Consider vitamin supplementation, since diets containing fewer than 1,400 calories/day may not meet the requirements for iron, thiamine, riboflavin, niacin, or vitamin E.

Patient Education: Dieting is based on the fact that 3,500 calories are needed to maintain 1 lb of body fat. Each week, by eating 7,000 calories less (1,000 calories less each day), 2 lb of body fat will disappear. However, patterns of weight loss vary from individual to individual and may fluctuate even though the caloric intake remains constant. This is because water accumulates in spaces where fat is lost and may cause temporary plateaus or gains in weight. This water is eventually eliminated, establishing a new weight level equilibrium. The patient should not become discouraged and waver from the diet at these times. A single high-carbohydrate meal may delay the loss of surplus water (and weight) for several days.

Keep a record of prediet and present calorie consumption such as:

Calories	Mon	Tues	Wed	Thur	Fri	Sat	Sun	Total
Original # Today's #								
Savings								

Chart daily weight loss toward ideal weight as follows:

Body weight																
200																
198																
196																
194																
↓																
176																
174																
172																
170																
Goal																
	1	2	3	4	5	6	7	8	9	10	11	12	13	14	15	16 days

Keep these general dieting guidelines in mind:

1. Plan a well-balanced diet based on lower-calorie foods and food preparations you like.
2. Learn to measure portions accurately, as well as the number of calories in everything you eat.
3. Stock up on low-calorie substitutes and do not keep high-calorie foods in the house.
4. Stay out of the kitchen when you are not preparing a meal.
5. Don't skip meals. It is easier to overeat if you are hungry.
6. If you become very hungry, control your appetite with a small "dose" of carbohydrate (2 soda crackers or a small glass of vegetable juice) one-half hour before mealtimes.
7. If you drink alcohol, have a glass of wine with dinner. It will slow eating and help satisfy hunger.
8. Always eat sitting down at the table.
9. Try using a smaller-sized dinner plate. Chew well. Eat slowly. Start the meal with a salad.
10. Learn to stop eating before you feel full. The slight hunger you feel will disappear half an hour after the meal.
11. Never take second helpings.
12. Budget calories to allow for extra eating on special occasions or weekends.
13. Increase your daily activity. Walk and use the stairs whenever you can. Try to adopt a regular exercise program.
14. Diet with a friend or join a support group.

Follow-up: Provide close support through weekly weight checks or phone conversations. Refer patients who need in-depth counseling to a registered dietitian. Encourage the use of group organizations whenever possible.

▸ *Support Groups for Weight Loss*

Laboratory Tests: None.

Therapeutic Measures: None.

Patient Education: Overeaters Anonymous
World Services Office
2190 West 190th Street
Torrance, California 90504

Follow-up: Help patients make contact as needed.

▸ *Hepatitis A Virus (HAV)*

Laboratory Tests: Chemical screening for liver enzymes (SGPT, SGOT) and bilirubin. Urine for bilirubin. Anti-HAV (IgM) or acute and convalescent titers of anti-HAV (IgG).

Therapeutic Measures: Use enteric precautions (see Chapter 4). Prescribe bed rest as needed during the acute illness, with a gradual return to normal activity. Food of the patient's choosing should be divided into five to six small meals (with the largest meal at breakfast, when nausea is least bothersome). Hard candy, fruit juices, and carbonated beverages are well tolerated and help fill caloric requirements. Protein restriction is required only with impending PSE. Emphasize that alcohol and other hepatotoxic agents must be eliminated during the acute illness. Evaluate the use of medications the patient is currently taking (including oral contraceptives, which are metabolized largely by the liver). Small amounts of alcohol may be taken during the convalescent period.

Patient Education: Explain the viral cause of the illness and the oral-fecal routes of transmission. Reassure the patient that the disease is self-limiting and that most courses are mild. Severe symptoms should be reported. Note specifically that HAV does not lead to chronic liver disease or to carrier states, but in rare cases enzymes remain elevated for 4–6 months after infection. Discuss ISG recommendations for contacts and travelers (see the next section).

Follow-up: As needed for work clearance (patients may return to work as tolerated once the acute illness is over).

▸ *Immune Serum Globulin*

Laboratory Tests: None.

Therapeutic Measures: Recommend ISG as follows:

1. To prevent or ameliorate disease among the close personal contacts (household or sexual) of a person sick with HAV or NANB, give ISG, 0.02 mL/kg IM within 2 weeks of exposure.
2. To prevent epidemic spread when a case is reported in settings predisposed to poor personal hygiene or fecal soiling (mental retardation homes, psychiatric institutions, day-care centers), give ISG, 0.02 mL/kg IM, within 2 weeks of single exposure and an additional 0.05 mL/kg every 4 months for repeated exposures. Prophylaxis is not effective in outbreaks from common sources such as contaminated food, water, and shellfish.
3. To prevent disease among travelers to endemic areas, give ISG at least 2 weeks after live attenuated vaccines are administered. The dose is based on the length of stay and the body weight as follows:

Length of Stay	Body Weight	IM Dose (mL)
Less than 3 months	Less than 50 lb or 23 kg	0.5
	50–100 lb or 23–43 kg	1.0
	More than 100 lb or 45 kg	2.0
More than 3 months*	Less than 50 lb or 23 kg	1.0
	50–100 lb or 23–43 kg	2.5
	More than 100 lb or 45 kg	5.0

*Repeat every 4–6 months for very prolonged stays. Check the most recent issue of *Health Information for International Travel* (see Chapter 4 for the address).

4. To offer some protection to persons exposed to hepatitis B when HISG is unavailable or unaffordable, give 0.06 mL/kg body weight IM immediately.

Patient Education: For persons exposed to hepatitis, ISG has its greatest value with early administration and is of no value after 2 weeks. It provides only passive, short-time immunity, so that travelers or persons with repeated exposures will require subsequent injections. Side effects of vaccination include a local reaction and, rarely, anaphylaxis. The cost is relatively low ($3–10 per injection).

Follow-up: None.

▸ *Hepatitis B Virus (HBV)*

Laboratory Tests: Chemical screening for liver enzymes (SGPT, SGOT) and bilirubin. Urine for bilirubin. HBsAg in early disease. HBcAg or HBeAg to show recent disease and continued infectivity. Anti-HBs with past disease and immunity.

Therapeutic Measures: Prescribe bed rest as needed during the acute illness, with a gradual return to normal activity. Food of the patient's choosing should be divided into five to six small meals (offer the largest meal at breakfast, when nausea is least bothersome). Hard candy, fruit juices, and carbonated beverages are well tolerated and help fill caloric requirements. Protein restriction is necessary only with impending PSE. Emphasize that alcohol and other hepatotoxic agents must be eliminated during the acute illness. Evaluate the use of medications the patient is currently taking, including oral contraceptives. Small amounts of alcohol may be taken during the convalescent period.

Patient Education: Explain the viral cause of the disease, routes of transmission, and expected course of the illness (3–16 weeks). Have patients report worsening symptoms immediately. Review recommendations for contacts (see the next section). Stress the need for careful hand washing and precautions when using needles. Close personal or sexual contact should be avoided during the acute illness.

Follow-up: Patients who become severely dehydrated or show signs of liver failure should be hospitalized. Patients treated at home should return for clinical evaluation and enzyme studies every week during the acute illness and then every month until they are normal. If enzymes remain elevated beyond 6 months, a chronic hepatitis work-up is necessary. Check HBsAg levels at 3, 6, and 12 months. If the patient remains HBsAg positive after 1 year, begin management for the carrier state (see the next section). Patients may return to work as tolerated after the acute illness is over.

▸ *Hepatitis B Carrier State*

Laboratory Tests: Liver enzymes (normal). HBsAg (positive for more than 6 months).

Therapeutic Measures: HBIG or hepatitis B vaccine for contacts as recommended in the next sections. There are no restrictions on work or school activities as long as careful hygiene is practiced.

Patient Education: Explain the antigenemia following a known or subclinical case of hepatitis B. Reassure patients that they have recovered from HBV without any damage to the liver and are immune to further infections. However, they are at increased risk for superinfection with hepatitis D virus. Furthermore, as carriers of virus particles, they may be a source of infection to other people. To reduce this risk, carriers should:

1. Never donate blood and avoid the common use of razors and instruments for IV drugs, ear piercing, acupuncture, or tattooing (transmission through blood).
2. Advise sexual partners about potential risks (transmission through semen, vaginal secretions, menstrual blood).
3. Arrange prophylaxis or vaccination for close contacts as needed.

4. Inform medical and dental workers before venipuncture, oral procedures, and so on so that gloves can be worn and other precautions taken.
5. Not be overly concerned about kissing, sneezing, or sharing cigarettes, drinking or eating utensils. Although the saliva, tears, nasopharyngeal secretions, and feces of carriers may contain small amounts of HBV, they are generally not a significant source of disease transmission.
6. Be tested for HBeAg if they are health care workers. If the test is positive, they should practice meticulous hygiene and wear gloves for any procedure that may expose their blood to the patient's blood or mucous membranes. Unless otherwise required, surgical gowns and masks are unnecessary.

Follow-up: None.

▸ *Hepatitis B Hyperimmune Globulin (HBIG)*

Laboratory Tests: Confirm the antigen status of the contact. R/O the carrier state (HBsAg) and immunity (anti-HBs) in the exposed patient, since HBIG is not indicated if these tests are positive.

Therapeutic Measures: Recommend the use of HBIG (e.g., HyperHep, Hep-B-Gammagee) for the following conditions or persons:

1. Exposure through mucous membranes or skin puncture to blood (on pipettes, hypodermic needles, tattooing or ear-piercing apparatus, surgical or dental instruments) or body secretions (semen, saliva, tears, but probably not feces) of an HBsAg-positive individual. Give 0.06 mL per kilogram of body weight immediately and a second dose (same amount) 1 month later.
2. Sexual contact with a person who has hepatitis B or is a carrier. Give HBIG, 0.06 mL per kilogram of body weight, within 7 days.
3. Infants born to mothers who are known to be chronic carriers or who contracted hepatitis B in the third trimester. Give 0.13 mL/kg IM at birth. For continued exposure and as long as the baby remains HBsAg negative, repeat the dose at 3 months. If baby is still negative at 6 months, give vaccine (see the next section).

Patient Education: HBIG has its greatest value during early administration and is indicated only within the first 7 days after exposure. It provides only passive, short-term immunity. ISG is preferred for travelers, 80% of related hepatitis being type A. Side effects of vaccination include a local reaction and, rarely, anaphylaxis. The cost is relatively high (approximately $40 for laboratory tests and $180 per injection).

Follow-up: None.

▸ *Hepatitis B Vaccine*

Laboratory Tests: R/O carrier state (HBsAg) and immunity (anti-HBs) in the proposed recipient. If either is present, use of the vaccine is not indicated.

Therapeutic Measures: Advise the use of the vaccine for the following high-risk populations: (1) health care workers, with priority for dialysis unit and laboratory workers, emergency room nurses, IV and blood bank teams, oral surgeons, and dental providers or intensive care unit and house staff, oncologists; (2) homosexual men; (3) drug addicts; (4) babies whose mothers are chronic carriers; (5) institutionalized residents, particularly if immunosuppressed (e.g., those with Down's syndrome); (6) military personnel or travelers spending prolonged periods in endemic areas; and (7) household or sexual contacts of chronic carriers. Due to lack of testing, administration has not been approved during pregnancy or lactation.

Vaccinate as follows:

For dialysis or immunosuppressed patients, give two series: two 1-mL injections IM at different sites followed by the same dose 1 month later.

For children over age 10 and adults, give three series: 1 mL IM followed by the same dose 1 month and 6 months later.

For children 3 months to 10 years old, give three series: 0.5 mL IM followed by the same dose 1 month and 6 months later.

Store the vaccine in a refrigerator, but avoid freezing.

Patient Education: Vaccine provides 80–95% protection from HBV infection. The duration of this protection is still unknown; further trials may indicate the need for boosters. The side effects are usually mild. They include soreness at the injection site, low-grade fever, malaise, fatigue, headache, nausea, dizziness, achiness, and rash during the first 48 hours.

Follow-up: For boosters, should they become recommended.

▸ *Non-A, Non-B (NANB) Hepatitis*

Laboratory Tests: Chemical screening for liver enzymes, bilirubin. Urine bilirubin. Anti-HAV (negative), HBsAg (negative).

Therapeutic Measures: Same as for hepatitis B. Consider ISG for contacts.

Patient Education: Same as for hepatitis B.

Follow-up: Patients who become severely dehydrated or show signs of liver failure should be hospitalized. Patients treated at home should return for clinical evaluation and enzyme studies every week during the acute illness and then every month until normal. If enzymes remain elevated beyond 6 months, a work-up for chronic hepatitis is necessary.

▸ *Alcoholic Hepatitis*

Laboratory Tests: Complete blood count, SMAC.

Therapeutic Measures: Strict avoidance of alcohol and hepatotoxic agents. Refer to the patient to Alcoholics Anonymous if he or she is willing. If there is no PSE, start the patient on a high-protein (1 g protein per kilogram of body weight), high-calorie (2,000–3,000) diet. For nausea or vomiting, advise small, frequent feedings with high-calorie snacks. Vitamin supplements, particularly vitamin B_1, should be given.

Patient Education: Explain the progressive nature of the disease. Stress the fact that no treatment will protect the liver from further damage if drinking continues.

Follow-up: Patients who have signs of ascites, impending liver failure, or withdrawal should be hospitalized. Visits should be scheduled every week during the acute illness and every 4–6 months thereafter for supportive care.

▸ *Laennec's Cirrhosis*

Laboratory Tests: Complete blood count, SMAC, prothrombin time, partial thromboplastin time. If the patient is young, check the serum ceruloplasmin and urine copper to rule out Wilson's disease.

Therapeutic Measures: Have patients discontinue alcohol use and avoid other hepatotoxins. Provide supportive care. Intervene for ascites and/or PSE as they develop. Otherwise, there is no specific therapy.

Patient Education: Explain the irreversible nature of the illness. For alcoholics, stress the fact that discontinuance of drinking halts disease progression, whereas continued drinking is fatal. Instruct patients to report hematuria, tarry stools, bleeding gums, easy bruisability, and hematemesis.

Follow-up: Every 4–6 months for supportive care.

▸ *Early Stages of PSE*

Laboratory Tests: Blood ammonia levels (do not always correlate with severity of encephalopathy). Psychometric testing (tests concentration, verbal fluency, visual motor reaction time). EEG.

Therapeutic Measures: Treat the underlying problem if possible. Discontinue the use of sedatives, tranquilizers, or other medicines that depend on hepatic metabolism if possible. Maintain a protein-restricted diet (40–60 g/day), with limited intake of red meats that are high in aromatic amino acids (AAA). However, give protein supplements rich in branch chain amino acids (BCAA), since increasing the BCAA:AAA ratio may improve symptoms. Start lactulose 20 cc qid (or amount needed to produce two to three bowel movements per day). This decreases the intestinal pH and increases the bowel transit time, both of which prevent NH_4 from leaving the gut. To reduce the amount of intestinal bacteria that produce cerebral toxins, give neomycin, 2 to 4 g/day (discontinue immediately if tinnitis develops).

Patient Education: Explain the etiology of the disease and the rationale for all treatments. Advise patients to decrease the intake of lactulose if diarrhea or constipation develops. Have them (or family members) report signs of infection or exacerbation (lethargy, fatigue, irritability, confusion).

Follow-up: Frequent visits are needed to monitor drug therapy, to repeat psychometric tests, and to provide support. Patients with acute exacerbations require hospitalization.

▸ *Ascites*

Laboratory Tests: SMAC; possible examination of ascitic fluid.

Therapeutic Measures: Treat the underlying cause if possible. Restrict sodium to 2 g/day. Provide a diet adequate in vitamins, minerals, and protein (make adjustments if there is coexisting PSE). To reduce the fluid load, use diuretics (potassium-sparing, with or without Lasix) with extreme caution. During diuresis, monitor blood urea nitrogen, electrolytes, and creatinine clearance. Ascites is rarely life-threatening, but overaggressive therapy can be.

Patient Education: Explain the etiology of the problem and the rationale for treatment. Teach patients to monitor their daily weight and abdominal girth. Note that the upright position may be the most comfortable during bed rest. Advise frequent change in positions while lying or sitting to prevent skin breakdown (tissue perfusion is compromised by increased intra-abdominal pressure and interstitial edema).

Follow-up: Monthly visits are needed to monitor weight, abdominal girth, and electrolytes. Severely compromised patients may need to be hospitalized for a peritoneal tap.

▸ *Gilbert's Syndrome*

Laboratory Tests: Liver enzymes (normal). Bilirubin (mildly elevated, unconjugated).

Therapeutic Measures: None. Avoidance of prolonged fasting may help avert episodes of jaundice. Treat any intercurrent illness that is present.

Patient Education: Explain the etiology and genetic predisposition (autosomal dominant trait). Reassure the patient that the condition is benign and does not result in chronic liver disease. Advise the patient that increased jaundice may indicate another illness or hemolysis and should be evaluated.

Follow-up: None required.

BIBLIOGRAPHY

Abramowicz M (ed.). Drugs for parasitic infections. *The Medical Letter on Drugs and Therapeutics,* (Dec.) 1979, 21(26):105–112.

Albanese AA. Nutrition in the elderly. *Physician Assistant and Health Practitioner,* (Aug.) 1980, 16–20.

Ali AS, Baig FN. Hepatorenal syndrome. *American Family Physician,* (June) 1982, 25(6):127–131.

Almy TP. Dietary fiber: Current role in therapy and preventive medicine. *PA Drug Update,* (Oct.) 1984, 16–24.

Anderson JW. High-fiber diets in diabetes. *Continuing Education,* (Apr.) 1981, 22–27.

Anderson JW. Fiber, carbohydrate, and diabetes. *Nutrition and the MD,* (July) 1981, 7(7):1–5.

Anderson JW, Sieling B. *HCF Diets: A Professional Guide.* University of Kentucky Diabetes Research and Education Fund, Lexington, Ky., 1979.

Bates B. *A Guide to Physical Examination.* Lippincott, Philadelphia, 1974.

Becker K. Hypoglycemia: Diagnosis and treatment. *The Female Patient,* (Oct.) 1979, 69–71.

Beeson P (ed.), et al. *Textbook of Medicine.* Saunders, Philadelphia, 1979.

Berkow RB (ed.). *The Merck Manual of Diagnosis and Therapy,* 14th ed. Merck, Sharp & Dohme Research Laboratories, Rahway, N.J., 1982.

Best C, Taylor N. *The Physiological Basis of Medical Practice.* Williams & Wilkins, Baltimore, 1966.

Bird WF Jr, et al. Make diabetes control a family affair. *PA Practice,* 1982, 1(2):4–6.

Blumberg BS. Introduction: The clinical laboratory diagnosis of viral hepatitis. Laboratory Management, (Jan.) 1983, 17–27.

Boyer TD. Variations in hepatic failure. *Emergency Medicine,* (Nov.) 1984, 97–112.

Brecher DB. Home glucose monitoring. *American Family Physician,* (Jan.) 1984, 29(1):241–244.

Brody J. *Jane Brody's Nutrition Book.* Norton, New York, 1981.

Brown AM, Stubbs DW (eds.). *Medical Physiology.* Wiley, New York, 1983.

Brownlee M, Vlassara H. Exercise and the diabetic patient. *Drug Therapy,* (Mar.) 1982, 66–72.

Bryan J. Viral hepatitis: Clinical and laboratory aspects and epidemiology. *Postgraduate Medicine,* (Nov.) 1980, 68(5):66–76.

Burke MD. Diabetes mellitus: Test strategies for diagnosis and management. *Postgraduate Medicine,* (Nov.) 1979, 213–218.

Cashman MD. Geriatric Malnutrition: Recognition and correction. *Postgraduate Medicine,* (Mar.) 1982, 71(3):185–194.

Cherner R. Diabetic patients: Check *all* the drugs they take. *Consultant,* (Oct.) 1979, 202–208.

Colwell JA. Specialized management of diabetes mellitus. *Continuing Education,* (June) 1982, 63–72.

Committee on Education for Diabetics of the American Diabetes Association. *Understanding Your Diabetes.* Pfizer Laboratories, New York, 1981.

Conn HF, Conn RB Jr (eds.). *Current Diagnosis.* Saunders, Philadelphia, 1980.

Crafts RC. *A Textbook of Human Anatomy,* 3rd ed. Wiley, New York, 1985.

Crouch JE, McClintic JR. *Human Anatomy and Physiology,* 2nd ed. Wiley, New York, 1976.

Davidson MB. How age affects carbohydrate metabolism. *Drug Therapy,* (Mar.) 1984, 83–105.

Derelian D, Schaefer D. Clinical use of the "four food groups." *Nutrition and the MD,* (Dec.) 1981, 7(12):1–5.

Devlin J, Horton E. Diet and exercise: Important therapeutic tools. *Drug Therapy,* (Mar.) 1984, 109–115.

Devlin J, Horton E. Diet and exercise: The keys to controlling type II diabetes. *Drug Therapy,* (Mar.) 1984, 135–136.

Dzik WH, Alter HJ. Hepatitis B viral infection, part II: Public health aspects. *American Family Physician,* (Sept.) 1982, 26(3):135–142.

Eastwood M. Nutrition: The changing scene. *Lancet,* (July) 1983.

Eddy LJ. Pharmacology of the agents used to treat diabetes mellitus. *Continuing Education,* (Feb.) 1980, 84–91.

Elias H, Pauly JE, Burns ER. *Histology and Human Microanatomy,* 4th ed. Wiley, New York, 1978.

Ellenberg M. Chronic complications of diabetes mellitus. *New York State Journal of Medicine,* (Dec.) 1979, 2005–2014.

Ellenberg M. Oral hypoglycemic agents: A status report. *Consultant,* (Mar.) 1980, 223–231.

Epstein M. A rational approach to the management of ascites. *Drug Therapy,* (Mar.) 1982, 167–176.

Epstein M. Renal complications of liver disease. *Clinical Symposia,* 1985, 37(5):3–32.

Farthing MJG. Hepatitis: A special problem, part 2: Chronic hepatitis. *The Female Patient,* (Oct.) 1984, 9:48–51.

Feinglos MN. When to prescribe sulfonylureas and insulin. *Drug Therapy,* (Mar.) 1984, 127–134.

Feng CS. Immunoglobulin prophylaxis for viral hepatitis. *The Journal of Family Practice,* 1982, 14(4):677–681.

Food and Nutrition Board. *Recommended Dietary Allowances,* 9th rev. ed. National Academy of Sciences, Washington, D.C., 1980.

Forsham PH. Diabetes mellitus. *Postgraduate Medicine,* (Mar.) 1982, 71(3):139–153.

Galambos, J. A five-level approach to treating ascites. *Consultant,* (Jan.) 1980, 89–95.

Galambos J, Hersh T. *Digestive Diseases.* Butterworth, Boston, 1983.

Genuth SM. Type II diabetes mellitus: Why the response to insulin is impaired. *Drug Therapy,* (Mar.) 1984, 64–80.

Gibson JC, Brown WV. The human plasma apolipoproteins: Assay methods, part I. *Laboratory Management,* (Mar.) 1983, 19–27.

Gibson JC, Brown WV. The human plasma apolipoproteins: Assay methods, part II. *Laboratory Management,* (Apr.) 1983, 27–35.

Gitnick G. Non-A, non-B hepatitis: Etiology and clinical course. *Laboratory Medicine,* (Nov.) 1983, 14(11):721–726.

Goldstein JL, Brown MS. Low-density lipoproteins and atherosclerosis. *Cardiovascular Reviews and Reports,* 1982, 17–22.

Goroll AH, May LA, Mulley AG. *Primary Care Medicine: Office Evaluation and Management of the Adult Patient.* Lippincott, Philadelphia, 1981.

Gotto AM Jr. The plasma apolipoproteins: Regulation of the structure and function of the plasma lipoproteins. *Cardiovascular Reviews and Reports,* 1982, 12–16.

Gray H. *Anatomy of the Human Body,* 29th American edition. (CM Goss, ed.). Lea & Febiger, Philadelphia, 1973.

Greenberger N. *Gastrointestinal Disorders.* Year Book Medical Publishers, Chicago, 1981.

Gregg B, Behm P. *High Protein, Low Carbohydrate Diet for Spontaneous Hypoglycemia.* Carnation Company, Pico Rivera, Calif., 1980.

Griber M, Nuwer N. Treating esophageal varices with sclerotherapy. *American Journal of Nursing,* (Aug.) 1982.

Grundy SM. Experience with individual lipid-lowering drugs: Clofibrate. *Cardiovascular Reviews and Reports,* 1982, 40–44.

Guthrie D. Helping the diabetic manage his self-care. *Nursing80,* (Feb.) 1980, 57–64.

Guyton AC. The liver and biliary system, in *Textbook of Medical Physiology,* 6th ed. Saunders, Philadelphia, 1981.

Hamburger SC, Rush DR. Pathogenesis and treatment of diabetic ketoacidosis. *Family Practice Recertification,* (Oct.) 1979, 1(6):45–65.

Hamby RI, Shermay L. Duration and treatment of diabetes: Relationship to severity of coronary artery disease. *New York State Journal of Medicine,* (Oct.) 1979, 1683–1692.

Harrington TM. Infection control. *The Physician Assistant Drug Newsletter,* 1983.

Havel RJ. Experience with individual lipid-lowering drugs: Nicotinic acid. *Cardiovascular Reviews and Reports,* 1982, 48–49.

Henry JB (ed.). *Todd-Sanford-Davidson Clinical Diagnosis and Management by Laboratory Methods,* 16th ed., Vols. 1 and 2. Saunders, Philadelphia, 1979.

Herbert PN. Experience with individual lipid-lowering drugs: Probucol. *Cardiovascular Reviews and Reports,* 1982, 38–39.

Herbert V. Facts and fictions about megavitamin therapy. *Resident and Staff Physician,* (Dec.) 1978, 43–50.

Hirschman SZ. The hepatitis B vaccine: Current recommendations for use. *PA Drug Update,* (May) 1983, 57–66.

Hoffnagle JH. Type A and type B hepatitis. *Laboratory Medicine,* (Nov.) 1983, 14(11):705–716.

Hoole AJ, Greenberg RA, Pickard CG Jr. *Patient Care Guidelines for Nurse Practitioners.* Little, Brown, Boston, 1982.

Howell D, et al. Current medical management of diverticular disease. *Consultant,* (Sept.) 1981.

Hunninghake DB. Experience with individual lipid-lowering drugs: Bile-acid sequestrants. *Cardiovascular Reviews and Reports,* 1982, 45–46.

Isselbacher KJ, et al. *Harrison's Principles of Internal Medicine,* 9th ed. McGraw-Hill, New York, 1980.

Jenkens DJA. Diabetes and hyperlipidemia: Dietary implications of treatment with fiber. *Practical Cardiology,* (Oct.) 1980, 6(11):123–134.

Kirschmann J. *Nutrition Almanac.* MaGraw-Hill, New York, 1979.

Koff RS. *Viral Hepatitis.* Wiley, New York, 1978.

Koivisto VA, Sherwin RS. Exercise in diabetes: Therapeutic implications. *Postgraduate Medicine,* (Nov.) 1979, 66(5):87–95.

Krause M, et al. *Food, Nutrition and Diet Therapy.* Saunders, Philadelphia, 1978.

Krugman S. Hepatitis B immunoprophylaxis. *Laboratory Medicine,* (Nov.) 1983, 14(11):727–732.

Krupp MA, Chatton MJ, Werdegar D (eds.). *Current Medical Diagnosis and Treatment 1985.* Lange, Los Altos, Calif., 1985.

Langley L, Telford I, Christensen J. Anatomy of the digestive system, in *Dynamic Anatomy and Physiology.* McGraw-Hill, New York, 1976, pp. 596–598.

Levy RI. The mechanisms of action of lipid-lowering drugs. *Cardiovascular Reviews and Reports,* 1982, 34–37.

Liebrandt T (ed.). *Diabetes.* Intermed Communications, Horsham, Pa., 1981, pp. 722–747.

Luckmann J, Sorensen KC. *Medical Surgical Nursing: A Psychophysiologic Approach,* 2nd ed. Saunders, Philadelphia, 1980.

Mahler RJ. Maturity onset diabetes: Current basis for treatment. *Consultant,* (Feb.) 1980, 23–30.

Mann JM, Ahtone JL. Prophylaxis for hepatitis A. *American Family Physician,* (Mar.) 1982, 25(3):129–132.

Manninen V. Clinical investigation of gemfibrozil: The treatment of dyslipidemia. *Cardiovascular Reviews and Reports,* 1982, 56–57.

Mayfield RK, Wohltmann HJ. New methods of managing the insulin-dependent diabetic patient. *Continuing Education,* (June) 1982, 55–62.

McFarland KF. Care of the pregnant diabetic. *Postgraduate Medicine,* (Nov.) 1979, 64–71.

Meddrey WC. When dry toxicity underlies hepatitis. *Patient Care,* (Nov.) 1979, 143–162.

Melnick DE. Future management of diabetes mellitus. *Postgraduate Medicine,* (Nov.) 1979, 66(5):101–110.

Miller D. Seroepidemiology of viral hepatitis. *Postgraduate Medicine,* (Sept.) 1980, 68(3):137–147.

Miller NE. Lipoproteins and atherosclerosis: Epidemiologic and metabolic considerations. *Cardiovascular Reviews and Reports,* 1982, 26–29.

Mirsky S. Hypoglycemia. *Physician Assistant,* (Dec.) 1983, 19–26.

Moss JM. New diagnostic classification of diabetes mellitus. *American Family Physician,* (Feb.) 1981, 23(2):179–181.

Munro HN. The ninth edition of recommended dietary allowances. *Nutrition and the MD,* (Feb.) 1980, 6(2):1–6.

Nanji AA. Hypoglycemia: When it's the real thing. *Diagnostic Medicine,* (Oct.) 1983, 60–70.

Nash DT. Clinical investigation of gemfibrozil: Gemfibrozil versus clofibrate. *Cardiovascular Reviews and Reports,* 1982, 58–60.

National Heart and Lung Institute. *The Dietary Management of Hyperlipoproteinemia.* Department of Health, Education, and Welfare, Bethesda, Md., 1976.

National Research Council. *Estimated Safe and Adequate Daily Dietary Intakes,* RDA 9th ed. Washington, D.C., 1980.

Newell J. Portal systemic encephalopathy. *Nurse Practitioner,* (July) 1984, 9(7).

Nyhan WL. Understanding inherited metabolic disease. (ME McKinsey, ed.). *Clinical Symposia,* 1980, 32(5):2–35.

Peabody HD Jr. Clinical investigation of gemfibrozil: The treatment of primary hyperlipoproteinemia. *Cardiovascular Reuiews and Reports,* 1982, 50–55.

Penn I. Management of the diabetic foot. *Continuing Education,* (Oct.) 1980, 37–44.

Pennwalt Corporation. *Are You Really Serious About Losing Weight?* 5th ed. Pennwalt Corp., Rochester, N.Y., 1982.

Peoples M. The dysvascular foot in diabetes mellitus. *PA Outlook,* (Nov.) 1983, 10–16.

Podolsky S. Pitfalls in managing the elderly diabetic. *PA Drug Update.* (Oct.) 1983, 36–44.

Polesky HF, Hanson M. Transfusion-associated hepatitis: A dilemma. *Laboratory Medicine,* (Nov.) 1983, 14(11):717–720.

Prosser PR. Diabetes mellitus: Diet therapy for the non-insulin-dependent patient. *Consultant,* (Feb.) 1982, 209–218.

Ranch J, McWeeny M. *Managing Your Diabetes.* Eli Lilly, Indianapolis, 1982.

Ross R. Lipoproteins, endothelial injury, and atherosclerosis. *Cardiovasclar Reviews and Reports,* 1982, 6–11.

Rubin JM. Food allergies. *Hospital Medicine,* (Mar.) 1982, 86–90.

Schaffner F. Remove the "rarity" label from PBC? *Patient Care,* (Dec.) 1979, 80–97.

Schiff L (ed.), et al. *Diseases of the Liver.* Lippincott, Philadelphia, 1982.

Schonfield LJ (AH Trench, ed.). Gallstones and other biliary diseases. Clinical Symposia, 1982, 34(4):2–32.

Seltzer HS. Evaluation of the patient with borderline glucose intolerance. *Practical Cardiology,* (Feb.) 1980, 6(2):55–65.

Shuman CR. Management of diabetes today. *Continuing Education,* (Oct.) 1982, 55–76.

Silverstein A. *Human Anatomy and Physiology.* Wiley, New York, 1980.

Sloan RW. Hyperlipidemia. *American Family Physician,* (Sept.) 1983, 28(3):171–182.

Sorting out heartburn's causes. *Acute Care Medicine,* (Jan.) 1984, 59–65.

Spiro H. *Clinical Gastroenterology,* 3rd ed. Macmillan, New York, 1983.

Steinberg D. High-density lipoproteins and atherogenesis. *Cardiovascular Reviews and Reports,* 1982, 23–25.

Stoerner JW. Neonatal jaundice. *American Family Physician,* (Nov.) 1981, 24(5):226–232.

Tideiksaar R. Factors that affect nutrition in the elderly patient. *Physician Assistant and Health Practitioner,* (Feb.) 1983, 23–28.

VonSeggen W. Portal-systemic encephalopathy: Recognition and management. *PA Outlook,* (Dec.) 1983, 5–11.

Watlington CO. The oral glucose tolerance test. *The Journal of Family Practice,* 1979, 9(5):915–919.

Weinstein I. Pharmacological treatment of abnormalities of lipid metabolism. *Continuing Education,* (Feb.) 1980, 55–60.

Weissman HM, Freeman LM. Evaluating hepatobiliary disease with cholescintigraphy. *Diagnostic Medicine,* (May/June) 1983, 32–46.

Wyngaarden JB, Smith LH Jr (eds.). *Cecil Textbook of Medicine,* 16th ed., Vols. 1 and 2, Saunders, Philadelphia, 1982.

Zimmerman HJ. Drugs that can cause icterus. *Consultant,* (Feb.) 1982, 76–89.

6

Cardiopulmonary System

Mary Alice Higgins Donius

Outline

Sarcoidosis
Fungal diseases (histoplasmosis, coccidioidomycosis, blastomycosis)
Opportunistic infections

Pulmonary Circulation

Pulmonary edema (initial phase, acute)
Acute respiratory distress syndrome (ARDS)
Pulmonary emboli

Protective Features (Chest Wall and Pleura)

Chest trauma
Pleurisy
Pleural effusion
Mesothelioma
Metastatic disease of the pleura
Pleurodynia

HEART

Myocardium and Heart Chambers

Congenital heart defects
Myocarditis
Rheumatic fever (RF)
Chronic rheumatic heart disease
Prevention of recurrent RF
Cardiomyopathies (primary, secondary, dilated, hypertrophic, restrictive)
► Congestive heart failure (CHF)
Cardiac overload

Electrical Control of Myocardial Contractions

Cardiac arrhythmias (atrial, junctional, ventricular)

Blood Flow Through the Heart Chambers and Great Vessels

Valvular disease
Chronic rheumatic heart disease
Mitral valve stenosis
P-mitrale
Mitral valve regurgitation
Papillary muscle dysfunction
Ruptured chordae tendinae
Mitral valve prolapse
Aortic stenosis
Idiopathic hypertrophic subaortic stenosis (IHSS)
Aortic regurgitation
Quincke's sign
Duroziez's murmur
Tricuspid valvular disease
Tricuspid regurgitation

Coronary Circulation

Coronary artery disease (CAD)
Arteriosclerosis
Atherosclerosis
► Reducing CAD risk factors
► Angina (stable, unstable, Prinzmetal's)
Myocardial infarction (MI)
Coronary artery bypass graft (CABG)
Percutaneous transluminal coronary angioplasty (PTCA)
Streptokinase
Plasminogen

Protective Features (Endocardium and Pericardium)

Infectious endocarditis (acute and subacute)
► Endocarditis prophylaxis
Acute pericarditis
Pericardial effusion
Ewart's sign
Cardiac tamponade
Chronic pericardial effusion
Constrictive pericarditis
Effusive-constrictive pericarditis

PERIPHERAL CIRCULATION

Arteries

► Essential hypertension
► Peripheral vascular disease
► Raynaud's disease
Takayasu arteritis
Acute arterial occlusion
Beurger's disease

Veins

► Varicose veins
Thrombophlebitis
Homan's sign
► Long-term anticoagulant therapy

LUNGS

Respiration

Air moves into and out of the lungs, as illustrated in Figure 6.1, by the processes of inspiration and expiration. In inspiration, intercostal muscle, rib, and diaphragm movements expand the thoracic cavity and reduce intrapulmonic pressure. Air enters the lungs. In quiet expiration, the diaphragm and intercostal muscles relax, the thoracic cavity reassumes its smaller size, and the lungs recoil. Air is passively expelled. Deep inspiration and expiration require additional muscle activity from diaphragm, intercostal, and abdominal muscles. The amount and force of air that can be inspired and expired provide various measurements of pulmonary function, as described in Table 6.1.

Neurologic centers in the brain, guided by input from peripheral chemoreceptors, control the respiratory process, as pictured Figure 6.2 and described in Table 6.2. They maintain normal ventilation in an adult that is characterized by diaphragmatic breathing at a regular, uninterrupted rate of 12–20 respirations per minute. Neurologic centers also make adjustments according to tissue demands for oxygen. The central and peripheral chemoreceptors initiate increased respiration as soon as blood levels of carbon dioxide rise. As discussed at length in a later section, the partial pressures of oxygen and carbon dioxide are normally balanced. Rising levels of P_{CO_2} occur during strenuous exercise when large skeletal muscles use 10–20 times more oxygen than normal and in conditions marked by lowered tissue perfusion such as reduced cardiac output, vascular insufficiency, or edema. Crossing from the blood to the cerebrospinal fluid (CSF), increased P_{CO_2} levels trigger a series of events. First, the CO_2 changes to carbonic acid (H_2CO_3) and then separates to form hydrogen ions (H^+ ions) and bicarbonate (HCO_3). The increase in H^+ ions, along with the increase in P_{CO_2}, lowers the pH of CSF and stimulates chemoreceptors. This activates the respiratory center to increase ventilation and the exhalation of CO_2.

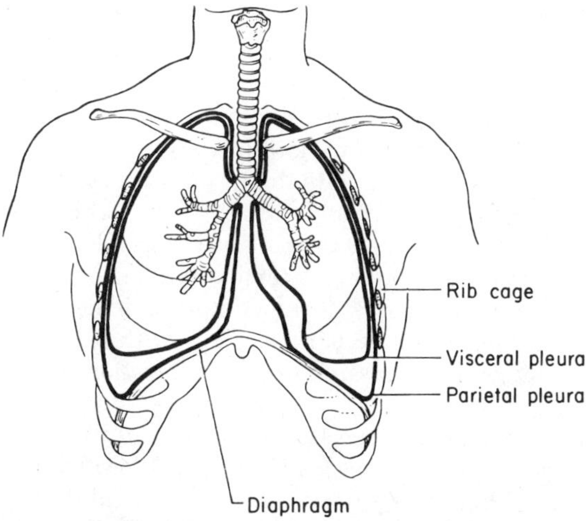

Figure 6.1 The lungs. (From Brown AM, Stubbs DW, *Medical Physiology,* copyright © 1983 by John Wiley & Sons, Inc. Reprinted by permission.)

TABLE 6.1 MEASUREMENTS OF PULMONARY FUNCTION

Term	Description
Ventilation	Movement of air into and out of lungs.
Tidal volume	Volume of air exchanged with each normal respiratory cycle (inspiration and expiration). Coded as VT, the tidal volume is normally 500 mL, 350 mL of air entering the alveoli and 150 mL remaining in the airways.
Expiratory reserve volume (ERV)	The largest volume of air that can be forcibly expelled after the tidal volume has been expired. The normal range is 1,000–1,200 mL. This volume is an index of the mobility and strength of thoracic and abdominal muscles.
Residual volume (RV)	The air remaining in the lungs after a forceful expiration, about 1,200 mL. This is the air remaining for ventilatory exchange at the alveolocapillary membranes between breaths.
Inspiratory reserve volume (IRV)	The volume of air that can be inspired above the tidal volume (usually 3,000 mL). It is an index of the muscle strength and elasticity of the lungs and thoracic wall.
Inspiratory capacity (IC)	Tidal volume and inspiratory reserve volume together. It is the largest volume of air inspirable after a normal expiration.
Functional residual capacity (FRC)	Expiratory reserve volume added to residual volume. It is the volume of air still in the lungs at the end of a normal expiration (normally 2,200–2,400 mL) When this value is increased, a state of hyperinflation exists, as in emphysema.
Vital capacity (VC)	The maximum air volume that can be expired after a maximum inspiration (normally, 4,800 mL). This figure is the sum of the tidal volume and the inspiratory and expiratory reserve volumes.
Total lung capacity (TLC)	The greatest air volume in the lungs after a maximum inspiration (normally, about 6,000 mL).
Forced vital capacity	Vital capacity with a forced maximum expiration.
Forced expiratory volume over 1 second	Timed forced vital capacity. Various time periods are used, but 1 second is most common.
Forced expiration flow	Measurement taken early, middle, or late in the determination of the forced vital capacity. Indicates flow ability in the large, smaller, and smallest airways.
Maximal voluntary ventilation	The volume of air expired during exercise over a specified period. This is a test of exercise tolerance.

Blood levels of PCO_2 and CSF levels of H^+ ions return to normal. The reverse occurs as the PCO_2 level decreases; breathing is inhibited and less CO_2 is exhaled. The peripheral chemoreceptors can stimulate the respiratory center of the medulla and take over if the central chemoreceptors fail to activate ventilation. These receptors respond to both PCO_2 and PO_2 levels in the blood, and respiration rates either increase or decrease to provide appropriate compensation.

Blood pressure also affects the respiratory rate and rhythm. A sudden rise in blood pressure acts on the peripheral baroreceptors, with resultant slowing of respiration. A sudden drop in blood pressure causes respiration to increase in rate and depth.

The Hering-Breuer reflex is a reaction by which inspiration is ended. The increase in lung volume stimulates the stretch receptors located in the small airways, and the afferent vagal impulses from these receptors inhibit the medullary and pontine centers, and as a result end inspiration. Other reflexes that directly affect

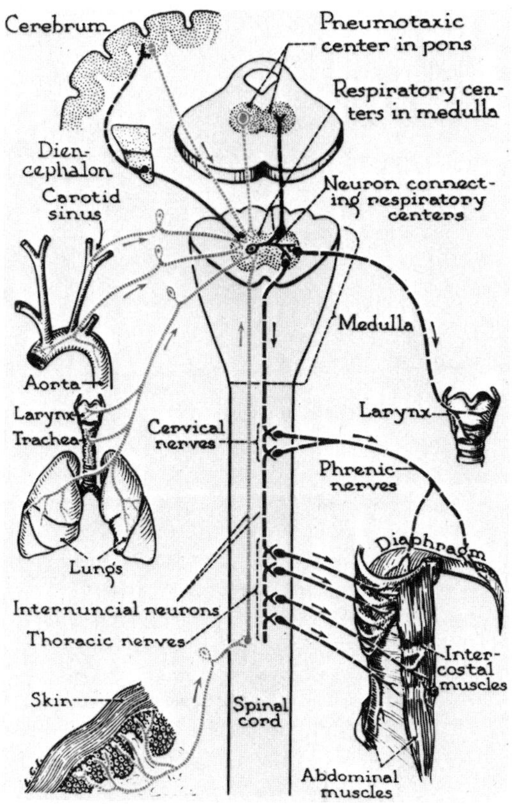

Figure 6.2 CNS control of respiration. (From Snyder M, *A Guide to Neurological and Neurosurgical Nursing,* copyright © 1983 by John Wiley & Sons, Inc. Reprinted by permission.)

the respiratory rate and rhythm include (1) irritant receptors (located in the large airways) that cause coughing, bronchoconstriction, and breath holding in response to particles, vapors, and smoke; (2) juxtacapillary receptors (J-receptors), that initiate tachypnea when the pulmonary microvasculature is distended or distorted (e.g., with emboli or vascular congestion from congestive heart failure); and (3) chest wall receptors that transmit afferent information and give rise to the feeling of dyspnea.

Dysfunction of respiratory control can cause minimal alteration in breathing patterns or complete respiratory failure. ***Cheyne-Stokes respiration*** is characterized by a regular pattern of alternating periods of apnea and hyperventilation. Occurring because of delayed feedback of impulses from peripheral chemoreceptors to the brain stem, it may be seen in CHF, central nervous system (CNS) depression from (CVA), or from high altitudes. ***Biot's breathing*** is characterized by irregular breathing with periods of apnea. It is associated with disease or injury to the brain. A more severe dysfunction of respiratory control includes the ***sleep apnea syndromes*** (see also Chapter 12). They result from loss of upper airway muscle tone

TABLE 6.2 RESPIRATORY CONTROL

Control Center	Response	Effect
Newial mechanism	Voluntary and involuntary.	Controls respiratory muscles.
a. Medullary center Aorsal respiratory group (DR6)	Processes input from vagal and glossopharyngeal nerves.	Transmits the impulses generated within the brain stem to the respiratory muscles. Primary rhythm generator.
Ventral respiratory group (VR6)	Receives impulses from DR6.	Stem to the respiratory muscles. Primary rhythm generator.
b. Pontine center Pneumotaxic center (PNC)	Adjusts respiratory system's sensitivity to stimuli.	Inhibits inspiration.
Apneustic center (APC)	Affects respiratory spinal motor neurons.	
c. Central chemoreceptors (located on or beneath ventral surface of medulla)	Controls respiration by CNS response to concentration of H^+ and CO_2.	H^+ has an indirect effect on the CNS, since it does not cross the blood–brain barrier. Increased levels stimulate respiration; decreased levels depress it. CO_2 crosses the blood–brain barrier, so its level has a direct effect on CNS chemoreceptors. Increased CO_2 levels stimulate respirations. Decreased HCO_3 acts as a buffer in CSF and stimulates respirations.
Peripheral receptors (carotid and aortic bodies)	Respond to changes in O_2 and H^+ concentration in arterial blood. O_2 levels monitored by carotid bodies, H^+ levels by both carotid and aortic bodies.	Decreased PO_2 and increased H^+ stimulate respiration.
Reflexes		
a. Stretch receptors (in small airways)	Stimulated by increased lung volume.	Hering-Breuer reflex.
b. Irritant receptors in large airways	Stimulated by inhaled smoke, noxious fumes, and particles.	Coughing, breath holding, bronchoconstriction.
c. Juxtacapillary receptors (in pulmonary microcirculation)	Stimulated by emboli or vascular congestion, which distend or distort microvasculature.	Tachypnea.
d. Chest wall receptors	Transmit afferent information about chest wall position and respiratory effort.	Sensation of dyspnea.

during rapid eye movement (REM) sleep. Usually the individual awakens and normal muscle tone returns. Complaints of chronic fatigue are associated with disrupted sleep patterns. Sleep apnea may also be related to reduced chemoreceptor sensitivity to O_2 and CO_2 that may be familial.

Pickwickian syndrome is characterized by massive hypoventilation, and daytime somnolence. The obesity promotes a form of restrictive lung disease and forces the inspiratory muscles to increase their work load. The increased CO_2 level induces somnolence and reduces chemoreceptor sensitivity. As a result, both hypercapnia and hypoxia are present. Immediate treatment centers on reversing these conditions. Treatment of the chronic condition centers primarily on weight reduction.

TABLE 6.3 CONDITIONS ASSOCIATED WITH HYPOVENTILATION

Depression of the respiratory center caused by: Drugs Injury Disease Infections	Neuromuscular or skeletal disease affecting the thorax Kyphoscoliosis Muscular dystrophy
Interruption of neural pathways to respiratory muscles from: High cervical trauma Polio Guillain-Barré syndrome	Decreased gas perfusion in the lungs Emphysema Chronic bronchitis Fibrosis Inflammatory disease Tumor Anatomic or physiologic shunts
Respiratory muscle fatigue/weakness from: Chronic lung diseases that increase the work of breathing Curare-like drugs	Anemia Hypokinetic anemia (decreased peripheral blood flow) Blood disorders affecting oxygen carrying capacity/release

Hypoventilation is defined as arterial hypoxia. Associated with respiratory center problems as well as other conditions listed in Table 6.3, it ultimately leads to an inadequate supply of oxygen to the body tissues. Depending on the rate of onset and the severity of hypoxia, patients present with fulminant, acute, or chronic symptoms of cyanosis, tachycardia, and tachypnea. Oxygen therapy, mechanical ventilation, or blood transfusions may be initiated to treat the acute hypoxia, but primary treatment focuses on the underlying pathology.

Hyperventilation is defined as arterial hypocapnia. It can be induced by a number of causes noted in Table 6.4, and is characterized by an increase in the rate and depth of respirations. Treatment depends on the underlying pathology. In cases of anxiety, patients may be taught to breathe into and out of a paper bag. By rebreathing exhaled CO_2, low levels of CO_2 can be corrected.

Bronchial Tree

Air enters the lungs through the upper airway (nasal cavities and pharynx), as described in Chapter 2. It is then drawn into the lower airway or bronchial tree, consisting of the trachea, bronchi, bronchioles, and aveoli (Figure 6.3). The trachea, 11 cm in length, extends from the cricoid cartilage in the neck into the lung. It

TABLE 6.4 CONDITIONS ASSOCIATED WITH HYPERVENTILATION

Pulmonary Interstitial lung disease Pulmonary emboli Pneumonia Atelectasis ARDS COPD	Metabolic Hypothyroidism Fever Bacteremia Shock Epinephrine Respiratory stimulants Salicylate intoxication
CNS Pontine lesions Meningitis Encephalitis	Psychogenic Pain Anxiety

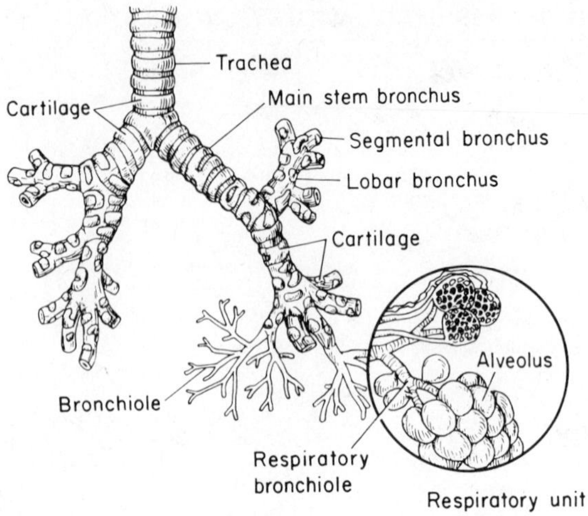

Figure 6.3 The bronchial tree. (From Brown AM, Stubbs DW, *Medical Physiology*, copyright © 1983 by John Wiley & Sons, Inc. Reprinted by permission.)

divides into the right and left mainstem bronchi, which in turn divide into five lobar branches, one into each lobe of the lung. The right lung has three lobes and the left, to allow space for the heart, has two (see Fig. 6.1). Smaller segmental bronchi (10 on the right, 8 on the left) branch off the 5 lobar bronchi. Each bronchus continues to divide into at least 50 terminal bronchioles. The terminal bronchioles subdivide even further into two or more respiratory bronchioles. The respiratory bronchioles open into an aveolar duct from which bud several aveoli. As discussed later, gas exchange and other functions are carried on by the aveoli.

Bronchial tubes are lined with columnar epithelium containing both goblet and ciliated cells. Mucus secreted by goblet cells traps particles and organisms that have gained entrance to the upper bronchi in inspired air. The cilia then propel the debris-laden mucus in a wavelike motion back up toward the oropharynx, where it can be coughed up or swallowed. Thus, irritating particles and infectious organisms are kept from reaching lung tissue. By the same token, macrophages in alveoli rapidly ingest microorganisms and debris in lung tissue. With pseudopodal action, they bring the phagocytized remains to bronchioles for mucociliary transport to the oropharynx. The debris is then swallowed and destroyed by gastric acid or expectorated.

Although the mucociliary system offers great protection, a number of irritants and microorganisms can affect the larger divisions of the bronchial tree. ***Allergic tracheobronchitis*** is an inflammatory reaction to inhaled allergens and is characterized by a cough that may not be productive.

Viral tracheobronchitis is commonly caused by adenovirus, influenza virus, and some echoviruses. Acute inflammation of the tracheobronchial tree from these agents may follow acute pharyngitis or laryngitis and is usually a mild, self-limited illness marked by low-grade fever, hoarseness, retrosternal discomfort, malaise, and a productive cough. Excess mucus and an inflammatory exudate cause reflex coughing that traumatizes tracheobronchial tissue.

Bacterial tracheobronchitis often develops in the wake of viral or allergic inflammation when respiratory defense mechanisms have been compromised and may prolong the symptoms. *Staphylococcus aureus,* stretococci, *Hemophilus influenzae,* and pneumococci account for most cases. Diagnosis is based on symptoms, rhonchi, and occasional wheezing on auscultation, and sputum culture. Treatment includes rest, fluid intake, and steam or cool mist inhalation. Medications include an antitussive (every 4 hours), oral theophylline (every 6 hours) if wheezing occurs, and antibiotics (every 6 hours) if indicated. Cough suppressants should be avoided in patients with chronic obstructive pulmonary disease.

Smoking alters the mucociliary transport mechanism in several ways. It damages cilia, stimulates excess mucus production, and promotes thickening of bronchial walls, reducing their elasticity. Excess mucus, which is not efficiently moved by damaged cilia, accumulates, irritating the trachea and bronchi. Coughing results. The thickened, inelastic membranes of the bronchial tree and aveoli inhibit ventilation and gas exchange. Dyspnea develops. Since stagnant mucus provides a breeding ground for infection and cellular invasion, patients become more prone to respiratory infections, acute at first and then chronic. In the latter case, they constantly cough up yellow, green, or brown sputum, which is most profuse in the morning after secretions have accumulated during sleep ("smoker's hack"). Irreversible pulmonary conditions, discussed in a later section, are not unlikely. Smoking increases the risk of chronic bronchitis and emphysema as much as 25 times. It is the primary cause of lung cancer, men who smoke 1 to 2 packs a day being 20 times more likely than nonsmokers to develop this malignancy. The risk of developing other types of cancers (oral, esophageal, pancreatic, bladder, pharyngeal) is also increased by smoking, especially in combination with chronic alcohol abuse. In addition, the relationship between smoking and coronary artery disease is well documented, with male smokers being twice as likely to die of coronary disease as nonsmokers. Smoking by pregnant women is associated with low birth weight babies and higher rates of miscarriage. Carelessness with lighted cigarettes is the direct cause of many automobile accidents, fires, and burns. Finally, cigarette smokers miss considerably more work than nonsmokers. Because of the undeniable health risks of smoking, primary care providers should take every opportunity to actively promote ▶ ***smoking cessation.*** Toward this end, routinely offered advise to quit smoking followed up with a variety of personal and/or group methods is helpful. Kits prepared by the American Cancer Society, support groups, nicotine substitutes, hypnosis, and behavior modification are some examples of the methods used.

The mucociliary system is also demaged in many ***occupational lung diseases.*** The inhalation of a variety of substances causes symptoms of pulmonary inflammation, fibrosis, and emphysema, depending on the causative agent and the amount of length of exposure. Table 6.5 lists several of these diseases and discusses each. A careful, detailed history of exposure is essential. Treatment is avoidance of offending substances. COPD interventions may be needed for some patients (see later section).

Both smoking and occupational exposure are major factors in the development of ***bronchogenic (lung) cancer*** (see Tables 6.6 and 6.7). Although some patients may be asymptomatic, others may present with a cough (usually nonproductive), localized wheezing, chest pain, rust-streaked or purulent sputum, hemoptysis, and/or dyspnea. Patients often have a history of unexplained weight loss and decreased energy. Physical exam may reveal rhonchi or absence of breath sounds due to obstruction. A secondary pulmonary infection (lung abscess, pneumonitis) occurring

TABLE 6.5 SOME OCCUPATIONAL LUNG DISEASES

Hazard	Discussion
Pneumoconiosis	General term referring to accumulation of dust in the lungs and the tissue reaction to its presence.
Noncollagenous changes of pneumoconiosis	Pneumoconiosis consisting mainly of a fibrous stromal reaction, with the alveolar architecture left intact. Sometimes reversible.
Coal workers' pneumoconiosis	Noncollagenous pneumoconiosis caused by exposure to coal dust. If exposure continues, it may progress to a profoundly disabling massive fibrosis.
Collagenous pneumoconiosis	Pneumoconiosis with permanent nodular or diffuse scarring of the lungs.
Silicosis	Crystalline dust of silica provokes nodular collagenous pneumoconiosis. The fibrogenic tissue response is unique in that it progresses through various immunologic steps to an onion-like fibrous nodule (silicotic nodule) that pervades the lymphatics and parenchyma.
Asbestosis	Diffuse collagenous pneumoconiosis caused by exposure to asbestos particles.
Occupational bronchitis	Chronic bronchitis with cough, sputum production, and eventual airway compromise associated with various occupational groups, notably miners. Smoking acts as a lethal adjunct, potentiating and/or exaggerating the effects of other inhalants.
Lipoid pneumonia (Inhalation of oil vapor/aspiration of oil liquid)	The inflammatory response differs according to the amount, variety, and circumstances surrounding the absorption of oil. In general, lipid-filled macrophages coalesce to form vacuoles and eventually granulomas that may look like tubercles or sarcoid.
Mushroom pickers' lung, bark strippers' lung, bird fanciers' lung, farmers' lung	Particles from mushrooms, bark, birds, and (in the case of farmers' lung) a mold (*Micropolyspora faeni*) that grows on wet or poorly stored hay are recognized as external antigens by pulmonary connective tissue (the interstitium). This results in hypersensitivity pneumonitis. The small airways may also react, adding an asthma-like picture. The inflammatory response can produce an acute clinical picture of dyspnea, cough, chills and fever, and malaise. A potential for chronic scarring exists. Acute airway reactions occur when inhaled particles provoke airway obstruction through immunologically mediated or nonimmunologic pathways (reflex constriction of airways from stimulation of cough and irritant receptors).
Byssinosis	Airway obstruction caused by a reaction to inhalation of cotton, linen, hemp, and jute fibers. Though exposure to these fibers may cause an acute atopic reaction, the disease is the eventually chronic condition in which cough, chest tightness, and dyspnea progress to COPD.

distal to a bronchial obstruction may complicate the diagnosis; any persistent or recurrent pulmonaray infection, or one that is incompletely responsive to therapy, should prompt a search for a possible neoplasm. Diagnosis is based on noninvasive techniques [sputum cytology, arterial blood gases, complete blood count (CBC), pulmonary function tests, chest-x-ray films, and computed tomography (CT) scan] as well as invasive procedures (bronchoscopy, mediastinoscopy for centrally located tumors, percutaneous needle biopsy, bronchial brush biopsy, and biopsy of palpable cervical or axillary lymph nodes or of sites of metastasis). The prognosis and treatment of choice are both influenced by the cell type and stage of the disease. Early surgical treatment (before metastases occur) is preferred if the tumor is primary, localized, and resectable. Radiotherapy or chemotherapy (or both) may be used in nonresectable localized tumors, in recurrent disease, or in metastatic disease as a

TABLE 6.6 LUNG CANCER RISK FACTORS

Male sex	Exposure to ionizing radiation
Smoking	Exposure to certain viruses
Older age	Family history of lung cancer
Urban living	Personal history of cancer
Occupational exposure to asbestos, coal tar, arsenic, nickel	Coagulation disorder

palliative measure. Careful follow-up of patients is essential to identify remission or progression of the disease, as well as to provide treatment of the symptoms related to the disease and its medical and/or surgical management.

At distal levels of bronchial divisions, the pseudostratified ciliated columnar epithelium found in the trachea and bronchi becomes simple ciliated columnar epithelium. Having fewer goblet cells to secrete mucus, bronchioles normally secrete a mucus-free, watery fluid. In some instance of bronchiolar inflammation, however, the rare goblet cells multiply and enlarge, secreting mucus that can obstruct the lumen, a condition referred to as ***bronchiolitis.*** Causes of inflammation in adults include respiratory syncytial virus and environmental exposure, especially to *Micropolyspora faeni* (farmers' lung) and nitrogen oxides. Bronchiolitis of small airways (less than 2 mm in diameter) seems to be an early consequence of smoking. In fact, bronchiolitis is felt to be a possible precursor of chronic obstructive pulmonary disease. Symptoms include increasing respiratory distress, tachypnea, tachycardia, paroxysmal cough, costal breathing, an expiratory wheeze, and elevated temperature. Diagnosis is based on arterial blood gas analyses and chest-x-ray films showing hyperinflated lungs and a depressed diaphragm. Bronchiolitis is treated with humidity (which may be combined with oxygen), increased fluid intake, and rest.

The cartilaginous rings that support the walls of larger bronchial tubes become progressively shorter and narrower along distal divisions and finally disappear. Thus, the walls of the smaller bronchioles are composed mainly of smooth muscle. Hyperactivity of the smooth muscle with spasmodic contractions, which occurs in ▶***asthma,*** is called ***bronchospasm or acute asthma attack.*** Bronchospasm is usually associated with excessive mucous production, mucosal swelling, and often eosinophil infiltration. Although the exact cause of an asthmatic attack is not clearly understood, certain precipitating factors and variations of the disease have been described (Table 6.8). Depending on its severity, patients present with variable degrees of shortness of breath, inspiratory and expiratory wheezing, cough, and sputum production. A mild attack (stage I) is marked by mild dyspnea, chest tightness, and diffuse wheezing. A moderate attack (stage II) is characterized by respiratory distress at rest, tachypnea, and marked wheezing. A severe asthmatic attack produces respiratory distress indicated by intercostal retractions, poor skin color, lethargy, confusion, and pulsus paradoxus (an abnormal decrease in systolic blood pressure during inspiration). It should be noted that absent or minimal wheezing does not always correspond to mild bronchospasm; in fact, it may be an ominous sign of complete airway obstruction. Furthermore, ventilatory deficits may persist after most symptoms clear. Bronchoconstriction of small airways may persist after larger airways have returned to normal, and often leads to a relapse within a week after acute attack has seemingly been brought under control. For this reason, blood gases and peak flow readings, rather than clinical symptoms alone, are often needed

TABLE 6.7 TYPES OF PRIMARY LUNG CANCER

Type	Features
Squamous cell (epidermoid) carcinoma	Centrally located lesion nearly always associated with cigarette smoking. May undergo cavitation. Early onset of symptoms leads to earlier diagnosis than other types and has a more favorable prognosis (some studies report a 50% survival rate). Accounts for approximately 60% of pulmonary cancers.
Adenocarcinoma a. Bronchogenic b. Acinar c. Papillary	Lung scarring (focal scars and chronic interstitial fibrosis) is a risk factor. Peripherally located lesion. Late diagnosis due to late onset of symptoms. This category accounts for approximately 15% of pulmonary cancers.
Anaplastic (undifferentiated) carcinoma, large and small cell a. Small cell (oat cell, fusiform cell, polygonal cell, and others) b. Large cell (solid with mucin-like content, solid without mucin-like content, giant cell, clear cell)	Occurs in relatively younger age groups than other types. Late diagnosis and rapid metastasis. Central and peripheral regions affected with about equal frequency. Occurs predominantly in men. About 20% of pulmonary cancers are in this category. Small cell anaplastic carcinomas have the worst prognosis of all pulmonary carcinomas, especially the oat cell variant. Oat cell carcinoma has been associated with multiple endocrinopathies.
Bronchioloalveolar carcinoma (alveolar cell or bronchiolar carcinoma)	Unifocal or multifocal origin (multifocal is more typical). Rarely extends beyond the lungs. May mimic a pneumonia. Relatively uncommon type (accounts for about 2% of lung cancers). Patient classically presents with bronchorrhea, dyspnea, and increasing hypoxemia and hypocapnia.
Bronchial adenoma (carcinoid bronchial adenoma)	Uncommon, malignant. Equal sex distribution. Affects somewhat younger age groups than other categories. Primarily central in location, with a prolonged course. Often associated with recurrent pneumonia within the same lung zone, hemoptysis, and localized overlying pleural pain. Metastasis (slow) occurs infrequently (5–10% of patients). Has been associated with multiple endocrinopathies. Diagnosis depends on bronchoscopic biopsy or exploratory thoracotomy, since exfoliation is rare, and sputum examination is not always useful.
Others (combined epidermoid and adenocarcinoma, mixed tumors and carcinosarcomas, unclassified tumors, sarcoma, mesotheliomas, melanomas, carcinoids, solitary lymphoma)	Variations and combinations of above.

to provide an accurate index of air exchange status. Severe or lasting compromise is indicated by low P_{O_2}, high P_{CO_2}, and peak flow rates ranging around 100.

Acute, mild attacks of asthma are usually controlled with elixophyllin elixir and/or bronchial inhalants containing isoproterenol, metaproterenol, or other sympathomimetic drugs. Moderate cases may require subcutaneous injections of epinephrine solution, 1:1,000. Patients with severe attacks or attacks that do not respond to the above measures require hospitalization. In addition to epinephrine, they are usually treated with intravenous (IV) aminophylline, 5–6 mg per kilogram of body weight over 20 minutes, and then 0.2–0.5 mg/kg/h. Extra fluids (initially in IV form) are given to correct dehydration and to thin mucus secretions. Promoting rest and decreasing anxiety are other important aspects of care, since asthma attacks are exhausting and frightening. Sedation, however, should be avoided, since it reduces respiratory drive.

TABLE 6.8 CLASSIFICATIONS OF ASTHMA

Classification	Discussion
Extrinsic	Former classification that included childhood-onset, allergen-induced disease.
Intrinsic	Former classification that included adult-onset disease unassociated with an identifiable allergen. Included asthma induced by exercise, anxiety, and upper respiratory infections.
Atopic disease	Identifiable allergens account for the major factor of disease in one-third of asthmatics and are thought to be related in another one-third. Some asthmatics identify specific allergens that inevitably lead to wheezing. IgE levels may be high.
Exercise-induced	Bronchospasm develops mainly with exercise or anxiety.
Sampter's syndrome	Occurs in asthma patients who have nasal polyps, hypersensitivity to aspirin and other nonsteroidal anti-inflammatory drugs.
Triple asthma	Asthma in patients who also have allergies to aspirin and penicillin.
Tokyo-Yokohama or New Orleans asthma	Asthma-bronchospasm in otherwise nonasthmatic patients when air pollution (inorganic pollutants as well as pollen and mold spores) and humidity are pronounced.
Recurrent endobronchial *Aspergillus fumigatus*	Asthma patients prone to chronic fungal endobronchitis marked by cough, fever, pleuritic pain, and eosinophils in blood and mucous plugs.
Beta-adrenergic blockers	The development of bronchospasm in previously nonasthmatic patients after treatment with beta blockers such as propranolol.
Environmentally induced disease	Bronchospasm resulting from inhaled agents (particles, fumes) in a wide variety of industrial settings.
Cardiac asthma	Wheezing secondary to heart disease.
Thymic asthma	Asthma precipitated in children by sudden closure of the pharynx. Thought to be due to sudden enlargement of the thymus gland.

Prophylaxic measures should be undertaken for patients with ***chronic asthma.*** These may include bronchodilators (carefully titrated) and/or beta-adrenergic receptor agonists. Cromolyn sodium may be given to patients with exercise-induced asthma. Inhaled topical steroids or even oral steroids may be needed in refractory cases, but these cases are best managed by the specialist. Some of the more common drugs used in the treatment of asthma are summarized in Table 6.9. In addition to pharmacologic agents, patient education about smoking, exercise, allergens, environmental temperatures, and humidity is extremely important.

Bronchiectasis is abnormal dilatation of the bronchi and bronchioles. It is permanent and radiologically visible. Most cases of bronchiectasis are the result of past pulmonary infections, commonly in childhood, that change to chronic, latent, infectious conditions. Other causes are cystic fibrosis, asthma, chronic bronchitis and emphysema, lung scarring usually from pulmonary tuberculosis, and bronchial obstruction from foreign bodies, tumor, or, rarely, mucous plugs. Clinical manifestations of bronchiectasis are cough, intermittent fever, and production of purulent, odorous sputum. Probably both obstruction and infection are necessary for the production of bronchiectatic dilatation. Obstruction may cause atelectasis, the collapse of lung tissue (see later section). Infection causes inflammation, weakening, and further dilatation of bronchial walls. Distal bronchi and bronchioles are most seriously affected. Dilatation, to as much as four times the normal size, can bring the airways out to the pleural surfaces. These dilated airways are filled with exudate

TABLE 6.9 DRUGS USED IN THE TREATMENT OF ASTHMA

Classification	Dose	Indication	Adverse Reactions
	Adrenergic Bronchodilators		
Ephedrine	*PO:* 25–50 mg two to four times daily (allow 4 hours between doses).	To treat and prevent mild asthmatic attacks.	*Cardiovascular:* tachycardia, flushing, diaphoresis *CNS:* restlessness, tremors, insomnia, vertigo, headache *Ocular:* visual changes, photophobia *Renal:* difficulty voiding *Respiratory:* dyspnea, chest pain
Terbutaline	*PO:* 2.5–5 mg every 6 hours, not to exceed 15 mg/day. *SC:* 0.25 mg into lateral deltoid area; repeat after 15–30 minutes if needed, but not to exceed 0.5 mg/4-hour period.	To prevent mild asthmatic symptoms from becoming severe.	
Ethylnor-epinephrine	*SC (or IM):* 0.5–1.0 mg, depending on severity of attack.	To treat acute attacks.	
Metaproterenol	*Inhalant:* 2–3 inhalations separated by 5-minute intervals; may be repeated every 3–4 hours. *PO:* 20 mg three to four times daily.	To provide symptomatic relief and prevent mild asthmatic symptoms from progressing to more severe forms.	
Albuterol	*PO:* 2–4 mg three to four times daily; may gradually increase (if needed and tolerated) to 8 mg four times daily. *Inhalant:* 1–2 inhalations every 4–6 hours.	To treat mild asthmatic attacks.	
Isoetharine	Based on severity of attack. *Inhalant:* 2–3 inhalations every 20 minutes prn initially, then every 4–6 hours.	To treat mild asthmatic attacks.	
Isoproterenol	*Inhalant:* 1 inhalation to start; repeat after 1 minute if necessary, not to exceed 5 doses/day, with doses not less than 3–4 hours apart. *Sublingual:* 10–15 mg (if needed, up to four times/day).	To treat mild to moderately severe asthmatic attacks.	
Epinephrine	*SC:* 0.2–0.5 mg, repeated every 20 minutes to 4 hours as needed; up to 1 mg/dose may be given in severe cases. *Inhalant:* 1:100 solution.	To treat acute asthmatic attacks. To treat mild attacks quickly.	
	Methylxanthine Bronchodilators		
Dosages are individualized and then adjusted to maintain therapeutic serum levels (10–20 μg/mL).			*Gastrointestinal:* nausea, vomiting, diarrhea, anorexia *CNS:* restlessness, insomnia, vertigo, tremors *Cardiovascular:* tachycardia, flushing, hypotension, heart failure *Respiratory:* tachypnea *Renal:* urinary frequency, albuminurea
Theophylline			
a. Anhydrous	*PO:* initially 100–200 mg every 12 hours, then adjusted according to serum levels.	Used alone or in combination with ephedrine to treat or prevent mild to moderate attacks.	
b. Sodium glycinate	*PO:* 300–600 mg three to four times daily is a typical adult dosage (adjusted according to serum levels).		
Aminophylline	*PO:* 200–400 mg three to four times per day; adjust dosage as needed.	To treat and prevent mild attacks.	

TABLE 6.9 *(Continued)*

Classification	Dose	Indication	Adverse Reactions
Aminophylline (Con't)	*PR:* 7 mg/kg to start; then 3.5 mg/kg every 6 hours for the next 12 hours, and then every 8 hours for maintenance.	For acute or chronic asthma.	
	IV: 6 mg/kg (preferably by infusion) to start, followed by 0.7 mg/kg/hr for next 12 hours and then 0.5 mg/kg/hr.	For acute attacks and status asthmaticus.	
Oxtriphylline	*PO:* 200 mg four times daily; adjust dosage as needed.	To treat mild to moderate attacks.	
Dyphylline	*PO:* 200–400 mg (or up to 15 mg per kilogram of body weight) every 6 hours as needed and tolerated. *IM:* 500 mg to start, followed, if needed and tolerated, by 250–500 mg every 2–6 hours, not to exceed 15 mg per kilogram of body weight every 6 hours.	To treat mild to moderate attacks.	
		Adrenocorticosteroids	
Used in combination with bronchodilators in severe illness and acute episodes, then gradually withdrawn.			*Metabolic:* cushingoid features, hyperglycemia, osteoporosis, peptic ulcer *Immunologic:* infections *Endocrine:* failure of growth in children *CNS:* initial euphoria, mood swings, behavioral changes, inability to cope with stress *Ocular:* glaucoma, cataracts
Hydrocortisone sodium succinate	*IM:* Start at 15–240 mg/day; then gradually reduce to lowest effective dose. *IV:* 100–500 mg to start; repeat (IV or IM) at intervals of 2, 4, or 6 hours according to response and clinical condition.	Status asthmaticus.	
Methylprednisolone sodium succinate	*IV:* 10–40 mg given over a period of 1 to several minutes to start; repeat IV or IM according to response and clinical condition.	Status asthmaticus.	
Prednisolone sodium phosphate	*IV:* Start at 4–60 mg/day, then gradually reduce to lowest effective dose.	Status asthmaticus.	
Triamcinolone acetonide	*Inhalant:* 2 inhalations three to four times daily.	To prevent asthmatic attacks.	
Beclomethasone dipropionate	*Inhalant:* 2 inhalations three to four times daily.	As a substitute for oral steroids for control of asthma (not for treatment of symptoms).	
		Miscellaneous	
Cromolyn sodium	*Inhalant:* contents of one 20-mg capsule or ampule four times daily.	To prevent asthmatic attacks; may reduce bronchodilator and steroid dosage.	Discontinue use if no effect is noted within several weeks or if an allergic response occurs.

under which desquamated or necrotic mucosa is found. Necrosis can progress to lung abscess when bronchiolar walls are destroyed. In less rapidly progressive cases, fibrotic changes can develop in the bronchiolar walls and peribronchial tissue. Even in cases where the chronic infection is stopped, dilatation and scarring remain. If epithelium does regenerate, there is a risk of squamous metaplasia.

Alveolar Units and Gas Exchange

Alveolar units (Fig. 6.3) include the respiratory bronchioles, alveolar ducts, and alveolar clusters—about 300 million in the average adult (70–80 m^2 of surface area).

Each alveolar unit is entwined by 9–11 pulmonary capillaries carrying unoxygenated blood pumped from the right ventricle of the heart. The blood meets air that has been inhaled into the lungs at the alveolar–capillary membrane, a layer of squamous epithelium about 1 (μm) thick. Oxygen in the inspired air diffuses across surfactant and endothelial layers of the alveolar membrane, into interstitial fluid, across the capillary membrane, into the plasma, and from there across the red blood cell (RBC) membrane. In the reverse process, carbon dioxide diffuses out of the RBC into the alveoli and is exhaled. The mechanism responsible for this directional diffusion is expressed by Dalton's law, which states that in a mixture of gases, the total pressure of the gases is the sum of the partial pressures of each gas. Exerting independent pressure, each gas moves from the area of higher partial pressure to the area of lower partial pressure across the alveolar–capillary membrane. After gas exchange takes place in the lungs, the partial pressures in both the alveoli and arterioles should be approximately the same, as noted in Table 6.10. The molecular weight and solubility of the gases also affect the diffusion rate. Both O_2 and CO_2 diffuse rapidly because of the weight of O_2 and the solubility of CO_2.

In addition to O_2 and CO_2, the lungs help regulate levels of hydrogen ion levels along with the kidney buffering system (see Chapter 7). The lungs excrete the volatile hydrogen ions of carbonic acid as carbon dioxide and water. In ***respiratory acidosis*** the hydrogen ion concentration is greater than normal, usually because insufficient carbon dioxide is being expelled. The P_{CO_2} is elevated in the alveoli and arterial blood. The H_2CO_3 is increased and the pH is decreased. Conditions that alter the structure or function of the lungs and do not allow for adequate ventilation (i.e., pneumonia, pulmonary edema, airway obstruction, chest trauma, and chronic obstructive pulmonary disease) may cause hypercapnia. Suppression of the respiratory reflexes by medications and anesthesia also cause respiratory acidosis. Symptoms include headache, dyspnea, fine tremors, tachycardia, elevated blood pressure, and vasodilatation. Arterial blood gases confirm the diagnosis, with a P_{CO_2} above 45 mm Hg and a pH below 7.35. If respiratory acidosis is not treated, it can lead to coma and death. Treatment consists of determining the condition associated with hypoventila-

TABLE 6.10 PARTIAL PRESSURES OF ALVEOLAR AND ARTERIAL GASES AFTER NORMAL DIFFUSION

	Alveolar (Pa)	Arterial (P)
O_2	100 mmHg	95 mmHg
CO_2	40 mmHg	40 mmHg

tion and treating it accordingly. General management includes oxygen therapy, bronchodilators given intravenously, administration of sodium bicarbonate, and hydration. Careful monitoring of respiratory, cardiovascular, and CNS function is essential. Some patients may require mechanical ventilation.

In ***respiratory alkalosis,*** carbon dioxide and water loss is too great and the hydrogen ion concentration is too low. The P_{CO_2} level is decreased and the pH is increased as a result of hyperventilation. The most frequent cause is anxiety. Pulmonary causes include asthma, pneumonia, and pulmonary vascular diseases. Other causes include aspirin toxicity, fever, metabolic acidosis, hepatic failure, and gram-negative septicemia. Diagnosis is confirmed by the finding of a P_{CO_2} level below 35 mm Hg and a pH that is greater than 7.45 and has risen in proportion to the fall of the P_{CO_2}. In the chronic phase, the pH is normal. Treatment of the underlying pathology is essential. Anxiety may be treated with medications and psychotherapy. Symptomatic treatment is managed by rebreathing exhaled air and prescribing sedatives to decrease the respiratory rate.

As might be expected, diffusion rates are directly related to alveolar surface area and inversely related to bronchiolar membrane thickness. In ***chronic obstructive pulmonary disease (COPD),*** the alveolar surface area is decreased (emphysema) and/or the bronchiolar membrane thickness is increased (chronic bronchitis). The "and/or" is important: although emphysema and chronic bronchitis are distinct diagnostic categories, the clinical presentation of each often includes features of both conditions. Furthermore, a number of subcategories have been described (Table 6.11). All types result from chronic irritation from respiratory infections, air pollution, occupational exposure, and, most notably, cigarette smoking.

In ▶ ***chronic bronchitis,*** irritant exposure causes the mucous glands to become hyperplastic and the cilia to be damaged. Failing to be cleared through cilial action, the excess mucus stagnates. Patients then develop a chronic productive cough

TABLE 6.11 SUBCATEGORIES OF COPD

Type	Characteristics
Bronchitis	
Simple chronic bronchitis	Mucous sputum.
Mucopurulent chronic bronchitis	Purulent sputum from local suppuration such as a bronchiectasis.
Obstructive chronic bronchitis	Pulmonary function shows decreased forced expiratory capacity.
Chronic asthmatic bronchitis	Patients have a long history of cough productive of sputum and late onset of wheezing.
Emphysema	
Panacinar (panlobular)	All parts of the acinus (respiratory bronchioles, alveolar ducts, and alveoli-filled clusters) are affected. Associated with a genetic deficiency of the antienzyme of alpha-atritrypsin, especially in early-age onset cases and familial groups.
Centroacinor (centrilobular)	Disease enlarges and eventually destroys the respiratory bronchioles and alveolar ducts. The peripheral acinus is relatively spared, leaving a rim of functioning lung parenchyma. Often seen in conjunction with chronic bronchitis. Most emphysematous lungs demonstrate both panacinar and centroacinar lesions on autopsy.

("smoker's cough") and recurrent respiratory infections (acute bronchitis, pneumonia, sinusitis). Eventually the bronchioles undergo structural changes such as edema, thickening, and loss of elasticity. Then even coughing is rendered ineffective as a cleaning technique; though the vagus nerve–mediated reflex may still be stimulated by tracheobronchial irritation, airway obstruction prevents inspiration that is large or fast enough to deliver air to the distal areas where retained matter lies. Diagnostic criteria for chronic bronchitis include sputum production and cough for 3 months for each of 2 consecutive years. The majority of patients are middle-aged, obsese, and have a long history of cigarette smoking. They display dyspnea, cyanosis, and characteristic changes in pulmonary function tests (normal total lung capacity, lowered FVC and FEV). Breath sounds may be normal or significant for rhonchi and wheezes. Chest x-ray films typically show increased bronchovascular markings and cardiac hypertrophy. Medical treatment includes the use of bronchodilators and intermittent antibiotics. However, to prevent further permanent damage to lung tissue, the heart of management is patient education concerning smoking withdrawal, pulmonary hygiene, and general health measures.

In ► ***emphysema,*** irritant exposure causes distention of air spaces distal to the terminal nonrespiratory bronchioles with destruction of alveolar walls. Obstruction by thick, excess, sluggish mucus, as well as by inflammation and infection, initiates the problem. This in turn leads to edema, more mucus production, bronchiolar spasm, and eventual fibrosis. With narrowing of the bronchioles, individual aveoli become hyperinflated and eventually perforate their walls. As the alveoli erode, the small blood vessels of the alveolar wall are lost, increasing pulmonary resistance to blood flood and raising pulmonary arterial pressure. In lung tissue, unlike other body tissue, hypoxia promotes vasoconstriction rather than dilatation. In healthy lungs, this process distributes blood to better-oxygenated areas and maintains circulatory exchange. In emphysematous lungs, however, a hypoxic response to vasoconstriction makes a bad situation worse. Increased pulmonary pressure and heightened cardiac output can lead to pulmonary hypertension and right heart failure. Furthermore, as aveolar destruction progresses, a state of relative carbon dioxide retention develops. Initially, central chemoreception of high carbon dioxide levels induces hyperventilation, but with time this respiratory drive becomes deadened. Respiratory stimulation then becomes dependent on the detection of hypoxemia by peripheral receptors. (For this reason, oxygen therapy must be given with caution and in low concentrations to patients with CO_2 retention; by correcting hypoxemia, O_2 inhalation can suppress respiratory drive.)

The clinical picture of emphysema includes insidious development of breathlessness progressing to dyspnea at rest. Most patients experience anorexia and weight loss. On exam, a wasted appearance, forward sitting, accessory muscle use, intercostal retractions, and grunting with prolonged expiration may be observed. The lungs are hyperresonant to percussion, with distant breath sounds. A right ventricular impulse may be present. Chest x-ray films reveal a flat diaphragm, hyperinflated lungs, interrupted peripheral vascular markings, and a narrowed, elongated cardiac silhouette. Total lung capacity and residual volume are increased on pulmonary function tests, while arterial blood gases show decreased Po_2 and increased Pco_2. Treatment is similar to that of chronic bronchitis. In addition, patients may benefit from the support and information available from various ► ***organizations for respiratory disorders.***

Cystic fibrosis is a chronic disease of the exocrine system in which an unknown defect causes the production of thick, sticky protein secretions that obstruct various ducts of the body. It is inherited in an autosomal recessive pattern. Previously limited to infants and children, cystic fibrosis is now being seen with some frequency in adults because advances in management have resulted in longer life spans. The major clinical features involve the pulmonary system (mucus secretion in the lungs) as well as the gastrointestinal tract (pancreatic insufficiency with steatorrhea, abnormal fecal accumulation with partial obstruction, biliary cirrhosis, cholelithiasis). The diagnosis is based on the health history, physical exam, positive sweat test, absence of pancreatic enzymes, and absence of trypsin in the stool. Although the gastrointestinal complications can be severe, it is the degree of pulmonary compromise that dictates the patients longevity. Occurring in 97% of patients with cystic fibrosis, pulmonary disease is manifested by sinusitis, chronic bronchitis, recurrent pneumonia, bronchiectasis, hyperaeration, and cor pulmonale. Sputum cultures, chest x-ray films, and arterial blood gases indicate its degree. Treatment of cystic fibrosis requires a multisystemic approach. Pancreatic enzymes as well as sodium must be replaced. Adequate hydration must be maintained to keep secretions as thin and loose as possible. Fat-soluble vitamins must be added to a diet high in protein, calories, and sodium but low in fat. Respiratory treatment includes regular postural drainage, percussion, and exercise, as well as the use of bronchodilators and antibiotics when needed. To minimize respiratory infections and bronchospasm, exposure to crowds of people and air pollutants (such as cigarette smoke) should be minimized.

Lung Parenchyma

The lung parenchyma is made up of aveolar units (acini), connective tissue, and blood vessels. Alveolar epithelium consists of two types of cells: type I, the cells that form the pulmonary surface epithelium, and type II, the cells that secrete pulmonary surfactant, a detergent-like phospholipid compound. Without surfactant, a thin layer of water could collect on alveolar surfaces, exerting enough surface tension to prevent aeration at birth (***atelectasis*** or collapsed lung). ***Acquired atelactasis*** is the collapse of previously inflated lung tissue. It may result from obstruction by secretions or exudates or by foreign bodies. Bronchitis, bronchial asthma, and bronchiectasis can lead to this situation. Bronchial neoplasia can also lead to this obstructive atelectasis, although the obstruction is most frequently partial. When complete obstruction from any cause occurs, oxygen trapped in the dependent airways is gradually absorbed, and the oxygen-deprived alveoli collapse. Blood flow, however, continues through the alveolar walls in obstructive atelectasis. In contrast to the obstructive form of acquired atelectasis, ***compressive atelectasis*** is the result of pressure on the lung parenchyma from the pleural space or the diaphragm. Blood clots, tumor, fluid, or air can fill the pleural space partially or completely, collapsing the lung tissue. Similar collapse occurs when an elevated diaphragm creates basal atelectasis, as in the recumbent patient with abdominal distention and a decreased ability to move secretions. Compressive atelectasis is frequently the result of hydrothorax (as from CHF), pneumothorax, pleural effusions from neoplasms and lymphatic obstruction, and hemothorax (e.g., rupture of a thoracic aneurysm). Even where atelectasis does not significantly deter ventilation, the collapsed tissue is at risk for superimposed infection.

The clinical manifestations of atelectasis depend on the site of collapse, the rate at which it occurs, and the presence or absence of infection. A range of symptoms include dyspnea, dyspnea on exertion (DOE), tachycardia, cyanosis, pleuritic chest pain, asymmetric movement of the ribs on inspiration, rales, and decreased or absent breath sounds over the affected area. A chest x-ray film may show the segment or lobe involved as densely consolidated and smaller than normal. The diaphragm may be elevated on the affected side, and in severe cases there may be a mediastinal shift toward that side. Medical management is determined by the underlying pathology.

As previously mentioned, infectious agents and physical irritants are normally cleared from lung tissue by macrophages in the aveoli and by the mucociliary action of the bronchial tree. If not, a number of ***inflammatory lung processes*** may develop.

► ***Pneumonia*** is a broad term covering a range of lung diseases, the most significant of which are described in Table 6.12 with recommended treatments (fungal processes and opportunistic infections are discussed in a later section). The basic pathophysiology, however, is relatively constant, involving an inflammatory reaction in the alveolar interstitium and exudative collections in the alveolar and even airway spaces. Solidification of lung tissue and subsequent loss of function may follow. Agents causing this reaction can reach the tissue in three ways: (1) by outside contact with lung tissue, from penetrating trauma or therapeutic and diagnostic invasion, for example, chest surgery; (2) by blood-borne spread of infection from another body source; and (3) by inhalation of elements such as environmental particulates, noxious fumes and smoke, infectious organisms, or aspiration of secretions or foreign matter. When foreign bodies enter the lung, they usually go to the right lung because of the straighter course and wider caliber of the right bronchus. Similarly, aspiration of liquid material (e.g., vomitus) also results in a right-sided pneumonia. Patients with reduced coughing ability (due to neuromuscular disorders, chronic pulmonary disease) are at increased risk for the development of pneumonia. So, too, are patients with damaged mucociliary/phagocytic capacity (smokers, drinkers, the immunosuppressed and the chronically ill).

The classic presentation of pneumonia includes fever, productive cough, chest wall pain, and malaise. Examination usually reveals dull percussion over infected areas, rhonchi, rales, and changes in transmitted sound. The CBC often shows an elevated white blood cell (WBC) count with a left shift. The clinical picture may vary depending on the causative agent (see Table 6.12). For example, patients with viral pneumonia typically develop symptoms more insidiously than those with bacterial infection. Respiratory complaints appear several days after the constitutional symptoms of headache, sore throat, and myalgias. Unlike many bacterial infections, viral pneumonia may neither raise the WBC count nor shift the differential to the left.

Confirming the diagnosis of pneumonia, x-ray changes are described by the distribution of disease through the lung anatomy. ***Lobular pneumonia*** (bronchopneumonia) is patchy consolidation distributed throughout several lobes. It may be seen with staphylococcus, streptococcus, and *H. influenzae*. Fungi, especially in the poorly resistant host, can also be causative. ***Lobar pneumonia*** is suppurative and fibrinous consolidation of an entire lobe (or most of it). Almost exclusively the result of pneumococcus, klebsiella, legionella, and aspiration, it is more severe than lobular pneumonia and is associated with more complications, including lung abscess and bacteremia. ***Interstitial pneumonia,*** in contrast to lobular and lobar disease, refers to inflammatory changes of the alveolar septa and interstitium. It occurs with multiple viruses (influenza, parainfluenza, respiratory syncytial forms, and rhinoviruses) and mycoplasma. It should be noted that x-ray changes often lag behind clinical symptoms. In addition to x-ray findings, exam of the sputum is another essential

TABLE 6.12 TYPES OF PNEUMONIA

Causative Agent	Etiology	Signs, Symptoms, and Complications	Diagnosis	Treatment
Gram-positive bacteria				
Pneumococcus	Most common; affects all age groups. Pneumococcus is present in normal flora of the respiratory tract; susceptibility to and development of infection result from impaired normal resistance. Predisposing conditions include viral infection, malnutrition, exposure to cold, noxious gases, depressed cerebral function caused by drugs, alcohol intoxication, and cardiac failure.	Sudden chills, fever (104–106°F), productive cough with rust-colored sputum (blood-tinged), chest pain (stabbing) that may be referred to the shoulder, abdomen, or flank, tachypnea (30–40 breaths per minute). Asymmetric diaphragmatic excursion, decreased breath sounds, rales, friction rub, and abdominal distention may present on physical exam. Signs of consolidation may appear later. Possible complications include pleural effusion, empyema, endocarditis, and meningitis.	Diagnosis is based on health history and physical exam. Laboratory findings include positive blood culture, leukocytosis, and positive sputum culture. Chest x-ray film may show haziness of the involved lung field at first; consolidation is noted later, with a lobar or patchy distribution.	Procaine penicillin, 600,000 units every 12 hours IM for moderate illness. Aqueous penicillin G, up to 1,000,000 units every 4 hours IV for severe cases. Penicillin V, 400,000 units every 4–6 hours once the response to treatment has been determined. Alternatives to penicillin include cephalexin or cephradine, 0.5 g every 4–6 hours by mouth, or cefazolin, 4 g IV daily. Supportive therapy includes O_2, increased fluid intake, and diet therapy. Other therapy includes symptomatic treatment of cough and pain, and prevention of complications of shock, pulmonary edema, and CHF in the elderly.
Streptococcus	Secondary to viral respiratory infection (i.e., influenza, measles) or associated with underlying pulmonary disease.	Same as pneumococcus.	Positive hemolytic streptococci in blood and sputum.	Penicillin G (see pneumococcus).
Staphylococcus	Secondary to viral respiratory infection and after antimicrobial drug therapy.	Headache and generalized pain prior to onset of symptoms (see pneumococcus); deep cyanosis. Complications include pleural effusion, empyema, and tension pneumothorax.	Positive *Staph. aureus* in sputum, pleural fluid, and blood; elevated WBC (20,000/μL). Chest x-ray film may reveal pyopneumothorax or cavities with air-fluid levels.	Nafacillin, 6–12 g daily, or vancomycin, 2 g daily, given in an IV bolus in divided doses. If the organism is penicillin sensitive, give penicillin G, 20–60 million units daily IV for several weeks.
Gram-negative bacteria				
Klebsiella	Relatively uncommon; occurs in persons over 40 years of age who have a history of debilitating disease, malnutrition, or alcoholism. May occur as a secondary infection following antimicrobial therapy for pneumonia or in patients hospitalized with serious illness.	Abrupt onset of chills, fever, dyspnea, cyanosis, and red, mucoid, sticky sputum that is difficult to expectorate. Infection may be fulminating and fatal. If subacute, it may cause necrosis of lung tissue and abscess formation.	Laboratory findings include a positive culture in sputum and blood for gram-negative bacteria, which appear short and encapsulated.	Cefotaxime (or a similar cephalosporin), 1–2 g IV bolus every 4–6 hours in combination with tobramycin, 5–7 mg per kilogram of body weight per day IM. Continue antimicrobial treatment for 2 weeks. Supportive therapy is the same as that for pneumococcus.
Legionella	These bacteria occur in the environment and are acquired from aerosols, via dust from air-conditioning units, water, and soil. Infection is not transferable from the patient to others. Asymptomatic infection is common in all age groups. Symp-	Malaise, myalgias, and headache, followed by high fever and chills, nausea, vomiting, and diarrhea. Symptoms progress to a cough, which may be slightly productive, dyspnea, hypoxia, and confusion. Possible complications include respi-	Laboratory findings include leukocytosis (10,000–20,000/μL), hyponatremia, abnormal liver function tests, possibly microscopic hematuria, and positive *Legionella pneumophila* isolated from sputum, bronchial washings, pleural	Erythromycin, 0.5–1 g every 6 hours IV or po for 2–3 weeks; alternatively, rifampin, 10–20 mg per kilogram of body weight daily, or doxycycline, 100–200 mg daily. Supportive measures are the same as for pneumococcal pneumonia.

TABLE 6.12 *(Continued)*

Causative Agent	Etiology	Signs, Symptoms, and Complications	Diagnosis	Treatment
	tomatic infection occurs in the elderly, smokers, and patients treated with hemodialysis or renal transplant. Incubation period is 2–10 days.	ratory failure, renal failure, shock, and disseminated intravascular coagulation.	fluid, blood, or lung biopsy.	
Hemophilus influenzae	Rare, primary form in adults occurring in the presence of chronic pulmonary disease, cardiac disease, and hypogammaglobulinemia.	Same as for other bacterial pneumonias.	Positive blood and sputum cultures.	Ampicillin, 12 g/day, or moxalactam, 150–200 mg per kilogram of body weight daily IV. As alternatives, chloramphenicol, 0.5 g po or IV every 6 hours, or trimethoprim with sulfamethoxazole may be tried. See discussion of pneumococcal pneumonia for supportive measures.
Mycoplasma	Infection is caused by bacteria occurring endemically, and is usually spread by respiratory secretions within a family, schools, and military populations.	Gradual onset of respiratory and influenza-like symptoms, with slowly rising temperature and a progressive cough that may be productive and painful. Patients usually do not appear to be seriously ill.	Chest x-ray films typically reveal greater involvement of the lungs than symptoms suggest, including consolidation with or without pleural fluid. Laboratory findings include WBC within normal range, *Mycoplasma pneumoniae* antibodies, and "cold agglutinins" in serum. Bacteria can be grown from throat swab or sputum on a special medium after extended incubation.	Severe cases may require treatment with tetracycline or erythromycin, 0.5 g po every 4–6 hours, but mild to moderative cases usually do not require antimicrobial therapy. Supportive measures are the same as those for pneumococcal pneumonia.
Mixed bacterial pneumonias	May occur as a complication of surgery, trauma, aspiration, or chronic illness. More severe and threatening in debilitated patients, the elderly, and the chronically ill.	Insidious onset with low-grade fever, productive cough, dyspnea, and possibly cyanosis. Sputum appearing green or yellow should suggest complicating pneumonia.	Culture and smear reveal several organisms, none of which can be identified as the causative agent. Leukocytosis may not be present in the debilitated or elderly patient. The chest x-ray film may reveal patchy, irregular infiltrations; abscess may be present.	Maintain airway and adequate oxygenation, and begin therapy with cefotaxime, 12 g/day IV, to be modified during the course of infection.
Viral and rickettsial pneumonias	Atypical because they resemble mycoplasma pneumonia. Usually occur in immunosuppressed persons. May begin as influenza and result in seconday bacterial pneumonia, or there may be a history of exposure to viruses or vectors.	Respiratory signs and symptoms are the same as those of mycoplasma pneumonia. Other features (e.g., rash) are specific to the underlying virus.	Diagnosis depends upon recognition of the underlying virus and/or positive antibody titers for specific organisms.	Treatment is symptomatic for viral pneumonia and is the same as for the related bacterial pneumonia if secondary infection develops. Initial treatment of rickettsial pneumonia may consist of 1 g tetracycline or chloramphenicol IV, followed by 0.5 g orally every 4–6 hours for 4–10 days (or 50 mg per kilogram of body weight daily).

TABLE 6.12 *(Continued)*

Causative Agent	Etiology	Signs, Symptoms, and Complications	Diagnosis	Treatment
Parasitic pneumonias				
Pneumocystis carinii pneumonia	Occurs in debilitated children and immunodeficient adults; common in AIDS patients.		With bronchoalveolar lavage or open lung biopsy, cysts of *P. carinii* can be demonstrated in smears stained with methenamine-silver.	Sulfamethoxazole-trimethoprim can be curative if given early.
Aspiration pneumonia	High mortality. Occurs following aspiration of gastric contents as well as normal respiratory secretions. Predisposing factors include inadequate cough reflex, dysfunction of the swallowing mechanism, impaired gastric emptying, and pulmonary injury from gastric secretions.	Bronchospasm; other signs and symptoms same as those of bacterial pneumonia.	Diagnosis is based on the history.	Treatment includes administration of prednisone, 100 mg po on first 2 days, as well as appropriate treatment of secondary bacterial infection if present.

aspect of diagnosis. Patients with bacterial infections are likely to have copious amounts of purulent-appearing sputum, the Gram stain of which reveals an abundance of neutrophils and a predominant, characteristic organism (see Table 6.12). Those with viral infections generally have little sputum, with neither bacteria nor neutrophils appearing on Gram stain. ***Aspiration pneumonias*** may produce infections of mixed organisms. Secretions from gingival and periodontal disease, as well as foreign body and toxic ingestions, may be involved. Gram stain revealing more than 10 epithelial cells per high-power field indicates an inadequate specimen (one produced from the oropharynx rather than the lower respiratory tract), and a new sample must be obtained.

Treatment of pneumonia includes antibiotics, fluids, and rest. The choice of antibiotics should be guided by the Gram stain and culture results. In most cases, pneumonia can be managed on an outpatient basis. However, anyone without dependable care at home should be admitted to a hospital. Hospital admission is also indicated for the elderly, the immunosuppressed, patients with gram-negative or aspiration pneumonia, and patients with signs of serious illness such as high fever, confusion, tachycardia, tachypnea, respiratory distress, or dehydration.

Influenza is sometimes thought of as a form of tracheobronchitis, but the respiratory symptoms (head congestion, nasal discharge, dry throat, cough) may be less prominent than the constitutional symptoms (headache, myalgia, fever and chills, and malaise). Respiratory complaints tend to be most significant as the constitutional symptoms recede during daily recovery. Pneumonia is the chief complication. The invasion of lung parenchyma in pneumonia (as opposed to the infection of the respiratory epithelium, which occurs almost exclusively in primary influenza) may be due to the original virus or a secondary bacterial infection, commonly from pneumococci and *Staph. aureus*. When an outbreak of influenza has been confirmed to be caused by a type A strain, the administration of an antiviral medication, amantadine, is quite effective in reducing the incidence of clinical disease in exposed, previously unvaccinated individuals if it is begun immediately and continued for 10 days. Administration of amantadine should supplement vaccination of exposed persons (see below).

Yearly vaccination with polyvalent ▶***influenza vaccine*** prior to the flu season (or immediately after exposure to the virus) is recommended for all patients over 65, particularly if they have a chronic or debilitating disease, and for younger patients with chronic disease, especially cardiopulmonary conditions, diabetes mellitus, or Addison's disease. The vaccine is usually administered in one dose, but depending on the current recommendations of the Center for Disease Control, two doses given 1 month apart may be required for immunization (this occurs when new viral strains arise). The intramuscular (IM) or subcutaneous (SC) injections of vaccine should be given in September or early October to allow sufficient time for development of the antibody response to the disease, which most typically occurs during the fall and winter months. The same high-risk patients may also be candidates for inoculation with ▶***pneumococcus vaccine*** to help protect them against the development of pneumococcal pneumonia and subsequent bacteremia (except pregnant patients, unless clearly indicated). Simultaneous administration of these two vaccines does not seem to result in an increased occurrence or severity of adverse reactions or an impaired development of immunity, but unless the likelihood of the patient returning for a second injection is questionable, it is recommended that these vaccines not be administered simultaneously in order to simplify the determination of the source of a possible hypersensitivity reaction.

Lung abscess develops when liquefaction occurs in an area of necrotizing pneumonia. The suppurative infection is recognized by radiographically visible cavities containing an air-fluid level. It usually follows aspiration pneumonia and is thus most common among patients with profound suppression of the cough or gag reflex (stuporous or comatose patients, stroke victims, substance abusers, epileptics, and patients with swallowing disorders and intestinal obstruction). However, lung abscess is not an uncommon sequela of pneumonia caused by gram-negative bacteria or staphylococcus. It is also seen in patients with periodontal or gingival disease, bronchial obstruction (atelectasis, foreign body, neoplasm), pulmonary infarcts, bacteremia, and septic emboli. In keeping with the anatomy of the lungs, the dependent segments of the lungs are most frequently involved—the posterior segment of the right upper lobe and the superior segments of the lower lobes. Development of empyema is often seen in lung abscess. ***Empyema*** is an accumulation of pus in the pleural cavity. It may be caused by bacterial pneumonia, posttraumatic infection, or postsurgical infection. The signs and symptoms may be masked by the primary infection but include fever and pleural pain following improvement of the infection. A purulent exudate from thoracentesis may be cultured for organisms. This condition may become chronic. Nonsurgical treatment includes thoracentesis and antibiotic therapy (penicillin, 600,000 units IM every 6 hours, or cephalothin, 8 g IV daily). If the pus has a foul odor, the condition may be secondary to an intra-abdominal infection. The treatment should include oral chloramphenicol, 50 mg per kilogram of body weight per day. Surgical drainage may be necessary.

Pulmonary tuberculosis (TB) is an acute or chronic communicable disease that causes an inflammatory lung reaction characterized by the formation of tubercles. The result of infection by *Mycobacterium tuberculosis* (a gram-positive, acid-fast bacillus), it is contracted almost exclusively by inhalation of bacillus-laden droplets produced by a person with infected sputum and spread via coughing, sneezing, or talking; alternatively, it may be contracted by drinking contaminated milk from infected cows (bovine TB is caused by *M. bovis*). The danger of contracting the disease from contaminated surfaces is negligible. Although the incidence of pulmonary TB has fallen dramatically in this country, certain groups are still at risk: American Indians and Eskimos, immigrants, alcoholics, the aged, the immunosuppressed or chronically ill, and inner-city residents.

The disease begins with the primary infection. The incubation period is about 4–8 weeks. It may progress fairly rapidly to active pulmonary TB, known as "primary progressive TB," the signs and symptoms of which are noted in Table 6.13, but this course is rather uncommon. Instead, with the development of tuberculin hypersensitivity in a matter of weeks, the infection is usually arrested and the disease enters a latent phase. Lesions occur most commonly in the lower two-thirds of the lung, with a consequent tissue reaction, granuloma formation, caseation (formation of a cheese-like substance), cavitation, and scarring. Calcification of the lesion occurs if the body's defenses are adequate. As long as the bacillus remains contained by body defenses, clinical disease does not develop and contagious spread is not a danger. This is the case for the majority of patients, no matter what the age of the primary infection. However, if at any time body defenses are compromised, the bacillus contracted in the primary infection becomes the source of active disease, even years later. Signs and symptoms of reactivation (described in Table 6.13) then develop. Risk factors favoring a conversion to overt disease include malnutrition, alcoholism, uncontrolled diabetes, measles, chronic corticosteroid administration, silicosis, pregnancy, old age, local injury (cancer, lung abscess, surgery, or local joint or back injury), gastrectomy, and general debilitation. In fact, the presence of any such factor in the face of clinical findings is one of the criteria for diagnosis. The diagnosis is further suggested by a positive tuberculin skin test (a skin reaction of greater than 10 mm of induration) and a chest x-ray film revealing cavitation, calcification, and/or pleural effusion. However, definitive diagnosis rests with the isolation of the mycobacterium bacillus. Toward this end, sputum specimens, tracheal washings with fiberoptic bronchoscopy, gastric washings, pleural biopsy, or mediastinal node biopsy may be required. Since prevention of the spread of TB includes isolation of the patient with a newly diagnosed or suspected active TB infection, hospitalization may be necessary initially to perform tests and begin treatment, as well as to isolate the patient.

The patient with active TB is usually best managed by an infectious disease specialist. Isoniazid (INH), considered the most effective antituberculin drug, is given, often in combination with rifampin, ethambutal hydrochloride, streptomycin sulfate, or para-aminosalicylic acid (PAS). Table 6.14 lists the antituberculin drugs, along with their usual dosages and side effects. Depending on the severity of the disease, the period of treatment may range from 18 to 24 months. However, isolation may be suspended as soon as sputum becomes negative. Finally, the patient and family must be informed that having an active disease does not confer immunity and that treatment does not produce a cure. Both reinfection (although this occurs rarely, if ever) and reactivation can occur. All persons in close contact with active TB patients should be tested with purified protein derivative (PPD) skin tests as soon as the TB is discovered. Positive tests should be followed by chest x-ray films and treatment appropriate to the findings (i.e., prophylaxis or treatment for active TB).

TABLE 6.13 SIGNS AND SYMPTOMS OF ACTIVE PULMONARY TB

PPD skin test	Positive (10 mm or more of induration after 24–72 hours) Questionable (5- to 9-mm) reactions may result from recent infections or partial anergy occurring in the presence of overwhelming TB infection, exanthematous diseases, corticosteroid treatment, sarcoidosis, debility, or advanced age. Anergy (reaction of less than 5 mm of induration in the presence of infection) may occur in the presence of one of the above conditions, but more predominantly in elderly or very ill patients.
Symptoms	Symptoms may initially be absent (for months or years), but insidious onset of nonspecific, slowly progressive *constitutional symptoms* eventually occurs. Malaise, lassitude, easy fatigability, anorexia, mild weight loss, low-grade afternoon fever, chills, night sweats, and wasting are common. *Pulmonary symptoms* also vary in degree of severity and time of onset. Mild to severe cough, sputum production (may be scanty and mucoid or copious and purulent), hemoptysis, dyspnea, shortness of breath, and chest pain may occur in advanced disease. In late, chronic disease, rupture of an artery within the fibrous walls of a cavity may produce sudden, copious hemorrhage (Rasmussen's aneurysm).
Clinical findings	Fine, persistent apical rales (best heard during inspiration after a slight cough) may occur in the early disease. An evanescent wheeze may be elicited if enlarged hilar nodes have resulted in compression of a bronchus (may occur in primary disease, but wheezing is a more common finding in advanced disease). Coarse rales or rhonchi, bronchial breathing, impaired percussion note, and signs of consolidation may be found in acute forms of TB. Chest wall retraction, deviation of trachea, dullness to percussion, coarse rales and rhonchi, and signs of pulmonary consolidation may be present in advanced disease. Egophony, whispered pectoriloquy, and tympany (signs of cavitation) are unreliable signs. Laryngeal involvement with hoarseness and dysphagia, painful pharyngeal ulceration, otitis media, or a perirectal abscess may develop in rare instances where treatment is not sought until late.
Sputum	Direct microscopic exam with acid-fast or fluorescent stain may reveal rods when the bacterial count is high. Demonstration of *M. tuberculosis* (or *M. bovis*) by culture of sputum or other specimens (obtained by bronchoscopic or tracheal washings or aspiration of gastric contents) is definitive proof of infection.
X-ray findings (lateral and PA films are standard)	*Primary disease:* X-ray films may be normal or reveal unilateral hilar adenopathy with or without parenchymal infiltration (occasionally bilateral). Most commonly, infiltrates are confined either to the anterior segment of the upper lobe or to the lower or middle lobe (usually on the right side, which has a larger respiratory surface). Involvement of the apical or posterior segments of the upper lobe or the superior segment of the lower lobe is less common in primary disease. Atelectasis with volume shrinkage and retraction of the lung to the side of involvement may be seen if compression of a bronchus has occurred. Calcification of the primary lesion may be seen if healing has occurred. *Postprimary disease:* Lesions (usually nodular or linear in character) are most typically seen in the atypical and posterior segments of the upper lobes or the superior segments of the lower lobes. Subsegments, segments, or an entire lobe may be involved. Bilateral involvement is common. Atelectasis with retraction of the hilum and deviation of the trachea may also be seen. Demonstration of cavitation (typically a thick-walled cavity surrounded by an area of pneumonitis) is presumptive evidence of TB activity; tomography may be necessary. Symmetric distribution of miliary nodules throughout both lungs is seen if hematogenous spread has occurred. Unilateral or bilateral pleural effusion may also occur (small or intrapulmonary effusions may require positioning of the patient on the involved side to permit visualization of fluid along the lateral chest wall (lateral decubitus film). Lower lung field involvement in the absence of upper lobe lesions occurs in only about 3% of all cases. Lobar consolidation may also occur.

TABLE 6.14 DRUGS USED IN THE TREATMENT OF TB

Drug	Classification	Side Effects	Dosage	Patient Education
Isoniazid (INH)	Antibacterial, tuberculostatic	Hepatotoxicity, hypersensitivity (fever, chills, skin eruptions, lymphadenitis), neurologic symptoms (e.g., visual disturbances), hematologic symptoms (e.g., aplastic anemia), metabolic and endocrine disorders (i.e., pyrodoxine deficiency, hyperglycemia), and GI symptoms.	300 mg/day orally (5 mg/kg/day); continue for 18–24 months for active TB.	Teach signs of side effects, especially hepatotoxicity, and instruct patients to stop medication if these develop until checked. Teach importance of uninterrupted medication therapy.
Rifampin	Antibacterial	Hypersensitivity (fever, pruritus, urticaria, skin eruptions, mouth and tongue soreness, acute renal failure), GI, CNS, and hematologic (e.g., thrombocytopenia) symptoms, hepatorenal syndrome.	600 mg/day orally (10 mg/kg/day); continue for 18–24 months.	Teach common side effects (i.e., red-orange color of urine, feces, sputum, sweat, tears). Stress importance of uninterrupted medication therapy. Instruct patients to take rifampin 1 hour before meals or 2 hours afterward. Discuss the purpose of periodic liver function tests. The use of rifampin (in combination with other anti-TB drugs) has been reported to interfere with the reliability of oral contraceptives in some patients; suggest that female patients switch to an alternative contraceptive method while taking rifampin. Discuss side effects and instruct patients to report hepatic (jaundice, etc.) and GI symptoms immediately.
Ethambutol	Tuberculostatic	Decreased visual acuity (unilateral or bilateral), hepatotoxicity (transient), CNS and GI symptoms, gout.	15 mg/kg/day orally; Continue for 18–24 months.	Instruct patients to report changes in vision immediately. Teach importance of uninterrupted medication therapy.
Streptomycin	Antibiotic, tuberculostatic	Hypersensitivity (skin rashes, pruritus, fever, stomatitis, blood dyscrasias), ototoxicity, neurotoxic effects (paresthesia, muscle weakness).	0.75–1.0 g/day orally; continue for up to 9 months if organism is sensitive.	Teach side effects and instruct patients to report any symptoms when they occur (report symptoms of ototoxicity immediately).
Pyridoxine hydrochloride	Vitamin B_6	Rare pyridoxine megavitaminosis has been associated with severe sensory neuropathy.	Initial therapy: 100 mg/day orally for 3 weeks. Maintenance therapy: 50 mg per day orally for 18–24 months (duration of INH therapy).	Teach need for vitamin B_6 for prevention of INH-induced deficiency. Stress importance of uninterrupted medication therapy.

All close contacts who are initially negative should have the test repeated in 2 months. If they are still negative, no further treatment is necessary. However, if they test positive at that time, and if chest x-ray films and other findings are negative for progressive TB, they should receive INH as a preventive treatment (see the next section).

▶ ***TB screening and prophylaxis*** is an important aspect of disease control. A positive reaction to the PPD skin test does not necessarily indicate active disease; it may mean only contact infection and subsequent immunologic recognition of the tubercle bacillus. The Mantoux test using an intradermal injection of intermediate-strength PPD (5 tuberculin units) is the standard test procedure for TB screening. The results are interpreted in 48–72 hours after the injection, using the diameter of the palpable induration rather than erythema for interpretation. Skin reactions of 5 mm of induration or less in a person with no known recent exposure indicate that a TB infection is unlikely. Reactions of 5–9 mm of induration in 24–72 hours necessitate a repeat test in 1 week and a chest x-ray film. Reactions of 10 mm or more are diagnostic of past or current infection and necessitate further evaluation (physical exam, chest x-ray film, CBC with differential, urinalysis, and SMAC) to exclude active infection. An increase of at least 6 mm of induration (from less than 10 mm to more than 10 mm) is termed a "conversion." Recent converters (persons in whom such a change has occurred within 2 years) are considered newly infected. Mishandling of the antigen or faulty administration may produce false-negative test results; therefore, transfer or tuberculin from one container or another, delay of administration after filling the syringe, and SC (rather than intradermal) injection should be avoided. False-negative results may also occur in the presence of overwhelming or advanced TB, exanthematous diseases, sarcoidosis, malnutrition, debility, corticosteroid therapy, or advanced age, and newly infected individuals may test negatively since tuberculin sensitivity does not develop until 2–10 weeks after the initial infection.

Prior vaccination with bacille Calmette-Guérin (BCG), an antituberculin vaccine made from a culture of *M. bovis,* will also cloud the results of PPD, since persons who have received the vaccine always test somewhat positive, and it is difficult to distinguish between a PPD skin reaction due to a suprainfection (BCG is not always effective in preventing TB infection) and a reaction due to persistent postvaccination sensitivity. Since the incidence of TB infection is considerably lower in the United States than in undeveloped countries, BCG vaccination is rarely given in this country, with the exception of certain PPD-negative individuals who are in well-defined high-risk communities or groups proven to contain an unusually high incidence of new TB infections, where the usual surveillance (routine PPD screening, etc.) and treatment programs are not accessible (e.g., in poverty-stricken rural areas) or effective (e.g., close contacts of patients with active disease who either refuse treatment or have had ineffective treatment). However, questioning patients about prior BCG vaccination, particularly immigrants, will reduce the chance of drawing improper conclusions from positive PPD reactions when such vaccination has been given. Previously vaccinated persons with skin reactions of 10 mm or more should be considered positive for past or present infection and treated in the same manner as unvaccinated persons (i.e., evaluated for active TB infection and treated according to the findings with preventive INH or combination drug therapy for active infection). However, PPD skin reactions in vaccinated persons that are less than 10 mm in diameter may be used as a baseline for routine screening in the future, since the size of the reaction can be expected to decrease with time. Any future increase in PPD reaction should be followed up accordingly. Multiple puncture tests (tine test, Mono-Vacc test) are not as reliable as intradermal tests. These may be used for screening when the latter is not feasible, but any positive test must be confirmed by intradermal PPD.

Patients with newly positive skin tests or those who have tested positive but have had no known previous testing should, as stated above, be evaluated further to rule out active disease. If the findings for active pulmonary TB are negative, chemoprophylaxis with INH may be considered for certain of these positive reactors. The following are candidates for preventive treatment with INH: (1) all recent converters of any age (conversion from negative to positive occurring within the past 2 years); (2) any positive reactors under the age of 35 who are otherwise healthy; (3) positive reactors who are close contacts of recently diagnosed TB patients (retest adults contacts who initially test negative to tuberculin in 2 months and begin preventive treatment at that time if test results become positive); (4) persons with positive skin tests alone or with x-ray findings suggestive of nonprogressive TB; and (5) positive reactors who are also in one of the high-risk groups for reactivation of latent TB (e.g., those with immunosuppression from medications or disease, silicosis, insulin-dependent diabetes mellitus, malnutrition, alcoholism, postgastrectomy patients), with the exception of pregnant women, since the potential risk to the fetus necessitates postponement of treatment until after delivery. Positive reactors over 35 years of age who are otherwise healthy may be considered for treatment on an individual basis, since the risk of developing hepatitis with INH therapy increases with age. Contraindications to INH prophylaxis include a history of severe adverse reactions to INH (e.g., hypersensitivity reactions including drug-induced hepatitis; other signs of INH-induced hepatic injury, such as drug fever, chills, arthritis), acute hepatic disease of any etiology, evidence or strong suspicion of progressive TB (positive chest x-ray film, bacteriologic findings), and a history of adequate treatment with INH.

►***Active pulmonary TB*** is treated with a combination of drugs (usually two or three, but sometimes more in infections caused by resistant organisms), the most commonly used being INH, rifampin, ethambutol, and streptomycin. The particular combination schedule chosen for treatment of an active infection depends on a number of factors, including the patient's reliability in complying with the chosen regimen (the medication must be taken daily in at least the early stages of therapy and sometimes throughout the course), whether any underlying liver dysfunction is present (both INH and rifampin have some potential for hepatotoxicity, which may be synergistic if they are used in combination), whether the patient is an alcoholic or will drink alcoholic beverages daily (daily alcohol use is associated with an increased risk for INH-induced hepatotoxicity), the potential for close supervision, and whether the infection is suspected or proven to be (by results of sensitivity studies) due to organisms resistant to the first-line agents. Table 6.15 lists the various combination drug therapy schedules commonly used in the treatment of active pulmonary TB, as well as the indications and advantages of each. In addition, to prevent the development of an INH-induced deficiency of pyridoxine (vitamin B_6), 50 mg of this vitamin is routinely prescribed as a daily oral dosage for all patients who are receiving treatment with INH (possibly more for alcoholics).

Sarcoidosis, a disease thought to be of autoimmune etiology, causes noncaseat-

TABLE 6.15 COMBINATION DRUG THERAPY SCHEDULES FOR THE TREATMENT OF PULMONARY TB

Combination Schedule	Uses
IA INH (300 mg/day), ethambutol (see "uses"), and streptomycin (1 g/day) IB INH (300 mg/day and ethambutol (as in IA)	Standard long-course regimen (total duration of IA and IB is 18–24 months) for moderate to mild pulmonary TB. Schedule IA is prescribed for 2 months (or until sputum is negative for severe disease), and then followed by schedule IB. Advantage is low toxicity, and can be used when opportunity for supervision is limited or for patients in whom hepatotoxicity is a risk (e.g., alcoholics and daily drinkers). Daily dosage for ethambutol is 15–18 mg per kilogram of body weight for outpatients or 25 mg/kg for patients under very close observation (usually on an inpatient basis).
II INH (300 mg/day) and rifampin (600 mg/day)	Prescribed for compliant patients with infections presumed to be caused by susceptible organisms. To be taken for a minimum of 9 months.
IIIA INH (300 mg/day), rifampin (600 mg/day), and ethambutol (15 mg/kg/day) IIIB INH (900 mg twice a week) and rifampin (600 mg twice a week)	For compliant patients. Schedule IIIA is prescribed for the first month (or 2 months), followed by a minimum of 7–8 months of schedule IIIB. The addition of ethambutol during the first stage of treatment allows for the possibility of resistant organisms pending the results of sensitivity tests. Advantage over schedule II is reduced cost of medication, but closer supervision and compliance in symptom reporting are necessary. Intermittent RIF use may cause influenza-like allergic reactions or (rarely) renal hypersensitivity reactions.
IV INH (300 mg/day), rifampin (600 mg/day), and streptomycin (0.75–1.0 g/day)	Prescribed for infections presumed to be due to resistant organisms (i.e., contact with a treatment-failure patient or an individual from an area with a high incidence of drug-resistant infections). Continue streptomycin while awaiting the results of sensitivity studies. If sensitivity tests prove that the organism is sensitive, switch to combination schedule I (above). If the organism is resistant, a more intensive treatment, using three or four primary or secondary drugs may be required, with careful monitoring.
V INH (900 mg twice a week), rifampin (600 mg twice a week), and streptomycin (1.0 g IM twice a week)	Prescribed for noncompliant patients with susceptible organisms following 2 months of daily therapy described in schedule IV. Total duration of treatment should be at least 9 months (or 6 months following change to negative sputum cultures). Offers advantage of full supervision during administration of medication.
VI INH (900 mg twice a week) with *either* ethambutol (50 mg/kg twice a week) *or* streptomycin (25–28 mg/kg twice a week)	Alternative intermittent regimen for alcoholics and patients with established liver disease. After 2 months of schedule IA (usually while hospitalized), patients are placed on a twice-weekly schedule. Offers the advantage of full supervision of administration, as with schedule V, but avoids the possible synergistic hepatotoxic effect possible with the combined use of INH and rifampin.

ing granuloma formation that may lead to scarring and loss of viable tissue in the lungs, the neighboring lymph system, and other organs. Usually appearing between the ages of 20 and 40, it is more common in blacks than in whites and in females than males. Disease onset is generally marked by spiking fever, weight loss, and fatigue. Otherwise, the clinical presentation depends on the systems affected. Uveitis, erythema nodosa, hepatomegaly, splenomegaly, peripheral adenopathy, hepatitis, salivary and lacrimal gland enlargement, and arthritis may be associated. Respiratory symptoms, the leading complaint of patients with sarcoidosis, initially include cough with minimal sputum production, chest pain, and dyspnea. In progressive disease, as ventilatory capacity is lost due to scar tissue formation (pulmonary fibrosis), severe complications such as hemoptysis, spontaneous pneumothorax, pulmonary insufficiency, cor pulmonale, and superimposed fungal, TB, or other infections may arise. Patients with sarcoidosis usually exhibit cutaneous anergy. The CBC often indicates anemia and a depressed WBC count, and SMAC is significant for elevation of serum calcium and serum globulins. The classical chest x-ray findings include enlarged lymph nodes and fibrosis. Arterial blood gases usually show decreased Po_2 and Pco_2, and pulmonary function tests indicate progressive decline. In milder cases, no treatment is necessary. Patients with progressive pulmonary disease are best managed by respiratory specialists using progressive corticosteroids. Although many patients with sarcoidosis may have recurrent or even permanent remission from disease, the chronic pulmonary fibrosis is associated with poor survival rates, with cor pulmonale or ventilatory insufficiency being the leading causes of death.

Several ***fungal diseases*** cause inflammatory lung changes. Among the more common are ***histoplasmosis, coccidioidomycosis, blastomycosis.*** Residing in soil and dust, fungal spores are inhaled into the lungs, causing an allergic response of variable significance. The diseases are endemic to a particular section of the United States and usually occur in patients who are sensitive to the spores, in immunosuppressed patients, and in the elderly and infants. They are not communicable among humans. Depending on the type of fungus involved, the clinical presentations range from asymptomatic disease to life-threatening changes in the lungs and other organs. They are described, along with mention of endemic areas and routes of transmission, in Table 6.16.

The respiratory system may also be affected by ***opportunistic infections.*** They usually occur in persons who are debilitated, malnourished, or immunosuppressed. Some of these infections are listed in Table 6.17.

Pulmonary Circulation

The pulmonary circulation is diagrammed in Figure 6.4. The pulmonary arteries and arterioles receive blood from the right ventricle and distribute it to the pulmonary capillaries for the exchange of oxygen and carbon dioxide. The pulmonary

TABLE 6.16 SIGNIFICANT FUNGAL DISEASE AFFECTING THE LUNGS

Fungus	Disease	Endemic Area	Transmission
Histoplasma capsulatum	Histoplasmosis	East, Midwest	Soil inhabited by infected chickens, birds, bats contains spores.
Coccidioides immitis	Coccidioidomycosis	Southwest	Inhalation of dust containing spores (arid regions).
Blastomyces dermatitidis	Blastomycosis	Central United States, Southeast	May possibly enter through skin or lungs.
Filobasidiella neoformans (Cryptococcus neoformans)	Cryptococcosis	Southeast	Inhalation of soil containing yeast buds. Also found in dried pigeon dung.
Sporothrix schenckii	Sporotrichosis	No particular region is endemic	Inhalation of spores through contact with plants, decaying wood, soil.

TABLE 6.17 OPPORTUNISTIC INFECTIONS OF THE LUNGS

Disease	Organism(s)
Cryptococcosis	*Filobasidiella neoformans (Cryptococcus neoformans)*
Aspergillosis	*Aspergillus fumigatus* and others
Candidiasis	*Candida albicans* and others
Phycomycosis (mucormycosis, zygomycosis)	Species of *Rhizopus, Absidia, Mucor,* or *Basidiobolus*
Nocardiosis	*Nocardia asteroides, N. brasiliensis*
Histoplasmosis	*Histoplasma capsulatum*
Pneumocystis infection	*Pneumocystis carinii*
Cytomegalovirus infection	Cytomegalovirus
Toxoplasmosis pneumonitis	*Toxoplasma gondii*

venules and veins then collect the blood, returning it to the left atrium for circulation to peripheral vessels. Compared to blood vessels of the systemic circulation, pulmonary vessels are shorter and thinner, contain less smooth muscle, and are more distensible, with less resistance to blood flow.

In addition to the primary function of gas exchange, the pulmonary circulation acts as a resevoir for the left ventricle. Normally, 10% of the total circulative blood volume is in the lungs. The high compliance of the pulmonary vessels allows the volume to vary greatly with relatively little change in pressure. Thus, discrepancies in volume output between the right and left ventricles can be accommodated by the pulmonary blood resevoir. However, in cases of CHF, severe lung disease, or any condition that causes increased pulmonary pressure (Table 6.18), fluid from the pulmonary circulation is forced into interstitial spaces, a condition known as ***pulmonary edema.***

The ***initial phase of pulmonary edema*** occurs when fluid that cannot be handled by the lymphatic system accumulates in the peripheral alveoli and small bronchi and begins to interfere with gas exchange. It is marked by a dry cough, dyspnea,

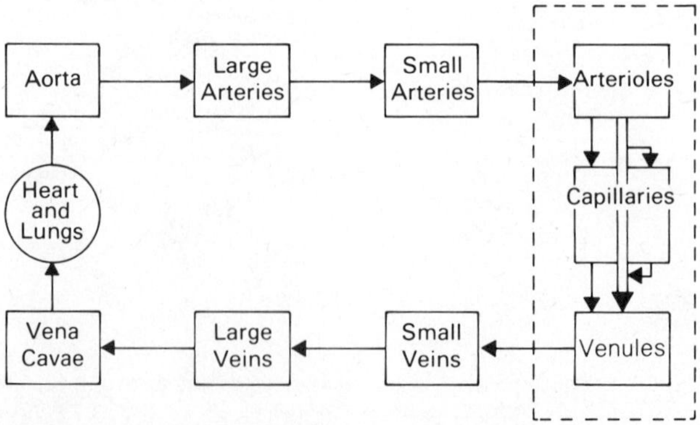

Figure 6.4 Pulmonary circulation. (From Brown AM, Stubbs DW, *Medical Physiology,* copyright © 1983 by John Wiley & Sons, Inc. Reprinted by permission.)

TABLE 6.18 CAUSES OF PULMONARY EDEMA

- Cardiac disease
- Severe pulmonary disease
- Postcardiopulmonary bypass (pump lung, postperfusion lung)
- Diffuse pulmonary infections (viral, bacterial, fungal, pneumocystis)
- Aspiration (gastric contents with Mendelson's syndrome, water with near drowning)
- Lymphatic drainage blockage (e.g., tumor)
- Drug reaction or overdose (e.g., nitrofurantoin, heroin, methadone, hydrochlorthiazide, propoxyphene, morphine, contrast media)
- Inhalation of smoke or toxic substances (e.g., chlorine gas, NO_2 as in silo filler's disease, ozone, high concentrations of O_2)
- Fluid overload
- Rapid ascent to altitudes above 3,000 m (10,000 ft)
- Massive nonthoracic trauma with hypotension (shock lung)
- Hypotension of any cause (continued hemorrhage)
- Severe CNS trauma (neurogenic pulmonary edema)
- Immunologic response to host antigens (e.g., Goodpasture's syndrome, systemic lupus erythematosus)
- Associated with systemic reactions to extrapulmonary processes (gram-negative septicemia, hemorrhagic pancreatitis, amniotic fluid embolism, fat embolism)

orthopnea, and paroxysmal nocturnal dyspnea (PND). PND is characterized by coughing, tachycardia with a gallop rhythm, diaphoresis, and a feeling of suffocation; it usually occurs after several hours of sleep. On auscultation of the chest, rales may be heard in the base of the lungs. In cases associated with heart failure, an S_3 or diastolic gallop (a faint, dull, low-pitched sound heard after S_2) may be noted. Blood pressure may be increased. Arterial blood gases show a decreased P_{CO_2}, along with a mild decrease in P_{O_2}. Diagnosis is confirmed by a chest x-ray film showing the presence of excess fluid. Treatment for the early stages of pulmonary edema may be undertaken on an outpatient basis. Furosemide is given to reduce fluid excess, and the underlying pathology (such as CHF) is corrected whenever possible.

If pulmonary pressure becomes high enough, fluid fills the entire bronchial tree, causing ***acute pulmonary edema.*** Experiencing respiratory distress, patients appear anxious or frightened and express a feeling of dread. They have severe shortness of breath and a productive cough that is typically marked by a frothy hemoptysis. Physical exam may reveal rapid, shallow respirations, cyanosis, diaphoresis, and tachycardia. Blood pressure is low. On auscultation of the chest, moist rales, rhonchi, and/or wheezing ("cardiac wheezing") may be noted. Diminished breath sounds and a rapid, irregular heartbeat are ominous signs. Similarly, the P_{CO_2}, which falls considerably below normal initially, becomes markedly elevated in end-stage disease. The chest x-ray film shows interstitial and alveolar infiltrates that may progress to areas of consolidation ("whiteout"). These patients require hospitalization. Treatment may include sedation (morphine sulfate is commonly used), supplemental oxygen, bed rest, bronchodilators, diuresis, digitalis therapy, phlebotomy, and rotating tourniquets.

In the ***acute respiratory distress syndrome (ARDS),*** pulmonary edema develops, with damage to the aveolar–capillary membrane. The damage may follow shock (from stress, trauma, or hemorrhage), toxin inhalation, narcotic overdose, oxygen toxicity, diffuse pulmonary infections, gram-negative sepsis, multiple transfusions, and hypersensitivity reactions to organic solvents or bone marrow (fat emboli). It leads to the development of hyaline membrane, the components of which (protein-rich fluid, fibrin, sloughed cytoplasm, and necrotic epithelium) move into interstitial and alveolar spaces. In addition to signs of progressive pulmonary edema (see the previous sections), patients may rapidly develop hypotension, mental confusion, and loss of consciousness. Arterial blood gases indicate hypoxia and hypocapnia; the chest x-ray film shows aveolar filtrates, and pulmonary function tests reveal decreases in both pulmonary compliance and residual capacity. Emergency treatment includes ventilatory support, oxygen therapy, and hemodynamic monitoring. Diuretics and fluid restriction may help to reduce circulating fluids. Medication to treat any underlying pathology is needed, as well as bronchodilators and corticosteroids as appropriate.

Because pulmonary and systemic vessels make up a continuous closed system, blood clots developing in peripheral vessels can break off and travel to the lung, resulting in ***pulmonary emboli.*** The cause of 50,000 deaths a year, pulmonary embolism is a major risk for patients who are prone to thrombus formation: bedridden, chronically ill, postpartum or postsurgical patients, as well as women taking birth control pills. Most clots affecting the lungs originate with phlebitis of the deep leg veins (see the later section on phlebitis). Small clots may pass easily through the heart and larger bronchial arteries. However, they eventually become lodged in smaller vessels, causing hemorrhage (if the bronchial arterial supply can maintain the circulation) or infarcts (if the alternative circulation is inadequate). Larger clots may occlude major pulmonary vessels, even the main pulmonary artery. A so-called saddle embolus straddles the bifurcation of the pulmonary artery.

The clinical manifestations of pulmonary embolism vary according to the size of the artery occluded and whether infarction has occurred. If the occlusion involves a small artery, dyspnea with or without pleuritic pain will be present. Occlusion of a main pulmonary artery will present with dyspnea, substernal chest pain, anxiety, and shock. Occlusion of lesser arteries involves a combination of the preceding symptoms. If infarction has occurred, hemoptysis develops 12–36 hours after embolization. Important laboratory tests include elevated WBC, elevated erythrocyte sedimentation rate (ESR), decreased PO_2 with normal or decreased PCO_2 on arterial blood gases, and elevated lactic dehydrogenase (LDH) on serum enzymes. While chest x-ray films are not helpful, a lung scan usually shows ventilation to be greater than perfusion. Pulmonary angiography provides the most specific test information, showing actual clots and obstruction. A fibrinolytic agent such as streptokinase may be useful within the first few hours of clot development. For the most part, however, treatment focuses on anticoagulant therapy (heparin or Coumadin) and preventive measures for venous stasis, as outlined for thromboembolic disease in a later section.

Protective Features (Chest Wall and Pleura)

The thorax is a bony cage that protects the vital organs of the cardiopulmonary system. A thin membrane or parietal pleura separates the mediastinum and the two pleural cavities, each of which contains one lung. The surface of the lung is in contact with the visceral or pulmonary pleura. The thoracic cavity and diaphragm are lined with the second layer, the parietal pleura. The space between the visceral and parietal pleuras is normally a potential, not actual, space, called the "pleural space." The two layers of the pleura are continuous with one another and form a closed unit. A thin coat of serous fluid, the pleural fluid, is present between them. It serves as both a lubricant (aiding easement of the two layers during chest expansion) and an adhesive (producing a tensile force that holds the lungs in expansion). The adhesive function of the plural fluid, along with subatmospheric intrapleural pressure and pulmonary surfactant (a detergent-like substance produced by type 2 acinar cells), prevents pulmonary tissue collapse.

Chest trauma may be categorized as either (1) penetrating injuries in which the pleural cavity is perforated, allowing air to enter, or (2) blunt trauma in which impact on the chest wall compresses the alveoli, damages lung tissue, and/or results in hemorrhage. A number of serious immediate or eventual complications may occur as a result of trauma to the chest, including pulmonary edema, traumatic pneumothorax (open or closed), hemothorax, pulmonary contusion, and empyema (from post-traumatic infection).

Pleurisy is inflammation of the pleural membrane of the lungs. It can be caused by all of the processes that affect the lung: bacterial, mycotic, or viral infections or systemic diseases such as rheumatic fever, lupus erythematosus, and typhoid, to name a few. If a fluid collection is present, the process is referred to as ***pleural effusion.*** It is further described according to the type of fluid produced: serous, fibrinous, serofibrinous, suppurative, and hemorrhagic. Suppurative pleuritis is empyema, or pus in the pleural space. Noninflammatory collections of fluid can also occur. These are hydrothorax (serous fluid in the pleural cavity from such causes as heart failure or ovarian tumor); hemothorax (the escape of whole blood into the pleural space; almost invariably from the rupture of a thoracic aneurysm); chylothorax (accumulation in the pleural space of chyle, the fatty, milky fluid usually produced by lymphatics blocked by malignancy); and pneumothorax (air or gas in the pleural space, either spontaneously, as from a ruptured lung abscess, or traumatically).

Patients who develop pleurisy and/or pleural effusion present with severe chest pain that may be characterized by a sharp, stabbing pain on either the right or left side of the chest and increased on deep inspiration, coughing, and sneezing. Shallow breathing, dyspnea, fever, cough with or without purulent sputum, malaise, and weight loss are other associated symptoms. Physical exam may show a friction rub and decreased or absent breath sounds. A chest x-ray film may reveal pleural fluid or, in cases of chronic adhesive pleuritis, pleural thickening. It may also show underlying malignancy, mediastinal shift, atelectasis, or empyema. To determine the etiology, cultures, Gram stains, and/or cytologic exam of sputum, aspirated pleural fluid, and pleural tissue may be needed. Treatment of pleurisy focuses on pain relief as well as the underlying pathology (i.e., pneumonia, viral infections, TB, CHF, pulmonary abscesses, pulmonary infarction, pulmonary edema, neoplasms, trauma). To relieve pain, analgesics and antitussives are prescribed, along with bed rest, chest splinting, and heat application. In severe cases, thorancentesis may be necessary.

Neoplastic changes may affect the pleura. Primary pleural cancer is called ***mesothelioma.*** Associated with asbestos exposure, this rare tumor spreads widely throughout the pleura, causing effusions and eventual invasion of the thorax. ***Metastatic disease of the pleura*** is far more common, with the lungs, breasts, and ovaries being the usual sources of the primary cancer.

Pleurodynia is an acute inflammation of the intercostal muscles and the muscular attachment of the diaphragm to the chest wall. The symptoms, which are aggravated by respiration and movement, include sudden severe pain and tenderness, fever, headache, and anorexia. There is no cough or pleural effusion, since the lungs are not involved.

HEART

Myocardium and Heart Chambers

The wall of the heart (myocardium) is formed by bundles of striated muscle fibers. The muscle is attached to a fibrous skeleton that divides the heart into right and left sides, as well as upper chambers (atria), and lower chambers (ventricles), as illustrated in Figure 6.5.

A number of ***congenital heart defects*** may alter cardiac function, including patent ductus arteriosus, atrial septal defect, ventricular septal defect, coarctation of the aorta, and tetralogy of Fallot. (These defects are discussed in Table 6.19.)

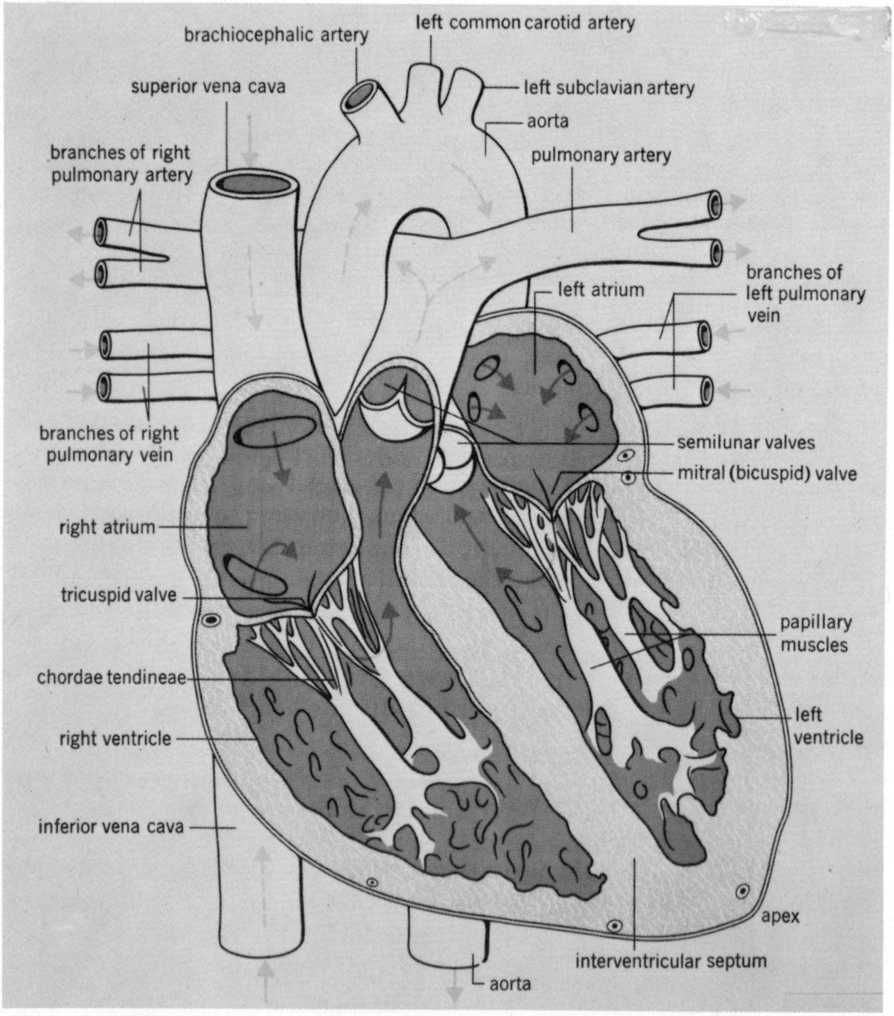

Figure 6.5 The heart. (From Crouch JE, McClintic R, *Human Anatomy and Physiology*, 2nd ed., copyright © 1976 by John Wiley & Sons, Inc. Reprinted by permission.)

TABLE 6.19 CONGENITAL HEART DEFECTS

Diagnosis	Etiology	Signs and Symptoms	Diagnosis	Treatment
Atrial-septal defect	Refers to the persistence of the ostium primum or ostium secundum (most common in the atrial septum). Rarely, a third form presents as the sinus venosus defect.	Slight or moderate defects are asymptomatic; larger defects produce dyspnea on exertion, visible and palpable right ventricular pulsations, a loud systolic ejection murmer, and a soft middiastolic murmer. S_2 is widely split.	ECG reveals right ventricular hypertrophy and complete or incomplete right bundle branch block. X-ray film reveals an enlarged right atrium and ventricle and large pulmonary arteries with increased vascularity. Diagnostic studies include cardiac catheterization and echocardiography.	Surgical closure in all but small defects.
Ventricular septal defect	Refers to the persistence of the opening between the upper interventricular septum and the aortic septum.	Clinical manifestations are in proportion to the size of the defect. A small or moderate defect produces a long, loud, harsh systolic murmur and thrill (third and fourth intercostal spaces adjacent to the sternum). A larger defect produces a pansystolic murmur, a middiastolic murmur, and a palpable right ventricular heave. Cardiac failure is common in infants.	ECG is normal or may reveal right and/or left ventricular hypertrophy. An enlarged right and/or left ventricle, left atrium, pulmonary arteries, and increased pulmonary vascularity may be seen on chest x-ray films. Diagnostic studies include cardiac catheterization and echocardiography.	Surgical repair.
Patient ductus arteriosus	Refers to the persistence of the embryonic ductus arteriosus between the pulmonary artery and the aorta.	Asymptomatic until ventricular failure results; then pulse pressure is wide and diastolic pressure is low. Other signs are a continuous, rough murmur, louder at late systole, thrills, and paradoxic splitting of S_2.	ECG may be normal or indicative of left ventricular hypertrophy. X-ray film shows a normal heart size with or without atrial and/or ventricular enlargement and prominence of the pulmonary artery, left atrium, and aorta. Diagnostic studies include cardiac catheterization.	For premature infants with cardiac failure, a trial of indomethacin. For older infants, surgical repair. For asymptomatic adults, no treatment is required.
Tetralogy of Fallot	Refers to pulmonary stenosis and a high ventricular septal defect.	Dyspnea, fatigue, cyanosis, clubbing, slight right ventricular heave, short, harsh systolic murmur and thrill at the left sternal border. S_2 may be split.	ECG indicates moderate right ventricular hypertrophy. X-ray film shows a heart of normal size, but boot-shaped due to blunting of the apex and the concave appearance of the pulmonary artery segment. Diagnostic studies include cardiac catheterization and echocardiography.	Surgical repair.
Coarctation of the aorta	Refers to localized stenosis of the aortic arch just distal or proximal to the ligamentum arteriosum.	Asymptomatic until complications of hypertension are evidenced by left ventricular failure or cerebral hemorrhage.	ECG findings may be normal or may reveal left ventricular hypertrophy. X-ray findings include notching of the ribs as a result of enlarged collateral vessels, enlargement of the left ventricle, and dilatation of the left subclavian artery and the poststenotic portion of the aorta. Diagnostic studies: cardiac catheterization.	Surgical repair recommended for all patients 20 or younger and for patients 20–35 years old with left ventricular hypertrophy.

TABLE 6.20 CAUSES OF MYOCARDITIS

Infectious
- Viral (including coxsackievirus A and B strains, poliomyelitis, influenza, rubeola, rubella, adenovirus, echovirus, and encephalomyocarditis or EMC virus)
- Bacterial (pneumococcus, diphtheria, meningococcal)
- Protozoal (*Trypanosoma cruzi, Toxoplasma gondii*)
- Fungal (*Candida, Aspergillus*)
- Others (Lyme disease, trichinosis, strongyloidiasis, leptospirosis, scrub typhus)

Toxic
- Drugs (e.g., sulfonamides, daunorubicin)
- Chemical (carbon dioxide)
- Exotoxin produced by *Corynebacterium diphtheriae*

Systemic disease
- Acute rheumatic fever
- Acute glomerulonephritis
- Connective tissue disorders (systemic lupus erythematosus, scleroderma, rheumatoid arthritis, sarcoidosis)

Radiation therapy

Unknown (idiopathic giant cell myocarditis or Fiedler's myocarditis; a viral etiology has been postulated)

Forming a functional syncytium, series of individual cardiac muscle fibers are connected at intercalated discs. As discussed later, action potentials are originated by a conduction system and sent from the atrial syncytium to the ventricular syncytium through these discs. The electrical impulses cause actin and myosin filaments within the muscle cells to slide together, bringing an all-or-nothing contraction in much the same manner as occurs in skeletal muscle (see Chapter 11). The chemical energy necessary for this process is derived from the aerobic metabolism of glucose, fatty acids, and other nutrients in myocardial cells. Inflammation or disease affecting the muscle cells can compromise the contractile process of the heart.

Myocarditis (carditis), inflammation of the myocardium, is most often the result of a bacterial or viral infection. It may also be associated with exposure to radiation, drugs, and chemicals, metabolic disorders, autoimmune disease, and other factors noted in Table 6.20. Pericarditis, CHF, and cardiomyopathy are possible complications (see later discussions). Patients may present with only vague complaints such as fatigue, dyspnea, palpitations, and precordial discomfort. Chest pain usually reflects associated pericarditis. Tachycardia is usual, as is fever. Heart sounds are muffled, and a gallop rhythm and/or transient apical systolic murmur may be heard. The most common electrocardiographic (ECG) changes are ST-segment and T-wave abnormalities, although arrhythmias [particularly ventricular, atrioventricular (AV) and intraventricular conduction defects and, rarely, Q waves] may also be seen. A chest x-ray film often reveals a normal or markedly enlarged heart and, in severe cases, pulmonary congestion. Isolating the causative agent often requires culturing of feces, mucosal secretions, or pericardial fluid. Endomyocardial biopsy may be necessary as a last resort. General treatment measures include management of cardiac failure, arrhythmias, and conduction defects. Immunosuppressive drugs combined with corticosteroids may be needed in severe cases marked by rapidly developing cardiac failure. In addition, specific treatment is undertaken for the underlying disease. For example, causative drugs or chemicals should be withdrawn immediately. Appropriate antimicrobial agents are given for diphtheria, pneumococcosis, candidiasis, and toxoplasmosis. Metabolic disorders should be corrected. Unfortunately, antiviral agents are not available. The long-term prognosis is variable and ranges from complete recovery to progressive cardiac failure and death.

TABLE 6.21 CLINICAL MANIFESTATIONS OF RF

Major Manifestation	Description
Fever	May be low-grade, continuous or intermittent.
Carditis	Evidenced by any of the following: 1. Pericarditis (fibrinous or serofibrinous): diagnosed by progressive increase in heart shadow on serial CXRs or by echocardiography. 2. Cardiac enlargement from dilatation of weakened, inflamed myocardium: diagnosed by serial CXRs. 3. CHF: right-sided heart failure, with liver engorgement particularly common in children. 4. Change in heart sounds: mitral or aortic diastolic murmurs developing from dilatation of a valve ring or valvulitis (especially Carey-Coombs short middiastolic murmer). Pansystolic apical murmur transmitted to the axilla that persists or intensifies during the course of the disease. S_3 gallop. 5. ECG changes: increase of the PR interval greater than 0.04 of baseline (returns to normal as rheumatic activity subsides). Changing contour of P waves or inversion of T waves. Sinus tachycardia out of proportion to degree of fever. Ectopy.
Erythema annulare	Slightly raised, rapidly enlarging macules characterized by crescent shape and central clearing. May be transient or persist for long periods.
Subcutaneous nodules	Small (usually less than 2 cm in diameter), firm, painless nodules attached to fascia or tendon sheaths over bony prominences. Rare in adults, they persist for days or weeks and are typically recurrent.
Arthritis	A migratory sequential polyarthritis (i.e., heat, redness, swelling, and pain subside in one joint, only to flare up in another). In children, affects the large joints, but in adults, small joints (or single joints) may be affected. Usually self-limiting in 1–5 weeks, with no residual joint deformities. Exception is a rare, persistent arthritis (Jaccoud's arthritis).
Sydenham's chorea	Involuntary, purposeless movement of the muscles of the trunk and extremities, impairment of speech and memory, and/or behavioral changes. Thought to be caused by an arteritis, it usually develops 2–3 months after other symptoms of RF and is more common in women than in men. May recur during pregnancy or with oral contraceptive use.

As the most common cause of carditis, ***rheumatic fever (RF)*** deserves further discussion. More prevalent in men than in women, it peaks between ages 5 and 15 and is rare before age 4 or after 50. A delayed immunologic response to group A streptococcal infections of the upper respiratory tract causes perivascular granulomatous lesions and vasculitis, which affect a number of systems. Typically, 1–4 weeks after a bout of tonsillitis, nasopharyngitis, or otitis, patients develop two or more of the manifestations described in Table 6.21. Laboratory findings include nonspecific evidence of inflammatory disease (i.e., elevated ESR and/or WBC), a moderate degree of anemia, and occasional proteinuria and hematuria. Evidence of a prior streptococcal infection is indicated by a high or increasing titer of antistreptolysin O (ASO). X-ray, ECG, and echocardiographic changes are described in Table 6.21.

Treatment of RF begins with bed rest until all signs of active disease have disappeared. Antibiotics are given to eradicate any existing streptococcal infection. While salicylates markedly reduce fever and relieve joint pain, there is no indication that they alter the natural course of the disease. By contrast, short-term corticosteroid therapy does seem to reverse some of the acute manifestations. Even with aggressive intervention, however, initial episodes last for months in children and for weeks in adults and are associated with a mortality of 1–2%. In addition, two-thirds of the survivors develop ***chronic rheumatic heart disease.*** The small pink granules that appear on the heart valves during the acute phase of RF fail to resolve or recur with subsequent attacks of RF. Causing subacute or chronic inflammation over months or years, they eventually lead to fibrosis and thickening of the cusps, commissures, or chordae tendinae (AV valves), as discussed in a later section. For this reason, ***prevention of recurrent RF*** is a primary concern in all cases. Adults should receive prophylactic therapy once a month for about 5 years after an acute attack or until about age 30 if they are exposed to a population with a high rate of streptococcal infection. Prompt, intensive treatment of future streptococcal infections is vitally important. Finally, general prophylactic measures should be instituted for dental work and urologic or surgical procedures (see the later section on endocarditis).

Myocardial diseases that are not the result of ischemia, hypertension, valve or pericardial disease, or congenital abnormalities are called ***cardiomyopathies.*** The chief causes of cardiomyopathy are listed in Table 6.22. ***Secondary cardiomyopathy*** accompanies a systemic disease, while ***primary cardiomyopathy*** is not part of a disorder affecting other organs. Three types have been identified: ***dilated cardiomyopathy, hypertrophic cardiomyopathy,*** and ***restrictive cardiomyopathy.*** They are described in Table 6.22, along with the signs and symptoms, diagnostic findings, and treatment. Close attention by a cardiac specialist is invariably required. The prognosis is generally poor, with many patients facing transplant surgery as their final hope in the later stages of disease.

Compromise of myocardial tissue for any reason can interfere with the heart's ability to supply sufficient blood to body tissues to meet metabolic demands. Whenever this occurs, a syndrome develops that is referred to as ▶***congestive heart failure (CHF).*** Physiologically, it evolves from three sequential conditions. The first condition is ***cardiac overload.*** This may be secondary to pressure overload (high afterload), volume overload, and/or loss of functional myocardial tissue, as described in Table 6.23. Four compensatory mechanisms develop in an attempt to increase cardiac performance and thereby maintain adequate cardiac output. Constituting the second condition in CHF, they include (1) ventricular dilatation, which increases the force of the contraction and thus the stroke volume and cardiac output (Frank-Starling principle); (2) sympathetic nervous system response (elevation of circulating catecholamines), which affects the heart by increasing the pulse rate and myocardial contractility, and affects the peripheral vascular system by increasing vasocontractility, causing renal retention of sodium and water to expand the volume; (3) ventricular hypertrophy, in which an increase in cardiac muscle mass helps boost ventricular contractility; and (4) an increase in oxygen extraction from circulating blood by various tissues so that less blood flow is needed to maintain the oxygen consumption level.

If these compensatory mechanisms are unable to mediate the overload or fail themselves, cardiac decompensation, the third sequential condition, occurs. Beginning with the left side of the heart only, the right side of the heart only, or the left and right sides of the heart in combination, it is responsible for the development of symptoms and signs that vary depending on the the underlying pathology and severity of failure. Patients may develop dyspnea, dyspnea on exertion (DOE), paroxysmal nocturnal dyspnea (PND), orthopnea, shortness of breath (SOB), or a dry cough. They may note problems related to fluid retention such as daytime oliguria, nocturia, and weight gain. Venous congestion may be marked by abdominal pain especially in the upper right quadrant, distention, bloating, anorexia, nausea, and con-

TABLE 6.22 TYPES OF CARDIOMYOPATHIES

Type	Description	Clinical Findings	Diagnosis	Treatment
		Acute		
Acute myocarditis	Inflammation of the myocardium, either focal or diffuse, which occurs during or after an infection or after administration of medications. The primary infection may be viral, bacterial, rickettsial, spirochetal, fungal, or parasitic. Causes include coxsackie B virus, acute rheumatic fever, diphtheria, scrub typhus, and Chagas' disease.	Acute febrile symptoms (i.e., fever, malaise, arthralgia). Chest pain, dyspnea, palpitations. Tachycardia greater than that associated with fever, systolic murmur or gallop rhythm with S_3. Possible complications include cardiac failure, ventricular arrhythmias, AV conduction defects, circulatory collapse, emboli, and sudden death.	ECG: nonspecific ST-T changes; conduction defects (if conduction system is affected by the inflammatory process). Chest x-ray film: nonspecific findings. Echocardiogram: enlarged left ventricle. Endomyocardial biopsy: should be done to identify the specific cause.	Administer specific drug therapy for causative organism. In severe cases, administer corticosteroids with immunosuppressive medication. Stop cardiotoxic medication. Manage symptoms and complications. Restrict vigorous activity.
		Chronic		
Idiopathic dilated congestive cardiomyopathy (primary cardiomyopathy)	Disease of the myocardium of unknown cause, but labeled based on clinical manifestations of cardiomegaly, increased cardiac volume, and CHF.	Exertional dyspnea, fatigue, nondescript chest pain, palpitations, vertigo, syncope. CHF. AV arrhythmias. Complications include pulmonary and systemic emboli.	ECG: Atrial or ventricular arrhythmias; left ventricular hypertropy; conduction defects; nonspecific ST-T changes. Chest x-ray film: Cardiomegaly (left ventricular); pulmonary congestion. Echocardiography: May help rule out pericardial effusion, aortic stenosis, and mitral valve disease.	Treat symptoms and complications.
Idiopathic hypertrophic (obstructive) cardiomyopathy a. IHSS b. Asymmetric septal hypertrophy	Genetic disease of unknown cause that results in a disproportionate hypertrophy of the ventricular septal wall and may obstruct left or right ventricular outflow.	Exertional dyspnea, chest pain, fatigue, vertigo, syncope. Pansystolic murmur. Complications include cardiac failure.	ECG: QRS and ST-T changes indicative of left ventricular hypertrophy; arrhythmias. Chest x-ray film: Cardiomegaly. Echocardiography: Disproportionate thickening of the ventricular septum.	Administer beta-adrenergic blocking agents (e.g., propranolol, verapamil). Treat arrhythmias. Myotomy and limited resection of hypertrophied muscle if symptomatic and unresponsive to propranolol.
Restrictive cardiomyopathy	Uncommon disease associated with diseases that impair left ventricular filling and emptying. May be associated with amyloidosis, endomyocardial fibrosis, hemochromatosis, or scleroderma.	Biventricular failure. Normal or slightly enlarged heart. Similar to congestive cardiomyopathy.	See congestive cardiomyopathy.	See congestive cardiomyopathy.

stipation. Symptoms of the peripheral vascular system that reflect systemic vasoconstriction include cold, pale extremities; cyanosis of the lips, nail beds and extremities; and increasing fatigue and muscle weakness. Cerebrovascular symptoms often result from decreased oxygenation of tissue and include irritability, restlessness, mental confusion, and syncope. Patients suffering from relatively acute CHF may appear anxious and apprehensive. By contrast, those with insidious onset of disease often shows signs of depression.

On physical exam, distended neck veins, hepatomegaly, hepatojugular reflex, ascites, and dependent pitting edema may be noted. Changes that may be heard

TABLE 6.23 TYPES OF CARDIAC OVERLOADING

Type	Cause
Pressure overload (from resistance in great vessels)	Aortic stenosis, pulmonary and/or systemic hypertension, CAD
Volume overload (from excessive filling of the ventricles during diastole)	Mitral regurgitation, aortic regurgitation, excessive venous return, and intracardiac shunt anomalies
Weakened pumping action (from loss of functional myocardial tissue)	Usually MI

on auscultation of the chest may include rales, rhonchi, friction rub, increased respiration rate, decreased breath sounds, muffled heart sounds, and increased heart rate. A murmur may be heard if the underlying cause of CHF is valvular disease. On a chest x-ray film the lung field may be hazy, the pulmonary vein distended, and the heart enlarged. Arterial blood gas studies may indicate decreased P_{O_2}, decreased P_{CO_2}, and increased pH. Serum levels of urea nitrogen, uric acid, and creatinine may be increased. Liver function tests may be abnormal. Results of routine urinalysis may show mild proteinuria. Treatment of CHF is based on three principles. First, there must be a decrease in excessive fluid retention (salt-restricted diet and diuretics). Second, there must be an increase in the effectiveness of myocardial contraction (digitalization). Third, the workload of the heart must be decreased (vasodilators, physical and emotional rest). Along with treatment of the CHF syndrome, the underlying cause of the heart failure should be treated (e.g., hypertension).

Electrical Control of Myocardial Contractions

Propagation of electrical stimuli through the myocardium initiates and controls myocardial contraction. It is influenced by potassium (K^+), sodium (Na^+), and calcium (CA^{2+}) ion concentrations as follows. Due to the high resistance of the muscle membrane (sarcolemma) to ion flow, resting cells have higher intracellular than extracellular K^+ concentrations and lower intracellular than extracellular Na^+ and Ca^{2+} concentrations. Calcium inside the cells is stored in the cisternae of the sarcolemma reticulum (SR). An electrical impulse traveling across cell membranes brings about an abrupt change in membrane permeability, allowing a rapid influx of Na^+ and a rapid efflux of K^+ (phases O and I). This initiates depolarization (phase II), represented as a spike on a recording graph. During the plateau stage (phase III) there is a slow inward flux of Ca^{2+} and a release of stored Ca^{2+}. The larger intracellular quantity of calcium blocks the action of troponin, a contraction-inhibiting protein, allowing actin and myosin to interact and produce a contraction. Repolarization (phase IV) and return to the resting state (phase V) are accomplished as K^+ reenters the cells and Na^+ and Ca^{2+} are expelled. The remaining intracelluar Ca^{2+} returns to the SR.

The impulses responsible for these synchronized cellular depolarizations originate in the sinoatrial (SA) node and are propagated through the specialized conduction system of the heart (see Fig. 6.6). Unlike the working myocardial cells, cells of these structures possess the property of automaticity and thus undergo spontaneous depolarization. Since the frequency of automatic impulse formation is greatest in the SA node, this node functions as the pacemaker of the heart.

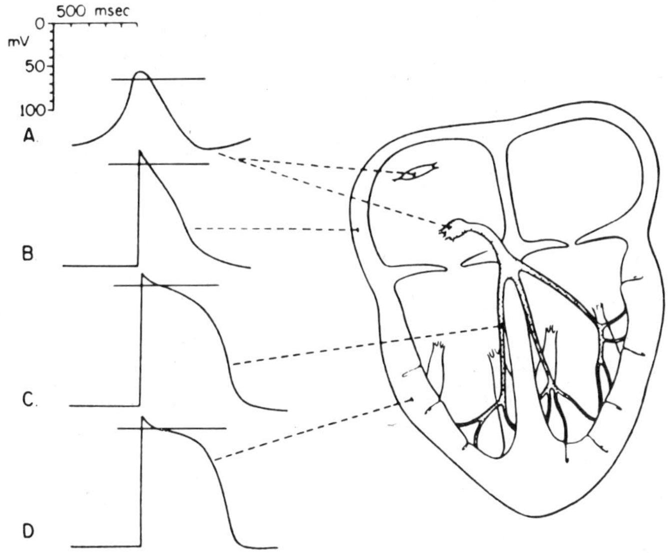

Figure 6.6 Conduction tissue of the heart. (From Brown AM, Stubbs DW, *Medical Physiology,* copyright © 1983 by John Wiley & Sons, Inc. Reprinted by permission.)

Atrial contractions begin when the automatic cells of the SA node depolarize, exciting adjacent cells in the atrial walls. The wave of depolarization moves downward and to the left, reaching the most distant portions of the atria in about 0.08 seconds. The impulse also travels along the specialized fibers of the conduction system to the AV node, the only normal avenue over which an impulse is transmitted from the atria to the ventricles. The impulse continues down the bundle of His, through its right and left bundle branches into the ventricular myocardium via the Purkinje fibers. This elaborate system of fibers finally merges with working myocardial muscle fibers.

The electrical currents generated by the conducting system of the heart spread throughout the surrounding tissues and to the surface of the body, where they can be picked up and amplified by an electrocardiograph. As demonstrated in Figure 6.7, each recorded wave traces the path of depolarization through the heart. Analyses of the P wave and the QRS complex, their rate, and their temporal relationship to each other are invaluable in diagnosing cardiac rhythm disturbances or localizing areas of injury or necrosis. In addition, deviations of the electrical axis and associated ventricular abnormalities can be determined from the standard lead ECG via vectorial analysis. Vectors are arrows that point in the direction of positive current flow. Their length is proportional to the generated voltage. Each of the standard leads (I, II, III) is actually a pair of electrodes connected to the body on opposite sides of the heart. The mean electrial axis (normally 59 degrees) is determined by averaging the vectors between each of the pairs. Under certain abnormal ventricular conditions, the direction of these vectors and thus the electrical axis is shifted to the left or right.

The normal rhythm is generated by the SA node and ranges from 60 to 100 regularly spaced beats per minute (sinus rhythm). ***Cardiac arrhythmias*** may be classified as ***atrial,*** AV nodal ***(junctional),*** or ***ventricular,*** as described in Table

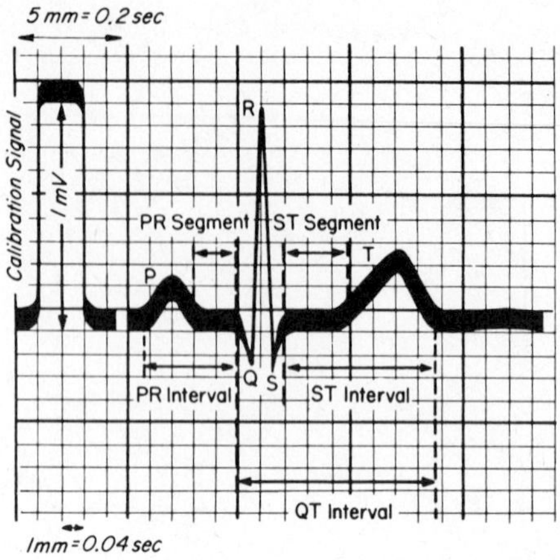

Figure 6.7 Cardiac contraction as recorded on ECG. (From Brown AM, Stubbs DW, *Medical Physiology,* copyright © 1983 by John Wiley & Sons, Inc. Reprinted by permission.)

6.24. Recent evaluations of cardiac electrophysiology have led to the reentry theory of arrhythmias. During normal sinus rhythm, conduction occurs along rapidly conducting pathways that require long refractory periods and along slow fibers with short resting intervals. Impulses traveling along the latter pathways end at their junction with the fast fibers, since the fast fibers, having already depolarized, are resting. If conduction is blocked in the fast pathway, impulses proceed along slow fibers to the junction and on to the distal portions of the system. In addition, impulses at the junction can travel in a retrograde manner in the fast pathway back to the SA node, leading to its early repolarization and an arrhythmia. Several important factors increase the likelihood of cardiac arrhythmias. Excess or reduced extracellular calcium (hypo- or hypercalcemia) and potassium (hypo- or hyperkalemia) concentrations also cause rhythm disruption. Hypoxia, hypercapnia, hyperthermia, and cardiac dilatation produce tachycardia and ectopic discharges from secondary pacemaker sites. Hypothermia leads to bradycardia. As automaticity increases in tissues bordering areas of injury or necrosis, ectopic rhythms are likely to occur. Finally, liberation of acetylcholine during increased vagal activity produces sinus slowing and allows secondary pacemakers to assume control.

Cardiac arrhythmias are best handled by the cardiac specialist. Diagnosis is based on the history, the physical findings, and the ECG. Ambulatory ECG monitoring (using a 24-hour cardiocorder) is invaluable for determining the presence and type of arrhythmias and evaluating treatment success. Several drugs, which are administered singly or in combination, are available for the treatment of a variety of cardiac arrhythmias. The ideal antiarrhythmic drug has a wide range of therapeutic activities in both atrial and ventricular arrhythmias with minimal side effects (both cardiac depressant and noncardiac), permits simple dosage schedules to facilitate compliance, and provides long-term prophylaxis. Antiarrhythmic agents have been classified according to their anatomic site of action and their electrophysiologic action on isolated cardiac fibers. Table 6.25 describes the leading drugs according to these guidelines. Cardioversion is an effective method of converting several types of

TABLE 6.24 CARDIAC ARRHYTHMIAS

Arrhythmia	Description	Treatment
	Atrial	
Sinus arrhythmia	Variable rate occurring as a normal phenomenon in children and young adults in relationship to respiration.	None necessary.
Sinus tachycardia	Rapid SA nodal activity produces a heart rate greater than 100 beats per minute. While tachycardia is a normal physiologic response to exercise, fright, stress, excitement, or emotional upset, it may also indicate pathology (fever, anemia, shock, hyperthyroidism, CHF, pulmonary embolism, acute MI, pericarditis).	Based on the underlying etiology. Sedatives and beta blockers may be necessary. Carotid massage will slow the rate, allowing return to sinus rhythm. In cases of CHF, digitalis is helpful.
Sinus bradycardia	Heart rate of less than 60 beats per minute. Common in young adults, trained athletes, and many elderly persons. May be caused by drugs (digitalis, beta blockers, morphine, reserpine, prostignine). May also accompany acute MI or heart block.	None necessary unless rate fails to increase with exercise, atropine, or treatment of the underlying condition, in which case a ventricular pacemaker is indicated.
Premature atrial contractions (PAC)	Ectopic atrial impulse that converts to the normal conduction path once it reaches the AV node. Most frequently associated with organic heart disease (notably disease or enlargement of the atria). May also be precipitated by fatigue, anxiety, and tobacco and caffeine use. Irregular heartbeat may be evident on exam. ECG shows an ectopic P wave followed by a pause prior to the next sinus beat. The P wave may be hidden by the T wave if it occurs too close to the preceding beat. Normal QRS complex.	If patient is symptomatic, digitalization may be required, as well as treatment of the underlying cause of the arrhythmia.
Atrial fibrillation	Loss of synchronized atrial contractions marked by extremely rapid and irregular atrial and ventricular rates. Usually associated with mitral valve disease, acute MI, atherosclerotic heart disease, hypertension, thyrotoxicosis. Less commonly associated with COPD, pulmonary embolism, and multiple atrial ectopic foci. Pulse is rapid and irregular. ECG shows an indistinguishable P wave that may be wavy and irregular or flat and straight. The PR interval is irregular, but the QRS complex is normal. Condition associated with decreased cardiac output, thrombus formation, and emboli.	Treatment of the underlying cause of the arrhythmia. Defibrillation in emergency situations. Verapamil or digitalis (except in Wolff-Parkinson-White syndrome, where these drugs may decrease AV conduction in normal pathways, enhancing aberrant pathways).
Atrial flutter	Atrial impulse rates of 250–350 beats per minute, with 2:1 ventricular conduction (ventricular rate around 150). Uncommon arrhythmia usually confined to patients with rheumatic heart disease, CAD, cor pulmonale, atrial septal defect, or quinidine effect.	DC countershock. If unavailable, digitalis as drug of choice. Beta blockers and calcium entry blockers also used. Quinidine sometimes given to digitalized, difficult-to-control patients.
Paroxysmal atrial tachycardia (PAT)	Episodes of tachycardia (rates typically 170–220 beats per minute) beginning abruptly, lasting for several hours, and ending abruptly. The rhythm is regular, and there are no associated symptoms, though dyspnea and chest tightness may occur with prolonged attacks, particularly in patients with underlying mitral stenosis or CAD. Often occurs in young patients with normal hearts or secondary to digitalis toxicity.	Mechanical stimulation of vagus nerve (arm/body stretching, lowering head between knees, Valsalva maneuver, induced vomiting, carotid massage). For prolonged attacks, verapamil, tensilon, pressor agents, procainamide, beta blockers, digitalis, or quinidine may be used.
Sick sinus syndrome	Due to abnormalities of sinus node and its AV conduction, patients develop alternate episodes of tachycardia and bradycardia, often resulting in failing ventricular function. Pathologic causes include CAD and fibrotic lesions of the cardiac conduction system.	Best managed with insertion of an artificial demand pacemaker into the right atrium, as well as antiarrhythmic drugs.

TABLE 6.24 (*Continued*)

Arrhythmia	Description	Treatment
	AV Nodal	
Junctional rhythm	Rather than originating from the sinus node, pacemaker activity arises from the atrial–nodal or nodal–His bundle junctions. Results in a passive escape rhythm with a rate of 40–60 beats per minute that increases normally with exercise. Occurs in patients with normal hearts as well as in those with myocarditis, CAD, or digitalis or quinidine toxicity.	Except for cases associated with drug toxicity, no intervention is necessary.
Junctional tachycardia	Tachycardia marked by rates of 140–240 beats per minute due to regular transmission of impulses originating in the AV node or His bundle to the ventricles. Common with cor pulmonale, digitalis toxicity, and serious myocardial disease. Sometimes benign. Besides tachycardia, ECG findings often include a QRS duration exceeding 0.14 second, left axis deviation, AV dissociation, monophasic or biphasic complexes in V_1, or a QR or QS complex in V_6.	Similar to that for atrial tachycardia. Refractory cases may require surgical correction of aberrent circuits.
Wolff-Parkinson-White syndrome	Impulses begin normally in the sinus node but then short-circuit the AV node via the bundle of Kent or the Mahaim fibers, resulting in preexcitation. Depending on the bypass tract, the disorder is grouped into two main and several complex subcategories. Type A (left accessory bypass) produces ECG findings consistent with right ventricular hypertrophy or right bundle branch block. Type B (right lateral accessory pathway) produces ECG tracings similar to those of left bundle branch block. Other characteristic ECG findings include a short PR interval, a wide QRS complex, and a slurred, short delta wave. Half of these patients remain asymptomatic, while the other half develop atrial arrhythmias (tachycardia, flutter, or fibrillation).	No treatment is necessary unless atrial arrhythmias develop (see preceding section). Drug selection must be based on refractory periods of both normal and aberrent pathways determined through His bundle recordings. Atrial pacemakers, DC cardioversion, or surgery may also be necessary.
First-degree heart block	Classified by severity, heart block is an anatomic or functional disturbance of an impulse through the conduction system that may be permanent or transient. First-degree block, the mildest and most common form, is characterized by an impulse that originates in the SA node and follows the normal conduction pathway through the AV node, but has a delay in conduction time. It is evidenced as a prolonged PR interval followed by a normal QRS complex on ECG. Causes are CAD, digitalis toxicity, or acute RF.	Usually asymptomtic; treatment is not advised.
Second-degree heart block	A conduction delay, usually within the AV node, that produces a partial and progressive AV block until an impulse is no longer conducted.	Careful observation. If weakness or cardiac failure results from bradycardia, a pacemaker is indicated.
Mobitz type I (Wenckebach)	A second-degree heart block characterized by a progressively increasing PR interval until the blocked P wave occurs. The next P wave is conducted, and the sequence begins again. May be associated with CHF and transient ventricular ectopic beats and syncope.	As above.
Mobitz type II	Another, less common type of second-degree heart block. Marked by a periodic blocked impulse in the bundle of His or the right and left bundle branches. Usually occurs as the result	Administration of atropine. Surgical insertion of a permanent pacemaker may be necessary.

TABLE 6.24 *(Continued)*

Arrhythmia	Description	Treatment
	of an MI. The ECG shows a PR interval that may be prolonged or normal. The blocked P wave may occur in an irregular or regular 2:1, 3:1, or 4:1 pattern. If the QRS complex is widened, it indicates a block below the AV node.	
Third-degree (complete) heart block	Inability of any impulse from the SA node to be conducted to the AV node and into the ventricles. Caused by any factors that affect the myocardial conduction system (congenital heart disease, valve disease, cardiac tumor, connective tissue disorders, myocardial ischemia, MI, hypokalemia, drug toxicity). The ECG reveals P waves with no relation to QRS complexes and a ventricular rate of 40 to 50 beats per minute. If the block occurs within the AV node, QRS is wide and bizarre.	Treatment of the underlying pathology is necessary to prevent complications, especially asystole or Adams-Stokes syncope (loss of consciousness due to slow heart rate). Insertion of a temporary or permanent pacemaker may be advisable.
	Ventricular	
Premature ventricular contractions (PVC)	Conduction of impulses that originate in either ventricle. May have a single focus or multiple foci. On ECG, the PVC is seen as a wide, bizarre QRS complex with no preceding P wave. A compensatory pause may follow the PVC, or the PVC may be interpolated between two normal beats with no change in rhythm. PVCs may be due to acute MI or any form of heart disease, open heart surgery, digitalis toxicity, or any serious illness. May also be precipitated by fatigue, anxiety, or tobacco or caffeine use. Complications include ventricular tachycardia and ventricular fibrillation.	Treatment is not usually necessary in healthy adults. However, if PVCs cause symptoms or occur in association with heart disease, digitalization may be required. If they occur in the presence of acute MI, lidocaine or procainamide should be administered.
Ventricular bigeminy	PVC occurring with every other beat.	As above.
Ventricular trigeminy	PVC occurring with every third beat.	As above.
Ventricular tachycardia	Ventricular rhythm with a heart rate of 130–250 beats per minute at predominantly regular intervals. It may occur in short runs of 3 or more beats or as the dominant rhythm. On ECG, the P wave, if present, has no relationship to the QRS complex or is indistinguishable because of the rapid rate. QRS complexes are wide and bizarre. Associated with any form of heart disease (notably CAD), digitalis toxicity, and one or more ectopic foci in either ventricle. Ventricular fibrillation, MI, cerebral ischemia, CHF, or shock may complicate this condition.	A medical emergency, it requires DC countershock. Lidocaine, procainamide, quinidine, Norpace, Dilantin, digitalis, amiodarone, or vasopressors also used. Treatment of the underlying pathology is crucial.
Accelerated idioventricular rhythm	Fast ventricular rates (usually around 100 beats per minute) caused by escape rhythm or short episodes of ventricular tachycardia with reentry. Ventricular fibrillation may follow.	As above.
Ventricular fibrillation	An uncoordinated, chaotic rhythm with no effective ventricular contraction. Impulses originate at multiple ectopic foci to spread simultaneously within the ventricular conduction system. Can result from severe myocardial damage, ventricular tachycardia, or drug toxicity related to digitalis, quinidine, or epinephrine. Unless corrected, cardiogenic shock and death rapidly ensue.	To prevent this medical emergency, preceding arrhythmias should be treated with lidocaine, procainamide, epinephrine, or isoproterenol. Defibrillation and cardiopulmonary resuscitation may be necessary.

TABLE 6.25 ANTIARRHYTHMIC MEDICATIONS

Name	Action	Indication	Dose	Side Effects
Bretylium tosylate	Increases conduction velocity and strengthens the heartbeat.	Life-threatening arrhythmias, such as ventricular tachycardia (if unresponsive to first-line antiarrhythmic agents such as lidocaine) or ventricular fibrillation.	*IV:* 5 mg/kg of body weight (bolus) initially; if patient is unresponsive to this or other treatment, give a repeat bolus of 10 mg/kg. *IM:* 5–10 mg/kg of body weight initially; may be repeated at 1- to 2-hour intervals if arrhythmia persists. Once arrhythmia has been corrected, give same dose as maintenance dose every 6–8 hours.	Hypotension, transient hypertension, increased frequency of arrhythmias, may aggravate digitalis toxicity. Avoid use in patients with decreased peripheral resistance unless as a last resort, since severe hypotension may result (administer vasoconstrictive catecholamines immediately if this occurs).
Disopyramide	Slows rate of conduction, increases effective refractory period of atrial and ventricular muscle cells, and decreases rate of spontaneous depolarization.	Ventricular tachycardia, PVCs, supraventricular and ventricular arrhythmias.	*PO:* Initial dose: 300 mg. Maintenance: 400–800 mg/day in divided doses (every 6 hours) *IV:* 2 mg/kg may be given as an alternative	Hypotension, CHF, and anticholinergic side effects (dry mouth, urinary retention, aggravation of sick sinus syndrome). Consider discontinuing drug if there is significant widening of the QRS complex or prolongation of the QT interval. Reduce dosage if first-degree heart block develops. Rarely, lowered blood glucose level may occur (monitor laboratory values).
Lidocaine	Depresses automaticity at ectopic sites.	PVCs, ventricular tachycardia, or ventricular arrhythmias associated with acute MI.	*IV:* 1 mg/kg bolus (50–100 mg for an adult) initially, which may be repeated at 5- to 10-minute intervals at 0.5 mg/kg bolus, the total not to exceed 225 mg. After initial bolus, begin IV infusion of 2 g in 500 mL of 5% dextrose at rate of 1–4 mg/min. *IM:* 300 mg is the average adult dose (4.3 mg/kg of body weight); may be given as a single IM injection in the deltoid muscle and repeated in 60–90 minutes if necessary. After initial injection, switch to IV infusion if possible.	CNS symptoms (e.g., lightheadedness, nervousness, apprehension), cardiovascular (hypotension, bradycardia, cardiovascular collapse, etc.) or allergic reaction (rare).
Phenytoin	Shortens the action potential and the effective refractory period, decreases automaticity, depresses rate of spontaneous depolarization, and increases conduction from the AV node through the ventricles.	PVCs and other ventricular arrhythmias (especially if caused by digitalis toxicity).	*IV:* 5 mg/kg or 100–500 mg as a slow bolus (not to exceed 50 mg/min). Discontinue administering bolus when arrhythmia ceases or if severe side effects develop (continue monitoring ECG and blood pressure throughout period of administration).	Contraindicated in sinus bradycardia, SA block, and advanced AV block.

TABLE 6.25 *(Continued)*

Name	Action	Indication	Dose	Side Effects
Procainamide	Depresses automaticity, reduces the rate of conduction, increases the refractory period, and has a vagus-blocking effect.	PVCs, ventricular tachycardia, supraventricular arrhythmias, atrial fibrillation, paroxysmal atrial tachycardia (PAT).	*PO:* Dosages may range from 0.5 to 1.5 g every 4–6 hours, depending on the particular arrhythmia. *IV:* 200 mg to 1.0 g is given as a slow bolus (not to exceed 50 mg/min). Discontinue administering bolus when arrhythmia ceases or if severe side effects develop (continue monitoring ECG and blood pressure throughout period of administration). After initial bolus, begin IV infusion of 2 g in 500 mL of 5% dextrose at rate of 1–4 mg/min. *IM:* 0.5–1.0 g every 4–8 hours until oral therapy is possible (0.1–0.5 g for arrhythmias associated with anesthesia and surgery).	GI, hematologic (e.g., agranulocytosis), cardiovascular (e.g., hypotension, ventricular asystole, or fibrillation), dermatologic (urticaria, pruritus, rash), and CNS (e.g., psychosis, hallucinations). Contraindicated in advanced AV heart block and myasthenia gravis.
Propranolol	Shortens the effective refractory period and decreases automaticity. A beta-adrenergic blocking agent.	Supraventricular and ventricular arrhythmias, atrial flutter, PAT, atrial fibrillation, digitalis toxicity.	*PO:* 10–30 mg three or four times daily. *IV:* 1–3 mg at a rate of no more than 1 mg/min; initial dose may be repeated after 2 minutes, but after the second dose wait 4 hours to repeat. Monitor ECG and central venous pressure continuously.	GI, respiratory (bronchospasm), CNS (mental depression), and cardiovascular (bradycardia, hypotension, further AV block, CHF). Contraindicated in sinus bradycardia, cardiogenic shock, bronchial asthma, advanced AV heart block, and overt CHF.
Verapamil	Calcium channel blocker. Decreases rate of conduction, conduction velocity, and contractility of smooth muscle, suppresses ectopic pacemaker, and causes vasodilatation.	Paroxysmal supraventricular tachycardia, slow ventricular rate associated with atrial fibrillation and atrial flutter, ventricular arrhythmias, ischemic heart disease (as a vasodilator).	*IV:* Average initial adult dose is 5–10 mg (0.075–0.15 mg/kg), given as a slow bolus over at least 2 minutes. Second dose (if needed, 30 minutes after initial dose): 10 mg (0.15 mg/kg). *PO:* Initial dose is 80 mg three to four times daily (total daily dosage for most patients averages 320–480 mg).	Hypotension, sinus bradycardia, severe tachycardia, dizziness, and headache are the most frequent side effects. Contraindicated in sick sinus syndrome, hypotension, advanced AV heart block, cardiogenic shock, and severe left ventricular dysfunction. Use with caution in patients with impaired hepatic or renal function.
Quinidine	Depresses the rate of spontaneous depolarization, automaticity, and conduction velocity, and increases the effective refractory period.	PAC, PVCs, PAT, atrial fibrillation and flutter; decreases paroxysmal ventricular tachycardia (without complete heart block), AV junctional tachycardia.	*For quinidine gluconate* *PO:* 324–648 mg (sustained release) every 8–12 hours. *IV:* 300–800 mg diluted in 50 mL of 5% dextrose, given at a rate of 1 mL/min. (Monitor ECG and blood pressure continuously.) *For quinidine sulfate* *PO:* 300–600 mg (sustained release) every 8–12 hours.	GI symptoms, allergic response, CNS reaction, cinchonism (ringing in the ears, visual disturbances, headache, decreased myocardial contractility, and peripheral vasodilation); contraindicated in heart block. Stop medication for all but mild GI symptoms.

arrhythmias to sinus rhythm. It includes atrial fibrillation, atrial flutter, paroxysmal atrial tachycardia (PAT), ventricular fibrillation, and ventricular tachycardia. Pacemaker insertion is utilized for patients with severe bradycardias, sick-sinus syndrome, and symptomatic AV block. Less frequently, cardiac pacing is used in the control of drug-resistant ventricular tachycardia or PAT.

Blood Flow Through the Heart Chambers and Great Vessels

Contractions of the myocardium are responsible for the circulation of blood as follows. Between contractions (diastole), deoxygenated blood from peripheral tissues fills the right atrium via the superior and inferior vena cavas, and oxygenated blood from the lungs fills the left atrium via the pulmonary vein (see Fig. 6.4). Due to the pressure gradient, this blood flows freely from the atria (areas of higher pressure) to the ventricles (areas of lower pressure) through the open AV valves (tricuspid and mitral). This is called the "period of rapid filling" of the ventricles. With myocardial contraction (systole), the atria contract first, forcing an additional quantity of blood into the ventricles. Almost immediately thereafter, the ventricles contract, causing an abrupt rise in pressure that forces the AV valves to close and the semilunar valves (pulmonary and aortic) to open. Blood is forced into the pulmonary, coronary, and systemic arterial systems. Finally, as the ventricles relax and their pressure is reduced, the semilunar valves close and the AV valves open, and another cycle begins (see Fig. 6.8).

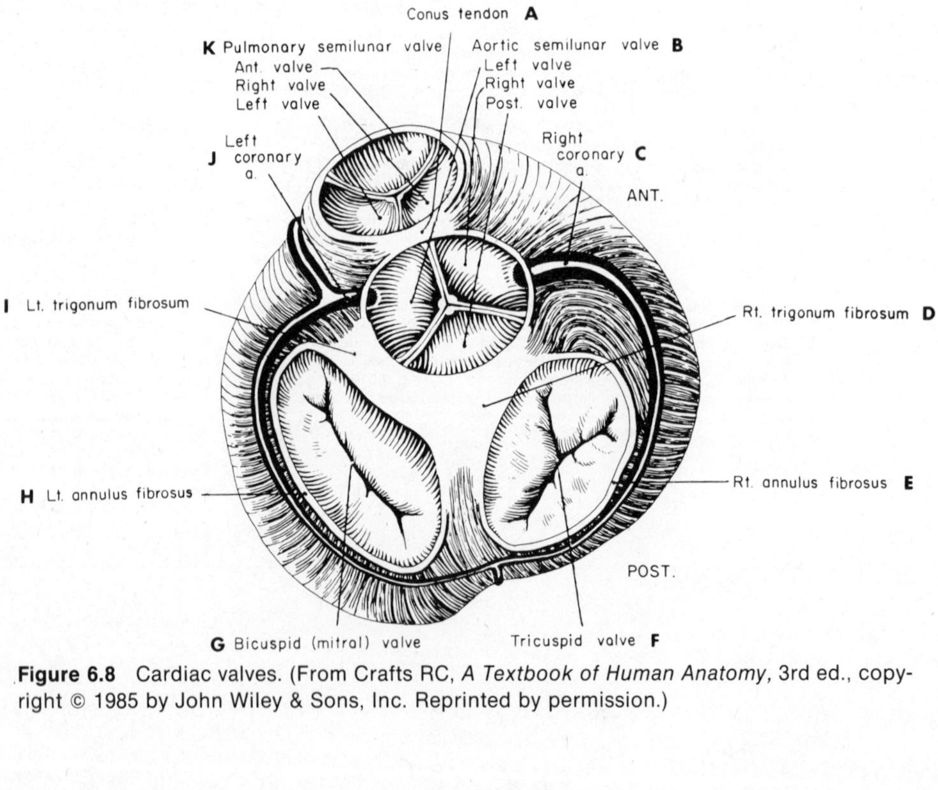

Figure 6.8 Cardiac valves. (From Crafts RC, *A Textbook of Human Anatomy,* 3rd ed., copyright © 1985 by John Wiley & Sons, Inc. Reprinted by permission.)

TABLE 6.26 HEART VALVES

Valve	Discussion
AV valves	The two valves (tricuspid and mitral) that close off the openings between the atria and the ventricles. Each consists of thin leaf-like cusps or flaps attached to fibrous rings (annula) rooted in the endocardium. The ends of each cusp project downward and are attached by fibrous tissue (chordae tendinae) to thick bands of muscle tissue (papillary muscle) on the inner wall of the ventricles. Shutting of the AV valves when the ventricles contract is largely responsible for the first heart sound.
Right AV valve (tricuspid)	The AV valve that closes off the right atria from the right ventricle. Having three cusps, it is also referred to as the "tricuspid" valve. When fully open, it is large enough to admit three or four fingertips.
Left AV valve (bicuspid or mitral)	The AV valve that closes off the left atria from the left ventricle. Having two cusps and shaped like a bishop's hat, it is alternately called the "bicuspid" or "mitral" valve. When fully open, it is only large enough to admit two fingertips. Although smaller than the tricuspid valve, it is stronger and thicker, and therefore able to withstand the more forceful pumping of the left ventricle.
Semilunar valves	The two valves (aortic and pulmonary) that close off the entrances to the great vessels. Each consists of three half-moon–shaped cusps (hence the name "semilunar") attached to a fibrous ring (annula) that is rooted in the endocardium. When the heart contracts (systole), a pulse of blood forces the valves open and spurts into the great vessels. When the heart rests (diastole), blood flow back in the vessels and fills the bowl-like cusps, causing them to shut. Shutting of the semilunar valves immediately after ventricular contraction produces the second heart sound.
Right semilunar valve (pulmonary)	The semilunar valve that closes off the entrance to the pulmonary artery.
Left semilunar valve (aortic)	The semilunar valve that closes off the entrance to the aorta. Larger and stronger than the pulmonary valve.

Passive action of the heart valves ensures the unidirectional movement of blood through the heart. As the backward pressure gradient pushes blood against the valves, they snap closed, preventing backflow. The AV valves prevent blackflow of the blood from the ventricles to the atria during systole, the semilunar valves keep blood from leaking into the ventricles from the aorta and the pulmonary arteries during diastole. Conversely, blood propelled by a forward pressure gradient forces the valves open. The thin, leaflike cusps of the AV valves require almost no backward flow to close them, while a rapid backflow is needed to shut the heavy half-moon-shaped semilunar cusps. Further description of the heart valves appears in Table 6.26.

Four distinct heart sounds are produced during each cardiac cycle by the opening and closing of the heart valves and the acceleration of the blood. The first heart sound (S_1) is produced by the closing of the AV valves and ejection of blood with the opening of the semilunar valves. The second heart sound (S_2) is created by the abrupt closing of the semilunar valves and sudden rebound of blood against them. It is heard as a short, low-frequency thump. Prominent in children and adolescents, the third heart sound (S_3) is believed to be caused by the vibration of the ventricle walls during the rapid filling period. Finally, the fourth heart sound (S_4) is associated with the acceleration of blood as it flows into the ventricles following atrial contraction.

Valvular disease refers to any structural damage to the cardiac valves. The damage may affect the valvular ring (annulus), the valvular leaflets (cusps), or the leaflet junctions (commissures). In the case of the AV valves, it may also affect the papillary muscles and their attachments, the chordae tendinae. These are auxiliary structures that check the upward movement of the valves and prevent them from flapping up to the atrium during forceful ventricular contractions. There are two types of valvular disease: stenosis, in which valve opening is hampered (forward blood flow is restricted), and regurgitation, in which valve closure is defective (backward blood flow is permitted).

The most common cause of valvular dysfunction is ***chronic rheumatic heart disease.*** As discussed in a previous section, the small pink granules that appear on the heart valves during the acute phase of RF fail to resolve or recur with subsequent attacks of RF. As a result, subacute or chronic inflammation over months or years eventually leads to fibrosis and thickening of the cusps, commissures, or chordae tendinae (AV valves). Other causes and the clinical presentations of valvular disease vary according to which valve is involved and to what extent. A comparison of heart sounds appears in Table 6.27.

TABLE 6.27 DISTINCTIVE HEART SOUNDS IN COMMON VALVULAR DISORDERS

Disorder	Heart Sounds
Mitral stenosis	Loud apical S_1. Narrow splitting of S_2. Diastolic opening snap. Diastolic rumbling murmer accentuated just before S_1; heard loudest at apex.
Mitral regurgitation	Pansystolic murmer heard loudest at apex and transmitted to base and axilla. Wide physiologic splitting of S_2. S_3 gallop. Short, early diastolic murmur extending from S_3 gallop.
Aortic stenosis	Harsh systolic ejection murmur loudest at aortic area and transmitted to neck. Soft S_2 that may be paradoxically split. Faint diastolic murmur in aortic area or at upper left sternal border. Apical S_4 gallop.
IHSS	Pansystolic or midsystolic ejection murmur heard over entire precordium. Increases with standing or Valsalva strain. Decreases upon squatting. Paradoxically split S_2 common. S_4 gallop common.
Aortic regurgitation	Systolic ejection murmur ending well before S_2. Loud at aortic post, soft at apex. Decrescendo diastolic blowing murmur at upper left sternal border. Diastolic rumble (Austin Flint murmur) often heard at apex. "Pistol shot" sounds over peripheral arteries.
Tricuspid regurgitation	Pansystolic murmur heard at lower left sternal border or below xiphoid. Intensifies during inspiration. S_3 gallop intensifying with inspiration. Short diastolic rumble extending from S_3 gallop. Also intensifies with inspiration.
Mitral valve prolapse	Midsystolic click heard at apex. May occur earlier with sitting or standing. Late systolic murmur at apex following click. May become louder and longer with sitting up or standing.

In ***mitral valve stenosis,*** the mitral valve orifice, normally 4–6 cm^2 wide, narrows to 1–2 cm^2. More prevalent among women than men, this problem is the direct result of fibrotic thickening or calcification of the leaflets (cusps) of the valve and chordae tendinae, as well as interadhesion of the commissures between the two major leaflets. This may be congenital or a complication or malignant carcinoid, systemic lupus erythematosus, rheumatoid arthritis, and mucopolysaccharidoses of the Hunter-Hurley phenotype. However, the most common etiology is acute RF (see the later discussion). Symptoms of rheumatic mitral stenosis develop no sooner than 2 years after the onset of acute RF, usually at age 30 or 40. With blood flow in the left side of the heart impeded, left ventricular function and cardiac output are preserved only at the expense of a markedly elevated left atrial pressure. This, in turn, leads to increased pulmonary artery pressure, right ventricular hypertrophy, tricuspid regurgitation, systemic venous congestion, and decreased cardiac output. The principal symptoms are related to CHF. Patients have dyspnea, fatigue, anorexia, chest or abdominal discomfort, and fluid retention. Hoarseness (Ortner's syndrome) may be present if the pulmonary artery is dilated. Patients with severe stenosis and low cardiac output often exhibit mitral facies, characterized by pinkish-purple patches on the cheeks. Exercise, emotional stress, infection, fever, sexual intercourse, pregnancy, or atrial fibrillation, all of which increase the amount of blood flow and decrease the available flow time across the mitral orifice, further elevate left atrial pressure, precipitating orthpnea, pulmonary edema, and hypertension.

A significant murmur is the earliest physical finding in mitral valve stenosis. Auscultation of heart sounds may reveal an intensified, snapping S_2 except in cases of marked calcification or thickening of the mitral leaflets (the sound is muffled). Intensification and later splitting of S_2 signals rising pulmonary artery pressure. The opening snap of the mitral valve is best heard at the apex, as is a low-pitched, rumbling diastolic murmur. The duration of this murmur is a guide to the severity of the mitral narrowing; the longer the murmur, the more significant the stenosis. Posteroanterior (PA) and lateral chest x-ray films demonstrate the extent of complications (enlarged left atrium, enlarged right ventricle, increased pulmonary artery prominences, increased pulmonary venous markings, and mitral valve calcifications). ECG may show right axis deviation and P waves that are broad and/or notched ***(P-mitrale),*** findings consistent with right ventricular hypertrophy and left atrial enlargement from pulmonary hypertension. It may also show atrial fibrillation and atrial flutter, conduction disturbances that often accompany mitral stenosis. An echocardiogram is specific and shows the limited mobility of the mitral valve. However, cardiac catheterization denotes the size of the orifice and evaluates the heart for associated and unassociated cardiac diseases.

The differential diagnosis includes primary pulmonary hypertension or that caused by severe chronic lung disease, left atrial myxoma, congenital cor triatriatum (a rare fibrotic malformation within the left atrium above the mitral valve), aortic regurgitation, and atrial septal defect. Oral diuretics and restricted sodium intake offer symptomatic improvement for many patients. Digitalis, while of no real value in the primary treatment of mitral stenosis, is helpful for complications of CHF. Since the possibility of systemic emboli is increased by leaflet calcification and backflow, preventive anticoagulant therapy is usually instituted. Antiarrhythmic drugs are effective in treating associated rhythm disturbances. Antimicrobial prophylaxis against streptococcal infections is indicated in some patients when there is a history of RF. With these interventions, patients may remain minimally symptomatic for a

TABLE 6.28 CAUSES OF MITRAL VALVE REGURGITATION

Mitral annulus (constriction, dilatation, calcification)
  Systemic hypertension
  Aortic stenosis
  Diabetes
  Hypertrophic obstructive cardiomyopathy
  Chronic renal failure with secondary hyperparathyroidism
Mitral leaflets (shortening, rigidity, deformity, retraction of one or both cusps)
  Chronic rheumatic heart disease
  Healing phase of endocarditis
  Penetrating and nonpenetrating trauma
	Chordae tendinae (stretching or rupture due to mechanical strain)
	  Infective endocarditis
	  Trauma
	  RF or other heart disease
	  Papillary muscle dysfunction
	Papillary muscles (ischemia or necrosis)
	  Acute MI

long period. However, once severe symptoms develop, mitral valve replacement or commissurotomy (incision of the adhesions on the valve leaflets) becomes necessary. Without it, complications rapidly progress and lead to death.

Mitral valve regurgitation (insufficiency) is the backward flow of blood from the left ventricle into the left atrium during ventricular systole. Regurgitation through the mitral valve begins in early systole, when the pressure in the left ventricle exceeds that in the left atrium, and continues until the aortic valve opens, allowing ejection (left ventricular pressure then decreases). As noted in Table 6.28, it may stem from abnormalities of the mitral annulus, the mitral leaflets, the chordae tendinae, and/or the papillary muscle ***(papillary muscle dysfunction).*** As in mitral valve stenosis, most cases of chronic disease can be traced to RF. By comparison, however, rheumatic mitral regurgitation occurs more commonly in men than in women, with signs (e.g., the murmer) developing during or soon after the acute episode rather than much later. The chronic regurgitation leads to several compensatory changes. The left atrium enlarges, with only a slight increase in left arterial pressure. Hypertrophy of the left ventricle results from a marked volume increase at the end of diastole. Since very little if any increase in end-diastolic pressure occurs, normal cardiac output is initially maintained. Frequently, patients remain asymptomatic for 10–20 years, or even for their entire life. Eventually, however, myocardial contractility is depressed and left ventricular end-diastolic volume and pressure are increased, leading to elevated left atrial pressure and hypertrophy and, finally, pulmonary hypertension. Once left ventricular failure begins, patients may complain of cardiac and respiratory symptoms. These include weakness, exertional fatigue, dyspnea and orthpnea, and palpitations (due to atrial fibrillation).

On exam, severe mitral regurgitation is often indicated by a sharp, abbreviated peripheral pulse. Precordial palpation reveals an enlarged left ventricle, a hyperactive and laterally displaced apex beat, and an apical systolic thrill. Rarely, a greatly enlarged left atrium is palpable. Auscultation of heart sounds reveals a characteristic high-pitched pansystolic murmur at the cardiac apex. Other findings include a soft S_1 sound, a loud ventricular diastolic gallop, a short early diastolic rumble, and wide splitting of S_2. X-ray findings include an enlarged left atrium and ventricle, pulmonary engorgement, and an enlarged right ventricle. The ECG may be nonspecific or may show evidence of left ventricular or biventricular hypertrophy. An echocardiogram is useful in detecting abnormal leaflets and ventricular hypertrophy. Cardiac catheterization in selected patients confirms the diagnosis and denotes the type of disease and the extent of incompetence. Careful work-up is important, since mitral regurgitation should be differentiated from ventricular septal defects, tricuspid regurgitation, aortic stenosis, and idiopathic hypertrophic subaortic stenosis. Medical therapy is similar to that for mitral stenosis. Diuretics and restricted sodium intake are important, as is antimicrobial and anticoagulant prophylaxis. Digitalis is indicated to control ventricular rate and contractility. If medical treatment is not successful, surgery for mitral valve replacement or reconstruction may be advised.

Ruptured chordae tendinae proves an exception to the slowly developing picture described above. Associated with ischemia and necrosis of the papillary muscle, it typically develops as an acute complication of MI. If the papillary muscle ruptures completely, sudden florid regurgitation quickly leads to severe pulmonary hypertension, left atrial hypertrophy (giant left atrium) with low mean left atrial pressure, and greatly decreased cardiac output and death.

Regurgitation may be absent, mild, or severe in patients with ***mitral valve prolapse*** ("floppy mitral valve", Barlow's syndrome). Particularly prevalent among women, this fairly common condition can be traced to excessive mitral valve tissue (particularly of the posterior cusp) and increased chordae tendinae length. Although the mitral valve leaflets close normally with the onset of ventricular contraction, decreasing cardiac volume causes their abrupt movement or prolapse into the left atrium and tensing of the chordae tendinae and other valvular structures. This results in a midsystolic click. Occasionally, backflow through the prolapsed leaflet follows. A number of patients remain asymptomatic. Others report nonexertional, prolonged chest discomfort or pain. In addition, they may complain of weakness, fatigue, palpitations, lightheadedness, and dyspnea. The hallmark physical finding is one or more midsystolic clicks, which generally occur 0.14 second or more after S_1. Occasionally, it is followed by a crescendo-decrescendo late systolic murmur that closely resembles the murmur associated with papillary muscle dysfunction, hypertrophic subaortic stenosis, hypertrophic cardiomyopathy, or asymmetric septal hypertrophy. The ECG is abnormal in a large number of patients with mitral valve prolapse. T-wave inversion in leads II, III, and aV_F, V_5, and V_6 are common. ST-segment abnormalities, sometimes seen on an exercise ECG, are not usually found on resting tracings. Associated rhythm disturbances include atrial fibrillation and supraventricular tachycardia, as well as atrial and ventricular ectopic beats. Abnormal movements of the mitral leaflets are readily shown on echocardiogram. Cardiac catheterization offers additional definition. Asymptomatic patients with no arrhythmias and without evidence of severe mitral regurgitation require no treatment. However, since infectious endocarditis is a complication of mitral valve prolapse, antibacterial prophylaxis is recommended for anyone with the latter condition. Antiarrhythmics should be appropriately prescribed. Chest pain and syncope are often relieved by propranolol. Rarely, surgical treatment is required for mitral valve prolapse with severe regurgitation.

Aortic stenosis is progressive narrowing of the aortic orifice from calcification, fibrosis, or fusion of the three aortic cusps (right, left, and posterior). It results from congenital anomalies (fused commissure or bicuspid valve) or sclerotic degeneration. More frequently, however, it is rheumatic in origin. Obstruction usually develops over a prolonged period, except in children with severe congenital defects. The earliest compensatory response is increased left ventricular diastolic volume, pressure, and fiber length. Gradually, hypertrophy develops to maintain left ventricular wall force. With hypertrophy, the oxygen demands of the myocardium exceed the supply offered by the coronary circulation, and myocardial ischemia develops. Finally, longstanding pressure overwork by the hypertrophic left ventricle leads to a severe decrease in cardiac output. As a reflection of these changes, the three major features of aortic stenosis are syncope, angina pectoris, and symptoms of CHF. Their onset is often delayed for many years due to the fact that cardiac output is usually well maintained by compensatory mechanisms. Once they do begin, however, the subsequent course is generally downhill with survival times as follows: syncope (6 years), angina (5 years), and CHF (18 months to 2 years).

The cardinal physical signs of aortic stenosis are a slowly rising arterial pulse, a sustained outward apical impulse, a loud, rough aortic systolic murmur, and a faint or inaudible aortic second sound. Abnormal ECG findings are universal and include voltage criteria for left ventricular enlargement and associated ST- and T-wave changes, along with left atrial enlargement. Occasionally, intraventricular conduction delay or bundle branch block is present. Atrial fibrillation is a late and uncommon finding. Complete heart block is rare. An echocardiogram will detect thickened aortic leaflets, a compromised valve opening, and left ventricular hypertrophy. With significant stenosis, left ventricular enlargement and displacement are demonstrated on an x-ray film. Cardiac catheterization, recommended for all patients with suspected stenosis, reliably determines the degree of mechanical obstruction and the need for surgical intervention. Patients with mild aortic stenosis must be followed carefully. Strenuous physical exertion should be prohibited. Antimicrobial prophylaxis is necessary for dental and surgical procedures. Aortic valve replacement is carried out in patients with symptoms of significant narrowing.

Idiopathic hypertrophic subaortic stenosis (IHSS) is a genetic obstructive hypertrophic cardiomyopathy of unknown cause that results from the disproportionate or asymmetric hypertrophy of the ventricular septum. As a result, the left ventricular cavity is misshapen and the papillary muscles are misaligned. Ultimately, this causes an obstruction of left ventricular outflow. The degree of obstruction varies depending on the contractile force of the left ventricle, systemic vascular resistance, competence of the mitral valve, and left ventricular diastolic volume. Obstruction of right ventricular outflow may also be present. The most common symptoms reported are chest pain similar to that of angina but not relieved by nitroglycerine and dyspnea on exertion. Other symptoms are often related to the degree of obstruction and include fatigue, vertigo, syncope, orthopnea, paroxysmal nocturnal dyspnea, ankle edema, and clinical signs of left ventricular failure. IHSS is often the cause of sudden death in young athletes. A systolic ejection murmur is heard, as well as a prominent S_4. There is an increase in the left ventricular apical impulse and a brisk carotid pulse. Signs of mitral regurgitation are also present. ECG findings are consistent with left ventricular hypertrophy and left atrial enlargement. Conduction disturbances such as left bundle branch block and Wolff-Parkinson-White syndrome may also be noted. A chest x-ray film shows cardiomegaly with left ventricular enlargement. Cardiac catheterization, angiography, and echocardiography will reveal the septal defect, obstruction, and its consequences. Treatment is often unsuccessful in preventing progression of the disease. Medications, such as propranolol to reduce left ventricular and diastolic pressure, or verapamil to improve left ventricular diastolic function, may be given. Surgical repair (left ventricular septal myotomy) may be advised in some cases.

Aortic regurgitation (insufficiency) is faulty closure and sealing of the aortic valve with backflow of blood into the left ventricle during diastole. It follows dilatation of the annulus or loss of aortic wall support to the valve from disease of the aortic root and the ascending aorta. As expected, the leading causes of aortic regurgitation are RF and congenital anomalies. It is also associated with syphilis, ankylosing spondylitis, rheumatoid arthritis, Marfan's syndrome, Hurler's syndrome, relapsing polychondritis, severe systemic hypertension, and infectious endocarditis. Retrograde blood leakage to the left ventricle during diastole increases the volume to be ejected during the next systole. Initially, the left ventricle responds to the overwork condition with increased force of contraction. As regurgitation becomes more severe, however, the left ventricle slowly dilates and then becomes hypertrophied. Long-standing overload leads to myocardial damage and depressed contractility. End-diastolic volume and pressure are increased, and symptoms of failure are manifested. The symptoms accompanying aortic regurgitation are the same as those of progressive cardiac enlargement and left ventricular failure. These are described in more detail in previous discussions.

A number of striking physical signs characterize aortic regurgitation. Head bobbing, a nodding head motion, accompanies each systole. Pulsations of the carotid arteries are visible, as is ***Quincke's sign,*** alternating nail bed blushing and blanching that occurs with each cardiac cycle. An abrupt, quickly rising and then collapsing arterial pulse (also called "water hammer pulse") is palpable. Auscultation reveals a pistol shot sound over the femoral arteries and ***Duroziez's murmur*** (a to-and-fro bruit over the femoral artery with slight compression of the stethoscope diaphragm). A decrescendo, blowing diastolic murmur at the left sternal border in the third and fourth intercostal spaces is diagnostic. In the early stages it is high-pitched, soft, and heard only in early diastole. Later it becomes rougher in quality and lasts throughout diastole. When regurgitation is severe, a systolic ejection murmur in the aortic area that is transmitted to the jugular notch and carotid arteries is heard. ECG shows left ventricular hypertrophy with associated ST-segment and T-wave changes. Late in the disease, left axis deviation, intraventricular conduction defects, or left bundle branch block may occur. Atrial fibrillation is a late and uncommon finding. X-ray findings include enlargement of the left ventricle and aorta. Marked dilatation or aneurysm of the ascending aorta indicates aortic root disease. The size of the aortic orifice and the left ventricular chamber may be determined by echocardiography. Cardiac catheterization is helpful in assessing ventricular function. Restricted physical activity is advised to reduce the likelihood of sudden arrhythmia. Antimicrobial prophylaxis is again recommended. Surgical intervention is necessary once signs of left ventricular failure become significant.

Tricuspid valvular disease occurs less frequently than the other valvular diseases. Tricuspid stenosis is usually associated with acute RF and resultant mitral stenosis or aortic valve dysfunction. Tricuspid regurgitation may be a primary valvular disease or dysfunction due to acute rheumatic fever, bacterial endocarditis, trauma, or tumor. Secondary sources of dysfunction include right heart conditions that cause right ventricular dilatation and heart failure such as pulmonic stenosis and primary pulmonary hypertension. Left ventricular failure associated with any pathology, but particularly mitral valve disease, may also result in right ventricular failure and ***tricuspid regurgitation.*** Clinical manifestations of tricuspid regurgitation reflect increased right-sided volume and pressure and generalized signs of heart failure, and may indicate whether the valvular dysfunction is primary or secondary. A pansystolic murmur that is increased on inspiration and a loud S_3 or S_4 or both may be heard on auscultation. A chest x-ray film shows an enlarged right atrium and ventricle, and ECG demonstrates this condition, as well as atrial fibrillation. Echocardiography, cardiac catheterization, and angiography are needed for definitive diagnosis. Medical management of the underlying pathology, along with the associated consequences and complications, is appropriate, including digitalis, diuretics, anticoagulants, and prophylactic antibiotics. Surgical tricuspid valvuloplasty or valve replacement may be indicated in some cases.

Coronary Circulation

Blood is supplied to the heart muscle itself through the coronary circulation (Fig. 6.9). The coronary arterial tree has two functional divisions: (1) the large coronary arteries, which serve as conduits for blood along the epicardial surface of the heart, and (2) the small arteries, which penetrate the myocardium for exchange of nutrients and wastes.

The large arteries consist of the right and left coronary arteries and their tributaries. The left coronary artery originates in the left aortic sinus. Passing left and downward, it divides into two main branches: (1) the anterior descending branch, which continues along the anterior interventricular groove, and (2) the circumflex branch, which continues along the AV groove. The anterior descending artery, the most conspicuous vessel on the surface of the heart, services the left atrium, both ventricles, and the interventricular septum. The circumflex artery supplies the adjacent section of the left ventricle, the left atrium, the septum, and the AV node. Together with its branches, the left coronary artery accommodates 60% of the total coronary arterial flow.

The right coronary artery originates in the anterior aortic sinus and continues along the AV groove to the posterior aspect of the heart, where it joins the left coronary artery. Along with its branches, it supplies about 40% of the total coronary flow. It carries blood to the right atrium, the right ventricle, and, in most persons (about 85% of the population), to a portion of the posterior left ventricle. In about 15% of the population, the posterior left ventricle is supplied by the left coronary artery. These anatomic variations give rise to the terms "right predominance" and "left predominance." They are somewhat confusing, since the left coronary artery always supplies the major portion of coronary blood.

From the main arteries on the epicardial surface, two types of small coronary arteries branch at right angles and descend vertically into the myocardium. The first type branches immediately. Forming a network of vessels that supply the outer part (epicardium) of the wall, they are called "epicardial vessels." The second type penetrates almost the entire thickness of the wall before branching. These arteries form a network just beneath the inner surface of the wall and are thus referred to as "subendocardial vessels." By constricting or dilating, the small coronary arteries regulate the flow of blood through the coronary circulation. Thus, they are the principal resistance vessels of the heart.

Coronary artery disease (CAD) is a general term referring to the development of ***arteriosclerosis*** or ***atherosclerosis*** within the coronary arteries. Causing vessel lumens to narrow, the two processes are described in Table 6.29. Actually, the principal cause of CAD is the development of atherosclerotic plaques in the larger arteries, but not the smaller arterioles. The plaques partially obstruct blood flow to the myocardium, causing intermittent myocardial ischemia and angina. By promot-

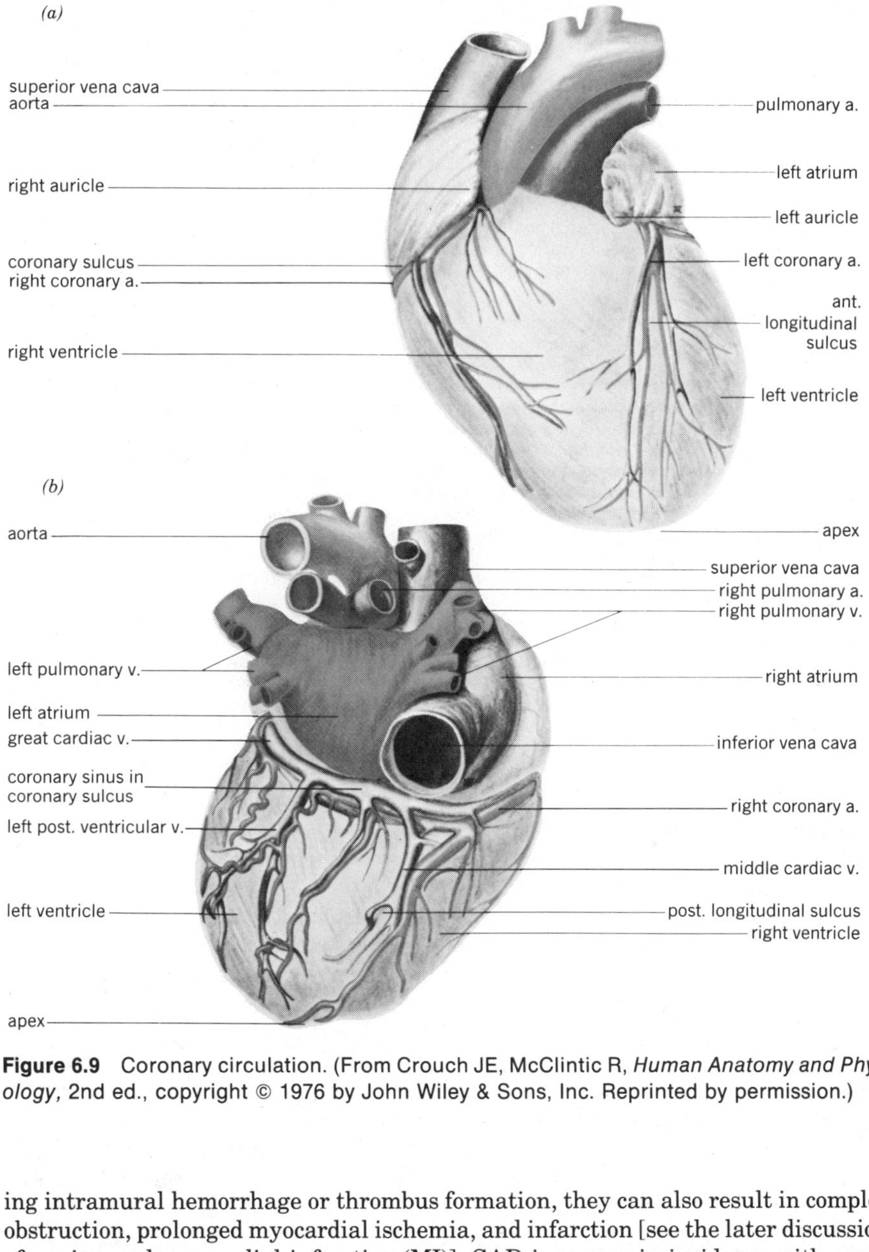

Figure 6.9 Coronary circulation. (From Crouch JE, McClintic R, *Human Anatomy and Physiology,* 2nd ed., copyright © 1976 by John Wiley & Sons, Inc. Reprinted by permission.)

ing intramural hemorrhage or thrombus formation, they can also result in complete obstruction, prolonged myocardial ischemia, and infarction [see the later discussions of angina and myocardial infarction (MI)]. CAD increases in incidence with age, is most often seen in men and postmenopausal women, and is prevalent in affluent societies, the United States ranking second only to Finland in the number of CAD-related deaths. Other risk factors are noted in Table 6.30. The consequences of the disease are devastating, and perhaps the greatest hope for averting them depends on ► ***reducing CAD risk factors.*** Toward this end, primary care providers play a key

TABLE 6.29 ARTERIOSCLEROSIS AND ATHEROSCLEROSIS

Process	Description
Arteriosclerosis	General term for the group of degenerative arterial diseases characterized by thickening and hardening of arterial walls. Most commonly manifested as gradual arterial narrowing leading to occlusion, but aneurysm (dilatation of an arterial segment from weakening of a wall) may occur with or without occlusive form of disease. Included in this category are atherosclerosis (below), Mönckeberg's arteriosclerosis (focal calcific arteriosclerosis), and arteriolosclerosis. Normal arterial changes associated with aging (including loss of elastic tissue, spotty calcification, gradually progressive, symmetric intimal thickening, and increased vessel rigidity) are sometimes included in this classification as well.
Atherosclerosis	A subtype of arteriosclerosis featuring the development of patchy nodular arterial lesions (atheromas). There are three types of lesions: fatty streaks, fibrous plaques, and complicated lesions. Fatty streaks are early, localized lesions that develop on the arterial intima as a result of irritative or mechanical forces. In response to the local injury, phospholipid production and fibrous tissue collection occur in the arterial wall. These lesions occur in various segments of the arterial tree, are usually asymptomatic, and cause little obstruction. With advancing atherosclerosis, fibrous plaques develop. These are firm, palpable, dome-shaped elevations representing areas of intimal thickening. They consist of a central core of lipid and necrotic cellular debris and an outer layer of smooth muscle cells and collagen, and favor certain segments, including the abdominal aorta, coronary arteries, and carotid arteries. Complicated lesions, frequently associated with symptoms, are calcified fibrous plaques with various degrees of necrosis, thrombosis, ulceration, and weakening of the arterial wall leading to rupture of the intima and creating a potential for aneurysm or hemorrhage. Arterial emboli, occlusion, and thrombus formation are also possible. Atherosclerosis is the underlying pathologic condition in coronary artery disease, aortic aneurysm, and arterial disease of the lower extremities. It is also involved in cerebrovascular disease. Predisposing factors include hyperlipidemic conditions, hypertension, diabetes mellitus, and smoking.

role. They should educate all patients about diet, weight, exercise, smoking, and stress reduction, and should advocate the use of screening tests for cholesterol levels. In addition, they should develop aggressive approaches to contributing medical problems such as diabetes, hypertension, and gout.

A major presentation of CAD is ▶ ***angina.*** A response to myocardial ischemia, it is pain or discomfort described as a retrosternal squeezing, gripping, strangling, burning, or vice-like sensation that may or may not radiate to the neck, jaw, teeth, or arms. It is usually accompanied by a sense of impending doom. In addition to CAD, pathologic conditions that contribute to ischemia, and therefore angina, are severe aortic stenosis or insufficiency, severe mitral stenosis or insufficiency, hypotension, hyperthyroidism, and marked anemia and polycythemia. Factors that decrease the amount of oxygen (O_2) delivered by the coronary arteries, increase the caridac workload, or increase the need of the myocardium for O_2 may precipitate the chest pain itself. They include physical and emotional stress, heavy exercise, cold, large meals,

TABLE 6.30 CAD RISK FACTORS

Age over 40	Gout	Obesity
Male sex	Prostaglandin production	Use of oral contraceptives
Family history of CAD	Hypercholesterolemia	Inability to handle stress
Hypertension	Hypertriglyceridemia	Sedentary job or lifestyle
Diabetes mellitius	Smoking	

extreme excitement, anger, and sexual activity. Once precipitated, angina is clearly self-limiting and subsides completely without residual discomfort. If it is precipitated by exertion and the patient immediately stops to rest, the attack typically lasts for less than 3 minutes (though it may seem infinitely longer). By contrast, attacks that follow a heavy meal or emotional upset may last for 15–20 minutes. Diagnostic information obtained from the history is essential. The description of the pain, its location, radiation, duration, and associated or precipitating factors are all indicative of the diagnosis. During ischemic episodes, the clinical findings resemble those of MI. However, findings between attacks may only reveal the presence of associated risk factors and atherosclerotic changes. The ECG may be normal or may reveal evidence of a previous MI. During an ischemic episode, changes in the ST or T wave may be noted. Comparison of both tracings may show subtle alterations. Other significant diagnostic studies to determine the extent of the disease and its effects include both invasive and noninvasive procedures (see Table 6.31).

Management of angina is aimed at reducing the pain and treating the underlying ischemic disease. Nitrates are the most common drugs prescribed. By producing

TABLE 6.31 CARDIAC TESTING

Type	Description	Use
	Noninvasive	
Exercise ECG (stress tests)	Serial graded exercise with ECG minitoring. a. Two-step exercise test. b. Multilevel treadmill exercise test.	Determines abnormal changes in cardic function during exercise.
Vectocardiogram	Recording of the electrical activity of the heart as referred to the body surface.	Provides same information as ECG and may be diagrammed simultaneously.
Echocardiogram	Ultrasonic visualization of the structure and motion of the heart.	Assesses the structure and function of the atrial and ventricular chambers, the septa, the valves, and the ventricular wall.
Nuclear studies	Scintigram monitoring of myocardial perfusion at the end of an exercise test following an IV injection of thallium-201.	Indicates areas of myocardial ischemia by failure of blood flow to deliver tracer uniformly to myocardial cells.
Serology tests	Measurement of serum levels of cardiac enzymes.	Indicates reversible ischemic disruption to myocardium if levels are normal.
Computed tomography (CT) scan	Visualization of underlying tissue.	Assesses the structure of the heart.
	Invasive	
Cardiac catheterization with angiography and arteriography	Visualization of the chambers of the heart, the valves, and the coronary arteries by injecting contrast material under fluoroscopy.	Assesses cardiac structures and function (pressures and blood flow) and facilitates the diagnosis of cardiac disease related to anatomic malfunctioning.
Cardiac and coronary cineangiography	Visualization of the chambers of the heart and coronary arteries using radiopaque contrast material at the time of catheterization and recorded on moving film.	Evaluates valvular lesions, intracardiac shunts, ventricular contraction, and coronary artery occlusion.

vasodilatation, they increase myocardial perfusion by the coronary arteries, decrease peripheral vascular resistance, and decrease cardiac output. Beta blockers and calcium antagonists are also employed. Beta blockers such as propranolol block beta-adrenergic stimulation, thereby decreasing the heart rate, myocardial irritability, and the force of contractions. Furthermore, they affect the conduction system by depressing the "automaticity" of the sinus node, depressing the source of ectopic beats, and decreasing the velocity of conduction between the AV and intraventricular pathways. Calcium antagonists dilate the coronary epicardial arteries and lower the blood pressure. Digitalization may be introduced to decrease the cardiac workload and to increase myocardial contractility. Further information about these drugs appears in Table 6.32. Besides pharmacology, treatment should focus on risk factors. A diet low in calories, cholesterol, and saturated fats should be prescribed. Planned programs of exercise and stress reduction should be developed.

Stable angina (exertional angina) is that which is well controlled by rest and medication. It sometimes evolves into ***unstable angina*** (crescendo angina), which is precipitated by minimal exertion or even at rest or during sleep. The pain increases in duration and changes in character. It is not relieved as promptly by nitroglycerine and gradually worsens. Diagnosis is based on the history and the results of studies (see the discussion of angina pectoris). Treatment is the same as for a small MI. It includes bed rest, nitrates (administered IV if necessary), beta-blocking agents, calcium antagonists, and psychological rest. More invasive treatment may be indicated if symptoms persist, such as percutaneous transluminal coronary angioplasty or bypass graft (both are discussed later).

Prinzmetal's angina (variant angina) is pain due to coronary artery spasm triggered by cold, a coronary angiogram, or drug toxicity. It occurs most often at rest during the day or night and may be associated with arrhythmias and conduction defects. Clinical distinction of Prinzmetal's angina is difficult; therefore, cardiac catheterization is required to determine the absence of atherosclerotic obstruction. Treatment with nitrates is the primary regimen. However, if the response is slow, calcium antagonists may be effective. Nonselective beta-adrenergic blocking agents should be avoided as they may potentiate the spasm.

Myocardial infarction (MI) is ischemic necrosis of the myocardial tissue due to an abrupt decrease in blood flow to the myocardium. As previously noted, it usually occurs as a result of CAD, that is, occlusion of one or more of the coronary arteries due to atherosclerotic plaque formation. However, MI may also result from the gradual development of sclerosis, embolism, hypertrophy of the heart muscle, myocardial aneurysm, or a temporary decrease in blood flow due to shock. The main symptom of MI is severe, prolonged substernal pain with or without radiation to the left arm, both shoulders, neck, jaw, and teeth. It may be accompanied by nausea, vomiting, low-grade fever, signs of left ventricular failure, and shock. Patients appear restless and anxious, and may express apprehension. Their skin is cold, clammy, and ashen. The ECG may be normal or show q-wave development or loss of the r wave, depending on the area of infarction. Some classic ECG changes are described in Table 6.33. Any patient with characteristic symptoms of MI should be hospitalized. Diagnostic findings include increased WBC, elevated ESR, and the changing serum enzyme levels of creatinine phosphokinase (CPK), LDH, and serum glutamic oxaloacetic transaminase (SGOT) described in Table 6.34. The goal of treatment is to increase myocardial profusion and minimize cellular damage. Patients are placed on bed rest, IV feeding, oxygen, and continuous cardiovascular monitoring. In addition

TABLE 6.32 SOME DRUGS USED IN THE TREATMENT OF ANGINA

Classification and Name	Dose	Indication	Action	Side Effects
		Beta-Adrenergic Blockers		
Nadolol	*PO:* Initial: 40 mg/day, gradually increased to 80–240 mg/day.	Ischemic heart disease, angina triggered by exertion, unstable angina.	Reduces the oxygen demand of the myocardium; reduces the heart's responsiveness to sympathetic stimulation, thus slowing the heart and lessening the force of the contraction.	Bronchospasm, vertigo, fatigue, GI symptoms, hypotension, left ventricular failure, sinus bradycardia.
Propranolol	*PO:* Initial: 10–20 mg three to four times per day, gradually increased to 160–320 mg/day in divided doses.			
		Calcium Channel Blockers		
Diltiazem	*PO:* Initial: 30 mg four times daily, gradually increased to 240 mg/day in divided doses.	Prinzmetal's angina, chronic stable angina.	Selectively blocks the calcium channels of the specialized tissue and muscle cells of the heart and smooth muscle, thus slowing the heart rate and decreasing myocardial contractility, conduction rate, and peripheral vascular resistance. Ultimately, cardiac workload and oxygen consumption are reduced. Also increases dilatation of coronary arteries and decreases coronary spasm.	Hypotension, bradycardia, vertigo, fatigue, GI symptoms. Cautious use advised with hepatic or renal dysfunction.
Nifedipine	*PO:* Initial: 10 mg three times daily, gradually increased to 120–180 mg/day in divided doses.			
Verapamil	*PO:* Initial: 80 mg three times daily, gradually increased to 240–480 mg/day in divided doses.			
		Nitrates and Nitrites		
Nitroglycerine	*Sublingual:* 0.15–0.6 mg every 5 minutes as needed for pain. *Topical:* 15–30 mg (1–2 in.) every 8 hours. *Transdermal:* 2.5–15 mg (1 pad daily). *Transmucosal:* 1 mg three times daily. *PO:* 1.3–9 mg (sustained release) every 8–12 hours. *IV:* dilute solution, 5 mg/min.	Angina pectoris: during acute attack, for immediate prophylaxis, and for sustained prophylaxis.	Relaxes smooth muscle, causing vasodilatation (nitrites) and reduction of myocardial oxygen need (nitrates).	Hypotension, weakness, vertigo, headache, postural hypotension, and reflex tachycardia. Should not be taken in conjunction with alcohol.
Isosorbide dinitrate	*Sublingual:* 2.5–10 mg as needed for pain or every 4–6 hours. *PO:* 5–30 mg as necessary or daily, or 40 mg (sustained release) every 6–12 hours.			
Erythrityl tetranitrate	*Sublingual:* 5–15 mg (immediate prophylaxis). *PO:* 10–30 mg three times daily.			
Pentaerythritol	*PO:* Initial: 10–20 mg three or four times daily, gradually increased to 40 mg four times daily, or 30–80 mg (sustained release) every 12 hours.			

TABLE 6.33 ECG FINDINGS IN ACUTE MI

Wave Changes	Interpretation
Q wave abnormal	Necrosis of myocardium
ST segment elevated	Injury to myocardium
T wave inverted	Ischemia of myocardium

Type	Leads	Changes
Transmural		Q wave present and abnormal ST segment large and elevated
Subendocardial		Q wave absent ST segment depressed T wave inverted
Anterior wall	I, aV_L, V_1, V_2, V_3, V_4	Q wave present and abnormal ST segment elevated T wave inverted
	II, III, aV_F	Q wave absent R wave taller ST segment depressed T wave taller
Posterior wall	V_1, V_2, V_3	Q wave absent R wave developing ST segment depressed T wave taller
Lateral wall	I, aV_L, V_4, V_5, V_6	Q wave present and abnormal ST segment elevated T wave inverted
	II, III, aV_F	Q wave absent R wave taller ST segment depressed T wave taller
Inferior wall or diaphragmatic	II, III, aV_F	Q wave present and abnormal ST segment elevated T wave inverted
	I, aV_L, V_4, V_5, V_6	Q wave absent R wave taller ST segment depressed T wave taller

to sedatives, analgesics, and vasodilators, they may be started on antiarrhythmic drugs, digitalis, and diuretics. The outcome depends on the location and extent of the infarction, the presence of previous MI, and the adequacy of collateral circulation. Complications of MI include arrhythmias, cardiac arrest, thromboembolism, mitral insufficiency, pericarditis, cardiac shock, ventricular aneurysm, CHF, acute renal failure, and cerebral infarction. Patients with uncomplicated cases progress on an activity tolerance schedule, moving from complete bed rest to resumption of the activities of daily living while in the hospital for 7–14 days.

Patients with uncontrollable angina or MI may be candidates for cardiac bypass. A ***coronary artery bypass graft (CABG)*** is the anastomosis of a saphenous vein autograft to an area proximal and distal to the coronary occlusion in one or more of the main coronary arteries. This procedure may be indicated depending upon which artery is occluded, the degree of occlusion, and the severity of symptoms.

Other invasive but nonsurgical treatments are ***percutaneous transluminal***

TABLE 6.34 ENZYME CHANGES IN ACUTE MI

Enzyme	Rise	Peak	Deviation
CPK	2–5 hours after infarction	Within 24 hours after infarction	4–6 days
LDH	12 hours after infarction	48–72 hours after infarction	7–9 days
SGOT	6–12 hours after infarction	24–35 hours after infarction	5–7 days

coronary angioplasty (PTCA) and streptokinase. PTCA involves the dilatation of the stenosed coronary artery by compression of the atherosclerotic material against the arterial lining. It is done during cardiac catheterization using a specially designed catheter directed under fluoroscopy. During MI or within 5 hours of the onset of symptoms, ***streptokinase*** may be administered via cardiac catheterization to dissolve the atherosclerotic material. Finally, ***plasminogen activator,*** a noninvasive drug treatment is now under investigation (timi study). Given I.V. soon after the onset of MI symptoms and signs, this anticoagulant dissolves coronary blood clots preventing or limiting ischemic damage to the myocardium.

Protective Features (Endocardium and Pericardium)

Within the heart, protection against infectious and toxic agents is provided by the endocardium. This thin, delicate membrane, composed of endothelial cells, lines the surfaces of each cavity, covers the valves, surrounds the chordae tendinae, and is continuous with the lining of the large vessels.

If endocardial defense mechanisms are compromised or overwhelmed by any of the factors listed in Table 6.35, ***infectious endocarditis*** may develop. Bacteria accounts for most cases, though any microorganism can cause the disease. In fact, the incidence of fungal infections has been on the rise due to the increasing use of prosthetic valves. Pathologically, endocarditis is characterized by the development of lesions (vegetations) that in the early stages are pink, red, yellow, or green but turn gray as they heal. The lesions collect around the heart valves and/or cordae

TABLE 6.35 PREDISPOSING FACTORS IN INFECTIOUS ENDOCARDITIS

Bloodstream invasion by organisms	Collagen-vascular disease
Transient bacteremias: follow various types of manipulations of areas in which organisms are normally found (mouth, upper airway, skin, external genitalia, intestine)	Preexisting renal failure
Cirrhosis	Treatment with corticosteroids
IV drug addiction	Antitumor chemotherapy and irradiation
Surgery (cardiac, prosthetic valve insertion, prolonged use of polyethylene catheters)	Perinephric abscess
Burns	Obstruction of common bile duct
Transvenous pacemaker	Bowel perforation
Nonmalignant blood disorders	Sternal wound infection
Neoplastic disease	Hyperalimentation (particularly fungal endocarditis)
Diabetes mellitus	Underlying heart disease (rheumatic fever, congenital defects, atherosclerosis and calcification, hypertrophic obstructive cardiomyopathy, Marfan's syndrome, mitral valve prolapse, MI)
Chronic viral hepatitis	

TABLE 6.36 ACUTE INFECTIOUS ENDOCARDITIS (AIE) AND SUBACUTE INFECTIOUS ENDOCARDITIS (SIE)

	AIE	SIE
Usual organisms	*Staphylococcus aureus, Streptococcus pneumoniae, Neisseria meningitides, N. gonorrhoeae, Streptococcus pyogenes, Hemophilus influenzae.*	*Streptococcus viridans, Strep. fecalis* (enterococcus), *Staphylococcus epidermis, Staph. aureus, Candida albicans.*
Manner and progression of infection	Intense bacteremia from IV drug abuse, surgery on infected tissues, urologic procedures, or insertion of prosthesis leads to the acute development of vegetations on normal, abnormal, or prosthetic valves. Typically large and friable, vegetations of AIE are associated with severe embolic episodes and metastatic abscess formation. The latter contributes to rapid perforation, tearing, or ruptured chordae tendinae of affected valves.	Mechanical stress from abnormal (usually regurgitant) or prosthetic valves is a critical factor. A "jet effect," produced as blood is driven from a high-pressure chamber through the faulty valve into a low-pressure chamber, and subsequent backflow traumatize endocardial surfaces. Invasive organisms, attracted to the platelet deposits on exposed collagen, adhere and begin to multiply over time.

tendinae, causing their eventual destruction. In the past, the valves on the left side of the heart (mitral and aortic) were most commonly involved. However, in recent years, because of the widespread use of IV drugs, the incidence of tricuspid valve involvement has increased. In addition to direct valvular damage, vegetations send off particles of infected debris that embolize to various organs.

Depending on the infection and its manner of invasion, ***acute infectious endocarditis (AIE)*** and ***subacute infectious endocarditis (SIE)*** have been described. The main differences between the two are compared in Table 6.36. The clinical manifestations are similar, those associated with AIE being more pronounced and accelerated. Fever is common in most cases, though it may be intermittent, particularly in the elderly. Anemia is also universal, the result of intravascular hemolysis (erythrocytes are broken apart by the turbulent flow of blood through affected valves). From it stem findings of tachycardia, pallor, pale mucous membranes, clubbing of fingers and toes, a yellowish-brown skin hue, and splenomegaly. Other signs and symptoms of endocarditis include fatigue, malaise, anorexia, weight loss, night sweats, shaking chills, myalgias, arthralgias, and redness or swelling of the joints. Embolization causes a variety of distinctive findings: petechiae, splinter hemorrhages, roth spots, and Janeway lesions. It may also lead to serious complications such as stroke, meningitis, renal failure, or immunologic disorders. A loud diastolic blowing murmur is outstanding in patients with AIE, particularly in cases associated with staphylococcus. Related to the development of aortic regurgitation, it may be recognized as a new murmur or as a change in the quality of a previously existing murmur. Although 50 years ago the abscence of a heart murmur ruled out endocarditis, today increasing numbers of patients have none during the initial exam. A murmur may develop during the course of treatment, 2 or 3 months after cure, or not at all. This decreased frequency of murmurs is explained in part by the higher incidence of tricuspid valve endocarditis.

The diagnosis of infectious endocarditis depends heavily on recovering the causative organism from the blood. Multiple blood cultures are the method most frequently used, although bone marrow cultures may be helpful when the blood is sterile. Exposure to antibiotics before endocarditis is suspected renders cultures useless. In these cases, therapy must be discontinued 24–48 hours before cultures are done, and the procedure must be repeated in 7–10 days if the blood is sterile. Technical factors may also yield falsely negative results. Additional laboratory tests assist in establishing the diagnosis. The ESR is usually elevated, and thrombocytopenia is present in both subacute and acute endocarditis. Anemia progresses slowly in subacute disease but rapidly in acute disease (it is pronounced within 1 or 2 weeks). In SIE, total WBC counts remain normal, while in AIE they are elevated (15,000–20,000 mm^3). In either case, there is a left shift. ECG changes are not diagnostic of endocarditis, but they may signal complications. Echocardiography plays an important role in determining the size of the vegetations and the state of valvular function. This technique is of less value in the presence of small vegetations. Scintillation scanning is sometimes helpful in locating vegetations.

Immediate hospitalization is indicated for all patients with infectious endocarditis. This is particularly important in AIE because of the rapidity with which ruptured chordae tendinae or abscess may occur. Other potential complications that may develop from infectious endocarditis are listed in Table 6.37. Specific antimicrobials are initiated as soon as blood cultures are available and are continued for 4–6 weeks. They must be given IV, since oral and IM therapy has limited success. Surgical placement or replacement of a prosthetic valve may be required as well. This is indicated for (1) the development of intractable cardiac failure due to disrupted valve leaflets, (2) a poor response to antibiotics, (3) repeated embolic occlusions, (4) the presence of an abscess, and (5) relapse suffered within 3 months of "cure." Despite the availability of effective antibiotics and surgical procedures, however, the prognosis for patients with infectious endocarditis is not good. The overall 5-year survival rate has been reported to range from 47 to 90%; of those who do survive, 15–25% are incapacitated by heart failure or by the sequelae of embolization.

Since this picture is so pessimistic, ▶ ***endocarditis prophylaxis*** is an important issue for the primary caregiver. A high-dose, short-term antibiotic regimen of penicillin, erythromycin, or vancomycin should be prescribed for high-risk patients prior to certain dental and medical procedures (Table 6.38). Dental and upper respiratory procedures carry the highest risk, since streptococcal strains most often affiliated with endocarditis reside in the mouth and nasal pharynx as flora. Prior to 1984, the

TABLE 6.37 COMPLICATIONS OF INFECTIOUS ENDOCARDITIS

Cardiac disease	Embolization
Heart failure	Neurologic disease
Pericarditis	Vascular phenomenon due to embolism
Myocarditis	Rupture of mycotic aneurysm
Mycotic aneurysm rupture	Acute meningitis or meningocerebritis
Aorta rupture	Arthralgia
Aneurysm of the sinus of Valsalva rupture	Kidney disease
Perivalvular abscess	Infarction due to embolism
Myocardium abscess	Interstitial nephritis
Pericardio-mediastinal fistula	Acute or chronic proliferative glomerulitis
AV ring abscess	Immunologic disorder
Prosthetic thrombosis	

TABLE 6.38 INDICATIONS FOR ENDOCARDITIS PROPHYLAXIS

Any patient with:
- Prosthetic heart valve, including biosynthetic
- Congenital cardiac malformation
- Surgically constructed pulmonary shunt
- Rheumatic[a] and other acquired valvular dysfunction
- Idiopathic hypertrophic subaortic stenosis
- Previous history of endocarditis
- Mitral valve prolapse with insufficiency

Undergoing:
- Any dental procedure likely to cause gingival bleeding, including detailed exams, routine professional cleaning, etc.[b]
- Oral surgery (e.g., biopsy, extraction)
- Tonsillectomy
- Adenoidectomy
- Rigid bronchoscopy and certain other invasive diagnostic procedures
- Biopsy of the respiratory mucosa
- Surgical implantation of prosthetic heart valves, intracardiac materials, or vascular prostheses (possibly antistaphylococcal)
- Obstetric delivery or abortion
- Insertion or removal of an intrauterine contraceptive device
- Urethral catheterization or dilatation, cystoscopy
- Any other surgical procedures involving the urinary, GI, or female genital tract
- Any surgical procedure involving infected soft tissues (e.g., drainage of abscess)

[a]Patients who have had RF are not at increased risk unless heart damage has occurred.
[b]Spontaneous loss of primary teeth, simple fillings above the gingival margin, and adjustment of orthodontic appliances do not involve a significant risk.

American Heart Association recommended that the drugs be given both before and several days after the procedure. The revised recommendation calls for single pre- and postprocedure doses. It reflects recent studies showing that bacteremia occurs and resolves within minutes of instrumentation. What counts, therefore, is the amount of antibiotic present at the time of the procedure and immediately afterward. Besides efficacy, the new guidelines are associated with better compliance.

The pericardium, a loose, two-layered, flasked-shaped sac, provides a protective cover for the heart. It has short tube-like extensions that also enclose the origins of (1) the aorta, (2) the aortic arch junction, (3) the pulmonary artery where it branches, (4) the proximal pulmonary veins, and (5) the venae cavae. A parietal (outer) layer, composed of collagen bundles and elastin fibers, separates the structures in the thoracic cavity and is adjacent to the parietal pleural of the lungs. The visceral (inner) layer adheres to the cardiac musculature and forms the epicardium (external surface) of the heart. Microvilli and long cilia project from the serous mesothelium of the visceral pericardium and the inner lining of the parietal pericardium. These special structures increase the surface area available for fluid transport, permit movement of the pericardial membrane over each other during each cardiac cycle, and allow the pericardium to accommodate changes in cardiac shape during contraction. The visceral pericardium supplies a clear fluid composed of electrolytes, protein, and albumin that acts as a lubricant.

The heart is fixed in place by the pericardium's firm ligamentous attachments anteriorly to the sternum and xiphoid process, posteriorly to the vertebral column, and inferiorly to the diaphragm. Thus, excessive motion of the heart with changes in body position is prevented. The pericardium also reduces friction between the heart and the surrounding organs and provides a barrier against contiguous spread of infection. Experimental evidence suggests that it also limits acute distention of the heart and contributes to diastolic coupling between the two ventricles.

Acute pericarditis, inflammation of the pericardium, results from viral, bacterial, tuberculin, fungal, or parasitic infection, as well as from acute MI, neoplasm, or trauma. The specific pathology varies somewhat according to the underlying cause. In general, however, there is polymorphonuclear invasion, increased vascularity, and fibrin deposition within the pericardium. The visceral pericardium may also react with increased fluid production (see the later discussion). Chest pain is the chief complaint of patients with acute pericarditis. Dull and oppressive, it is often localized to retrosternal and left precordial regions and radiates to the trapezius ridge and neck. Occasionally, it may be localized to the epigastrium or radiate to the left arm. The pain is aggravated by lying supine, inspiring deeply, coughing, and swallowing. It may be relieved by sitting up or leaning forward. Other symptoms—dyspnea, cough, sputum production, weight loss, fever, pallor, anxiety, and restlessness—are often due to the underlying systemic disease. A pericardial friction rub, heard as a scratching, grating, or high-pitched sound on auscultation, arises from friction between the roughened pericardial and epicardial surfaces or in the presence of a scant or large fluid buildup. Consisting of three components related to cardiac motion (atrial systole, ventricular systole, and rapid ventricular filling in early diastole), it often changes in quality from one exam to the next. Therefore, if acute pericarditis is strongly suspected, repeated exams in a quiet room are necessary if a true three-component rub is not readily detected.

On exam, a single-component rub may be mistaken for a systolic murmur or mitral regurgitation. A classic, four-stage evolution of ECG changes may be also be noted (Table 6.39). Rhythm disturbances—sinus tachycardia or bradycardia, intermittent atrial fibrillation, SVT, and atrial flutter—occur infrequently. The chest x-ray film may be normal or may show cardiac dilatation. The echocardiogram is a valuable tool for the detection and quantification of pericardial fluid. Cardiac isoenzymes are usually normal, but the ESR and WBC count are elevated. Observation in the hospital is advised to rule out MI and prevent complications. Determining the underlying systemic disease is of vital importance. Antibiotics are given only when purulent pericarditis is confirmed. Anti-inflammatory agents are administered for pain. Severe, unresponsive pain can be treated on a short-term basis with corticosteroids. Rarely, total pericardectomy is necessary in patients with recurrent, disabling pericarditis who cannot be weaned off steroids.

TABLE 6.39 FOUR-STAGE EVOLUTION OF ECG CHANGES IN PERICARDITIS

Stage	ECG Change
I	ST-segment elevation is concave upward and usually present in all leads except aV_R and V_1 (ST segment is often depressesd in these leads), and T waves are usually upright.
II	Several days later, ST segments return to baseline, accompanied by T-wave flattening.
III	Inversion of the T waves, generally present in most leads. Inversion is not associated with the loss of R-wave voltage or the appearance of Q waves.
IV	Reversion of T-wave changes to normal. Return to normal usually occurs within weeks or months. In cases of pericarditis associated with TB, uremia, or neoplasm, T-wave inversion persists indefinitely.

Pericardial effusion, the accumulation of excessive fluid in the pericardial sac, often accompanies acute pericarditis. Normally, the pericardial space contains 15–50 mL of fluid. When fluid accumulates slowly, the sac stretches to accommodate up to 1 or 2 L without elevation of intrapericardial pressure. However, the pericardium can accommodate the rapid addition of only 80–200 mL without increased pressure. In addition, excessive pericardial stiffness due to fibrosis or tumor infiltration further limits the toleration of excess fluid. Patients who develop pericardial effusion without increased intrapericardial pressure may have no symptoms or may complain of a constant, oppressive, dull ache or pressure in the chest. Larger effusions cause mechanical compression of adjacent structures, giving rise to dysphagia, cough, dyspnea, hoarseness, nausea, or abdominal fullness. They also result in muffled or distant heart sounds. Compression of the base of the left lung is signaled by ***Ewart's sign,*** a patch of dullness on auscultation beneath the angle of the left scapula. Rales are also heard over the lungs secondary to compression. Abnormalities of the arterial and jugular venous pulses and blood pressure are not present without significant elevation of intrapericardial pressure. The cardiac silhouette does not appear enlarged on a chest x-ray film until at least 250 mL of fluid has accumulated. At that time, it may appear globular or water-bottle shaped, with blurring of the left cardiac border and hilar vessels. Marked separation of the pericardial fat lines, normally separated by 1–2 mm, may be noted. Nonspecific ECG changes include lowered QRS voltage and flattening of the T waves. Echocardiography remains the most accurate, rapid, and widely used technique for evaluating the extent of the effusion. Primary treatment of acute pericarditis usually leads to the resolution of pericardial effusion. In some cases, however, pericardiocentesis is indicated to establish the diagnosis or to relieve pressure on adjacent structures.

Increased intrapericardial pressure secondary to fluid accumulation results in compression of the heart and ***cardiac tamponade.*** Initially, this condition limits cardial filling and therefore cardiac output. These limitations, in turn, lead to decreased arterial pressure, coronary artery filling, compromise of myocardial function, and, finally, severe myocardial ischemia. Identifying physical manifestations of cardiac tamponode are a decline in systemic arterial pressure, elevation of systemic venous pressure, and "a small, quiet heart." In addition to or in the absence of these signs, identification of pulsus paradoxus (weakening or disappearance of the arterial pulse during inspiration) is important. Jugular venous pressure is usually markedly elevated, and jugular venous distention is common. Precordial heart activity is not usually palpable, heart sounds are distant or inaudible, extremities are cold and clammy, and anuria is present. Patients with chronic tamponade experience weight loss, anorexia, and profound weakness.

The diagnosis of tamponade begins with a chest x-ray film suggesting the presence of a large pericardial effusion, as discussed above. ECG changes include those of acute pericarditis and effusion, as well as phasic alterations of R-wave amplitude (electrical alternans). Alternans of the P wave, QRS complex, and T wave rarely occurs and is limited to extreme tamponade. The echocardiogram rapidly differentiates cardiac tamponade from other causes of systemic venous hypertension and hypotension (constrictive pericarditis, cardiac muscle dysfunction, and right ventricular infarction). Cardiac catheterization provides absolute confirmation of tamponade, quantifies the magnitude of hemodynamic compromise, detects coexisting problems, and guides treatment. Pericardial effusion with tamponade is considered a medical emergency. Pericardiocentesis is immediately performed to reduce fluid accumulation, and to prevent venous congestion and possible shock. Pericardiectomy and pericardiotomy may be necessary in severe cases.

Chronic pericardial effusion is effusion that persists for more than 6 months. It may accompany any form of pericardial disease, particularly previous idiopathic or viral pericarditis, uremic pericarditis, and pericarditis secondary to myxedema or neoplasm. Surprisingly, many cases are discovered when a routine chest x-ray film reveals an enlarged cardiac silhouette. Treatment depends on the etiology. Stable, nonsymptomatic idiopathic effusions require no treatment except for avoidance of anticoagulants. Those due to TB, neoplasm, purulent infection, or hemorrhage, which usually progress, necessitate periocardiocentesis, partial pericardiotomy, or total pericardiectomy.

Pericarditis with fibrin deposition and effusion may be followed by slow reabsorption of the fluid and chronic inflammation. This, in turn, leads to symmetric thickening and fibrosis or calcification of the pericardial membrane, which restricts diastolic filling of the heart. Known as ***constrictive pericarditis,*** it is most apt to follow pericardial inflammation associated with TB, chronic dialysis, connective tissue disorder, or neoplastic infiltration. It may also be induced by mediastinal irradiation therapy or by drugs such as methysergide, hydralazine, and procainamide. Slowly developing symptoms reflect the progressive nature of the disease. Edema, abdominal swelling and discomfort, and difficulty in breating due to ascites or hepatic congestion are frequent complaints. Postprandial fullness, indigestion, flatulence, and anorexia may be reported, along with exertional dyspnea, cough, and orthopnea. Severe fatigue, weight loss, and muscle wasting suggest fixed or reduced cardiac output. Atrial arrhythmias and CHF are possible complications.

An important diagnostic physical finding with constrictive pericarditis is an abnormal contour of the jugular vein and elevation of jugular venous pressure. A "pericardial knock" or a loud, sharp S_3 may be heard on auscultation along the left sternal border in rigid constrictive pericarditis. Hepatomegaly is usually present and may be accompanied by ascites. The heart appears small, normal, or enlarged on chest x-ray films. Cardiac enlargement is due to coexisting effusion or preexisting cardiac disease. Engorgement of the superior vena cava and left atrial enlargement are often seen. Calcification of the pericardium is often detected in the AV groove or along the anterior and diaphragmatic surfaces of the right ventricle on lateral x-ray films. Left atrial abnormalities (notched P waves) and atrial arrhythmias (often fibrillation), low QRS voltage, and T-wave inversion or flattening are identifying ECG changes. AV block, intraventricular conduction defects, and pseudoinfarction patterns with deep, wide Q waves are related to severe calcification. Cardiac catheterization and angiography are used to assess ventricular compromise and differentiate constrictive pericarditis from restrictive cardiomyopathy. Early or mild constrictive pericarditis may respond to diuretics. Progressive disease may require surgical stripping of the pericardium (pericardiectomy). Patients with underlying TB are additionally treated with multidrug anti-TB therapy for 2–4 weeks prior to surgery and 6–12 months afterward.

Effusive-constrictive pericarditis is characterized by pericardial effusion with visceral pericardial constriction and continued elevation of right atrial pressure after pericardiocentesis. It probably represents a stage in the development of classic constrictive pericarditis. Indeed, the clinical presentation and treatment for the two disorders are similar.

PERIPHERAL CIRCULATION

Arteries

With systole, oxygenated blood is pumped through the aorta and into the peripheral circulation (Fig. 6.10). Main arteries (e.g., cerebral, mesenteric, hepatic, renal, and iliofemoral) feed major organs, the separate circulatory systems of which are discussed in specific chapters throughout the book.

Having thick, muscular walls, arteries transport blood rapidly, under high pressure. They bifurcate into smaller vessels (arterioles), which in turn branch into capillaries (Fig. 6.11). Capillaries are thin-walled vessels about one cell thick where oxygen and nutrients are delivered to the tissues and where carbon dioxide and wastes are picked up.

Primary or ► ***essential hypertension*** is a sustained or intermittent increase in both systolic and diastolic blood pressure (greater than 140/90 mm Hg) with no well-defined etiology. It is the leading cause of morbidity in the United States. Benign essential hypertension is defined as hypertension with a gradual onset and prolonged course. Malignant essential hypertension is diagnosed by its abrupt occurrence and its short, dramatic course. It is fatal if untreated. Though the etiology is undetermined, theories being investigated include the correlation of a defect in the renal hormonal regulation and hypertension, and the antihypertensive effects of prostaglandins. The incidence of primary hypertension increases with age (with onset between 25 and 55 years of age), and it is more prevalent in postmenopausal women and blacks. Other contributing factors include the family history, increased sodium intake, obesity, stress, inactivity, smoking, atherosclerosis, and diabetes, Underlying changes include an increase in cardiac output with normal peripheral vascular resistance or a normal cardiac output with increased peripheral vascular resistance.

The signs of essential hypertension include a gradual or abrupt rise in blood pressure (above 140/90 mmHg) taken on three separate occasions after the patient has rested for 20 minutes or more in quiet surroundings. Retinal changes using the Keith-Wagener classification correlate well with the clinical course and have prognostic significance (Table 6.40). Assessment of heart sounds may reveal a loud aortic S_2 and an early systolic ejection click. As left ventricular enlargement and failure occurs, pulmonary rales, a gallop rhythm, and pulsus alterans are evident. Blood pressure should be taken in both arms and legs, and bilateral comparison of all peripheral pulses should be made. Complications are caused by an acceleration in the development of atherosclerosis in the major arteries, increased peripheral vascular resistance by fibrotic narrowing of the smaller arteries in the systemic circulation, and hypertrophy of the left ventricle with a cyclic consequence of higher systemic pressures. Complications that can range from minor disabilities to death include CHF, arteriosclerosis, MI, cardiovascular accident, renal failure, and ophthalmic damage. Laboratory studies include CBC and serum electrolytes and urinalysis to evaluate the extent of disease. The ECG, echocardiogram, and chest x-ray film denote left ventricular function and structure. Other specific tests to rule out causes of secondary hypertension (e.g., hyperaldosteronism, Cushing's disease, renal artery stenosis, hyperthyroidism) are indicated. Pharmacologic treatment focuses on control, since the cause is unknown and cannot be cured. Medications include diuretics, sympathetic blocking agents, and vasodilators. In addition, a low-sodium diet,

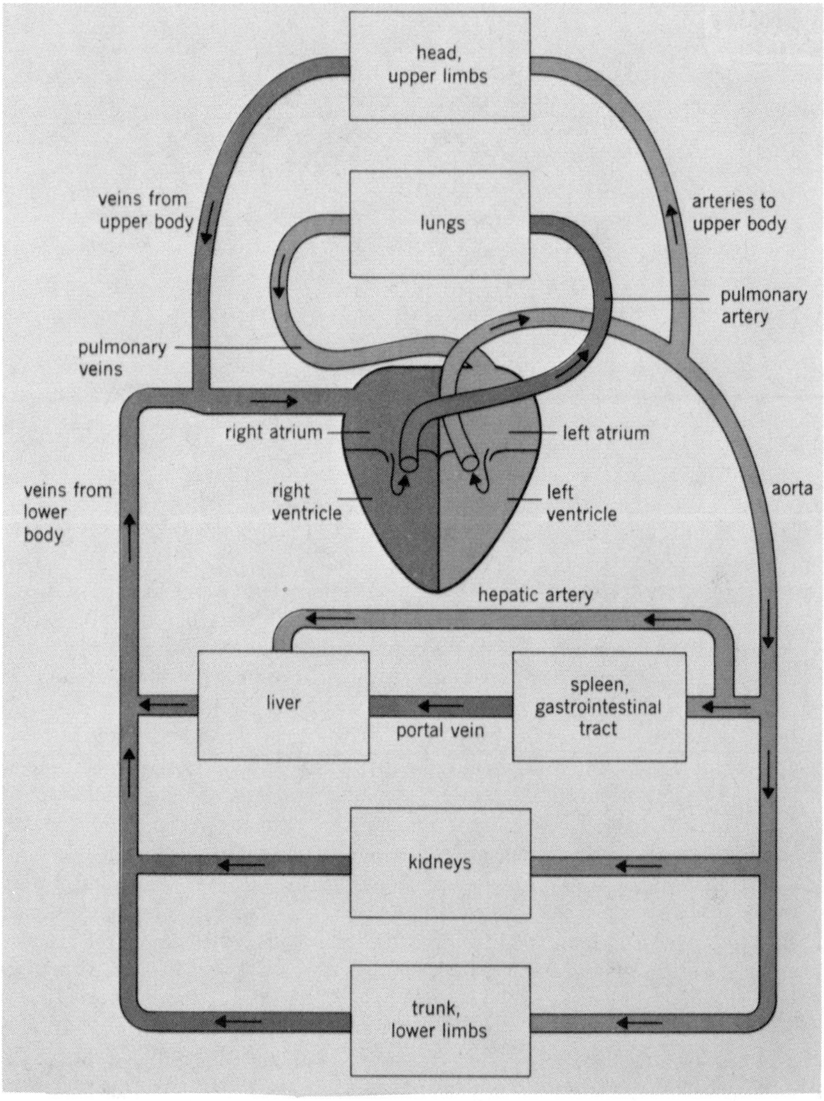

Figure 6.10 Schematic representation of the circulatory system. (From Crouch JE, McClintic R, *Human Anatomy and Physiology,* 2nd ed., copyright © 1976 by John Wiley & Sons, Inc. Reprinted by permission.)

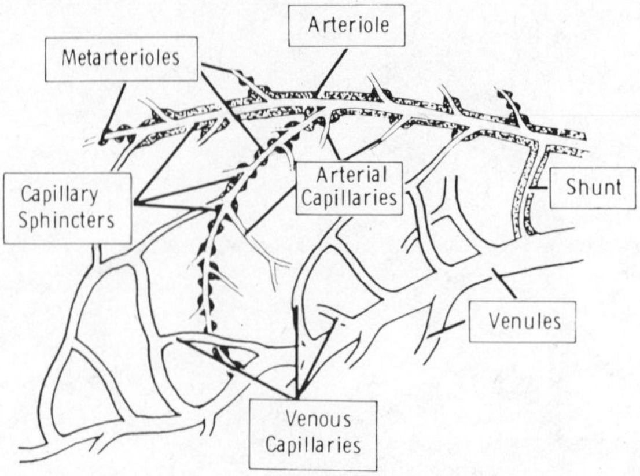

Figure 6.11 Arterioles, capillaries, and venules. (From Brown, AM, Stubbs, DW, *Medical Physiology,* copyright © 1983 by John Wiley & Sons, Inc., New York.)

relaxation techniques, reduction of stressors, and modifications of appropriate risk factors are needed.

▶ ***Peripheral vascular disease*** occurs with decreased arterial compliance from either atherosclerosis or arteriosclerosis, two processes described in Table 6.29. The risk factors are the same as those for coronary artery disease. The primary symptom is claudication, which may be identified as intermittent heaviness, numbness, weakness, aching, or cramping in the muscles distal to the site of obstruction. Other symptoms include pain at rest, diminished or absent peripheral pulses below the site of occlusion, and cool, dry, shiny skin, which may appear cyanotic or pale when elevated and reddened when dependent. Because of decreased circulation, the skin atrophies, there is loss of hair on the extremities, and the nails become hard and thickened. The patient may experience delayed healing of minor lesions, diminished or absent sensory and motor functions, edema, ulceration, or superficial gangrene. Diagnostic studies should include oscillometric readings, skin temperature studies, and ultrasound or Doppler studies. Treatment begins with measures to prevent further progression of disease. Smokers must stop smoking forever. Blood sugar, cholesterol, and triglyceride levels and weight should be controlled. A carefully monitored exercise program should be initiated to promote collateral circulation. Finally, vasodilators may be given to improve blood flow and reduce painful claudication. In addition, anticoagulant therapy may be initiated to prevent thrombus

TABLE 6.40 KEITH-WAGENER SCALE OF RETINAL CHANGES ASSOCIATED WITH HYPERTENSION

Classification	Signs
KW1	Minimal narrowing and irregularity of arteries.
KW2	Increased narrowing of arteries and AV nicking.
KW3	Flame-shaped or round hemorrhages and fluffy "cotton wool" exudates.
KW4	Any of the above with papilledema (optic disk elevation, physiologic cup obliteration, blurred disk margins). Malignant hypertension is always classified in this category.

formation. If a thrombus does develop, fibrinolytics may prove helpful. Vascular bypass or endarterectomy (the surgical excision of the tunica intima of an artery thickened by atherosclerosis) are other alternatives in management.

Reduction of the blood supply to the extremities as a result of arterial spasm results in ► ***Raynaud's disease.*** Typically appearing before age 40, this disease occurs almost exclusively in women, especially in smokers. The etiology is unknown. Symptoms, which may be precipitated by emotional stress and cold, begin with pallor and cyanosis, which are most evident in the hands and/or feet. After the spasm abates, vasodilatation occurs and rubor develops. The diagnosis is based primarily on the symptoms. In mild cases, no treatment is necessary other than education and reassurance. Patients with more asymptomatic cases may respond favorably to tranquilizers or vasodilators. Smoking and cold should be avoided.

Takayasu arteritis is an occlusive polyarteritis of unknown cause that occurs most commonly in oriental persons and young women. The clinical manifestations of the disease depend on the vessels occluded. Surgical bypass grafting to provide adequate blood flow is the only effective treatment.

Blockage of a large or small peripheral artery is referred to as ***acute arterial occlusion.*** It may be caused by atheromatous plaque formation within the vessel, or by embolization or a thrombus originating either from the left side of the heart or from an aneurysm. Predisposing factors include atrial fibrillation, MI, mitral valve disease, valvular replacement, endocarditis, and CHF. Usually the patient experiences sudden pain distal to the site of occlusion that may be preceded by numbness and paresthesias and increased by movement. Decreased peripheral vascular circulation and ischemia of the lower extremities are evidenced by pallor, cyanosis, cold skin, absent or diminished pulses distal to the occlusion, and bruits over the abdomen or groin. Complications that may occur as a result of decreased blood flow to the extremities include arterial ulcers and gangrene. The diagnosis is confirmed by arteriography. Patients should be hospitalized for anticoagulant therapy, intra-arterial administration of vasodilators, and observation. They should be kept on bed rest and given heat applications to promote vasodilatation. If these measures prove ineffective, embolectomy or vascular bypass may be undertaken. Extremities affected by gangrene may have to be amputated.

Inflammatory obstruction of arteries (and veins) leads to ***Beurger's disease.*** Occurring most frequently in young men, the disease is particularly prevalent among Jews and is rare among blacks. It is episodic and occurs in the limbs. The specific cause has not been identified, but known contributing factors include smoking, infections, toxic agents, and hypercoagulability of the blood. Symptoms usually begin in the feet and move up the legs, then to the upper extremities. Their severity depends on the vessel involved, the extent of the involvement, and the presence of collateral circulation. Severe cases may be marked by infection and tissue necrosis. These changes are aggravated by cold temperatures, smoking, and tension. Kidney involvement is not uncommon (see Chapter 8). The treatment is similar to that employed for Raynaud's disease and involves methods to increase vasodilatation and peripheral circulation.

Veins

After blood vessels passes through the capillaries, it enters venules, the smallest branches of the venous system (see Fig. 6.11). Venules converge, eventually forming larger vessels known as "veins." Veins are responsible for transporting blood back to the heart, but in contrast to arteries, they have thin, muscular walls. For this reason, the movement of blood through veins depends on contraction of surrounding muscle tissue. In the extremities, it is aided by valves that help counteract the gravitational backflow of blood.

▶ ***Varicose veins*** is a condition stemming from incompetent valves along the greater and lesser saphenous veins and their tributaries in the lower extremities. Congenital weakness of the veins, pregnancy, obesity, prolonged standing, and tall stature are the main contributing factors. Secondary causes include thrombophlebitis, arteriovenous fistula, and pressure on the inferior vena cava or iliofemoral vein. In response to one or more of these conditions, the leaflets of the valves fail to close, and backflow and pooling are permitted. The vessels become dilated, elongated, and tortuous. Venous stasis and increased venous pressure interfere with the muscular compression of the deep veins, and pooling occurs in these vessels as well. Patients complain of swelling, an aching sensation, muscle cramps, or fatigability in the legs. On exam, the skin over the lower legs appears brownish, the result of erythrocytes in surrounding tissue. The diagnosis is usually based on the presence of symptoms and contributing factors. It may be confirmed by phlebography and retrograde filling tests. Treatment begins with measures to reduce venous stasis (elastic stockings, elevation of legs, avoidance of prolonged standing, exercise). Affected vessels may also be injected with sclerosing solutions to obliterate the varicosity and the communicating vein. Alternatively, they may be removed surgically (stripping).

Thrombophlebitis is the inflammation of a vein wall with clot formation. Venous stasis, traumatic, bacterial, or chemical injury to the vein, hypercoagulable states (including birth control pills), and a previous history of the condition are risk factors. The occurrence of thrombophlebitis is usually sudden. The severity of symptoms depends upon the location and extent of involvement of the vein. The calf is usually affected. Symptoms include localized pain, tenderness, redness, warmth, and edema. Pain may be increased by dorsiflexion of the foot (positive ***Homan's sign***). The diagnosis is confirmed by isotope studies, phlebography, and ultrasonic studies. Pulmonary embolization, a condition discussed in a previous section, is always a worrisome possibility. For this reason, patients are usually hospitalized for anticoagulant therapy, heat applications, bed rest, and observation. Elastic stockings may be used following the acute phase, and analgesics and antibiotics (for cases associated with bacterial infection) may be employed as well. Once the acute phase has resolved, patients may be discharged on ▶ ***long-term anticoagulant therapy.*** Since they are at risk for recurrence, preventive measures such as exercise, elevation of extremities, and proper use of elastic stockings should be taught.

Details of Management

▸ *Smoking Cessation*

Laboratory Tests: None needed.

Therapeutic Measures: While some smokers have been able to cut back gradually on the number of cigarettes smoked per day until they finally quit, it is usually preferable for smokers to stop at once, since the gradual reduction approach usually causes the person to think constantly about how many cigarettes are allowed each day, when the next cigarette may be smoked, and so on, making an obsession of the idea and the behavior he or she is trying to eliminate. With the patient's help, devise an acceptable quitting plan that includes choosing a day on which to quit (and circling it on the calendar). One should not choose a time of high stress for quitting, since there is a greater chance that such an attempt will fail. The quitting day should be about 2 or 3 weeks off to allow patients time to study their smoking habits. Self-evaluations focusing on why and when they smoke may help patients discover the factors involved in their own addiction and provide possible strategies for each type of smoker trying to quit. The American Cancer Society's (ACS) "I Quit" kit (contact the ACS at 90 Park Avenue, New York, New York 10016 or call 212-599-8200) and the National Institutes of Health (NIH) pamphlet "Why Do You Smoke?" (NIH Pub. No. 81-1822) both contain such questionnaires. Another helpful pamphlet is "Clearing the Air: A Guide to Quitting Smoking" (NIH Pub. No. 83-1647). Have patients compile a list of reasons for quitting, including all the positive results that will come of it, and read through the list at least once daily until the quitting day arrives. Suggest that the patient spend the first nonsmoking day with a friend who knows about the quitting and plan to fill the time with enough enjoyable activities to remain occupied, thereby limiting the amount of empty time for thinking about smoking. A nicotine substitute (e.g., Nicorette) may be prescribed as a temporary aid for some patients who have been repeatedly unsuccessful in their attempts to quit smoking and whose nicotine dependence is primarily physical. However, it is preferable that patients use other nonchemical means to fill the behavioral void that quitting leaves. For example, a new hobby or sport may be tried, or another behavior may be chosen to replace smoking, such as drinking a glass of seltzer with a straw, doodling with a pencil, or opening and chewing a stick of gum. However, discuss the tendency for many quitters to replace smoking with eating, with the common result of unwanted weight gain, and suggest a few relaxation exercises that may be practiced whenever the patient feels the need for a cigarette to "relieve tension" (see "Stress Reduction"). Nicotine substitutes should never be prescribed for pregnant women (a pregnancy test is recommended prior to instituting this therapy), and female patients should be advised to avoid pregnancy for the duration of therapy. Other patients who should not use nicotine substitutes are those recovering from a recent MI, those with life-threatening arrhythmias or angina pectoris that is severe or worsening, or those with active temporomandibular joint dysfunction. (See the manufacturer's inserts for other relative contraindications, dosage, information on patient selection, and signs and symptoms of toxicity). Hypnosis, behavior modification, group therapy, acupuncture, and aversive stimulus therapy have all been used to assist persons in quitting smoking, with varying degrees of success. Some patients may wish to be recommended to a specialist for one of these therapies.

Patient Education: Ask all patients whether they smoke, and encourage all smokers to quit. Emphasize the importance of quitting (not just reducing the number of cigarettes, cigars, or pipes smoked), relating smoking to the patient's and his or her family's personal health experience and to the increased risk of developing disease. Suggest that the patient team up with a friend, roommate, or family member to quit, since success will be more likely if a smoking partner also quits. It may be helpful for some patients to avoid activities or environments that they associate with smoking (e.g., bars, movie theaters) at first, but reassure them that they can expect to lose their intense craving for tobacco after about 8 weeks. Discuss increased appetite and diet changes with patients, and provide a list of low-calorie foods and drinks that can be snacked on whenever they feel compelled to nibble. If necessary, create a diet plan and discuss an enjoyable exercise program if weight gain becomes a problem (i.e., if more than a few pounds are gained or if weight gain persists beyond the first few weeks). Discuss with patients for whom you prescribe nicotine substitutes their proper use, as well as the signs and symptoms of toxicity. Discuss pregnancy prevention with female patients using the substitutes and instruct them to discontinue using them if they suspect that they may be pregnant until that possibility has been ruled out. Check local listings for a support group that interested patients can be referred to or contact:

Smoke-Enders
525 Prospect Street
Memorial Parkway
Phillipsburg, New Jersey 08865
Tel.: (201) 454-4357

Office of Cancer Communications
National Cancer Institute
National Institutes of Health
Bethesda, Maryland 20205
Tel.: (800) 638-6694

Office on Smoking and Health
U.S. Department of Health and Human Services
5600 Fishers Lane
Park Bldg., Room 110
Rockville, Maryland 20857
Tel.: (301) 443-5287

American Cancer Society
777 Third Avenue
New York, New York 10017
Tel.: (212) 371-2900

American Heart Association
7320 Greenville Avenue
Dallas, Texas 75231
Tel.: (214) 750-5300

American Lung Association
1740 Broadway
New York, New York 10019
Tel.: (212) 315-8700

Follow-up: Follow-up is essential in order to check on the patient's progress and reinforce success. Discuss relapses and offer encouragement, reminding patients that a relapse does not equal a failure and that successful cessation requires practice. Patients using a nicotine substitute should be seen at regular intervals and the product gradually tapered. Any female patient using a substitute should be questioned about the possibility of pregnancy at every office visit. Assist interested patients in making contact with a support group or specialist for an appropriate therapy (hypnosis, behavior modification, etc.).

▶ *Asthma*

Laboratory Tests: Diagnosis is usually based on clinical findings, but pulmonary function tests and arterial blood gas studies may be used to determine the effectiveness of treatment. Serum levels of theophylline should be measured regularly to ensure maintenance of therapeutic levels.

Therapeutic Measures: For mild attacks, isoproterenol or beta$_2$-adrenergic isoetharine may be given in a nebulizer with normal saline, or metaproterenol may be given via inhaler. (See Table 6.9 for dosages.) For moderate to severe attacks, give 1:1,000 epinephrine, 0.2–0.5 ml SC, repeated at 20-minute intervals up to 3 doses (do not use epinephrine for hypertensive or elderly patients or those with angina). The patient with severe wheezing that persists in spite of the above medications should be referred to the hospital. There, a loading dose mg of 250–500 mg aminophylline (in a 50-mL normal saline solution) may be dripped IV over 15 minutes if epinephrine is not effective and the patient is not already taking a theophylline medication. Severe attacks unresponsive to epinephrine and aminophylline may require corticosteroids. Administer 250 mg hydrocortisone sodium succinate IV (in a single dose) and 40–60 mg oral prednisone (in divided doses) for 1 day. Continue the oral prednisone, gradually tapering the dosage over the next 7–10 days until none is given. Oxygen may be administered via mask or nasal prongs for moderate to severe wheezing (in concentrations sufficient to relieve hypoxemia).

If necessary (i.e., for the status asthmaticus patient), the initial loading dose of aminophylline may be followed by a continuous drip of aminophylline in 5% dextrose to attain and maintain therapeutic blood levels. The dosages are as follows:

Patients with CHF or liver failure	0.5 mg/kg/h for the first 12 hours, then 0.1–0.2 mg/kg/h*
Elderly patients or those with cor pulmonale	0.6 mg/kg/h for the first 12 hours, then 0.3 mg/kg/h*
Healthy adults (nonsmokers)	0.7 mg/kg/h for the first 12 hours, then 0.5 mg/kg/h*
Children and young adults who smoke	1.0 mg/kg/h for the first 12 hours, then 0.8 mg/kg/h*

Adjust the subsequent dosage as needed to maintain therapeutic serum levels (10–20 μg/mL). Patients who are already receiving a theophylline preparation should have the initial loading dose reduced or eliminated by determining the time and amount of the last medication taken (1 mg theophylline is equivalent to 1.2 mg aminophylline). If the amount and time are not known, give 2.9 mg/kg aminophylline as a loading dose and then continue the maintenance dose as above. Hydrocortisone sodium succinate or methylprednisolone sodium succinate (125 mg) may be given IV every 4 hours until improvement occurs, with a gradually tapered course of oral prednisone as described above (or methylprednisolone, 16 mg orally four times a day to start, then tapered over 7–10 days). Intravenous fluid replacement should be given as needed for dehydration.

For management of chronic asthma, long-acting theophylline preparations may be used in dosages that will maintain serum levels within the therapeutic range (usually 300 mg twice daily). For mild asthma, oral beta-adrenergic stimulators may be effective (albuterol is also available as an inhaled aerosol); the dosage terbutaline sulfate (Brethine, Bricanyl) is 2.5–5.0 mg three times daily, and for albuterol sulfate (Ventolin, Proventil) it is 2–4 mg three to four times daily, gradually increased to 8 mg four times daily if necessary. Isoproterenol, metaproterenol, and isoetharine in a hand bulb or pressurized nebulizer may be used to relieve or prevent mild wheezing; two inhalations separated by a 5-minute period will produce maximum benefit (see information on individual dosages for the recommended frequency of use). If these measures are not sufficient to keep patients relatively symptom free, long-term corticosteroid therapy may be employed. The initial dosage should be 10 mg three to four times per day, which may be reduced gradually to the lowest effective maintenance dose that is able to prevent symptoms (preferably using an alternate-day schedule). As an alternative, aerosolized beclomethasone dipropionate in a nebulizer may be given with virtually no systemic absorption or side effects, but it is not effective in acute attacks since it must be deposited deep in the bronchial tree. It may be used, however, to reduce or eliminate the required systemic steroid dose once wheezing has been controlled with other medications. Deeper deposition of beclomethasone may be achieved by using it after nebulized isoetharine or albuterol (rapidly acting bronchodilators). Start patients on two inhalations (separated by a 5-minute interval) of beclomethasone four times per day and gradually decrease to the lowest effective dose. If necessary, beclomethasone may be used up to eight times per

*Since theophylline does not penetrate fatty tissue, base calculations for obese patients on ideal rather than actual body weight.

day, but isoetharine or albuterol may not be used more often than every 4 hours. This schedule should be discussed carefully with patients who are using both types of aerosolized preparations.

Patient Education: Focusing treatment on self-care will help to provide patients with a sense of personal control. This is especially valuable for patients with chronic illnesses, since it helps to lessen the normal reactions of fear and dependency. Personal measures that should be discussed with patients include:

Adequate hydration (2–3 quarts of water per day) to keep secretions liquefied.

Quitting smoking.

Attaining and maintaining ideal body weight.

Staying active and participating in some form of regular exercise. Self-paced sports like swimming or walking are recommended, since major exertion or excessive fatigue may precipitate an attack.

Learning about the drugs the patient uses so that he or she may understand how to vary dosages and drugs according to the symptoms. Emphasize keeping appointments for blood tests to monitor theophylline levels.

Avoidance of known precipitants and pulmonary irritants, such as cigarette smoke and other types of smoke, fumes, spray deodorants, hair sprays (and other sprays), seasonal allergens, house dust, animal dander, certain foods, and so on.

Environmental measures to be discussed include:

The use of cotton or synthetic materials for clothing, bedding, and floor and furniture coverings rather than wool, fur, silk, or woven grass (e.g., mats) if there seems to be a sensitivity to these materials. Feather pillows and down-filled comforters and sleeping bags should be avoided, and some patients may have trouble with horsehair stuffing, which is found in some furniture and car seats.

Bed linens should be aired daily and household dust controlled by frequent damp-cloth dusting. Objects that collect dust, such as thick carpeting, bedspreads, heavy drapes, and knicknacks should be avoided or cleaned frequently, preferably by a nonasthmatic family member, and the patient should remain out of the room for at least an hour after completion of the cleaning. A vacuum cleaner should be used to reach dust in crevices, and close attention should be paid to the control of mold growth in bathrooms, closets, and basements.

Family pets may cause a problem for asthmatics; not only are allergies to furred and feathered animals (particularly cats) common, but the animals also shed and trap dust. If possible, pets should be kept outside to help protect the patient.

The temperature of the home should be kept relatively constant and warm. Home air should be humidified during the heating season (use a furnace humidifier and a separate cold-mist humidifier in the bedroom), and the heating system filtered and cleaned yearly. Air conditioning during summer months is helpful, particularly when the pollution level or pollen count is high, but extremes of temperature should be avoided.

Instruct patients in breathing exercises (see "Emphysema") and advise them to practice them at least once daily and whenever they experience dyspnea. The pursed-lip breathing technique provides patients with a sense of control over the breathing process, which helps to prevent a panic response and counteracts the tendency to hyperventilate. Teach postural drainage and cupping and clapping techniques (with extra attention to the lower lobes) to a family member, to be performed twice daily when patients are producing a significant amount of sputum. Provide information about organizations and support groups of asthmatics (see "Organizations for Respiratory Disorders").

Follow-up: Arrange office visits as needed to provide symptomatic treatment, check serum medication levels, and monitor the status or progression of the disease and the medical management. Assist the patient in locating and contacting support groups.

▸ *Chronic Bronchitis*

Laboratory Tests: Tests of sputum include culture (*H. influenzae* and *Streptococcus pneumoniae* are commonly found), sensitivity, and cytology (during infection). Chest x-ray films reveal hyperinflation of lungs with an increase in the anteroposterior diameter, a flattened diaphragm, increased retrosternal air space and bronchial markings at the base of the lungs, and bullae of varying sizes in the upper lung fields. CBC may reveal secondary polycythemia. Arterial blood gas studies show low Pa_{O_2} and low, normal, or elevated Pa_{CO_2}. Even in cases of chronic hypercapnia, most patients are well compensated and pH levels remain near normal. Acidemia of any degree is always a poor sign (indicating end-stage disease or acute illness). Pulmonary function tests reveal obstruction of expiratory air flow, and atypical results of liver function tests (SGOT, alkaline phosphatase, bilirubin, etc.) are not unusual if right ventricular failure and hepatic congestion are present.

Therapeutic Measures: If infection is present, administer ampicillin, 250–500 mg every 6 hours for 5–7 days, or erythromycin, 500 mg every 6 hours for 5–7 days. Also, give oral aminophylline, 250–500 mg four times daily, or 200 mg twice daily of a sustained-release preparation (to sustain a blood theophylline level of 10–20 μg/mL). Inhaled bronchodilators (e.g., metaproterenol), 2 to 3 puffs, three or four times daily, or oral metaproterenol sulfate, 10–20 mg three to four times daily, may be helpful for chronic management. For acute bronchospasms, inhaled metaproterenol may be administered every 4 hours, but the total daily dose should not exceed 12 inhalations. The use of corticosteroids for chronic bronchitis is controversial, but it is often used as a last resort in patients with severe disease. Urge all patients who smoke to quit. Immunization against influenza and pneumococci is important, especially in chronically ill or elderly patients (see "Influenza Vaccine" and "Pneumococcus Vaccine"). If acute respiratory distress ensues, provide necessary emergency treatment (ventilatory support, low-flow oxygen therapy with nasal prongs or Venturi mask) and arrange for immediate hospitalization (see "Acute Respiratory Distress Syndrome"). Manage the signs and symptoms of associated cardiac dysfunction (i.e., right or left ventricular dysfunction) with diuretics, and treat CHF (see the section on CHF) if this develops.

Patient Education: Discuss the association of this illness with chronic inhalation of pulmonary irritants and assist patients in quitting smoking (see the section on "Smoking Cessation"). Instruct patients in the proper use of inhaled and oral medications, and discuss with them the rationale for therapy, expected results, side effects, and possible signs of toxicity. Encourage discussion of any questions or concerns your patients have, and urge them to notify you immediately about the development of any side effects or signs of acute exacerbation (increased cough, increased dyspnea, change in sputum, fever, etc.). Discuss ways of avoiding and preventing respiratory infections and other personal and environmental measures (see the section on "Asthma") that may be applicable to patients (e.g., avoidance of allergens or inhaled irritants, maintenance of ideal body weight, etc.). Discuss the importance of adequate hydration and encourage patients to drink 2–3 quarts of water daily. Humidification of the indoor environment is advisable, and regular inhalation of steam, even in the form of a cup of hot tea, is useful practice. Teach breathing exercises (see the section on "Emphysema") for patients to use during periods of dyspnea to help reduce the tendency to panic and hyperventilate. Also, teach coughing and postural drainage exercises. For coughing, the patient should be seated in a comfortable position and should lean slightly over a pillow held in front of the abdomen. Have him or her take several slow, relaxed, deep breaths through the nose, hold them for a few seconds, and then exhale through the mouth with the lips pursed to slow the exhalation and avoid the use of accessory muscles. Even if mucus is felt in the airways, the patient should suppress the coughing response until several slow breaths have been taken. Then, the patient should focus on breathing abdominally (the pressure of the expanding abdomen against the pillow is a good cue), lean forward against the pillow, and cough softly in a series of short, rapid coughs. Postural drainage, and cupping and clapping, are helpful when sputum production is significant. Instruct a family member in the proper positioning and technique, paying particular attention to the lower lobes, and suggest that this exercise be performed about twice daily. When patients become comfortable with the controlled breathing exercises, they may be encouraged to begin a graduated exercise program; walking is probably the best choice, since it is self-regulated. Discuss the need for patients to avoid respiration-depressing sedatives and narcotics. Provide information about support organizations (see "Organizations for Respiratory Disorders") and assistance patients in making contact.

Follow-up: As needed for treatment of exacerbations and to monitor the progression of disease, the medical regimen, and serum theophylline levels.

▸ *Emphysema*

Laboratory Tests: Pa_{O_2} is lowered and Pa_{CO_2} may be low, normal, or high. The serum bicarbonate level is elevated, expiratory air flow obstruction is present, and total lung capacity and residual volume are increased (seen in pulmonary function studies). Many patients have a hereditary deficiency of serum alpha$_1$-antitrypsin (normal levels are greater than 180 mg/dL). Liver function tests may be abnormal due to deposition of alpha$_1$-antitrypsin granules in liver parenchyma.

Therapeutic Measures: There is no medical treatment capable of halting the progression of the underlying disease process, but symptomatic treatment measures may provide subjective improvement in the patient's quality of life and appropriate treatment of exacerbations may slow the process and prolong the patient's life. Treatment of bronchospasm with bronchodilators (e.g., theophylline-type methylxanthines or beta-adrenergic sympathomimetics in inhaled or oral form) may be helpful. It is critical that all patients, regardless of the severity of their disease, be urged to quit smoking and to avoid other pulmonary irritants (e.g., aerosol cleaners and deodorants, hair sprays, spray paints, insecticides). Initiation of a course of antibiotics at the first sign of respiratory infection (e.g., an increased amount or a change in the color of sputum, fever, dyspnea) is recommended. Ampicillin, 250–500 mg every 6 hours for 1 week, or erythromycin, 500 mg every 6 hours for 1 week, are the drugs of choice. Tetracycline (250–500 mg every 6 hours for 1 week) or trimethoprim-sulfamethoxazole combinations (160 mg trimethoprim and 800 mg sulfamethoxazole twice a day for 10 days) are also used. Some experts recommend prophylactic antibiotic therapy during the winter months to prevent exacerbations, but this is controversial. Vaccination against respiratory pathogens is important for all patients because of the greatly increased risk of developing respiratory failure with even minor respiratory infections (see "Influenza Vaccine" and "Pneumococcus Vaccine"). Episodes of acute respiratory distress are common in emphysema patients, requiring emergency ventilatory support, low-flow oxygen therapy (1–2 L/min via nasal prongs or at a concentration of 24–28% via Venturi mask), and hospitalization for treatment. Some patients may require occasional home oxygen therapy for severe symptoms of respiratory distress or during vigorous activity producing dyspnea; this should be administered via nasal cannula at a rate of 1–2 L/min, using any portable oxygen delivery system. However, the use of oxygen to treat episodes of dyspnea is controversial, since this form of therapy readily encourages habituation, increasing the tendency toward invalidism. Patients with severely incapacitating hypoxia may be candidates for chronic oxygen therapy, administered during sleep and continued for up to 18 hours per day. However, one should *never* attempt oxygen therapy without first establishing that the patient does not retain CO_2 and determining the optimal flow rate by arterial blood gas analysis.

Patient Education: Emphasize the importance of stopping smoking, and provide patients who smoke with instructions and encouragement (see "Smoking Cessation"). Patients should drink at least 2–3 quarts of water daily in addition to other fluids. Humidification of the indoor environment is advised, and regular inhalation of steam, even in the form of a cup of hot tea, is a useful practice. Provide instruction in breathing exercises, especially for patients who panic and hyperventilate readily when they experience dyspnea. Patients should relax and inhale slowly and deeply through the nose, hold the breath for a few seconds (if possible without causing discomfort), and then exhale through pursed lips (as if blowing out a candle). As patients become more comfortable with the exercises, have them concentrate on breathing abdominally. If breathing exercises are done in a reclining position, a box of facial tissues or a light book can be placed on the abdomen so that the patient can observe abdominal movement during inhalations and exhalations. This controlled breathing technique provides the patient with a sense of control over this own breathing and induces a more relaxed respiratory pattern. In addition, pursed-lip breathing eliminates the forceful exhalation through inelastic airways that may lead to airway collapse and further distal air trapping (retained pressure in the airways produced by the slowed respiration helps to prevent expiratory collapse).

Once control of breathing through this technique is gained, a graduated exercise training program to improve exercise tolerance should be begun. Walking is a good choice, since it can be self-regulated. Teach effective coughing technique (see "Chronic Bronchitis"). Emphasize good oral hygiene, since aspiration of infected sputum from the mouth (e.g., due to periodontal disease) may lead to a life-threatening respiratory infection. Counsel patients to avoid fatigue by not attempting overly strenuous activities and by planning their days so that most of their work may be accomplished when their energy level is highest (e.g., at the beginning of the day). Discuss the need for a nutritious, balanced diet and suggest eating several small meals, since their preparation, consumption, and digestion tend to be less tiring than those involving large meals. Discuss good sleep practices and counsel patients on dealing with insomnia. Stress the importance of avoiding respiration-depressing sedatives and narcotics. Discuss other practical measures for avoiding infection (e.g., avoidance of known infectious persons and crowds, humidification of home air during the heating season). Patients should avoid temperature and climate extremes, known allergens, and inhaled irritants (smoke, dust and dust traps, powders, sprays, pollutants), and the home furnace should be kept filtered and clean.

Follow-up: Every 2–3 months as needed to monitor the progression of disease and medical management. Periodically discuss the patient's personal exercise program and emphasize the need for regular exercise to prevent excessive disability that can result from prolonged inactivity. Patients who are severely disabled may need to be referred to a physical therapist for trained supervision in this area. Assist patients in making contact with a local support group by consulting local listings or getting contacts though national organizations (see below).

▸ *Organizations for Respiratory Disorders*

Laboratory Tests: None.

Therapeutic Measures: None.

Patient Education: Discuss the purpose of organizations and support groups for various disorders and assist patients in making contact with appropriate ones. Consult local listings or contact:

American Lung Association
1740 Broadway
New York, New York 10019
Tel.: (212) 315-8700

Emphysemics Anonymous, Inc.
P.O. Box 66
Fort Meyers, Florida 33902

Asthma and Allergy Foundation of America
1835 K Street, NW
Washington, D.C. 20006
Tel.: (202) 293-2950

National Jewish Hospital National Asthma Center
1400 Jackson Street
Denver, Colorado 80206
Tel.: (800) 222-LUNG

▸ *Pneumonia*

Laboratory Tests: Based on the history and physical exam, a WBC count and differential, sputum smear and culture, blood culture, and chest x-ray films (PA and lateral) should be obtained. Gram stain, culture (including cultures for anaerobic bacteria and mycobacteria), and determination of protein, glucose, and LDH concentrations may also be done on pleural fluid obtained via thoracentesis if there is evidence of pleural effusion and a sufficient volume is present. Leukocytosis (polymorphonuclear) is more common in bacterial than in viral pneumonias, although a high leukocyte count may occur with viral infections, while overwhelming bacterial infections or infections in elderly or debilitated patients may be associated with a low or normal WBC count. A good sputum sample is necessary for gross and microscopic exams and culture. If the patient cannot produce an adequate sample, aerosolization of warm saline or intermittent positive-pressure breathing with humidified air may be helpful. A sputum sample containing many squamous epithelial cells (more than 10 cells per high-power field on Gram stain) is not adequate for examination, since this represents heavy contamination by oral secretions and flora. Nasotracheal suction may be necessary. However, this is not a first resort, since attempts to pass the catheter beyond the vocal cords of an alert patient may be not only futile but also distressing to an already ill patient. Transtracheal aspiration should be considered if all attempts by other means to obtain the necessary sputum sample fail or if anaerobic infection is suspected, but because of the risks involved, only a person who is experienced in the procedure (or who is overseen by an experienced person) should attempt it. An anaerobic culture should be done only if the sample was obtained transtracheally, since contamination by pharyngeal organisms may produce a false-positive result (anaerobic cultures should be obtained whenever sputum is foul-smelling). Sputum and blood cultures should be done promptly and administration of antibiotics delayed until the results are obtained, since transient bacteremias occur frequently (especially with pneumococcal infection) and it is not always possible to grow an organism from the sputum culture. Infiltration and signs of consolidation may be seen on x-ray films, but these findings may be minimized by dehydration.

Therapeutic Measures: Appropriate antibiotic therapy should be instituted (see Table 6.12) as soon as the results of cultures are obtained. Rest and adequate hydration should be emphasized. Any undue disturbances should be avoided initially (except for routine blood pressure, respiratory rate, and urinary output evaluations), fluid intake should be sufficient to maintain a total daily output of at least 1,500 mL of urine, and attention should be given to local airway humidification. Patients who are treated early and respond readily may be allowed to increase their activity gradually after they have been afebrile for a few days. In general, younger patients who do not have signs of serious illness (e.g., high fever, tachycardia, tachypnea, severe dyspnea, confusion, dehydration) may remain at home for treatment, but those whose condition is more serious (i.e., exhibiting any of the above signs) should be hospitalized, as should older patients or those with gram-negative pneumonias, aspiration pneumonia, or signs of serious illness, or persons who are unable to be cared for adequately at home. Humidified oxygen should be administered to patients with severe infection, severe dyspnea, circulatory disturbances, asthenia, delirium, or cyanosis with Pa_{O_2} less than 60. It may also relieve excessive coughing and restlessness, but periodic arterial blood gas determinations should be made, particularly for patients with underlying COPD (who receive low concentrations), to monitor the efficacy of the oxygen therapy. In general, the use of antipyretics should be avoided because these interfere with the use of temperature variations as a means of monitoring progress. However, if control of fever seems necessary, aspirin or acetaminophen may be given on a regular, frequent dosage schedule (to avoid subjecting patients to temperature fluctuations and associated periods of heavy perspiration that may result from intermittent, haphazard administration). To treat severe chest pain or respiratory fatigue resulting from severe coughing attacks, especially during the acute phase, 15–30 mg of codeine phosphate may be given every 3–4 hours or as necessary for pain. As an alternative for temporary relief of mild pain, a local anesthetic may be injected into the areas of greatest pain to anesthetize the involved dermatomes, or ethyl chloride may be sprayed over the painful area for about 60 seconds. Meperidine, 50–100 mg SC, or morphine sulfate, 10–15 mg SC, may be given for very severe pain, but patients must be carefully monitored for respiratory depression and excessive suppression of cough. Antitussive medications are generally not recommended unless a persistent cough is interfering with sleep and rest, in which case codeine (as mentioned above) or a terpin hydrate and codeine elixir (4 mL every 3–4 hours as needed) may be prescribed. Expectorants (e.g., acetylcysteine, guaifenesin, terpin hydrate) may be useful in some patients for loosening sputum, although adequate hydration and humidification of inhaled air is generally considered better. Postural drainage and/or suction may also be helpful. A liquid diet may be preferred by patients initially, but a normal diet may be resumed as soon as patients are able to tolerate it.

Patient Education: Instruct patients who are treated at home (or responsible family members) in proper antibiotic use, emphasizing the timing of doses and the necessity of finishing the medication. Instructing patients to take each tablet or capsule with two glasses of water will help ensure adequate hydration. Steam inhalation in the form of a hot cup of tea is a simple and soothing way to provide airway humidification. Discuss humidification of the home environment as well. Discuss other medications and the rationale for their controlled use (e.g., the need to avoid cough suppression unless coughing is interfering with sleep or causing extreme pain), and suggest ways to avoid excessive use (e.g., by limiting the use of codeine, if possible, to small doses at bedtime). Encourage patients (or a responsible family member) to contact you if there are any questions about medications or concerns about the response to treatment.

Follow-up: A resurgence of fever after an afebrile period and decline in the patient's condition may signal the development of a suprainfection following antibiotic treatment, necessitating reculture of sputum and blood. The emergence of a drug allergy may also necessitate discontinuation or substitution of the antibiotic. For all patients, a repeat exam and Gram stain of sputum should follow completion of antibiotic therapy, and a follow-up chest x-ray film should be performed in 6 weeks to 2 months, since pneumonia may be the presenting feature of a malignancy. Any underlying disease (e.g., COPD) or risk factors (e.g., smoking) that may have contributed to the development of the infection should be discussed and an appropriate plan for management of these issues discussed.

► *Influenza Vaccine (Types A and B)*

Laboratory Tests: None.

Therapeutic Measures: Recommended for patients who are elderly or who have a chronic or debilitating illness (especially chronic respiratory conditions or cardiac disease). Polyvalent influenza virus vaccine (inactivated) given in the fall prior to the flu season or after exposure to the virus will provide partial immunity to the virus for a few months to 1 year. The vaccine should be given IM or SC, usually in one dose, but, depending on the current Center for Disease Control recommendations, a second booster injection given 1 month after the first may be required for immunization (this occurs when new viral strains arise). A single dose consists of 0.5 cc of vaccine (see the package insert for dosage recommendations and formulation). Whole (whole virion) and split virus (subvirion) preparations are available, but for use in adults, both types of vaccine are comparable. The composition of the vaccine is changed yearly according to the serotypes predicted to be most prevalent during the next season, but the vaccine almost always contains one or two strains of influenza A virus and one strain of influenza B virus. If an epidemic of type A influenza is confirmed in a community, supplementary administration of an antiviral medication (amantadine) may be effective in reducing the incidence of clinical disease in exposed, previously unvaccinated individuals if it is begun immediately and continued for 10 days. The dosage for amantadine hydrochloride is 200 mg by mouth daily (or 100 mg by mouth every 12 hours). This drug may be particularly useful for protecting elderly patients exposed to influenza A during nursing home outbreaks, but the risk of CNS toxicity should be weighed against the risk of exposure to influenza or its complications in these patients. Amantadine does not protect against other types of influenza or other viral infections. If any person in this high-risk group contracts the flu, antibiotic therapy should also be instituted to reduce the incidence of a secondary bacterial infection, especially pneumonia.

Patient Education: Instruct high-risk patients (persons over 65 years of age or those with chronic disease) about the importance of receiving the vaccine annually or immediately following exposure. They should also be taught how to avoid and prevent respiratory infections, and, if indicated, encouraged to receive pneumococcal vaccine as well. Potential side effects of influenza vaccine to be discussed include local reactions (redness and induration lasting for 1–2 days occur in a small percentage of patients receiving the vaccine) and the development of fever and other constitutional symptoms (in 1–2% of patients, beginning 6–12 hours after vaccination and lasting for 1–2 days). Immediate hypersensitivity reactions (extremely rare) presumably reflect a sensitivity to a component of the vaccine, probably egg protein;

therefore, use of the vaccine is contraindicated in persons with a history of anaphylactic-type sensitivity to eggs.

Follow-up: Since immunity is temporary, patients should return yearly for vaccination prior to the flu season.

▸ *Pneumococcus Vaccine*

Laboratory Tests: None.

Therapeutic Measures: Persons at high risk for contracting pneumococcal pneumonia and subsequent bacteremia should receive this vaccine. This group includes elderly persons who travel (especially if they also have COPD or other chronic debilitating illnesses), debilitated persons, immunosuppressed patients, alcoholics, and those with COPD, cirrhosis, diabetes mellitus, Hodgkin's disease, multiple myeloma, chronic cerebrospinal fluid leakage, sickle cell anemia, asplenia (anatomic or functional), or functional impairment of the cardiac or renal system. Administer a single 0.5-mL dose of 23-type pneumococcus vaccine IM or SC (several weeks prior to departure for patients who are planning to travel). Do not inject it IV, and avoid intradermal administration, since this may cause severe local reactions. Patients with Hodgkin's disease should receive the vaccine only if it can be given at least 10 days prior to treatment (preferably at least 14 days prior to radiation therapy or chemotherapy for a maximum antibody response). Do not administer this vaccine to adult patients who have been previously immunized with any polyvalent pneumococcus vaccine, since repeat injections have been associated with an increased incidence and severity of adverse reactions in healthy adults and since the data suggest that such reinjections do not result in increased antibody titers. Use of the vaccine is also contraindicated in persons with a known hypersensitivity to any of the vaccine's components (including thimerosal), and for all patients epinephrine injection (1:1,000) should be available for immediate use in the event of an anaphylactoid reaction. Reasons for delaying vaccination include pregnancy, lactation, or the presence of any febrile illness or active respiratory infection; vaccination when any of these conditions is present should be done only if clearly necessary.

Patient Education: Instruct patients in high-risk groups and elderly patients planning to travel regarding the importance of receiving this vaccine. Discuss its potential side effects, including local soreness of the injection site within 3 days after vaccination and low-grade fever (less than 100°F) with mild myalgia during the first 24 hours. Rare adverse reactions include rash and arthralgia, fever over 102°F with marked local swelling, a relapse in thrombocytopenia in patients with otherwise stabilized idiopathic thrombocytopenic purpura (2–14 days after vaccination and lasting for up to 2 weeks), and anaphylactoid reactions. Encourage patients to bring to your attention any unusual symptoms.

Follow-up: As needed. Remind patients that they should not receive this vaccine again (especially important for patients who may move or change primary care providers).

▸ *TB Screening and Prophylaxis*

Laboratory Tests: Intradermal PPD, if positive (i.e., skin reaction of more than 10 mm of induration), should be followed with a chest x-ray film, SMAC (particularly liver alkaline phosphatase), CBC with differential, and urinalysis to rule out active TB infection as well as acute liver disease, which are contraindications for INH prophylaxis. (See Table 6.13 for findings in active TB infection; for therapeutic measures, see the discussion of active pulmonary TB.) Patients with skin reactions of 5–9 mm of induration in 24–72 hours should have a repeat test within 1 week and a chest x-ray film. If PPD results are still questionable and the chest x-ray film is negative, the PPD test should be done again in 3 months. Skin reactions of 5 mm induration or less are considered negative unless there is a history of recent exposure or clinical findings are strongly suggestive of TB.

Therapeutic Measures: The standard PPD test procedure is the Mantoux test using an intradermal injection of intermediate-strength PPD (5 tuberculin units). Multiple puncture tests such as the tine test are not as reliable as the intradermal test, and should therefore be used for screening only when the latter is not feasible; any positive test must be confirmed by intradermal PPD. Test results are interpreted 48–72 hours after the injection by measuring the diameter of the palpable induration (not erythema). Prophylactic therapy with INH to prevent the development of active disease should be considered for positive reactors (10 mm or more of induration) once active TB infection has been excluded. Treat all recent tuberculin converters (i.e., those whose skin reaction to PPD has increased by 6 mm or more within 2 years), and positive reactors who are: under age 35, close contacts of patients with recently diagnosed active TB, and members of a high risk group for reactivation of latent TB (e.g., postgastrectomy and immunosuppressed patients, insulin-dependent diabetics, malnourished persons, alcoholics, patients with silicosis, leukemia, or lymphoma). Give INH, 300 mg by mouth in a single morning dose for 1 full year (dosage for adolescents and adults). Also, prescribe pyrodoxine (vitamin B_6), 50 mg/day, to prevent INH-induced deficiency. Patients who are over 35 years of age and have a positive PPD but do not have any of the additional risk factors mentioned above (i.e., close contact with an active TB patient, recent conversion, high-risk patients) may be considered for this preventive therapy on an individual basis, weighing the predicted risk of developing active TB (and the likelihood of serious consequences) against the risk of developing INH-induced hepatitis, which increases with age, particularly after 35. The annual risk for patients with previously known but presently inactive TB who have not been adequately treated with INH is about 1 in 75, while the risk of developing hepatitis with INH therapy is about 12 per 1,000 in persons 35–49 years of age, 23 per 1,000 in persons 50–64 years of age, and 8 per 1,000 in older persons. An important factor that may favor the treatment of some of these patients is the likelihood that they may later enter a high-risk group in which reactivation of latent TB infections is common. Examples include the possibility that corticosteroid therapy may be required in the future for patients with asthma or chronic bronchitis, the possibility of a future pregnancy that may activate a latent infection, and the potential for individuals in known acquired immune deficiency syndrome (AIDS) high-risk groups (eg, IV drug users, homosexual men, or incarcerated men). Treating such persons with INH prophylaxis at their present age may entail fewer risks than waiting until one of these other factors become prominent, because by that time (i.e., when the patient is older), the risk of developing hepatitis from INH prophylaxis (or from treatment of active TB infection) may be even greater. Preventive treatment should be deferred in persons with acute hepatic disease and in pregnant women. Patients who have previously had adequate treatment with INH, those with evidence or findings strongly suggestive of progressive TB infection, or those with a history of adverse reactions to INH (e.g., hypersensitivity reaction, such as a skin eruption or drug-induced hepatitis, or other signs of INH-induced liver damage, such as drug fever, chills, or arthritis) should not receive INH prophylaxis.

Patient Education: Once active TB infection has been excluded, patients who have positive PPD tests should be reassured. The rationale and expected benefits, as well as the risks, of preventive therapy with INH should be carefully explained to them so that they may participate in the decision about initiating therapy. Patients should also be warned that the risk of developing severe (and sometimes fatal) hepatitis as a result of INH therapy is increased with daily alcohol consumption. It is especially important to stress that the medication must be taken continuously for 1 full year, despite the fact that the patient may never have experienced any symptoms of infection. Caution patients about possible symptoms of INH toxicity (e.g., unexplained fever, abdominal distress and other gastrointestinal symptoms, rash) or prodromal symptoms of hepatitis (e.g., weakness, malaise, fatigue, anorexia, nausea, or vomiting), and advise them to discontinue the medication and report such symptoms immediately. Patients who decide against INH prophylaxis should be warned about the possibility of later activation of TB and advised to notify any future care providers that they have had a positive PPD test but have not received preventive treatment, so that any medical or surgical decisions (e.g., initiation of immunosuppressive therapy, gastric resection) may be made with this in mind.

Follow-up: Patients receiving preventive therapy should be seen after the first month on medication to monitor compliance, discuss alcohol intake, and check for hypersensitivity reactions or signs or symptoms of toxicity. If patients report any such symptoms, repeat blood and liver function tests and check for enlarged, tender liver and other signs (see Chapter 5 for a discussion of INH hepatitis). Any signs or symptoms suggestive of liver damage necessitate immediate discontinuation of INH until that possibility has been ruled out. If patients report no symptoms, repeat blood tests and liver function tests are not necessary (mild, transient SGOT elevations can be expected to develop in 10–20% of patients receiving INH, usually during the first 3 months of therapy, but these will usually return to normal despite continuation of therapy and are of no clinical significance). Patients may be seen every 3 months thereafter. Write prescriptions for 100 tablets to last until the patient's next visit, but encourage patients to return at once if any questionable symptoms develop. Patients who drink alcohol daily, who have current chronic liver disease or severe kidney dysfunction, or who are receiving concurrent phenytoin therapy require more frequent and careful monitoring (phenytoin excretion may be decreased or its effects enhanced by INH). Patients who have a positive PPD test and negative chest x-ray film, but who decide against INH prophylaxis, require additional x-ray films only if they are symptomatic (e.g., if they develop a persistent cough, fever, sputum production, pleuritis chest pain, liver or spleen enlargement). Future PPD testing should not be done on patients who have tested positive, whether or not they have received preventive INH therapy, since they will remain PPD positive. Patients should be advised of this and of the fact that once they have completed an adequate course of therapy, there is no need for further treatment.

▸ *Active Pulmonary TB*

Laboratory Tests: A positive PPD test must be followed by a chest x-ray film (more than one may be required) and SMAC, CBC with differential, ESR, and sputum tests for acid-fast bacillus strains and culture. Since a positive diagnosis requires culture of *M. tuberculosis,* every effort should be made to obtain adequate specimens. In addition, more than one sputum sample (at least six is typical) should be obtained and sent for testing, since isolation of the organism may be difficult and the length of time required to grow the organism is so great (4–6 weeks). Direct microscopic exam of sputum may reveal acid-fast rods when the bacterial count is high, but this finding is not diagnostic, since other mycobacteria may be present. Positive smears should be confirmed by culture for *M. tuberculosis* using fresh sputum (early morning collection is best). If spontaneous sputum production is not present, inhalation of heated aerosolized saline (5%) or intermittent positive-pressure breathing to induce sputum, or tracheal or bronchoscopic washings with saline may be used to obtain specimens for culture. If these methods are not successful, or if patients are unable to cooperate (e.g., children, senile patients), aspiration of gastric contents immediately upon awakening and after 8–10 hours of fasting may produce a specimen for culture (collection bottles for gastric aspirates should contain sodium bicarbonate or a similar buffer, since gastric acid is toxic to mycobacteria). Sensitivity testing should be done on specimens as well to determine whether the infection is due to resistant organisms requiring a more intensive and carefully monitored therapy. When sputum is negative, provisional diagnosis may be facilitated by fiberoptic bronchoscopy with lung biopsy, although negative findings on biopsy do not necessarily rule out TB. If lung or other tissue shows histologic evidence of tubercle formation, TB should be suspected. However, this finding is not conclusive evidence of *M. tuberculosis* infection, since non-TB mycobacteria may also cause such changes. Unless lesions are hidden behind anatomic structures (i.e., the heart, ribs, diaphragm), chest x-ray films will reveal disease in almost all cases, but more than one film is usually necessary for diagnosis. (See Table 6.13 for findings in active pulmonary TB infection.)

Therapeutic Measures: Treat patients with combination therapy using INH plus one or more of the other anti-TB agents listed in Table 6.14 (rifampin, ethambutol, streptomycin). Table 6.15 lists various possible combination schedules (with dosages) used to treat active pulmonary TB, and the advantages and possible indications for each. Treatment with ethambutol, particularly long-term treatment with doses greater than 15 mg/kg/day, can result in reversible optic neuropathy demonstrated by loss of visual acuity and color discrimination. Pretreatment testing for visual acuity (Snellen chart) and color discrimination is recommended for all patients who require prolonged treatment with this drug, followed by periodic reexaminations for the duration of ethambutol therapy. A balanced diet should be maintained (small, frequent meals may be helpful), and adequate rest and a moderate, progressive exercise program encouraged. Prescribe pyrodoxine (vitamin B_6), 50 mg/day, to prevent INH-induced deficiency. Isolation is important during the initial phase of therapy while patients are still infectious, so a short-term admission to the hospital for this period is recommended to minimize the risk of spread. Reliable and clinically stable patients may usually be discharged in 2–3 weeks for continued therapy on an outpatient basis. If signs or symptoms suggestive of liver damage or a hypersensitivity reaction develop with therapy, discontinue all medications at once. Particularly at this point, an infectious disease specialist should be called in, since treatment will have to be altered if INH is not tolerated, and this is best managed by such a specialist. Patients in whom INH is contraindicated (i.e., those with active hepatitis or a history of severe adverse reaction to the drug) should also be referred to a specialist, as should pregnant women who require treatment for active TB (INH and ethambutol, which seem to be well tolerated by both mother and fetus, are the preferred drugs in this case). Report all cases of active TB infection promptly to public health authorities.

Patient Education: Teach the medication regimen, including doses, routes, times, and side effects. Stress the importance of taking all prescribed medication continuously and for the recommended period of time. During the initial stages of therapy while patients are still contagious, they should be taught to cover the mouth and nose effectively with a disposable tissue while coughing or sneezing, and to wear a mask whenever they are outside of their isolation room or when other persons (e.g., hospital personnel) are present. Advise them to practice healthful behaviors, including adequate rest, moderate exercise, and a proper diet. Instruct patients to report any symptoms of increasing respiratory distress (i.e., dyspnea, hemoptysis, chest pain) as soon as they occur. Discuss other symptoms of drug toxicity or hypersensitivity that they should also bring to your attention at once (e.g., neurologic symptoms, fever, rash, abdominal distress, jaundice, rheumatic syndromes, symptoms of hepatitis), and warn patients about the increased risk of developing INH hepatitis, which is associated with daily alcohol consumption. Warn patients taking rifampin to expect a reddish-orange discoloration of urine, tears, saliva, sweat, and feces that is clinically insignificant. All family members and other close contacts of patients should be tested with intradermal PPD and treated prophylactically if they test positive (see "TB Screening and Prophylaxis"). Reassure patients and family members, since many people still associate a diagnosis of TB with a social stigma and a poor prognosis. Stress the fact that patients are not infectious after the first few weeks of adequate chemotherapy, that those who are asymptomatic and are being managed with an adequate medical regimen may resume normal activities throughout the course of therapy, and that an adequate course of therapy will produce a lasting cure in about 95–100% of cases of initially treated pulmonary TB infection.

Follow-up: Follow-up should be done on a routine basis while treatment is in progress in order to monitor compliance and to check for the development of hypersensitivity or drug toxicity reactions, but no follow-up is necessary after adequate treatment. Short visits may be arranged on a monthly basis initially during therapy, but if no problems develop with medications and the patient is clinically stable, less frequent visits may be necessary. Periodic testing if visual acuity and color discrimination (possibly best handled by a specialist) should be performed on all patients receiving ethambutol for comparison with pretreatment test results to evaluate patients for changes in vision associated with optic neuropathy. This testing should be performed at least monthly for patients taking dosages greater than 15 mg/kg/day. If significant changes in visual status occur, these effects are generally reversible with prompt discontinuation of ethambutol. Question all patients periodically about blurred vision and other subjective eye symptoms that may be related to the development of visual abnormalities. Routine SGOT determinations are not recommended by the U.S. Public Health Service for monitoring of INH therapy in patients who are reliable and able to understand and comply with directions for taking medications and reporting symptoms, particularly since mild, transient elevations in SGOT occur as a predictable and clinically insignificant response in about 10–20% of patients who receive INH, especially during the first 3 months of therapy. However, patients whose reliability is questionable, who appear to require the reassurance of close follow-up, who are concurrently taking phenytoin, or who have chronic liver disease or severe renal dysfunction may require more frequent and careful monitoring. Monthly SGOT determinations during the first 3 months of therapy will detect most abnormalities. Patients with symptoms suggestive of liver damage and elevated SGOT should have the drug discontinued, and liver function tests should continue to be monitored. Asymptomatic patients with mild SGOT elevations (possibly up to 100 units) may continue to receive the medication. However, weekly determinations should be made for 3–4 weeks, and if SGOT does not revert to normal by that time, discontinuation of INH should be considered. An asymptomatic patient with even a single substantial elevation (i.e., above 200 units) may also need to be taken off INH. However, the exact details of management of these situations should be determined on an individual basis, and probably with the consultation with an infectious disease specialist.

▸ *Congestive Heart Failure*

Laboratory Tests: Serum levels of sodium, potassium, blood urea nitrogen (BUN), uric acid, and creatinine should be determined (sodium, potassium, CO_2, and chloride will be within normal limits before initiation of diurectic therapy in normal CHF, but BUN may be elevated due to reduced renal flow). Urinalysis often reveals mild to significant proteinuria and an increase in specific gravity. Arterial blood gas studies show a decrease in Pa_{CO_2} and an increase in pH. Cardiomegaly, hazy lung fields, and distended pulmonary veins are seen on chest x-ray films, and a echocardiogram may demonstrate changes in the ventricular mass and volume and in the ejection fraction. ECG may demonstrate ventricular hypertrophy.

Therapeutic Measures: Determine, whenever possible, and treat or eliminate the precipitating cause of CHF (e.g., overexertion, respiratory or other infection, pulmonary infarction, increased intake of sodium, discontinuation of medication, HTN, arrhythmias, MI, and anemia). Administer oxygen as needed for hypoxemia and restrict activities to reduce the cardiac workload and promote sodium diuresis. Meals should be small and frequent (four to six per day) at the onset of therapy, and should be bland, low-calorie, low-sodium, low-residue, and accompanied by vitamin supplements. Whenever possible, it is preferable to attempt early treatment of CHF with rest and sodium restriction alone in order to avoid the potential side effects of diuretic therapy. However, most patients find a low-sodium diet difficult to maintain, and reliance on a strict low-sodium intake as the sole means of management is not advisable; therapy with an oral diuretic (intermittent or long-term, depending on the need) may be necessary. Examples of diuretics include the thiazides (hydrochlorothiazide, 50 mg once daily), furosemide (40–80 mg/day), or aldosterone antagonists (spironolactone, 25 mg four times daily). If only potassium-depleting diuretics are utilized, potassium supplementation will be needed to prevent an imbalance and decrease the risk of digitalis toxicity if that medication is used as well. If diuretic therapy does not promptly relieve the condition, and especially if cardiac failure is accompanied by sinus rhythm (controversial) or atrial fibrillation, begin digitalis administration (dosages are individualized). Vasodilator therapy may be indicated for severe cardiac dysfunction not relieved by the above methods, but this should be used with caution while monitoring the hemodynamic result.

Patient Education: Restriction of activities should be maintained long enough to allow the heart to regain strength, but a progressive ambulation schedule should be begun as soon as compensation occurs. Instruct patients in passive or active leg exercises to prevent the development of phlebothrombosis from extended bed rest. Teach low-sodium diet (see the section on "Low-Sodium Diet") and fluid restriction if indicated. Discuss the medication regimen, including the rationale for therapy, proper administration, expected effects, side effects, and toxic effects. If diuretics are used in treatment, discuss the potential for dehydration, and electrolyte imbalance, as well as the signs and symptoms of these conditions, daily intake and output assessment, and routine blood tests for electrolyte levels and renal function. If a digitalis preparation is used in treatment, give careful instructions regarding its potential toxicity (i.e., signs and symptoms, the need for routine determination of serum electrolyte and digitalis levels, and pulse rate assessment prior to administration). Discuss the rationale for and importance of an activity level that will not increase cardiac output and a planned program for increased activity. Teach stress-reduction and relaxation techniques (see the section on "Stress Reduction"). Identify and counsel patients on needed lifestyle changes to accommodate the medical regimen for this chronic illness.

Follow-up: Every 3–6 months for evaluation of the illness and serum level assessment.

▸ *Reducing CAD Risk Factors*

Laboratory Tests: Screening tests include serum level determinations of cholesterol, triglycerides, glucose, and uric acid, as well as blood pressure assessments. Also, check for evidence of contributing factors such as anemia, renal disease, myxedema, syphilis, or other cardiac disorders. ECG, exercise stress tests, and a chest x-ray film may be done, and if symptoms warrant investigation, an echocardiogram and/or cardiac catheterization should be performed.

Therapeutic Measures: Prescribe medications as indicated for existing cardiovascular conditions (e.g., digitalis preparations, nitrates, beta blockers, calcium antagonists, antihypertensives) and for treatment of other conditions associated with an increased risk of CAD (e.g., diabetes, gout, hypercholesterolemia). The diet should be low in salt, cholesterol, and fat. If diabetes or gout is present, prescribe an appropriate diet for these conditions. Obese patients should be placed on a low-calorie weight reduction diet, and attainment and maintenance of optimal weight and physical fitness should be encouraged for all patients. Active patients who have been seriously disabled by angina pectoris not adequately responding to medical treatment may be candidates for CABG or PTCA.

Patient Education: Assist patients in accepting personal responsibility for maintaining their health by practicing behaviors that will reduce the risk and/or effects of this chronic, progressive disease. Identify and discuss the risk factors for each individual, and teach ways to reduce their influence. Urge patients who are smokers to quit (see "Smoking Cessation"). Discuss diet therapy, an active exercise program (have patients gradually progress to walking 2 mi/day), and techniques for stress reduction and relaxation (see "Stress Reduction"). Discuss the medication regimen, including the rationale, expected results, and side effects. Discuss birth control with female patients over 35 years of age who have a family history of CAD; such women, particularly if they also smoke, should not use oral contraceptives.

Follow-up: Every 4–6 months for evaluation or as necessary when symptoms of disease are experienced.

▸ *Angina*

Laboratory Tests: Diagnostic studies as described in Table 6.31. SMAC, CBC as a baseline for drug treatment and to identify CAD risk factors such as hyperlipidemia and diabetes.

Therapeutic Measures

General: Avoidance of obvious precipitating factors such as smoking, emotional stress, cold temperatures, and heavy meals. Control of CAD risk factors, particularly hypertension and hypercholesterolemia.

Drug selection: *No associated conditions.* Nitrates are the drugs of choice unless angina is secondary to coronary artery spasm. In the latter case, calcium channel blockers should be considered. They are also preferable for resting/nocturnal angina. Nonselective beta blockers may be used as second-line agents, particularly in younger patients who lead active lives and are subjected to high levels of emotional stress. If beta blockers are used in patients with coronary artery spasm, cardioselective agents should be used to avoid spasm exacerbations secondary to the alpha-adrenergic effect of nonselective beta blockers. *Associated with hypertension.* Beta blockers (cardioselective if the patient's history suggests coronary artery spasm) and calcium channel blockers prove quite effective. In elderly patients, calcium channel blockers are generally better tolerated. If beta blockers are used for these patients, water-soluble agents such as atenolol or nadolol are preferable (lipid-soluble beta blockers such as propranolol may produce significant CNS side effects including disquieting dreams, depression, or mental obtundation). *Post–acute MI.* By helping to preserve uninjured myocardium, beta blockers given during the post-acute MI period have been shown to reduce the overall incidence of sudden death. Caution must exercised when they are used in the presence of left ventricular dysfunction. In such cases, addition of nitrates or nifedipine may be necessary to prevent significant depression of cardiac output. *Associated with CHF.* Nifedipine, which significantly reduces the preload and afterload with a net improvement in left ventricular contractile function and cardiac output, is the drug of choice. Verapamil may further depress left ventricular contractility and lead to progressive decompensation. Beta blockers should never be prescribed for patients with CHF. On the other hand, patients already taking beta blockers who develop CHF should be carefully weaned (abrupt withdrawal may result in worsening of angina). *Associated with sick sinus syndrome and AV blocks.* Nitrates in combination with nifedipine is the preferred therapy. Both agents have a negligible effect on SA automaticity and AV conduction. By contrast, beta blockers, verapamil, and diltiazem may adversely affect SA automaticity and AV nodal conduction and should be avoided. *Associated with supraventricular tachyarrhythmias.* Beta blockers or verapamil should be used to decrease conduction at the AV nodal level and control the ventricular rate. Angina related to an increased oxygen demand by the myocardium secondary to tachycardia therefore improves. *Associated with IHSS.* By improving left ventricular diastolic compliance, calcium channel blockers are quite effective in this setting. Beta blockers, which reduce left ventricular wall stress due to their negative inotropic effect, provide sustained relief of symptoms in one-third of patients. Nitrates are contraindicated; they reduce venous return to the heart and lead to a decrease in left ventricular volume. *Associated with COPD.* Calcium channel blockers and nitrates may be used, since they have no deleterious effect on the bronchial muscle (calcium channel blockers produce bronchodilatation and may have a salutary effect on pulmonary vascular resistance). Beta blockers, even cardioselective agents, are considered hazardous, since they may trigger bronchospasm. *Associated with peripheral vascular disease.* Calcium channel blockers are the preferred drugs, since they have been shown to improve peripheral circulation. Nitrates may also be used. Beta blockers have the potential to facilitate alpha-adrenergic vasoconstriction and are contraindicated. *Associated with insulin-dependent diabetes.* Calcium channel blockers and nitrates are the preferred choices. They interfere with neither hypoglycemic symptoms (as may beta blockers) nor glucose tolerance (as may diuretics). *Associated with chronic renal failure.* Nitrates (metabolized by the liver) should be used as the sole therapy whenever possible. If additional control is required, a lipid-soluble beta blocker or diltiazem may be used, since they too are cleared predominantly by the liver. *Associated with hepatic dysfunction.* Use with caution those agents metabolized by the liver (nitrates, lipid-soluble beta blockers, diltiazem). To avoid further liver damage and drug toxicity, the doses of such agents should be reduced. *Associated with depression.* Nitrates and calcium channel blockers are the best choices in this setting, since they do not produce mood swings or worsening of depressive symptoms. By the same token, beta blockers should be used with caution, lipid-soluble agents being particularly hazardous. *Associated with impotence.* Not shown to cause impotence, nitrates and calcium channel blockers are the preferred drugs.

Drug prescription: Appropriate drugs as outlined above may be given alone or in combination. Studies have shown that (1) beta blockers with nitrates produce a better effect than either drug alone and (2) nifedipine with propranolol may be especially effective for chronic stable angina. These drugs should be used in the maximum tolerated doses for the best effect (see Table 6.23).

Surgical treatment: If the extent of disease and the degree of disability are severe and the drug response is poor or associated with intolerable side effects, patients should be referred for surgical evaluation. The decision to perform coronary artery bypass may then depend on the age and general condition of the patient. In some cases, a partially obstructed artery can be dilated with balloon catheterization.

Patient Education: Use a diagram of the heart and coronary arteries to explain the etiology of angina. Emphasize the importance of reducing CAD risk factors (see the sections on "Hypertension," "Smoking Cessation," "Weight Reduction," "Exercise Prescribing," and "Stress Reduction"). Teach the rationale, proper use, and side effects of the medication. Instruct patients to report any episode of angina that lasts longer than 5 minutes, any increase in the number of pain episodes, and any new onset of nighttime or resting angina. Review the warning signs of MI.

Follow-up: Stable patients should be seen every 3–4 months for symptom and medication review.

▸ *Endocarditis Prophylaxis*

Laboratory Tests: As needed to confirm valve disorder.

Therapeutic Measures: In indicated cases (see Table 6.38), the new standard recommendation for endocarditis prophylaxis is as follows:

DENTAL AND UPPER RESPIRATORY TRACT PROCEDURES

Penicillin V 500 mg, 2 g (4 pills) 1 hour before treatment and 1 g (2 pills) 6 hours later.

or

For penicillin-allergic patients, erythromycin 500 mg, 1 g (2 pills) 1 hour before treatment and 500 mg (1 pill) 6 hours later

or

For any prosthetic valve patient, parenteral therapy consisting of procaine penicillin G 600,000 U IM 1–2 hours before the procedure plus aqueous penicillin G 600,000 U IM just prior to the procedure, followed by procaine penicillin G 600,000 U IM once daily for 2 days. Gentamycin or streptomycin with the penicillin may be advisable.

SURGERY/INSTRUMENTATION OF THE GENITOURINARY TRACT, GASTROINTESTINAL TRACT, OR INFECTED SOFT TISSUE

Give IM aqueous penicillin G 5,000,000 U and gentamycin 3 mg/kg 1–3 hours before the procedure and once a day for 2 days.

Patient Education: Explain the pathologic process of endocarditis and the importance of prophylaxis. Note that high levels of antibiotics must be present at the time of and immediately after procedures associated with bacteremia to be preventive.

Follow-up: None.

▸ *Essential Hypertension*

Laboratory Tests: Urinalysis. SMAC, CBC. Baseline ECG and CXR. Tests as indicated by the history and physical findings to rule out secondary hypertension.

Therapeutic Measures: Prescribe a diet low in sodium (350 mg or less of sodium per day; see "Low-Sodium Diet"). A weight reduction diet and an exercise program should be initiated as necessary. Instruct patients on reduction of stressors and relaxation techniques (see "Stress Reduction"). For patients with moderate hypertension or mild hypertension not controlled with the above measures, initiate stepped-care drug therapy. Increase the doses and/or substitute drugs every 2—4 weeks until blood pressure is controlled (diastolic pressure less than 90 mmHg) as follows:

STEP I

Diuretic at less than full dose (e.g., thiazide type or beta blocker):

- Hydrochlorothiazide, 25 mg daily
- Chlorthalidone, 25 mg 5 days/week
- Bendrofluazide, 2.5 mg daily
- Benzthiazide, 25 mg daily
- Chlorothiazide sodium, 250 mg daily
- Cyclothiazide, 1 mg daily
- Hydroflumethiazide, 25 mg daily
- Indapamide 2.5, mg daily
- Methyclothiazide, 2.5 mg daily
- Metolazone, 2.5 mg daily
- Polythiazide, 2 mg daily
- Quinethazone, 50 mg daily
- Trichlormethiazide, 2 mg daily

Loop diuretics (reserve for patients with renal failure)

- Bumetanide, 0.5 mg daily
- Ethacrynic acid, 50 mg daily
- Furosemide, 40 mg daily

Potassium-sparing drugs (for treatment of diuretic-induced hypokalemia)

- Amiloride hydrochloride, 5 mg daily
- Spironolactone, 50 mg daily
- Triamterene, 50 mg daily

Diuretic at full dose (e.g., thiazide type) or add or substitute beta blocker

- Hydrochlorothiazide, 50 mg daily
- Chlorthalidone, 50 mg daily

- Bendrofluazide, 5 mg daily
- Benzthiazide, 50 mg daily
- Chlorothiazide sodium, 500 mg daily
- Cyclothiazide, 2 mg daily
- Hydroflumethiazide, 50 mg daily
- Idapamide, 5 mg daily
- Methyclothiazide, 5 mg daily
- Metolazone, 5 mg daily
- Polythiazide, 4 mg daily
- Quinethazone, 100 mg daily
- Trichlormethiazide, 4 mg daily

Loop diuretics (reserve for patients with renal failure)

- Bumetanide, 2 mg daily
- Ethacrynic acid, 200 mg daily
- Furosemide, 80 mg daily

Potassium-sparing drugs (for treatment of diuretic-induced hypokalemia)

- Amiloride hydrochloride, 10 mg daily
- Spironolactone, 100 mg daily
- Triamterene, 100 mg daily

STEP II

Add small dosage of adrenergic-inhibiting agent. If necessary, continue the diuretic and substitute a different adrenergic-inhibiting agent

- Reserpine, 0.10–0.25 mg daily
- Propranolol, 40–80 mg bid
- Propranolol LA daily
- Atenolol, 25–50 mg daily
- Metoprolol, 50–300 mg daily
- Nadolol, 20–160 mg daily
- Timolol, 10–30 bid
- Acebutolol, 200–800 daily
- Pindolol, 10–30 mg bid
- Alpha-methyldopa, 250–500 mg bid
- Clonidine, 0.2–0.4 mg bid
- Clonidine-TTS, 0.1, 0.2 or 0.3 mg, one patch/week
- Guanabenz, 4–8 mg bid
- Prazosin, 2–5 mg bid

STEP III

Substitute vasodilators, angiotensin-converting enzyme (ACE) inhibitors, or calcium-entry blockers

- Hydralazine, 25–50 mg bid for prazosin (75–80% of patients with mild to moderate hypertension will respond).
- Captopril, 25–150 mg bid or tid as the step II or step III drug if blood pressure is not lowered or if side effects limit the use of other agents.
- Diltiazem, 30–60 mg bid to tid (maximum, 120 mg bid) as the step II or step III drug or verapamil, 80 or 120 mg bid or tid given in ranges of 240–480 mg as the step II or step III drug.

Nifedipine, 10 mg given in ranges of 30–90 mg divided into two or three doses as the step II or step III drug.

A potassium supplement may be necessary if hypokalemia develops secondary to diuretic therapy (see "Hypokalemia"). Treat and/or prevent cardiac, cerebral, and renal complications of hypertension.

Patient Education: Identify the personal risk factors of all patients. Teach the importance of reducing risk factors through smoking cessation, weight reduction, maintenance of a low-sodium, low-fat, low-cholesterol diet, increasing exercise and avoiding a sedentary lifestyle, reducing stress and performing relaxation exercises, and preventing and/or managing related medical conditions (e.g., atherosclerosis, diabetes). Discuss the medication regimen, including the rationale for therapy, proper administration, expected results, side effects (e.g., impotence in men, dehydration), and toxic effects, and encourage patients to bring any questions or side effects to your attention as soon as they occur. Inquire about any other medications patients may be taking, and discuss potential drug interactions (e.g., monoamine oxidase inhibitors should never be used in combination with antihypertensive medications because of the risk of provoking a hypertensive crisis). Discuss the implications of the hereditary nature of the disease, as well as the importance of screening family members and promoting behaviors that will reduce the risk factors for them. It may be helpful to suggest that patients purchase a sphygmomanometer and offer instruction in its use so that family members may assess their blood pressure routinely.

Follow-up: Every 2 weeks until blood pressure is controlled. Then schedule visits 3–6 months for stable patients to monitor the effectiveness of medication, discuss its side effects, and ask questions about success in other efforts (diet, stress reduction techniques, etc.). Periodic ophthalmoscopic studies, blood tests, urinalysis, ECG, and CXR.

▸ *Peripheral Vascular Disease*

Laboratory Tests: Diagnosis is usually based on the symptoms (i.e., exercise–pain–rest cycle with pain disappearing after a few minutes of rest) and clinical findings, but angiography may be used to reveal the extent and exact location of the obstruction and collateral circulation if surgery is being considered. Retrograde filling tests and ultrasound or Doppler studies may be useful. Serum lipid level determinations should be done on all patients with arteriosclerosis, since this disorder may be treatable. Screening for diabetes and hypertension is also recommended.

Therapeutic Measures: Treat related disorders (i.e., diabetes, hyperlipidemia, hypertension). All smokers should be urged to quit at once. Weight reduction in overweight patients with only intermittent claudication and normal-appearing limbs will enable them to walk further without pain by reducing the workload involved and the metabolic demands on the extremities. A rigorous program of frequent daily exercise is an important aspect of the treatment of intermittent claudication, since it helps to stimulate the development of collateral circulation and increase walking distances. Patients should be instructed to walk repetitive distances (on level terrain) of about 75% of the claudification distance (that distance required to induce pain), interspersed with 1- to 2-minute periods of rest. It is easier for patients to measure walking distances in units of time (i.e., minutes) rather than actual units of length. Walking up hills or stairs will shorten the claudication distance, so the timing of rest periods should be adjusted. If pain develops, patients should stop and rest until the pain has totally disappeared, and then begin walking again. The total exercise time may be about 15 minutes at first, and can be gradually increased (over a period of 4–6 weeks) to a total of 45 minutes to 1 hour if tolerated. On a weekly basis, the maximum walking distance (length of time the patient can walk until pain develops) should be reassessed and daily walking distances adjusted accordingly. This daily exercise should be continued for the rest of the patient's life if improvement is to be maintained. Buerger's foot exercises are also helpful for promoting peripheral circulation: While seated, the patient should hold the feet elevated for 1 minute, dependent for 3 minutes, and then horizontal for 6 minutes, wiggling the feet gently for the entire 10 minutes. This cycle should be repeated three to six times daily. Careful attention to foot care is imperative (see below), especially when there is a coexisting decrease in peripheral sensation. Calcium channel blocking agents (e.g., diltiazem) have been shown to improve peripheral circulation, and may be prescribed if symptoms persist and there are no contraindications (e.g., sick sinus syndrome, concomitant use of beta blockers in patients with AV node conduction abnormalities). Patients with advanced ischemia resulting in gangrene, nonhealing ischemic ulceration, or ischemic pain at rest should be referred for surgical consultation (inflatable balloon catheterization, surgical reconstruction, or possibly amputation may be required). Also, some patients who have claudication without any of the other developments may occasionally require surgical referral if the pain is unrelenting and an inability to walk far seriously impairs the patient's lifestyle or livelihood. Preganglionic lumbar sympathectomy may be of limited benefit in some cases where there is pain on rest or small areas of ulceration or gangrene if presurgical testing can demonstrate that the sympathetic nervous system in the extremity is intact.

Patient Education: Explain the necessity of quitting smoking (tobacco use causes cutaneous vasoconstriction via the sympathetic nervous system) and help all patients who smoke to quit (see "Smoking Cessation"). Discuss a diet to assist overweight patients lose excess weight and remind them that the daily exercise program that is prescribed will further aid them in obtaining and maintaining their proper weight. Discuss possible complications of injuries to the feet or legs. Teach a daily exercise program, foot exercises, and proper care of the legs and feet (it may be helpful to provide patients with written instructions on all of these topics). Proper foot hygiene includes daily gentle washing with a soft washcloth, lukewarm water, and mild soap. Excessive soaking should be avoided, since it may lead to maceration. Thorough drying, especially between the toes, with a soft absorbent towel should be done using pressure, not excessive friction. After careful drying, a mild talcum powder may be applied between the toes to discourage fungal infections. To prevent the development of cracks and fissures, patients should apply a bland lubricating cream (lanolin or petroleum jelly) to the tops and bottoms of the feet (but not between the toes), and gently but thoroughly massage it into the skin (patients whose feet are normally moist may have to dust powder over the entire foot surface instead of using a lubricating agent). No medication should be applied to the feet or legs without first checking with the care provider. Toenails should be carefully cut (in good light) straight across and even with the end of the toe (never close to the skin), leaving them long at the corners to prevent the development of hangnails. Emery boards should be used with extreme care. Treatment of corns and calluses and, if at all possible (especially for patients who are unable to take proper care of their own toenails), nail care should be done by a podiatrist. Teach patients to inspect their feet carefully at least daily (preferably in the morning and at night), particularly between toes, around nail beds, and on heels, for any cuts, scratches, blisters, drainage, dryness, cracking, fissures, calluses, or changes in color or temperature and to report any changes to their provider. A hand mirror should be used for any hard-to-observe spots. Socks or stockings should fit snugly but not tightly over the foot, calf, and upper thigh and should be changed at least daily. Circular garters, which may constrict blood flow, should never be worn. Thin socks of a wool-cotton-nylon blend are best for everyday wear, since they are cool and absorbent. Shoes should be comfortable, properly fitted, and of soft leather. The toe section should be sufficiently high to accommodate the toes without causing rubbing (it is especially important to check for this in the case of hammer toes or bunions). Specially made shoes may be necessary for patients unable to find a good-fitting size. Heels of everyday shoes should be no more than 1.5 in. in height, and shoes should be carefully checked before wearing for any defects or foreign objects that may cause skin irritation. Any unavoidable friction points (e.g., backs of ankles, bunions) should be padded with moleskin. New shoes should be broken in gradually, using shorter strides for the first day or two. Wet shoes should never be worn. Extremes of temperature (hot baths, hot water bottles, heating pads, excessively cold environmental temperatures) and walking barefoot should be avoided. Teach patients not to cross the legs and to avoid sitting in a manner that causes excessive pressure on the portion of the thigh comes in contact with the chair edge (lower chairs or chair cushions may help). Teach patients never to elevate their legs (many patients feel that this will ease their symptoms, but instead it further reduces peripheral circulation). Elevation of the head of the bed, using 6- to 8-in. blocks, may benefit patients with more advanced ischemia and rest pain at night. Discuss the side effects of all medications and symptoms that should be brought to your attention.

Follow-up: Patients receiving medications may be seen about every 3–4 months, or sooner if problems develop. (See other sections for discussions about routine monitoring of patients with other conditions such as diabetes or hypertension.) Do periodic liver function tests for patients who receive calcium antagonists. Patients who are on a weight reduction or smoking cessation program may also need to be followed up more frequently at first. Other patients may be seen every 6 months to 1 year unless their condition changes.

▶ *Raynaud's Disease*

Laboratory Tests: The history and clinical findings are usually sufficient to make a diagnosis, but specific tests may be done to rule out other disorders associated with Raynaud's disease if these are suspected (e.g., temporal cell arteritis, rheumatoid vasculitis, thoracic outlet syndrome, carpal tunnel syndrome, systemic lupus erythematosus, scleroderma).

Therapeutic Measures: Most cases of Raynaud's disease are benign, and general measures are sufficient (see below), but rapid progression with severe, disabling pain, limitation of motion, and secondary distal joint fixation may occur rarely, requiring vasodilators or other measures (e.g., local IV injection of reserpine, IV infusion of prostaglandin E, or sympathectomy). Calcium channel blockers are being used and show great promise. Patients who smoke should be advised to quit.

Patient Education: Patients should be advised to keep the entire body warm, and especially to protect the hands from cold exposure and injury. Gloves or preferably mittens should be worn whenever the patient is outdoors in cold weather. Protective rubber gloves should be used whenever prolonged or repeated exposure to water, detergents, or irritating chemicals is necessary (for housecleaning, dish washing, etc.) Patients should also wear protective cotton gloves when doing gardening or yard work. Any development of sores, blisters, cracking, fissures, and so on should be reported to the health care provider. No topical medications should be applied to the hands without first checking with the provider. Question all patients about smoking and explain that peripheral vasoconstriction caused by tobacco use contributes to this condition. Provide patients who smoke with instructions for quitting and encouragement (see "Smoking Cessation").

Follow-up: As needed for treatment of symptoms.

▶ *Varicose Veins*

Laboratory Tests: Diagnosis is usually based on the clinical findings, but venography or Doppler studies may be useful in ruling out suspected thrombosis or other disorders.

Therapeutic Measures: General measures include the use of proper medium- or heavyweight elastic support hose and periodic elevation of the involved extremity during the day. Properly fitted surgical stockings, which may be obtained from a surgical supply company, are probably best. They should be high enough to provide external support to the proximal foot and leg up to (but not including) the knee. Thigh-height stockings are usually difficult to keep up and do not achieve proper compression of the thighs. As an alternative, good medium- to heavyweight support panty hose (available in most department stores) may be used, but these should be the correct size and should be put on properly to avoid causing constriction of superficial venous return at the level of the thigh. Wrapping the legs with ace bandages should be discouraged, since these are not only cumbersome but are also often improperly applied, resulting in a tourniquet effect at the level of the knee. The use of birth control pills is best avoided by women with varicose veins. Patients with severe symptoms may be referred for surgical consultation. Vein stripping and the use of sclerosing agents have obtained good results, with relief of symptoms in many cases.

Patient Education: All patients should be instructed to avoid the use of tight garments that constrict the thigh (e.g., circular garters, tight underwear, panty girdles) and prolonged periods of standing whenever possible. Patients should be encouraged to attain and maintain ideal weight. Hot tub baths or the application of heat in any form will cause relaxation of blood vessels and should be avoided. Teach patients the signs and symptoms of thrombophlebitis (heat, redness, slight swelling, spasm, and tenderness particularly with dorsiflexion of the foot). Women should be particularly encouraged to wear supportive stockings during pregnancy in order to prevent the further development of varicosities.

Follow-up: None needed.

▸ *Long-Term Anticoagulant Therapy*

Laboratory Tests: Tests necessary to rule out contraindications to therapy should be done. Such contraindications include severe hypertension, blood dyscrasias, hemophilia, purpura, thrombocytopenia, hepatic disease with hypoprothrombinemia, vitamin K deficiency, leukemia with bleeding tendencies, suspected intracranial hemorrhage, suppurative thrombophlebitis, inaccessible ulcerative lesions (especially gastrointestinal), subacute bacterial endocarditis, acute nephritis, impaired renal or hepatic function (relative contraindication), and increased capillary permeability (e.g., in ascorbic acid deficiency). (Other contraindications include recent eye, brain, or spinal cord surgery, threatened abortion, alcoholism, the presence of drainage tubes in any orifice, open wounds, extensive areas of skin denudation, and usually pregnancy.)

Therapeutic Measures: Since heparin acts quickly, it is the drug of choice for short-term therapy and for initiation of long-term anticoagulant therapy (to be followed by prothrombin depressant anticoagulant drugs). Hospitalization is necessary for administration, since it can only be given parenterally. After 7–14 days (sometimes longer), the switch to oral prothrombin depressant drugs for maintenance therapy can be made. Of the prothrombin depressant drugs available, warfarin (Coumadin) is the most commonly used. Begin with a single loading dose of 40–60 mg (20–40 mg in elderly or debilitated patients) or 10–15 mg/day for 2–3 days. In either case, this is followed by a maintenance dose of 2–10 mg/day, adjusted according to prothrombin time determinations.

Patient Education: Discuss possible drug interactions with patients and stress that patients must not use any medication that is not first cleared with the provider supervising the anticoagulant therapy. Emphasize that many nonprescription drugs, including aspirin, alcohol, and preparations high in vitamin K, may interact with anticoagulants. Tell patients that a change in diet or physical state may alter the effect of the anticoagulant, and instruct them to report any illnesses promptly to their care provider. Teach the signs of excessive bleeding to report, including bleeding gums, bruising or petechiae, hematuria, tarry stools, hematemesis, or any sudden joint pain, including lumbar pain. Women should be advised to avoid pregnancy while taking anticoagulant therapy. If the patient is unable to understand the therapy or cannot be relied on to take medication without supervision (such as elderly senile, mentally disabled, or alcoholic patients), it is essential that a responsible family member or care taker receive these instructions and be actively involved in reporting adverse effects and ensuring that patients keep all appointments for blood tests. All patients should be encouraged to wear a Medic-Alert bracelet or necklace stating that they are taking anticoagulant therapy in order to alert emergency or other medical personnel in the event of an accident or excessive bleeding incident or if surgery is required. At the very least, they should carry a card, although this is less likely to be discovered early in the event of an emergency if the patient is unable to communicate.

Follow-up: Initially, prothrombin times should be determined daily and each subsequent dose should be withheld until the results of the preceding day's tests are obtained. Therapy should be aimed at maintaining prothrombin times at 1.5–2.5 times control values. Weekly to monthly determinations may be adequate for well-stabilized patients. Closer monitoring may be required when patients are receiving a drug known to interact with anticoagulants and in premenopausal girls around the time of menstruation. Since the use of warfarin is contraindicated during pregnancy, female patients should be questioned at each visit about the possibility of pregnancy; if their status is uncertain, pregnancy testing should be done.

BIBLIOGRAPHY

Abramowicz M. *Handbook of Antimicrobial Therapy,* rev. ed. The Medical Letter, New Rochelle, N.Y., 1980.

Alderman MH, Stanback ME. Preventive cardiology: The state of the art. *Cardiovascular Reviews and Reports,* (Mar.) 1981, 2(3):247–252.

Alpert JS, Rippe JM. *Manual of Cardiovascular Diagnosis and Therapy.* Little, Brown, Boston, 1980.

Altrose MD (B Bekiesz, ed.). The physiological basis of pulmonary function testing. *Clinical Symposia,* 1979, 31(2):2–39.

American Lung Association. *Bronchiectasis: The Facts About Your Lungs.* ALA pamphlet #0091. March 1977.

American Lung Association. *Asthma: Facts About Your Lungs.* ALA pamphlet #0052. August 1979.

American Lung Association. *Emphysema: The Facts About Your Lungs.* ALA pamphlet #0301. September 1979.

Amsterdam EA. Optimal medical therapy for angina pectoris. *Practical Cardiology,* (Sept.) 1982, 8(10):41–48.

Anderson JL. Managing cardiac arrhythmias: An empiric approach. *Modern Medicine,* (Nov.) 1981, 78–94.

Athanasiou R, Cameron CTM. Hyperventilation syndrome: A sheep in wolf's clothing. *Physician Assistant and Health Practitioner,* (Oct.) 1982, 52–62.

Bacterial endocarditis guidelines revised: Less postoperative medication recommended. *ADA News,* (Dec.) 1984.

Balmes J, Cullen MR, Matthay RA. Occupational and environmental lung disease. In: George, Lingt, and Matthey (eds.), *Chest Medicine.* Churchill Livingston, London, 1983.

Bates B. *A Guide to Physical Examination,* 3rd ed., Lippincott, Philadelphia, 1983.

Berkow RB (ed.). *The Merck Manual of Diagnosis and Therapy,* 14th ed. Merck Sharp & Dohme Research Laboratories, Rahway, N.J., 1982.

Berte JB. Management of bronchospasm. *Practical Cardiology,* (Dec.) 1979, 5(12):31–44.

Bloomberg AE. Carcinoma of lung: Indications for surgery. *New York State Journal of Medicine,* (Dec.) 1979, 2033–2038.

Bone RC. *Pulmonary Disease Reviews.* Wiley, New York, 1981.

Brigham KL, Newman JH. The pulmonary circulation. *Basics of RD,* (Sept.) 1979, 8(1):

Brodoff AS (staff ed.). When asthma causes "moderate" trouble. *Patient Care,* (Nov.) 1981, 143–187.

Brown AM, Stubbs DW (eds.). *Medical Physiology.* Wiley, New York, 1983.

Brown ML. *Occupational Health Nursing.* Springer, New York, 1981.

Burrows B. Management of chronic obstructive lung disease. *PA Drug Update,* (June) 1982, 52–56.

Cassell GH, Cole BC. Mycoplasmas as agents of human disease. *New England Journal of Medicine,* (Jan.) 1981, 80–88.

Chobanian AV. Hypertension. (AH Trench, ed.). *Clinical Symposia,* 1982, 34(5):3–32.

Christlieb AR. Diabetes and hypertension. *Cardiovascular Review and Reports,* (Nov.) 1980, 1(8):609–616.

Cody RJ Jr. Chronic heart failure: Specific therapy for vasoconstrictor mechanisms. *PA Drug Update,* (Aug.) 1983, 17–22.

Conn HF, Conn RB Jr (eds.). *Current Diagnosis.* Saunders, Philadelphia, 1980.

Conn R (ed.). *Current Therapy.* Saunders, Philadelphia, 1983.

Corday E, Swan HJC, Corday SR. Medical versus surgical treatment of coronary artery disease—1981. *Cardiovascular Reviews and Reports,* (Mar.) 1981, 2(3):281–287.

Cotes JE. *Lung Function,* 4th ed. Blackwell, Oxford, 1979.

Crafts RC. *A Textbook of Human Anatomy,* 3rd ed. Wiley, New York, 1985.

Cressman MD, Gifford RW Jr. New approaches to initial drug therapy of mild hypertension. *Practical Cardiology,* (May) 1986, 12(5):83–92.

Cressman MD, Gifford RW Jr. Use of calcium-channel blockers in antihypertensive therapy. *Practical Cardiology,* (May) 1986, 12(5):95–103.

Crouch JE, McClintic JR. *Human Anatomy and Physiology,* 2nd ed. Wiley, New York, 1976.

Davis FB, Sczupak CA. Outpatient oral anticoagulation: Guidelines for long-term management. *Postgraduate Medicine* (July) 1979, 66(1):100–109.

Decker EL, Anderson ER. Antifungal agents for systemic mycoses. *Therapeutics,* 1982,

Deedwania PC, Carbajal E. Current trends in antianginal therapy. *Therapaeia,* (May–June) 1986, 22–35.

Dietrich EB. *Advances in Cardiovascular Nursing.* Robert J. Brady, Bowie Md., 1980.

Disch JM. *Diagnostic Procedures for Cardiovascular Disease.* Appleton-Century-Crofts, East Norwalk, Conn., 1979.

Edwards JE Jr. Update on systemic fungal infections—part 2. *Physician Assistant,* (July) 1983, 129–140.

Elias H, Pauly JE, Burns ER. *Histology and Human Microanatomy,* 4th ed. Wiley, New York, 1978.

Ellis EF. The thin line of asthma therapy. *Emergency Medicine,* (Feb.) 1981, 25–35.

Fekety R. Office treatment of infection, part 1: Respiratory infections. *Postgraduate Medicine,* (Feb.) 1980, 67(2):74–83.

Fenster PE, Kern KB. Common drug interactions with digoxin. *PA Drug Update,* (Sept.) 1983, 42–48.

Ferrer MI. The sick sinus syndrome. *Hospital Practice,* (Nov.) 1980, 79–89.

Finnerty FA Jr. Clinical factors affecting the choice of drugs at step 2 control of hypertension. *Practical Cardiology,* (Nov.) 1980, 6(12):35–41.

Freitag JJ, Miller L (eds.). *Manual of Medicine Therapeutics,* 23rd ed. Little, Brown, Boston, 1980.

Gardner AW. *Current Approaches to Occupational Medicine.* Yearbook Publishers, Chicago, 1979.

Geelhoed GW. Prevention of thromboembolism. *American Family Physician,* (Mar.) 1979, 19(3):147–153.

Gelfant B. Hypertension protocol. *Nurse Practitioner,* (Sept.) 1983, 25–74.

Gentry LO. Pneumonia and bronchitis: Causes, diagnosis, and treatment. *Consultant,* (Mar.) 1980, 161–165.

Giudice JC, Komansky HJ, Kaufman J. Pulmonary thromboembolism, part 2: New trends in prophylaxis and therapy. *Postgraduate Medicine,* (May) 1980, 67(5):81–89.

Goldstein S. Beta-blockers after MI: 10 questions physicians often ask. *Consultant,* (June) 1983, 93–100.

Goroll AH, May LA, Mulley AG. *Primary Care Medicine: Office Evaluation and Management of the Adult Patient.* Lippincott, Philadelphia, 1981.

Grayboys TB, Poser R. Can sudden cardiac death be prevented? *PA Drug Update,* (Jan.) 1983, 26–33.

Gray H. *Anatomy of the Human Body,* 29th American ed. (CM Goss, ed.). Lea & Febiger, Philadelphia, 1973.

Guyton AC. *Textbook of Medical Physiology,* 6th ed. Saunders, Philadelphia, 1981.

Harper RW. *A Guide to Respiratory Care: Physiology and Clinical Applications.* Lippincott, Philadelphia, 1981.

Hauser CJ, Shoemaker WC. Volume therapy, part 2: Treatment of hypovolemia. *Physician Assistant and Health Practitioner,* (May) 1981, 44–55.

Higgins JR, Ports TA. Mitral valve prolapse: A review. *Continuing Education,* (June) 1982, 83–90.

Hirschmann JV, Lipsky BA. Pneumococcal vaccine in the United States: A critical analysis. *Journal of the American Medical Association,* (Sept.) 1981, 246(13):1428–1431.

Holloway NM. *Nursing the Critically Ill Adult.* Addison-Wesley, Menlo Park, Calif., 1979.

Holverson HE. *Myocardial Infarction: Diagnostic Challenges.* Healthways Communications, Union, N.J., November 1982.

Hoole AJ, Greenberg RA, Pickard CG Jr. *Patient Care Guidelines for Nurse Practitioners.* Little, Brown, Boston, 1982.

Horwitz LD. Congestive heart failure: An overview of drug therapy. *Postgraduate Medicine,* (Aug.) 1984, 76(2):187–193.

Hurst JW (ed.). *The Heart.* McGraw-Hill, New York, 1978.

Isselbacher KJ, et al. *Harrison's Principles of Internal Medicine,* 9th ed. McGraw-Hill, New York, 1980.

Jacob W, Francone CA, Lossow W. *Structure and Function in Man,* 5th ed. Saunders, Philadelphia, 1982.

Judge RD, Zuidema GD. *Methods of Clinical Examination: A Physiologic Approach,* 3d ed. Little, Brown, Boston, 1974.

Kandel G, Aberman A. Asthma: Diagnostic and therapeutic strategies that work. *Consultant,* (June) 1983, 143–160.

Kannel WB, Lerner DJ. Present status of risk factors for atherosclerosis. *Medical Times,* (Sept.) 1984, 33–45.

Kaplan LA, Stein EA. In search of biochemical markers for acute MI. *Diagnostic Medicine,* (Feb.) 1985, 25–33.

Karus CA. Tuberculosis: An overview of pathogenesis and prevention. *Nurse Practitioner,* (Feb.) 1983, 21–28.

Kasanof DM (staff ed.). Common infections: Current care for the flu syndrome. *Patient Care,* (Dec.) 1980, 115–131.

Kasanof DM (staff ed.). Common infections: Current care for pneumonia. *Patient Care,* (Dec.) 1980, 135–151.

Kaufman CE Jr. Essential hypertension: Essentials of management. *Hospital Medicine,* (May) 1982, 93–104.

Kross DE, Effmann EL, Putman CE. Adult aspiration pneumonia. *American Family Physician,* (July) 1980, 22(1):73–78.

Krupp MA, Chatton MJ, Werdegar D (eds.). *Current Medical Diagnosis and Treatment 1985.* Lange, Los Altos, Calif.,

Kupersmith J, Wolfson M. Digoxin–drug interactions. *Physican Assistant,* (Nov.) 1983, 66–71.

Landesman SH. Who should receive the pneumococcal vaccine? *PA Drug Update,* (Feb.) 1983, 38–49.

Last JM (ed.). *Maxcy-Rosenau Public Health and Preventive Medicine,* 11th ed. Appleton-Century-Crofts, New York, 1980.

Laxarus A. Pulmonary function tests in upper airway obstruction. *Basics of RD,* (Jan.) 1980, 8(3).

Levy JM, et al. Digital subtraction angiography. *Continuing Education,* (Oct.) 1982, 27–39.

Loebl S, Spratto G. *The Nurse's Drug Handbook,* 3d ed. Wiley, New York, 1983.

Luckmann J, Sorensen KC. *Medical Surgical Nursing: A Psychophysiologic Approach,* 2nd ed. Saunders, Philadelphia, 1980.

Mahoney E. Pieri-Flynn J. *Handbook of Medical-Surgical Nursing.* Wiley, New York, 1983.

Mandell GL, Douglas RG Jr, Bennett JE. *Principles and Practice of Infectious Diseases,* Vols. 1 and 2. Wiley, New York, 1979.

Maseri A, et al. The role of spasm in angina pectoris and infarction: Indications for future research and therapy. *Practical Cardiology,* (Mar.) 1981, 7(3):29–40.

Massaro D. Clinical implications of the effect of breathing pattern on the lung. *Basics of RD,* (Nov.) 1979, 8(2):

Maxey K, Rosenau M (J Last, ed.). *Public Health and Preventive Medicine,* 11th ed. Appleton-Century-Crofts, New York, 1980.

McAuley BJ, Ginsburg R. Varian angina: Update on diagnosis and current therapy. *Consultant,* (June) 1983, 166–179.

McHenry MC. The infectious pneumonias. *Hospital Practice,* (Dec) 1980, 41–52.

McIntyre KM, Lewis AJ (eds.). *Textbook of Advanced Cardiac Life Support.* American Heart Association, New York, 1983.

Meltzer AH, et al. Congestive heart failure following upper respiratory infection. *Physician Assistant,* (Nov.) 1983, 57–65.

Milhorn HT Jr. Understanding pulmonary function tests. *American Family Physician,* (Nov.) 1981, 24(5):139–145.

Morady F, Scheinman M. Electrophysiologic testing: In-depth study of severe arrhythmias. *Consultant,* (Feb.) 1982, 91–112.

Moritz ED, Matthay RA. Cor pulmonale: Diagnosis and management. *The Journal of Respiratory Diseases,* (May) 1980, 34–55.

Moser M. *High Blood Pressure and What You Can Do About it.* Benjamin, Elmsford, N.Y., 1982.

Moser M. When does mild hypertension warrant treatment? *Journal of Cardiovascular Medicine,* (Oct.) 1982, 7(10).

Moser M. Stepped-care approach to hypertension: Is it still useful? *Physician Assistant,* (Feb.) 1986, 63–68.

Moss AJ, Milner M. Nifedipine: A calcium antagonist for treating angina pectoris and other cardiovascular disorders. *Cardiovascular Reviews and Reports,* (May) 1981, 2(5):487–494.

Mudge GH Jr. Coronary spasm: Rationale for therapy. *PA Drug Update,* (June) 1981, 21–29.

Murphy CA, et al. Anti-smoking resources. *Physician Assistant,* (July) 1983, 125–126.

National High Blood Pressure Conference, 1984. Recommendations for treatment of hypertension.

Niarchos AP. Pathophysiology, diagnosis, and treatment of hypertension in the elderly. *Cardiovascular Reviews and Reports,* (Nov.) 1980, 1(8):621–627.

Petty TL. COPD: A new look at Dx and Rx of an old problem. *Modern Medicine,* (Feb.) 1985, 128–136.

Pingleton SK. Rational drug therapy for asthma. *Family Practice Recertification,* (May) 1980, 2(5):21–34.

Pinneo R. *Congestive Heart Failure.* Appleton-Century-Crofts, East Norwalk, Conn., 1978.

Pope JC III. Congestive heart failure: Management update. *Physician Assistant,* (May) 1983, 26–38.

Ravel R. *Clinical Laboratory Medicine: Clinical Application of Laboratory Data,* 3d ed. Year Book Medical Publishers, Chicago, 1978.

Reichel J. Pulmonary emphysema. *Hospital Medicine,* (Feb.) 1980, 8–21.

Robbins SL, Cotran RS. *Pathologic Basis of Disease,* 2nd ed. Saunders, Philadelphia, 1979.

Rodman M, Karch AM, Boyd EH, et al. *Pharmacology and Drug Therapy in Nursing,* 3d ed. Lippincott, New York, 1985.

Russell SL, Canedo MI, Watkins LO. Cardiac catheterization: Indications, procedure, and interpretation. *Physician Assistant and Health Practitioner,* (Feb.) 1983, 77–94.

Sahn SA. Pleural manifestations of pulmonary disease. *Hospital Practice,* (Mar.) 1981, 73–89.

Scheidt S (W Heidel, ed.). Basic electrocardiography: Leads, axes, arrhythmias. *Clinical Symposia,* 1983, 35(2):2–32.

Schwaber JR. Pulmonary neoplasms. *Hospital Medicine,* (Oct.) 1980, 55–64.

Scoggin CH. Practical new strategies for managing COPD. *Modern Medicine,* (Feb.–Mar.) 1981, 42–48.

Sexton DL. *Chronic Obstructive Pulmonary Disease.* Mosby, St. Louis, 1981.

Silverstein A. *Human Anatomy and Physiology.* Wiley, New York, 1980.

Sklar T, Sy M. Asthma diagnosis and management. *Health Practitioner and Physician Assistant,* (June) 1979, 43–54.

Slonim NB, Hamilton LH. *Respiratory Physiology.* Mosby, St. Louis, 1981.

Sly RM. Management of exercise-induced asthma. *Drug Therapy,* (Mar.) 1982, 95–101.

Smialowicz CR. Clinical and bacteriological evaluation of cefaclor and tetracycline in acute episodes of bacterial bronchitis. *Clinical Therapeutics,* 1982, 5(2):113–118.

Smith BR. Pneumonia. *The Physician Assistant Drug Newsletter.* Healthways Communications, Union, N.J., 1982.

Sokolow M, McIlroy MB. *Clinical Cardiology,* 3d ed. Lange Medical Publications, Los Altos, Calif., 1981.

Sonnenblick EH, Frishman WH. The role of beta-adrenergic blockers in the treatment of angina pectoris. *Cardiovascular Reviews and Reports,* (May) 1981, 2(5):439–443.

Spector SL. Management of chronic symptoms in the asthmatic patient. *Hospital Medicine,* (Aug.) 1979, 16–26.

Staub NC. Lung structure and function 1982. *Respiratory Care,* (Dec.) 1982, 27(12):1550–1556.

Steere AC, et al. Lyme carditis: Cardiac abnormalities of Lyme disease. *Annals of Internal Medicine,* (July) 1980, 93(1):8–16.

Stellman SD, Stellman JM. Women's occupations, smoking, and cancer and other diseases. *Ca—A Cancer Journal for Clinicians,* (Jan.–Feb.) 1981, 31(1):29–40.

Still J, Mannion M. Smoking and pregnancy. *Physician Assistant,* (July) 1983, 114–120.

Tattersall SF. How to avoid some common errors in asthma management. *Modern Medicine,* (Oct.) 1979, 59–71.

Teirstein AS, Kleinerman J. Diffuse interstitial lung disease. *Hospital Practice,* (June) 1981, 126–136.

Thompson JM, McFarland GK, Hirsch JE, et al. *Clinical Nursing.* Mosby, St. Louis, 1986.

Tockman MS. Lung cancer: Early diagnosis. *Hospital Medicine,* (May) 1981, 51–63.

U.S. Department of Health and Human Services. *Health information for international Travel 1985.*

Varkey B, Politis J. Pulmonary tuberculosis: A multifaceted disease. *Postgraduate Medicine,* (Jan.) 1981, 69(1):117–126.

Weber MA, Drayer JIM. Treating hypertension via selective blockade of the renin axis. *PA Drug Update,* (July) 1982, 30–34.

Weil H. Occupational lung diseases. *Hospital Practice,* (Apr.) 1981, 65–81.

Wenger NK, Hurst JW, McIntyre MC. *Cardiology for Nurses.* McGraw-Hill, New York, 1980.

Wenger NK. The coronary patient: Interactions of cardiovascular drugs and exercise. *Drug Therapy,* (Mar.) 1982, 59–63.

Williams MH Jr. Severe asthma: Prevention and treatment. *Consultant,* (Mar.) 1980, 292–294.

Wyngaarden JB, Smith LH Jr (eds.). *Cecil Textbook of Medicine,* 16th ed., Vols 1 and 2. Saunders, Philadelphia, 1982.

7

Blood and Immunology

Carla Greene

Outline

BLOOD-FORMING CELLS

Extramedullary hematopoiesis
Acute myelogenous leukemia (AML)
Acute lymphoblastic leukemia (ALL)
Chronic myelogenous leukemia (CML)
Chronic lymphocytic leukemia (CLL)
► Leukemia organizations
Lymphomas
Non-Hodgkin's lymphomas
Sézary's syndrome
Hodgkin's disease
Chronic myeloproliferative disorders
Polycythemia vera
Agnogenic myeloid metaplasia
Primary thrombocytopenia
Pancytopenia
Aplastic anemia
Fanconi's anemia

RED BLOOD CELLS (RBCs)

Erythropoiesis

Reticulocytosis
Poikilocytosis
Microcytes
Macrocytes
Anisocytosis
Normochromic
Hypochromic
Hyperchromic
Anemia as a general term
Megaloblastic anemia
► Folic acid deficiency
Vitamin B_{12} deficiency
► Vitamin B_{12} deficiency related to diet
► Vitamin B_{12} deficiency due to malabsorption
Immerslund-Grasbeck syndrome
Pernicious anemia

Heme Complex

Sideroblastic anemias
► Pyridoxine-responsive anemias
Acute and chronic lead poisoning
Porphyrias

Hemoglobin

Hemoglobinopathy
Heterozygous

Hemizygous
Homozygous
Double heterozygous
Beta-thalassemia
Cooley's trait
Cooley's anemia
Alpha-thalassemia
Hydrops fetalis
Hemoglobin H
Alpha-thalassemia minor
Alpha-thalassemia silent carrier
► Sickle cell trait
Sickle cell disease
Sickle crisis
► Sickle cell organizations
Hemoglobin C
Sickle cell-hemoglobin C disease
Unstable hemoglobin variants
Stable hemoglobin variants

Oxygen Transport and Cellular Metabolism

Enzyme deficiencies
Glucose-6-phosphate dehydrogenase (G-6-PD) deficiencies
Mosaicism
Heinz bodies
Methemoglobinemia

RBC Life Cycle

Intramedullary hemolysis
Extravascular hemolysis
Intravascular hemolysis
Hemolytic anemia
Hemoglobinemia
Hemosiderinuria
Hemoglobinuria
Hereditary spherocytosis
Hereditary elliptocytosis
Hemoglobinopathies
Immune hemolytic anemias
Paroxysmal nocturnal hemoglobinuria (PNH)
Traumatic hemolysis

Iron Balance

► Iron deficiency anemia
Hemosiderosis
Iron overload
Hemochromatosis
Idiopathic hemochromatosis

MYELOGENOUS WHITE BLOOD CELLS (WBCs)

Neutrophils

Arthus reaction
Fever
Right shift
Left shift
Neutrophilia
Physiologic leukocytosis
Leukemoid reaction
Neutropenia
Agranulocytosis
Toxic granulation
Dohle inclusion bodies
May-Hegglin anomaly
Alder-Reilly anomaly
Pelger-Huet anomaly
Chediak-Higashi syndrome
Auer rods

Basophils and Eosinophils

Basophilia
Eosinophilia
Parasite infections
Acquired toxoplasmosis
Toxoplasmic chorioretinitis
Congenital toxoplasmosis
Trichinosis
Malaria
► Malaria prophylaxis for travelers
Bebesiosis
Hypereosinophilic syndrome

Monocytes

Monocytosis
Monocytopenia

LYMPHOCYTES AND SPECIFIC IMMUNITY

B Lymphocytes and Humoral Immunity

Hypersensitivity reaction
Infectious mononucleosis

Cytomegalovirus (CMV)
Congenital CMV
CMV mononucleosis or CMV hepatitis
Antibody deficiency disorders
Plasma cell dyscrasias
Macroglobulinemia of Waldenström
Heavy chain diseases
Multiple myeloma
Amyloidosis
Primary amyloidosis
Secondary amyloidosis
Cutaneous amyloidosis

T Lymphocytes and Cellular Immunity

Type IV hypersensitivity reactions
T-cell deficiencies
AIDS
▶ AIDS organizations
Combined immune deficiency disorders

Allogens

Blood types
Blood transfusions
Transfusion reaction
Erythroblastosis fetalis
▶ Rhogam administration
Organ transplantation
Rejection reaction
Autoimmunity

HEMOSTASIS

Primary hemostasis

Thrombocytopenia
Thrombocytosis
Hemorrhagic thrombocytosis
Qualitative platelet disorders
Vascular abnormalities

Secondary Hemostasis

Coagulation disorders
Hemophilia A
Hemophilia B
▶ Hemophilia organizations
Acquired coagulation disorders
Vitamin K deficiency and liver dysfunction
Disseminated intravascular coagulation (DIC)

BLOOD-FORMING CELLS

Mature circulating blood cells are depicted in Figure 7.1. Erythrocytes, platelets, neutrophils, monocytes, eosinophils, and basophils are produced in the bone marrow (myeloid tissue). They arise from a constant self-renewing pool of pluripotent stem cells called "colony-forming unit-spleen (CFU-S)" cells. CFU-S cells turn into committed stem cells (BFU-E, CFU-MG, CFU-D, CFU-EO) that proliferate along the specific lineages illustrated in Figure 7.2. CFU-D cells give rise to both monocytes and neutrophils and CFU-EO cells to both eosinophils and basophils. While they also originate in myeloid tissue, pluripotent lymphoid cells differentiate along two pathways outside bone marrow: in the lymph organs, thymus gland, and parts of the intestinal tract. Under the influence of the thymus, one pathway produes T lymphocytes. Under the influence of the bone marrow, the other pathway produces B lymphocytes, which, in turn, form plasma cells.

Myeloid tissue is composed of reticular meshworks and vascular channels called "sinusoids." Throughout the myeloid tissue are blood cells of all types in all stages of production. Although physical groupings do not actually exist, it is useful to think that cells are produced and distributed within distinct "pools." The first pool contains the uncommitted cells that are normally present in small numbers and have a slow

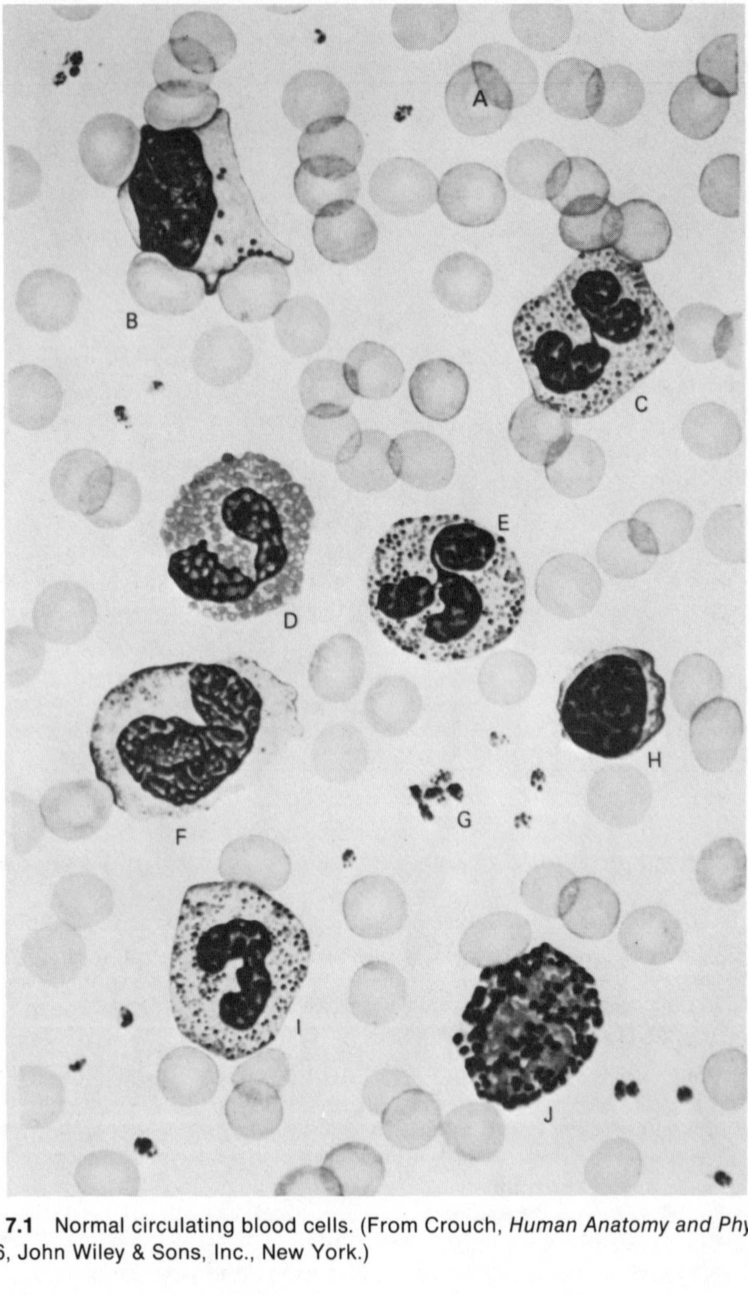

Figure 7.1 Normal circulating blood cells. (From Crouch, *Human Anatomy and Physiology*, © 1976, John Wiley & Sons, Inc., New York.)

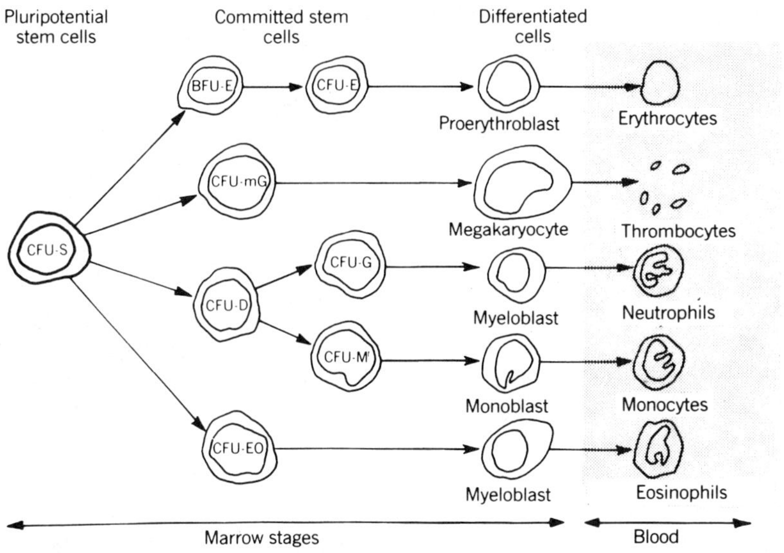

Figure 7.2 Stem cells. (From Sultan, *Manual of Hematology,* © 1985, John Wiley & Sons, Inc., New York.)

rate of turnover. For reasons that are not clear, these cells continually differentiate into the exact number and type of precursor cells required to meet the body's needs. Committed cells move to the second "mitotic pool," where they divide repeatedly and begin to mature. They decrease in size, undergo internal changes, and become more flexible. Having completed their divisions, the cells enter a third "postmitotic" pool, where they continue to mature and await delivery into the bloodstream. When called on, mature cells advance through openings in the marrow sinusoids. Picked up by venous capillaries, the newly released cells enter the circulatory system. Some of them travel in the main bloodstream ("circulating pool"), while others become sequestered along the vessel walls ("marginal pool"). Cells in the marginal pool act as a reserve supply.

In the adult, myeloid tissue is confined to the cancellous spaces of the ribs, vertebrae, sternum, pelvis, skull, and long bones. Under conditions of extreme stress, tissues in other organs (e.g., yellow marrow, liver, spleen, lung or kidneys) undergo myeloid metaplasia and produce blood cells in a process referred to as ***extramedullary hematopoiesis.*** Some causes of extramedullary hematopoiesis are listed in Table 7.1.

Acute myelogenous leukemias (AML) (acute nonlymphocytic leukemia, ANLL) is a malignant change in myeloid stem cells. Subclassifications have been described according to the characteristics of the predominant cells (Table 7.2). AML is the most common leukemia in infants. Its incidence decreases in childhood, rises slightly from adolescence through adulthood (15 cases per million), and peaks after age 55 (55 cases per million by age 75). The exact cause of this malignancy is unknown. However, genetic predisposition, viruses, radiation exposure, chemicals, and drugs have been correlated with it. These factors have the potential to cause marrow aplasia, compromise immune surveillance systems, and/or induce chromo-

TABLE 7.1 CONDITIONS ASSOCIATED WITH EXTRAMEDULLARY HEMATOPOIESIS

Severe hemolytic anemias

Hodgkin's disease

Metastatic neoplasms to the bone marrow

Bone marrow infections (notably tuberculosis)

Bone marrow toxicity
- Fluorine
- Phosphorus
- Benzol
- Strontium

Bone marrow fibrosis
- Chronic illness
- Irradiation
- Myeloproliferative disorders

somal breaks. As a result, leukemic cells neither respond to the normal controlling mechanisms for division nor follow normal routes for development. For example, normal myeloblasts generate in 24–48 hours and proceed through limited stages of cell division, whereas leukemic myeloblasts generate in 15–60 hours and divide indefinitely. Furthermore, leukemic cells can pass from the bloodstream into the tissues, replicate, and reenter the bloodstream.

Clinical and laboratory manifestations of acute leukemia are related to the invasion of organs by leukemic cells and to the reduced number of normal blood cells. Patients usually present with sudden onset of weakness, intermittent fever, infection, and signs of bleeding abnormalities. Physical exam may reveal hepatosplenomegaly, adenopathy, bone tenderness, petechiae, and ecchymosis. Anemia, an elevated white count with an abnormal differential, and thombocytopenia are common laboratory findings. As many as 10% of patients have normal complete blood counts

TABLE 7.2 FAB CLASSIFICATIONS OF AML

Type	Description
M1 Acute myeloblastic leukemia with little differentiation	Varying from 15 to 25 μm in size, cells have a round or oval nucleus with one or two nucleoli. Auer bodies seen in majority of blasts. Mature granulocytic elements absent or markedly diminished.
M2 Acute myelobalstic leukemia with maturation	Though more than 50% of cells are myeloblasts, granulocytic maturation to progranulocyte stage or above occurs. Mature cells have a number of abnormalities such as poor nuclear segmentation (pseudo–Pelger-Huet) and scant or absent granules. May be difficult to differentiate from myeloid dysplasias.
M3 Hypergranular or promyelocytic leukemia	Majority of cells are promyelocytes containing numerous atypical granules (large, fused, rose red or purple colored). Auer bodies seen in bundles ("faggots"). M3 variant characterized by cells with kidney-shaped or bilobed nucleus. Recognition of both M3 and M3 variant is important because intravascular coagulation is often associated.
M4 Myelomonocytic leukemia	Same as M2 except that monocytes or promonocytes constitute more than 20% of cells (peripheral blood characteristically contains more than 5,000/μL).
M5 Acute monocytic leukemia	Bone marrow almost completely replaced by two types of monocytic cells. In subtype M5a, monoblasts predominate. They have abundant cytoplasm containing prominent nucleoli and pseudopods. In subtype M5b, there may be promonocytes and monocytes as well as monoblasts. Auer rods generally absent in both subtypes. Diagnosis confirmed by a positive esterase reaction that is inhibited by sodium fluoride.
M6 Erythroleukemia	Erythrocytic cells predominate (myeloblasts, promyelocytes, erythroblasts, micromegakaryocytes, giant platelets). Circulating erythrocytes are markedly abnormal and include erythroblasts.

(CBCs) initially. Later, blasts appear in the peripheral circulation, many of them containing red-staining, rod-like inclusions ***(auer bodies).*** Auer bodies are pathognomic for AML. Patients with these signs and symptoms should be referred to a hematologist for definitive diagnosis based on bone marrow aspiration. The specimen typically shows hypercellular changes, with 60–100% blast cells. Most patients are hospitalized for aggressive chemotherapy to suppress malignant stem cells so that normal cells can reestablish. The agents routinely used (combinations of daunorubicin, doxorubicin, 6-thioguanine, cytosine arabinoside, and others) induce profound marrow aplasia. The specific treatment and survival expectancy vary with the subclassification. In general, 75% of these patients may be expected to achieve remission lasting for 1.5–2 years with extended use of cytotoxic agents. Even so survival beyond 3 years is uncommon.

Acute lymphoblastic leukemia (ALL) is due to a malignant change in lymphoid stem cells. Subdivisions are described by the morphologic characteristics of malignant cells as well as by T-cell or B-cell predominance (Table 7.3). As in AML, the exact etiology is unknown. However, inciting factors such as radiation and viral infections have been well established. A genetic predisposition and chromosomal abnormalities (Down's syndrome, neurofibromatosis) are also associated with ALL. Its incidence peaks by age 5 (50 per million cases) and then declines for all other age groups (10–15 cases per million.) The disease develops insidiously. Symptoms begin with anorexia, irritability, and malaise. Patients have low-grade fevers with intermittent temperature spikes that may or may not be accompanied by infection. Recurrent infections are the rule, particularly those of the urinary tract. Migratory arthritis (joints are notably painful, swollen, and tender) is common.

Physical exam reveals pallor, hepatosplenomegaly, and lymphadenopathy. There may also be signs of abnormal bleeding such as petechiae and ecchymosis of the skin and mucous membranes. The initial laboratory tests reveal anemia, thrombocytopenia, either leukopenia or leukocytosis, and the presence of blast cells on the

TABLE 7.3 CLASSIFICATIONS OF ALL

Type	Description
	By Morphologic Definition (FAB Classification)
L1	Most frequent type seen in children. Cells are homogeneously small, with large nuclei and a poorly defined nucleolus.
L2	Most frequent type seen in adults. Cells are variably sized, many being twice as large as normal lymphocytes. They have cleaved or folded nuclei with well-defined nucleoli.
L3	Cells are homogeneously large. They contain round nuclei with well-defined nucleoli. Vacuoles usually present in the abundant cytoplasm.
	By Cell Type
T-cell ALL	Blasts form spontaneous rosettes with sheep RBCs.
B-cell ALL (also called "Burkitt cell ALL" or "ALL3")	Blasts do not form rosettes with sheep RBCs.
Non-A, non-B ALL	Clear characteristics of neither T cells nor B cells. Heavy chains often present in cytoplasm. Two subtypes of classification: *common ALL,* in which the blasts react with anti-ALL non-T, non-B serum, and *null cell,* in which they do not.

peripheral smear. CXR may reveal thymic or mediastinal infiltration, particularly in cases of T-cell ALL. Lactic acid dehydrogenase (LDH), uric acid, and blood urea nitrogen (BUN) are increased. The definitive diagnosis is based on bone marrow biopsy showing massive proliferation of primitive malignant cells. Peroxidase-staining cytoplasmic granules are absent (this distinguishes ALL cells from AML cells). On the other hand, an antigen marker, called the "common acute lymphoblastic leukemia antigen (CALLA)," is found in the majority of cases. Patients are initially treated with systemic drugs (vincristine, prednisone, mercaptopurine, and methotrexate), intrathecal methotrexate dissolved in spinal fluid, and/or central nervous system (CNS) radiation. This is followed by long-term maintenance with cytotoxic agents. The purpose of such rigorous therapy is to attack the leukemic cells in different phases of mitotic division. The goal is total eradication of malignant cells. Apparent cures are being achieved in one-third of patients.

Chronic myelogenous leukemia (CML) has been traditionally classified as a myeloproliferative disorder. However, unlike myeloproliferative cells, typical CML cells have a distinct cytogenic abnormality and are more likely to undergo further malignant change. Chromosome 22 loses large fragments, which attach to other chromosomes. Known as the "Philadelphia chromosome (Ph^1)," this abnormality is demonstrable in 90% of cases and is probably acquired, since it affects only myelogenous cells. The etiology of the disease is unknown. While its association with chemicals or drugs is ill-defined, high-dose radiation exposure, a heterozygous state for glucose-6-phosphate dehydrogenase (G-6-PD) deficiency, and chromosome mosaicism are definite risk factors. The incidence of the disease is 1.5 per 100,000, about 15% of all leukemias. It strikes men slightly more often than women, most cases appearing between ages 30 and 60. Since CML cells function normally and proliferate slowly, the early stages of the disease are often asymptomatic. Eventually, bone marrow hyperplasia leads to anemia, leukocytosis, thrombocytosis, and splenomegaly. This, in turn, is responsible for symptoms of fatigue, poor exercise tolerance, headaches, fever, bone pain, hemorrhagic manifestations (bleeding mucosa, ecchymoses, petechiae, retinal hemorrhages, hematuria), abdominal fullness, and left upper quadrant pain. High uric acid levels may cause gouty arthritis or renal problems. Chronic infections and thrombosis (splenic infarction, myocardial infarction, phlebitis) are common in advanced cases.

The diagnosis of CML should be suspected whenever unexplained leukocytosis is found in conjunction with splenomegaly. For the 10% of patients who are negative for the Ph^1 chromosome, mild leukocytosis associated with more pronounced anemia and/or thrombocytopenia is common. CML is confirmed by (1) bone marrow aspiration showing hypercellularity and an increased granulocyte/erythroid ratio, (2) blood detection of the Ph^1 chromosome, and (3) decreased leukocyte alkaline phosphatase (LAP) score. Staging systems have not been developed, and treatment is generally withheld in asymptomatic disease. The clinical disease is managed with cytotoxic drugs (usually busulfan) and irradiation (local or total body). Purine and pyrimidine antagonists and hydroxyurea may be used for maintenance and to control chronic phases. Although there is no cure, patients under treatment can lead normal lives for 10 or more years. Most patients die from transformation to AML (myeloblastic transformation) after many years. The prognosis is most guarded for those who are Ph^1 negative.

Chronic lymphocytic leukemia (CLL) is characterized by the slow proliferation of long-lived, mature lymphocytes (predominantly B lymphocytes). More common than CML, its average annual incidence is 3 per 100,000, or 25% of all leukemias. CLL usually develops after age 50 and strikes men twice as often as women. The exact cause is unknown. A genetic predisposition seems likely, since CLL is the most frequent type of leukemia occurring in multiple family members. However, no correlation with radiation exposure, chemicals, or drugs has been shown. Unlike ALL, the fraction of proliferating cells remains low. Although infiltration of bone marrow occurs, it interferes little with normal hematopoiesis until the disease is quite advanced. On the other hand, CLL cells are immunologically defective, responding sluggishly or not at all to immunologic stimuli and failing to differentiate into plasma cells (which are responsible for antibody production).

The early stages of CLL are unassociated with symptoms and, in fact, 25% of these cases are discovered by the finding of lymphocytosis on routine blood tests. White blood cell (WBC) counts range from slight elevations to over 1 million per cubic milliliter. Patients in advanced stages present with malaise, fatigue, anorexia, weight loss, and undue infections. Sinusitis, pneumonia, herpes zoster, a hyperactive reponse to insect bites, skin infections, low-grade fevers, and/or night sweats are common. Exams reveal progressive enlargement of the lymph nodes, liver, and spleen. As leukemic cells collect in the skin, eye orbits, conjunctivae, pharynx, lungs, pleura, heart, and gastrointestinal (GI) tract, exams reflect other changes in these organs as well. Enlarging lymph nodes compress bile ducts, causing jaundice, or venous return, causing priapism, pedal edema, and/or thrombophlebitis. Compromised bile and venous circulation also leads to the formation of anasarca and ascites. Thrombocytopenia produces bruising and other bleeding manifestations. Patients with signs or symptoms of CLL should be referred to a hematologist.

The definitive diagnosis of CLL is based on persistent absolute lymphocytosis and characteristic cell marker studies on lymph node biopsy. There is an increased percentage of small lymphocytes with round nuclei on bone marrow aspiration, though bone marrow studies are not usually required for diagnosis. Patients are staged according to one of the classifications noted in Table 7.4. Treatment in the early stages is not advocated. Symptomatic cases are managed with radiation therapy, chemotherapy (chlorambucil or cyclophosphamide), and corticosteroids (prednisone). As with all types of leukemia, ▶***leukemia organizations*** can offer patients and family invaluable support and information.

Malignant changes of stem cells in lymphocyte organs are responsible for the ***lymphomas. Non-Hodgkin's lymphomas*** are the most common, with 15,000–23,000 new cases being reported annually (3% of all new cancer diagnoses). A classification of their subtypes is based on the disease distribution and histologic features of the predominant cells (Table 7.5). The disease may also be divided into T-cell types and B-cell types (most common). Non-Hodgkin's lymphomas are found in children under age 2 but appear with increasing frequency after age 50. The etiology is unknown, though there has been some association with viruses, radiation exposure, immunodeficiency disorders, both genetic (ataxia telangiectasia, Wiskott-Aldrich syndrome, congenital sex-linked agammaglobulinemia, Chediak-Higashi syndrome) and acquired (renal allografts, immunosuppressive therapy, Sjögren's syndrome). The majority of patients present with painless enlargement for several months of one or more peripheral lymph nodes.

One-third of patients with non-Hodgkin's lymphomas (particularly those with diffuse histiocytic variants) present with extranodal disease, the GI tract being the most common primary site. They have symptoms of malabsorption, GI obstruction,

TABLE 7.4 CLL STAGING

Stage	Description
	Binet System (1978)
O	Absolute lymphocytosis greater than 15,000/mL^3
I	Stage O plus adenopathy
II	Stage O plus hepatosplenomegaly with or without adenopathy
III	Stage O with adenopathy and splenomegaly
IV	Stage O with anemia and/or thrombocytopenia (hemoglobin less than 10 g/dL, platelet count less than 100,000/mL).
	Rai's System (1975)
O	Absolute lymphocytosis greater than 15,000/mL^3
I	Stage O plus adenopathy
II	Stage O plus hepatomegaly and/or splenomegaly with or without adenopathy
III	Stage O plus anemia (hemoglobin less than 11 g/dL in men, 10 g/dL in women) with or without adenopathy, splenomegaly, or heptomegaly
IV	Stage O plus thrombocytopenia (platelet count less than 100,000/mL^3) with or without adenopathy, splenomegaly, or hepatomegaly

bleeding, or perforation. Other primary sites include bone (usually lytic lesions of the femur, tibia, humerus, scapula, or pelvis), thyroid, testes, female genital organs, and salivary glands. Primary lung lesions are rare, but metastases are quite common. The skin may be either a primary site or involved as part of the generalized disease. Extradural tumors may cause neurologic manifestations, while parenchymal infiltration, hypercalcemia, and hyperuricemia may seriously impair renal function. Fever, weight loss, night sweats, and other systemic manifestations are uncommon. Furthermore, peripheral blood smears are typically normal in the early disease, though lymphocytosis may be seen with the differentiated lymphomas and characteristic notched cells with the nodular, poorly differentiated lymphomas. However, as the disease progresses or bone marrow infiltration occurs, anemia, hepatosplenomegaly, hemorrhage, and other hematologic abnormalities may prevail. Hemolysis and liver changes often result in severe itching. Frank leukemic conversion is rare in adults but occurs in 25% of children. ***Sézary's syndrome,*** diffuse infiltration of the dermis with chronic erythroderma and abnormal lymphocytes on peripheral blood smears, characterizes a T-cell variant.

TABLE 7.5 NON-HODGKIN'S LYMPHOMAS: MAJOR DIVISIONS AND SUBTYPES

- Follicular (nodular) malignant lymphomas
  - With small lymphoid cells
  - With large lymphoid cells
  - With mixed cell types
- Diffuse malignant lymphomas
  - Well differentiated
  - With small, atypical or poorly differentiated lymphoid cells
  - With large lymphoid cells
    - Regular
    - Irregular
    - Immunoblastic
    - True histiocytic (very rare)
  - With small and large lymphoid cells mixed
  - Lymphoblastic
  - Burkitt's lymphoma—associated with t(14) chromosome translocations
  - Mycosis fungoides
  - Undifferentiated

TABLE 7.6 ANN ARBOR STAGING SYSTEM

Stage	Description
I	Malignancy confined to one lymphatic site or one extralymphatic site
II	Malignancy evident in two or more lymphatic areas, with or without involvement of a single extralymphatic area on the same side of the diaphragm
III	Lymphatic sites on both sides of the diaphragm, plus involvement of spleen and/or extralymphatic sites
IV	Diffuse involvement of extralymphatic sites, with or without lymphatic involvement

The diagnosis of non-Hodgkin's lymphoma is confirmed by lymph node biopsy. Patients should be referred to an oncologist. To determine the best mode of treatment, the specialist must carefully type and stage the disease, usually employing the Ann Arbor system (Table 7.6). Treatment centers on radiation therapy and/or chemotherapy, with various protocols depending on the variant and stage of disease. The outlook for patients with stage I and II disease is quite favorable. It has also improved for those with more advanced disease.

Hodgkin's disease is a fairly uncommon malignancy, with only 7,000 new cases being reported annually. Lymphocytes, histiocytes, eosinophils, and abnormal Reed-Steinberg giant cells proliferate in areas of T-lymphocyte concentration and then spread to contiguous structures. Cell type is used to classify Hodgkin's disease into four subtypes: lymphocytic predominance, nodular sclerosis (most common), mixed cellularity, and lymphocytic depletion. The incidence of the overall disease is bimodal, the first and highest peak occurring between ages 20 to 40 and the second over age 60. Asymmetric lymphadenopathy is the usual presentation. Any regional nodes may be affected, the cervical, axillary, and inguinal ones being the most common. Rubbery and nontender, the nodes may be matted, or discrete and freely movable. Occasionally, mediastinal nodes noted on routing chest x-ray films may be the initial clue. Fever, night sweats, fatigue, weight loss, and itching mark more advanced disease. A cyclic fever ***(Pel-Ebstein or Murchin type)*** is unusual but particularly significant. Developing every evening for several days, it disappears for days or weeks at a time, only to return. Recurrent bouts are progressively longer and more severe. Pain developing in a Hodgkin's region within a few minutes of alcohol ingestion is another striking symptom (mechanism unknown).

If unarrested, Hodgkin's cells spread first to adjacent lymph nodes and then to contiguous structures. The rates of spread and proliferation vary from months to years. Involvement of the pleura, lung parenchyma, and/or pericardium results in cardiopulmonary complications. Bone marrow and spleen infiltration leads to a number of hematologic abnormalities. Mild microcytic anemia and elevated counts of neutrophils, eosinophils, and thrombocytes may be seen initially. Absolute lymphopenia, which occurs in a small number of patients, is a poor prognostic sign. Spread from the bone marrow results in multiple osseous lesions characterized by either an osteoblastic or osteolytic x-ray appearance. Although painful, these bone lesions rarely lead to fractures. Disease of the spleen may be associated with progressive infiltration of portal spaces in the liver. Intrahepatic biliary obstruction and severe hepatic dysfunction follow. Peripheral neuropathies may develop as a direct result of tumor growth within epidural regions. Because such lesions may quickly transect the spinal cord or cauda equina, symptoms of back or neck pain, numbness, tingling, or weakness of an extremity, as well as bladder or bowel dysfunction, must be investigated as a medical emergency.

Finally, Hodgkin's disease is associated with immunologic abnormalities. Delayed hypersensitivity (cutaneous anergy) and an abnormal serum factor that is thought to interfere with T-cell function have been demonstrated. These changes undoubtedly contribute to the development of noncaseating granulomas in 20% of patients and to the risk of infection during immunosuppressive treatment. On the other hand, statistics show that the relatively well patient with Hodgkin's disease is no more susceptible to infections of any kind than the population at large.

The diagnosis of Hodgkin's disease is based on lymph node biopsy. Once it is established, the disease is staged according to the Ann Arbor classification (Table 7.6) to determine the best mode of treatment. The process begins with a careful history and physical exam, chest x-ray film, lower extremity lymphangiogram, liver-spleen scans, bone marrow biopsy, erythrocyte sedimentation rate (ESR), CBC, and liver and renal function tests. Depending on the results of these tests, computed tomography (CT) scans of the lungs, abdomen, and/or bone may be ordered. Exploratory laparotomy and splenectomy are done routinely if stage I or II is suspected, though both practices are under current review. In the past, treatment was quite specific for each of the staging categories as follows: I, IA—extended-field radiation to the affected nodal regions and subtotal lymphoid radiotherapy; IB—involved-field radiotherapy plus chemotherapy; IIIA—total nodal irradiation or combined chemotherapy and involved-field radiotherapy; IIIB—total nodal irradiation plus chemotherapy; IV—combination chemotherapy or chemotherapy plus radiation. For a while, oncologists were using combination radiation and chemotherapy (e.g., MOPP) no matter what the stage. However, this practice increased the number of patients who later developed frank myelogenous leukemia and pancytopenia. Today, stage specific treatment is again in vogue. Chances of cure are 75%–85% (95% in early stages).

The development of clone cells that have an abnormal tendency to proliferate but produce relatively functional cells leads to a group of closely related syndromes referred to as ***chronic myeloproliferative disorders.*** Included in the group and described in Table 7.7 are ***polycythemia rubra vera, agnogenic myeloid metaplasia,*** and ***primary thrombocytopenia. Chronic myelogenous leukemia*** has also been included in this classification, but since CML cells are associated with a distinct cytogenic abnormality (the Ph^1 chromosome), it is also classified as a leukemia (see the previous discussion). Arising autonomously, clones responsible for myeloproliferative disorders divide at much faster rates than normal, flooding the peripheral circulation with excess cells. If the clone has departed from an undifferentiated cell, proliferation of all of the cells lines occurs (polycythemia vera and agnogenic myeloid metaplasia). On the other hand, if it has departed from more committed stem cells, only one series predominates (primary thrombocythemia).

In any of the myeloproliferative diseases, a hypermetabolic state due to increased cell turnover may produce symptoms of fever, weight loss, sweating, or bone pain. For the same reason, uric acid levels often become elevated, contributing to the frequent occurrence of gout and kidney stones. Increased neutrophil alkaline phosphatase and increased vitamin B_{12} binding capacity in serum reflect the high rate of granulocyte turnover and are diagnostically important. Hypercellular activity in the bone marrow stimulates an overproduction of fibrous material. Fibrotic changes can be extensive enough to cause marrow failure. Marrow failure explains other variable

TABLE 7.7 CHRONIC MYELOPROLIFERATIVE DISORDERS

Disorder	Pathophysiology and Epidemiology	Signs and Symptoms	Diagnostic Findings and Treatment
Polycythemia rubra vera (Vaquez's disease)	Autonomous, abnormal clone emerges from a single multipotential stem cell, resulting in overproduction of the entire myeloid cell series (erythrocytes, megakaryocytes, granulocytes). Factors responsible for clone development are unknown. Common disease with a slight preference for men of Jewish descent.	Headaches, weakness and weight loss. Pruritis (aggravated by bathing) and facial "rubor." Manifestations of hyperviscosity including thrombosis, vertigo, tinnitis, paresthesias, cerebral ischemia. Ulcers and GI bleeds common. Splenomegaly present in 75% of cases.	Significant elevation of RBCs in peripheral blood, along with some increase in platelets and WBCs (except lymphocytes). Bone marrow is hypercellular, with low fat content. Uric acid and usually serum vitamin B_{12} are increased. Serum iron is normal unless there has been blood loss. Treatment consists of phlebotomies to maintain hematocrits below 50%. Eventually chemotherapy or ^{32}P may be needed.
Agnogenic myeloid metaplasia	Lung, kidney, liver, spleen, and other tissue having the embryonic potential become stimulated to resume active hematopoiesis. This usually follows fibrosis of bone marrow. The cause is unknown, though immune complex damage to bone marrow or development of an abnormal stem cell clone have been proposed. Strikes men and women equally. Occurs mainly in older age groups (two-thirds of patients are between ages 50 and 70).	Insidious development of weakness is the major symptom. Patients may also have gout, hearing impairment, and abdominal pain. Signs include pedal edema, and enlarged liver, spleen, and lymph nodes. Bleeding disorders common.	Diagnosis based on bone marrow biopsy. Early disease shows hyperplasia of erythrocytic, granulocytic, and particularly megakaryocytic series, with increased fibroblasts and reticulin fibers. Later there is diminished cellularity, dense fibrosis, dilated sinuses, and new bone formation. Ph^1 is absent. Uric acid and serum vitamin B_{12} are increased. Treatment is symptomatic, since chemotherapy is poorly tolerated.
Primary thrombocythemia	Abnormal clone emerges from a megakaryocyte stem cell, causing overproduction of platelets. The cause is unknown. Men and women are affected equally, with the peak incidence of disease occurring after age 50.	Deterioration in general health accompanied by coagulation disorders (both bleeding and thrombosis). Slight splenomegaly found on exam.	Platelets increased (usually more than 1,000,000/μL), with abnormal morphology (bizarre shapes and giant size). WBC count elevated (particularly neutrophils), but hemoglobin and hematocrit normal unless hemorrhaging has occurred. Bone marrow shows hypercellularity (predominance of megakaryocytes and platelets) and disappearance of fat cells. Platelet studies are abnormal. Uric acid and vitamin B_{12} are increased. Ph^1 chromosome absent. ^{32}P or chemotherapy required for treatment.

TABLE 7.8 FACTORS ASSOCIATED WITH THE DEVELOPMENT OF APLASTIC ANEMIA

Medical	Gold salts	Chlorpromazine
Pregnancy	Indomethacin	Meprobamate
Thymoma	Chloramphenicol	Chlordiazepoxide
Paroxysmal nocturnal hemoglobinuria (PNH)	Sulfamides	Antithyroid preparations
Idiopathic factors	Tolbutamide	Colchicine
Viral hepatitis	Chlorpropamide	Chemicals
Drugs	Methicillin	Benzene
Phenylbutazone	Hydantoins	Insecticides
	Phenothiazines	Radioactive materials

findings such as bizarrely shaped cells, anemia, leukopenia, and bleeding problems. Extramedullary hematopoiesis may develop, leading to hepatosplenomegaly and adenopathy. It is most extensive in agnogenic myeloid metaplasia, in which hematopoietic tissue develops indiscriminately in the spleen, liver, and lymph nodes, as well as the lungs, adrenal glands, kidneys, and other organs. Spleen enlargement can be extensive enough to produce symptoms of dyspepsia, abdominal pain, or fullness. The diagnosis of myeloproliferative disorders is based on the symptoms and findings outlined in Table 7.7. Treatment centers on controlling the cell masses with phlebotomies, chemotherapy, or radiation therapy. Complications from bleeding problems, hypermetabolic states, or marrow failure must also be managed.

Damage to the marrow or stem cells can inhibit the production of entire myelogenous series (erythrocytes, polymorphonucleocytes, monocytes, and thrombocytes). This condition is known as ***pancytopenia*** or, in severe cases, as ***aplastic anemia.*** A number of factors have been implicated in the development of aplastic anemia (Table 7.8). Many cases follow exposure to radiation, chemicals, drugs, or other diseases, but at least 50% have no explanation. The onset of disease may be marked by little more than pallor, weakness, and fatigue. If thrombocytopenia is severe, there may be ecchymosis, petechiae, or bleeding from mucous membranes. Fever without infection is common, although lymphadenopathy and splenomegaly are notably absent. CBCs may reveal severe granulocytopenia and thrombocytopenia, as well as severe anemia without reticulocytosis. Leukocyte alkaline phosphatase and serum iron levels rise. Bone marrow biopsy reveals focal areas of normal cellularity or even hypercellularity. Overall, however, there is a marked decrease of hematopoietic tissue, with an increase in iron storage and a high percentage of lymphocytes, although absolute lymphocyte counts are often decreased.

The first measure in the treatment of aplasia is to identify and remove any toxic agents. Hospitalization is necessary for blood transfusions, androgen/corticosteroid stimulation of residual marrow, and control of bleeding. Optimal treatment consists of marrow transplant with human leukocyte antigen (HLA)-compatible tissue from a sibling. When neutrophil counts fall below 500/mL, patients must be protected from infection. This entails reverse isolation, as well as measures to reduce normal bacterial colonies residing in the nasopharynx and GI tract. Patients should receive mouth and dental care, bowel preparations containing nonabsorbable antibiotics, and food with low bacterial contents. Systemic antibiotics are avoided unless there is an established infection.

Fanconi's anemia is a congenital form of aplastic anemia that is usually diagnosed in early childhood. In addition to pancytopenia, these patients often have underdeveloped kidneys and spleens, as well as a number of skeletal abnormalities.

RED BLOOD CELLS (RBCs)

Erythropoiesis

In the bone marrow, erythropoiesis begins when committed stem cells (BFU-E and CFU-E) differentiate to the proerythroblast (see Fig. 7.1). The proerythroblast passes through a series of internal alterations that are marked by a changing affinity for certain dyes described in Figure 7.3. During these stages, four divisions take place at daily intervals, resulting in a 16-fold increase in number. Even under normal conditions, about 10% of RBCs die before reaching the peripheral circulation as a result of intramedullary hemolysis or ineffective erythropoiesis. Those that survive produce increasing amounts of hemoglobin, protein chains that contain the oxygen-carrying heme complexes. Hemoglobin and heme complexes are discussed subsequently. During early maturation, cell size decreases but prominent nuclei remain.

When the cytoplasm of the forming red cell becomes one-third filled with hemoglobin, the cell's nucleus breaks apart. The fragments, which form a "reticulum" of ribosome strands, give the still immature cell the name "reticulocyte." Reticulocytes spend 3 days in the marrow and then pass through the marrow sinusoids into the circulation. Within the first 24 hours, vestiges of the reticulum disappear and the

STAGES OF ERYTHROPOIESIS

ERYTHROPOIESIS (MORPHOLOGIC CHARACTERISTICS OF CELL STAGES)

Cell Type (Size in μm)	*Nucleus*		*Cytoplasm*	
	Chromatin	*Nucleolus*	*Color*	
Proerythroblast (15 to 20)	Very fine	Visible	Basophilic	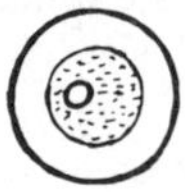
Basophilic erythroblast (12 to 18)	Fine	Absent	Basophilic	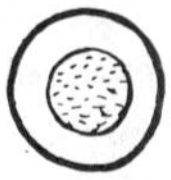
Polychromatophilic erythroblast (12 to 15)	Clumped	Absent	Polychro-matophilic	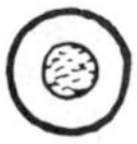
Acidophilic erythroblast (8 to 12)	Very dense	Absent	Red to purple	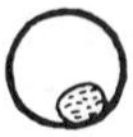
Reticulocyte (8 to 10)	No nucleus		Red, + reticulin	
Erythrocyte (7 to 8)			Red	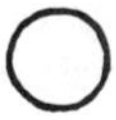

Figure 7.3 Erythropoiesis. (From Sultan, *Manual of Hematology,* © 1985, John Wiley & Sons, Inc., New York.)

cells become fully mature erythrocytes. Normally, the number of reticulocytes remains between 0.5 and 1.5% of the total RBC count. A higher percentage, referred to as ***reticulocytosis,*** may indicate that erythropoiesis has been stepped up to meet an increase in body need. However, to make this assumption, an absolute reticulocyte count, not merely a percentage, must be used. This is calculated by multiplying the reticulocyte percentage by the erythrocyte count. It must also be considered that in times of increased cell production, immature reticulocytes (known as "stress reticulocytes") are thrown into the circulation. Having a longer maturation period in the blood, these cells falsely boost the reticulocyte count. In anemic states, this increased maturation time should be taken into consideration when considering reticulocyte counts.

The mature RBC has a number of morphologic characteristics that are best studied on specially stained slides made from smears of peripheral blood samples (hence the term "peripheral smear"). In a healthy person, erythrocytes appear as homogeneous circular discs, the presence of abnormal shapes or structures being referred to as ***poikilocytosis.*** Normal cells have uniform sizes ranging from 6 to 8 μm in diameter. Small cells are called ***microcytes,*** large cells ***macrocytes,*** and size variations ***anisocytosis.*** Besides their appearance on peripheral smears, size variations may be indicated by mean cell volume (MCV). The MCV is calculated from the hematocrit and RBC count. Staining intensities provide a rough guide to the amount of hemoglobin contained by the cells, the center of each cell normally being somewhat paler than the periphery ***(normochromic).*** With diminished hemoglobin, the central area is broader and considerably paler ***(hypochromic).*** Increased hemoglobin is characterized by deeper staining and less central pallor ***(hyperchromic).*** Hemoglobin content is further assessed in terms of mean cell hemoglobin (MCH) and mean cell hemoglobin concentration (MCHC). The MCH is the hemoglobin weight of an average cell, and the MCHC is the concentration of hemoglobin in a volume of packed cells. Both indices are generally low in microcytic anemias. In macrocytic anemias, MCH is high but MCHC remains normal or decreased except in spherocytosis. These and other morphologic characteristics of RBCs are noted in Table 7.9.

Anemia as a general term is considered to be present if the hemoglobin concentration or the hematocrit falls below normal levels. Anemias are classified by morphology (macrocytic, normocytic, microcytic) or by the pathophysiologic mechanism involved (impaired production, accelerated destruction, blood loss). In some cases, several processes occur simultaneously. Classic signs and symptoms result from the diminished delivery of oxygen to the tissues but vary with a number of coinciding factors. These include the underlying disease process and its complications; the metabolic requirements of the tissues as conditioned by the illness; the capacity of the cardiovascular system to compensate; and the rate at which the anemia develops. When anemia develops slowly, it can be surprisingly well tolerated. In general, the anemic patient demonstrates the signs and symptoms noted in Table 7.10.

When DNA is impaired, cells neither divide nor mature properly, and the result is ***megaloblastic anemia.*** Only 4 macro-ovalocytes (large, oval-shaped cells) develop instead of 16 normocytes. To compensate for this low number, the marrow increases the production of red cell precursors. The ratio of megaloblasts to white cell precursors, usually 1:3, approches 1:1. As a result of this hyperplastic change (known as "megaloblastic"), white cells overmature. Hypersegmented neutrophils with six or more lobes appear in the peripheral circulation before anemia develops in 98% of cases. The anemia is described as macrocytic: MCV between 100 and 140, an

TABLE 7.9 SOME MORPHOLOGIC CHARACTERISTICS OF RBCs

Characteristic	Description	Significance
Size		
Macrocytes	Abnormally large cells.	Deficiencies of vitamin B_{12}, folic acid, copper, and/or ascorbic acid.
Microcytes	Abnormally small cells.	Iron deficiency, sideroblastic anemia, anemia of chronic disease.
Normocytic	Cells uniformly of normal size (roughly same as small lymphocyte, i.e., 6–8 μm in diameter)	Normal. Also found in anemia of chronic disease, aplastic anemia, and myeloproliferative disease.
Color		
Anisochromia (double population)	Presence of normochromic and hypochromic cells on same slide.	Sideroblastic anemia, posttransfusion, posttreatment in iron deficiency.
Hypochromia	Cells have decreased staining due to low hemoglobin content.	Iron deficiency, sideroblastic anemia, anemia of chronic disease.
Normochromia	Cells display normal staining (darker shading at periphery, with small central area of lighter shading).	Normal. Also found with anemia of chronic disease, aplastic anemia, myeloproliferative disease.
Polychromasia	Due to variation in RNA content, cells stain different colors (RNA-rich cells stain blue or purple).	Implies reticulocytosis from hemolysis or acute blood loss.
Shape		
Acanthocyte	Round cell with bulbous projection radiating from the cell membrane.	Abetalipoproteinemia, liver disease.
Burr cells	Irregular cells with prominent spicules radiating from the cell membrane.	Intravascular hemolysis.
Crenated cells	Round cells with sharp spicules radiating from the cell membrane.	Artifact, hyperosmolarity.
Elliptocytes	Oval-shaped cells. If there are less than 10%, considered normal.	Iron deficiency anemia, myelofibrosis, megaloblastic anemia, and sickle cell disease. Hereditary syndrome (hereditary elliptocytosis).
Helmet cells	Cells shaped like a helmet.	Intravascular hemolysis.
Poikilocytosis	Cells of varying shape noted on the same slide.	Megaloblastosis.
Schistocytes	Due to fragmentation, cells are variably sized, with an angular shape.	Intravascular hemolysis.
Sickle cells	Cells become elongated and doubled over in a C shape.	Sickle cell anemia.
Spherocytes	Spherical cells lacking a central depression.	Hereditary syndrome (hereditary spherocytosis), acquired hemolysis.
Stomatocytes	Central depression is shaped like a mouth.	Rh null cells, hereditary syndrome (hereditary stomatocytosis).
Target cells	Cells have bull's-eye appearance.	Obstructive jaundice, hypochromia (e.g., thalassemia, hemoglobin C).
Internal structure		
Basophilic Stippling	Scattered throughout the cytoplasm are fine, bluish-colored granules.	Fine stippling seen with increased production of RBCs. Coarse stippling with impaired hemoglobin synthesis, megaloblastosis.
Cabot rings	Within the cells can be seen rings, figure-eights, or loops that stain red or purple.	Abnormal erythropoiesis.
Heinz bodies	Hemoglobin precipitates within blood cells.	Oxidant stress.
Howell-Jolly bodies	Cells contain smooth, round chromatin residues.	Megaloblastic anemia, hemolytic anemia, postsplenectomy.

TABLE 7.10 GENERAL CHARACTERISTICS OF ANEMIA

Symptoms	Pale conjunctiva
Easy fatigability	Tachycardia
Dyspnea on exertion	Systolic murmur
Palpitations	Low blood pressure
Headache	Pronounced hypostatic tachycardia/hypotension
Dizziness	Dependent edema
Tinnitis	CHF
Signs	Fever
Pallor	Leukocytosis

elevated MCH, a normal MCHC, and macro-ovalocytes on peripheral smear. Serum iron is elevated or normal. Since large numbers of the abnormal megaloblasts are destroyed in the marrow, unconjugated bilirubin and LDH may be elevated. These two findings often lead to the mistaken diagnosis of hemolytic anemia.

DNA synthesis requires the enzyme tetrahydrofolate. Because tetrahydrofolate is reduced from circulating folic acid, megaloblastic anemia can develop from ▶ ***folic acid deficiency.*** The body converts properties found in fruits, vegetables, dairy products, and yeast into folic acid. These properties are measured as folacin, and though food concentrations are rather low, so are body requirements. As described in Table 7.11, pregnancy, infections, malabsorption syndromes, hemolysis, certain drugs, and other conditions increase folic acid requirements or change its utilization. Body stores (primarily the liver) last for only 3 months, and therefore, anemia develops relatively fast. Once serum levels of folate fall, hypersegmented neutrophils appear by 11 weeks, macro-ovalocytes by 18 weeks, and anemia within 3–6 months. Persons with folate deficiency anemia can be asymptomatic or note fatigue, dizziness, or weakness. If severely malnourished, they may also have diarrhea, cheilosis, or glossitis. The diagnosis is based on findings of megaloblastic anemia, normal vitamin B_{12} levels, and low serum folate levels. The latter is often less than 2 ng/mL. Because neurologic complications of vitamin B_{12} deficiency can be complicated by folic acid replacement, vitamin B_{12} assays must be included as part of the work-up. It should also be noted that serum levels of folate can be subnormal even though stores are adequate. Therefore, a low serum level without a finding of hypersegmented neutrophils or macrocytic anemia does not indicate a deficiency. Treatment consists of improved diet and daily supplements of folic acid. If possible, any folic acid antagonist, such as methotrexate, pyrimethamine, or trimethoprim, should be discontinued.

The circulating form of folic acid cannot be used for DNA synthesis until it is converted to tetrahydrofolate. The conversion is made by the enzyme homocystine methyltransferase, which is vitamin B_{12} dependent. Thus, ***vitamin B_{12} deficiency*** leads to megaloblastic anemia. Since this vitamin is needed for the high turnover of cells in the GI tract, the anemia is often accompanied by anorexia, weight loss, constipation, or sometimes diarrhea. The tongue becomes swollen and sore, with a smooth, beefy red appearance. Besides anemia, a serious consequence of vitamin B_{12} deficiency is demyelination of nerve tissue. The spinal cord, cerebrum, and/or peripheral nerves can be affected. Degenerative changes develop in the dorsal and lateral columns of the spinal cord, producing the so-called subacute combined system disease. The first symptoms are numbness and tingling of the extremities, followed later by weakness, poor coordination, sphincter disturbance, and altered reflexes.

TABLE 7.11 FACTORS ALTERING NORMAL BODY USE OF FOLIC ACID

Poor dietary intake	Amyloidosis affecting the bowel
Increased requirements	Diabetic enteropathy
Pregnancy	Bowel resections
Severe hemolysis	Drug interference with folic acid metabolism
Long-term hemodialysis	Methotrexate
Decreased absorption	Trimethoprim
Tropical sprue	Pyrimethamine
Nontropical sprue (gluten sensitivity)	Phenytoin
Crohn's disease	Ethanol
Lymphoma	Antitubercular drugs
	Oral contraceptives

Mentation changes vary from irritability and forgetfulness to acute psychosis. It is important to note that neurologic disease can devleop while the hematocrit is still normal. If the vitamin B_{12} deficiency is not corrected in its early stages, the changes are irreversible.

As one of the few mammals that does not synthesize vitamin B_{12}, man must acquire it through diet. In the United States, ▶ ***vitamin B_{12} deficiency related to diet*** is rare. However, strict vegetarians are at risk because the vitamin (also called "extrinsic factor") is made by intestinal bacteria and found only in animal products: meat, fish, eggs, and dairy. Megaloblastic anemia due to vitamin B_{12} deficiency can be readily identified by taking a careful diet history and checking serum levels of folate and vitamin B_{12}. The treatment consists of increasing the food sources of the vitamin or providing supplements. A number of breakfast cereals are now fortified with vitamin B_{12}, and slight amounts can be obtained from vegetables grown in fresh manure. The belief that yogurt is a good source is not true (it would take 10 lb to supply the recommended daily amount).

▶ ***Vitamin B_{12} deficiency due to malabsorption*** is more common. Certain intestinal problems may cause this problem because the vitamin is absorbed principally from the lower small bowel. These conditions include celiac disease, tropical sprue, fish tapeworm, bacterial proliferation (bacteria ingest large amounts of vitamin B_{12}), terminal ileum resection, and inflammatory diseases. Primary failure of the intestine to absorb the vitamin is called ***Immerslund-Grasbeck syndrome,*** but this is quite rare. Malabsorption of vitamin B_{12} is demonstrated by the Schilling test. If it is present, vitamin B_{12} injections may help correct the deficiency.

Vitamin B_{12} deficiency from lack of intrinsic factor ***(pernicious anemia)*** is a third cause. Intrinsic factor is a protein produced by gastric parietal cells. In the acid environment of the stomach, it binds vitamin B_{12} for passage to the small bowel. In the intestine, the vitamin is absorbed into the blood and given up to a group of transporting proteins (transcobalamin I, II, and III). It is carried by transcobalamin II to the liver, where it is converted to an active form used to reduce folic acid to tetrahydrofolate. Lack of intrinsic factor interrupts the entire process. It results from gastrectomy or damage to the gastric mucosa from corrosive agents. It is also thought that parietal cells are destroyed by an autoimmune reaction, since 80% of patients have antibodies to parietal cells and 50% to intrinsic factor. Furthermore, many of them have Graves' disease, myxedema, thyroiditis, myasthenia gravis, hypothyroidism, or other immune disorders. Gastric atrophy involving only the acid- and pepsin-secreting portion of the stomach is a characteristic finding.

Occurring in all ethnic groups, pernicious anemia affects men as often as women. It is rarely seen in persons below age 30 and most often occurs after age 60. Because the liver stores enough vitamin B_{12} to last for several years, anemia develops slowly and can be surprisingly well tolerated. It is not uncommon for hematocrits to fall below 20% before patients present with symptoms of pallor, weakness, dizziness, palpitations, or congestive heart failure (CHF). Premature gray hair and mild jaundice may be noted. The anemia is often accompanied by GI symptoms including anorexia, weight loss, constipation, or sometimes diarrhea. The tongue may be swollen and sore, with a smooth, beefy red appearance. Pernicious anemia is diagnosed from the Schilling test, along with findings of megaloblastic anemia, serum levels of vitamin B_{12} below 100 mg/mL, and normal or high folate levels. The histamine achlorhydria test demonstrates gastric atrophy. Some patients with pernicious anemia require hospitalization for blood transfusions and CHF management. In less severe cases, treatment can be initiated on an outpatient basis. Cyanocobalamin, a form of vitamin B_{12}, is given IM on a weekly basis for 4 weeks and then monthly for life. The response is dramatic, with clinical symptoms improving in the first few days, reticulocytosis peaking within a week, and anemia clearing over the next couple of months. Hypokalemia and salt retention can develop early in the course of treatment and should be watched. With ongoing replacement, patients have no further problems with anemia. However, 1–2% develop carcinoma of the stomach. Cancer screening is therefore an important aspect of follow-up care.

Heme Complex

The heme complex contains a single atom of iron bound to four atoms of nitrogen by a system of porphyrin rings. The complicated synthesis (Fig. 7.4) takes place in most body cells, but mainly in erythroid precursors. It begins with the formation of aminolevulinic acid (ALA). This vital building block is condensed by a mitochondrial reaction that requires vitamin B_6 (pyridoxine) as a cofactor. Two molecules of ALA are condensed to form porphobilinogen. Four molecules of porphobilinogen are joined to form a tetrapyrole ring that is converted in stages to protoporphyrin. The porphyrin ring receives iron as the final step in heme formation. By transferring electrons, the iron atom can bind and release an oxygen molecule.

If ALA synthesis is defective, iron fails to be incorporated into the porphyrin ring during RBC formation. It collects in granules (siderin) around the blast's nucleus. The abnormal cell (sideroblast) characterizes a group of disorders known as the ***sideroblastic anemias.*** They may be hereditary, acquired, or secondary to drugs or toxins, as noted in Table 7.12. Hereditary forms often follow an X-linked pattern that affects mostly men. Acquired disorders are associated with underlying illnesses such as malignancy, inflammatory diseases, or drugs that interfere with vitamin B_6 metabolism. Sideroblastic anemias are diagnosed by the presence of a normochromic or hypochromic, normocytic anemia and the finding of a large number of sideroblasts upon iron staining of bone marrow specimens. Because iron is not being incorporated into the cells, serum iron levels increase and iron-binding proteins remain completely saturated. Excess stores of iron may lead to deposition in the skin or in organ parenchyma. The latter may lead to hypersplenomegaly or damage to the pancreas or heart. Indirect bilirubin increases in the blood and fecal urobilinogen occur. Only a few inherited forms of sideroblastic anemia respond to vitamin B_6. Treatment for secondary sideroblastic anemia centers on the underlying cause. In some cases,

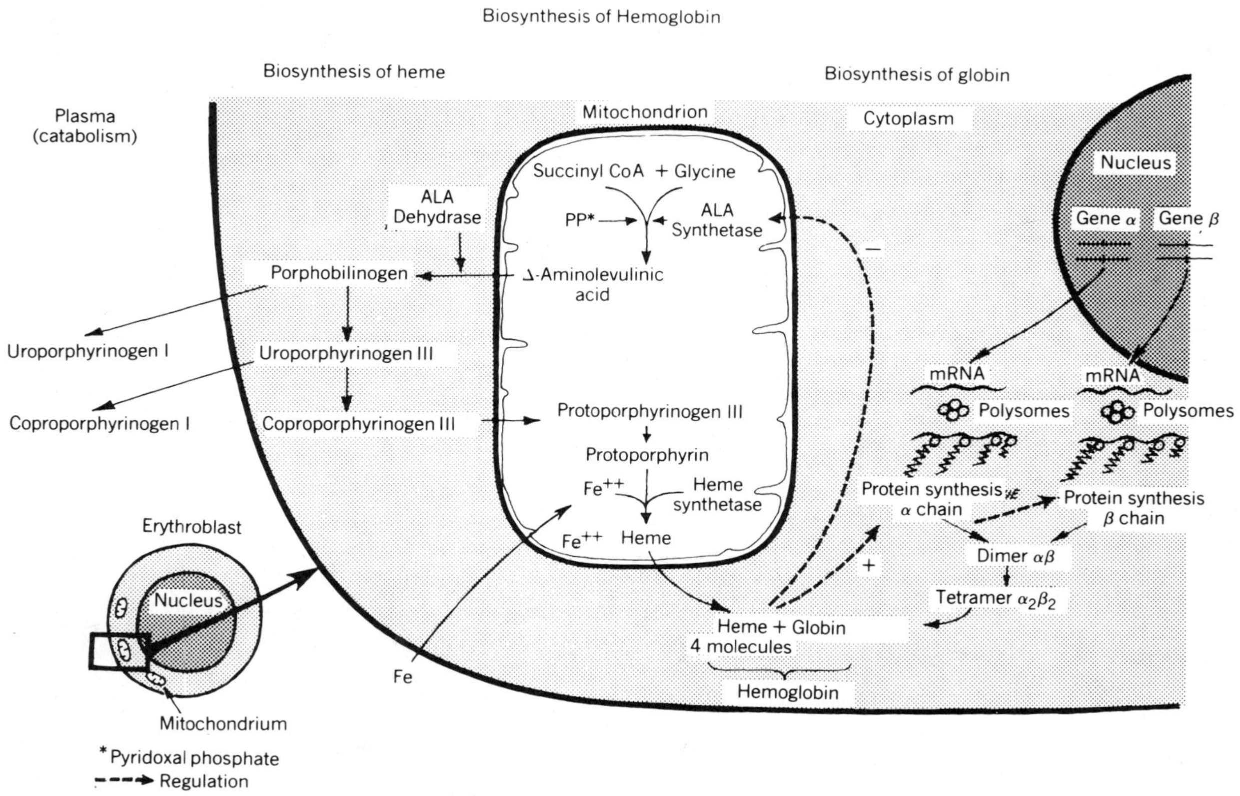

Figure 7.4 Heme synthesis. (From Sultan, *Manual of Hematology,* © 1985, John Wiley & Sons, Inc., New York.)

TABLE 7.12 SIDEROBLASTIC ANEMIAS

Inherited
  Sex-linked sideroblastic anemia
    Pyridoxine-responsive
    Non-pyridoxine-responsive
  Thalassemic syndromes and related hemoglobinopathies
 	
Acquired
  Associated with:
    Agnogenic myeloid metaplasia
    Erythrocytic hyperplasia (idiopathic sideroblastic anemia or AISA)
    Myelodysplasia
    Myeloma and other neoplasms
    Granulomatous diseases
    Rheumatoid arthritis
	Secondary to drugs or toxins
	  Chloramphenicol
	  Alkeran, cytoxin
	  Cytosine arabinoside
	  Androgen therapy
	  Chlorambucil
	  Phenacetin
	  Antitubercular therapy
	  Lead intoxication
	
	Secondary to vitamin deficiencies
	  Vitamin B_{12}
	  Folate

withdrawing an offending drug [notably alcohol or isoniazid (INH)] or correcting the underlying disease process may lead to resolution of the anemia. If not, patients should be given vitamin B_6, and folic acid supplements for a 2-month trial period and, failing that, androgen therapy. Idiopathic cases are only rarely corrected by either vitamin B_6, folate, or androgen therapy, and 10% of these patients develop acute myelogenous leukemia. Continuous follow-up is important even though the anemia remains stable. In all cases of sideroblastic anemia, iron-containing medications are contraindicated. If iron deposition occurs, chelating agents may be necessary in selected patients.

Those conditions improving with B6 therapy are referred to as ▶***pyridoxine-responsive anemias.*** Patients with inherited enzyme disorders that interfere with B6 metabolism require treatment of life (pyridoxine dependent). Those with acquired problems usually respond to a two-month course of the vitamin along with correction of underlying disorders (pyridoxine deficient). In both cases, diet and patient education are important as well.

Lead blocks the synthesis of ALA. ***Lead poisoning*** therefore interferes with heme formation and normal erythropoiesis. ***Acute lead poisoning*** is seen in children (mostly due to eating chips of lead-based paint) but is nonexistent in adults, in whom lead absorption is slow. Adults, however, may develop ***chronic lead poisoning*** from prolonged exposure to solders, paint sprays, remelting processes, or fumes from burning storage batteries. Chronic lead poisoning has also been traced to food cooked and served in homemade pottery and the ingestion of "moonshine" whiskey. Lead levels rise slowly, but once toxic levels are reached, signs and symptoms develop suddenly. Patients may experience agonizing abdominal pain (painter's cramps) or neuritis with paralysis of frequently used muscle groups. Wrist and foot drop is common. Lead sulfide concentrations may appear along the gums, leaving a characteristic grayish "lead line" just above the teeth. This sign is absent in persons who maintain good oral hygiene, as well as those who are edentulous. Lead poisoning is diagnosed from blood tests showing increased lead levels. Anemia tends to be mild, but peripheral smears show large numbers of microcytic, normochromic cells with basophilic stippling. Treatment in all cases begins with identifying and removing the source of lead contamination. Patients with mild cases are given an iron-rich diet and iron supplements. Those with encephalopathy, neuropathy, or abdominal

TABLE 7.13 PORPHYRIAS

Erythropoietic Gunther's disease (congenital erythropoietic porphyria) PROTO (excess protoporphyrin) Hepatic with neurologic manifestations Acute intermittent porphyria	Hereditary COPRO (excess coproporphyrin) Variegate porphyria Hepatic without neurologic manifestations Porphyria cutanea tarda Hepatotoxins (e.g., fungicides, industrial chemicals)

symptoms must be hospitalized and treated with chelating agents (dimercaprol, calcium disodium edetate, and/or D-penicillamine).

Abnormal porphyrin synthesis is responsible for a number of inherited or acquired disorders called the ***porphyrias.*** These disorders are divided into erythropoietic and hepatic groups according to the major site of error (Table 7.13). Each is defined by a unique pattern of overproduction, accumulation, and excretion of porphyrin or porphyrin precursors—alpha aminolevulinic acid (ALA), porphobilinogen (PBG), uroporphyrin (URO), coproporphyrin (COPRO), and protoporphyrin (PROTO). Due to the chemical properties of porphyrin, spectacular changes in blood and urine may be noted. Immature erythrocytes fluoresce in the dark, while urine darkens visibly to a deep red color when exposed to light. Patients with PROTO develop cutaneous photosensitivity. Within minutes of sunlight exposure, the skin burns, itches, and becomes erythematous ("solar urticaria"). Although the attack subsides spontaneously, repeated episodes may lead to thickening of the skin ("solar eczema"). Whenever plasma levels of ALA and PGB increase in certain hepatic porphyrias, patients may suffer neurologic problems such as seizures, psychosis, paresis, respiratory paralysis, electrolyte imbalances, and neurogenic bowel. Episodes may be exacerbated by the drugs listed in Table 7.14. Patients with accumulations of other products develop liver dysfunction, as well as severe skin changes marked by bullae, vesicles, and ulcers. Further discussion appears in Chapters 5 and 10.

If iron is unavailable for heme construction during erythropoiesis, iron deficiency anemia develops. This is discussed in a later section.

Hemoglobin

During RBC formation, four types of globin chains (alpha, beta, delta, and gamma) are manufactured along with heme complexes (see Fig. 7.4). During the final stages of cell maturation, four globin chains enfold four heme groups to form a single molecule of hemoglobin. The heme groups appear on the surface of the chains, where they can readily combine with oxygen. Normally, three types of hemoglobin are found in every adult: HbA, HbF, and HbA2. Made from two identical alpha chains and two identical beta chains, HbA is the most abundant (98% of total hemoglobin). HbF is the major hemoglobin of the fetus and newborn. It is similar to HbA except that gamma chains are found in place of beta chains. After birth, the gamma chains convert to beta chains and HbF becomes HbA. By adulthood, only trace amounts of HbF are left (less than 0.5%). HbA2 consists of two alpha chains and two delta chains. It constitutes only 2% of the total hemoglobin.

Hemoglobinopathy results from malformation of one or more globin chains. Mutations (often the substitution of a simple amino acid) are usually inherited as a

TABLE 7.14 DRUGS THAT MAY PRECIPITATE AN ATTACK OF PORPHYRIA

Antimicrobials	Glutethimide
Chloroquine	Methsuximide
Griseofulvin	Methyprylon
Sulfonamides	Ergot preparations
Seizure, migraine, and psychiatric medications	Miscellaneous
Barbiturates	Chlorpropamide
Hydantoins	Dichloralphenazone
Imipramine	Methyldopa
Meprobamate	Estrogens
Chlordiazepoxide	Ethanol

dominant trait, giving rise to variable expressions of disease. There may be ***heterozygous, hemizygous, homozygous,*** or ***double heterozygous*** disease, as noted in Table 7.15. There are more than 400 hemoglobinopathies. A few are listed in Table 7.16.

The ***beta-thalassemias*** develop from a mutation in the gene directing the production of beta globin. Beta chains fail to replace gamma chains after birth, and large amounts of HbF remain. Persons who have inherited the mutation from only one parent have beta-thalassemia minor ***(Cooley's trait).*** Blood studies show an elevation of HbA2 and HbF, with mild hypochromia and microcytosis, but patients are rarely anemic. Persons who inherit the mutation from both parents express a pure form of disease known as ***Cooley's anemia.*** The two variations are described in Table 7.17.

Normally, production of alpha globin is directed by four genes, two from each chromosome 16-pair. The ***alpha-thalassemias*** develop from deletions of one, two, three, or all four of the genes directing the production of alpha globin. If four abnormal genes are passed on, death occurs in utero from a severe homozygous disease called ***hydrops fetalis.*** If three abnormal genes are passed on, the patient has a milder form of homozygous disease, ***hemoglobin H. Alpha-thalassemia minor*** and ***silent carrier*** are heterozygous expressions. All types are described in Table 7.18.

The most common hemoglobinopathy in the Untied States is the heterozygous condition called ▶ ***sickle cell trait*** (HbSA). As a result of valine replacement on the surface of the beta chain, the abnormal hemoglobin (HbS) is subject to polymerization and crystal formation when O_2 is extremely low. Becoming rigid, HbS causes the cell to deform into a sickle shape. Sickled cells are vulnerable to trauma in the bloodstream and are readily trapped by the spleen. This leads to hemolysis and

TABLE 7.15 EXPRESSIONS OF HEMOGLOBINOPATHIES

Heterozygous: Gene mutation inherited as a dominant trait from one parent. Associated with few or no symptoms.

Hemizygous: Gene mutation inherited as a dominant trait in a sex-linked pattern.

Homozygous: If both parents are heterozygous, each of their children has a 25% chance of being homozygous. In other words, the child inherits two abnormal genes (one from each parent) and expresses a pure form of the disease.

Double heterozygous: Trait for one type of hemoglobinopathy inherited from the mother and trait for an entirely different trait inherited from the father.

TABLE 7.16 SOME HEMOGLOBINOPATHIES

Hemoglobin S (sickle cell) disease
  Sickle cell trait
  Sickle cell disease
	Iwate
	Saskatoon
	Hyde Park
	Milwaukee

Hemoglobin C disease	

Hemoglobin S-C disease	Unstable hemoglobinopathies
	  Hammersmith
	  Zurich
	  Sydney
	  Philly
	  Genova
	  Sabine
	  Bushwick

Thalassemias
  Cooley's anemia
  Beta-thalassemia trait
  Alpha-thalassemia trait
  Hydrops fetalis
  Hemoglobin H
  Silent carrier	

Hemoglobin S-beta thalassemia	Abnormal hemoglobins with altered oxygen affinity
	  Kempsey
	  Kansas

Hemoglobin M Boston	

anemia. Such biologic transformation probably evolved as a protective response to malaria. Sickling, occurring with oxidative stress produced by parasite invasion, results in cellular destruction, thereby shortening one of the propagation stages. In patients with sickle cell trait, HbS represents 30–45% of HbA. These amounts are sufficient to cause sickling in conditions that alter oxygen tension, such as high altitudes, air travel, respiratory infection, anesthesia, or acidosis. Even in these cases, sickling usually has relatively few consequences. An impaired ability to concentrate urine and hematuria from papillary necrosis are the most common complications. For the most part, patients with sickle cell trait remain asymptomatic. Cell counts and peripheral smears are usually normal. Patients are diagnosed on the basis of positive sickle cell preparations and solubility tests. Electrophoresis typically shows 50–70% HbA, 30–45% HbS, normal HbF, and normal to slightly increased HbA2. Specific treatment for sickle cell trait is usually not necessary. However, screening, education about the disorder, and genetic counseling are quite important.

In contrast, ***sickle cell disease*** (homozygous HbSS) is a serious disorder inherited by 0.1–0.2% of U.S. blacks. Clinical manifestations appear early in life. Sickling

TABLE 7.17 BETA-THALASSEMIAS

Subtype	Pathogenesis	Clinical Course
Beta-thalassemia trait	Heterozygous for an abnormal gene governing the synthesis of beta globin chains	Mild anemia with microcytosis and hypochromia.
Cooley's anemia	Homozygous for an abnormal beta globin gene with pure form of disease; marked deficiency of beta globin synthesis, but normal synthesis of alpha globin.	From birth, severe anemia, growth retardation, hepatosplenomegaly, bone marrow expansion. Eventual development of bone deformities. Divided into two subgroups: Patients with *thalassemia major* must have constant transfusions for survival. Patients with *thalassemia intermedia* are able to maintain hemoglobin levels above 6 g without transfusions.

TABLE 7.18 ALPHA-THALASSEMIAS

Type	Pathogenesis	Clinical Course
Alpha-thalassemia	Heterozygous for gene deletion from chromosome 16 (normally four genes govern the synthesis of alpha globin).	Mild microcytic, hypochromic anemia.
Hydrops fetalis	Homozygous expression whereby all four genes are missing.	Death in utero.
Hemoglobin H	Homozygous for one chromosome with two deleted genes and the other with one deleted gene.	Variable expression. Patients usually have moderately severe hemolytic anemia, icterus, and splenomegaly.
Silent carrier	Heterozygous for one normal chromosome and one with a deleted gene (inherited from a parent with hemoglobin H disease).	No hematologic symptoms.

occurs even at physiologic O_2 tensions, so that hemolysis is chronic. To compensate for the continual destruction of cells, the marrow becomes hyperplastic, resulting in a number of bone changes. Marrow spaces expand, the cortex thins out, and radial striations appear on skull films (the "hair-on-end" sign). Even with hyperplastic marrow activity, however, patients remain anemic. The anemia may be protective in that it limits the number of sickle cells in the blood. More important, it reduces viscosity, or the "Trojan horse" phenomenon. A normally shaped cell enters a capillary, where it sickles. Cells pile up behind it, cutting off the O_2 supply to the tissue. This causes debilitating episodes of bone, joint, or abdominal pain ***(sickle crisis).*** Tissue infarctions follow. Along with hemolysis, they are responsible for the clinical signs and symptoms noted in Table 7.19.

In addition to the striking clinical manifestations, the diagnosis of sickle cell disease is based on a number of distinct laboratory findings. Although erythrocytes are usually normocytic and normochromic, normoblasts, target cells (up to 30%), Howell-Jolly bodies, and sickle cells are regularly present. Osmotic fragility is decreased, while mechanical fragility is increased. There may be leukocytosis, which is not necessarily indicative of infection. Electrophoresis shows over 80% HbS, no HbA, 1–20% HbF, and 2–4.5% HbA2. Patients with sickle cell disease should be handled by a specialist. No treatment is currently available for sickle cell disease, although multivitamins and 1 mg of folic acid may be given daily to avoid megaloblastic impairment. Treatment of sickle crisis includes rest, hydration, pain control, and electrolyte corrections. Severe crisis necessitates exchange transfusions or plasmapheresis. Most patients face a long and difficult course. ▶ ***Sickle cell organizations*** can offer guidance, support, and encouragement.

Hemoglobin C is present in 2–3% of U.S. blacks. Cells containing this insoluble form of hemoglobin are relatively rigid. As a result, they become fragmented and lose membrane material noted on peripheral smear as target cells and/or microspherocytes. Both heterozygous and homozygous forms are asymptomatic, though homozygous disease may be marked by mild hemolytic anemia and splenomegaly. The diagnosis is supported by finding hemoglobin C crystals in erythrocytes that have been dehydrated (by incubation or hypertonic solutions) and then stained. It is confirmed by hemoglobin electrophoresis. No therapy is necessary.

Sickle cell-hemoglobin C disease may result from double heterozygous expres-

TABLE 7.19 SIGNS AND SYMPTOMS OF SICKLE CELL DISEASE

Hemolytic anemia	Hyperviscosity with tissue infarctions
Heart murmurs	Abdominal and limb pain
Cardiomegaly	Autosplenectomy with increased susceptibility to infections (notably pneumococcus and hemophilus influenza)
Dyspnea on exertion	Damage to renal vasculature (inability to concentrate urine, hematuria)
Palpitations	Damage to retinal vessels (repeated vitreous hemorrhage)
Delayed skeletal and sexual maturation	Leg ulcers
Jaundice and cholelithiasis	CNS infarctions with seizures, hemiparesis, or severe brain damage
Splenomegaly	
Nontender hepatomegaly	
Aplastic crisis	
Folic acid deficiency	

sion. Occurring with some frequency (in 0.1–0.2% of U.S. blacks), this variant is characterized by almost equal amounts of HbS and HbC, 1–2% HbF, small amounts of HbA2, and an absence of HbA. Except for splenomegaly, most patients remain asymptomatic, unless surgery or another medical crisis precipitates sickling and hemolysis. On the other hand, some have a more severe course than patients with sickle cell disease. The diagnosis is suggested by finding both target cells and sickle cells on peripheral smear. It is confirmed by hemoglobin electrophoresis. Management of sickle cell-hemoglobin C disease is similar to that of sickle cell disease.

Some of the hemoglobinopathies affect the structural stability of the molecules and are thus known as ***unstable hemoglobin variants.*** Often the heme complex dislodges. Should this happen, the hemoglobin chain collapses and its debris leaves an intracellular precipitate, the Heinz body. Erythrocytes with large concentrations of Heinz bodies are destroyed by reticuloendothelial cells, and hemolytic anemia may result. Small amounts of the precipitate are sometimes removed in a process called "pitting," and the cell is spared. Hemolytic crisis with jaundice can develop with exposure to oxidant drugs such as sulfa, nitrofurantoin, or nalidixic acid. Such drugs should be avoided as the main aspect of treatment.

In the ***stable hemoglobin variants,*** the heme complex remains secure, but its functional behavior is altered and the molecule has an abnormal affinity for O_2. Some variants have an increased affinity, resulting in abnormal unloading of O_2 into the tissues and chronic hypoxia. Ironically, hematocrit levels are usually high, since the hypoxia stimulates erythropoiesis. Other than a ruddy complexion, patients are generally unaffected. Other variants have decreased O_2 affinity. They cause a cyanotic appearance due to partially unsaturated arterial blood. The appearance looks more serious than it is; other blood functions and values remain normal.

Oxygen Transport and Cellular Metabolism

During respiratory exchange in the lungs, electrons from iron atoms of the four heme complexes partially transfer to oxygen, binding four oxygen molecules to each hemoglobin chain. With 280 million hemoglobin chains, a single RBC has an enormous oxygen-carrying capacity. Erythrocytes carry O_2-laden hemoglobin (oxyhemoglobin) throughout the body. The reaction between O_2 and hemoglobin is reversible, O_2 diffusing out of the cell and into the tissues wherever O_2 pressure is low. The lower the pressure, the more readily O_2 is given up. This fact is reflected by the oxygen dissociation curve. Oxygen reversibility also depends on the electron transfer of iron atoms in heme complexes. If iron is in a ferric rather than a ferrous state, oxygen fails to dissociate. Each day, 3% of hemoglobin remains fixed in an oxidized form called "methemoglobin." However, most of this methemoglobin is eventually reduced back to hemoglobin.

Deoxygenated hemoglobin combines with CO_2 (carbinohemoglobin). Carbinohemoglobin transports about 30% of the CO_2 back to the lungs for elimination. By carrying another 60% of the CO_2 in the form of intracellular potassium bicarbonate, erythrocytes provide the main source of transport for CO_2 wastes. For this reason and because hemoglobin has a high affinity for H^+ ions, erythrocytes play an important role in acid-base balance as well as oxygen transport.

Oxygen transport and delivery depend on cellular metabolism. Having no nucleus, ribosomes, or mitochondria, RBCs have the capacity for neither cell division, protein synthesis, nor oxidative phosphorylation. They have a simple metabolic scheme fueled only by glucose. Through enzyme activities, 90% of the glucose is metabolized along the Embden-Meyerhof pathway and the remaining 10% along the hexose monophosphate shunt. The products of these pathways (Fig. 7.5) are crucial to RBC function. Listed in Table 7.20, ***enzyme deficiencies*** along the Embden-Meyerhof pathway affect deformability or oxygenation/deoxygenation. Those along the hexose-monophosphate shunt leave RBC membranes unprotected from the oxidizing effect of certain drugs and toxins.

The ***gluocose-6-phosphate dehydrogenase (G-6-PD) deficiencies*** are due to mutations of the erythrocytic G-6-PD enzyme. While such mutations have been discovered in all ethnic groups, the highest incidence occurs in populations from malaria endemic areas. As with sickle cell anemia, such biologic transformations probably evolved as a protective response. Unable to withstand the oxidative stress produced by malarial invasion, RBCs lacking G-6-PD hemolyze prematurely, shortening one of the propagation stages of the malaria parasite. The deficiency is inherited as a sex-linked trait. With the genetic coding located on the X chromosome, the

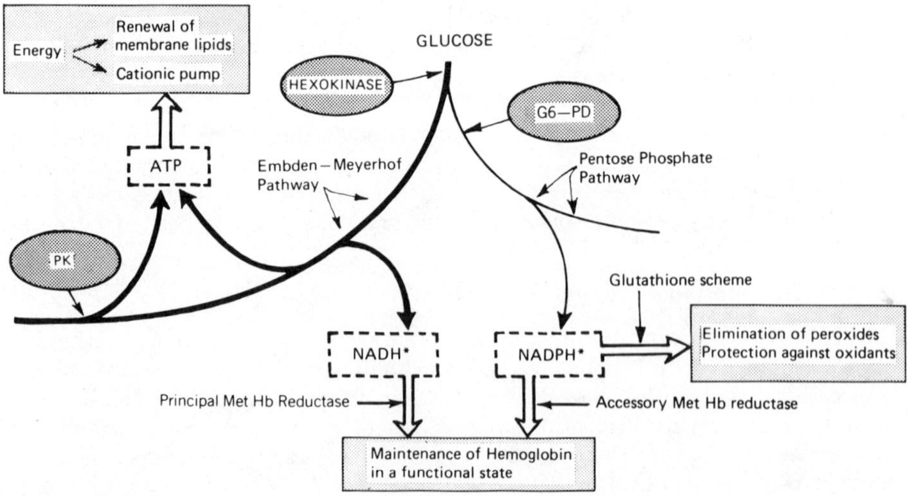

Figure 7.5 RBC glycolysis: Emboden-Meyerhof and pentose phosphate pathways. (From Sultan, *Manual of Hematology,* © 1985, John Wiley & Sons, Inc., New York.)

TABLE 7.20 SOME ENZYME DEFICIENCIES

Along the aerobic pathway	Along the anaerobic pathway
G-6-PD	Pyruvate kinase
Glutathione synthetase	Hexokinase
Glutathione reductase	Triose phosphate isomerase
Glutathione peroxidase	3-Phosphoglycerate

defect may be expressed fully in male hemizygotes and female homozygotes but variably in female heterozygotes (see Table 7.15). Furthermore, in heterozygous cases, two populations of RBCs (normal and G-6-PD deficient) may exist in varying proportions, a condition known as ***mosaicism.*** This is the most common expression of the disease. In white and Oriental populations, severe deficiencies are the rule (enzyme activity ranging from 0 to 5%).

U.S. blacks, however, have universally mild disease (enzyme activity 85–100% for most affected women and 85% for most affected men). In such cases, RBCs function perfectly well under normal circumstances. However, when exposed to the oxidative stress of ketoacidosis, or any of the drugs or infectious agents listed in Table 7.21, they may not be able to generate sufficient amounts of the reducing substance nicotinamide adenine dinucleotide (NADH) to prevent oxidation. First, ferrohemoglobin oxidizes to methemoglobin. Eventually, sulfhydryl groups oxidize hemoglobin, causing hemoglobin chains to break apart and form precipitates known as ***Heinz bodies.*** Assuming coccoid shapes, Heinz bodies attach to the inner surface of the RBC membrane, limiting its ability to deform. Following a lag period of 2–3 days after the triggering stress, explosive destruction of circulating blood cells occurs. The hemolysis is typically short-lived, since new RBCs with nearly normal G-6-PD activity replace the older, more deficient cells being destroyed. However, this is not true for nonblack patients with more severe disease. They can have acute, life-threatening episodes of hemolysis that follow exposure to offending drugs or illness, superimposed on chronic hemolytic anemia that exists in the absence of a specific stress. During acute episodes, patients present with hemoglobinemia and hemoglobinuria. Generally, the spleen is not enlarged. The diagnosis is confirmed by measuring low G-6-PD activity at a time when the patient is stable or normal G-6-PD levels following marked hemolysis (when the ensuing reticulocytosis would normally coincide with elevated G-6-PD activity). The major aspect of treatment consists of reduc-

TABLE 7.21 AGENTS PRECIPITATING HEMOLYSIS IN G-6-PD DEFICIENCY

Antimicrobials
- Nitrofurans
- Sulfonamides
- Chloroquine
- Chloramphenicol
- Paraquine
- Primaquine
- Quinacrine
- Para-aminosalicylic acid (PAS)
- Methylene blue
- Nalidixic acid

Analgesic, anti-inflammatory, uricosuric agents
- Aspirin (large doses)
- Probenecid
- Phenacetin (acetophenetidide)

Nutritional supplements and hypoglycemic agents
- Tolbutamide
- Vitamin K
- Ascorbic acid
- Nitrates

Miscellaneous
- Lead
- Fava beans
- Naphthalene
- Dimercaprol (British anti-lewisite)

TABLE 7.22 METHEMOGLOBINOPATHIES

Hereditary	Drug-induced
Defective NADH diaphorase	Sulfones
Abnormal M	Phenacetin
Boston	Nitrites
Iwate	PAS
Saskatoon	Antimalarials (primaquine, chloroquine)
Hyde Park	Caine derivatives (prilocaine, benzocaine, lidocaine)
Milwaukee	Menadione (vitamin K_3)
Acquired	Naphthalene
Reduced NADH diaphorase from dietary excess of nitrates	Resorcinol
	Phenylhydrazine

ing future episodes. This centers on aggressive control of acidosis, uremia, and infection, as well as avoidance of offending drugs.

As mentioned previously, 3% of hemoglobin remains fixed in an oxidized form called "methemoglobin." Several enzymes, particularly nicotinamide adenosine dinucleotide phosphate (NADPH)-dependent methemoglobin reductase, are crucial to methemoglobin reduction. ***Methemoglobinemia*** results from one of the inherited or acquired conditions listed in Table 7.22 that interfere with these enzymes. Although some patients are asymptomatic, most display some degree of cyanosis without hypoxia. They appear considerably blue without being sick and without having evidence of cardiopulmonary disease or clubbing. However, severe acute methemoglobinemia from drugs or toxins can cause collapse and coma. Reddish-brown in appearance, drawn blood fails to turn bright red when exposed to oxygen. The diagnosis is confirmed by methemoglobin assays. Levels greater than 60–70% can cause death. Treatment consists of administration of methylene blue solution and ascorbic acid.

RBC Life Cycle

A mature RBC circulates for 90–120 days. Cells with any abnormality in size or shape, or any membrane defect, may be destroyed by reticuloendothelial cells in the marrow ***(intramedullary hemolysis)*** or in the spleen ***(extravascular hemolysis).*** In peripheral capillaries, they may become frayed and break apart ***(intravascular hemolysis).*** Lysis of small numbers of abnormal cells is normal. Furthermore, all senescent cells are selectively destroyed by the spleen. The signal for removal is uncertain, though it is likely that the surface of aging cells becomes coated with autoantibodies or loses deformability due to a reduced sialic acid content.

Hemolytic anemia may develop whenever there is chronic or massive destruction of young and old cells alike. The specific types of hemolytic anemia are listed in Table 7.23. Some elements of the clinical picture vary with the specifics of disease, while others are universally related to the pathophysiology of hemolysis. To begin with, hemolysis stimulates erythropoiesis and is usually marked by reticulocytosis (previously discussed). Since RBCs have relatively high concentrations of LDH, accelerated cell lysis causes serum levels of LDH to rise as well. It also releases hemoglobin. Hemoglobin released within reticuloendothelial cells during extravascular lysis is cleared directly. However, hemoglobin released into the plasma with intravascular hemolysis combines with the protein haptoglobin to form hemoglobin–

TABLE 7.23 TYPES OF HEMOLYSIS

Inherited RBC abnormalities	Acquired RBC abnormalities
Hereditary spherocytosis (Minkowski-Chauffard)	Parasites
Hereditary elliptocytosis	Cell membrane defects
Hereditary acanthocytosis	Autoimmune damage
Hereditary stomatocytosis	Dysplastic alterations
Erythropoietic porphyria	Chemical and drug damage
Hemoglobinopathies	Septicemia
Thalassemic syndromes	Mechanical trauma
Sickle cell	Defective heart valves
Hemoglobins C, D, E, and unstable hemoglobin	Hemolytic uremic syndrome
Enzyme defects	Malignant hypertension
G-6-PD deficiency	Eclampsia
Pyruvate kinase deficiency	Graft rejection
	Cavernous hemangioma
	Sequestration

haptoglobin complexes that are then picked up by reticuloendothelial cells. These cells degrade hemoglobin into iron, globin, and PROTO. Iron and amino acids from the globin are recycled for body use. PROTO is processed into urobilinogen and bilirubin (see Chapter 5).

A normally functioning liver can conjugate excess bilirubin with no problem, and though a rise in unconjugated bilirubin may occur with severe hemolysis, it rarely exceeds 4 mg%. In such cases, bilirubin measurements (including the catabolites urinobilinogen and stercobilin) may be of little value in assessing the presence of hemolysis. On the other hand, severe elevations of bilirubin may be noted in the presence of any form of liver impairment. For these reasons, some persons with hemolytic anemia have jaundice. Because the spleen bears most of the responsibility for processing hemoglobin, many patients develop splenomegaly as well. As might be expected, levels of serum haptoglobin are reduced in cases of intravascular hemolysis. When haptoglobin becomes saturated by released hemoglobin, free hemoglobin accumulates in the plasma ***(hemoglobinemia).*** Filtered by glomerular membranes, small amounts are reabsorbed by the proximal tubules and catabolized into ferritin and hemosiderin. As cells of the proximal tubule are sloughed, ***hemosiderinuria*** may be noted with Prussian blue stains of the urinary sediment. Large amounts of filtered hemoglobin exhaust the mechanisms for reabsorption, and free hemoglobin then appears in the urine ***(hemoglobinuria).*** Both hemosiderinuria and hemoglobinuria represent large sources of iron loss, and hemolytic anemia may then be complicated by iron deficiency and reduced erythropoiesis.

In ***hereditary spherocytosis,*** a genetically determined abnormality of the erythrocyte membrane is passed on as a dominant trait. The defect permits sodium to enter the cell at an enhanced rate, causing a hypertonic state, and as water is drawn in, the discoid shape become spheroid. Sodium-potassium pumps are activated to rid the body of excess sodium, an effort that utilizes increased amounts of adenosine triphosphate (ATP). As a result, the cells may become metabolically depleted. Furthermore, the bloated cells are either delayed or destroyed in the spleen. This leads to splenomegaly and ongoing symptoms of jaundice, with the possible development of gallstones. Splenic rupture sometimes occurs, and patients run a high risk of developing marrow aplasia. The diagnosis is usually made in childhood on the basis of anemia with spherocytes on the peripheral smear, reticulocytosis, high bilirubin counts, and positive osmotic fragility tests. The treatment consists of splenectomy. Splenectomy prevents many of the clinical manifestations of hemolytic anemia, including aplastic crisis. ***Hereditary elliptocytosis*** is a variant of hereditary spherocytosis. Patients who inherit the trait for disease display elliptocytes on peripheral smear but rarely experience clinical problems. Associated with a number of cell alterations, the ***hemoglobinopathies*** are also characterized by hemolysis. They were discussed in a previous section.

The ***immune hemolytic anemias*** account for many instances of hemolysis. Due to an immunologic mistake or change, antigens on RBC surfaces interact with IgG or IgM antibodies. Interaction with IgG incites phagocytes: neutrophils and monocytes in the spleen attack and totally ingest or fragment the RBC, resulting in extravascular hemolysis. These immunologic abnormalities can be detected by Coombs' serum, which reveals IgG in the patient's serum (indirect Coombs' test) or on RBC surfaces (direct Coombs' test). Alternatively, interaction of surface antigens with either IgG or IgM can activate a complement cascade, with subsequent damage to the cell (see the later discussion). Screening is usually performed with the Coombs' reagent and followed by immunoglobin or complement components of Coombs' sera to define the specific pattern of RBC sensitization. Treatment is directed to the underlying cause, beginning with the discontinuation of suspect drugs. High-dose prednisone may also be initiated and then tapered over the course of a few days. If the response is good, alternate-day maintenance may be continued for several months. Other therapeutic modalities that may be effective include splenectomy or cytotoxic drugs such as cyclophosphamide or azathiopurine.

Paroxysmal nocturnal hemoglobinuria (PNH) is an acquired dysplastic disorder of unusual but not rare incidence. It is most common among young adults and in patients with other stem cell dysplasias (aplastic anemia, myeloproliferative disease). In PNH, abnormal clones of stem cells produce granulocytic populations of cells with membrane defects. Symptoms include intermittent hemoglobinuria, which, in spite of the condition's name, is not necessarily nocturnal. Episodes of thromboembolism developing in the hepatic, portal, splenic, or cerebral veins are common. Embolic phenomena in smaller vessels may also occur during acute hemolysis and are thought to explain the GI symptoms, particularly the esophageal spasm, experienced by many patients. Back pain is another frequent complaint; its etiology is unknown.

PNH should be considered in patients with pancytopenia accompanied by hemolysis, iron deficiency, and reticulocytosis. It is confirmed by several tests that watch for cell changes once serum complement has been activated. Complement may be activated by acidifying the serum (Ham's test), by substituting sucrose for salt (sucrose lysis test), or by using antibodies (e.g., complement lysis sensitivity test). Although Ham's test is the most widely used, it is neither as sensitive nor as accurate as most antibody tests. For treatment, iron replacement is necessary, but this may promote hemolysis by increasing the delivery of new cells to the circulation. To minimize this problem, iron replacement is often preceded by transfusion and by prednisone therapy. Prednisone diminishes the degree of hemolysis by PNH cells, and high alternate-day doses are used during acute episodes. Androgens (fluoxymesterone, oxymetholone) are often given to increase the hematocrit response. Patients with thromboembolic complications require high doses of heparin (low doses may increase hemolysis) or Coumadin. The prognosis is extremely variable. Patients may die within a short time of diagnosis, survive for many years, or revert to normal erythropoiesis following spontaneous loss of the abnormal clone.

Traumatic hemolysis (microangiopathic hemolytic anemia) includes the various types of disorders noted in Table 7.23. Due to excessive shear or turbulence in the blood vessels, RBCs become torn or fragmented. The appearance of triangular, helmet-shaped, or burr-like cells on peripheral smear is the main clue to the diagnosis, along with other signs of intravascular hemolysis. The superimposition of iron deficiency anemia can result from hemosiderinuria, in which case iron supplements may be beneficial. Otherwise, there is no specific treatment. If the underlying process cannot be corrected, hemolysis continues. It is often attended by the development of small thrombi in arterioles, thrombocytopenic purpura, and some degree of disseminated intravascular coagulation. Chronic cases have a poor prognosis.

Iron Balance

Senescent and damaged RBCs supply most of the iron needed by the body. The cells are removed from circulation by the spleen, which degrades hemoglobin into PROTO, globin, and iron. PROTO is processed by the liver into waste products (urobilinogen and bilirubin) that can be excreted by the kidneys and gut (see Chapter 5). The amino acids from globin enter the amino acid pool. Iron is picked up by the protein transferrin and transported back to the marrow, where it is incorporated into a new generation of erythrocytes. About 90% of the iron salvaged from degraded hemoglobin is reused by erythrocytes. The other 10% is used by myoglobin and heme enzymes. Thus, iron is found in virtually every body cell.

If all body cells could be recycled, there would be no need for exogenous iron. However, cells lost from the body take iron with them. Epithelial cells normally shed from the skin, gut, lungs, and genitourinary tract account for a daily loss of 1 mg of iron. This amount must be replaced by the diet. Since only 10% of ingested iron is absorbed, diets containing 5–10 mg/day are needed by men and nonmenstruating women. Iron is also lost through bleeding (1 mg of iron per milliliter of RBCs). Women in the child-bearing years generally need dietary intakes of more than 20 mg/day to offset menstrual blood losses and fetal requirements during pregnancy. The iron deficit in a normal pregnancy ranges from 440 to 1,050 mg. Finally, iron is lost during lactation but may be balanced by associated amenorrhea.

Although the iron in red meats is absorbed directly as an intact heme molecule, iron from other food sources must first be reduced in the acid environment of the stomach to a ferrous form (ferrous gluconate or ferrous sulfate). Regulated by mucosal cells of the intestine, reduced ferrous iron binds to the protein transferrin for transport in the plasma. Transferrin is measured indirectly by the amount of iron it readily binds and is thus called the "total iron-binding capacity (TIBC)." Transferrin is capable of binding an additional amount of iron, which is measured as the "unsaturated iron-binding capacity (UIBC)." In laboratory terms, the TIBC equals the UIBC plus the serum level of iron. This expression is more usefully expressed as the "percent saturation." Serum iron levels and the TIBC fluctuate rather predictability in a number of conditions and can offer important diagnostic information when considered together.

Once transferrin is saturated, leftover iron combines with the protein apoferritin and forms ferritin. Ferritin levels thus provide an execellent reflection of body iron stores. In contrast, serum levels of iron cannot be used to monitor changes in storage because they are altered by food intake and are subject to significant diurnal variations (they are one-third higher in the morning than at night).

TABLE 7.24 CAUSES OF IRON DEFICIENCY

- Inadequate iron intake
  - Poor diet
  - Malabsorption
  - Pregnancy
- High output
  - Female reproductive organs
    - Heavy menstrual periods
    - Blood loss from childbirth, gynecologic procedures, cancer
  - GI tract
    - Ulcers
    - Esophageal bleeds
    - Polyps
    - Cancer
    - Hemorrhoids
    - Diverticulosis
    - Aspirin abuse
    - Gastritis
    - Ulcerative colitis
    - Hemorrhagic telangiectasia
  - Phlebotomy
    - Repeated diagnostic tests
    - Blood donations
  - Hemolysis (when there is hemosiderosis)
  - Trauma

The average U.S. diet provides 15–18 mg of iron a day; if needed, the body can absorb up to 6 mg of this amount for use. When iron loss exceeds absorption, stores become drained, leading to the first stages of ▶***iron deficiency anemia.*** At this point, most diagnostic tests are normal and patients are asymptomatic. Hemoglobin below 6 g/dL may be attended by symptoms of severe anemia, described previously in Table 7.10. Cheilosis and koilonychia (spooning of the nails) may be present. Pica (compulsive eating of ice, clay, laundry starch, and paper) occurs in about 50% of patients. The diagnosis is based on findings of microcytic, hypochromic anemia, high iron-binding cpacity, a low percentage of iron saturation, low serum iron, and low ferritin levels. Once it is made, blood loss must be assumed and the cause determined. Inquiring about more common sources of bleeding (heavy menstrual flow, recent pregnancy or childbirth, bleeding hemorrhoids) provides the answer in many cases. If not, bleeding from the GI or urinary tract should be ruled out, since iron deficiency anemia accompanies a number of serious diseases (Table 7.24). Most cases of iron deficiency anemia are successfully treated with supplements of ferrous sulfate or ferrous gluconate. Symptomatic improvement may be noted within 1 or 2 weeks and correction of iron imbalance within 3 months. Lack of response could indicate an incorrect diagnosis (iron deficiency anemia is the only anemia that responds to iron). More often, however, it results from failure of the patient to follow through with a complete course of medication. Oral iron frequently causes diarrhea, constipation, or GI upset, and noncompliance rates are high. Bothersome side effects can be minimized by slowly increasing the dose and by instructing patients to take the pills with food. Parenteral iron should be limited to patients whose iron requirement exceeds the amount that can be given by mouth. Both expensive and dangerous, transfusions are rarely justified for the correction of iron deficiency anemia.

In contrast to iron-deficient states, iron stores are abnormally high in cases of ***hemosiderosis*** (siderosis). In milder forms, extra iron is laid down in storage compartments, a condition known as ***iron overload*** (absolute siderosis). In more severe forms, iron in the form of hemosiderin deposits in joints, or in parenchyma of the liver, pancreas, heart, adrenals, testes, and/or kidneys. This general deposition is referred to as ***hemochromatosis.*** As noted in Table 7.25, three types of iron overload are described. ***Idiopathic hemochromatosis*** affects 20,000 people in the United States. As with other types, it is most common among men and typically develops after age 50. Symptoms relate to affected organs. Patients present with joint pain, hepatic dysfunction, hypogonadism, diabetes, and/or cardiac changes (ar-

TABLE 7.25 HEMOCHROMATOSIS (HEMOSIDEROSIS)

Idiopathic
Acquired
  Increased iron uptake
    Iron supplements
    Repeated transfusions
    Excess alcoholic beverages
	Focal
	  Renal hemosiderosis
	  Pulmonary hemosiderosis
	  Porphyria cutanea tarda

rhythmias and refractory CHF). "Bronzing of the skin" due to melanin excess occurs in over 90% of patients. Ascorbic acid deficiency and osteoporosis are other common associations. Most patients are afflicted with combined problems, the classic tetrad being liver disease, heart failure, diabetes, and skin changes.

The diagnosis is based on laboratory findings of elevated plasma iron concentrations, iron-binding capacity, and, most important, serum ferritin. Normally between 50 and 200 μg/L, the latter may be elevated into the thousands. The diagnosis is confirmed by liver biopsy showing heavy parenchymal deposits of hemosiderin with fibrous reactions. Chemical estimations of iron concentrations can also be made of organ specimens taken by needle biopsy. In order to deplete iron stores, 500 ml of blood are phlebotomized on a weekly basis, sometimes for 2–3 years. Less frequent maintenance phlebotomies are then required for life. The chelating agent deferoxamine may also be employed. Care of hepatic, renal, or diabetic complications is undertaken as necessary. In cases of genetic disease, affected relatives (particularly siblings) should be screened. Early treatment can prevent massive iron overload and organ damage.

MYELOGENOUS WHITE BLOOD CELLS (WBCs)

Neutrophils

Neutrophils are the most abundant of the WBCs. They constitute the body's first line of defense against infectious diseases. Within 24 hours of release from the marrow, neutrophils randomly migrate from the bloodstream into tissue spaces. Having receptors for IGa and C3, they draw to and bind organisms that have been tagged with corresponding components by the immune system. The neutrophil forms a vacuole around the invading organism and releases bactericidal enzymes in a process known as "degranulation." These enzymes are powerful enough to cause tissue necrosis if degranulation takes place outside the vacuole ***(Arthus reaction).***

In addition to bactericidal enzymes, neutrophils release a pyrogen that produces ***fever*** by influencing the hypothalamus to elevate the body's thermostat. Fevers are discussed in Chapter 10.

Neutrophils pass through five mitotic divisions, the final three occurring in the myelocytic stages (Fig. 7.6). Throughout these stages, cytoplasmic granules containing bactericidal enzymes are formed. The first stage of postmitotic development is the metamyelocyte. It is called a "band" because of its single kidney-shaped nucleus. During final maturation, sections of the band-like nucleus split into two or more segments. The mature cells are thus called "segmented neutrophils," "polymorphonuclear leukocytes," or "polys." The more lobes there are, the more mature the

GRANULOCYTE MORPHOLOGY

		Nucleus			Cytoplasm		Granulations	
Cells	*Size (μm)*	*Shape*	*Chromatin*	*Nucleoli*	*Quantity*	*Color*[a]	*Number*	*Type*
Myeloblasts	18 to 22	Round or oval	Delicate, fine	Two or three visible	$N > P$[b]	Basophilic	None visible or rare	Primary Azurophilic
Promyelocyte	15 to 20	Oval, eccentric	More clumped	Faint or not visible	$N > P$	Basophilic	Abundant	Primary Azurophilic
Myelocytes	12 to 15	Oval	Coarsely clumped	Not visible	$N \leqslant P$	Rose Violet	Abundant Abundant Abundant	neutrophilic secondary eosinophilic basophilic
Metamyelocytes	12 to 15	Horseshoe Two lobes	Coarsely clumped	Absent	$N < P$	Rose Lilac	Abundant	"
Polynuclears	10 to 15	Polylobed Three to five lobes	Coarsely clumped	Absent	$N < P$	Rose Lilac	Abundant	"

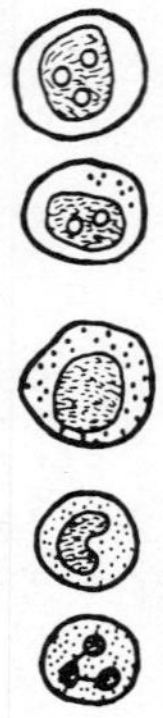

[a]Color with May-Grünwald-Giemsa.
[b]N: size of nucleus; P: size of cytoplasm.

Figure 7.6 Neutrophil stages. (From Sultan, *Manual of Hematology*, © 1985, John Wiley & Sons, Inc., New York.)

cell; this fact is an important index of cell production. Normally, 35% of these cells have two lobes, 41% have three lobes, 17% have four lobes, and no more than 3% have five lobes. In cases of folic acid or vitamin B_{12} deficiency, neutrophils tend to hypermature; the result is a higher percentage of cells with four and five lobes ***(right shift).*** Cells developing six or more lobes are called "hypersegmented neutrophils" (megaloblastic leukocytes). The presence of a single hypersegment neutrophil should raise the suspicion of megaloblastic anemia.

In a ***left shift*** there is an increase of immature neutrophils (bands and segmented cells with only two lobes). This develops whenever a large number of leukocytes are called out of the bloodstream to the site of infection or tissue damage. The mass exodus would cause a serious depletion of the circulating pool except that the bone marrow responds by releasing cell reserves. Due to overcompensation, the neutrophil count actually rises above the normal range. This response, called ***neutrophilia,*** occurs in a number of conditions (see Table 7.26). It tends to be more pronounced in children, localized infections, and infections from pyogenic bacteria but impaired in cases of iron, folate, and vitamin B_{12} deficiency and marrow failure. A brisk elevation of neutrophils actually demonstrates good resistance. Conversely, a left shift in the presence of a normal or falling WBC count signifies that marrow production is being severely stressed and is an ominous sign.

Physiologic leukocytosis occurs in the absence of infection or tissue damage. Strenuous exercise, pain, epinephrine, and corticosteroids are a few of the factors that stimulate cells from the marginal pool to flood the circulation. This influx,

TABLE 7.26 CONDITIONS CHARACTERIZED BY ABNORMAL NEUTROPHIL COUNTS

Neutrophilia
- Convulsions
- Blood disorders
  - Hemolysis
  - Hemorrhage
  - Polycythemia vera
- Malignancies
  - Leukemia
  - GI tract
  - Liver
- Drugs
  - ACTH
  - Adrenalin
  - Digitalis
  - Phenacetin
- Poisons
  - Camphor, tetrachlorethane, benzene, turpentine
  - Arsenic, carbon monoxide, lead
  - Venoms
- Infections
  - Tuberculosis
  - Bacterial
- Toxemias
  - Diabetic acidosis
  - Eclampsia
  - Gout
  - Uremia

Neutropenia
- Blood disorders
  - Genetic agranulocytosis
  - Chediak-Higashi syndrome
  - Megaloblastosis
  - Splenic neutropenia
  - Myeloproliferative disorders
- Ionizing radiation
- Drugs
  - Cancer chemotherapeutics (nitrogen mustard, cyclophosphamide, chlorambucil, busulfam, vinblastine, vincristine, cytosine arabinoside, methotrexate, 6-mercaptopurine, azathioprine)
  - Analgesics and antiarthritic agents (phenacetin, gold salts, colchicine, indomethacin, phenylbutazone)
  - Antibiotics (chloramphenicol, sulfonamides)
  - Antiarrhythmic agents (procainamide, quinidine)
  - Anticonvulsants and psychiatric drugs (phenothiazines, dibenzazepines)
- Benzene
- Antithyroidal agents
- Quinine

Infections
- Viral
- Severe bacterial

Pseudoneutropenia (shift from circulating to marginal pool)
- Endotoxins
- Anesthetic agents (ether, pentobarbital)

which is brief and without a left shift, can double the WBC count within a few minutes.

Most of the conditions listed in Table 7.26 have WBC count elevations ranging from 10,000 to 24,000/mm^3. Persistent neutrophilia with counts between 30,000 and 50,000/mm^3 is called a ***leukemoid reaction.*** This occurs with certain infections (whooping cough, infectious mononucleosis, tuberculosis), in blood dyscrasias, and advanced cancer. Unlike leukemia, the neutrophils seen in leukemoid reactions are predominantly mature. Furthermore, erythrocytes and platelet counts are fairly normal. If an underlying cause is not established, the patient should be evaluated by a hematologist to rule out leukemia.

Neutropenia is a reduction in the absolute neutrophil count, with ranges below 2,000/mm^3 for whites and 1,300/mm^3 for blacks. It is seen in a wide variety of disorders listed in Table 7.26. The neutropenia that characterizes certain infections (measles, typhoid, brucellosis, mononucleosis, hepatitis, and malaria) is generally mild and probably due to a shift of cells into the marginal pool. However, neutropenia following an overwhelming infection (gram-negative bacteremia, pneumococcal pneumonia, miliary tuberculosis) signals a dangerous depletion of marrow stores.

Severe neutropenia is called ***agranulocytosis.*** It can occur as a reaction to innumerable drugs, with phenothiazines, quinines, and hydantoins being common culprits. From weeks to months after drug initiation, the patient becomes acutely ill with fever, sore throat, and/or oral or perianal ulcerations. Both the peripheral blood and the bone marrow lack any sign of neutrophils, and the total WBC count may drop below 2,000/mm^3. With discontinuation of the drug and hospital support, marrow recovery is the rule. Some drugs, notably phenothiazines, carbamazepine, and propylthiouracil, cause gradual neutropenia and should be stopped if WBC counts fall below 3,000/mm^3.

The cytoplasm of the mature neutrophil, in itself colorless, is packed with tiny granules that normally stain tan to pink. However, granules in immature or damaged cells retain a basophilic staining (dark blue or purple) known as ***toxic granulation.*** This is seen in severe infections, toxic reactions, and leukemic states. Other morphologic changes such as ***Dohle inclusion bodies, May-Hegglin anomaly, Alder-Reilly anomaly, Pelger-Huet anomaly, Chediak-Higashi syndrome,*** and ***auer rods*** are described in Table 7.27.

Basophils and Eosinophils

Although eosinophils and basophils seem to arise from the same marrow stem cell (CFU-EO), they are different in both structure and function (Fig. 7.7).

Basophils are the least numerous of the WBCs produced in bone marrow. Little is known about the activity of basophils in the blood, and even less is known about their fate in the tissue. The cells have a partially segmented nucleus and cytoplasmic granules that stain red-purple due to a high heparin content. In addition to heparin, basophils manufacture factors involved in hypersensitivity reactions and platelet activity. Thus, ***basophilia*** (WBC counts above 2,000/mm^3) is most commonly seen in allergic reactions such as asthma or contact dermatitis. It is also seen in chicken pox, myeloproliferative disorders, hypothyroidism, chronic hemolytic anemia, and following radiation therapy or splenectomy.

In a 2-week process, eosinophils mature in a manner similar to that of neutrophils

TABLE 7.27 MORPHOLOGIC CHANGES OF WBCs

Change	Description
Auer rods	Red-purple–staining rod-like inclusions found in myeloblasts or promyeloblasts. Found in the majority of cases of AML and sometimes in myelomonocytic leukemia, erythroleukemia, and leukemoid reactions. Almost never seen in any other conditions.
Toxic granulation	Advanced-stage cells (metamyelocytes, bands or neutrophils) retain purple-staining granules in the cytoplasm (normally, only granules in blast stages stain purple, while those in mature stages stain tan or pink). Occurs with severe infections or other toxic conditions.
Dohle inclusion bodies	Mature cells (polymorphonuclear cells) have pale blue–staining bodies in cytoplasm. The inclusion bodies look like micrococci or small rods. Often accompany toxic granulation. Seen with infectious diseases (notably scarlet fever), burns, aplastic anemia, and exposure to toxins.
May-Hegglin anomaly	Neutrophils as well as eosinophils, basophils, monocytes, and megakaryocytes contain cytoplasmic inclusions that resemble large Dohle bodies. The anomaly characterizes a rare inherited condition associated with thrombocytopenia.
Alder-Reilly anomaly	All WBCs contain dense blue granules in cytoplasm similar to toxic granulation. Occurs as a feature of genetic mucopolysaccharide disorders (notably Hurler syndrome). Also seen in healthy persons.
Pelger-Huet anomaly	Nuclei of granulocytes fail to mature and large numbers of bands occur in peripheral circulation. Occurs as a hereditary autosomal dominant condition.
Chediak-Higashi syndrome	Containing large cytoplasmic granules (probably lysosomes), all WBCs function subnormally. A rare autosomal recessive disorder, the syndrome is marked by partial albinism as well as the leukocyte abnormality. Patients develop lymphadenopathy, hepatosplenomegaly, pancytopenia, and lymphoid infiltrates and die at an early age.

but develop fewer nuclear lobes. They contain two types of cytoplasmic granules that stain a characteristic red-orange color. Mature eosinophils circulate in the blood for less than 8 hours before moving to the tissue. Representing 4–8% of the total WBC count, peripheral numbers rarely exceed 5,000/mm^3. Tissue cells, however, are 100 times more numerous with the highest concentrations found in epithelial surfaces of the skin, respiratory tract, and gut.

Eosinophil function is only partially understood. During the immune response mediated by IgE, chemotactic factors are released that attract eosinophils. This explains why ***eosinophilia*** occurs in atopic diseases, allergies, and hypersensitivity reactions. Eosinophils also protect the body against invading parasites by both cytoxic action and the transfer of passive immunity.

In ***parasite infections,*** eosinophil counts often rise when parasites first invade body tissue but may return to normal in other stages of the parasitic life cycle. Although protozoa, nematodes, trematodes, and cestodes all cause human disease, their incidence in the United States is quite low due to good sanitation and host controls. Most parasites cause GI disturbances and are discussed in Chapter 4. However, a few affect primarily blood and lymph.

Acquired toxoplasmosis affects 1% of the U.S. population. After ingestion of infected, uncooked meat (pork and lamb more than beef) or hand contamination with feces of birds and animals (particularly cats), cysts of the protozoa enter the human digestive tract. They produce trophozoites that enter host cells by endocytosis. Trophozoites may be transmitted directly through accidental inoculation, organ

COMPARISON OF STRUCTURE AND FUNCTION

	Eosinophils	*Basophils*
Secondary granules (structure on electron microscopy)	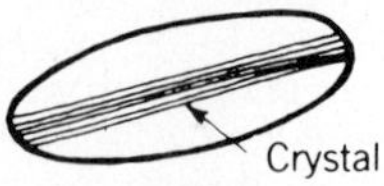	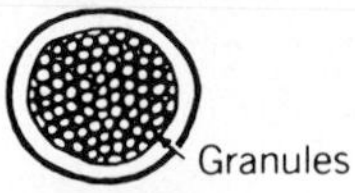
Contents of granules	Peroxidase Arylsulfatase Specific basic protein	Histamine Heparin Serotonin Bradykinin Platelet activating factor
Membrane		Receptor for IgE
Functions shared with neutrophils		
Chemotaxis	+	+
Phagocytosis	+	±
Bacterial killing	±	−
Specific functions	Role in the immediate hypersensitivity reaction	Effector cells in the immediate hypersensitivity reaction by liberation of granule contents

Figure 7.7 Eosinophils and basophils. (From Sultan, *Manual of Hematology,* © 1985, John Wiley & Sons, Inc., New York.)

transplants, or blood donations, but this is rare. For a period of 1–2 weeks, they divide until they cause host cells to rupture. This cell rupture, quickly repeated in adjacent cells and then distant sites, causes variable amounts of tissue necrosis and inflammation. Many patients exhibit no clinical symptoms. Others develop low-grade fever, marked fatigue, muscle discomfort, and lymph node enlargement. The nodes are typically nontender and rubbery, and the spleen may be enlarged. Sore throat, headache, and a maculopapular rash are not uncommon. Encephalitis, myocarditis, myositis, pneumonitis, or hepatitis may occur when organ involvement is severe. Infection of the eye causes inflammatory retinal lesions, episodes of posterior uveitis, and progressive loss of vision known as ***toxoplasmic chorioretinitis.*** Serious complications are unusual in otherwise healthy persons but frequently occur in immunosuppressed patients.

The diagnosis of toxoplasmosis is confirmed by isolation of the virus from tissue cultures or by titers of antitoxoplasma antibodies. Serial tests showing a rise or fall in titers, a single titer of 1:1,024 or higher, and positive IgM or enzyme-linked immunosorbent assay (ELISA) tests may all be considered evidence of active disease. Recovery is spontaneous. Although fever disappears within days, fatigue and lymphadenopathy may persist for months. To shorten this period, symptomatic patients are treated with combinations of Daraprim, sulfadiazine, and folinic acid for 1 month. Because the antimicrobials have been associated with marrow toxicity, platelet counts and WBC counts should be done regularly during treatment. Following disease, antibody titers decrease slowly over a period of 2–4 years. Stable titers ranging from 1:16 to 1:256 remain for a lifetime.

If a woman contracts toxoplasmosis during pregnancy, the baby may suffer from ***congenital toxoplasmosis.*** Being immunologically underdeveloped, the fetus is likely to suffer from severe organ involvement, mentioned above. This results in permanent damage, particularly to the brain and eyes. Many babies are born with micro-ophthalmia, microcephaly, or hydrocephalus, seizures, and retardation. Furthermore, they carry cysts in various tissue sites that rupture later in life, causing transient episodes of active disease and creating a potential for transmission. Thus, treatment must be undertaken as soon as the disease is diagnosed. For prevention, screening tests to detect immunity or disease in pregnant women are usually performed as part of prenatal care.

Trichinosis is caused by a tissue nematode that enters the body through ingestion of inadequately cooked, contaminated meat (chiefly pork, bear, or walrus). With a 4.5% incidence in U.S. autopsy studies and 100,000 cases annually, the problem is fairly common. Once ingested, the cysts are broken down in the stomach, releasing immature trichinella. At maturity, each female trichinella burrows into intestinal walls, where she deposits over 100 larvae. The larvae reach the blood through lymphatics and the portal circulation and from there travel to target organs (notably muscle tissue). The clinical course depends on the number of invading larvae, the tissues affected, and the physiologic condition of the patient. Most patients have a subclinical course. Others experience GI upset and slight fever 1 or 2 days after eating the contaminated meat (intestinal phase). Systemic signs (larval stage) may develop 7–15 days later. Heralded by edema of the upper eyelids, they are characterized by profuse sweating, fever, chills, and severe myalgia. The muscles most affected are the ocular, diaphragm, intercostal, tongue, pharyngeal, and masseter muscles. As a result, patients may have visual disturbances, respiratory distress, and/or difficulty in talking, swallowing, chewing. If larvae disseminate outside striated muscle, patients may develop lymphadenitis, encephalitis, meningitis, pneumonitis, pleurisy, or myocarditis. Laboratory tests are likely to show elevated creatine phosphokinase (CPK), LDH, serum glutamic oxaloacetic transaminase (SGOT), serum glutamic pyruvic transaminase (SGPT), and a marked reversal of the albumin/globulin ratio. Serum aldolase may be very high, though ESR remains low. CXR during acute phases often reveals disseminated or localized infiltrates. Eosinophilia and leukocytosis, which are important diagnostic signs, develop 2 weeks into the disease. Muscle biopsy (of gastrocnemius or pectoralis muscle) confirms the diagnosis but is unlikely to provide a yield until 4 weeks into the disease. Serologic tests are also available. However, positive titers may be the result of old disease and are helpful only if changes can be documented. Skin tests are of little value.

Mild cases of trichinosis resolve spontaneously and require no treatment. Thiabendazole is given before the development of systemic signs to patients exposed to contaminated meat. It has also been given during acute illness, but with equivocal effectiveness. While corticosteroids are contraindicated in the intestinal stage, high doses are recommended in the larval stage of severe infections. Hospitalization may be required in severe cases.

Four strains of parasites belonging to the plasmodium family may affect humans, causing ***malaria.*** Disease is spread through the bite of an infected anopheles mosquito, the transfusion of infected blood, or the use of a contaminated drug syringe. After an incubation period of 9–30 days, patients develop a 2- to 3-day prodrome marked by intermittent low-grade fever, headache, and myalgia that is often mistaken for the flu. The primary attack follows. It is characterized by an enlarged

TABLE 7.28 TYPES OF MALARIA

Type	Incubation Period	Characteristics of Infected RBC	Clinical Course
Plasmodium falciparum	9–12 days	Normal size with Maurer's dots. Two or more parasites per cell. A small ring and one or two chromatin dots mark trophozite stage.	Lasting for 20–36 hours, paroxysms (rigors) characterized by chilly sensations rather than typical shaking chills and gradual rise in temperature (may reach 104°F). They are associated with severe prostration and headaches. Patients are also quite sick, with low-grade fevers during the intervals between paroxysms (36–72 hours). Very high parasitemia not uncommon. May result in severe anemia, renal failure, cerebral dysfucntion, pulmonary edema, and death.
P. vivax	13–15 days	Enlarged and pale with Schüffner's dots. Uncommon to find more than one parasite per cell. In trophozite stage, large ameboid rings occupy the entire cell.	Primary paroxysm begins abruptly with shaking chills, followed by fever and sweats. After a week of irregular fever, a typical paroxysmal pattern recurring every 48 hours is established: a short period of headache or malaise precedes a chill, which is followed by 1–8 hours of fever. The patient does not feel particularly sick between paroxysms.
P. ovale	13–15 days	Enlarged, pale, and oval, with Schüffner's dots. Uncommon to find more than one parasite per cell. In trophozite stage, ring occupies one-third of cell.	Same as for *P. vivax*.
P. malariae	30 days	Normal size. Rare to find more than one parasite per cell. Pigmented band characterizes trophozite stage.	Abrupt onset of paroxysms that recur at 72-hour intervals. Parasitemia is usually limited. Chronic disease is common.

spleen and a pattern of chills and fever that varies with the type of malarial infection, as noted in Table 7.28. Many patients recover spontaneously. Others develop persistent disease characterized by jaundice, hepatosplenomegaly, and recurrent attacks of fever and chills. Diagnosis is made by identifying the parasite on stained blood smears. *Plasmodium malariae* can be treated with chloroquine alone. *P. vivax* and *P. ovale* are treated with chloroquine followed by primaquine. Frequently resistant to chloroquine, *P. falciparum* may require quinine and pyrimethamine/sulfadoxine (Fansidar). Due to the increase in foreign travel and immigration, malaria is now being seen with some frequency in the United States. Thus, ▶***malaria prophylaxis for travelers*** is an important concern for primary care providers. It involves education as well as the prescription of antimalarial drugs.

A protozoon of the genus *Babesia* may be transmitted through tick bites or blood transfusions to infect RBCs in much the same manner as malaria. The disease is called ***babesiosis.*** Most cases are acquired on offshore islands of New York and Massachusetts. Many individuals remain asymptomatic or experience a mild, indolent illness characterized by myalgias and fatigue. Others develop a hemolytic anemia or an acute febrile illness 1–6 weeks after inoculation. Splenectomized or immunocompromised persons suffer severe cases. Preceded by several days of anorexia and general malaise, fevers (to 40°C) develop, along with drenching sweats and chills. Nausea and vomiting, emotional lability, and hyperesthesias are not uncommon. Though splenomegaly may be noted on exam (it occurs in 25% of cases), rash and lymphadenopathy are absent. The CBC shows anemia, reticulocytosis, and thrombocytopenia, but a normal WBC. There may be proteinemia and slightly elevated LFT's. The diagnosis is confirmed by thick and thin peripheral smears showing typical intraerythrocytic organisms. When smears are inconclusive but the suspicion of disease is high, inoculation of laboratory rodents or serologic tests can be undertaken. Mild cases require no treatment. However, patients with significant illness should be given a trial of pentamidine isethionate IM, 4 mg/kg daily for 10 days (clindamycin and quinine have been described as potentially effective as well). Splenectomized or otherwise immunodepressed patients require hospitalization and possibly exchange transfusions as a lifesaving measure. For prevention, persons staying in endemic areas should practice tick control measures (see Chapter 10); residents should not donate blood.

A persistently high eosinophil count with an unproven cause is the main criteria for ***hypereosinophilic syndrome.*** The disorder is thought to be either a preleukemic state or the result of a chronic hypersensitivity reaction. In addition to eosinophilia, patients often have circulating myeloblasts and elevated serum vitamin B_{12} levels, along with low neutrophil alkaline phosphatase levels. Hepatosplenomegaly may be present. By some unknown mechanism, large numbers of circulating eosinophils damage vital organs, particularly the heart. For this reason, multispecialty management is often required and the mortality is high. There may be a response to corticosteroids or hydroxyurea.

Monocytes

Monocytes share the same progenitor cells as neutrophils (CFU-MG). In fact, monoblasts cannot be distinguished from myeloblasts in normal marrow tissue. As illustrated in Figure 7.8, the promonocyte, the first recognizable stage, is somewhat layer than the myeloblast, with an oval-shaped nucleus. It divides twice within 56–60 hours. At maturity, the cell's nucleus develops a lobulated or horseshoe appearance and the nucleoli become obscure. Although it is classified as an agranulocyte, its cytoplasm contains an abundance of fine, blue-staining granules filled with degradative enzymes. The monocyte has a diameter two to three times larger than that of an erythrocyte and can be recognized as the largest cell on a peripheral smear (see Fig. 7.1).

Monocytes remain in the blood with a half-life of over 8.4 hours. They then move to tissues and transform into larger cells (macrophages) that maintain the general ability to divide. They also acquire certain characteristics unique to the different sites of differentiation. For example, macrophages in lung alveoli develop metabolisms that utilize oxidative phosphorylation, while those in the peritoneum develop a system that uses glycolysis. Monocytes and macrophages make up the monocyte–macrophage system (formerly called the "reticuloendothelial system"). This system removes from tissue, foreign matter such as bacteria, fungi, and abnormal or senescent cells. In addition to their phagocytic functions, monocytes play a complicated role in the immune response. They have receptors for IgG, IgM, and complement. They also synthesize components for the complement system and process antigens

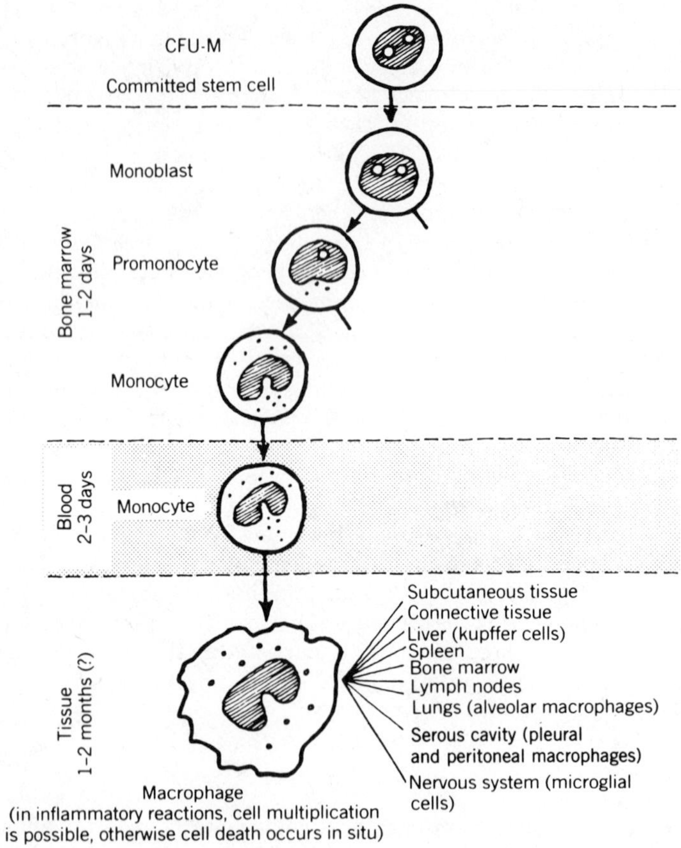

Figure 7.8 Monocytopoiesis. (From Sultan, *Manual of Hematology,* © 1985, John Wiley & Sons, Inc., New York.)

for lymphocyte-mediated immunity. Accordingly, monocyte counts fluctuate in response to certain disease states. Conditions associated with ***monocytosis*** and ***monocytopenia*** are listed in Table 7.29.

LYMPHOCYTES AND SPECIFIC IMMUNITY

B Lymphocytes and Humoral Immunity

B lymphocytes mature under the influence of bone marrow. Upon entering the bloodstream, these small cells become known as "resting" B lymphocytes. They migrate to lymphoid tissues and collect in germinal centers of lymph nodes, follicles of the spleen, Peyer's patches of the intestinal tract, tonsils, adenoids, and the appendix. There they may be exposed to an antigen (e.g., a virus, bacteria, or toxin) that has invaded the body for the first time. If so, the B lymphocyte reacts by developing surface receptors (marker) explicit for that antigen. The markers they form are antibodies. They give the cells a hairy appearance under the electron microscope.

TABLE 7.29 CONDITIONS ASSOCIATED WITH ABNORMAL MONOCYTE COUNTS

Monocytosis
- Infectious (rare)
  - Recovery phase of acute infections, agranulocytosis
  - Worsening tuberculosis
  - Subacute endocarditis
  - Systemic mycotic infections
  - Rickettsial disease
  - Protozoan infections
  - Viruses
- Hematologic/malignancies
  - Monocytic or granulocytic leukemia
  - Lymphoma (particularly Hodgkin's disease)
  - Multiple myeloma
  - Myeloproliferative disorders
  - Other malignancies
- GI and hepatic diseases
  - Ulcerative colitis
  - Regional enteritis
  - Nontropical sprue
  - Cirrhosis

Monocytopenia (poorly studied)
- Prednisone therapy (transient)
- Hairy cell leukemia

Antibodies are complex protein structures also known as "immunoglobulins." There are five classes: IgG and subclasses, IgA and subclasses, IgM, IgD, and IgE. Figure 7.9 depicts them in more detail. As noted, a four-chain structure is basic to each: two heavy and two light. The chains are formed from specific sequences of amino acids—about 450 in heavy chains and 200 in light chains. The chains fold back and forth upon themselves, forming hollows, clefts, and bumps that create a "lock" configuration for the "key-like" fit of the antigens. The point of lock and key fit is referred to as a "combining site."

Initial lymphocyte exposure to an antigen evokes a "primary response" as follows. The differentiation of surface antibodies takes 2–4 days (latent period). As soon as it is completed, the lymphocyte differentiates into a plasma cell, which produces large quantities of IgM for the next 10–12 days. In the absence of continued antigenic stimulus, the plasma cell switches production to IgG for the next 4–days and thereafter to specific IgG antibodies.

Once formed, antibodies enter the bloodstream. The response that follows is thus referred to as "humoral immunity." In the bloodstream, antibody surface markers lock with antigens that have a matching chemical profile. Antigen–antibody complexes are formed. The complexes stimulate complement, a series of nine enzymatic proteins that then interact in a cascade fashion to bring about cell lysis. Since the individual components of complement were named in the order of their discovery, C4 is out of sequence. This makes the order of activation (C1, C4, C2, C3, C5, C6, C7, C8, and C9) a bit confusing. Furthermore, C1 has three separate proteins (C1q, C1r, and C1s).

Classic activation of the cascade begins when C1q binds to combining sites on either a single molecule of IgM or two closely spaced molecules of IgG_1, IgG_2, or IgG_3. The binding of C1q induces C1r to activate C1s and then C4. Activation continues in the sequence pictured in Figure 7.10. It generally involves the cleavage of each component into two fragments. The larger fragment combines with the preceding component, producing enzymatic activity needed to cleave the next component. Cleavage of C2 and C4 produces kinin-like activity that contracts smooth muscle and increases vascular permeability without causing histamine release. Combining C5, C6, and C7 is chemotactic for neutrophils. Furthermore, the small fragments, particularly those produced during C3 and C5 activation, are capable of initiating inflammatory processes of their own. Called "anaphylatoxins," the fragments C3a and C5a stimulate the release of histamines from mast cells, causing further in-

PRINCIPAL PHYSICAL AND BIOLOGICAL PROPERTIES OF DIFFERENT CLASSES OF IMMUNOGLOBULINS

	IgG	*IgA*
Light chain	κ or λ	κ or λ
Heavy chain	γ	α
subclasses	γ_1 γ_2 γ_3 γ_4	α_1 or α_2
Other chains		J chain (polymers) and secretory component (in secretions only
Structure ▲ J chain △ Secretory piece	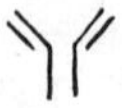	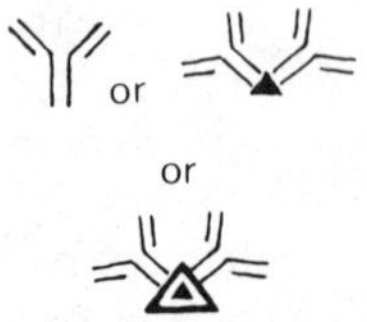
Molecular weight	150,000	152,000 to 385,000
Serum concentration (adult) mg/dl	650 to 1,500	80 to 440
Percent of Ig	80	13
Carbohydrate content (%)	2.5	5 to 10
Half/life	23 days	4 to 6 days
Principal biologic properties	Principal Ig synthesized in the secondary response Diffusion into extravascular spaces: Act against microorganisms or toxins Binding of complement (γ_1 γ_2 γ_3) Binding on Fc receptors of macrophages and neutrophils (γ_1 γ_3) Placental transfer (γ_1 γ_2 γ_4) Passage in milk	Ig in external secretion Inhibits the adherence of microorganisms to mucosal surfaces Passage in milk

Figure 7.9 Immunoglobulins. (From Sultan, *Manual of Hematology,* © 1985, John Wiley & Sons, Inc., New York.)

IgM	*IgD*	*IgE*
κ or λ	κ or λ	κ or λ
μ	δ	ε
J chain		
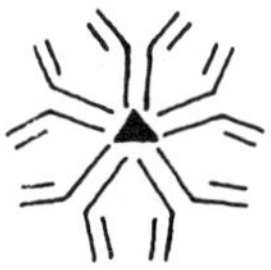	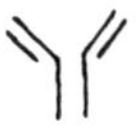	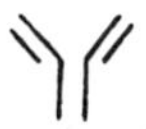
900,000	175,000	190,000
50 to 200	0.3 to 14	0.006 to 0.6
6	1	0.002
5 to 10	5 to 10	11.5
4 to 8 days	2 to 8 days	
First immunoglobulin to appear in the immune response Predominately intravascular Agglutinating properties: role in case of bacteremia		Cytophilic: bind to mast cells and basophils Role in anaphylaxis

Figure 7.9 *(Continued)*

creases in vascular permeability and smooth muscle contraction. They also attract neutrophils into the area (neutrophils accumulating within the area of myocardial infarction do so in direct response to C3a). In addition to the classic pathway just described, the complement system can be activated by an alternative properdin system (see Fig. 7.10). The cascade itself is quite similar except that C1, C4, and C2 are bypassed. Also, activation is stimulated by the Fab portion rather than the Fc portion of the antibody and by aggregates of IgG_1 to IgG_4, IgA, and IgE. It may also be triggered by bacterial endotoxins, bacterial cell walls, and polysaccharides.

Antibodies produced during the primary response to a given antigen circulate in blood, lymph, colostrum, and saliva, as well as GI and urinary tracts. In a second attack, they bind to that antigen, removing it directly from circulation. Antigens that are not bound to circulating antibodies are picked up by antibody surface markers of "sensitized" lymphocytes, and a "secondary response" follows. The lymphocytes differentiate into plasma cells that use the surface markers as a replica for specific IgG antibody production. As a result of such counterattacks, antigens are cleared before infections take hold. Known as "immunity," this state can be achieved by natural means or by vaccination methods.

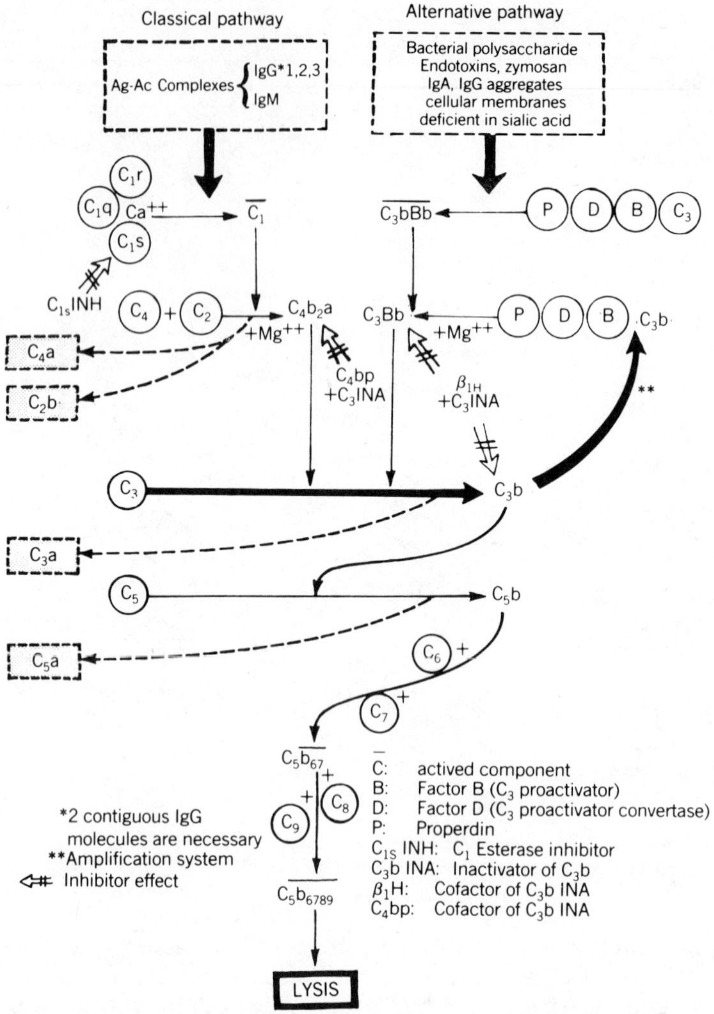

Figure 7.10 Complement cascade. (From Sultan, *Manual of Hematology,* © 1985, John Wiley& Sons, Inc., New York.)

Secondary responses are always immediate and normally controlled. If they are uncontrolled, a ***hypersensitivity reaction*** may develop. Type I (immediate), type II (cytotoxic), and type III (immune complex) are described in Table 7.30. Atopy (eczema, asthma, anaphylaxis), Goodpasture's syndrome, arthritis, glomerulonephritis, Farmer's lung, hepatitis, and many other disorders result. Each is discussed under the affected system.

An increase in atypical lymphocytes is the hallmark of ***infectious mononucleosis.*** It is caused by the Epstein-Barr virus (EBV); intimate contact is usually required for its transmission. Outbreaks are common in families, educational institutions, and military facilities. Young members of lower socioeconomic groups are particularly susceptible. Mononucleosis can also occur following blood transfusions.

TABLE 7.30 HYPERSENSITIVITY REACTIONS

Reaction	Example[a]	Mechanism
Type I (immediate)	Seasonal allergies, atopy, anaphylaxis	Mast cells of patients have IgE attached to the surface. If antigen exposure occurs, the antigen cross-links two IgE molecules, thereby triggering the release of vasoactive substances and symptoms (sneezing, runny nose and eyes, wheezing, and/or eczema skin rashes). When the allergen is removed, symptoms subside, though IgE remains attached to mast cells.
Type II (cytotoxic)	Transfusion reaction	Circulating antibodies attach to antigens on the surface of the patient's own cells, causing their destruction.
Type III	Arthus reaction, serum sickness, streptococcal disease, SLE, farmer's lung hepatitis B	Immune complexes formed in the course of antigen exposure cause damage to tissues in several ways. Complexes of "critical size" penetrate blood vessel walls and lodge in basement membranes. Complement attaches to the complexes, attracting neutrophils that release inflammatory products, causing vasculitis and tissue damage.
Type IV	Drug allergies, insect bites, autoimmune disease, contact dermatitis, graft rejection	T lymphocytes become sensitized to antigen with first exposure. Two days following a subsequent exposure, they mediate the activity of lymphokines and macrophages, which not only destroys the antigen but harms surrounding tissue.

[a] Many conditions reflect combined reactions.

The incubation period is 10–50 days, and the period of communicability is unknown. The onset of symptoms is sudden. The patient complains of sore throat, fever, chills, fatigue, malaise, and loss of appetite. Enlarged lymph glands in the anterior and posterior cervical areas, axilla, and groin are important clinical findings. Petechiae of the palate, a false pharyngeal membrane, splenomegaly, and hepatomegaly are common. The diagnosis is confirmed with differential blood counts and the monospot test. Antibiotic treatment is necessary for superimposed streptococcal infection, which occurs in 15–30% of cases due to lowered resistance. If tonsils are enlarged enough to obstruct the throat and cause dehydration, a short course of steroids is beneficial. Patients, particularly those with an enlarged liver or spleen, should be advised to avoid contact sports, roughhousing, or vigorous lovemaking for 6 weeks. Otherwise, activity can be pursued to toleration. Kissing should probably be avoided during acute illness, but more stringent measures for infection control are not necessary. The disease confers lifelong immunity.

Closely related to EBV, ***cytomegalovirus (CMV)*** is ubiquitous. Infections can be acquired in utero or during childbirth ***(congenital CMV),*** or in later life from infected secretions (urine, semen, cervical mucus, feces, milk, blood). Presentation of the congenital infection ranges from asymptomatic carriers to miscarriage or postnatal death. Infants with severe nonfatal disease are likely to have liver dysfunction, hemorrhagic disorders, and CNS damage (psychomotor retardation, spasticity, blindness, deafness, seizures). Their prognosis is guarded. Usually developing in early childhood, acquired infections are facilitated by close living arrangements, such as schools and institutions. By adulthood, 60–90% of the population has evidence of disease. Among homosexuals, the incidence approaches 95%. Most cases are asymptomatic. However, some patients experience an acute febrile illness marked by hepatitis with or without jaundice ***(CMV mononucleosis*** or ***CMV hepatitis).*** Atypical lymphocytosis is characteristic. Occasionally, rash may develop. The diag-

TABLE 7.31 ANTIBODY DEFICIENCY DISORDERS

X-linked infantile agammaglobulinemia	Transient hypogammaglobulinemia of infancy
Common variable immunodeficiency	Antibody deficiency with nearly normal immunoglobins
Selective IgA deficiency	X-linked lymphoproliferative disease (Duncan's disease)
Secretory component deficiency	
Selective IgM deficiency	
Immunodeficiency with elevated IgM	

nosis is confirmed by culturing the virus from urine, blood, cervical mucus, or other tissues. Rising or falling titers on paired serologic tests are also diagnostic. There is no treatment.

Antibody deficiency disorders occur as a congenital or acquired disease. Various types are listed in Table 7.31 according to the immunoglobulin class affected. All are quite rare, and most are manifested in early life. The clinical signs and symptoms vary somewhat with the disease. The most universal characteristic is recurrent bacterial infections, primarily of the skin and respiratory tract (with the exception of hepatitis and enterovirus, viral infections are not a major problem). A high incidence of autoimmune disorders (arthritis, systemic lupus erythematosus, autoimmune hemolytic anemias, pernicious anemia) and malignancies is also associated. The diagnosis is based on the finding of an antibody deficiency in serum and secretions. It is important to note that a specific deficiency can still exist in the presence of normal or nearly-normal total serum immunoglobulin secretions. Immunoglobin replacements are given in most instances, and if infections can be controlled, many patients live into adulthood.

Increased antibody production characterizes the ***plasma cell dyscrasias*** noted in Table 7.32. Due to a dysplastic (often malignant) transformation, plasma cells fail to act in the normal polyclonal fashion whereby measured amounts of the various antibodies are manufactured. Instead, they behave in a monoclonal fashion, producing large quantities of a whole antibody (IgG, IgA, IgD, IgE), light chain portions (Bence Jones protein), or heavy chain portions. In addition, the neoplastic plasma cells usually secrete an M-component immunoglobulin, the amount of which varies with the tumor buron. Appearing as a "spike" on protein electrophoresis, M-component provides a crucial marker for the diagnosis, growth, and regression of disease. ***Macroglobulinemia of Waldenström*** and ***heavy chain diseases*** are rare. However, multiple myeloma and amyloid occur with some frequency and deserve further discussion.

Multiple myeloma accounts for 1% of all forms of cancer. It usually appears in

TABLE 7.32 PLASMA CELL DYSCRASIAS

Multiple myeloma	Secondary amyloidosis
Macroglobulinemia of Waldenström	Chronic inflammation (tuberculosis, leprosy, RA)
Heavy chain diseases	Neoplasms (notably Hodgkin's disease)
Gamma chain disease	Cytotoxic drugs
Alpha chain disease	Monoclonal gammopathies of undetermined significance
MU chain disease	
Primary amyloidosis	

middle and old age, striking men slightly more often than women. Due to malignant transformation of plasma cells in bone marrow, "monoclonal" production of IgG, IgA, IgD, IgE, or light chain portions of antibodies (Bence Jones protein) occurs. The cause of the disease is unknown, though genetic predisposition, chronic antigenic or inflammatory stimuli, and oncoviruses have all been implicated. The neoplasm appears to originate from a single transformed stem cell at a single location. Having a rapid doubling time, the tumor stem cell floods the marrow in that location with malignant clones, which are then spread by blood to distant sites.

Clinical signs and symptoms of multiple myeloma are related to tumor growth and activity. As marrow spaces become crowded, normal hematopoiesis is disrupted and contiguous bone invaded. Tumor cells secrete large quantities of M-components, causing hyperviscosity syndromes and osteoclast-activating factor (OAF), which stimulates bone resorption and uric acid production. Patients typically present with weakness and fatigue due to anemia and/or bone pain from osteolytic lesions and pathologic fractures. Many have recurrent infections, renal failure with hypertension, and hypercalcemia with confusion, polyuria, and constipation. Other than pallor and bony tenderness, the exam is unremarkable. Occasionally, lymphadenopathy and splenomegaly may be present. However, laboratory tests show an elevated ESR, rouleaux formation on blood smear, low hemoglobin and hematocrit, and high serum calcium levels. The total serum immunoglobulin is usually elevated, but a normal level does not rule out disease. Electrophoresis of serum and a 24-hour urine specimen typically reveal a spike (the result of M-component). Bence Jones proteins may or may not be detected on special urine analysis. X-ray films may show osteopenia resembling osteoporosis or extensive "swiss cheese" lesions. Definitive diagnosis requires the demonstration of plasma cells in marrow or soft tissue. Once it is made, patients should be referred to an oncologist for staging and treatment. In addition to chemotherapy, patients usually require medical treatment for hypercalcemia, anemia, renal failure, and infection. Tumors causing intractable bone pain may be reduced with radiotherapy. Those causing spinal cord compression are treated on an emergency basis with radiotherapy, high-dose steroids, and/or surgery.

In ***amyloidosis,*** plasma cells produce large quantities of a fibrillar protein (amyloid). ***Primary amyloidosis*** is a rare inherited disorder. ***Secondary amyloidosis*** develops in the wake of long-standing inflammatory processes and is seen with some frequency. It may follow tuberculosis, bronchiectasis, osteomyelitis, rheumatoid arthritis, or Crohn's disease, as well as multiple myeloma, Hodgkin's disease, and other tumors. It is also associated with adult-onset diabetes and aging. The clinical picture depends on the target area of amyloid infiltration. Skin thickening, waxy papules, and purpura mark ***cutaneous amyloidosis.*** Nerve and artery damage leads to a variety of neuropathies and ischemic conditions, particularly of the bowel. Other manifestations are nonspecific: fever, weakness, weight loss, lymphadenopathy, and congestive heart failure. Changes of the liver, spleen, kidney, and adrenal glands are particularly common. Amyloid should be suspected when any patient with a chronic disease develops cutaneous findings, hepatosplenomegaly, or albuminuria. The diagnosis is confirmed if tissue sections stained with Congo red dye show green birefringence under the polarizing microscope. The highest yield on a screening biopsy comes from rectal mucosa, though tongue and buccal mucosa provide other easily accessible sites. If underlying disorders can be controlled, amyloid deposition may be arrested. Otherwise, there is no cure. Corticosteroids and immunosuppressive agents have only occasionally proven useful.

T Lymphocytes and Cellular Immunity

T lymphocytes (T cells) originate from marrow stem cells but mature under the direction of the thymus gland. In the cortex of the gland, the earliest forms of the cells (thymocytes) divide rapidly and migrate toward the medulla. Before reaching the medulla, the T lymphocytes mature and enter the bloodstream for their first pass in a long, unique pattern of recirculation from blood to lymph nodes to the thoracic duct and back to the blood. During their stay in the lymph nodes, the cells migrate to areas unoccupied by B lymphocytes. Whereas B lymphocytes reside in the germinal centers, the T lymphocytes concentrate in the deep cortex and areas between germinal centers (thymic-dependent areas). Like B lymphocytes, T cells develop surface markers that are capable of recognizing antigens. These markers consist of two linked chains of amino acids that are imperceptible under the electron microscope. Compared to the hairy surface of B lymphocytes, T lymphocytes appear smooth. However, when sheep blood is mixed with human blood, sheep erythrocytes attach to surface markers of T lymphocytes in rosette fashion. They do not form a rosette around B lymphocytes, a fact used to separate and study the two cell populations.

T lymphocytes interact with antigens inside cells, antigens that are inaccessible physically and architecturally to antibodies. The response effected by T lymphocytes is thus referred to as "cellular immunity." It is initiated by the binding of an antigen to the surface marker of a sensitized T lymphocyte. Occurring directly or through macrophage mediators, antigen binding stimulates the T lymphocyte to differentiate into one of two main groups of cells. The first group includes (1) cells that release interferon (proteins that defend against viral infection), (2) cells that release lymphokines (chemical substances that recruit and stimulate macrophages), and (3) cytotoxic T lymphocytes (which destroy target cells, virus-infected cells, and tumor cells). The second group includes (1) helper cells (which bolster B-lymphocyte activity and antibody production) and (2) suppressor cells (which shut off B-lymphocyte activity when antibody production has reached sufficient levels). As might be expected, cellular immunity defends against infections established inside cells, particularly viruses. It is also responsible for the surveillance and destruction of cancer cells.

Cellular immunity is less immediate than humoral immunity, with responses lagging behind antigenic exposure by approximately 2 days. As in humoral immunity, protective effects may be offset by damaging effects. For example, granuloma formation in cases of tuberculosis infections is meant to wall off bacilli and prevent dissemination. In some instances, however, it creates large caseating abscesses that damage the lung itself. Furthermore, uncontrolled responses cause the ***type IV hypersensitivity reactions*** described in Table 7.30. Related problems are discussed under the affected system in other chapters.

T-cell deficiencies are listed in Table 7.33. Manifested in early life, all are quite rare. Although serum immunoglobulins are usually normal, B-cell function is somewhat compromised due to depletion of helper T cells. The most universal characteristic of these diseases is recurrent infections of the opportunistic agents such as fungi, viruses, and *Pneumocystis carinii*. As a result, patients display retarded growth and wasting. They have cutaneous anergy, chronic diarrhea, and high rates of malignancy. Fatal reactions may follow immunization with live viruses or bacilli Calmette Guérin (BCG), while graft-versus-host (GVH) disease threatens all transfusion and transplant procedures. Depending on the disorder, treatment involves

TABLE 7.33 T-CELL AND COMBINED DEFICIENCIES

T-cell deficiencies	X-linked recessive SCID
Thymic hypoplasia (diGeorge's syndrome)	SCID with leukemia (reticular dysgenesis)
Cellular immunodeficiency with immunoglobins (Nezelof's syndrome)	Partial combined immune disorders
Cellular immunodeficiency with nucleoside phosphorylase deficiency	Immunodeficiency with thrombocytopenia and eczema (Wiskott-Aldrich syndrome)
Severe combined immune disorders (SCIDs)	Ataxia telangiectasia
Autosomal recessive SCID	Immunodeficiency with short-limbed dwarfism
SCID with adenosine deaminase (ADA) deficiency	Immunodeficiency with thymoma
	Hypergammaglobulinemia E syndrome
	Chronic mucocutaneous candidiasis

thymic transplantation, transfusions, enzyme replacements, and/or bone marrow transplant. Survival to adulthood is rare.

AIDS (acquired immune deficiency syndrome) arises from the total destruction of a subset of helper T cells known as "T4 cells." A new disease, it was first described in the summer of 1981 when the Center for Disease Control (CDC) began to investigate the emergence of opportunistic infections in otherwise healthy homosexual men. Within five years, over 15,000 cases had been reported with nearly 7,000 deaths (AIDS is now a leading cause of natural death among prisoners). Caused by a retrovirus, human T-cell leukemia virus type III (HTLV-III), the disease was first seen almost exclusively among Haitians, homosexuals, homosexual contacts, IV drug users, prostitutes, and persons undergoing transfusions of blood products, particularly hemophiliacs. Recently, increasing numbers of persons who do not fall into the above categories have also contracted AIDS. In fact, it is estimated that 500,000 to one million people in the United States have been infected. The clinical disease is manifested in a variety of ways. Some patients experience a prodrome marked by persistent, unexplained fatigue and a "wasting syndrome triad" (lymphadenopathy, unexplained weight loss, and fever). Known as AIDS Related Condition (ARC), this may last for months to years before the development of the disease. The latter is signaled by the onset of hairy glossitis, Kaposi's sarcoma, or one of the opportunistic infections and cancers noted in Table 7.34. Haitians most commonly present with disseminated tuberculosis or an atypical mycobacterium.

If the suspicion of AIDS is high, patients should be referred to an infectious disease specialist or AIDS center for diagnosis. Many laboratory findings are characteristic. Blood chemistry tests are significant for mild elevations of SGOT, SGPT, triglycerides, and mild to severe hypoalbuminemia. There are no characteristic radiographic findings. The CBC commonly reveals mild anemia, leukopenia, and a normal to reduced platelet count. Bone marrow biopsy is negative except for mild hypoplasia. Lymph node biopsy may also be unremarkable. However, lymphocyte studies show lymphopenia related to reduced helper cells. The ratio of helper to suppressor cells (normally 2:1) is reversed (1:2). T-cell function is altered both in vivo and in vitro. This, in turn, accounts for a number of B-cell abnormalities noted on testing: increased numbers of immunoglobulin-secreting cells, elevated levels of serum immunoglobulins and circulating immune complexes, and poor B-cell activation including failure to respond to new antigens. With dysfunction of both humoral and particularly cellular immunity, cancers and opportunistic infections overwhelm the body. At present, there is no means of restoring the damaged immunologic function. Investigators are attempting therapy with agents that interfere with

TABLE 7.34 INFECTIONS AND CANCERS CHARACTERISTIC OF AIDS

Respiratory infections	CNS and eye infections
Pneumocystis carinii	Cryptococcal meningitis
Cytomegalovirus	Cerebral toxoplasmosis
Cryptococcus neoformans	Cytomegalovirus retinitis
Legionnaire's disease	GI infections
Fungal pneumonia	Candida esophagitis
Mycobacterium avium-intracellulare	Enteric cryptosporidiosis
Activated tuberculosis	*Giardia lamblia*
Mucocutaneous and disseminated infections	*Entamoeba histolytica*
Cytomegalovirus	*Shigella* and *Salmonella* species
Mycobacterium avium-intracellulare	Cancers
Herpes simplex virus I & II	Kaposi's sarcoma
Epstein-Barr virus	Lymphoma
	Carcinoma of tongue
	Anal and rectal carcinoma

HTLV-III's reproductive abilities (HPA-23, suramine, compound S, rebavirin) and with agents that increase the immune system's effectiveness (isoprinosine, imreg-1, interleukin-2). All of these experimental drugs have serious side effects. Although antimicrobial drugs are given for various infections, most patients die within 18–48 months from the time of diagnosis. Supportive care for victims is essential. Toward this end, important information can be gained from various ▶ ***AIDS organizations.*** As an important preventive step, a serologic marker is being used to screen all donated blood products and for patient screening. It should be noted that researchers estimate only 10% of patients with positive HTLV-III antibodies will develop the disease.

Combined immune deficiency disorders are characterized by depression of both humoral and cellular immunity. Various types are also listed in Table 7.33. Patients are at risk for recurrent bacterial and/or opportunistic infections and malignancies. They often require interdisciplinary care by various medical specialists.

Allogens

Antigen surface markers (allogens) exist on body cells to ensure recognition of self by the immune systems. There are erythrocyte and tissue antigens.

Erythrocyte antigens, which are genetically determined, include predominantly the ABO and Rhesus (Rh) groups. They may also include uncommon groups such as the RHo variant (Du), Kell (K), Duffy (Fya), and hr′ (c). The ABO and Rh groups give rise to the major ***blood types,*** which are listed in order of frequency in Table 7.35. Blood type is determined by routine antibody testing, in which (1) anti-A and/or anti-B reagents react with A or B surface antigens, confirming their presence or absence (cell or forward typing); (2) A and/or B RBCs react with serum containing anti-A or anti-B antibodies (serum or reverse typing); and (3) typing shows Rh factor to be present (Rh positive) or absent (Rh negative). The uncommon groups are determined by multiple agglutination tests using a pool of group O Rh-positive and Rh-negative RBCs that contain almost all important RBC antigens.

Typing is mainly needed for ***blood transfusions.*** Recipient blood must be matched to donor blood (cells and serum are tested for similar ABO, Rh, and any

TABLE 7.35 FREQUENCY OF ABO BLOOD TYPES

	Type O	Type A	Type B	Type AB
Whites	45%	40%	11%	4%
Blacks	49%	27%	20%	4%
Orientals	40%	28%	27%	5%
Americans	79%	16%	4%	<1%

Source: Statistics from Todd, Sanford, Davidson, *Clinical Diagnosis and Management.* Saunders, Philadelphia, 1979.

uncommon antigen types). It must also be cross-matched to determine the presence of IgG or IgM antibodies capable of reacting with transfused RBCs. Cross-matching is done with high-protein, enzyme-modified RBCs and indirect antiglobulin procedures. Ideally, only matched and cross-matched blood should be used for transfusions. In urgent situations, patients with any of the blood types may receive type O blood and patients with AB blood may receive type A or type B blood (never both). Although Rh-positive or Rh-negative blood may be given to an Rh-positive patient, Rh-negative blood must never be given to an Rh-negative patient except in life-threatening cases.

Transfusion reaction is characterized by hemolysis of recipient or donor RBCs during or following the administration of incompatible blood products (plasma, whole blood, or blood components). Fever, urticaria, pruritis, vasospasm, or sepsis may also occur. The worst and most common reactions occur when donor RBCs are hemolyzed by antibodies in the recipient's plasma. The severity of the reaction also depends on the degree of incompatibility, the amount of blood given, and the rate of administration, as well as the status of the patient's heart, kidneys, and liver. Some cases are mild enough to cause few if any symptoms. Usually, however, patients develop sudden anxiety followed by flushing, fever, chills, a bursting sensation in the head, and difficulty in breathing. Chest, neck, and low back pain may be severe. Within an hour, there may be progression to shock, marked by a rapid feeble pulse, cold clammy skin, nausea, and vomiting. Other than immediate discontinuation of the transfusion and supportive intervention, there is no specific treatment.

Erythroblastosis fetalis is a form of transfusion reaction resulting from an incompatibility of maternal and fetal blood. During gestation and particularly at the time of delivery, fetal blood cells enter the maternal circulation. If they are incompatible with the mother's blood type, maternal antibodies develop. The most common source of the problem is an Rh-negative mother/Rh-positive fetus or type O mother/type A, B, or AB fetus. Unless the mother was previously sensitized by transfusion, abortion, or miscarriage, the first born is rarely affected. During subsequent pregnancies, however, maternal antibodies may cause fetal hemolysis with anemia. Fetal bone marrow responds with reticulocytosis and the release of erythroblasts (immature RBCs), and further hemolysis ensues. Bilirubin rises. It is cleared in utero by crossing the placenta into the maternal circulation. However, in the newborn, bilirubin is not readily cleared and excess amounts deposit in the basal ganglia of the brain, producing kernicterus (a syndrome of poor feeding, flaccidity, opisthotonus, seizures, and apnea). During a pregnancy complicated by erythroblastosis fetalis, fetal bilirubin concentrations may be monitored by serial amniocentesis. Dangerously elevated bilirubin levels indicate the need for intrauterine transfusions every 2 weeks during gestation and immediate exchange transfusions at birth. The most important intervention, however, is prevention. Pregnant women should be blood typed. Those who are Rh negative should receive high-titer anti-Rh y-globulin (Rhogam) within 72 hours of delivery or abortion whenever the fetal blood type is unknown or known to be Rh positive. While ► ***Rhogam administration*** is usually performed by an obstetrician and at abortion clinics, it is also an important consideration in cases of spontaneous miscarriage, which are often seen in primary care settings.

The tissue or HLA antigens are coded in a locus of chromosome 6 called the "major histocompatibility complex (MHC)." At least five closely linked but separate loci are known to exist (A, B, C, D, and DR), each having a number of alternative forms (alleles). Antigens coded by A, B, or C loci are found on all nucleated cells except erythrocytes. They can be determined by serum studies and are referred to as the "serologically determined (SD) antigens." Antigens coded by D and DR loci exist only on B lymphocytes, monocytes, and epidermal and endothelial cells. Best studied by mixed lymphocyte culture reactions, they are often referred to as "mixed lymphocyte reaction (MLR)" antigens or LD "lymphocyte-determined (LD) antigens."

Certain alleles were recognized before the establishment of their loci. This resulted in the nonconsecutive numbering of A and B alleles and a confusing HLA nomenclature. To minimize future problems with nomenclature, a World Health Organization committee meets periodically to assign universally accepted designations to the rapidly growing number of HLA antigens now being recognized through research. Well-established antigens are given permanent names such as HLA-A1 or HLA-B5. Provisionally recognized antigens are given a workshop number such as HLA-Cw1 or HLA-Dw2.

Knowledge of tissue antigens and histocompatibility is central to ***organ transplantation.*** Typing donor and recipient tissues and matching HLA antigens as closely as possible has significantly improved the outcome of both sibling and cadaver transplants by reducing the ***rejection reaction.*** As described in Table 7.36, several types of rejection reactions can occur. In addition to tissue matching, they are minimized by suppressing the recipient's own immune system before and after transplantation. Immunosuppressive drugs (azathioprine, cyclophosphamide, prednisone, cyclosporin A), total body irradiation, total lymphatic irradiation (TLI), antilymphocyte serum (ALS), antilymphocyte globulin (ALG), and hybridized cells to eliminate specific lymphocyte subpopulations have been used for this purpose. In

TABLE 7.36 TYPES OF REJECTION REACTIONS

Type	Description
Hyperacute rejection	Graft never takes. Is quickly destroyed due to widespread vascular occlusion caused by presence of previous antibodies.
Acute rejection	Cell-mediated response (T lymphocytes) causes rejection 2–4 weeks after transplant.
Chronic rejection	Slight tissue incompatibility produces a weak immune response that causes rejection months or even years after transplant.
GVH	In bone marrow transplants, the immunocompetent cells of the donor attack tissue of the recipient. The graft recipient experiences skin rashes, weight loss, and diarrhea and may die if the grafted tissue is not removed.

addition, monoclonal antibodies and plant substances called "lectins" are being used to pretreat donor bone marrow. By selectively inhibiting T-cell activity, these procedures have significantly reduced GVH disease even in poorly matched tissue. In many cases, organ transplants are the last hope for a better quality of life or for any life at all. Unfortunately, organ banks are unable to meet transplant needs. Primary care providers can help reduce this shortage by offering important ***information about organ donations*** (see Chapter 1).

When allogens stimulate humoral or cellular immune systems to attack body cells in much the same way that they attack foreign substances, ***autoimmunity*** develops. The exact cause of misrecognition is unknown, but some kind of alteration in either allogens or the immune response is suspected. Alteration is thought to follow a traumatic or infectious process occurring in a genetically susceptible host. This supposition arises from associations of autoimmune disorders with HLA antigen types (Table 7.37). Autoimmune disorders are covered in other chapters where the target organs most affected are discussed.

HEMOSTASIS

Primary Hemostasis

As depicted in Figure 7.11, hemostasis is a series of events that arrests bleeding from damaged blood vessels. The initial physiologic response (primarily hemostasis) involves an interaction between vessel walls and platelet activities. Platelets (thrombocytes) are tiny discoid units without nuclei that arise from the marrow stem cell (CFU-MG). Thrombopoiesis involves the differentiation of committed stem cell

TABLE 7.37 HLA ASSOCIATIONS

Disorder	Antigen Association	Disorder	Antigen Association
Musculoskeletal		Endocrine	
Ankylosing spondylitis	B27	Graves' disease	Dw3, Bw35
Reiter's syndrome	B27	Hashimoto's disease	DR3
Psoriatic arthritis	B27	Addison's disease	Dw3
Yersinia and *Salmonella* arthritis	B27	Juvenile diabetes	Dw3, Dw4
Juvenile arthritis	B27	de Quervain syndrome	Bw35
Rheumatoid arthritis	DR4	Vascular	
SLE	DR2	Takayasu's disease	Bw5
Lyme arthritis	DRw2	Buerger's disease	B12
CNS		Hematologic	
Multiple sclerosis	Dw2	Hodgkin's disease	A1
Myasthenia gravis	Dw3	Acute lymphoblastic leukemia	A2, B12
Mucocutaneous and skin		Hemochromatosis	A3
Behçet's disease	B5	Renal	
Pemphigus vulgaris	DR4	Goodpasture's syndrome	DR2
Psoriasis	Cw6	Idiopathic membranous nephropathy	DR3
Dermatitis herpetiformis	Dw3	Liver and GI	
		Chronic active hepatitis	DR3
		Gluten-sensitive enteropathy	Dw3

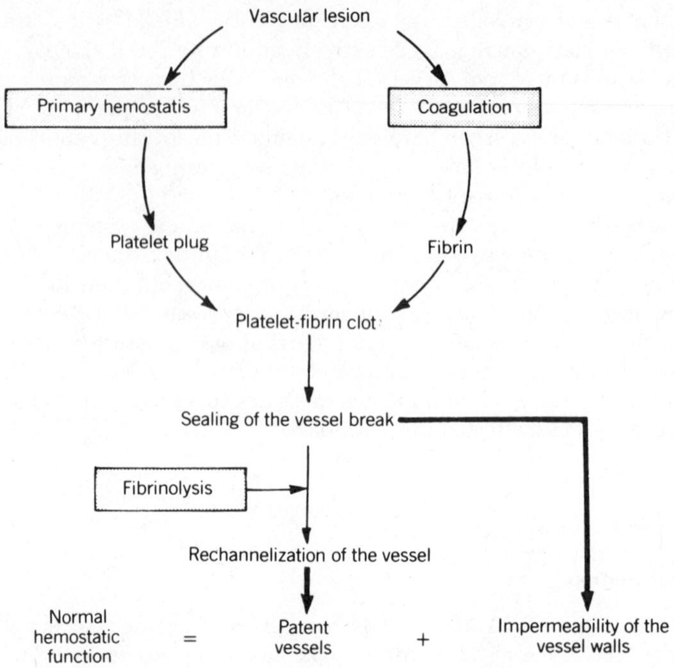

Figure 7.11 Hemostasis. (From Sultan, *Manual of Hematology,* © 1985, John Wiley & Sons, Inc., New York.)

into a megakaryocyte. During maturation in bone marrow, cytoplasm of the megakaryocyte develops demarcation membranes within which form granules, tubules, and canal systems of future platelets. Eight to 10 days later, the mature megakaryocyte extends a pseudopod into the circulation and breaks along demarcation membranes. Clumps of platelets are released into the blood, where they circulate with a life span of 10 days. When vascular injury occurs, smooth muscle in the vessel walls contracts to expose collagen fibers of the endothelium. Undergoing a change in shape, passing platelets adhere to the collagen fibers and release intrinsic adenosine diphosphate (ADP), which, in a complicated series of events, stimulates other platelets to aggregate at the wound site (Fig. 7.12). Aggregation results in the formation of a plug and the release of other substances that initiate coagulation (secondary hemostasis).

A reduced platelet count or ***thrombocytopenia*** alters primary hemostasis. It may be associated with problems resulting in decreased platelet production or increased platelet destruction, as noted in Table 7.38. In all cases, the hallmark is a prolonged bleeding time. The cardinal symptom is the presence of petechiae, pinpoint skin lesions that signify increased permeability of small blood vessels. Confluent petechiae (purpuric lesions) may develop, particularly along mucous membranes. Frank bleeding may follow from membrane linings of the nose, gums, hemorrhoids, vagina, or uterus. If extravasated blood traverses fascial planes, ecchymoses develop. However, their presence usually suggests a defect of secondary hemostasis. Whenever any of these symptoms are present, abdominal palpation or

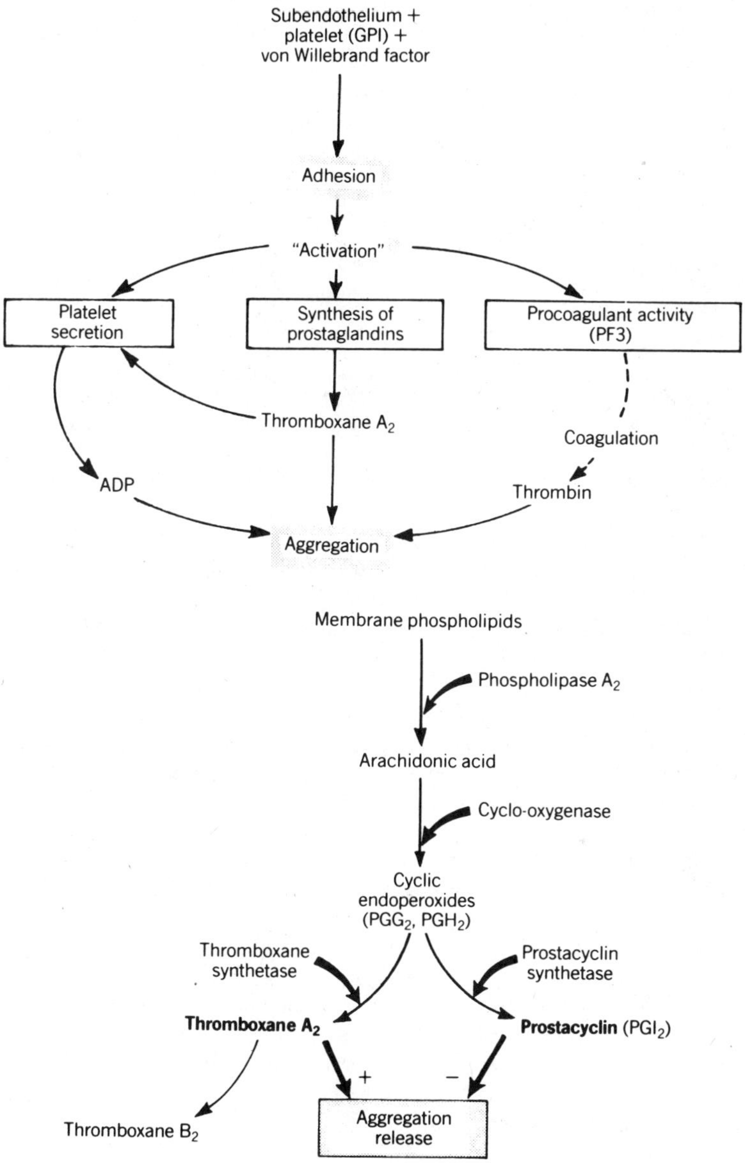

Figure 7.12 Platelet aggregation. (From Sultan, *Manual of Hematology,* © 1985, John Wiley & Sons, Inc., New York.)

TABLE 7.38 CONDITIONS ASSOCIATED WITH THROMBOCYTOPENIA

Decreased platelet production
- Aplastic anemia
- Leukemia
- Lymphoma
- Megaloblastosis
- Drug-induced suppression

Increased platelet destruction
- Cavernous hemangioma (Kasabach-Merritt syndrome)
- Infection (associated with endotoxins)
- Splenomegaly
- Idiopathic thrombocytopenic purpura (ITP)
- DIC
- Lymphoid malignancies
- SLE
- Hemolytic uremic syndrome (Gasser's syndrome)
- Cardiac prosthesis
- Evan's syndrome
- Thrombotic thrombocytopenic purpura (TTP)
- Postimmune purpura
- Drug-induced cell destruction
- Dilutional (transfusions of RBCs and/or plasma without platelets)

bimanual or rectal exams should be carefully conducted. Rough exam of an enlarged spleen is particularly dangerous and could lead to bleeding and rupture. The diagnosis is confirmed by reduced platelet counts. In addition to the bleeding time and platelet count, the work-up usually includes a thorough history with a search for genetic or drug connections, CBC, bone marrow aspiration, prothrombin time and partial thromboplastin time, Coombs' test, antinuclear antibodies (ANA), and ESR. The specific treatment depends on the cause. It may involve involve prednisone, splenectomy, and/or platelet transfusions. Related drugs must be discontinued. All patients should be protected from trauma; those with a platelet count of less than $20{,}000/mm^3$ are usually hospitalized.

An increased platelet count, or ***thrombocytosis,*** is another cause of altered primary hemostasis. Three forms occur (Table 7.39). They may be associated with thrombosis resulting from the physical presence of platelet masses or from the increased thromboxane production by excess platelets. As noted in Figure 7.12, thromboxane A2 stimulates vasoconstriction and platelet aggregation. Since cardiopulmonary embolism is the most clinically significant outcome, thrombus formation is covered in Chapter 6. Paradoxically, thrombocytosis may also be associated with the hemorrhagic changes described under thrombocytopenia. Referred to as ***hemorrhagic thrombocytosis,*** this phenomenon develops when platelet proliferation is accompanied by platelet dysfunction. It is encountered in chronic myelogenous leukemia, polycythemia vera, and agnogenic myeloid metaplasia, disorders mentioned at the beginning of this chapter. Thrombocytosis is diagnosed by increased platelet counts. It should be noted that a normal or low count does not rule out disease, since automated devices may mistake large platelets for erythrocytes. Thrombocytosis is also associated with spuriously high serum levels of potassium,

TABLE 7.39 CONDITIONS ASSOCIATED WITH THROMBOCYTOSIS

Primary thrombocythemias
- Essential or hemorrhagic thrombocythemia
- Chronic myelogenous leukemia
- Polycythemia vera
- Agnogenic myeloid metaplasia

Transitory thrombocytosis (following exercise or stress)

Epinephrine (transitory)

Reactive thrombocytosis
- Infections
- Hemolysis
- Hemorrhage
- Inflammatory disease
- Carcinomas
- Lymphomas
- Splenectomy

TABLE 7.40 QUALITATIVE PLATELET DISORDERS

Bernard-Soulier syndrome (giant platelet syndrome) Von Willebrand's disease Thrombasthenia (Glanzmann's disease) Release Reaction Defects Primary "Aspirin-like" disorder Associated with Hermansky-Pudlak, Wiskott-Aldrich syndrome, Chediak-Higashi syndrome, and type I glycogen storage disease	Acquired dysfunctions Uremia Paraproteinemia Acute and chronic leukemias SLE Pernicious anemia Scurvy Hepatic cirrhosis DIC

acid phosphatase, lactic acid dihydrogenase, uric acid, and zinc (all are normal on plasma determination). Treatment aims at lowering platelet production. Platelet pheresis is indicated for cases complicated by brisk spontaneous hemorrhage or repeated thrombotic episodes. However, most cases are managed with intermittent alkylating therapy (melphalan or busulfan for 4–6 weeks), aspirin (325 mg daily), and dipyridamole (200–400 mg daily).

Prolonged bleeding in the presence of normal platelet numbers occurs in ***qualitative platelet disorders.*** The various types (Table 7.40) evolve from either a congenital or an acquired dysfunction of specific platelet action—adhesion, aggregation, or release. Patients present with the same symptoms as those suffering from thrombocytopenia. The work-up is similar except that tests of platelet function must also be undertaken. The treatment is specific for the disease.

Vascular abnormalities may also affect primary hemostasis. Vasculitis, a variety of vascular purpuras, and hereditary hemorrhagic telangiectasia are characterized by prolonged bleeding times. These problems are discussed in Chapter 6.

Secondary Hemostasis

As depicted in Figure 7.13, secondary hemostasis (coagulation) is a complicated sequence of events that involves about 20 substances, most of which are plasma proteins. Coagulation substances have been assigned Roman numerals and/or named after the patients in whom they were first discovered. They circulate in blood in precursor forms (zymogens) or as cofactor proteins until activated. The precise mechanism for activation is debated but has traditionally been divided into extrinsic and intrinsic pathways. A substance not readily available within the vascular system is required to initiate the extrinsic pathways. Called "tissue thromboplastin" ("tissue factor"), it is contained in all body tissues. Upon contact with blood, it forms a complex with and thus activates factor VII. By contrast, mechanisms that occur within the vasculature activate the intrinsic pathway. They include changes initiated by primary hemostasis (direct activation of platelets, platelet aggregation on damaged endothelial tissues, and activation of factor XII). Extrinsic and intrinsic pathways converge in a common pathway that culminates in the formation of thrombin and thus a clot. To prevent excessive clotting, antithrombotic activities also occur. First, the liver removes activated clotting factors, while antithrombin III and other coagulation inhibitors neutralize activated clotting enzymes. Then clotting factor intermediates stimulate the conversion of plasminogen to plasmin. Plasmin

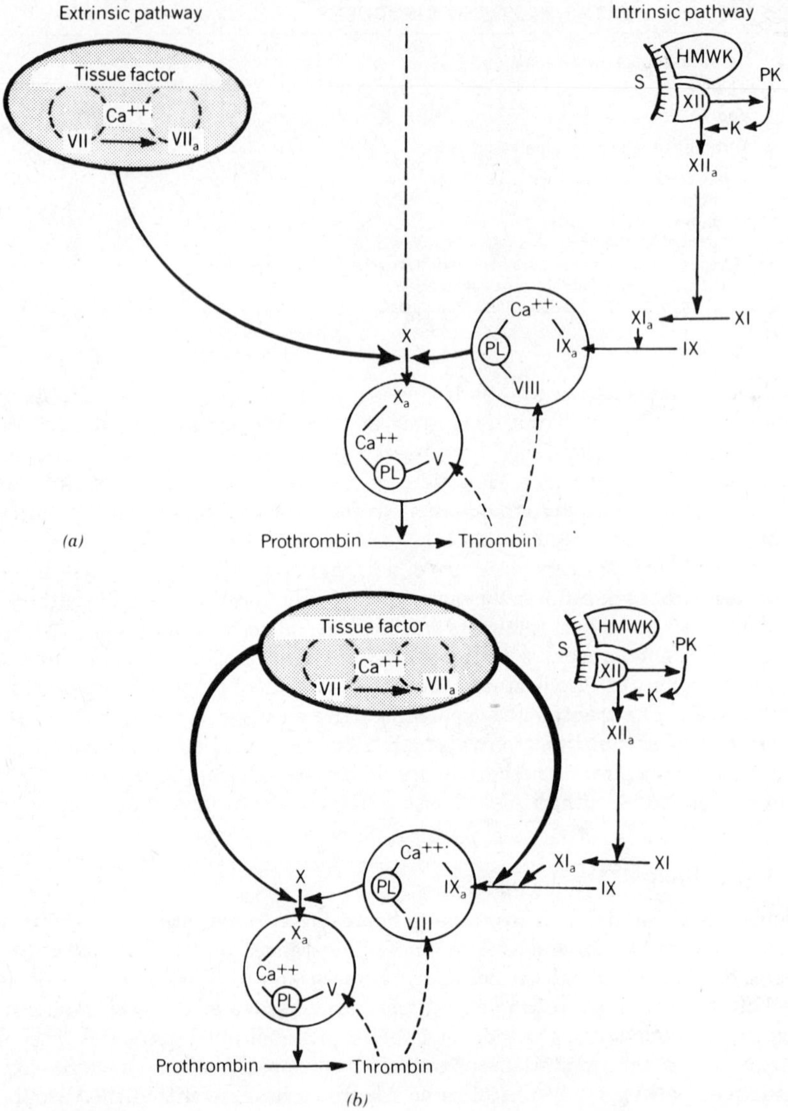

Figure 7.13 Coagulation. (From Sultan, *Manual of Hematology*, © 1985, John Wiley & Sons, Inc., New York.)

digests fibrinogen and lyses fibrin thrombi into fibrin split products, which further interfere with coagulation.

Defective structure or abnormal synthesis of clotting substances characterizes the ***coagulation disorders.*** Listed in Table 7.41, a number of types exist depending on which factor is disturbed and the genetic pattern of transmission. More than 90% of all cases are due to a deficiency of factor VIII ***(hemophilia A)*** and factor IX ***(hemophilia B).*** Inherited as a sex-linked recessive trait, the hemophilias are manifested

TABLE 7.41 COAGULATION DISORDERS

Inherited	Acquired
Hemophilia	Vitamin K deficiency
Von Willebrand's disease	Deficiency in the newborn
Factor XII (Hageman factor) deficiency	Malabsorption syndromes
Prekallikrein deficiency (Fletcher trait)	Coumarin anticoagulants
High molecular weight kininogen deficiency (Fitzgerald, Williams, or Flaujeac trait)	Liver disease
Factor XI deficiency	Renal disease
Factor IX deficiency	Acquired factor X (Stuart-Prower) deficiency with amyloidosis
Factor VII deficiency	DIC
Factor X (Stuart-Prower) deficiency	Fibrinolysis
Prothrombin deficiency	Inherited
Factor V deficiency	Secondary (obstetric complications, prostatic metastases, AML)
Factor XIII (fibrin-stabilizing) deficiency	Localized
	Anticoagulants
	Heparin
	Factor VIII inhibitors
	Associated with SLE and other conditions

almost exclusively in men. However, mild bleeding problems may be seen in female carriers who have an inactivated X chromosome (Lyon hypothesis). The clinical picture varies with the disease. Patients usually present early in life with hematomas from bleeding into muscles and soft tissues. Bleeding into joints, particularly knees, elbows, and ankles, also marks coagulation dysfunction. Hemarthrosis is accompanied by considerable pain and eventual joint deformities. While nosebleeds are uncommon, pharyngeal, retroperitoneal, and GI bleeding can be severe and life-threatening. Episodes of bleeding are usually spontaneous and often related to stress such as school or family problems. Those following trauma may be delayed, since primary hemostasis remains intact. Depending on the specific disorder, laboratory tests show varying patterns of prolonged prothrombin time and/or partial thromboplastin time, corrected or uncorrected with stored plasma. Treatment consists of replacing the missing factor with plasma or plasma fractions. Immune assays used to quantify the various factors identify carrier states for the purpose of genetic counseling. ▶***Hemophilia organizations*** offer special services and support.

Acquired coagulation disorders are also listed in Table 7.41. Bleeding episodes are clinically similar to those seen in the inherited disorders, except that they develop in patients with no prior personal or family history of bleeding tendencies. ***Vitamin K deficiency and liver dysfunction*** are related because the synthesis of factors VII, IX, X, and prothrombin occurs in the liver and requires vitamin K, a fat-soluble vitamin whose absorption depends on bile salts. ***Disseminated intravascular coagulation DIC*** is the widespread activation of clotting mechanisms triggered by tissue and bacterial products. Developing in the wake of abruptio placenta, placenta previa, metastatic carcinoma, ischemic tissue (acute injury or shock), endotoxins, gram-negative sepsis, meningococcemia, and RBC or platelet destruction, it is a life-threatening condition that usually responds best to treatment of the underlying disorder.

DETAILS OF MANAGEMENT

▸ *Leukemia Organizations*

Laboratory Tests: None.

Treatment Measures: None.

Patient Education: National Leukemia Association
Roosevelt Field
Garden City, New York 11501
Tel.: (516) 741-1190

Follow-up: Help patients or family members make contact as needed.

▸ *Folic Acid Deficiency*

Laboratory Tests: CBC. Vitamin B_{12} and folic acid assays.

Therapeutic Measures: Wherever possible, discontinue any drugs that may interfere with folic acid absorption (see Table 7.11). Start folic acid, 1 mg po daily. If the patient has severe malabsorption syndrome, start folinic acid (Leucovorin), 3 mg IM daily. Increase the dietary intake as follows:

RECOMMENDED DAILY ALLOWANCES FOR FOLACIN

Males (11 years and older)	400 UG
Females (11 years and older)	400 UG
Pregnant women	800 UG
Lactating women	500 UG

Continue therapy until anemia resolves. In chronic cases, continue the maintenance dose (folic acid, 1 or 0.25 mg) as needed.

Patient Education: Explain the need for folic acid as a substance for building RBCs. Review the medication schedule and diet. Note that actual folic acid in food loses potency in the body; therefore, the Food and Drug Administration lists food sources in terms of an equivalency substance (folacin). Emphasize the importance of vegetables as a main source. Provide a list as follows:

FOODS HIGH IN FOLACIN

Food	mg/100 g	Food	mg/100 g
Brewer's yeast	2.0	Alfalfa	0.80
Soybeans	0.69	Endive	0.47
Chickpeas	0.41	Oats	0.39
Lentils	0.34	Beans	0.31
Wheat germ	0.31	Liver	0.29
Split peas	0.23	Barley	0.21
Rice	0.17	Sprouts	0.14
Asparagus	0.12	Green peas	0.11
Sunflower seeds	0.10	Collard greens	0.10
Spinach	0.08	Kale	0.07
Brussel sprouts	0.05	Almonds	0.05
Bran	0.04	Beef	0.04

Follow-up: Repeat blood tests every month until the blood picture returns to normal. Chronic patients receiving maintenance doses should be seen every 6 months for review, medication renewal, and CBC.

► *Vitamin B_{12} Deficiencies Related to Diet, Malabsorption, and Pernicious Anemia*

Laboratory Tests: (SMAC) (look for LDH, bilirubin elevations). CBC, reticulocyte count. Folate, vitamin B_{12} assays. Schilling test with and without intrinsic factor.

Therapeutic Measures

General: Hospitalize severely anemic patients presenting with CHF. Transfusions are needed only if the HgB level is below 5 g or the patient is in cardiovascular distress. Treat moderately anemic patients as outpatients depending on the cause. In the beginning, watch for and correct hypokalemia, which may accompany vitamin B_{12} administration.

Diet deficiency: Start vitamin B_{12} oral supplements, 100 μg daily. For all patients except strict vegetarians, increase the dietary intake as follows:

RECOMMENDED DAILY ALLOWANCES FOR VITAMIN B_{12}

Males (11 years and older)	3.00 UG
Females (11 years and older)	3.00 UG
Pregnant women	4.00 UG
Lactating women	4.00 UG

Continue supplements until the blood picture returns to normal. Keep strict vegetarians on 10 μg daily for maintenance.

Malabsorption and pernicious anemia: Correct the underlying disorder wherever possible. Start vitamin B_{12} injections as follows: cyanocobalamin, 1,000 UG IM daily for 1 week, or weekly for 6 weeks or until the blood picture returns to normal. Once the anemia has been corrected, maintain patients on cyanocobalamin, 1,000 UG at monthly intervals, for life.

Patient Education

General: Explain the ongoing need for vitamin B_{12} as a substance for developing blood, epithelial cells, and nerve cells. Note that symptoms of anemia can be expected to resolve in about 6 weeks but that neural symptoms may take up to 18 months to improve. Also, in some cases, damage may be permanent.

Diet deficiency: Emphasize that the only significant food sources are animal products. Review the medication schedule. Provide a list of foods such as the following:

FOOD SOURCES OF VITAMIN B_{12}

Food	µg/100 g	Food	µg/100 g
Liver	0.86	Sardines	0.34
Clams	0.20	Mackerel	0.10
Snapper	0.088	Flounder	0.064
Salmon	0.047	Lamb	0.031
Swiss cheese	0.021	Eggs	0.020
Beef	0.015	Liverwurst	0.014
Lobster	0.013	Egg yolk	0.012
Chicken	0.0050	Turkey	0.0042
Milk	0.0040	Cream	0.0035
Buttermilk	0.0022	Butter	0.0010
Yogurt	0.00006	Vegetables	0.00000
Fruits	0.00000	Nuts	0.00000
Oils	0.00000	Yeast	0.00000

Malabsorption: Review specific problems the patient has with vitamin B_{12} absorption. Note that injections are necessary, since the vitamin is not being absorbed from the gut.

Pernicious anemia: Explain the relationship of vitamin B_{12} absorption to intrinsic factor and gastric parietal cells. Note the association of decreased intrinsic factor to autoimmune disease and gastric atrophy. Given the association of pernicious anemia with the development of gastric cancer, emphasize the importance of cancer screening. Teach the warning signs of gastric cancer.

Follow-up

General: Weekly appointments for injections. Hematocrit and hemoglobin tests every month until blood pictures return to normal.

Diet deficiency: As needed.

Malabsorption: Monthly appointments for injections. Hematocrit and hemoglobin tests every month until anemia resolves, then every 6 months for the first year, then yearly.

Pernicious anemia: Monthly appointments for injections and follow-up of symptoms. As soon as the anemia is stabilized, arrange for an upper GI series to rule out gastric cancer and do hemoccult screening every 6 months. Hematocrit and hemoglobin tests every month until the anemia resolves, then twice a year for the first year, then yearly.

▸ *Pyridoxine-Responsive Anemias*

Laboratory Tests: Diagnostic for sideroblastic anemia (CBC, reticulocyte count, peripheral smear, iron stain of bone marrow specimen, serum iron studies, bilirubin studies).

Therapeutic Measures

Dependency: For maintenance, adults require vitamin B_6, 200–600 mg daily.

Deficiency: Whenever possible, correct the underlying causes of inactivation or malabsorption. Give vitamin B_6, 50–100 mg po daily for 2 months. In addition to medication, increase dietary sources of vitamin B_6 as follows:

RECOMMENDED DAILY ALLOWANCES FOR VITAMIN B_6

Males (15 to 18 years)	2.0 mg
Males (19 + years)	2.2 mg
Females (15 + years)	2.0 mg
Pregnant women	2.6 mg
Lactating women	2.5 mg

Patient Education

General: Explain the need for vitamin B_6 as a substance for building RBC formation. Because lack of this vitamin renders cells incapable of incorporating iron, iron overload may result. Warn patients not to take iron supplements in any form. Review prescriptions for vitamin B_6 supplements.

Dependency: Explain that the problem is due to a genetic enzyme dysfunction that prevents normal utilization of vitamin B_6.

Deficiency: Review the causative factors such as poor diet, overuse of alcohol or drugs, and so on. Provide a list of foods such as the following:

DIET SOURCES OF PYRIDOXINE (VITAMIN B_6)

Food	mg/100 g	Food	mg/100 g
Brewer's yeast	4.0	Rice	3.6
Wheat	2.9	Soybeans	2.0
Rye	1.8	Lentils	1.7
Sunflower seeds	1.1	Tuna	0.90

DIET SOURCES OF PYRIDOXINE (VITAMIN B_6)

Food	mg/100 g	Food	mg/100 g
Bran	0.85	Peas	0.67
Liver	0.67	Avocados	0.60
Shrimp	0.60	Beans	0.57
Peanuts	0.40	Turkey	0.40
Oats	0.40	Chicken	0.40
Beef	0.40	Lamb	0.32
Banana	0.32	Pork	0.32
Corn	0.30	Spinach	0.28
Eggs	0.27	Green peppers	0.26
Barley	0.21	Potatoes	0.20
Pecans	0.18	Fruits	0.080
Cheeses	0.080	Milk	0.040

Follow-up

Dependency: Routine follow-up.

Deficiency: Return appointment in 2 months for repeat CBC. If anemia has not improved, refer the patient to a hematologist for further evaluation and possible androgen therapy.

▸ *Sickle Cell Trait*

Laboratory Tests: Sickle cell screen for patients with black or Hispanic parents. If positive, do hemoglobin electrophoresis, CBC.

Therapeutic Measures: In cases of gross hematuria, increase fluid intake; watch for and treat iron deficiency. In pregnancy, watch for an increased incidence of urinary tract infections and treat them accordingly.

Patient Education: Explain the difference between sickle cell trait and sickle cell disease. Reassure patients that the effects are limited but may include hematuria, increased urinary tract infections during pregnancy, and some degree of sickling under circumstances of reduced oxygenation (high-altitude flying, congestive failure, acute alcoholism, shock). Counsel on genetic implications.

Follow-up: As needed. Refer couples in which both the man and woman have sickle cell trait/and or disease for professional genetic counseling.

▸ *Sickle Cell Organizations*

Laboratory Tests: None.

Therapeutic Measures: None.

Patient Education: National Association for Sickle Cell Disease
3460 Wilshire Blvd., Suite 1012
Los Angeles, California 90010
Tel.: (213) 731-1166

Follow-up: Help patients make contact as needed.

▸ *Iron Deficiency Anemia*

Laboratory Tests: CBC with reticulocyte count and RBC indices. Serum ferritin or serum iron/iron-binding capacities (less significant than ferritin). Tests (particularly GI work-ups) as needed to identify the source of blood loss.

Therapeutic Measures: Start ferrous sulfate, 300 mg tid. Give ferrous gluconate, 300 mg tid, to patients who experience gastric irritation from ferrous sulfate. It is more expensive and provides less iron but is better tolerated. Absorption is greatest on an empty stomach. Continue iron preparations for 3 months. For cases refractory to oral iron, give a course of parenteral iron (Imferon) as follows: First, calculate the total dose (250 mg for every gram of hemoglobin deficit, i.e., below 14 g for men and below 12 g for women). Give 50 mg (1 mL) the first day and 100–250 mL daily until the total dose had been reached. To minimize tissue discoloration, use a 5-cm needle and inject the solution, after pulling the skin to the side (Z-technique), into the upper outer quadrant of the buttock. Observe for anaphylaxis and have injectable epinephrine on hand for emergency use. In addition to medication, increase the dietary sources of iron as follows:

RECOMMENDED DAILY ALLOWANCES FOR IRON

Males (11 to 18 years)	18 mg
Males (19 + years)	10 mg
Females (11 to 50 years)	18 mg
Pregnant women	*
Lactating women	†

*Iron requirements during pregnancy cannot be met through the diet. Daily supplements (30–60 mg) are recommended to prevent deficiency.
†Iron needs during lactation revert back to the nonpregnant state. However, continued supplementation for 2–3 months after childbirth is advised to replenish stores depleted by pregnancy and delivery.

Patient Education: Explain the need for iron as a building material for RBCs. To minimize gastric irritation, advise patients to take supplements after meals for the first week. Therefter (providing there are no problems), they should take the pills one-half hour before meals, since there is better absorption on an empty stomach. Warn patients that iron can cause constipation and a black appearance of the stool. Advise the use of Metamucil for constipation, since antacids can reduce iron absorption. Provide a list of foods such as the following:

DIETARY SOURCES OF IRON

Food	mg/100 g	Food	mg/100 g
Kelp	370	Seaweed	90
Bone meal	82	Brewer's yeast	17
Pumpkin seeds	11	Wheat germ	9.4
Blackstrap molasses	9.1	Liver	8.8
Pistachio nuts	7.2	Egg yolk	7.2
Mature sprouts	7.2	Chickpeas	6.9
Lentils	6.7	Walnuts	6.0
Mussels	5.8	Parsley	5.0
Oats	4.5	Clams	4.1
Rye	3.7	Wheat	3.5
Veal	3.2	Beef	3.1
Spinach	3.1	Pork	2.9
Barley	2.7	Beans	2.7
Peanuts	2.1	Corn	2.1
Turkey	2.1	Chicken	1.8
Peas	1.7	Coconut	1.7
Rice	1.6	Salmon	1.4
Tuna	1.3	Maple syrup	1.2
Potatoes	1.1	Berries	1.0
Cheeses	0.80	Milk	0.04

Follow-up: CBC and reticulocyte count in 2 weeks, monthly until corrected, then in 3 months as follow-up.

▸ *Malaria Prophylaxis for Travelers*

Laboratory Tests: None.

Therapeutic Measures: Advise appropriate prophylaxis for any patient planning to travel to a malarious area. Contact Parasitic Disease Division, Center for Infectious Disease directly (404-329-3670), or check the yearly edition of *Health Information for International Travel,* obtained from the U.S. Department of Health and Human Services, Public Health Service, Center for Disease Control, Atlanta, Georgia 30333). For patients who are traveling to areas reporting chloroquine-sensitive strains of *P. falciparum,* prescribe chloroquine phosphate,* 500 mg (300-mg base) po once a week for 1 week prior to arrival, during their stay, and for 6 weeks after departure. For patients who are traveling to areas reporting chloroquine-resistant strains (e.g., parts of Africa and Oceania) and who plan to stay for longer than 3 weeks, start chloroquine phosphate, 500 mg, and pyrimethamine, 25 mg/sulfadoxine 500 mg (Fansidar),† 1 tablet each, once a week prior to arrival, every week during their stay, and every week for 6 weeks after departure.

*Chloroquine is contraindicated in G-6-PD deficiencies.
†Fansidar should not be taken during pregnancy or by patients who are allergic to sulfa or pyrimethamine.

Patient Education: To reduce the risk of contracting malaria, advise travelers to (1) remain in well-screened areas when possible, particularly during evening, night, and early morning hours; (2) use mosquito repellents at all times; (3) wear long pants and long-sleeved shirts; and (4) sleep under mosquito netting. Inform patients about drug side effects and complications. Those taking Fansidar should be instructed to watch for mucocutaneous skin lesions, pharyngitis, and/or fever, and to discontinue the drug immediately if these conditions develop. Note that chloroquine use within a year is a contraindication to donating blood. Warn patients that even with prophylaxis, delayed malarial attacks sometimes occur several months to a year later.

Follow-up: None.

▸ *AIDS Organizations*

Laboratory Tests: None.

Therapeutic Measures: None.

Patient Education: National Gay Task Force
80 Fifth Ave.
New York, New York 10011
Tel.: (800) 221-7044

American Social Health Association
National STD/VD Hotline
Tel.: (800) 227-8922

Follow-up: As needed.

▸ *Rhogam Administration*

Laboratory Tests: Maternal blood typing for Rh factor.

Therapeutic Measures: Unless the father's blood type or products of conception are conclusively shown to be Rh negative, primary care providers should be sure that immune globulin has been given to the Rh-negative woman as follows:

Amniocentesis, miscarriage, abortion, ectopic pregnancy at or beyond the 13th week—Rhogam, one vial IM within 72 hours.

Amniocentesis, miscarriage, abortion, ectopic pregnancy prior to 13 weeks—Micrhogam, one vial IM within 72 hours.

Patient Education: Explain isoimmunization, the risk to future babies, and the preventive role of Rhogam.

Follow-up: None.

▶ *Hemophilia Organizations*

Laboratory Tests: None.

Therapeutic Measures: None.

Patient Education: National Hemophilia Foundation
110 Green Street
New York, New York 10012
Tel.: (212) 219-8180

Follow-up: As needed.

BIBLIOGRAPHY

Ambramowicz M (ed.). Drugs for parasitic infections. *The Medical Letter on Drugs and Therapeutics,* (Dec.) 1979, 21(26):105–112.

Alli BA. Malaria and antimalarial therapy. *Continuing Education,* (July) 1981, 37–43.

Allison JG. The role of surgery in the management of lymphoma. *Journal of the American Medical Association,* (Dec.) 1981, 246(24):2843–2848.

Amin NM. Malaria: Prevention and treatment. *Family Practice Recertification.* (Feb.) 1985, 7(2):45–78.

Bakerman S. Metal poisoning: The laboratory detection of lead, arsenic, and mercury. *Laboratory Management,* (Apr.) 1983, 13–17.

Bates B. *A Guide to Physical Examination.* Lippincott, 3rd ed., Philadelphia, 1984.

Berkow RB (ed.). *The Merck Manual of Diagnosis and Therapy,* 14th ed. Merck, Sharp & Dohme Research Laboratories, Rahway, N.J., 1982.

Blood products. *The Medical Letter on Drugs and Therapeutics,* (Nov.) 1979, 21(23):93–96.

Bock GH, Vernier RL. Immunologic kidney disease. *American Family Physician,* (Nov.) 1980, 22(5):87–96.

Brown AM, Stubbs DW (eds.). *Medical Physiology.* Wiley, New York, 1983.

Camitta BM. *Childhood Anemia.* Monograph. American Academy of Family Physicians, Kansas City, Mo., June 1978.

Conn HF, Conn RB Jr (eds.). *Current Diagnosis.* Saunders, Philadelphia, 1980.

Crafts RC. *A Textbook of Human Anatomy,* 3rd ed. Wiley, New York, 1985.

Crosby WH. Iron deficiency: Seven rules for corrective therapy. *Consultant,* (Jan.) 1980, 49–50.

Crosby WH. Red cell mass: Its precursors and its perturbations. *Hospital Practice,* (Feb.) 1980, 71–81.

Crosby WH. Iron storage disease: Hemochromatosis. *Continuing Education,* (Jan.) 1981, 56–61.

Crosby WH. Hypersplenism: What causes it? Should you treat it? *Consultant,* (June) 1983, 103–110.

Crouch JE, McClintic JR. *Human Anatomy and Physiology,* 2nd ed. Wiley, New York, 1976.

Dixon FJ. Murine SLE models and autoimmune disease. *Hospital Practice,* (Mar.) 1982, 63–72.

Durant JR. The medical management of Hodgkin's disease. *Continuing Education,* (July) 1981, 57–61.

Eichelberger JW. *Fundamentals of Thrombokinetics.* Bio/Data Corp., Horsham, Pa. 1979.

Eipe J, Green D, Sussman I. Disseminated intravascular coagulation: When DIC threatens your patient. *Patient Care,* (May) 1980, 120–130.

Elias H, Pauly JE, Burns ER. *Histology and Human Microanatomy,* 4th ed. Wiley, New York, 1978.

English E, Finch CA. The clinical approach to anemia. *Physician Assistant and Health Practitioner,* (Mar), 1980, 18–25.

Frank E, Landesman SH. Acquired immune deficiency syndrome: Lessons learned and questions unanswered. *Drug Therapy,* (Sept.) 1983, 169–176.

Freedman SO, Gold P (eds.). *Clinical Immunology,* 2nd ed. Harper & Row, New York, 1976.

Friedman EW. Reticulocyte counts: How to use them, what they mean. *Diagnostic Medicine,* (July) 1984, 29–33.

Fry J. Infectious mononucleosis: Some new observations from a 15-year study. *Journal of Family Practice,* 1980, 10(6):1087–1089.

Fuller E. SLE: "Wolf" in sheep's clothing. *Patient Care,* (Mar.) 1984, 134–174.

Goldman JN, Goldman MB. What the clinician should know about the major histocompatibility complex. *Journal of the American Medical Association,* (Aug.) 1981, 246(8):873–876.

Goldsmith JC, et al. T-lymphocyte subpopulation abnormalities in apparently healthy patients with hemophilia. *Annals of Internal Medicine,* (Mar.) 1983, 98(3):294–296.

Goroll AH, May LA, Mulley AG. *Primary Care Medicine: Office Evaluation and Management of the Adult Patient.* Lippincott, Philadelphia, 1981.

Gray H. *Anatomy of the Human Body,* 29th American ed. (CM Goss, ed.). Lea & Febiger, Philadelphia, 1973.

Guttmann RD (ed.). *Immunology.* Upjohn Co., Kalamazoo, Mich., 1981.

Guyton AC. *Textbook of Medical Physiology,* 6th ed. Saunders, Philadelphia, 1981.

Hancock SL, Glatstein E. Hodgkin's disease: Radiation vs. chemotherapy as the treatment of choice. *Primary Care and Cancer,* (Nov.) 1984, 4(11):31–42.

Henley WL. Genetic predisposition to autoimmune disorders. *Pediatric Annals,* (Apr.) 1982, 11(4):369–374.

Henry JB (ed.). *Todd-Sanford-Davidson Clinical Diagnosis and Management by Laboratory Methods,* 16th ed., Vols. 1 and 2. Saunders, Philadelphia, 1979.

Herbert V. The nutritional anemias. *Hospital Practice,* (Mar.) 1980, 65–89.

Hoole AJ, Greenberg RA, Pickard CG Jr. *Patient Care Guidelines for Nurse Practitioners.* Little, Brown, Boston, 1982.

Isselbacher KJ, et al. *Harrison's Principles of Internal Medicine,* 9th ed. McGraw-Hill, New York, 1980.

Jackson JE, Bressler R. Prescribing tricyclic antidepressants, Part I: General considerations. *Drug Therapy,* (Dec.) 1981, 87–94.

Kaplan SA. Anaphylaxis: Diagnosis, prevention, and treatment. *Continuing Education,* (July) 1980, 13(1):27–32.

Kelley WN, et al. *Textbook of Rheumatology,* Vols. I and II. Saunders, Philadelphia, 1981.

Khan FA, Wollschlager CM. Acquired immune deficiency syndrome: A deadly new disease. *Postgraduate Medicine,* (Aug.) 1983, 74(2):180–191.

Kirkwood E, Lewis C. *Understanding Medical Immunology.* Wiley, New York, 1983.

Kitchens CS. The evaluation and treatment of thrombocytopenia. *Continuing Education,* (Nov.) 1980, 73–84.

Krupp MA, Chatton MJ, Werdegar D (eds.). *Current Medical Diagnosis and Treatment 1985.* Lange, Los Altos, Calif., 1985.

Kunkel HG. The immunopathology of SLE. *Hospital Practice,* (Nov.) 1980, 47–56.

Lacher MJ. Hodgkin's disease: Historical perspective, current status, and future directions. *Ca—A Cancer Journal for Clinicians,* (Mar.–Apr.) 1985, 35(2):88–93.

Lai PK. Infectious mononucleosis: Recognition and management. *Hospital Practice,* (Aug.) 1977, 47–52.

Lazerson J. The problem patient: Easy bruising but normal platelets in an old woman. *Hospital Practice,* (Nov.) 1984, 56A–56F.

Lubin BH, Kleman K, Pennathur-Das R. Sickle cell disease and the thalassemias: Diagnostic assays. *Laboratory Management,* (Aug.) 1980, 38–47.

Luckmann J, Sorensen KC. *Medical Surgical Nursing: A Psychophysiologic Approach,* 2nd ed. Saunders, Philadelphia, 1980.

Macher AM, Masur H, Lane HC, et al. *AIDS: Diagnosis and Management.* Burroughs Wellcome Co., Research Triangle Park, N.C., April 1984.

Malcolm Z, Rimland D. Acquired immune deficiency syndrome. *Physician Assistant,* (Oct.) 1983, 31–43.

Mandell GL, Douglas RG Jr, Bennett JE. *Principles and Practice of Infectious Diseases.* Wiley, New York, 1979.

Marchand A. Immune hemolytic anemia, part 2: Test procedures and strategy. *Diagnostic Medicine,* (Mar.–Apr.) 1983, 25–34.

Meuwissen HJ. Evaluating patients with suspected immunodeficiency: Guidelines for clinical and laboratory diagnosis. *Postgraduate Medicine,* (Nov.) 1979, 66(5):116–131.

Moake JL, Funicella T (AH Trench, ed.). Common bleeding problems. *Clinical Symposia,* 1983, 35(3):2–32.

Moake JL, Levine JD (AH Trench, ed.). Thrombotic disorders. *Clinical Symposia,* 1985, 37(4):3–32.

Muller-Eberhard HJ. Chemistry and function of the complement system. *Hospital Practice,* (Aug.) 1977, 33–43.

Nagel RL, Fabry ME, Kaul DK. New insights on sickle cell anemia. *Diagnostic Medicine,* (May) 1984, 26–33.

Neilan BA. Late sequelae of splenectomy for trauma. *Postgraduate Medicine,* (Sept.) 1980, 68(3):207–210.

New York State Department of Health. *15 Things You Should Know About Sickle Cell.*

Pearson HA. Splenectomy: Its risk and its roles. *Hospital Practice,* (Aug.) 1980, 85–94.

Peter JB. Acquired immune deficiency syndrome: A new medical mystery. *Diagnostic Medicine,* (Jan.–Feb.) 1983, 1–8.

Pinkel D, Silver RT, Simone JV, et al. Exploring current leukemia therapies. *Patient Care,* (Dec.) 1979, 54–78.

Pitchenik AE, et al. Opportunistic infections and Kaposi's sarcoma among Haitians: Evidence of a new acquired immunodeficiency state. *Annals of Internal Medicine,* (Mar.) 1983, 98(3):277–286.

Poon M-C, Landay A, Prasthofer EF, et al. Acquired immunodeficiency syndrome with *Pneumocystis carinii* pneumonia and *Mycobacterium avium-intracellulare* infection in a previously healthy patient with classic hemophilia. *Annals of Internal Medicine,* (Mar.) 1983, 98(3):287–293.

Prchal JT. Red cell enzymes: An overview. *Continuing Education,* (July) 1980, 41–50.

Sams WM Jr. Allergic vasculitis. *Continuing Education,* (May) 1982, 69–74.

Schafer AI. Bleeding disorders: Finding the cause. *Hospital Practice,* (Nov.) 1984, 88K-HH.

Schatz IJ. The coagulation of blood disorders and drugs. *Emergency Medicine,* (Mar.) 1981, 24–36.

Scott RB, Castro O. Screening for sickle cell hemoglobinopathies. *Journal of the American Medical Association,* (Mar.) 1979, 241(11):1145–1147.

Sell S. How the immune system works. *Medical Times,* (Dec.) 1980, 108(12):60–76.

Sheehy TW. Alcohol: Its effects on the hematopoietic system. *Continuing Education,* (Oct.) 1980, 71–78.

Silverstein A. *Human Anatomy and Physiology.* Wiley, New York, 1980.

Sloan RW. Antiplatelet therapy. *American Family Physician,* (Oct.) 1981, 24(4):129–134.

Sultan C, Gouault-Heilmann M, Imbert M. *Manual of Hematology.* Wiley, New York, 1985.

Tannenbaum S. Blood: Which component and why? *Physician Assistant,* (Nov.) 1983, 133–150.

Tips to prevent AIDS. *Your Patient and Cancer,* (June) 1983, 46–48.

Ultmann JE, Jacobs RH. The non-Hodgkin's lymphomas. *Ca—A Cancer Journal for Clinicians,* (Mar.–Apr.) 1985, 35(2):66–85.

Ward PA. The immunopathology and immunoprophylaxis of malaria. *Infectious Diseases,* (Oct.) 1978, 8(10):4–31.

Williams RC Jr. Immune complex–mediated rheumatic diseases. *Postgraduate Medicine,* (Nov.) 1980, 68(5):124–131.

Wormser GP, et al. Acquired immunodeficiency syndrome in male prisoners: New insights into an emerging syndrome. *Annals of Internal Medicine,* (Mar.) 1983, 98(3):297–303.

Wyngaarden J, Smith L Jr (eds.). *Cecil Textbook of Medicine,* 16th ed., Vols. 1 and 2. Saunders, Philadelphia, 1982.

Young N, Henry W, Nienhuis AW. Treatment of primary hemochromatosis with deferoxamine. *Journal of the American Medical Association,* (Mar.) 1979, 241(11):1152–1154.

8

Urinary Tract

Carla Greene

Outline

Dialysis
Dialysis dementia
► Organizations for renal patients
► Considerations for patients with renal failure
Kidney transplant

Glomerular Membranes

Glomerulonephridites
Immune complex disease
Antibody-mediated response
Postinfectious glomerulonephritis
Rapidly progressive glomerulonephritis (RPGN)
Chronic glomerulonephritis
IgA nephropathy
Nephrotic syndrome

URINE FORMATION

Tubules and Interstitium

Tubulointerstitial disease
► Acute pyelonephritis
Chronic pyelonephritis
Noninfectious tubulointerstitial disease
Acute noninfectious tubulointerstitial nephritis (TIN)
Chronic TIN

Water Balance and Volume Control

Syndrome of inappropriate antidiuretic hormone (SIADH)
Nephrogenic diabetes insipidus
Diabetes insipidus
Volume dipletion

Salt Regulation

► Salt-restricted diet
Hypernatremia
Hyponatremia
Acute hyponatremia
Chronic hyponatremia

Potassium Regulation

Sick cell syndrome
Hyperaldosterone conditions
Hypoaldosterone conditions
Hyperkalemia
► Hypokalemia

Bicarbonate and Hydrogen Ion Concentration

Metabolic acidosis
Metabolic alkalosis
Milk-alkali syndrome
Contraction alkalosis
Bartter's syndrome
Renal tubular acidosis
Proximal renal tubular acidosis (Type II)
Distal renal tubular acidosis (Type I)
Renal tubular acidosis (Type IV)

Glucose and Amino Acid Reabsorption

Glucosuria
Hyperosmolar diuresis
Renal glycosuria
Aminoaciduria
De Toni-Debre (Fanconi) syndrome

Uric Acid Clearance

Hyperuricemia
Gouty nephropathy
► Mild hyperuricemia
► Significant hyperuricemia

URINE ELIMINATION

Ureters

Congenital anomalies
Renal stones
Renal colic
Obstructive nephropathy
Hydronephrosis
Dietl's crisis
Retroperitoneal fibrosis

Bladder

Vesicoureteral reflux
Structural abnormalities of the bladder
Bladder (vesicle) stones
Cystitis
Interstitial cystitis
Schistosoma haematobium
Renal tuberculosis
Hemorrhagic cystitis
► Acute bacterial cystitis
Cystitis emphysematosa

Recurrent or chronic bacterial cystitis
Cystitis cystica (vesicular cystitis)
Bladder cancer

Urethra

Hypospadias
Phimosis
Balanitis
Male urethritis
Urethral gland abscess
Female urethritis
Honeymoon cystitis

Micturition

Micturition syncope
Urinary retention
Retention with overflow
Urinary incontinence
Enuresis
Stress incontinence
Urgency incontinence
Paradoxical incontinence
Continuous incontinence
Aging changes
Neurogenic bladder
Upper motor neuron bladder
Lower motor neuron bladder
Cord bladder
Autonomic hyperreflexia

The urinary tract consists of the kidneys, ureters, bladder, and urethra. Complicated in structure, the kidneys are responsible for filtering blood and forming urine. The ureters, bladder, and urethra all play a part in urine elimination.

KIDNEY STRUCTURE

Size and Position

The kidneys lie against the posterior abdominal wall, occupying a space behind the peritoneum. Due to the position of the liver, the right kidney is normally lower than the left, and its caudal pole may be slightly palpable. Each bean-shaped organ can be measured radiographically in relation to body habitus. The entire kidney normally occupies 3.5 times the distance from the top of L1 to L2. Average numerical measurements are 12.8 cm right kidney, 13.3 cm left kidney for men, and 12.3 cm right kidney, 12.8 cm left kidney for women.

Malformations of the kidney occur with some frequency. Sometimes the two kidneys are fused together. They may be joined together with a thick mass of renal tissue at their lower ends ***(horsehoe kidney)*** or completely united ***(disk-like kidney).*** Though such kidneys remain functionally normal, they are at higher risk for the development of stones and infection because the ureters emerge at abnormal angles, promoting urinary stasis.

A ***third kidney*** may be present, or one kidney may show ***congenital atrophy.*** Although very small, the atrophied kidney is usually normal in structure. About one in 1,000 individuals is born with an ***isolated kidney.*** In meeting the functional needs of the body, the single kidney may become hypertrophied, presenting in later life as an abdominal mass. Work-ups must be carefully managed, since a single kidney should not be subjected to the possibility of acute renal failure from an intravenous pyelogram (IVP) or hemorrhage from a percutaneous biopsy. Once the hypertrophied kidney extends beyond the protective confines of the rib cage, it is at increased risk for traumatic injury.

Ectopic kidneys are situated too high, too low, or too far forward in reference to the vertebral column. They are due to abnormal ascent from the pelvis during embryonic development. Movement within layers of the peritoneum enveloping ectopic kidneys creates the condition known as ***floating kidney.*** Ectopic kidneys occurring in the pelvis between the rectum and bladder or beside the uterus may be particularly prone to intercurrent infections.

Renal Zones

In transverse section, each kidney displays an outer zone (cortex), a middle zone (medulla), and a central zone (pelvis), as illustrated in Figure 8.1. The cortex and medulla contain specific portions of the functional unit of the kidney, the nephron. Nephrons originate in the cortex with a capillary bed called the "glomerulus." Surrounding the glomerulus is Bowman's capsule. It constitutes the beginning of the nephron's tubule system, parts of which are labeled in Figure 8.2. Although the proximal convoluted tubule remains in the cortex, the loop of Henle descends into the medulla. It is divided into descending and ascending limbs, the latter having thin and thick sections. Some nephrons have loops that descend a short distance to the junction between the outer and inner medullas (superficial or cortical nephrons). Others have loops that descend deep within the inner medulla (juxtamedullary nephrons).

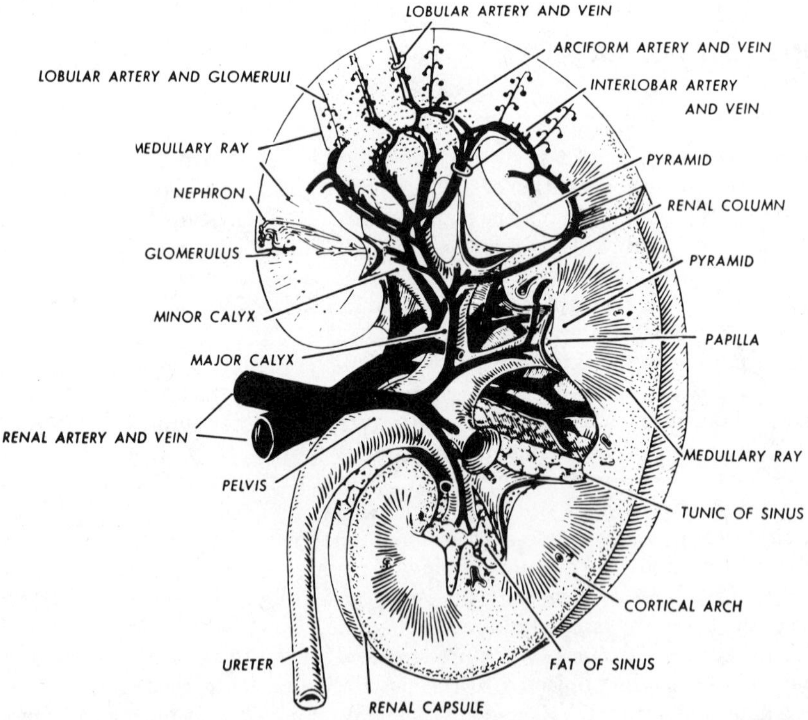

Figure 8.1 Renal zones and circulation. (From Brown, *Medical Physiology,* © 1983, John Wiley & Sons, Inc., New York.)

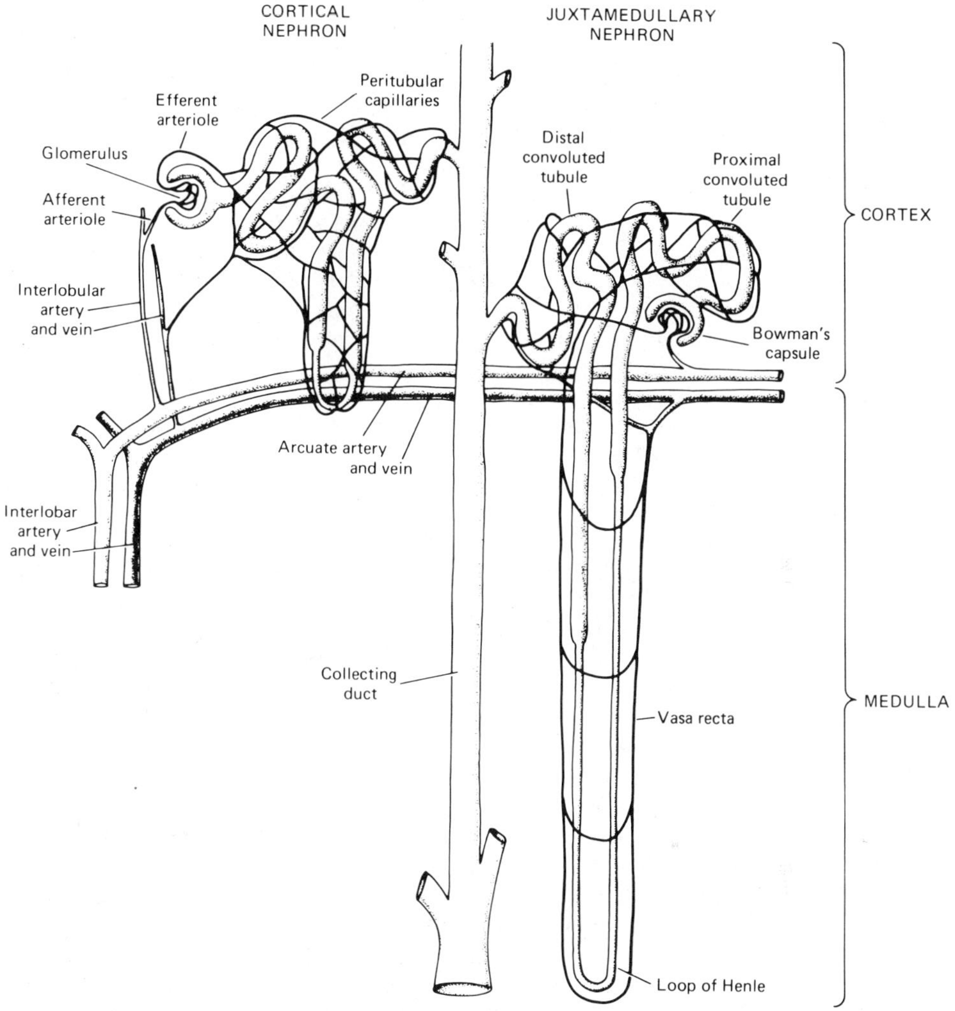

Figure 8.2 Nephron. (From Muir, *Pathophysiology: An Introduction to the Mechanisms of Disease,* © 1980, John Wiley & Sons, Inc., New York.)

A portion of the thick ascending limb of Henle's loop reenters the cortex. Here densely packed small cells (the macula densa) brush against specialized muscle cells (juxtaglomerular cells) contained in the wall of an afferent arteriole. At the point of contact, mesangium penetrates the arteriole and tubule walls, creating a channel of communication between the two types of modified cells. Together, juxtaglomerular cells, macula densa cells, and mesangial tissue make up the juxtaglomerulus apparatus.

The end of the macula densa marks the beginning of the distal convoluted tubule, structures of which fuse into the collecting tubule. Collecting tubules containing 3,000–5,000 nephrons converge to form a single collecting duct. Several ducts (each with its thousands of nephrons) create a striated segment of tissue known as the "renal pyramid." There are normally 8–18 pyramids per kidney, each coming to a tip (papilla) in the deepest region of the medulla. At the papilla, the collecting ducts terminate and urine generated by the tubules empties into the calices, cup-shaped areas that join together and form the renal pelvis (see Fig. 8.1).

The pelvicaliceal system also serves as an inner foyer for the hilum, where the renal artery enters the kidney and the renal vein and ureter exit. It parallels the psoas muscle. Thus the margin of the psoas can be clearly delineated on x-ray films unless there is some dilatation of the pelvicaliceal system. Referred to as the "renal mantle," the cortex and medulla together constitute the distance between the lateral outline and the nearest laterally directed calyx. The normal renal mantle measures 2.5 cm.

Cystic disease of the kidney may cause significant deformity. Several variations exist, as described in Table 8.1. Transmitted as an autosomal dominant trait, ***adult polycystic kidney disease (APDK)*** is the most common, affecting 1 in 500 persons. The exact cause of the disease is unclear. According to early investigators, APDK represented the failure of nephron tubules to communicate with the urinary space, either because of obstruction due to uric acid salts or as a developmental abnormality, but this theory was disproved by later studies. More recent proposals suggest altered compliance of tubular basement membranes and partial obstruction. Whatever the pathogenesis, the effect is sporadic development of cysts along all portions of the nephron in genetically predisposed kidneys. Originally appearing normal in structure and function, the kidney becomes enlarged and distorted over time. A similar process may occur in the liver due to noninvolution of intrahepatic bile ducts (polycystic liver disease) or in the vessels of the brain (berry aneurysms). Cysts have also been documented in the thyroid, lung, pancreas, spleen, ovary, testis, epididymis, uterus, and bladder. In the kidney, they fill with blood, serous fluid, or urine. Areas of normal and abnormal tissue intermix in both the cortex and the medulla. Although malformations are bilateral, cyst development may be asymmetric or unilateral. It may also advance at varying rates, causing problems as early as childhood, or not until the eighth decade. Most patients remain asymptomatic until age 40 or 50 and then present with flank pain, gross hematuria, and/or polyuria. Symptoms are often related to obstruction of the pelvicaliceal system by the cysts themselves or to the associated formation of stones and blood clots. Rupture of a cyst may be the origin of pain or hematuria. Clinical findings may include hypertension, proteinuria, enlarged palpable kidney, and elevated blood urea nitrogen (BUN) and creatinine.

Renal ultrasound for APKD reveals multiple round lucencies throughout an irregularly outlined renal margin ("Swiss cheese" or "cellulose sponge" appearance). Sonograms, which are extremely sensitive to early changes, pick up replacement of normal central medullary echo patterns with multiple rounded echo patterns. Sonography is currently considered the best and safest screening method for polycystic kidney disease. IVP and angiographic studies carry greater risk, particularly when renal function is impaired. Retrograde pyelography should almost never be performed due to the high incidence of subsequent infection. Concerning management, careful control of any associated hypertension helps to minimize the acceleration of renal damage. However, since there is no way to prevent progression of the underlying pathology, APKD invariably leads to renal insufficiency and the need for dialysis. It is also associated with complications such as calculi, pyelonephritis, abscess formation, cyst infection or rupture, and hemorrhage, requiring immediate

TABLE 8.1 CYSTIC DISEASES OF THE KIDNEY

Disease	Description
Simple cyst	Single or multiple thin-walled structures (filled with plasma filtrate) arising as a degenerative process. Usually bulges from the kidney surface. Common in the elderly but rare in younger age groups. Cysts are typically small and asymptomatic but can reach significant size. May be confused with polycystic or multicystic kidney disease. Possible site for malignancy. X-ray film shows visible calcification of walls ("eggshell" calcification). Aspiration reveals straw-colored fluid with low concentrations of LDH, fat, and protein and an absence of malignant cells. Injected with contrast medium following aspiration, cysts fill completely and demonstrate smooth walls. Treatment usually unnecessary.
Congenital multicystic kidney (CMK)	Obstruction (such as ureteral atresia or stenosis) during embryonic development disturbs cell formation (renal dysplasia). Cysts, mesenchyme, strangely branching tubules lined with atypical epithelium, and fatty, cartilaginous, or hematopoietic tissue forms within normal renal tissue. Bilateral diffuse disease is incompatible with life. Unilateral or segmental forms in adults have an excellent prognosis. Disease may be detected during work-up for abdominal mass, infection, hemorrhage, or hypertension. X-ray film shows a nonfunctioning segment or a mass of renal tissue with a poor or absent arterial supply and interrupted ureteral drainage. Rim-like calcifications of cyst walls may be present. Urinalysis, BUN, and creatinine remain normal. Except for complications of infection or trauma, no treatment is necessary. Malignant changes are not associated.
Childhood polycystic kidney disease (CPKD)	Rare disease inherited as a recessive trait. Causes dilation of collecting ducts in the kidneys and abnormal bile duct formation in the liver. Perinatal, neonatal, infantile, and juvenile variants have been described according to the clinical presentation and the ratio of kidney to liver involvement. While patients with mild renal dysfunction and portacaval shunting may live to adulthood, most die from renal failure or hepatic fibrosis in infancy or childhood.
Adult polycystic kidney disease (APKD)	Common disease inherited as a dominant trait. Causes cyst formation in the kidneys. May be associated with cystic changes in the liver but not fibrosis. Kidney pain and enlargement may precede dysfunction. Renal insufficiency progresses at varying rates, but most patients eventually require dialysis.
Nephronophthisis (cystic renal medulla complex)	Rare renal/retinal complex with variable presentations: isolated cases, recessively inherited cases, and dominantly transmitted disease. Retinal pathology (usually retinitis pigmentosa) may or may not be present. Kidney lesions are characterized by tubular atrophy, periglomerular fibrosis, and small medullary cysts. They invariably lead to decreased concentrating ability, salt wasting, and finally, renal insufficiency. Hypertension is rare, nephromegaly does not occur, and cyst formation in other organs is not associated. Diagnosis is made from the family history, arteriography or tomography, and biopsy.
Medullary sponge kidney (MKS)	Common disorder thought to be caused by in utero obstruction of the distal nephron by salt deposits. Expressed in adulthood when collecting ducts dilate into cysts and interstitium becomes infiltrated by inflammatory cells. Diagnosis is based on the history and IVP. Kidneys remain normal in size but are prone to infection and lithiasis.

control. Stone removal, antibiotics, and/or cyst drainage (to relieve the obstruction or loculated infection) may be needed intermittently. Unrelieved pressure from cysts or abscesses may lead to ischemia of functioning tissue and early fatality. Berry aneurysms are responsible for death in 10% of the cases.

Medullary sponge kidney (MSK) is another relatively common cystic disease. Obstruction by uric acid deposits along medullary portions of collecting tubules, possibly genetic in origin, has been proposed as the pathogenesis. Evidence of chronic infection is a frequent finding on pathology reports, but this is thought to be a secondary feature. Unlike APKD, MSK usually remains normal in size. If enlargement does occur, it is slight. The cysts, which are actually dilated collecting ducts, spare the cortex and appear only in the medulla (hence the name). They may develop in one or all pyramids in either or both kidneys. Patients with few cystic changes often remain asymptomatic. Those with more extensive disease tend to develop infections and stones, complications responsible for presentions anywhere from age 3 weeks to age 70. Men and women are equally affected. Renal colic, hematuria, and symptoms of urinary tract infections are the most common complaints. The ability to concentrate urine may be impaired, but acidification remains normal. Hypercalciuria and mild salt wasting may be present. Hypertension and renal insufficiency are uncommon. During careful execution of an IVP, contrast medium fills cystic tubules and persists in these spots after other areas have emptied. Diffuse persistence of dye (pyramidal blush) may also be noted. Some experts believe this to be a sign of early disease, while others consider it a normal variation. Although MSK usually runs a nonprogressive, benign course, 1 patient in 10 will be plagued by repeated hospitalizations for lithiasis and UTI.

Various types of ***renal tumors*** are listed in Table 8.2. The most common malignancy, ***renal cell carcinoma,*** may arise in any portion of the renal parenchyma. Affecting men three times more often than women, it usually appears in the sixth decade. Cortical adenoma is frequently associated with the disease and is thought by many experts to represent a premalignant lesion. The etiology is unclear, though animal studies suggest a relationship with certain chemicals (aromatic hydrocarbons, aflatoxins, *b*-anthraquinolines, dimethylnitrosamine, and lead compounds). Such studies have also implicated hormones, tobacco use, and viruses. Although considered classic, the triad of pain, gross or microscopic hematuria, and a palpable renal mass occurs in only 5–15% of patients. Those with pain describe a dull, constant discomfort in the flank or back. Alternatively, patients may complain of anorexia, nausea, vomiting, constipation, weakness, and lassitude. Before seeking medical attention, one-third of them will have developed metastases, the most frequent sites being regional lymph nodes, lungs, liver, bone, brain, or adrenal glands.

TABLE 8.2 TUMORS OF THE KIDNEY

Benign	Malignant
Vascular tumors	Nephroblastoma (Wilms' tumor)
Cystic lesions	Transitional cell carcinoma
Benign neoplasia of renal capsule, renal parenchyma, mesenchyme	Squamous cell carcinoma
Hydronephrosis	Renal cell carcinoma
Papilloma	Adenocarcinoma
	Papillary cystadenocarcinoma
	Myeloma
	Metastic lesions

TABLE 8.3 RENAL CANCER STAGING

Stage	Confines of Tumor
I	Limited to the kidney
II	Invasion of renal pedicle and/or renal fat pad
III	Local involvement
A	Renal vein or vena cava
B	Immediate lymph nodes
C	Regional blood and lymph vessels
IV	Advanced disease
A	Spread to adjacent organs
B	Distant metastases

For this reason, clinical findings can be extremely variable. Microscopic hematuria or flank pain are the first signs in 30–60% of patients. In addition to fever, hypertension, proteinuria, anemia, polycythemia, hypercalcemia, and renal insufficiency, there may be pulmonary lesions, pathologic fracture, hepatic dysfunction, varicocele, cardiac failure, amyloidosis, and/or neuromyopathy.

The diagnosis of renal cell carcinoma is based on an IVP showing a space-occupying lesion or calcifications. Lesions may be further investigated by nephrotomograms, ultrasonograms, computed tomography (CT) scans, angiograms, biopsy, or surgical exploration. If a malignancy is detected, metastatic bone series, chest x-ray films, bone and liver scans, blood and liver chemistry studies, electrolyte tests, and a complete blood count (CBC) may be done for staging purposes, those proposed by Robinson et al. being the most commonly used (Table 8.3). In stages, I, II, and IIIA, definitive treatment is possible by removing the tumor-bearing kidney within its perinephric fat, along with the adrenal and regional lymph nodes (radical nephrectomy). Tumors in more advanced stages require multimodal approaches involving chemotherapy and radiation. Nephrectomy is undertaken mainly for palliative purposes in cases of severe bleeding or pain and is usually preceded by arterial occlusion (angioinfarction). It is also done in stage IV disease with a single resectable metastasis, but not if multiple metastases are evident.

Wilms' tumor is a highly malignant mixed embryoma that may lie dormant for some time but becomes evident almost exclusively before age 6. Early metastasis to lungs, liver, and brain is common. The diagnosis is made when the child develops an abdominal mass, pain, anorexia, fever, nausea, vomiting, and/or hematuria. The problem is of interest to adult medicine because 50% or more of these patients are now being cured if they begin treatment before the tumor metastasizes. Treatment consists of nephrectomy followed by local irradiation and chemotherapy (usually with dactinomycin).

Protective Features

The kidneys are suspended in position by the large renal arteries and veins and by the renal fascia. The fascia forms a fibrous encasement packed with fat tissue (adipose capsule). Each kidney has a clear, smooth, adherent membrane (true capsule) as well. When there is loss of fat with emaciation, particularly in women, the kidney may slip around within the adipose capsule. This condition, referred to as ***movable***

kidney, should be distinguished from the congenital anomaly, floating kidney, previously described.

While these structural features are highly protective, ***kidney trauma*** is common. Contusions from a blow or fall, lacerations from a stab wound, rupture from a gunshot injury, and fragmentation from crush injuries may occur. They are frequently associated with damage to the colon, liver, spleen, and pancreas. Unless the pelvis is involved, the ureters and bladder are usually spared. Kidney trauma may produce hemorrhage, shock, extravasation of urine, and infection. Renal failure from acute tubular necrosis or infarction is a frequent complication. Obstruction secondary to clots in the ureter may also occur. Patients with any history of injury accompanied by flank pain and/or hematuria should be referred to a surgeon or urologist for immediate evaluation.

BLOOD FILTRATION

Renal Blood Flow and Glomerular Filtration Rate (GFR)

Nearly 20% of the total cardiac output goes to the kidney (renal fraction). The blood volume passing through the kidney is therefore three to five times higher than that passing through the heart, brain, liver, or other organs. It enters the large renal artery and passes through the interlobar, arcuate, and interlobular arteries into the cortex (see Fig. 8.1). There interlobular arteries branch into afferent arterioles, each ending in dozens of capillary loops haphazardly wound into the "glomerular tuft." Within the tuft, the capillary loops reconvene and emerge as the single "efferent arteriole." Branches of the efferent arterioles form the "peritubular capillary plexuses," which in turn send "vasa recta" (straight vessels) deep into the inner medulla. Efferent capillaries twist around nephron tubules in vine-like fashion, supplying tubules and interstitium with oxygen and nutritional substances. They are also instrumental in the processes of reabsorption and secretion, discussed in the later section on urine formation. Having followed the trelliswork of a nephron tubule back to the cortex, efferent vessels continue down the collecting tubules and end in a venous plexus.

As blood passes from afferent to efferent arterioles, hydrostatic pressure forces 19% of its plasma (the filtration fraction) across glomerular walls into the tubules. As explained later, this "plasma filtrate" contains water, nutrients, electrolytes, and metabolic waste products, which will be separated out in the renal tubules during urine formation.

The quantity of glomerular filtrate formed each minute by the two kidneys is called the "glomerular filtration rate (GFR)." The GFR remains remarkably constant under normal physiologic conditions, even through swings in systemic blood pressure between 80 and 200 mm Hg. This is because the kidneys have several mechanisms to "autoregulate" blood flow. To begin with, whenever blood flow to the glomerulus alters, the afferent and efferent arterioles change vascular tone. By constricting or dilating, they maintain a steady "flow velocity" across the glomerulus. This holds the GFR at a rate of 125 mL/min even when renal perfusion changes in response to systemic blood pressure, cardiac outflow, sympathetic stimulation, or volume status.

However, the arterioles cannot maintain steady flow velocity in the event of pronounced or prolonged changes in renal perfusion. In such cases, a second autoregulatory mechanism comes into play. As blood passes through the glomerular capillaries, hydrostatic pressure decreases because the volume within the vessel falls as plasma is lost into Bowman's capsule. Meanwhile, oncotic pressure rises. Barred from passage across the glomerular membrane, proteins remain in the vascular space, their concentration rising as the plasma volume falls. At the point where falling hydrostatic pressure comes into equilibrium with rising oncotic pressure, filtration ceases. When the arterioles are unable to compensate for changes in renal perfusion, the point of equilibrium shifts.

When flow velocity falls, the point of equilibrium shifts closer to the beginning of the capillary and the amount of filtrate decreases. A decreased amount of filtrate flows through the tubules at a slower rate than usual, allowing plenty of time for extra amounts of salt to permeate across tubule walls back into the blood. This, of course, directly expands the circulating volume. Furthermore, whenever the macula densa senses a low salt content in tubular fluid, it signals the juxtaglomerular cells to release renin, an enzyme that converts angiotensin I to angiotensin II. Angiotensin II, the most powerful vasopressor made in the body, constricts arteriolar flow to other parts of the body, making extra blood available to the kidney. Renin also stimulates the release of aldosterone from the adrenal cortex. As discussed later, aldosterone incites the kidney tubules to exchange sodium for potassium, thus sending even more sodium back into circulation.

When flow velocity steps up, the opposite set of events occurs. The point of hydrostatic/oncotic pressure equilibrium shifts toward the efferent end of the glomerular capillaries. The increased amount of filtrate entering Bowman's capsule flows quickly through the tubules, sweeping salt along at a pace that precludes its passage across the tubular walls and back into the blood. The hypertonic filtrate draws water from the interstitium, increasing urinary output. Increased salt and water excretion helps to reduce the circulating volume. Furthermore, sensing a high salt content in tubular fluid, the macula densa signals juxtaglomerular cell to refrain from releasing renin.

The GFR is adversely affected by any condition causing a prolonged or significant reduction in renal blood flow. In ***renal artery stenosis,*** narrowing or partial occlusion of the renal artery or its major branches results from ***atherosclerosis*** or ***fibromuscular dysplasia.*** Atherosclerosis accounts for most cases in men, the incidence increasing with age over 50 and in patients with a history of diabetes or hypertension. Causing inflexible thickening of the arterial walls, fibromuscular dysplasia is 10 times more common in women than in men. Unlike atherosclerosis, the process affects younger adults (30 to 40 years of age) and may extend deep within the arterial tree. Tending to be bilateral, both processes lead to a gradual decrease in the arterial blood entering the kidney. Reduced flow in the afferent arteriole incites the renin-angiotensin-aldosterone system, causing renovascular hypertension and fluid retention. At first, these compensatory mechanisms help maintain the GFR and the metabolic needs of kidney structures. Eventually, however, they contribute to nephron injury and renal failure.

Renal artery stenosis should be suspected in any patient below 30 or over 50 who presents with a new onset of hypertension. It should also be considered in patients with severe hypertension who respond poorly to drug therapy. An important suggestive sign is unexplained hypokalemia. An abdominal bruit (best heard with a stethoscope placed just lateral to the epigastrium) is particularly significant, occurring in

40–50% of patients with renovascular lesions. Confirmation of stenosis is often difficult and may require several expensive tests. Rapid-sequence intravenous urography can detect differences in renal size, unilateral delay of opacification, unilateral hyperconcentration of dye, and ureteral notching, all of which are consistent with the disease. Ureteral notching indicates collateral circulation. Although hypertensive IVP is often ordered as the first step in the work-up, it is helpful only in fairly advanced disease. On the other hand, significant lesions are rarely missed by renal angiography. Because some lesions occur without causing hypertension, renal vein renin assays should also be ordered. An aggressive attempt to control blood pressure is the first step in treatment. Beta-adrenergic blockers and inhibitors of angiotensin-converting enzyme have proven particularly useful. When medical measures fail, vascular surgery should be considered, particularly if the ratio of the preoperative renal vein renin measurement of the affected to the nonaffected side is greater than 1.5:1 under conditions of renin stimulation (upright position, diuretics, salt restriction). A graft is created from the aorta hepatic, splenic, or hypogastric arteries to bypass the obstruction. It is a wise intervention for patients with a high degree of bilateral atherosclerosis because the process tends to be progressive. Fibrous dysplasia is also progressive, but lesions tend to involve distal segments and branches of the renal artery. Bypass surgery can be technically difficult and is often held in reserve. A new technique, transluminal renal angioplasty, may prove useful in such cases. A balloon catheter is positioned in stenotic portions of the artery and inflated under pressure.

Renal artery occlusion implies an acute, complete obstruction of the main artery or major intrarenal branches. The cause is clot formation following embolism or blunt trauma to the abdomen or back. Emboli usually originate from a cardiac complication such as infective endocarditis, arterial fibrillation, mitral stenosis, myocardial infarction, or arteriosclerosis of the aorta. Due to ischemia, the tissue supplied by the obstructed artery becomes necrotic, creating a wedge-shaped area of renal infarction. The clinical features depend on the size of the infarct, which in turn depends on the level of the occlusion. Small infarcts involving intrarenal branches within the cortex can occur unnoticed. However, larger infarcts cause sudden pain in the flank or upper abdomen. Sharp and unremitting, the pain may be associated with fever, leukocytosis, and elevations of plasma lactic dehydrogenase (LDH). Proteinuria and microscopic hematuria are typical findings, but gross hematuria is rare. Hypertension, if it occurs at all, tends to be transient. The change in renal function is variable, depending a great deal on the previous health of the two kidneys. Occlusions of a sole functioning kidney may lead to acute oliguric failure. On the other hand, BUN and creatinine may remain within normal ranges, even with total infarction of one kidney, as long as the other kidney remains healthy. In such cases, there is a doubling of the renin and creatinine, which return to normal as soon as the remaining kidney begins to compensate. This response occurs to a reduced extent and at a slower rate in the elderly.

Total destruction of the kidney occurs within hours of a main artery occlusion. Therefore, emergency angiography is indicated for patients with acute signs and symptoms. If it shows collateral filling of the arterial tree, the kidney may still be saved with surgical embolectomy or dislodgement of the clot with a Fogarty catheter. Anticoagulants are also used and may be continued prophylactically in patients with emboli related to cardiac disease. Administration of anticoagulation or thrombolytic agents (streptokinase) is the treatment of choice for unilateral embolism since surgery adds to the risk of losing the kidney and the use of Fogarty catheters requires further study. Without treatment, restored kidney function is extremely rare. However, it has been reported in patients who have had previous partial occlusions resulting in collateral blood supplies.

Long-standing blood pressure elevations can affect renal circulation. Common among older persons with arteriosclerosis, it causes small afferent arterioles to become thickened and stenotic, a pathologic change called ***benign nephrosclerosis*** (nephroangiosclerosis, arteriolar nephrosclerosis). Narrowing or obliteration of the vessel deprives the nephron of its blood supply, leading to gradual reduction in renal function. Referred to as ***hypertensive kidney disease,*** the process is completely different from renovascular hypertension, discussed previously.

Malignant nephrosclerosis is the consequence of malignant hypertension. Concentric layers of collagen develop within interlobular arteries, virtually obliterating the vascular lumen. Dependent vessels become ischemic and ***fibrinoid necrosis*** of the arterioles, the hallmark of malignant hypertension, quickly develops. There may be proliferation of glomerular cells and formation of epithelial "crescents." Rapidly progressive disease can cause severe vascular thickening and hemorrhages resembling endarteritis. In addition to cardiovascular and neurologic signs of malignant hypertension, patients demonstrate varying degrees of renal insufficiency. Urine shows proteinuria (sometimes in nephrotic ranges) and microscopic hematuria. Granular cell casts are common, red cell casts less so. Broad waxy casts signify far advanced renal damage. Extremely high levels of renin and aldosterone are classic signs. Unless the blood pressure is brought under control, patients are likely to die within 6 months (40% from uremia). Treated patients who recover without significant renal failure have the best prognosis. Even then, many show signs of progressive renal failure and soon require dialysis.

Renal cortical necrosis is an unusual form of arterial infarction. Lesions resembling a Schwartzmänn reaction produce necrotic changes in the cortex but spare the medulla. Over half of the cases are associated with abruptio placenta and a high number with sepsis. Nephrotoxins, renal ischemia, intravascular coagulation, and renal allograft rejection are other predisposing conditions. Patients present with acute renal failure. Gross hematuria and flank pain are invariable, and fever and leukocytosis are common. Initial enlargement of the kidneys is quickly followed by atrophy and calcification. Within 6–8 weeks the kidneys may be reduced to 50% of their normal size and display linear calcification, which is most pronounced at the corticomedullary junction. The diagnosis is confirmed by biopsy. Patients require dialysis and other supportive treatment for acute renal failure. Although residual function is sometimes recovered, this is not the rule. Most patients face chronic dialysis or transplantation.

Renal vein thrombosis is associated with the conditions listed in Table 8.4. It may lead to an acute hemorrhagic infarction or a slow, unnoticed reduction in GFR. The clinical picture depends on the involvement of one or both kidneys, with either partial or complete occlusion. It is also influenced by the development of collateral circulation, recanalization of the thrombus, and previous kidney function. An acute process produces kidney enlargement, whereas progressive disease leads to atrophy. The diagnosis can be made with IVP (which shows nonexcretion of contrast material) or phlebography (which shows a filling defect of the renal vein or filling of the collateral system). The usual treatment is anticoagulation, which not only improves renal function but also lowers the incidence of pulmonary embolism.

TABLE 8.4 CONDITIONS ASSOCIATED WITH RENAL VEIN THROMBOSIS

Renal	Extrarenal
Nephrotic syndrome	Acute volume contraction
Membranous glomerulonephropathy	CHF
Focal sclerosing glomerulopathy	Pregnancy
Lupus nephritis	Constrictive pericarditis
Amyloidosis	Extreme obesity
Nil disease (rare association)	
Diabetic nephropathy (rare association)	
Trauma	

Clearance

A prime function of the GFR is renal clearance, whereby body wastes and toxins are removed from the blood and eliminated in the urine. It may involve tubular secretion as well as glomerular filtration. Clearance may also take place via gastrointestinal (GI), hepatic, respiratory, or other routes. Renal clearance is expressed as the amount of blood (in milliliters) that can be cleared of a specific substance (in milligram percent) within a given time (minutes). Clearance rates normally differ from substance to substance, being high when the kidneys can clear large amounts of blood and vice versa. If endogenous substances (such as metabolic wastes) are cleared at the same rate they are produced, or if exogenous substances (such as drugs) are cleared at the same rate they are introduced, a steady state exists.

Clearance of exogenous substances such as inulin and *p*-aminohippuric acid (PAH), which depends exclusively on glomerular filtration, can be used as a precise measurement of GFR. Such testing involves radioactive tracers or samples of blood from the renal vein. Less precise but extremely important clinical reflections of GFR can be determined by serum levels of creatinine (a breakdown product of muscle) and BUN (a waste product of protein metabolism). BUN and creatinine are produced and excreted at a fairly constant rate, promoting a serum ratio of less than 20:1 under normal circumstances. If kidney failure occurs, serum levels of creatinine and BUN usually rise proportionately. An increase in BUN out of proportion to creatinine is referred to as ***prerenal azotemia.*** It may occur with abnormally high production of urea from a large intake of dietary protein or accelerated catabolism of body proteins (in trauma, GI bleeding, chronic disease). In such cases, the kidney clears urea at its usual rate but cannot keep up with excess amounts. The problem is also seen with any condition that reduces urine flow through the tubules [prostate or other types of obstruction, dehydration, venous stasis with congestive heart failure (CHF)]. Again, urea is successfully cleared in the filtrate, but because of sluggish flow, it has time to diffuse across tubular walls back into the blood. By contrast, increased creatinine production occurs only with massive breakdown of muscle, a rare event. Furthermore, although creatinine can be secreted into tubular fluid, it cannot permeate out. Whatever is cleared in the glomerular filtrate or secreted into the tubules will be eliminated in the urine. Unlike BUN, rising levels of creatinine almost always indicate reduced renal clearance. It is important to note that by the time serum concentrations of creatinine exceed normal ranges, kidney function has fallen by at least 50%.

Azotemia refers to elevations of BUN and creatinine indicating ***renal insufficiency (failure).*** Progressive azotemia characterizes ***acute renal failure.*** Although exact definitions are difficult, a daily rise in creatinine by 0.5 mg/L and BUN by 10 mg/L is indicative. ***Oliguria,*** a decline in urine production, is typical of acute renal failure. Generally, urine flow of less than 400 mL/day represents decreased output, since individuals with normal renal function excrete at least 400–500 mL of urine daily even when dehydrated. ***Nonoliguric acute renal failure*** may also occur. ***Chronic renal insufficiency*** results from any condition causing gradual loss of nephron function. Since undamaged nephrons assume larger work loads, few changes may be noted initially. However, subsequent loss of overproductive nephrons increases the dysfunction logarithmically, which accounts for the "doubling time" pattern of many renal diseases. Suppose, for example, that the original doubling of creatinine (from a normal of 1.0 to 2.0) took place in 5 years. Creatinine can then be expected to double every 5 years, reaching 4.0 by year 10 and 8.0 by year 15. Renal failure may follow inadequate blood perfusion (prerenal cause), disease or damage to kidney structures, or urinary tract obstruction (postrenal cause). Acute renal failure, the causes of which are listed in Table 8.5, is sometimes reversible.

In addition to azotemia, there are many manifestations of both acute and chronic renal insufficiency (Table 8.6). Some vary with the specific disease process, as noted throughout this chapter. The effects of renal insufficiency also depend on the degree of protein catabolism. In hypercatabolic states (tissue trauma, sepsis, hemorrhage), BUN may increase by as much as 100 mg/L/day, and hyperkalemia may progress rapidly. Under any condition, salt and water overload may lead to edema—peripheral, pulmonary, and/or cerebral. Metabolic acidosis, hyperphosphatemia, hypocalcemia, and hypoalbuminemia are other consequences. They contribute to cardiac arrhythmias and CHF. Hypertension is common. So too are anorexia, nausea, vomiting, abdominal distention, ileus, and other GI disturbances. Ulcerations develop in the mouth, stomach, or colon and sometimes hemorrhage. Bleeding may be aggravated by a variety of hematologic changes (suppressed erythropoiesis, hemolysis, decreased platelet count, decreased coagulation factors, and capillary defects). Neuromuscular manifestations include hyperreflexia, muscle twitching, and asterixis, as well as lethargy, confusion, stupor, and coma. Agitation and abnormal behavior may also occur. Some of these latter findings may lead to the clinical diagnosis of ***uremia,*** that is, end-stage toxicity.

Dialysis is necessary for the survival of uremic patients. A solution (dialysate) is

TABLE 8.5 CAUSES OF ACUTE (POSSIBLY REVERSIBLE) RENAL INSUFFICIENCY

Toxins	Ischemia
Antibiotics (aminoglycosides, penicillins, tetracyclines, amphotericin)	Bilateral renal vein thrombosis
Other drugs (phenytoin, phenylbutazone)	Renal arterial occlusion
Radiographic contrast materials	Massive hemorrhage (postpartum, trauma, GI, etc.)
Anesthetic agents	Septic shock
Heme pigments (hemoglobin, myoglobin)	Transfusion reaction
Metabolic wastes (uric acid, calcium)	Cardiac dysfunction
Heavy metals (mercury, arsenic, lead, bismuth, uranium, cadmium, gold)	Surgery (especially cardiac, aortic, biliary)
Organic solvents (carbon tetrachloride, ethylene glycol, phenol, methyl alcohol)	Dehydration (pancreatitis, gastroenteritis)
Pesticides	Glomerular insult
Systemic allergens (allergic response to insect bites, drugs)	Acute poststreptococcal glomerulonephritis
	Pregnancy (abruptio placenta, abortion, postpartum renal failure)
	Subacute bacterial endocarditis
	Malignant hypertension
	Collagen disease

TABLE 8.6 MANIFESTATIONS OF RENAL FAILURE

Feature	Mechanism
Mild insufficiency	
Azotemia	Decreased clearance of metabolic wastes
Nocturia, polyuria	Impaired concentrating ability
Mild normochromic, normocytic anemia	Decreased erythropoiesis
Carbohydrate intolerance	Peripheral resistance to insulin
Hypertriglyceridemia	To replace protein lost in urine, liver steps up activity and overproduces lipids
Hyperuricemia	Decreased clearance
Hyperamylasemia	Decreased clearance
Hypermagnesemia	Decreased clearance
Moderate insufficiency	
Sexual dysfunction	Decreased well-being, altered pituitary, gonadal, and thyroid hormones
Hypocalcemia	Reduced conversion of hydroxycholecalciferol by kidney, phosphate retention
Secondary hyperparathyroidism	Initiated by hypocalcemia
Hyperphosphatemia	Decreased phosphate excretion due to decreased GFR
Metabolic bone disease	Secondary hyperparathyroidism
Acidosis	Reduced ammonia conversion by renal tubules, bicarbonate loss, decreased excretion of fixed acids
Pruritis and skin excoriations	Calcium reabsorption from bone and deposition in skin, sensory neuropathy
Tissue calcifications	Calcium reabsorption from bone, deposition in tissues
Early uremia	
Anorexia, nausea, vomiting	Accumulation of metabolic toxins
CHF	Fluid retention
Progressive hypertension	Renin and fluid retention
Uremic fetor	Accumulation of metabolic toxins
Metallic taste in the mouth	Enzymes in mouth split excess urea
Bleeding tendencies	Abnormal platelet function
Pulmonary edema	Hypertension, CHF, abnormal membrane diffusion
Pericarditis, pleuritis	Unknown
Pericardial, pleural effusions	Abnormal membrane diffusion
Muscle cramps	Osmolality changes
Sensory neuropathy and mild CNS changes	Altered neuromuscular transmission due to imbalances of calcium, magnesium, salt, potassium, and phosphate toxin accumulation
Advanced uremia	
Asterixis	Metabolic toxins
Uremic frost	Urea in sweat crystallizes on skin
Motor neuropathy	Advanced changes in neuromuscular transmission
Hyperkalemia	Reduced urinary output, severe acidosis
Cardiac arrhythmias	Hyperkalemia
GI bleeds/ulceration	Platelet dysfunction, increased gastrin production, irritation from toxins
Lethargy, psychosis, coma	Profound CNS abnormalities

continuously diffused across a semipermeable membrane that separates out toxic elements. The dialysate mimics the electrolyte composition of interstitial fluid, except for being potassium free and containing lactate or acetate substitutes for bicarbonate. The patient's own peritoneal membrane is used in peritoneal dialysis and a synthetic cellophane membrane in hemodialysis. Two other techniques, hemofiltration and hemodiafiltration, are based on convective transport rather than diffusion of dialysate. Although they are costly, their use during the first hour of hemodialysis enhances removal of large molecular weight solutes and fluids, thus reducing the disequilibrium, hypotension, and cramps experienced by many patients during the session. They can also be used alone for hypertension control.

Some cases of acute renal failure and certain types of drug overdose respond to short-term dialysis. However, patients with end-stage renal failure face chronic dialysis. Life for them is literally tied to machine treatments lasting for 4–8 hours, three to four times a week. The financial, psychologic, social, and physical costs are enormous. Patients often require public assistance to meet the expenses of ongoing medications and procedures. Their regular employment and leisure activities may be precluded by the travel and time required for dialysis sessions. Relationships with family and friends may change. Physical bearing declines due to the manifestations of kidney disease (Table 8.6) and problems associated with dialysis (e.g., access surgery, needle marks, anticoagulation therapy, hepatitis). A peculiar neurologic syndrome called ***dialysis dementia*** has been associated with high concentrations of aluminum in the brain, possibly from the high aluminum levels in the dialysate. It is characterized by progressive dementia, facial grimaces, myoclonic seizures, and specific electroencephalographic changes. Schizophrenia, manic depression, and maladaptive coping behaviors are also common among dialysis patients.

Renal patients require management by experts. Interdisciplinary teams usually include nephrologists, dialysis nurses, social workers, and psychiatric personnel. Since the best programs ensure as much patient independence as possible, home hemodialysis, home peritoneal dialysis, self-care or passive-care dialysis (performed in hospital centers by the patient with limited supervision), and continuous ambulatory peritoneal dialysis (CAPD) are gaining popularity. ▶ ***Organizations for renal patients*** provide support, information, and research. Finally, primary care providers may be called on for general health maintenance or episodic illnesses. For this reason, ▶ ***considerations for patients with renal failure*** must be kept in mind. Medication contraindications and adjustments are particularly important. Literature concerning all drugs (prescribed as well as over-the-counter) should be carefully reviewed for information about renal clearance. For many substances, doses should be reduced or intervals of administration extended according to the GFR status. Examples of antibiotic considerations appear in Table 8.7.

For a number of dialysis patients, ***kidney transplant*** offers hope for an improved quality of life. In some instances, organs are received from living relatives, but more often they come from persons who have arranged for organ donations after death (see Chapter 1). Suitable kidneys for transplant may come from anyone free from hypertension, diabetes, or malignant disease. For their own protection, living donors must also display normal overall health, bilateral renal function, and emotional stability. Tissue matching has been improved with blood typing and leukocyte typing for histocompatibility antigens. Experimental use of pretransplant blood transfusions and approved use of drugs (azothioprine, cyclophosphamide, steroids, antilymphocytic globulin, cyclosporin A) are being used to suppress immunity. Together, tissue matching and immunosuppression have lowered rejection rates, greatly improving the statistics for transplant success. Now 42% of compatible cadaver kidneys and 70% of compatible relative kidneys are still functioning after 3 years.

Glomerular Membranes

Filtration depends not only on renal blood flow but also on the glomerular membranes. Twenty-five times more permeable than those of other capillaries, glomeru-

TABLE 8.7 ANTIBIOTIC ADJUSTMENTS FOR RENAL INSUFFICIENCY

Drug	Adjustment Required	Special Renal Concerns
Aminoglycosides	Interval extension or dose reduction; loading dose required	Nephrotoxic
Amoxicillin/ampicillin	Interval extension	Nephritis, coagulopathy
Amphotericin B	Interval extension	Nephrotoxicity, hypokalemia
Cephalosporins	Dose reduction	Possibly nephrotoxic
Chloramphenicol	None	Ineffective for urinary tract infection when GFR <40 mL/min
Chloroquine	None	Alkaline urine enhances excretion
Clindamycin	None	None
Cloxacillin/dicloxacillin/nafcillin/oxacillin	None	Nephritis, coagulopathy
Erythromycin	None	More toxic, ototoxic in renal failure
Ethambutol	Interval extension	None
Isoniazid	None in mild failure; dose reduction in severe failure	
Mendalamine	None in mild failure; avoid in advanced failure (ineffective, exacerbates uremic GI symptoms)	Works only when urine pH is low; hemorrhagic cystitis
Miconazole	None	Hyponatremia
Nalidixic acid	None in mild failure; avoid in advanced failure (metabolites accumulate)	Metabolic acidosis; resistance high
Nitrofurantoin	Same as above	Ineffective when GFR <40 mL/min; spurious elevations of BUN, creatinine; cystitis
Penicillin	Interval extension	Potassium salts contain 1.7 meQ/million units
Quinine	Interval extension	None
Sulfamethoxazole/trimethoprim	Interval extension	Half-life reduced in alkaline urines; creatinines; nephrotoxic
Sulfisoxazole	Interval extension	Half-life reduced in alakaline urines; rare crystalluria
Tetracyclines	Interval extension	Potentiation of acidosis; catabolic effects; ineffective when GFR <20 mL/min

lar membranes act as a molecular sieve, allowing only substances lighter than plasma proteins to pass through. This ability stems from modifications of endothelial, basement membrane, and epithelial layers. Lining the lumen, the endothelium contains a number of fenestra (pores) covered by thin diaphragms. The basement membrane has three distinct "lamina" that serve as a second-line filter. Lamina are made up of collagen and glycoprotein, substances particularly suitable for this purpose. The epithelial lining possesses podocytes, large cells with foot processes that extend into the lamina externa of the basement membrane. Between the foot processes are spaces known as "slit pores" (filtration slits). Each is covered by a "slit diaphragm," a structure containing rectangular pores arranged in zipper-like fashion. Slit pores comprise 3% of the total surface area of the glomerular membrane.

Due to its filtering function and high blood flow, glomerular membranes are subject to a number of injuries referred to as ***glomerulonephridites.*** Various types are described in Table 8.8. Since most result from an immunologic process, immune reactions are being used for classification purposes (Table 8.9). In ***immune complex disease,*** antigens or antibodies (from bacterial or viral infections, drugs or chemicals, tumors, thyroglobulin, or circulating DNA) form antigen–antibody complexes in the blood. During blood filtration, the complexes permeate through glomerular membranes, becoming trapped. Immunofluorescent methods and electron microscopy have been used to identify lumpy deposits of IgG, IgM, IgA, and C3 between the epithelial cells and basement membrane in the mesangium. Once activated, C3 attracts leukocytes, which further damage glomerular tissue by releasing lysosomal enzymes. In the ***antibody-mediated response,*** glomerular tissue serves as the direct antigenic stimulus for antibody attack. Such injuries alter the permeability of the glomerular capillary. Protein, blood, and casts pass into the urine as hallmarks of the disease. Protein levels range from 1+ to 3+ on Dipstick and up to 3.5 g over a 24-hour period. Hematuria can be gross or microscopic, often causing urine to look pink, frankly bloody, or (when acidic) smoky and brownish. Casts appear in the form of red blood cell (RBC), hemoglobin, renal tubular cell, white blood cell (WBC), and/or a granular type, as described in Table 8.10. The presence of all types at the same time is referred to as "telescopic sediment." Hypertension, fluid retention, and altered GFR and clearance may be noted to variable degrees. There may be decreased tubular function (poor urine concentration and faulty ammonia excretion) if disease processes have disturbed the interstitium.

Glomerular diseases may be acute, rapidly progressive, or chronic. Glomerular disease of acute onset is typified by ***postinfectious glomerulonephritis,*** which develops from an immune complex reaction initiated by several organisms (Table 8.11). Glomerular inflammation can evolve during active infection but more often appears 1–6 weeks after all symptoms have cleared. If it is mild, it may go unnoticed. Usually, however, patients develop frank renal insufficiency with edema, hypertension, and gross or microscopic hematuria and feel quite sick. Proteinuria varies from 0.5 to almost 2 g/day but rarely reaches nephrotic ranges (2–3 g/day). Urinary sediment contains RBCs, WBCs, and casts (RBC casts identified in the wake of an infection strongly suggest an acute renal process). With appropriate treatment, renal function usually returns to normal within 3 months, but proteinuria may persist for a year and microscopic hematuria for several years.

Rapidly progressive glomerulonephritis (RPGN) results from both immune complex disease and antibodies directed against basement membranes. An initiating cause cannot be found in 40% of cases. Henloch-Schönlein purpura, polyarteritis nodosa, Wegener's granulomatosis, and systemic lupus erythematosus (SLE) are known associations. About 50% of these patients have a history of influenza-like symptoms occurring the month before presentation. Surprisingly enough, the onset of renal symptoms in RPGN is insidious. It may be marked by weakness, malaise, nausea, vomiting, and anorexia. Hypertension is uncommon and, when it does occur, is rarely severe. However, many patients are oliguric and azotemic by the time they are seen. Hematuria (typically microscopic) and anemia are invariable findings. Leukocytosis is common. Urine sediment always contains RBC casts; WBC, granular, waxy, and broad casts may also be noted. Renal failure reaches terminal stages

TABLE 8.8 GLOMERULAR INJURIES

Type	Etiology	Pathology	Typical Presentation	Treatment and Outcome
Minimal change (Nil disease)	Idiopathic. Secondary to Hodgkin's disease. Associations with atopy. HLA-B12 histocompatability antigen, recent immunization, or URI.	Diffuse effacement of epithelial foot processes but minimal change in glomerular capillaries. Absent or irregular deposits of immunoglobulin and complement.	Usually before age 8. Overt nephrotic syndrome with normal blood pressure, and GFR. Hematuria variable. Normal serum complement except for slight reduction in Clq. IgM increased. IgG depressed during relapses.	Steroids and cyclophosphamides. Excellent prognosis.
Focal sclerosis	Idiopathic (possibly a stage of Nil disease). Seen in SLE, Hodgkin's disease, diabetes, nail patella syndome, multiple myeloma, amyloidosis. Similar lesions associated with heroin abuse, vesicoureter reflux, and renal allograft.	Sclerosis and hyalinization of some but not all glomerular tufts. Affected tufts demonstrate collapse of basement membranes, denudement of epithelial surface, and effacement of foot processes. Lesions contain granular deposits of IgM and C3.	Hypertension, reduced GFR, abnormal tubular function, and variable proteinuria. Normal serum levels of C3 and reduced IgG. Urine sediment unremarkable.	Steroids of minimal value. Progressive renal failure is the rule. Lesions may recur in transplanted kidneys.
Membranous	Idiopathic. Also associated with RA, SLE, Sjögren's syndrome, sarcoidosis, malaria, hepatitis B, sickle cell disease, diabetes, tumors of the lung or colon, melanoma, gold and penicillamine therapy, mercury poisoning.	Irregular, electron-dense deposits of IgG in subepithelial space. All glomeruli affected. Coalescence of deposits leads to thickening of capillary walls. Basement membrane materials project between deposits toward Bowman's capsule ("spike" formations). Little proliferation of mesangial or endothelial cells.	Nephrotic syndrome in majority of cases. Blood pressure, GFR, and urine sediment normal in early disease. Normal serum complement, depressed IgG.	Spontaneous remissions fairly common. Steroid use controversial. Cytotoxic agents of no value. Fifty percent of patients die within 10 years of diagnosis. Recurrence in transplanted kidneys is rare.
Membranoproliferative (pure, focal, crescentic)	Idiopathic. Seen in hemolytic-uremic syndrome, transplant rejection, postinfectious conditions, Alport's syndrome, Fabry's disease, Goodpasture's syndrome, polyarteritis, Wegener's granulomatosis, rheumatoid vasculitis, temporal arteritis, Takayasu's syndrome, allergic vasculitis (Churg-Strauss syndrome), and SLE vasculitis. Also seen in cryoimmunoglobulinemia, sarcoidosis, chronic active hepatitis, diabetes, sickle cell disease.	Due to capillary necrosis and to deposits of IgG, IgM, and/or complement components, mesangial tissue proliferates and extends into glomerular membranes. This stimulates three patterns of change in glomerular membranes: mild, diffuse thickening (pure membranoproliferative); patchy, dense thickening (focal membranoproliferative); and extension of membranes into the urinary space to pack the crescent-shaped area outlined by Bowman's capsule (crescentic membranoproliferative).	No typical presentation. Full-blown nephrotic syndrome in 50% or more of cases. Microscopic hematuria of variable range. Blood pressure, GFR, urine sediment usually abnormal. Serum C3 often reduced, but Clq, C4, and C2 normal. C3 nephritic factor and circulating immune complexes are common findings.	Long-term alternate-day steroids may delay progression. Poor prognosis, especially with crescentic types. Lesions often recur in transplanted kidneys but may be less severe.

TABLE 8.8 *(Continued)*

Type	Etiology	Pathology	Typical Presentation	Treatment and Outcome
IgA nephropathy	Idiopathic (Berger's disease). Similar lesions in Henoch-Schönlein purpura.	Membranoproliferative changes distinguished by diffuse mesangial deposition of IgA and by lesser amounts of IgG, C3, properdin, and fibrin antigens. Clq and C4 absent.	Berger's disease as recurrent episodes of macroscopic hematuria following flu-like illness or vigorous exercise, particularly in young men. No skin rash, arthritis, or abdominal pain. Absent or mild proteinuria, normal blood pressure and GFR in early stages. Henoch-Schönlein purpura occurs as hematuria and proteinuria in the presence of thrombocytopenic purpura, arthralgias, and abdominal pain.	Berger's disease tends to progress slowly, with 50% of patients developing end-stage renal failure in 25 years. Intermittent steroids may reduce episodes of hematuria. Henoch-Schönlein purpura usually benign. Rare developments of RPGN treated with plasma exchanges, immunosuppressive drugs, and antithrombotic agents.

TABLE 8.9 IMMUNE REACTIONS AS A CLASSIFICATION OF GLOMERULAR DISEASE

Type	Description	Example
I (anaphylactic)	Hypersensitivity response mediated by the action of IGE on basophils and mast cells after contact with specific antigens. Vasoactive substances trigger platelet-mediated coagulation, causing thrombosis and fibrin deposition.	Minimal change (Nil disease) Malignant hypertension
II (cytotoxic)	Cytotoxic antibodies fix in smooth linear fashion to kidney tissue, activating complement and immune inflammatory reactions.	Anti-glomerular basement membrane disease Antitubular basement membrane disease Hyperacute renal allograft rejection
III (immnune complex)	Antigen–antibody complexes deposit in "lumpy-bumpy" fashion along mesangium, interstitium, and/or glomerular membranes. Localized within kidney tissues, the complexes activate complement and cause injurious inflammatory reactions.	Postinfectious glomerulonephritis Serum sickness Hepatitis B SLE
IV (cell-mediated)	Body becomes sensitized to kidney cells that act as antigens, triggering infiltration by monocytes and lymphocytes. In diffuse granular patterns, the latter release tissue destroying enzymes.	Chronic renal allograft rejection Chronic glomerulonephritis
Direct complement mediated	Deposition of C3 and properdin in mesangium and glomerular membranes directly activates alternate complement pathways. The cause is unknown, but a number of patients have a C3 factor (called "C3 nephritic factor") capable of spontaneous cleavage to an activating step (C3b) in the complement cascade. Complement activation leads to proliferation of renal cells and thickening of glomerular membranes.	Membranoproliferative glomerulonephritis

TABLE 8.10 URINARY CASTS

Type	Description	Associated with:
Bacterial	Bacteria bound within protein matrix	Bacterial pyelonephritis
Epithelial cell	Tubular cells bound within protein matrix	Acute tubular injury, glomerulonephritis, nephrotic syndrome
Fatty	Fat droplets and/or tubular cells bound within protein matrix	All types of nephritis, particularly nephrotic syndrome, Fabry's disease
Granular	Hyaline cast containing tubular protein droplets	Tubular injury
Hyaline	Mucoprotein matrix	Normal urine, low urinary flow
Mixed	Hyaline cast containing mixture of RBCs, WBCs, and tubular cells	Proliferative glomerulonephritis
Pseudocasts	Clumped urates, WBCs, bacteria, artifacts	Lower tract infection, normal urine
RBC	RBCs bound within protein matrix	Proliferative glomerulonephritis, acute tubular injury, cortical necrosis
Waxy	Serum proteins bound within mucoprotein matrix	Advanced renal failure
WBC	WBCs bound within protein matrix	Proliferative glomerulonephritis, interstitial nephritis

within several months. Without dialysis, patients quickly die. Patients with RPGN related to multisystemic or infectious disease may improve with appropriate treatment even though the histologic changes remain. However, the patient with an idiopathic occurrence has little chance for any kind of remission and will probably remain on dialysis permanently.

Chronic glomerulonephritis is associated with a number of systemic disorders (see Table 8.8). A history of acute glomerular disease is uncommon, and infectious or toxic agents are rarely implicated. The insidious nature of chronic glomerulonephritis makes the onset difficult to determine. Since patients are asymptomatic for years, the first indication of disease is often proteinuria or hematuria found incidentally during routine medical examination. Although renal function deteriorates slowly, there may be intermittent periods of accelerated injury marked by nephrotic syndrome or gross hematuria. The latter is particularly common in ***IgA nephropathy*** (Berger's disease). Whatever the etiology, when 50% or more of the nephrons become

TABLE 8.11 CAUSES OF POSTINFECTIOUS GLOMERULONEPHRITIS

- Bacteria
  - Streptococcal infections
  - Infective endocarditis
  - "Shunt" nephritis
  - Sepsis
  - Pneumococcal pneumonia
  - Typhoid fever
  - Secondary syphilis
  - Meningococcemia
- Virus
  - Hepatitis B
  - Infectious mononucleosis
  - Mumps
  - Measles
  - Chickenpox
  - Vaccinia
  - Echovirus
  - Coxsackie
- Parasites
  - Malaria
  - Toxoplasmosis
- Miscellaneous
  - Guillain-Barré syndrome
  - (DPT) vaccine
  - Serum sickness

dysfunctional, azotemia develops. Further progression leads to overt signs of renal insufficiency.

Patients suspected of having glomerular disease of any type should be referred to a nephrologist. Radiographic, isotopic, and ultrasonic evaluation should be undertaken before IVP, since IVP dye in the presence of severe proteinuria or marginal dehydration could cause acute renal failure. In early processes the kidneys appear enlarged, but with persistent disease they become progressively smaller. Specific blood studies may help establish the exact diagnosis. In cases of immune complex disease, antibody titers to the infectious organism (e.g., antistreptolysin, antihepatitis B antigen) rise in 1–2 weeks of the initiating illness. Cryoglobulinemia and circulating immune complexes may also be identified in the early stages. During this time, complement levels (C3, C4) are typically diminished (hypocomplementemia). In anti-(GBL) processes, hypocomplementemia rarely occurs, but anti-GBL antibodies can sometimes be identified. In most cases of glomerulonephritis, biopsy is required to specify the type and extent of tissue pathology. It should be done early in the course of the disease, before kidney tissue become scarred and atrophied. The findings may be crucial for diagnosis and transplant decisions, since some processes (notably IgA nephropathy and focal sclerosing glomerulonephritis) have a tendency to recur in donated organs. The therapy and prognosis for the various types of glomerulonephritis are outlined in Table 8.8.

Whatever the cause of glomerular disease, if proteinuria is severe or prolonged, ***nephrotic syndrome*** may develop. This problem also develops from severe right-sided heart failure and myeloma. From 2 to 3.5 g of protein are lost daily in the urine. To replenish these losses, the liver steps up protein production and, in the course of heightened activity, produces excess lipids as well. This explains the hyperlipidemia that accompanies nephrotic syndrome. Lipid levels up to 10-fold of normal can be identified by serum studies or by the presence of lipiduria (oval fat bodies and fatty granules in casts). If hepatic production of protein cannot keep pace with urinary loss, hypoalbuminemia develops and oncotic pressure falls. Along with abnormalities of the renin-angiotensin-aldosterone system, and of sodium and volume control, it leads to edema. Patients first experience mobile edema, consisting of eyelid swelling in the morning and ankle swelling in the afternoon. They later develop laryngeal edema, pleural effusion, pericardial fullness, ascites, scrotal swelling, or hydrarthrosis. Edematous extremities may develop "stretch marks" and fingernails may show white parallel lines. Shortness of breath and anorexia are common complaints. Patients with nephrotic syndrome should consult a nephrologist. The underlying glomerular disease should be diagnosed and treated if possible. Steps should also be undertaken to minimize the effects of metabolic changes. These include moderate salt restriction, a high-protein diet, judicious rest, and selective use of diuretics. Slow infusions of albumin and anabolic hormones (steroid trials) are sometimes very useful. If hypertension coexists, it can usually be controlled with beta blockers or renin-inhibiting drugs.

URINE FORMATION

Tubules and Interstitium

Filtrate passing through glomerular membranes enters Bowman's capsule and funnels into the tubular system. Now known as "tubular fluid," it begins flowing through three functional areas: the proximal tubule (initial and distal convoluted segments and straight segment); the loop of Henle (descending limb, thin and thick ascending limbs); and the distal nephron (distal convoluted tubule, cortical collecting tubule, and medullary collecting duct). The anatomy of a nephron tubule is illustrated in Figure 8.2.

Filtrate entering the tubules contain water, ions, and molecules of various substances referred to as "solutes." Some of these solutes are toxic wastes (e.g., urea, uric acid, creatinine) to be eliminated from the body. Others are metabolically useful substances (sodium, chloride, calcium, magnesium, phosphate, glucose, amino acids, and bicarbonate) that must be returned to the circulation according to body needs. Separation takes place in the complicated process of urine formation. It involves the selective passage of water and solutes through tubular walls into a space known as the "interstitium." Composed of reticular fibers and interstitial cells, the tissue here is scanty, particularly in the cortex, but does contain lymphatics and motor and sensory nerves. It also houses branches of the efferent arteriole that form the peritubular capillaries in the cortex and the vasa recta in the medulla. These vessels follow the course of the tubules. Blood within them "reabsorbs" needed substances that have passed from tubular fluid into the interstitium. It releases substances into the interstitium that can then be "secreted" back into the tubular fluid.

Reabsorption and secretion of various substances take place in specific portions of the tubules. They are controlled by (1) the flow rate of fluid through the tubule (tied to the GFR); (2) permeability of tubular walls to the substance; (3) changing osmolality of the tubular fluid and interstitium with flow from one segment to the next (osmotic gradient); (4) hormones (aldosterone antidiuretic hormone); and (5) systemic blood osmolality and volume. Both active mechanisms (transport pumps, carriers) and passive mechanisms (oncotic pressure, osmotic gradients, "solvent drag") are involved. For flexible regulation, some substances are subject to both reabsorption and secretion.

Tubulointerstitial disease (nephritis, nephropathy) refers to any condition in the kidney that affects mainly the tubules and interstitium. These conditions may be divided into infectious and noninfectious processes, the former encompassing acute and chronic pyelonephritis.

► ***Acute pyelonephritis*** is usually the result of a urethral or bladder infection ascending through the ureters to the renal pelvis and into the parenchyma. Its occurrence is facilitated by urinary stasis due to an obstruction (strictures, calculi, tumors, prostate enlargement, neurogenic bladder, or pregnancy). Procedures involving instrumentation, such as catheterization or cystoscopy, may injure or contaminate urinary tract structures. Immunodeficiency (due to diabetes, extended use of antibiotics, treatment with corticosteroids or immunosuppressive drugs) also leaves renal tissues susceptible to colonization. Finally, a systemic infection may be blood borne to the kidney. This is highly uncommon except for staphylococcal bacteremia, which leads to cortical and perinephric abscesses with some consistency.

Whatever the cause, infection develops in wedge-shaped regions of cortical interstitial tissue, tubule walls (particularly collecting ducts), and pelvic and caliceal epithelium. In a striking and characteristic way, it does not spread to contiguous areas, hence the patchy nature of the disease. Polymorphonuclear leukocytes, which initially invade the wedge-shaped regions, are replaced within a few days by chronic inflammatory cells. Tissues become necrotic, abscesses form, and the kidney enlarges. Symptoms develop rapidly. Patients often experience headache, malaise, nausea, and vomiting. High fevers, shaking chills, flank pain, and bladder irritation with frequency and urgency of voiding are typical. On exam the abdomen may be rigid and the costovertebral angle extremely tender. If rigidity and guarding are minimal, an enlarged kidney can sometimes be palpated. Leukocytosis with a marked shift to the left is likely. Analysis of a clean voided urine specimen shows pyuria, minimal proteinuria, and occasionally hematuria. Although WBC casts are pathognomonic of renal inflammation, they are not limited to infectious processes. Unspun urine or Gram stain thereof shows bacteriuria and more than 100,000 organisms on culture. The presence of antibody coating on the organisms has been used as an indication of upper genitourinary tract infection. However, positive tests for antibody coating have been shown to occur in cystitis (9%), acute hemorrhagic cystitis (67%), and prostatitis (67%). The diagnosis is therefore clinical in most cases. Once it is made, antibiotics should be started at once, guided by culture and sensitivity, and continued for a minimum of 10–14 days. In the event of recurrence, patients should be evaluated for an obstruction or reflux.

Most patients recover from acute pyelonephritis with no residual effects. However, those who are inadequately treated or who develop recurrent episodes may develop ***chronic pyelonephritis.*** Repeated inflammation produces interstitial scarring and atrophy. Adjacent papillae retract, and if there is obstruction anywhere along the tract, the calices become dilated. Scarring of the overlying cortex may also occur, with eventual shrinking of the entire kidney. Symptoms are vague and inconsistent. Patients may or may not experience fever, flank pain, and bladder irritation. On exam, there is less likely to be the abdominal rigidity or costovertebral angle tenderness seen with acute pyelonephritis. Pyuria and mild proteinuria are invariably present, but hematuria is less common. Typically scanty, the sediment may contain renal epithelial cells, granular casts, and occasionally WBC casts. Unspun urine or Gram stain thereof shows bacteria and more than 100,000 organisms on culture. While bacteriuria is necessary to make the diagnosis, it is not diagnostic of upper urinary tract infection and may be due instead to cystitis, prostatitis, or urethritis. Localization studies such as antibody coating tests or cultures following bladder washouts with neomycin-fibrinolytic enzyme solutions may be needed. An abnormal urogram showing a dilated caliceal system with overlying scar tissue formation is diagnostic.

The main goal of treatment of chronic pyelonephritis is correction of any obstruction. Obstruction damages tissues both indirectly by predisposing to infection and directly by increasing the pressure within the renal pelvis. Whenever possible, calculi, an enlarged prostate, or tumors should be removed and anatomic defects or strictures repaired. Overt infections should be aggressively treated (see the discussion of acute pyelonephritis). If the obstruction cannot be eliminated and infections recur, long-term antimicrobial drugs are useful. Patients with chronic pyelonephritis may have normal renal function for 20 years or more. However, once there is significant scarring, the concentrating ability decreases and hyperchloremic acidosis develops. This precedes azotemia and reduced clearance. End-stage renal failure is not uncommon. In fact, chronic pyelonephritis accounts for 10–15% of all dialysis patients.

As noted in Table 8.12, most cases of ***noninfectious tubulointerstitial disease*** (tubulointerstitial nephritis or TIN) are related to toxins (exogenous, metabolic, or immunologic). Because of high blood flow, kidney structures are exposed to more circulating toxins than those of other organs. Transport processes contribute to local accumulation of toxins in the tubules, and urine-concentrating mechanisms estab-

TABLE 8.12 NONINFECTIOUS TUBULOINTERSTITIAL DISEASES

Secondary to:	Examples
Medical treatment	Antimicrobials—sulfonamides, methicillin, ampicillin, aminoglycosides, polypeptides, amphotericin, bacitracin, rifampin, chlortrimoxazole, cephalothin, trimethoprim/sulfonamide, outdated tetracycline Analgesics (*analgesic nephropathy*)—phenacetin, acetaminophen, aspirin, all nonsteroidal anti-inflammatory agents Diuretics—thiazides, furosemide Radiation therapy—penicillamine, gold salts Antihypertensives—captoprel Diagnostic agents—bunamiodyl, iodides, all radiographic contrast materials Antiepileptics—trimethiadone, paramethadione Anticancer drugs—cisplatinum, nitrosoureas adriamycin, daunorubicin, *Corynebacterium parvum,* immunosuppressives Radiation (*radiation nephritis*)
Metabolic toxins	Hyperuricemia (*uric acid nephropathy*) Uric acid crystals (*gouty nephropathy*) Hypercalcemia (*hypercalcemic nephropathy*) Hypokalemia (*hypokalemic nephropathy*) Hyperoxaluria Cystinosis Fabry's disease
Environmental toxins	Lead (*lead nephropathy*) Other heavy metals—lead, mercury, cadmium, bismuth, uranium, gold, copper, arsenic, iron, thallium Solvents—carbon tetrachloride, methanol, glycols, trichloroethylene, other hydrocarbons Oxalosis-inducing agents—oxalic acid, methoxyflurane, ethylene glycol, antirust substances Herbicides/pesticides—paraquat, cyanide, dioxin, diphenyl Unidentified toxin endemic to Balkan Islands (*Balkan nephropathy*)
Other	Vasculitis Arteriolar nephrosclerosis Atheroembolic disease Sickle cell disease Chronic obstruction Glomerulonephritis Alport's syndrome Medullary cystic disease Medullary sponge disease Amyloid (*renal amyloidosis*) Myeloma (*myeloma kidney*) Urinary tract obstruction (*obstructive nephropathy*)

lish high levels in the medulla and papillae. Furthermore, the mildly acid pH of the fluid in certain sections of the tubules affects the ionization characteristics of many compounds, enhancing toxicity. The exact cause, pathologic picture, and clinical presentation depend on whether the course is acute or chronic.

Drug exposure is the main cause of ***acute noninfectious tubulointerstitial nephritis (TIN).*** Offending substances are listed in Table 8.12, antimicrobials leading the list. Aminoglycosides are particularly nephrotoxic. Accumulating in proximal tubular cells, they injure tissues by increasing urinary enzymes and protein. Colistin, polymyxin, bacitracin, and amphotericin B and outdated tetracycline are directly cytotoxic. Penicillins and sulfa drugs can cause TIN in hypersensitive individuals, as can phenacetin in patients with glucose-6-phosphate dehydrogenase (G-

6-PD) deficiency. Halogenated anesthetics and other inhaled solvents (methanol, carbon tetrachloride) are other sources. Radiographic contrast agents have also been implicated, although the mechanism of injury is poorly understood. Their use is most risky when associated with intra-arterial administration, patient age greater than 60, dehydration, existing renal insufficiency, solitary kidney, diabetes, myeloma, huperuricemia, CHF, and multiple, closely timed exposures. These factors should certainly be considered by primary care providers before any tests using contrast agents are ordered. In addition to drugs, any type of systemic hypersensitivity reaction may be associated with acute TIN. These reactions may occur in response to bacteria, viruses, spirochetes, pollens, or bee stings. Histologic changes include interstitial edema and infiltration by lymphocytes, plasma cells, or eosinophils. In contrast to infectious processes, polymorphonuclear leukocytes are present only in small numbers. The glomeruli usually remain normal, but patchy areas of tubular necrosis mark the disease.

Patients with acute TIN present with sudden renal failure, with or without oliguria. The signs and symptoms of acute renal failure were discussed previously. They occur anywhere from 5 days to 5 weeks after drug exposure, sooner in cases of hypersensitivity reactions. If urine is produced, it contains protein, WBCs, and RBCs. The absence of bacteria and the presence of eosinophils in blood or urine are important diagnostic findings. So too are systemic signs of hypersensitivity such as fever, lymphadenopathy, and skin rash. Although the kidneys show diagnostic enlargement on IVP, contrast dye used in the test may cause further injury. Avid uptake of radioactive material appears on gallium scan, but the rigorous preparation required for several days of testing may be poorly tolerated by acutely ill patients. For these reasons, physicians often rely on the history and the clinical picture to make the diagnosis. Withdrawal of the toxic agent is the first step in treatment. In addition, many specialists advocate corticosteroid therapy. Patients with anuria or prolonged oliguria require management for acute renal failure. Although complete recovery of renal function is the rule, irreversible cases necessitating lifetime dialysis have been reported.

Chronic TIN may also be associated with the factors noted in Table 8.12, particularly overuse of analgesics. It is characterized histologically by monocyte infiltration, interstitial fibrosis, and widespread tubule changes. The latter include atrophy, luminal dilatation, and thickened basement membranes. Papillary necrosis is pathognomonic and can be demonstrated by the "ring sign" on IVP (radiolucency at the base of the papilla). However, in many cases, renal pelvices are not affected. Clinical signs include impaired concentrating ability (polyuria, nocturia), diminished acid-base regulation (metabolic acidosis), and decreased reabsorption of filtered solutes (wasting of salt, amino acids, phosphate, chloride, potassium, and urates). Because the glomeruli are secondarily affected, a progressive reduction in GFR and overlapping symptoms of glomerular dysfunction are common. Symptoms such as hypertension, edema, proteinuria, and hematuria may then appear but are uncommon in the early disease. Patients with evidence of chronic TIN should be referred to a nephrologist. The diagnosis can often be made on the basis of the history and routine blood tests. Attention should focus on occupational hazards, radiation exposure, and pica and drug use. A history of gout and/or findings of hyperuricemia, hypercalcemia, or hypokalemia may be significant. So, too, is the presence of certain systemic diseases and inherited disorders of metabolism. Biopsy is not needed in most cases. Treatment centers on eliminating additional exposure to injurious substances whenever possible. If this is done in the early stages, renal damage can often be reversed or progression prevented.

Water Balance and Volume Control

Protein in blood leaving the glomerulus creates a high enough oncotic pressure to draw 70% of filtrate water entering the proximal tubule. The water carries sodium chloride and other solutes with it (solvent drag). Its reabsorption thus begins in a passive manner, intimately connected with sodium. In the loop of Henle, reabsorption continues through the use of an active mechanism (transport pumps) and a passive mechanism (osmosis). The two mechanisms act in a synergistic manner referred to as the "countercurrent multiplier" (Fig. 8.3).

Because of the hairpin arrangement of the loop of Henle, fluid flows in opposite (countercurrent) directions in the two closely approximated limbs. Solutes (mainly sodium chloride) are actively pumped through tubule walls of the ascending limb, creating an area of high osmotic pressure in the interstitial space between the U tube. Water from the descending limb is drawn into the space. Thus, active pumps of the ascending limb help passively to multiply the concentration of solutes (osmolal-

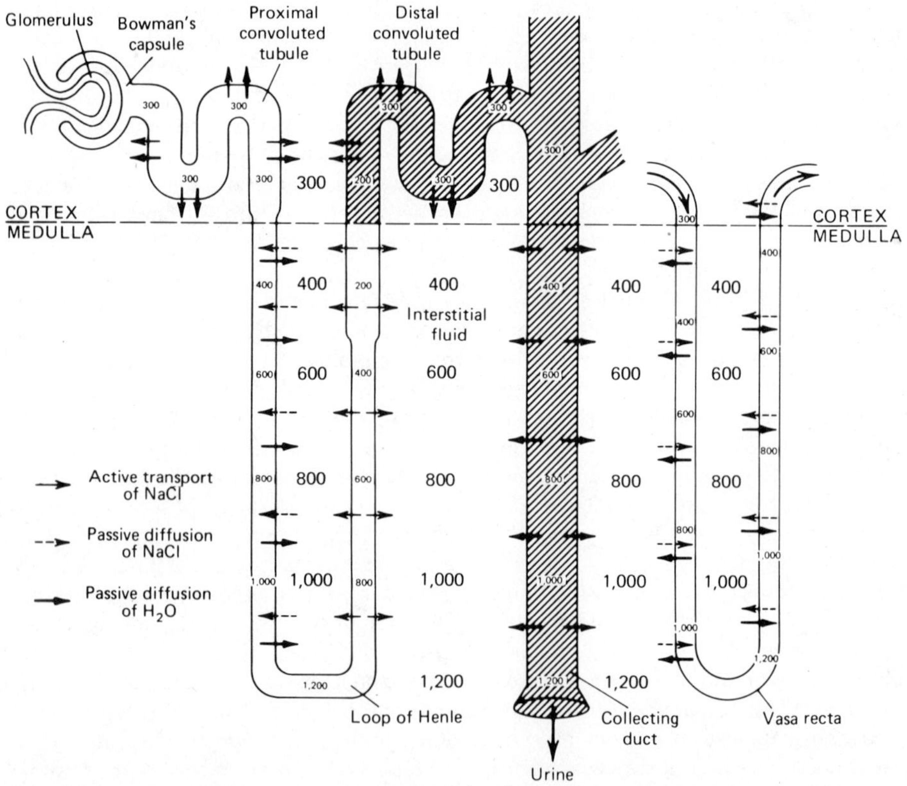

Figure 8.3 Urine-concentrating mechanism. (From Muir, *Pathophysiology: An Introduction to the Mechanisms of Disease*, © 1980, John Wiley & Sons, Inc., New York.)

ity) in the descending limb while sending another 20% of the filtrate's water back into circulation. Unlike the proximal tubule, water reabsorbed here is clear of solutes (free water).

Water remaining in the tubular fluid after it passes through the loop of Henle (about 15% of filtered water) is influenced by antidiuretic hormone (ADH). In the presence of ADH, skeletal proteins in membranes of the distal tubule and collecting duct aggregate, creating pores through which water can be reabsorbed. In the absence of ADH, the proteins dissociate and the pores close. Water cannot escape from the tubular fluid and is excreted.

Synthesized by nerve cells of the hypothalamus, ADH is liberated from terminals in the posterior lobe and pituitary stalk. With slight reductions in volume, solutes in the extracellular fluid (ECF), particularly sodium chloride and inert hexoses, become relatively concentrated. The hyperosmolality activates osmoreceptors in the brain to stimulate the release of ADH (osmotic secretion). Concentrations of urea and glucose may also contribute to hyperosmolality, but for some reason, these solutes have less influence on ADH stimulation. Within a few minutes, the hormone brings about membrane changes in the distal nephron, allowing reabsorption of water. Added to the ECF, this water helps to normalize osmolality and ADH is promptly removed from circulation.

With severe reductions in circulating volume (10% or more), ADH release is stimulated by baroreceptors (stretch receptors) in arterial walls (nonosmotic secretion). The hormone level thus increases with upright posture, positive pressure respirator breathing, hemorrhage, or reduced blood pressure. Activation of baroreceptors is potentiated by circulating catecholamines, angiotensin II, nicotine, and prostaglandins. Prostaglandins have an added effect. By acting on smooth muscle, they offset the vasoconstrictor action of norepinephrine and angiotensin II and help protect renal blood flow. Very high levels of norepinephrine and angiotensin II override prostaglandin protection, resulting in constriction of the afferent arteriole and renal ischemia.

ADH is stimulated whenever baroreceptors in the heart sense a decrease in effective circulating volume. Secretion thus occurs in CHF, cirrhosis of the liver, nephrotic syndrome, and hypoproteinemia. Although appropriate, it contributes to sodium and water retention, which complicate such disease processes.

By contrast, inappropriate secretion results from disruption of osmoreceptors in the brain. Occurring with certain drugs, pulmonary disease, central nervous system (CNS) disease, and other conditions listed in Table 8.13, it leads to the ***syndrome of inappropriate antidiuretic hormone (SIADH).*** The problem is characterized by a revolving sequence of events beginning with the retention of free water due to the vasopressin effects of ADH. This not only dilutes body fluids, producing hyponatremia and hypo-osmolality, but also expands the circulating volume. As a result, vascular volume receptors are activated and urinary excretion of sodium increases, worsening the hyponatremia. The diagnosis of SIADH rests on specific criteria: (1) hyponatremia with corresponding hypo-osmolality of plasma; (2) urine osmolality disproportionately high in relation to plasma osmolality; (3) excessive renal excretion of sodium; (4) absence of CHF, cirrhosis, hypoproteinemia, or nephrotic syndrome; (5) normal renal function; and (6) normal adrenal function. It should be emphasized that a urine osmolality above 100 mOsm/kg is entirely compatible with the diagnosis of SIADH even if it is lower than plasma osmolality. Most cases of SIADH respond to fluid restriction (500–1,000 mL/day). Because such limitations

TABLE 8.13 CAUSES OF SIADH

Idiopathic	Pneumothorax
CNS	Asthma
Neonatal hypoxia	Positive-pressure breathing
Meningitis	Malignancies
Encephalitis	All pulmonary
Hydrocephalus	Duodenum
Tumor	Pancreas
Abscess	Bladder
Cavernous sinus thrombosis	Ureter
Trauma	Prostate
Subarachnoid hemorrhage	Ewing's sarcoma
Cerebellar and cerebral atrophy	Surgical stress/anesthesia
Delirium tremens	Drugs
Acute psychosis	Vasopressin
Pulmonary	Oxytoxin
Oat cell carcinoma	Antineoplastic agents
Mesothelioma	Chlorpropamide
Thymoma	Thiazide diuretics
Lymphoma	Phenothiazines
Pneumonia	Monoamine oxidase inhibitors
Tuberculosis	Carbamazepine
Empyema	Clofibrate
Cystic fibrosis	Nicotine

may be difficult to enforce over long periods of time, chronic cases are often managed with either lithium or demeclocycline. These drugs leave the distal nephron somewhat refractory to the effects of ADH. In cases of severe hyponatremia (<110 mEq/L) accompanied by CNS symptoms, hypertonic saline may be needed in addition to fluid restriction.

In contrast to the clinical picture of excessive ADH secretion is ***nephrogenic diabetes insipidus,*** in which renal tubules are resistant to the vasopressor effects of ADH. Because the disease has an X-linked recessive pattern of expression, affected men demonstrate complete and heterozygous women partial unresponsiveness. While other tubule functions and GFR remain normal, there is varying inability to concentrate urine. Patients develop polydipsia, polyuria, and hypotonic urine soon after birth. As long as water intake remains adequate, the sequelae of dehydration and hypernatremia can be averted. Nonetheless, excessive thirst and urination plague most patients for life. Paradoxically, thiazide diuretics may be helpful. However, unlike ***diabetes insipidus,*** ADH substitutes are of little use. Diabetes insipidus is a temporary or chronic disorder of the neurohypophyseal system causing ADH deficiency. It is discussed in Chapter 12.

With significant volume reductions, renin is released in conjunction with ADH. Renin leads to the formation of angiotensin II and III. Both hormones act as potent vasoconstrictors (preventing systemic blood pressure from falling) and as thirst stimulators (ensuring restoration of body water). In the kidney, angiotensin II in low concentrations causes vasoconstriction of the efferent arteriole and helps maintain GFR without ischemia. It also prompts secretion of aldosterone. As noted later, this hormone influences the conservation of sodium and therefore of water.

When noting all of the mechanisms designed for volume preservation, the devastating effect of ***volume depletion*** is easy to surmise. The problem may be associated with renal or extrarenal losses of salt and water, as noted in Table 8.14. Those

TABLE 8.14 CAUSES OF VOLUME DEPLETION

Failure to replace normal losses	Blood loss /or fluid shifts
Disorders of the thirst mechanism	Hemorrhage
Coma or other alterations in mental status	Trauma
Lack of food/water sources	Burns
Loss of GI fluids	Shock
Vomiting	Abnormal urinary losses
Diarrhea	Diabetes insipidus (nephrogenic, pituitary)
Sequestration due to obstruction or peritonitis	Osmotic diuresis (diabetes, urea diuresis)
Paracentesis	Aldosterone insufficiency (Addison's disease, hyporeninemic hypoaldosteronism, interstitial nephritis)
GI fistulas	Renal tubular acidosis
Tube drainage	Bartter's syndrome
Excessive loss of sweat and respiratory secretions	Diuretic abuse
Strenuous exercise	Postobstructive diuresis
Fever	Acute TIN, diuretic phase
Hyperventilation	Chronic renal failure
Prolonged environmental exposure to heat, cold, high altitude	

conditions marked by loss of solute free water will suffer less disturbance of circulating volume than those with a combined deficit of sodium and water. Symptoms of volume depletion are nonspecific and include weakness, postural dizziness, nausea, headache, and thirst. Stimulation of sympathetic nerves results in associated tachycardia and peripheral vasoconstriction with cool, dry extremities. When volume contraction is moderate, recumbent blood pressure is normal and postural hypotension may be present. When it is severe, recumbent hypotension and shock develop. Decreased skin turgor and dryness of mucous membranes are valuable signs, particularly in children. There is a reduction in urine output and sodium excretion, except in cases of diabetes insipidus and renal salt wasting, respectively. Sodium excretion may also be increased in cases associated with vomiting or gastric drainage due to metabolic alkalosis.

Patients with severe volume contraction should be hospitalized for fluid replacement and close observation. Invasive monitoring may be needed for patients who are hemodynamically unstable (acute heart failure, septicemia, noncardiogenic pulmonary edema) or who may undergo large shifts of fluids between body compartments (trauma or burns). This involves measurement of pulmonary capillary wedge pressure with a Swan-Ganz (flow-directed) catheter. Central venous pressure correlates poorly with cardiac output and pulmonary vascular volume. Even the Swan-Ganz catheter may give normal readings when blood volume has been reduced by 5–10%, but the deficit may be determined by a fluid challenge. Decisions about the type and amount of fluid, and the route and rate of administration, vary with the particular circumstance. For example, potassium, sugar, water, and salt all need to be replaced in cases of cholera and are best given in oral solutions (see Chapter 4). Intravenous (IV) normal saline may be sufficient for the patient with a mild GI bleed, whereas whole blood is needed for massive hemorrhaging.

Salt Regulation

By increasing or decreasing the amount of salt excreted in urine, the kidneys adjust for wide variations in dietary intake. This is extremely important because salt, as the principal cation in plasma, interstitial fluid, and lymph (ECF) must be carefully regulated. The osmolality it creates in the ECF maintains equilibrium with that created by potassium in the intracellular fluid (ICF). Consequently, ECF is assured one-third of the total body water and ICF two-thirds. This important ratio remains steady even though cell membranes are freely permeable to water and fluids are continually exchanged between the two compartments.

The average American consumes about 170 mEq of salt daily, the kidneys excreting about 98% of this amount. When a healthy individual increases the intake of salt much beyond this amount, ECF becomes hypertonic, drawing water into the vascular space and interstitial fluid. As circulating volume expands, GFR and the flow of tubular fluid through the tubules increase. The fast flow of tubular fluid leaves no time for salt reabsorption, and sodium levels in the urine increase. In this manner, urinary excretion offsets high intake, but not for 3–4 days. During the interval of adjustment, positive sodium balance results in retention of water and consequent gain in body weight. When salt intake is reduced, the opposite effect is observed. This explains the rationale behind a ▶ ***salt-restricted diet.*** It may be prescribed for patients with premenstrual syndrome, CHF, HTN, or ascites from cirrhosis of the liver.

Low salt intake stimulates the adrenal cortex to produce aldosterone, a steroid that acts on the distal tubule and cortical collecting duct to cause an exchange of potassium for sodium. Sodium is reabsorbed and potassium excreted. Aldosterone promotes the same action in the epididymus, small and large intestines, and ducts of the salivary and sweat glands. It is further discussed in the next section.

Due to kidney regulation, serum sodium is normally kept within a very close range (136–146 mmol/L). ***Hypernatremia*** develops whenever water intake fails to offset water loss (Table 8.15). Due to the exquisite sensitivity of thirst mechanisms, it is rare in conscious patients. However, it is sometimes seen with excessive water loss from sweating, diabetes insipidus, or osmotic diuresis (e.g., hyperglycemia, mannitol use). Administration of large amounts of hypertonic solutions (notably sodium bicarbonate) is another cause. Furthermore, essential hypernatremia may develop from a central defect, either of the thirst center or of the osmoreceptors. This may be a congenital or acquired abnormality, the latter often associated with histiocytic infiltration of the CNS. In either case, elevations of serum sodium are mild, and both thirst and antidiuresis are stimulated when volume contraction occurs. Clinical manifestations of hypernatremia are produced by brain cell shrinkage from increased osmolality of the ECF. They depend on the degree of hypertonicity and the rate at which it developed. Acute hypernatremia causes somnolence, confusion, coma, respiratory paralysis, and death, while chronic hypernatremia may be accompanied by few CNS symptoms because brain cells have time to accumulate iogenic osmoles, minimizing shrinkage. Treatment consists of the slow administration of dilute solutions (e.g., one-half normal saline or 2.5% dextrose in one-fourth normal

TABLE 8.15 ABNORMALITIES OF SERUM SODIUM

Hypernatremia	Hyponatremia
Excessive salt intake without access to water	Essential (sick cell syndrome)
Excessive water loss (insensible, burns, diabetes insipidus, osmotic diuresis)	Dehydration (loss of salt and water)
Adrenal hyperfunction (Cushing's disease, primary hyperaldosteronism)	Dilutional (edema, adrenal insufficiency, SIADH)

saline). For thc first 2 days, replacement should be regulated to reduce serum sodium by no more than 1 mEq/L every 2 hours. More rapid reduction of serum sodium could cause brain swelling from the iogenic osmoles.

Volume contraction accounts for most cases of ***hyponatremia*** (Table 8.15). It stimulates ADH (returns water to the circulation) and reduces the delivery rate of sodium to the collecting ducts (prevents urine dilution). Hyponatremia is also a common feature of Addison's disease, intractable heart failure, advanced ascites, and the use of drugs that stimulate ADH release or enhance its action. Due to the redistribution of sodium from ECF to ICF, it may occur in the "sick cell syndrome" seen in severe debilitating illness.

Acute hyponatremia produces brain swelling. With dilution of ECF, there is an efflux of water into the CNS cells when serum sodium falls to 125 mEq/L or less. Beginning with lethargy, somnolence, and weakness, the clinical manifestations rapidly progress to seizures, coma, and death. Thus, the problem is an indication for immediate hospitalization. In volume-contracted states, serum sodium is raised to 125 mEq/L over a 6-hour interval using isotonic saline IV solutions. In volume-expanded states, water restriction or isotonic saline in combination with furosemide is usually required. Initially, levels raised higher than 125 mEq/L may be hazardous; they may be relatively hypertonic to brain cells that have been depleted of potassium in the development of hyponatremia.

Chronic hyponatremia may be associated with very few CNS manifestations, even with serum sodium levels as low as 110 mEq/L. Slow reduction of sodium in the ECF is accompanied by an equal loss of potassium from the ICF; because the ratio of intracelluar to extracellular solute remains fixed, sudden osmotic shifts of fluid do not occur and brain swelling remains minimal. Chronic hyponatremia can usually be corrected by discontinuation of the causative drugs (e.g., diuretics) or careful management of the underlying disorder (CHF, ascites). When associated with SIADH, it can be corrected by restricting water intake to 800–1,000 mL daily. Alternately, lithium or demeclocycline (drugs that interfere with the renal tubular effects of ADH) may be given. A high-protein diet to produce osmotic diuresis from urea loading may also be useful.

Potassium Regulation

About 3,500 mEq of potassium are found in the body, 98% of which is taken up by the cells. This makes potassium the principal cation of ICF. Serum levels, which measures the small amount of potassium found in ECF, are influenced by a number of "effector mechanisms." One of the most important mechanisms stems from the fact that cell membranes are partially permeable to both potassium and sodium (the latter is the principal cation of ECF). As a consequence, sodium continually leaks into the ICF and potassium into the ECF. Known as the "Donnan distribution," this passive movement would quickly cause the intracellular cations to exceed the extracellular ones; water would be drawn osmotically into the cells, and lysis would occur. To prevent this, transport pumps reverse the tendency to leak by creating constant sodium efflux to the ECF and potassium influx to the ICF. They are mediated by membrane-bound ATPase, whose energy expenditure accounts for more than 50% of the basal caloric consumption. Impairment of transport pumps is thought to cause the cellular swelling ***(sick cell syndrome)*** seen in many debilitated states.

Osmolality is a second effector mechanism controlling cellular uptake of potassium and thus influencing its level in the serum. With hypertonicity, water is drawn out of the cells, raising the concentration of intracellular potassium. To correct this situation, potassium enters the ECF and serum levels rise. Although it may seem contradictory, chronic hypotonicity causes potassium loss from brain and renal tubular cells. In such cases, potassium efflux helps to balance ECF and ICF osmolality in the presence of reduced ECF sodium and to minimize tissue swelling. However, since muscle cells (which account for most of the body's ICF potassium) do not behave in this manner, chronic hypotonicity has little effect on serum potassium levels.

Insulin is still another effector mechanism. It promotes the transfer of potassium from ECF to ICF independent of glucose uptake. In fact, hyperkalemia is thought to be the sensor that stimulates insulin release. Beta-adrenergic agents such as epinephrine and isoproterenol also promote cellular uptake of potassium, as do plasma bicarbonate concentrations and/or systemic alkalosis. By contrast, respiratory and metabolic acidosis promote cellular efflux of potassium. Generally, every 0.1 pH unit reduction is accompanied by a 0.6 mEq/L serum potassium increase, and vice versa. The mechanisms behind the inverse relationship between potassium and pH change are not clear.

Nearly all dietary potassium (50–150 mEq/L daily) is absorbed from the gut. Whatever is absorbed must be eliminated by the kidneys to maintain external balance. Fecal excretion also occurs but accounts for only 10 mEq/day unless diarrhea is present. In the kidney, potassium is filtered into the tubular fluid but is then reabsorbed (70% in the proximal tubule and the remainder in the loop of Henle). It is both reabsorbed and secreted in the distal nephron, the balance between the two processes determining the final amount excreted in the urine. The rate of secretion is influenced by aldosterone, acid-base changes, flow rate, and sodium reabsorption.

Aldosterone, a mineralocorticoid produced by adrenal glands, is apparently the only hormone responsible for maintaining ECF concentrations of potassium. It does so via a simple feedback loop, an increase in serum potassium stimulating aldosterone release. The hormone acts on the distal tubule to increase potassium secretion into the urine. With influx of the strong cation to tubular fluid, the surrounding interstitium becomes relatively electronegative. Sodium passes out of tubular fluid to balance the anion gap and is reabsorbed. In this way, aldosterone influences sodium reabsorption as well, thus playing an important part in salt and volume control. It increases in response to four factors: (1) increased plasma potassium concentrations, (2) increased plasma angiotensin II concentrations, (3) adrenocorticotropic hormone stimulation, (4) a low-salt diet. ***Hyperaldosterone conditions*** produce salt reabsorption with volume overload, hypertension, and excessive potassium loss. ***Hypoaldosterone conditions*** are associated with salt wasting and hyperkalemia (see Chapter 13).

Hyperkalemia may be associated with any of the conditions listed in Table 8.16. Since the diagnosis is usually based on serum potassium levels, one must consider the possibility of a sampling artifact. Erythrocytes contain significant amounts of potassium, which is released when the blood sample hemolyzes. Unless separated promptly from the red cell mass, serum may accumulate potassium from hemolyzed erythrocytes, giving a falsely high result. Platelets and leukocytes are also rich in potassium, and if they are present in large numbers (e.g., in thrombocytosis, leukemia), excessive potassium will be released during coagulation of the sample. In these cases, plasma from heparinized blood may be needed to give an accurate

TABLE 8.16 CAUSES OF POTASSIUM ABNORMALITIES

Hyperkalemia	Hypokalemia
Increased intake (rare unless renal failure is present)	Inadequate intake
High-dose potassium penicillins	Starvation
Excessive intake of oral supplements (including salt substitutes)	IV fluids without potassium supplements
Rapid infusion of IV solutions with potassium supplements	Excessive loss
Inadequate excretion	Excessive sweating (including cystic fibrosis)
Renal failure	Diuretics
Adrenal insufficiency	Diabetic ketoacidosis
Potassium-sparing diuretics	Adrenal steroid excess (including excessive licorice ingestion)
Shift of potassium out of cells	TIN (Fanconi's syndrome, pyelonephritis, RTA)
Acidosis	Diarrhea, chronic laxative abuse, villous adenoma of the colon
Crush injuries	Vomiting, GI suction
Burns	Transfer of potassium ions into cells
Internal bleeding	Parenteral nutrition
	Insulin administration
	Familial periodic paralysis
	Acute alkalosis

account of potassium levels. Symptoms of hyperkalemia are related to abnormal neuromuscular function (see Chapter 12). Patients may initially experience weakness, abdominal distention, and diarrhea. Paralysis develops in severe cases. As potassium increases, the electrocardiogram reflects the developing impairment in heart muscle conduction: peaked T waves of increased amplitude, atrial arrest, spread in the QRS, biphasic QRS-T complexes, and finally, ventricular fibrillation. Death occurs from cardiac arrest. Patients usually require hospitalization for close observation and treatment. Potassium in all forms is withheld, and measures are employed to drive the cation into the ICF. The latter may include administration of Kayexalate (an exchange resin), insulin in combination with glucose, and sodium bicarbonate. In the presence of kidney failure, dialysis may be necessary.

Associated with conditions noted in Table 8.16, ▶***hypokalemia*** is defined as a serum potassium level of 3.0 mEq/L or less. However, symptoms may develop at higher levels. They include muscle cramps, fatigue, and lethargy. Cardiac irritability and life-threatening arrhythmias may occur, particularly in patients with diabetes or CHF treated with digitalis. Patients taking diuretics have more potassium wasting if they ingest excessive amounts of sodium, which increases the tubular exchange for potassium. For them, treatment begins with a diet high in potassium and moderately low in salt. Strict salt restriction may actually produce hypokalemia due to aldosterone secretion. Adjustment of medication is also important, large doses of long-acting diuretics increasing the severity of hypokalemia. If these measures fail to correct the problem, potassium-sparing diuretics or potassium supplements are indicated.

Bicarbonate and Hydrogen Ion Concentrations

About 4,500 mmol of bicarbonate (i.e., most of the filtered amount) are quickly reabsorbed from the proximal tubule. Bicarbonate reabsorption is crucial to the acid-base balance, since the end products of metabolism are a number of weak organic acids. Without the CO_2-HCO_3 buffering system activated by kidney tubules, the constant generation of these acids would threaten the normal pH range of blood (7.35–7.45). The buffering process begins with CO_2 accumulation in proximal tubular walls. The CO_2 either permeates into the tubular walls (from tubular fluid or the interstitium) or is generated by tubular cells (cellular metabolism). Under the influence of carbonic anhydrase, it combines with H_2O, forming carbonic acid (H_2CO_3). Almost as soon as it is formed, carbonic acid dissociates into hydrogen ion (H^+) and bicarbonate (HCO_3). H^+ moves into the tubular fluid and HCO_3 is reabsorbed, a process that acidifies the urine but does not significantly change the pH of body fluids.

However, the addition of H^+ to tubular fluid enables the formation of new HCO_3, later reabsorption of which does help to alkalinize body fluids. It also helps to titrate acids formed by phosphates (filtered into tubular fluid) and ammonia (produced in tubular cells by the transamination of amino acids). Most of the filtered phosphate is reabsorbed from the proximal tubule in the form of HPO_4. The small amount that escapes reabsorption accepts a single hydrogen ion and becomes H_2PO_4. This alters its permeability, "fixing" the acid in the urine for excretion. NH_3 undergoes the same process. Once it combines with H^+ in the tubular fluid, it becomes NH_4, which cannot permeate across tubular walls and is therefore excreted in the urine. The NH_3-NH_4 buffer pair is particularly important because the rate of ammonia production is tied to the body's acid-base status. When the pH of body fluids drops, kidney tubules step up the production of ammonia. The excess ammonia ties up hydrogen ions, ensuring excretion. When the pH rises, ammonia production falls to zero. Lack of ammonia acids in the urine not only minimizes H^+ loss but also interferes with bicarbonate reabsorption. With the help of these tubular mechanism, pH changes can often be corrected.

A drop in blood pH below 7.35 marks the development of ***metabolic acidosis.*** The causes are listed in Table 8.17. The cardinal sign is hyperventilation, which in severe cases may be manifested as Kussmaul respiration (slow, deep breathing). These respiratory effects are an attempt to lower the H^+ level by blowing off CO_2. The fall of CO_2 below normal marks the development of respiratory alkalosis, a problem discussed in Chapter 6. In addition to the pulmonary effects, metabolic acidosis diminishes the cardiac response to catecholamines, causing negative inotropism. This sets up a potentially lethal chain of events: decreased tissue perfusion, lactic acid production, increased acidosis, and a further fall in cardiac function. Severe acidosis may also reduce the 2,3-diphosphoglycerate (2,3-DPG) in RBCs; an increase is needed to shift the oxyhemoglobin dissociation curve to the right, permitting delivery of oxygen to poorly perfused tissue. Failure of this compensatory mech-

TABLE 8.17 MAJOR CAUSES OF METABOLIC ACIDOSIS/ALKALOSIS

Acidosis	Alkalosis
Hydrogen ion accumulation (elevated ion gap)	Bicarbonate accumulation
Renal failure	Milk alkali syndrome
Diabetic ketoacidosis	Antacid therapy
Lactic acidosis	RTA
Poisons (notably aspirin)	Increased steroids (Cushing's disease, hyperaldosteronism, steroid drug therapy)
Bicarbonate loss (normal ion gap)	Diuretics
Through stool (diarrhea, ileostomy, colostomy)	Hydrogen ion loss
Tubulointerstitial disease (RTA)	Vomiting
	Gastric suction

anism (Bohr effect) aggravates the situation and furthers the fall of pH. Best handled by a clinician well versed in fluid and electrolyte problems, treatment depends on whether excess bicarbonate loss or H+ accumulation is the cause. Distinction between the two processes can be made by applying the "anion gap" formula to the patient's serum electrolytes:

$$\text{anion gap} = [Na^+] - ([HCO_3^-] + [Cl^-]) = 8\text{–}12 \text{ meq}$$

An increased gap (greater than 12 mEq/L) points to H+ accumulation. Very high gaps are life-threatening. They are usually associated with ketoacidosis or lactoacidosis. A normal gap (8–12 mEq/L) indicates bicarbonate loss, while a decreased gap (less than 8 mEq/L) may occur with elevations of monoclonal immunoglobulins that have isoelectric points higher than that of the serum pH. Patients with acute or severe problems require hospitalization, while those with mild or chronic changes may be managed as outpatients.

Associated with the conditions listed in Table 8.17, ***metabolic alkalosis*** is defined as a rise in pH above 7.45. Due to the efficiency of tubular excretion, it is nearly impossible to arrive at this state by excessive dietary intake of antacids. Patients who have hypercalcemia and secondary renal dysfunction are an exception. When they ingest calcium and absorbable antacids, both serum calcium and pH rise sharply. Known as ***milk-alkali syndrome,*** this problem may also be the consequence of ulcer therapy. Transient alkalosis occurs with excess loss of hydrogen ions from the body or from delayed conversion of accumulated organic acids. Sustained metabolic alkalosis is related to either increased reabsorption or increased generation of bicarbonate by the renal tubules. This, in turn, can be traced to one of four effector mechanisms: (1) volume contraction, (2) increased delivery of salt to the distal nephron, (3) potassium depletion, and (4) mineralocorticoid excess. Mild volume contraction favors metabolic alkalosis by increasing the threshold for bicarbonate reabsorption in the proximal tubule.

Severe volume contraction adds to the problem by enhancing sodium reabsorption. At first, potassium bicarbonate is excreted to maintain the urinary pH in the face of reduced sodium excretion. However, this leads to a potassium deficit and the eventual reabsorption of both potassium and sodium. Aciduria develops even though plasma pH and bicarbonate are elevated, a condition referred to as ***contraction alkalosis*** (paradoxical aciduria). As might be expected, renal tubular disease or hyperaldosteronism also leads to metabolic alkalosis. Both are present in ***Bartter's syndrome,*** a disorder appearing in childhood and characterized by the unlikely combination of salt wasting in the presence of high aldosterone secretion and normal blood pressure despite high levels of renin and angiotensin. There are no specific signs and symptoms of metabolic alkalosis, though severe cases can lead to cardiac arrhythmias and hypoventilation, particularly in patients with reduced renal function. However, since chronic cases are usually attended by hypokalemia, muscle weakness and hyporeflexia are actually more common. Suggested by an elevated bicarbonate level and a reduced potassium level on serum electrolyte measurements, the diagnosis of metabolic alkalosis can be confirmed with arterial blood gas measurements. Treatment for most cases focuses on volume expansion with saline solutions and potassium replacement.

Renal tubular acidosis stems from defective H^+ generation and/or exchange. Several types are described depending on the specific location of dysfunction. ***Proximal renal tubular acidosis (type II)*** can be traced to deficient production of H^+

ions by proximal tubule cells. The problem is usually genetic but may also be secondary to acetazolamide therapy. Without sufficient H^+ in the tubular fluid, new bicarbonate cannot be formed for reabsorption. As plasma bicarbonate diminishes, less bicarbonate is filtered, setting up an equilibrium that actually limits the degree of metabolic acidosis. However, reduced bicarbonate reabsorption is accompanied by increased chloride reabsorption. Furthermore, to correct the anion gap created by reduced H^+ in the tubular fluid, potassium is secreted into the urine and lost. The resulting hypokalemia stimulates aldosterone release, and hyperaldosteronism may develop. Also, since H^+ is needed to fix phosphate and ammonia for excretion, lack of the ion allows these substances to remain free for reabsorption, the consequences being azotemia, hypophosphaturia, and hyperphosphatemia. Sharing an inverse relationship to calcium, hypophosphaturia leads to hypercalciuria and hyperphosphatemia leads to hypocalcemia. These imbalances are associated with nephrocalcinosis and metabolic bone disease. As might be expected, type II acidosis tends to be severe and progressive, and should be handled by the specialist. Lifelong therapy with $NaHCO_3$ or Shohl's solution (sodium citrate and citric acid) and potassium supplements are usually required, along with emergency intervention during exacerbations. Hydrochlorothiazide therapy may also be helpful.

Distal renal tubular acidosis (type I) develops from any circumstance that lowers the amount of H^+ in distal fluid. Without H^+ to form new bicarbonate for reabsorption, metabolic acidosis develops. The problem may be genetically transmitted or associated with sickle cell disease, a variety of autoimmune diseases, chronic pyelonephritis, urolithiasis, or cirrhosis. It may also result from the use of amphotericin B, analgesics, and other drugs. Although moderate, type I acidosis is associated with hypokalemia and hyperchloremia. Treatment consists of replacing bicarbonate and potassium either in the form of $KHCO_3$ or Shohl's solution. As long as the acidosis remains corrected, patients do well.

Renal tubular acidosis (type IV) is related to a reduction in aldosterone activity, either from lack of the hormone's secretion or from failure of the hormone to regulate sodium/potassium exchange in the distal tubule. Such dysfunction reduces the amount of H^+ and potassium normally cleared in the urine, resulting in the development of acidosis and hyperkalemia. Acidosis is usually mild and can be corrected by small doses of sodium bicarbonate. Hyperkalemia is managed with a low-potassium diet, potassium-binding resins, and loop diuretics. Fluorocortisone is also used.

Glucose and Amino Acid Reabsorption

Under normal conditions, 100% of the glucose filtered by the glomerulus is reabsorbed from the proximal tubule and none appears in the urine. ***Glucosuria*** usually signals hyperglycemia from diabetes mellitus. The rate of glucose transport (by carrier proteins) across tubular walls is inversely related to plasma glucose levels. Reabsorption increases when plasma glucose is low. It ceases when blood saturation rises above 160 mg%, allowing excretion of glucose in the urine, but always at a lower than filtered rate. When urinary excretion is high, the added osmolality of glucose molecules in the tubular fluid interferes with water reabsorption, causing ***hyperosmolar diuresis.*** This explains the polyuria and the constant danger of dehydration experienced by patients with uncontrolled hyperglycemia.

Sometimes the proximal tubule is relatively unable to transport glucose, which appears in the urine even though plasma levels remain low. Referred to as ***renal glycosuria,*** this harmless condition is easily diagnosed by normal glucose tolerance testing and the absence of ketosis. No treatment is necessary, though there should be periodic retesting, since renal glycosuria may precede the onset of true diabetes. Diabetes is discussed in Chapter 5.

Like glucose, 100% of filtered amino acids are normally reabsorbed from the proximal tubule. Both carrier proteins and active transport are involved. ***Aminoaciduria*** occurs only when there is some defect, either of tubular transport or of amino acid generation. The most common congenital cause is cystinuria, an amino acid defect characterized by systemic accumulation of cystine crystals in tissue. Another notable cause is ***De Toni-Fanconi-Debre (Fanconi) syndrome,*** in which congential or acquired changes sometimes leave the proximal tubule thin and foreshortened ("swan neck deformity"). Acquired Fanconi syndrome results from creosol or heavy metal poisoning (cadmium, lead, copper, uranium, mercury); the use of outdated tetracycline; galactosemia; dysproteinemia; nephrotic syndrome; and amyloidosis. The problem is marked not only by aminoaciduria but also by glucosuria, phosphaturia, osteomalacia, and renal tubular acidosis. Patients should be closely followed by a nephrologist. Treatment consists of correcting the acidosis with bicarbonate or citrate and replacing phosphate, potassium, calcium, and other electrolyte losses. Vitamin D therapy is helpful. Any primary cause must also be addressed.

Uric Acid Clearance

Nucleic acids (DNA, RNA) are present in body cells and food (particularly organ meats and yeast). They are degraded into purines and then converted to uric acid by the enzymatic action of xanthine oxidase, predominantly in the liver. Of the uric acid that accumulates each day, approximately two-thirds is eliminated via the kidney and one-third via the GI tract. Renal excretion is a complicated process. Freely filtered across the glomerular membrane, plasma urate is almost completely reabsorbed in the proximal tubule. It is then secreted back into the tubule at a more distal site and partially reabsorbed a second time.

Urate clearance normally averages 6–12% of plasma clearance, keeping serum levels within a narrow range (6.9–7.5 mg/dL in men and 5.7–6.6 mg/dL in women). In measuring serum levels, it should be noted that methods based on the reducing ability of uric acid are subject to error. Underestimation results with protein precipitation and overestimation with the presence of high glucose concentrations, ascorbic acid, salicylates, caffeine, theophylline, theobromine, L-dopa, and other substances. Enzymatic assays, which are not affected by such variables, should be employed if a question of accuracy exists.

▶ ***Hyperuricemia*** may result from reduced renal clearance or excessive synthesis of uric acid (determined by clearance studies). Having primary or secondary origins as noted in Table 8.18, the problem may lead to gouty arthritis and tophus formation (discussed in Chapter 12) or to three types of kidney disease: (1) ***gouty nephropathy*** from deposition of urate crystals in the interstitium of the medulla, (2) acute renal failure from intratubular precipitation of uric acid, and (3) kidney stones from uric acid as the predominant stone material or as a nidus to calcium stones. These consequences are more likely to develop if obesity, diabetes, hyper-

TABLE 8.18 CAUSES OF HYPERURICEMIA

Idiopathic	Cytotoxic drug therapy
Genetic	Paget's disease
Lesch-Nyhan syndrome	To reduced clearance
GP-ribose-P synthetase deficiency	Renal disease
Glycogen storage diseases	Hyperthyroidism
Cystinuria	Adrenal insufficiency
Down's syndrome	Hyperoxaluria
Secondary	Acidosis
To excessive synthesis	Thiazides
Active psoriasis	Low-dose ASA
Proliferative blood diseases (e.g., multiple myeloma, polycythemia vera, leukemia)	Nicotinic acid
Soft tissue malignancies	Pyrazinamide
Sickle cell anemia	Ethambutol

lipidemia, and/or hypertension coexist. Because the exact cause–effect relationship between hyperuricemia and clinical manifestations is unclear, treatment remains controversial. Most experts feel that ▶ ***mild hyperuricemia*** (asymptomatic or associated with a history of mild, infrequent attacks of gout) should be managed with attention to the underlying causes and diet. ▶ ***Significant hyperuricemia*** (a history of renal complications, tophi, and uncontrolled gouty arthritis) warrants drug therapy (uricosuric agents or xanthine oxidase inhibitors).

URINE ELIMINATION

Ureters

From the renal pelvis, urine passes out of the kidneys through the ureters (see Fig. 8.3). The ureters are 25–30 cm long. In women, they run near the ovarian border and close to the cervix, and are thus at risk for injury during gynecologic procedures. Although one ureter normally exists from the hilus of each kidney, ***congenital anomalies*** are relatively common. Listed in Table 8.19, many of these conditions impede urine outflow and require surgical repair.

Ureteral tubes are made up of three layers: outer fibrous, middle muscular, and inner mucosal. The muscular layer contracts, creating peristaltic waves that perpetuate continual movement of urine into the bladder. However, the lumen is nar-

TABLE 8.19 CONGENITAL ANOMALIES OF THE URETERS

Atresia	Lower tract implantation to:
Complete duplication	Lateral bladder wall
Unilateral or bilateral	Bladder neck
Upper or lower pole (rare)	Along trigone
Ectopia	Female urethra
Right retrocaval (behind the right cardinal vein)	Vagina
Left retrocaval (behind the left cardinal vein, usually with inversus situs only)	Uterus
	Male urethra
	Prostate
	Seminal vesicles
	External body

row (4–5 mm in diameter) and relatively constricted at three locations: (1) the junction of the renal pelvis, (2) the crossing of the iliac artery, and (3) the entrance into the bladder. These areas are likely places for ***renal stones*** (calculi) to lodge. Various types of renal stones are described according to their composition and underlying cause (Table 8.20). If one does become lodged, it causes a severe, stabbing flank pain known as ***renal colic.*** Patients with renal colic typically writhe in bed or pace the floor, attempting to find a comfortable position. Alternatively, they may have lower abdominal or groin pain. Paralytic ileus, diminished bowel sounds, abdominal distention, nausea, and vomiting may be associated. Acute CVA tenderness and hematuria are common findings on exam.

The work-up for renal stones begins with urine culture, KUB (x-ray film of the kidney, ureter, and bladder), and IVP. X-ray studies are important because they (1) offer a baseline for subsequent evaluation, (2) determine the extent of disease, and (3) reveal predisposing factors such as malformations or anatomic obstructions. A careful medical history, simple blood tests (e.g., SMAC), and a 24-hour urine sample (analyzed for calcium, phosphorus, uric acid, cystine, and creatinine) should also be obtained to identify predisposing metabolic factors. The passage of small, nonobstructing stones can sometimes be forced with hydration. IV fluids and theophylline (which acts as a diuretic and relaxes the smooth muscle in ureteral walls) may be given for this purpose. Analgesics are inevitably required. During such treatment, all urine should be strained. Stones that cannot be cleared or that cause infection must be surgically removed. Retrieved stones should be sent to the laboratory for analysis. Identification of stone makeup and predisposing factors provides the basis for medical maneuvers in the event of recurrence and for preventive measures (Table 8.20).

If a kidney stone blocks urine flow, ***obstructive nephropathy*** may occur. This problem may actually be caused by any type of obstruction in the renal pelvis, ureter, bladder, or urethra, as noted in Table 8.21. Symptoms of obstructive nephropathy include low back pain, abdominal pain, and anuria or sometimes polyuria. If renal function has been affected, there may be symptoms of renal insufficiency. The kidney may also enlarge from fluid backup, a condition known as ***hydronephrosis.*** If it develops slowly, the complication may be attended by few symptoms. However, acute hydronephrosis produces excruciating pain from sudden expansion of the renal capsule ***(Dietl's crisis).*** Acute obstructive nephropathy is a critical condition, not only because it can lead to urosepsis with fever and prostration but also because immediate intervention may save the kidney. Therefore, patients should be referred to a urologist. If hydronephrosis is present, intervention should be done on an emergency basis. The work-up may include renal ultrasound, IVP, cystoscopy, retrograde pyelography, and/or radioisotope scans. Treatment begins by controlling the infection and problems related to renal insufficiency. In some cases, this may necessitate a temporary nephrostomy. Once patients are stabilized, surgical correction of the primary disorder is undertaken. If it is successful, the prognosis is good.

One cause of obstructive nephropathy ***retroperitoneal fibrosis*** warrants further note. It stems from chronic inflammation (retroperitoneal fasciitis or fibroplasia) of the retroperitoneal tissues surrounding the lower lumbar vertebrae. Such inflammation may be the result of drugs (methysergide, beta blockers), Hodgkin's disease, lymphomas, or metastatic tumors. Unless the drugs are stopped and the underlying disease is controlled, scar tissue may form and compress one or both ureters, with subsequent dilatation of the renal pelvis and collecting ducts. A similar effect may

TABLE 8.20 TYPES OF KIDNEY STONES

Stone Composition	Etiologic Description	Acute Treatment	Preventive Measures
Calcium (related to absorptive hypercalcemia)	Most common form of renal stones. Increased absorption of calcium from the gut occurs either from absolute increase in or increased sensitivity to vitamin D metabolite, 1,25-dihydroxycholecalciferol.	Surgical removal	Dietary restriction of sodium (100 mEq/day) and calcium (400 mg/day). Dietary phosphate supplements may also prove beneficial and are usually given in the form of orthophosphate, 250 mg qid to start, increasing to 500 mg qid. However, they are contraindicated in patients who have a tendency to form stones containing magnesium ammonium phosphate.
Calcium (related to renal leak hypercalciuria)	Inadequate reabsorption of calcium in the renal tubule with calcium loss in the urine results in low serum levels of calcium and increased production of parathyroid hormone.	Surgical removal	Hydrochlorthiazide, 50 mg bid. Also, sodium/calcium dietary restriction and dietary phosphate supplementation (see above).
Calcium (related to resorptive hypercalciuria)	Hyperparathyroidism (usually from parathyroid adenoma) causes both bone resorption and increased calcium absorption from the gut.	Surgical removal	Excision of parathyroid tumors.
Struvite	Caused by infection with urea-splitting organisms (notably *Proteus*).	Surgical removal of infected stones and antibiotic therapy.	Prompt treatment of urinary tract infections and correction of conditions contributing to urinary stasis.
Uric acid	Stones form in acidic urine that contains an increased concentration of uric acid.	Stones can often be dissolved with hydration (2 L/day), allopurinol (300 mg/day), and sodium bicarbonate to maintain urine pH between 6.5 and 6.8. Surgery may be needed.	Same as acute treatment.
Cystine	Forms only in patients with homozygous cystinuria.	High doses of sodium bicarbonate to keep urine pH at 7.5 or higher. Penicillamine may also be useful. Surgery may be needed.	Alkalinization of urine.

TABLE 8.21 CAUSES OF URINARY TRACT OBSTRUCTION

Renal pelvis and ureters	Bladder and urethra
Necrotizing papillitis	Tumors of the pelvic viscera
Congenital anomalies of the ureters	Tumors of the bladder
Renal calculi	Myogenic bladder
Ureteral compression from intrinsic or extrinsic tumors	Bladder neck anomalies
Retroperitoneal fibrosis	Prostatic enlargement
Secondary fibrosis (surgery, radiation)	Urethral stricture
Ureterocele	Urethral malformation
Accidental surgical ligation of ureter	Spinal cord injuries
Myogenic ureter	Anticholinergic drugs
Chronic vesicoureteral reflux	
Pregnancy	

occur in major blood vessels, notably the vena cava and sometimes the aorta. For this reason, patients with retroperitoneal fibrosis may present with a palpable mass over the sacrum, claudication, weakness of the legs, and impotence, as well as renal obstruction. Surgical treatment may be necessary.

Bladder

Ureters enter the bladder at the vesicoureteral junction. Here a segment of the ureter, several centimeters long, runs under the bladder epithelium. Its compression when the bladder is full prevents backflow of urine during urination. If urine from the bladder does wash back into the ureter, the problem is referred to as ***vesicoureteral reflux.*** Usually caused by misimplantation of the ureter into the bladder, it predisposes the patient to urinary tract infections. Because clubbing of the calices and renal scarring may evolve, the diagnosis is important and should be suspected whenever an infection develops early in life or recurs. If initial testing (with a radionuclide scan using ^{99m}Tc instilled into the bladder) is positive, a voiding cystourethrogram and IVP should be obtained to evaluate the anatomy further. Surgical reimplantation of the ureter into the bladder is usually advocated to prevent renal damage.

Hollow and pear-shaped, the bladder is located in the pelvis behind the symphysis pubis. Bladder walls are composed of three layers of smooth muscle. Fibers of the inner and outer layers tend to run longitudinally, while those of the middle layer are circular. The mesh-like arrangement of all three layers makes up the detrusor muscle, which is extremely elastic and strong. ***Structural abnormalities of the bladder*** (Table 8.22) are rare.

Foreign bodies within the bladder (e.g., a small kidney stone or debris from urinary tract infection) can serve as the nucleus (nidis) for ***bladder (vesicle) stones,*** but under normal conditions they are eliminated in the urine. Thus, most

TABLE 8.22 ANOMALIES OF THE BLADDER

Agenesis	Exstrophy (failure of bladder to close)
Hypoplasia	Cloacal exstrophy (failure of bladder and rectum to close)
Duplication	
Congenital diverticula	

vesicle stones form only in the presence of urinary retention (obstruction of the bladder neck or urethra, neurogenic bladder, diverticula), whereby a foreign body remains in residual urine long enough to collect deposits of calcium phosphate, calcium oxalate, uric acid, or magnesium phosphate. Patients present with symptoms of dysuria, frequency, and urgency. If the stone occludes the urethra in a man, pain in the penis and disruption of the urinary stream may be noted. The exam should include inspection for distended bladder, cystocele, or prostatic enlargement. Very large stones can sometimes be palpated. The urine inevitably shows signs of infection and RBCs. Patients with signs and symptoms of a bladder stone should be referred to a urologist for immediate evaluation. The KUB test may reveal the presence and location of calcified stones, and an IVP can show upper urinary dilatation from long-standing back pressure and lower urinary tract obstruction. Sometimes a direct cystoscopic exam is required. Treatment centers on surgical removal of the stone. In addition, analgesics are given to control pain and antibiotics to clear associated infections. The underlying causes should be corrected whenever possible.

A special form of epithelium, found only in urinary passages, lines the bladder walls. Called "transitional epithelium," it is composed of two underlying layers of large cells and a surface layer of smaller cells. Slippery and flexible, each surface cell is capable of contracting when the bladder is empty and extending when it is full. Inflammation of the bladder lining is called ***cystitis. Interstitial cystitis*** (Hunner's ulcer) is an unusual form affecting mostly middle-aged women. It is marked by unifocal or multifocal ulceration and scarring of the bladder mucosa, which eventually leads to contraction of the detrusor muscle and diminished urinary capacity. The exact cause is unknown. Autoimmune disease, an allergic response, an infectious agent still to be identified, and therapy with radiation or cytoxic drugs have been proposed.

Most other types of cystitis are infectious. ***Schistosoma haematobium*** may be the source in patients with a history of travel to Egypt, Africa, or the Middle East. The adult fluke matures in the venous plexuses of the bladder, prostate, and uterus. Eggs are passed in the urine or retained in the tissue walls, where they produce not only chronic cystitis but also fibrosis, ulceration, granuloma, papilloma formation, and bladder wall calcification. Seen on KUB, the last is an important diagnostic finding. Schistosomiasis is discussed in Chapter 4.

Cystitis with sterile pyuria (urine containing WBCs but no organisms on bacterial culture) suggests ***renal tuberculosis.*** Through hematogenous spread from lungs, lymph nodes, bone, or other sites, mycobacteria gain access to the cortex of the kidney. Beginning as a small focus, the infection spreads into the medulla and downward to the bladder. Though IVP shows signs of pyelonephritis and renal calcification in long-standing disease, patients typically remain in surprisingly good health. The diagnosis is confirmed by urine cultures for acid-fast bacilli. The primary site should be identified and treated accordingly (see Chapter 6 for a thorough discussion of tuberculosis).

Fungal agents are rare sources of cystitis except in patients immunosuppressed by chronic antibiotic therapy, antineoplastic drugs, steroids, or repeated catheterization. Similarly, while viruses may be responsible for immune complex nephritis, few are associated with bladder infection. One exception is adenovirus type II, which causes ***hemorrhagic cystitis*** in children. Characterized by gross hematuria, hemorrhagic cystitis may also be seen with bacterial infections in adults, especially women.

►***Acute bacterial cystitis*** is the most common of all types. The usual organisms are aerobic members of fecal flora, pure anaerobic infections being rare. In rare cases, infection with gas-forming bacilli produces ***cystitis emphysematosa,*** which causes foamy urine (pneumaturia) as well as bladder irritation. Bacterial cystitis is particularly prevalent in women because the female urethra is short and straight, allowing organisms to gain relatively easy access to the bladder. Furthermore, the meatus lies between the clitoris and the vaginal opening. Irritation from diaphragm rings, douches, deodorized tampons, spermatocides, or bubble baths often reduces the immunologic activity of urethral cells. During sexual activity, bacteria from the hands, vagina, or perineum can be rubbed into the urethra and ascend to the bladder. This may also follow improper toilet habits (notably, wiping forward). Most cases of bacterial cystitis in men are secondary to infection in the urethra or prostate. In both men and women, urethral instrumentation may be at fault.

The classic symptoms of acute bacterial cystitis are frequency, urgency, and/or dysuria. Fever, chills, flank pain, nausea, and vomiting are usually absent when the infection is localized to the lower urinary tract. However, patients often have discomfort in the low back or suprapubic regions. They may describe a constant desire to urinate even though the bladder contains only a few milliliters of urine. Some note a specific change in the urine—foamy, cloudy, bloody, darkened color, or a strong odor. Given such symptoms, the problem may be diagnosed if the urine sediment (a clean midstream specimen) shows WBCs and bacteria on microscopic exam or 100,000 bacteria per milliliter on culture. The importance of such quantitative measures is discussed in the next section. Treatment includes antibiotics guided by culture sensitivity tests, increased fluid intake, and analgesics. Aggressive management is particularly important in pregnant women, 15% of whom develop upper urinary tract infections in the third trimester. Extension is related to ureteral dilatation from hormonal changes and from pressure of the enlarging uterine fundus on the ureters (particularly the right).

Recurrent or chronic bacterial cystitis represents either relapses from an acute infection or reinfection. Relapse is highly likely if symptoms return within a few weeks of the initial treatment and the same organism is isolated on reculture. It may signal an inadequate course of therapy, emergence of resistant organisms, upper urinary tract infection, or underlying urologic abnormalities. Furthermore, it may lead to changes in the bladder lining. The development of submucosal cysts produces negative filling defects on urograms called ***cystitis cystica (vesicular cystitis).*** The presence of epithelialized spaces beneath the mucosa may be noted on histologic exam ***(cystitis glandularis).*** Finally, chronic cystitis is associated with the development of both bladder stones and bladder cancer. Therefore, in addition to extended courses of antibiotics (4–6 weeks), urologic referral is advised. The presence of reflux, obstruction, bladder stones, and/or pyelonephritis must be identified and treated, and patients should be screened for malignancy.

Most cases of ***bladder cancer*** arise from the transitional epithelium, although some originate as squamous cell carcinoma, adenocarcinoma, or rhabdomyosarcoma. Whatever the histologic picture, bladder cancer is the most frequent malignancy of the urinary tract. Responsible for 3% of all cancer deaths, it strikes men twice as often as women and usually appears between the fifth and seventh decades. Many etiologies have been proposed. A high percentage of workers exposed to aniline dye and other chemicals used in the manufacture of rubber, cable, textile, and leather goods have developed the malignancy. Therapy with cyclophosphamides, azathioprine, and pelvic radiation also seems to be associated. Phenacetin abuse and certain artificial sweeteners (saccharine and cyclamate) have been under suspicion for several years (the U.S. government banned the use of cyclamates in 1969). Smoking is another likely predisposing factor. Chronic cystitis was previously mentioned. Occurring in 75% of patients, hematuria is the most frequent first sign of bladder cancer. Because it is painless and tends to be intermittent in the early stages, there may be an unfortunate delay by patients in seeking medical attention or by providers in pursuing further evaluation. Thus, many cases are not diagnosed until complications of advanced disease such as obstruction, fistula formation, or recurrent infection with frequency and dysuria have developed. If the tumor encroaches on the bladder neck, patients may complain of a diminished stream, and, if it extends beyond the bladder, of suprapubic pain. Patients with tumors blocking a ureter may present with hydronephrosis.

The physical exam is typically unremarkable, though tumors may sometimes be noted on abdominorectal/abdominovaginal exam. Blood tests may reveal only anemia, but urinalysis shows RBCs, WBCs, bacteria, and a high concentration of epithelial cells. Urine for cytology may or may not reveal any cell changes, and a negative report does not rule out malignancy. In many cases, IVP, cystoscopy with biopsy, and bimanual exam under anesthesia are required. These procedures are used not only to confirm the diagnosis but also to grade and stage the tumor. "Grades" refer to cell type and "stages" to the depth of bladder wall invasion. Tumors confined to superficial layers (stages O, A, and B_1) can be removed by transurethral resection. Those extending into bladder walls (B_2, C) necessitate cystectomy and a urinary diversion procedure. After the bladder is removed, the ureters are usually anastomosed to an isolated loop of ileum (uteroileostomy) or sigmoid colon, which is then used to form an osteomy. Patients with metastatic disease do not usually undergo cystectomy. They are treated with radiation, thiotepa bladder instillations, and chemotherapy.

Urethra

A narrow tube, the urethra, eliminates urine stored in the bladder from the body (see Fig. 8.3). Composed of smooth muscle walls lined by a mucous membrane, it exits the bladder neck at a point called the "internal urethral orifice." A dense mass of circular detrusor muscle surrounds this orifice and forms the internal sphincter. The internal sphincter remains contracted until an accumulation of urine in the bladder stimulates the parasympathetic nervous system to initiate its relaxation and micturition. A short distance away, within the urethra itself, is an "external" sphincter of striated muscle. Under sympathetic control, the external sphincter can be voluntarily contracted to suppress urination momentarily. Micturition is a complicated process discussed in the following section.

There are several differences between the male and female urethras. The male urethra serves as a conduit for the reproductive tract as well as the urinary tract. About 20 cm in length, it threads through the prostate gland (prostatic portion), between two sheets of fibrous tissue connecting the pubic bones (membranous portion), along the penis (cavernous portion), and opens at the meatus. The meatus may be affected by congenital malpositioning ***(hypospadias),*** foreskin closure ***(phimosis),*** or local skin infection ***(balanitis).*** Because this long, tortuous path thwarts the ascension of infectious agents, cystitis in men is unusual. ***Male urethritis,*** however, is quite common. These problems are discussed in Chapter 9.

The female urethra remains separate from the reproductive passages. Only 3 cm in length, it runs a straight course behind the symphysis pubis, opening between the clitoris and the vaginal vestibule. The female meatus is surrounded by a complex network of urethral glands. Producing lubricants for the mucous lining, these glands may become infected, with the development of ***urethral gland abscess. Female urethritis*** may also occur secondary to sexually transmitted infections. Furthermore, sexual activity, diaphragm rings, douches, deodorized tampons, spermatocides, bubble baths, or other irritants may reduce lubrication by the urethral glands and/or the immunologic activity of the urethral lining. Bacteria from the hands, vagina, or perineum then gains entrance to the urethra and ascends the short distance to the bladder, quickly establishing cystitis. The same irritants can produce localized inflammation of the urethra in the absence of infection known as ***honeymoon cystitis.*** These problems are discussed in Chapter 9.

Urine produced in the kidney is sterile and remains so until micturition. It then picks up thousands of microbes from the normal flora inhabiting the distal urethra, which must be differentiated from pathogenic microbes whenever there is a question of urinary tract infection. Quantitative measures are used for this purpose. To be useful, the specimen must be taken from a midstream void following careful cleaning of the urethral meatus. Urinary tract infection may then be diagnosed if a single microbe in unspun urine or more than three to five microbes in spun urine can be noted on Gram stain or cover slip investigation under a high-power field. The same principle applies to cultures. The infection is confirmed if 1 mL of unspun urine produces 100,000 organisms. However, a negative culture does not necessarily rule out urinary tract infection.

Micturition

Bladder muscles are innervated by the hypogastric sympathetic, pelvic parasympathetic, and pudendal somatic nerves. Concentrated around ureteral and urethral insertions, the ganglia of these nerves function in a coordinated manner under the direction of both the sympathetic and parasympathetic nervous systems. The result is the complicated process of micturition (emptying of the bladder). It is the culmination of bladder filling as follows.

Through peristaltic action of the ureters, urine manufactured by the kidneys is continuously delivered to the bladder. With collection of the first 25 mL, there is a slight increase in intrabladder (intravesical) pressure. After that, pressure remains fairly stable until 400–500 mL of urine have accumulated. As the bladder fills, the detrusor muscle expands and stimulates stretch receptors, which produce an urge to void. The first urge is usually felt when 150 mL have collected. Beyond 500 mL, intravesicular pressure rises sharply, leading to an uncomfortable feeling of fullness. At this tolerance point (which can be increased or decreased by habit patterns), impulses are sent to the sacral portion of the spinal cord, initiating the micturition reflex. The bladder contracts, and as it pulls down, it pushes urine toward the urethra. At the same time, the urethra opens and shortens. Unless the urethra's external sphincter is voluntarily contracted, urination occurs immediately. The female urethra then empties by gravity and the male urethra by several contractions of the bulbocavernous muscle. ***Micturition syncope*** is an unusual side effect that sometimes follows. The person (typically a young, healthy man) arises from bed in the early morning or evening to void. During urination or immediately afterward, he becomes lightheaded and faints. The etiology of the episode is unclear but is thought to be related to vagal stimulation during bladder contraction. Postural hypotension, epileptic phenomena, and the Valsalva maneuver have also been proposed.

Impulses initiating urination are sent to the cerebral cortex as well as the spinal cord. Because of this "higher" order, toddlers can be toilet trained. They learn to constrict the external urethra voluntarily and postpone urination if the time or place seems inappropriate. By the same token, the cerebral cortex allows them to initiate the micturition reflex before the bladder is full.

Urinary retention occurs when urine continues to be produced by the kidneys but fails to be released from the bladder (see Table 8.21). Obstruction at or below the bladder outlet accounts for most cases. Telling signs are an absence of voided urine and the presence of a distended bladder. The latter can be percussed (producing a kettle drum sound) above the symphysis pubis, either midline or displaced to the side. The patient may complain of increasing discomfort and the need to urinate. As the bladder continues to fill, intravesicular pressure may overcome urethral restraint, causing the patient to void 25–50 mL of urine every hour or more. This is known as ***retention with overflow.*** Although continuously voiding, the patient complains that the bladder feels full. The first step in the management of urinary retention is to empty the bladder. Cases associated with muscle tension often respond to simple, noninvasive techniques. The power of suggestion may be elicited by sounds of running tap water or a flushing toilet, just as it may be inhibited by lack of privacy, cold bed pans, and a prone position. Dabbling hands under the faucet, pouring warm water over the perineum, or sitting in a warm bath may relax the external sphincter. Cholinergic medications such as bethanechol chloride and neostigmine can be used to stimulate bladder contraction. However, due to the danger of reflux or rupture, they must never be given if any mechanical obstruction is suspected. If these measures prove useless, the bladder must be catheterized. Once it has been emptied, the cause of retention must be found and, if possible, corrected.

In contrast to retention, ***urinary incontinence*** is uncontrolled passage of urine from the body. ***Enuresis*** occurs in the absence of any anatomic/physiologic dysfunction, generally at night. Although resolution before the end of childhood is the rule, the problem persists into adulthood in 1–3% of cases. Boys are affected much more frequently than girls. The exact etiology is unknown, but genetic predisposition, delayed development, parental failure, toilet training difficulties, sleep disorders, and food allergies have all been suggested. Psychotherapy such as behavior modification and conditioning alarm systems have been used in treatment. Physical measures such as fluid restriction after supper, waking the child to void during the night, and keeping the room warm have also been advocated. Tricyclic drugs, which are thought to relax the detrusor muscle, increase sphincter tone, and/or alter sleep patterns, are sometimes given.

Stress incontinence is most common in women with cystoceles but also occurs in men with prostatic hypertrophy. Characterized by dribbling of urine whenever patients cough, sneeze, or laugh, these problems are discussed in Chapter 9. ***Urgency incontinence*** is marked by the inability to hold back urine flow long enough to reach the bathroom once the urge to void is perceived. It is a common symptom of urinary tract infection. For some reason, it may also plague women who are free of infection a few days prior to the onset of each menstrual period. ***Paradoxical incontinence*** refers to the urine loss that occurs in cases of bladder retention with overflow (see the previous section).

Continuous incontinence occurs in patients who cannot exercise voluntary control over the external sphincter and urinate whenever the micturition reflex is stimulated. In toddlers before toilet training, it is the expected norm, but in older persons it can be a devastating condition invoking feelings of embarrassment, helplessness, and frustration. Some of these feelings may be alleviated by explaining the ***aging changes*** that affect urination. Because the surrounding connective tissue shrinks and loses elasticity, the bladder takes on a funnel shape. The smooth muscle comprising bladder walls displays less ability to elongate, decreasing bladder capacity to half that of younger adults. At the same time, the muscle becomes more irritable, increasing urgency. Cystoceles in women and prostatic hypertrophy in men alter the urethral-vesicle angle, lessening external sphincter control.

Either incontinence or retention may occur with ***neurogenic bladder,*** a problem caused by lesions of the central or peripheral nervous system. Lesions occurring above the sacral segments of the spinal cord produce a dysfunction referred to as ***upper motor neuron bladder.*** Lesions occurring below this area are called ***lower motor neuron bladder*** (see Chapter 12). ***Cord bladder*** describes problems resulting from acute injury or disease of the spinal cord. In the acute stage, the bladder is atonic or flaccid. This period, known as the "spinal shock phase," necessitates catheterization and may last for weeks to months. Hopefully, it is followed by a "recovery stage" in which the motor and sensory functions of the bladder begin to return. Rehabilitation may then be accomplished. It centers on a bladder training program, which attempts to schedule emptying of the bladder in the absence of sensory and/or motor control. Intermittent catheterization, chemotherapy, and surgical intervention may be employed. In addition, trigger points can be stimulated to help initiate and maintain micturition. Patients learn to pinch, stroke, or apply ice to specific areas on the abdomen, inner thigh, or pubis. Some may be taught to innervate the pudendal nerve through digital stretching of the anal sphincter. Others may learn to augment contraction of the detrusor muscle by placing external pressure on the abdomen (bending at the waist, tightening a corset, or taking a deep breath). The "Crede maneuver" (placing fingers over the bladder and using a downward milking action) is particularly effective for this purpose, but must be used with caution since it may led to urethral dyssynergia, retention, and subsequent reflux.

During bladder training in patients with upper motor neuron lesions, an excessive autonomic response may occur from stimulation of a distended bladder. This leads to the potentially life-threatening complication of ***autonomic hyperreflexia*** (autonomic dysreflexia). Visceral distention and stimulation of pain receptors in the skin may also initiate the condition. Patients experience a sudden onset of throbbing headache, blurred vision, nasal congestion, and nausea. Flushing, pilomotor spasm, diaphoresis below the spinal cord lesion, and bradycardia may be noted. Blood pressure skyrockets and, unless controlled immediately, leads to seizures and/or stroke. Patients should be taught to recognize the symptoms of autonomic hyperreflexia and to summon immediate help. Obviously, the problem warrants treatment as a medical emergency.

Details of Management

▸ *Organizations for Renal Patients*

Laboratory Tests: None.

Therapeutic Measures: None.

Patient Education: National Kidney Foundation
2 Park Avenue
New York, New York
Tel.: (212) 889-2210

Follow-up: Help patients make contact as needed.

▸ *Considerations for Patients with Renal Failure*

Laboratory Tests: Coordinate with nephrologist. Urine analysis, urine cultures, SMAC, CBC should be done on stable patients every 3–6 months.

Therapeutic Measures

Diet: Must be tailored to the changes created by the disease. For example, salt, potassium, and/or protein may be needed by the patient with a wasting syndrome. Sodium may be restricted in patients with increased blood pressure, but not too rigidly, since salt wasting and volume depletion can develop. Potassium is typically restricted to 40 mEq/day. Aluminum hydroxide (Amphojel) is given to bind phosphates if hyperphosphatemia occurs. Any antacids containing magnesium should be avoided due to the danger of magnesium toxicity.

Blood pressure: Monitor regularly and treat elevations aggressively. Beta blockers should be used with caution, since they reduce renal blood flow. Captopril is contraindicated.

Fluid retention: Maintain optimal weight, the weight at which the patient has no edema and normal electrolytes and demonstrates the lowest possible creatinine level in a BUN:creatinine ratio of 10:1. In this state, renal blood flow, cardiac output, and total body water are balanced. Optimal weight is best maintained by monitoring daily weight and administering a loop diuretic (e.g., furosemide) whenever it goes up. Potassium-sparing diuretics (triampterene, spironolactone, ameloride) should be avoided. If patients become hypokalemic, potassium supplements must be given with caution and electrolytes monitored closely. Since serum potassium is affected by pH, volume, and sodium delivery to the distal nephron, sudden and dramatic hyperkalemia can develop in patients with renal changes.

Illness: Episodic infections should be promptly treated, particularly if the patient is receiving immunosuppressive therapy. Cultures are imperative. Only sensitive antimicrobials should be used and the doses adjusted according to the GFR status (see "Medication adjustments"). Chronic diseases such as diabetes, RA, or CHF complicate the picture dramatically. Patients taking digitalis, insulin, and other long-term medications must be closely monitored for signs and symptoms of toxicity.

Medication adjustments: Literature concerning all drugs (prescribed as well as over-the-counter) should be carefully reviewed for contraindications and information about renal clearance. For many drugs, the doses should be reduced or intervals of administration extended according to the GFR status. Such information can be found in the *Physician's Desk Reference* and in articles such as that by Bennett et al. (see Bibliography). Some considerations regarding antimicrobials are noted in Table 8.7.

Patient Education: Assess the patient's understanding of the disease and its management. Review this information if necessary.

Follow-up: Refer any patient with unexpected deterioration in renal function or an unfavorable course of an episodic illness to the appropriate specialist.

▸ *Acute Pyelonephritis*

Laboratory Tests: U/A (dipstick and microscopic). Urine culture and sensitivity test.

Therapeutic Measures: Start ampicillin, 250–500 mg qid, or Bactrim DS bid pending culture reports. If needed, give Pyridium, 200 mg tid for 1–2 days, as a urinary tract analgesic. Continue the sensitive antibiotic for 10–14 days. Give Tylenol or acetylsalicylic acid (ASA) q4h for fever. Increase fluid intake (6–8 full glasses of water or citrus juice per day).

Patient Education: Explain the infectious nature and upper urinary tract location of the problem. Stress the importance of using antibiotics to prevent kidney damage. Note that Pyridium will cause the urine to turn red. This is a natural reaction, and there is no cause for alarm. Advise patients to rest during the acute phase of the illness. Have them report continued fever, chills, renal colic, and/or decreased urine output.

Follow-up: Repeat urinalysis in 4 days. If bacteriuria persists, reculture and change antibiotics accordingly. Arrange a urologic referral for men with persistent bacteriuria or for any patient with prolonged renal colic. Reexamine the urine 2 and 6 weeks after the completion of treatment.

▶ *Salt-Restricted Diet*

Laboratory Tests: None.

Therapeutic Measures: Start a no-salt-added-diet, which provides about 4 g of sodium a day.

Patient Education: Instruct family meal preparers to cook and serve the patient's food without added salt. Provide specific information such as the following:

SEASONING AND ADDITIVES

High in Salt—Avoid	Low in Salt—Use Freely
Baking powder	Allspice/cloves/ginger
Brine	Anise seed
Monosodium glutamate	Basil/marjoram/oregano
Sodium bicarbonate	Bay leaf
Sodium chloride	Caraway seed
Sodium in any combination	Cardamom
Bouillon cubes	Chives/onions
Catsup	Cinnamon
Celery salt/flakes	All peppers
Chili sauce	Coriander
Garlic salt	Cumin
Flavored gelatin	Curry
Salted horseradish	Fennel
Mayonnaise	Garlic bud/chips/powder
Meat extracts	Ginger, nutmeg
Meat tenderizers	Plain horseradish
Molasses	Mint/juniper
Prepared mustard	Dry mustard
Olives	Lemon/lime/orange peel
Onion salt	Rosemary/thyme/tarragon
Pickles	Powdered mushrooms
Relish	Paprika
Rennet tablets	Sesame seed
Soy sauce	Sage/saffron/savory
Worcestershire sauce	Poultry seasoning
Prepared salad dressings	Tumeric

FOODS WITH HIGH SALT CONTENT—AVOID OR LIMIT

Beverages, Soups, and Vegetables	
Chocolate milk	Milk shakes
Hot chocolate mixes	Malted milk
Tomato juice	Cup-a-Soup
All canned soups	Instant broths
All canned vegetables	Baked beans

Dairy Products, Meats, and Meat Substitutes

All canned meats/soups/stews	Bacon
Bologna	Brains
Chipped beef	Corned beef
Hot dogs	Ham
Kidneys	Liverwurst
Smoked/pickled/salted meat	Salami
Salt pork	Sausage
Fast food hamburgers	Fast food chicken
All canned/salted/smoked fish	All shellfish
Caviar	Anchovies
Cheeses	Butter

Vegetables, Snacks, and Desserts

Chips	Pretzels
Popcorn	French fries
Onion rings	Crackers
Salted nuts	Ice cream/sherbet
Instant puddings/Jello	Cookie/cake mixes

Follow-up: Reinforce the diet at each visit. Refer to a nutritionist patients requiring more severe salt restriction (1–2 g/day), which can be difficult to tolerate and can easily result in deficiencies of other nutrients.

▸ *Hypokalemia*

Laboratory Tests: Serum potassium levels.

Therapeutic Measures: If the patient is taking a diuretic, reinforce the importance of a salt-restricted diet (it minimizes potassium losses). Reduce the dose of the diuretic as much as possible. Switch from a long-acting drug (e.g., chlorthalidone) to a shorter-acting drug (e.g., hydrochlorothiazide). Increase the amounts of potassium-rich foods in the diet. If these measures fail to normalize serum potassium levels (particularly in digitalis patients), add 20–80 mEq/day of potassium supplements in divided doses. Supplements may be given in the form of powders (e.g., potassium chloride) or slow-release tablets (e.g., Slow-K or K-Tabs) according to the patient's preference. As an alternative to supplements, diuretic patients can be given potassium-sparing preparations (triamterene/spironolactone), either alone or in combination with other drugs.

Patient Education: Note that potassium, a mineral, is essential for fluid balance and neuromuscular activity and that body levels may become depleted from strenuous exercise and certain medications (particularly diuretics). For patients taking digitalis, point out that potassium depletion increases the risk of toxicity. Explain that salt restriction minimizes potassium losses from diuretics and that lost potassium can often be replaced by adding high-potassium (expressed in terms of milliequivalents and milligrams, 1 mEq equaling 75 mg) foods to the diet. Provide a list such as the following:

POTASSIUM, SODIUM, AND CALORIC CONTENT OF POPULAR FOODS

Food	Potassium (mg)	Sodium (mg)	Calories
Beverages			
Apricot nectar (6 oz)	279	1	105
Buttermilk (1 c)	388	212	92
Unsweetened orange juice ($\frac{2}{5}$ c)	186	1	45
Prune juice (1 c)	235	2	77
Unsweetened grapefruit juice	400	2	101
Grape juice (1 c)	293	5	167
Coffee (1 c)	65	2	2
Fruits and vegetables			
Apricots (2–3)	281	1	105
Avocado (1 c)	920	6	254
Banana (1 large)	720	2	170
Cantaloupe ($\frac{1}{4}$ melon)	251	12	30
Dates (1 c)	1,150	2	488
Orange (1 medium)	300	2	73
Raisins ($\frac{5}{8}$ c)	763	27	289
Artichoke (1 whole)	301	30	44
Lima beans ($\frac{5}{8}$ c)	422	1	111
Carrots (1 raw)	341	47	42
Celery (1 c)	341	126	17
Lettuce ($3\frac{1}{2}$ oz)	264	9	18
Potato (1 med.)	407	3	76
Tomato (1 med.)	366	4	33
Meats and fish			
Hamburger ($\frac{1}{4}$ lb)	382	40	224
Turkey (white meat, 2 slices)	349	70	150
Steak ($3\frac{1}{2}$ oz)	479	53	274
Lamb ($3\frac{1}{2}$ oz)	369	61	242
Chicken livers (1 c)	211	85	231
Pork (6 oz)	500	52	314
Veal ($3\frac{1}{2}$ oz)	466	49	318
Flounder (3 oz)	498	201	171
Cod (3 oz)	345	93	144
Herring ($3\frac{1}{2}$ oz raw)	420	74	98
Tuna ($3\frac{1}{2}$ oz canned in water)	279	41	127

To obtain a pad of tear-off sheets with similar information, request "Everyday Foods High in Potassium" from the CIBA Pharmaceutical Company, 556 Morris Avenue, Summit, NJ 07901. Give careful mixing instructions for powdered supplements to prevent GI upset. Warn patients who are using potassium-sparing preparations never to take potassium supplements and to avoid substances that contain large amounts of potassium chloride such as salt substitutes, Gatorade, and/or health foods. Have all patients report increasing symptoms of lethargy, muscular weakness, nervous irritability, or irregular heartbeat.

Follow-up: Diuretic and digitalis patients with a history of hypokalemia should have serum potassium checks every 4–6 months. Stable patients taking diuretics should be checked at least yearly.

▸ *Mild Hyperuricemia (Asymptomatic or a History of Mild, Very Intermittent Gout)*

Laboratory Tests: SMAC.

Therapeutic Measures: Whenever possible, correct the causative factors (see Table 8.18). For overweight patients, start a weight reduction diet (see Chapter 5). Otherwise, advise a well-balanced diet divided into frequent meals. The patient should avoid fasting. Ongoing purine-restricted, alcohol-free diets do little to correct hyperuricemia.

Patient Education: Describe uric acid, hyperuricemia, and associated clinical problems. Use the results of laboratory tests to explain overproduction or underexcretion as a cause of hyperuricemia. Review diet guidelines. Note that although ongoing, severe restriction is unnecessary, overindulgence in alcohol and high-purine foods can precipitate clinical problems for persons with hyperuricemia. Provide a list such as the following:

FOODS WITH HIGH PURINE CONTENT—AVOID OVERINDULGENCE

Yeast	Anchovies
Liver	Herring
Mackerel	Kidneys
Sweetbreads	Heart
Scallops	Wild game
Goose	Tongue
Meat broths/extracts	Meat gravies/drippings
Mincemeat	Sardines

Follow-up: Check uric acid levels yearly.

▸ *Significant Hyperuricemia (History of Renal Involvement, Tophi, Recurrent Gout)*

Laboratory Tests: Same as for mild hyperuricemia.

Therapeutic Measures: Same as for mild hyperuricemia. In addition, start and titrate drugs as follows:

Anti-inflammatory agent

Indocin, 25 mg bid for 1 month, then decrease to 25 mg daily for 2–3 months. *In conjunction with:*

Uricosuric agent (contraindicated in patients with a diagnosis of renal stones)

Benemid, 0.5 g/day for 3 weeks. For maintenance, increase the dose to 1–2 g/day.

Or

Sulfinpyrazine (Anturane), 100 mg/day for 3 weeks. For maintenance, increase the dose to 200–400 mg/day.

And/or

Xanthine oxidase inhibitor (for cases complicated by renal stones)

Zyloprim, 200–400 mg/day.

Patient Education: Same as for mild hyperuricemia. Review the possible side effects of drugs and signs and symptoms to report (check *Physician's Desk Reference*). In addition, instruct patients taking uricosuric drugs to maintain high fluid intake (6–8 glasses of water per day) and avoid using salicylates (uric acid antagonists).

Follow-up: Recheck uric acid levels every month. Titrate drugs until uric acid levels fall to normal ranges. Once the maintenance doses have been determined, arrange visits every 4–6 months for medication review and refill.

▸ *Acute Bacterial Cystitis*

Laboratory Tests: Midstream clean catch urine for analysis, culture, and sensitivity.

Therapeutic Measures: To patients who are experiencing the first episode, give ampicillin, 500 mg qid, or trimethoprim/sulfa DS (Bactrim DS, Septra DS), bid for 3 days. For patients with a history of urinary tract infections in the past, give ampicillin, 250 mg qid, or trimethoprim/sulfa DS, bid for 10 days. For pregnant women, give ampicillin, 250 mg qid, or cephalexin (Keflex), 250 mg qid (very expensive) for 10 days. If needed, give Pyridium, 200 mg tid for the first 2 days, as a urinary tract analgesic. Increase fluids to 6–8 glasses per day. Once the culture report is available, switch to a sensitive antibiotic if necessary. In cases of alkaline urine, lowering the pH by taking 250 mg vitamin C, or a large glass of citrus juice four to six times a day helps to reduce the bacterial load.

Patient Education: Explain the location of the infection within the bladder and the importance of antibiotics to prevent the involvement of the kidney. Warn patients that Pyridium produces a reddish-orange–colored urine. Note that cystitis in women is related to the urethral location and anatomy and that recurrence can be prevented by following these instructions: Drink plenty of fluids. Empty the bladder regularly, specifically before and after engaging in sexual intercourse. To minimize urethral irritation, avoid (1) deodorized tampons, perfumed soaps, powders, lotions, douches, and bubble baths; (2) ill-fitting diaphragms; and (3) extended periods of diaphragm placement. To guard against introducing fecal bacteria into the urethra, (1) always wipe from the vagina toward the anus after using the toilet and (2) never engage in vaginal intercourse after anal intercourse unless condoms are changed or the skin is thoroughly cleansed.

Follow-up: Microscopic exam of the urine in 4 days. Reculture 2 weeks after completion of antibiotics. Arrange a urology referral for women with multiple recurrences and for all men.

BIBLIOGRAPHY

Abramowicz M. *Handbook of Antimicrobial Therapy,* rev. ed. The Medical Letter, New Rochelle, N.Y., 1980.

Ali AS, Baig FN. Hepatorenal syndrome. *American Family Physician,* (June) 1982, 25(6):127–131.

Bates B. *A Guide to Physical Examination.* Lippincott, Philadelphia, 1974.

Bennett WM, et al. Drug therapy in renal failure: Dosing guidelines for adults, part 1: Antimicrobial agents, analgesics. *Annals of Internal Medicine,* 1980, 93(1):62–89.

Berkow RB (ed.). *The Merck Manual of Diagnosis and Therapy,* 14th ed. Merck Sharp & Dohme Research Laboratories, Rahway, N.J., 1982.

Brown AM, Stubbs DW (eds.). *Medical Physiology.* Wiley, New York, 1983.

Conn HF, Conn RB Jr (eds.). *Current Diagnosis.* Saunders, Philadelphia, 1980.

Crafts RC. *A Textbook of Human Anatomy,* 3rd ed. Wiley, New York, 1985.

Crouch JE, McClintic JR. *Human Anatomy and Physiology,* 2nd ed. Wiley, New York, 1976.

Cunha BA. Single-dose treatment of urinary tract infections. *Physician Assistant,* (Aug.) 1983, 105–111.

Densmore M. Incontinence in the female patient. *The Journal of Family Practice,* 1982, 14(5):935–948.

Denver DP, Weintraum M, Linke CA. Preventing diuretic-associated urinary stones. *Drug Therapy,* (Dec.) 1983, 211–226.

Desrochers RD. Magnesium imbalance: A review. *Physician Assistant and Health Practitioner,* (Nov.) 1982, 57–66.

Edsall RL (staff ed.). Probing the causes of hypercalcemia. *Patient Care,* (Jan.) 1982, 41–59.

Edsall RL (staff ed.). When you suspect hypercalcemia. *Patient Care,* (Jan.) 1982, 14–37.

Elias H, Pauly JE, Burns ER. *Histology and Human Microanatomy,* 4th ed. Wiley, New York, 1978.

Epstein M. Renal complications of liver disease. *Clinical Symposia,* 1985, 37(5):3–32.

Fischer RG. Managing diuretic-induced hypokalemia in ambulatory hypertensive patients. *The Journal of Family Practice,* 1982, 14(6):1029–1036.

Goodall WM. Cystitis in women: Common mistakes in recognition and treatment. *Consultant,* (June) 1983, 195–201.

Goroll AH, May LA, Mulley AG. *Primary Care Medicine: Office Evaluation and Management of the Adult Patient.* Lippincott, Philadelphia, 1981.

Gray H. *Anatomy of the Human Body,* 29th American ed. (CM Goss, ed.). Lea & Febiger, Philadelphia, 1973.

Guyton AC. *Textbook of Medical Physiology,* 6th ed. Saunders, Philadelphia, 1981.

Harrison LH, Kelly JH. How to individualize medical therapy for nephrolithiasis. *PA Drug Update,* (Feb.) 1983, 17–32.

Hauser CJ, Shoemaker WC. Volume therapy, part 2: Treatment of hypovolemia. *Physician Assistant and Health Practitioner,* (May) 1981, 44–55.

Henry JB (ed.). *Todd-Sanford-Davidson Clinical Diagnosis and Mangement by Laboratory Methods,* Vols. 1 and 2, 16th ed. Saunders, Philadelphia, 1979.

Hoole AJ, Greenberg RA, Pickard CG Jr. *Patient Care Guidelines for Nurse Practitioners.* Little, Brown, Boston, 1982.

Isselbacher KJ, et al. *Harrison's Principles of Internal Medicine,* 9th ed. McGraw-Hill, New York, 1980.

Jones GW. Renal cell carcinoma. *Ca—A Cancer Journal for Clinicians,* (Sept./Oct.) 1982, 32(5):280–285.

Juan D. Vitamin D metabolism: Update for the clinician. *Postgraduate Medicine,* (Nov.) 1980, 68(5):210–218.

Kannangara DW, Lefrock JL. Drugs for urinary tract infections in women. *American Family Physician,* (Dec.) 1981, 24(6):160–163.

Khachadurian AK. Hyperuricemia and gout: An update. *American Family Physician,* (Dec.) 1981, 24(6):143–148.

Krupp MA, Chatton MJ, Werdegar D (eds.). *Current Medical Diagnosis and Treatment 1985.* Lange, Los Altos, Calif., 1985.

Kutcher R. Recognition of adult renal polycystic disease. *Hospital Medicine,* (May) 1981, 37–50.

Lancaster LE. *The Patient with End Stage Renal Disease.* Wiley, New York, 1979.

Lazarus JM. Uremia: A clinical guide. *Hospital Medicine,* (Jan.) 1984, 175–195.

Luckmann J, Sorensen KC. *Medical Surgical Nursing: A Psychophysiologic Approach,* 2nd ed. Saunders, Philadelphia, 1980.

Mandell HN. Gases and 'lytes without anguish: A simplified framework. *Postgraduate Medicine,* (Feb.) 1981, 69(2):67–74.

Marsh DJ. *Renal Physiology.* Raven Press, New York, 1983.

Melikian DM. Anti-infective therapy in renal disease. *Therapeutics,* 1983, 3–11.

Navarro RP, et al. Diuretic induced hypokalemia in the elderly. *The Journal of Family Practice,* 1982, 14(4):685–689.

Panwalker AP. Modern management of urinary tract infections. *PA Drug Update,* (June) 1981, 11–17.

Reynolds LR, Flueck JA. Evaluation of the hypercalcemic patient. *American Family Physician,* (Apr.) 1981, 23(4):105–111.

Schaeffer AJ. Minimizing drug resistance to urinary infections. *Acute Care Medicine,* (Jan.) 1984, 66–68.

Silverstein A. *Human Anatomy and Physiology.* Wiley, New York, 1980.

Stein JH. The kidney in health and disease, part 12: Hormones and the kidney. *Hospital Practice,* (July) 1979, 91–105.

Tretbar HA. The diagnosis of hypercalcemia. *Continuing Education,* (Oct.) 1981, 43–46.

U.S. Department of Health, Education, and Welfare. *What You Need to Know About Cancer of the Kidney.* NIH publication #80-1569. Washington, D.C., January 1980.

Valva JR, et al. Diagnosis and initial management of genitourinary trauma. *Physician Assistant,* (Oct.) 1983, 15–30.

Vetrosky DT, Carson CC III. Hematuria: A guide to evaluation. *Physician Assistant and Health Practitioner,* (Nov.) 1982, 11–23.

Walking away with dialysis. *Emergency Medicine,* (Nov.) 1984, 85–91.

Waltzer WC. Acute renal failure. *American Family Physician,* (Sept.) 1982, 26(3):173–178.

Ward PCJ. Renal dysfunction, part 1: Urea and creatinine. *Postgraduate Medicine,* (May) 1981, 69(5):93–104.

Whittier FC. Proteinuria: Incidental finding or tip of an iceberg? *Consultant,* (Feb.) 1982, 151–156.

Wright DN, Matsen JM. Diagnosing urinary tract infection. *Diagnostic Medicine,* (June) 1984, 44–53.

Wyngaarden JB, Smith LH Jr (eds.). *Cecil Textbook of Medicine,* Vols. 1 and 2, ed. Saunders, Philadelphia, 1982.

Zerbe RL. Inappropriate antidiuretic hormone secretion. *Hospital Medicine,* (Jan.) 1984, 241–256.

9

Reproductive Tract

Ellen Rich, Ann Elizabeth Greig, and Carla Greene

Outline

MALE GENITAL TRACT

Male Hormones and Spermatogenesis (Testes)

Cryptorchidism
Testicular torsion
Precocious puberty (true, idiopathic)
Hypogonadism (hypergonadotropic, hypogonadotropic, eunuchoidism)
Delayed adolescence
Orchitis
Hydrocele
Chronic hydrocele
Hematocele
Spermatocele
Varicocele
Testicular cancer
► Testicular self-exam

Sperm Maturation and Storage (Epididymis)

Congenital abnormalities of the epididymis
► Epididymitis
Chronic or relapsing epididymitis
Epididymal tumors

Vas Deferens, Spermatic Cord, and Seminal Vesicles

Deferentitis
Funiculitis
Chronic and subacute funiculitis
Spermatic cord neoplasms
Inguinal hernia (indirect, direct)
Strangulated hernia
Seminal vesicle cyst
Tumors of the seminal vesicles
Vesicle and duct adenocarcinoma
Seminal vesiculitis (vasitis)

Prostate

Prostatitis
► Acute bacterial prostatitis
Prostatic abscess
► Chronic bacterial prostatitis
► Nonbacterial prostatitis

Prostatic calculi
Benign prostatic hypertrophy (BPH)
Cancer of the prostate

Urethra and Penis

Circumcision
Balanitis
Balanoposthitis
Phimosis
Paraphimosis
Urethritis
Peyronie's disease (acute cavernositis)

FEMALE GENITAL TRACT

Female Sex Hormones and Oogenesis (Ovaries)

Pseudoprecocious puberty
True precocious puberty
Delayed puberty
Turner's syndrome
Mittelschmerz
Ovarian cyst (follicular, corpus luteum, hemorrhagic)
Polycystic ovary syndrome (PCO)
Ovarian cancer

Fallopian Tubes

Salpingitis
Pelvic inflammatory disease (PID)
Fallopian tube carcinoma

Uterus

Uterine displacement (retroversion, retroflexion)
Uterine prolapse
Fibroids
Amenorrhea
Primary amenorrhea
► Secondary amenorrhea
► Dysfunctional uterine bleeding (DUB)
► Primary dysmenorrhea
Secondary dysmenorrhea
► Premenstrual syndrome (PMS)
Endometriosis
Adenomyosis
Endometrial cancer

Cervix

Nabothian cysts
Acute cervicitis
Chronic cervicitis
Cervical carcinoma
Carcinoma in situ
► Pap smear screening
Diethylstilbestrol (DES) exposure
► Screening women exposed to DES
► DES information/organizations

Vagina

Imperforate hymen
Hematoculpos
Vaginitis
Toxic shock syndrome (TSS)
► Measures to minimize the danger of TSS
Vaginal hernias (cystocele, urethrocele, rectocele, enterocele)
Vaginal carcinoma

Vulva

Clitoritis
► Acute bartholinitis
Chronic bartholinitis
Bartholin's cyst
Bartholin's abscess
Sebaceous cysts and other benign lesions of the vulva
Vulvar carcinoma

Menopause

► Surgical menopause
► Natural menopause
Vasomotor instability
Atrophic vaginitis

BREASTS

Male Breast

Witch's milk
Gynecomastia
Pubertal gynecomastia
Adult-onset gynecomastia
Male breast cancer

Female Breast

Aplasia
Hypoplasia
Breast hypertrophy
► Breast self-exam (BSE)

MALE GENITAL TRACT

Male Hormones and Spermatogenesis (Testes)

Organs of the male genital tract are illustrated in Figure 9.1. Spermatogenesis and hormone production take place in the testes. Each testes is composed of interstitial tissue, Leydig cells, and seminiferous tubules. Located in the interstitial tissue and constituting 5% of the total testicular volume, Leydig cells produce and secrete male sex hormones (androgens). The adrenal gland also produces androgens—at least

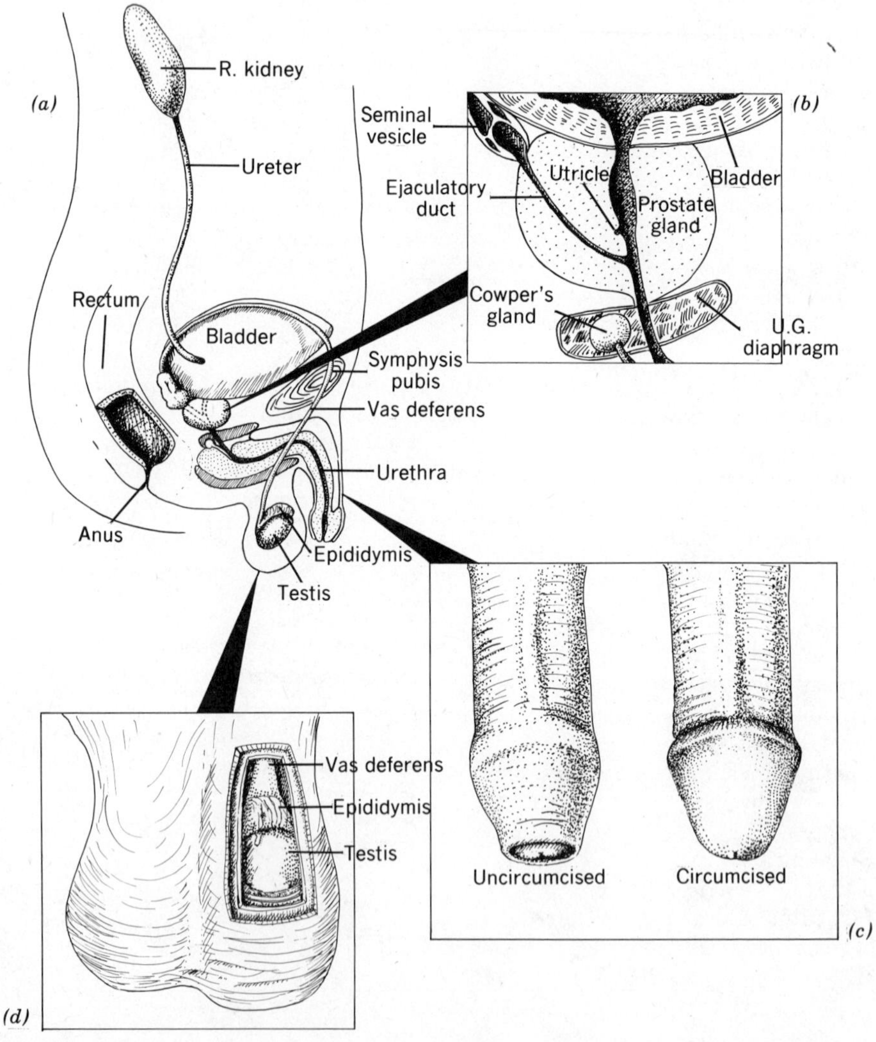

Figure 9.1 Male genital tract: (*a*) lateral view; (*b*) lateral view detail of the prostate gland; (*c*) detail of the glans penis; (*d*) scrotum (anterior view).

TABLE 9.1 HOW TESTOSTERONE INFLUENCES BODY SYSTEMS

Systems	How Influenced
Sex organs	Development of male sex organs in fetus. Provides stimulus for testicular descent. Responsible for pubertal changes—prostate becomes palpable, penis and scrotum enlarge, scrotal skin develops dark pigmentation and pronounced rugae.
Hair	With puberty, causes hair growth over pubis (in a diamond-shaped pattern that may extend upward along the linea alba, sometimes to the umbilicus and above), on face, axilla, chest, and sometimes back and/or perianal region. After puberty, contributes to decreased hair growth on the top of the head (may contribute to baldness in genetically predisposed men).
Larynx	Causes hypertrophy of laryngeal mucosa and enlargement of larynx, resulting in deepening of voice at puberty.
Skin	At puberty, responsible for thickening of skin, deepening of skin hue (from melanin deposition), and increased rate of sebaceous gland secretions (hypersecretions lead to acne).
Musculoskeletal	Increases muscle strength and mass. Influences high rate of calcium retention and subsequent density of bone matrix (bone mass greater in men than in women). Responsible for growth spurts an epiphyseal closure.
Hematopoietic	Increases erythropoiesis.
Metabolic	Increases basal metabolic rate by as much as 15%. Increases reabsorption of sodium by distal renal tubules.
Psychiatric	Contributes to aggressiveness and development of libido.

five, poorly understood types that seem to have mild effects. The major androgen produced by the testes is testosterone, the functions of which are noted in Table 9.1. Testosterone secretion is controlled by the hypothalamic-pituitary-gonadal axis, a negative feedback system. Beginning before birth and continuing throughout life, gonadotropin hormone releasing hormone (GnRH) is sent by the hypothalamus to the anterior pituitary to stimulate the synthesis and release of luteinizing hormone (LH). Once in general circulation, LH goes to the testes, binds to receptors on the Leydig cell membranes, and stimulates conversion of testosterone from cholesterol in several enzyme steps. Production continues until testosterone and other androgens reach optimal blood serum levels. This, in turn, inhibits GnRH and LH secretion (suppressive phase of negative feedback). Prolactin at high levels also inhibits the secretion of LH and follicle-stimulating hormone (FSH), Leydig cells having prolactin-specific receptors. When levels of testosterone fall, GnRH and LH are again released (recovery phase of negative feedback).

Enclosed in a capsule composed of three distinct layers (tunica vasculosa, tunica albuginea, and tunica vaginalis), the testes form in the peritoneal cavity. They descend through a peritoneal opening (the inguinal canal) into the scrotal sac, beginning around 8 months of fetal life. In the scrotum, the two testes are separated by a partition (the dartos). Made up of elastic fibers, smooth muscle, and a rich blood supply, the dartos is attached to scrotal skin. When exposed to cold, it contracts, thereby raising the testes closer to the heat radiated by the pelvis. For the most part, however, the scrotal sac protects the testes from body temperatures that are too high for normal spermatogenesis. Hanging outside the body, it maintains a relatively cool environment of 92–97°F.

The initiating signal for testicular descent is not known, though it is believed that pituitary hormones and testosterone are involved. A membrane called the "tunica vaginalis process" surrounds the fetal testes. Extending through the inguinal canal, it attaches to the scrotal floor via a ligament (gubernaculum testes). As the fetal body grows, the gubernaculum shortens and gradually pulls the testes into the scrotum.

Occasionally, testicular descent is delayed until shortly after birth or until 1 year of age. Testicular maldescent, ***cryptorchidism,*** may be caused by absence or abnormality of the gubernaculum, obstruction of the inguinal canal, a congenital gonadal defect that makes the testicle insensitive to gonadotropins, or lack of adequate maternal gonadotropins. Cryptorchidistic testes may be situated in the abdomen or in an ectopic position outside the scrotum. The majority, however, are within the inguinal canal. Unilateral arrest is more common than bilateral arrest, the latter most probably due to hormonal deficiency. Patients may complain of pain from trauma if the testis is in a vulnerable position. Scrotal examination, conducted both seated in a low chair before the standing patient and while he is lying down, reveals an empty, poorly developed, or atrophic scrotum. The testis is either not palpable or can be felt external to the inguinal ring. The exact location can be determined by ultrasound.

Treatment of cryptorchidism depends on the age at which diagnosis occurs. A trial of hormone therapy may be given to young patients. If this fails, the testis should be made to descend surgically (orchiopexy). Correction of the problem at the onset of puberty can preserve testicular function in up to 80% of cases of bilateral cryptorchidism (results are less satisfactory in unilateral cryptorchidism). After that time, chronic exposure to body heat causes atrophic changes, which not only cause infertility but also increase the risk of malignant change. Thus, an undescended testis discovered after the age of puberty should be removed (orchiectomy). For the same reasons, testicular biopsy should be performed at the time of orchiopexy and 2 years later to assess the degree of spermatogenesis. In unilateral cryptorchidism, if the repositioned testicle is not functional 2 years after surgery, it should be removed because of a high associated incidence of testicular malignancy.

To prevent injury from involuntary movement, the testes are suspended in the scrotal sac by a tough fibrous sheath called the "spermatic cord." The spermatic cord also acts as a conduit for important connecting structures: the vas deferens, the spermatic artery and veins, and the cremastic muscle. It attaches via a ligament to the outermost layer of the testicular capsule, the tunica vaginalis. If the attachment is unstable or high on the cord, the testis may twist. Known as ***testicular torsion,*** this problem usually afflicts prepubertal boys, though 2–25% of cases have been reported in men over age 21. Twisting occurs as a result of spontaneous cremastic muscle spasm. The mechanism that triggers this action is not known. While physical and sexual activity may predispose to and aggravate the condition, torsion also occurs when the patient is sleeping, sitting down, or otherwise inactive. If rotation of the testis exceeds 90 degrees, the blood supply is compromised. Patients present with rapid onset of severe testicular pain and swelling accompanied by reddened scrotal skin, nausea, vomiting, abdominal pain, and sometimes fever. Examination reveals a swollen, tender organ retracted upward in the scrotum and perhaps lying horizontally. Torsion causes the left testis to rotate counterclockwise and the right one clockwise. Urinalysis is almost always normal, though leukocytosis may develop. With acute onset of scrotal pain, torsion must be suspected and the patient sent for surgical evaluation. If the testicle is being strangled, the tissues become severely

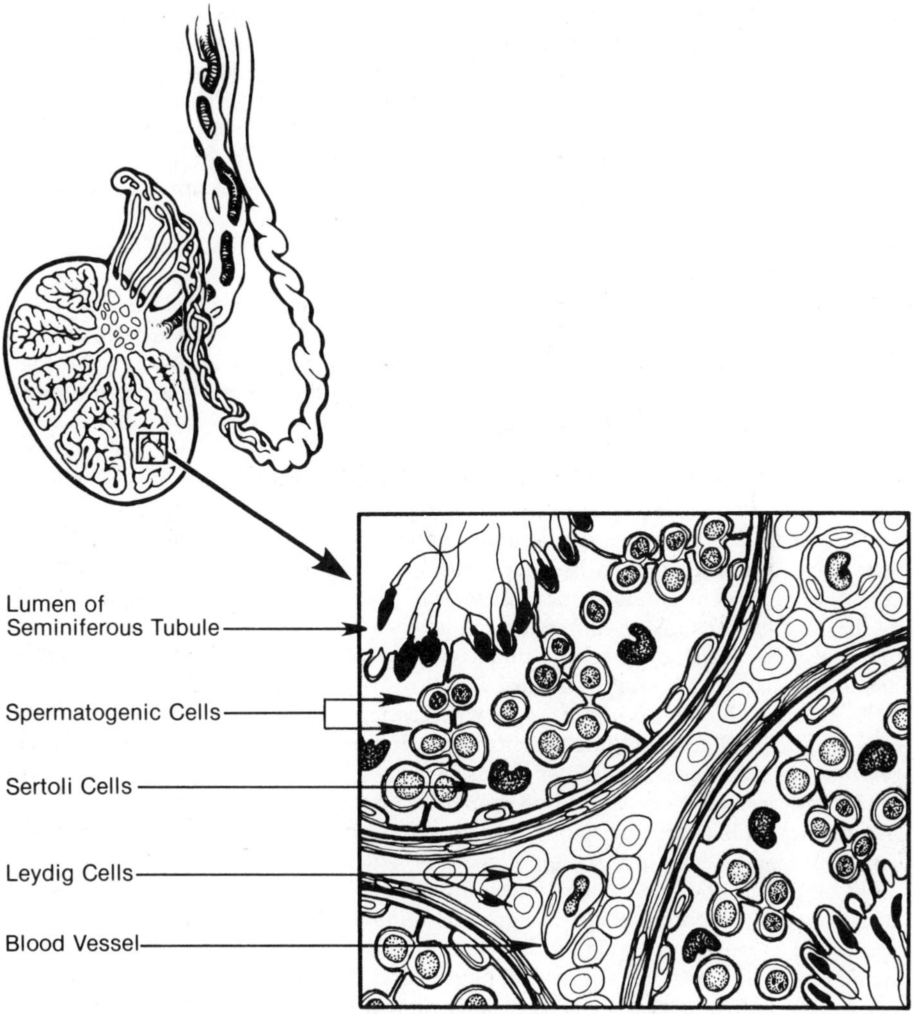

Figure 9.2 Cross section of the seminiferous tubule. (From Butnarescu, *Maternity Nursing: Theory to Practice,* © 1983, John Wiley and Sons, Inc., New York.)

damaged within 12 hours. Unless there is surgical intervention within 24 hours, preservation of the organ is doubtful and gangrene becomes a risk. Beyond 48 hours, orchiectomy is advised.

Having a volume of 2 mL or less, the testes in the prepubertal boy have a soft, rubbery consistency. However, soon after age 10, the hypothalamic-pituitary-gonadal loop becomes activated, initiating puberty. The testes undergo a period of rapid growth. Leydig cells mature and spermatogenesis begins. The latter takes place in the complex loops of the seminiferous tubules (Fig. 9.2). Tubular walls contain two specialized types of cells, Sertoli and germinal epithelial. Projecting from basement membranes, the large Sertoli cells have receptors specific for FSH. At the time of puberty, FSH binds to the receptors, initiating mitotic division of the least mature germinal epithelial cells (spermatogonia). The mitosis produces an enlarged cell, the primary spermatocyte. Through meiotic division, the primary spermatocyte forms two secondary spermatocytes, each with 23 chromosomes (haploid). These secondary spermatocytes undergo mitosis to become spermatids. The spermatids, in turn, develop into spermatozoa by undergoing dramatic structural modification and acquiring mechanisms permitting independent directional movement. Throughout the process, the lipid- and glycogen-rich Sertoli cells provide nourishment to developing sperm. Having phagocytic properties, they also identify and destroy abnormally developing sperm.

During the pubertal period, skeletal development accelerates and secondary sex characteristics appear. ***Precocious puberty*** is marked by the appearance of masculine characteristics and rapid skeletal growth with epiphyseal fusion before age 10. ***True precocious puberty*** results from some disorder of the posterior hypothalamus or, more rarely, from a tumor of testicular interstitial cells. In such cases, abnormal activation of the hypothalamic-pituitary-gonadal loop produces early masculinization as well as diabetes insipidus, bulimia, obesity, somnolence, emotional lability, and/or disturbance of temperature regulation. Occurring in the absence of an identifiable organic abnormality, ***idiopathic precocious puberty*** may be transmitted via a sex-linked gene. It is associated with seizure disorders and abnormal electroencephalograms. All types of precocious puberty are diagnosed on the basis of physical exam and increased levels of urinary and serum testosterone, LH, and FSH. Depending on the underlying cause, treatment may involve endocrinologic, neurologic, and/or surgical measures in boyhood.

By contrast, ***hypogonadism*** occurs with testicular failure ***(hypergonadotropic hypogonadism)*** or hypothalamic-pituitary abnormality ***(hypogonadotropic hypogonadism).*** Specific syndromes are described in Table 9.2, along with the clinical characteristics and therapies. If hypogonadism develops before puberty, ***eunuchoidism*** results. It is characterized by a high voice, female hair distribution, musculoskeletal changes (long arm to height span, broadened pelvis, and decreased muscle mass, strength, and endurance), and infantile genitalia. If hypogonadism develops after puberty, patients experience a gradual regression in secondary sex characteristics and a decrease in libido, with eventual impotence and infertility. Slight decreases in pituitary-gonadal function have been associated with genetic predisposition, inadequate diet, marked obesity, or chronic illness. This functional decrease, in turn, may cause ***delayed adolescence.*** Sexual and skeletal development eventually occurs, but at a later than usual age. Although benign, the condition can be the source of great psychologic stress to the patient and his parents. Correction of any basic disturbance and support of the patient and family are in order.

Following the onset of puberty, the testes reach full maturity in about 4 years. The adults testis is an ovoid, soft, tender body measuring roughly 4.5 cm in length, 2.5 cm in width, and 3.5 cm in diameter. Although the two testes are equal in size, the left one hangs slightly lower than the right.

Inflammation of the testes, ***orchitis,*** is rare in the United States. Mumps is the most well-known cause, with 30% of boys who contract it after age 10 developing orchitis. Other diseases that may result in orchitis are syphilis, tuberculosis, brucellosis, glanders, filariasis, and schistosomiasis. The acute form of orchitis, as noted in mumps infection, is characterized by testicular pain and swelling. Unilateral involvement is most common. Approximately 30% of cases involve both testes; in these

TABLE 9.2 CAUSES OF HYPERGONADOTROPIC AND HYPOGONADOTROPIC HYPOGONADISM IN THE MAN

Cause	Description
Hypergonadotropic	
Cryptorchidism	Degeneration of undescended testes from body heat.
Mumps orchitis (adults)	Virus causes testicular degeneration from progressive tubular sclerosis and hyalinization.
Testicular cancer therapy	Irradiation and chemotherapy destroy germinal epithelium.
Myotonia dystrophia	Associated with hyalinization and fibrosis of germinal epithelium.
Klinefelter's syndrome	Genetic defect (XXY karyotype) associated with seminal tubule/Leydig cell deficiency. Patients are typically tall with feminine features, skull changes, and gynecomastia. Testicular degeneration occurs after puberty with increased FSH and LH levels.
Male Turner's syndrome	Genetic defect associated with undescended testes and hypoplasia of seminal tubules.
Reifenstein's syndrome	Genetic defect associated with abnormal androgen production and genital development.
Sertoli cell only syndrome	Genetic defect characterized by damage to germinal cells.
Hypogonadotropic	
Delayed puberty	Patients display immature development, which resolves spontaneously. Familial tendency.
Eunuchoidism	Genetic defect characterized by arm span twice height (normally, about equal), increased depth of crotch, female hair distribution, high-pitched voice, infantile genitalia, poor muscle development, cleft palate; craniofacial asymmetry, poor or absent sense of smell.
Pasqualini syndrome	Hypothalamic dysfunction due to LH deficiency leads to testicular androgen deficiency, incomplete spermatogenesis, and varying degrees of eunuchoidism.
Pituitary/primary testicular failure	Eunuchoidism to varying degrees.
Adrenal hyperplasia	Full masculinization but azospermia.
Chlorpromazine toxicity	Impotence, ejaculatory failure.

instances, severe oligospermia or aspermia can result. Chronic orchitis, caused most frequently by syphilis, manifested as a painless, hard or nodular enlargement of the testicles. When signs and symptoms of orchitis are evident, the underlying systemic illness must be diagnosed and treated accordingly. In addition, bed rest, scrotal support, cold application, and possibly steroids may be beneficial. If severe pain is present, narcotics or local anesthesia with lidocaine injections may be necessary.

As noted earlier, each testis is surrounded by a capsule composed of three layers (tunicas). The outermost layer, the tunica vaginalis, secretes a fluid that is reabsorbed at a constant rate by venous and lymphatic systems of the spermatic cord. Accumulation of fluid between capsular layers (even along the cord, if the tunica vaginalis extends that far) is called ***hydrocele.*** It results from increased production of fluid due to trauma or inflammation (epididymo-orchitis). Hydrocele may also arise when there is decreased reabsorption due to venous or lymphatic obstruction (inguinal hernia, intra-abdominal or pelvic mass). Finally, it can be congenital or idiopathic. Hydrocele is painless unless accompanied by acute epididymal infection.

However, its bulk or weight can cause considerable discomfort. On visual exam of the scrotum, one side appears larger than the other. A rounded, cystic-feeling testicular mass can be palpated and transilluminated. Although some hydroceles reabsorb spontaneously, most should be aspirated to reduce the mass and to evaluate the fluid. Treatment is particularly warranted for a very tense hydrocele that may compromise the circulation to the testicle or for a large, bulky hydrocele that is unsightly and uncomfortable to the patient. After aspiration, the fluid often recollects over a period of 6–20 weeks ***(chronic hydrocele).*** Repeated aspiration or permanent cure via hydrocelectomy may then be required.

Collection of blood between the layers of the testicular capsule is called ***hematocele.*** It usually results from trauma, though carcinoma of the testes is another possible etiology. If it occurs secondary to trauma, the patient will present with testicular pain and tenderness and scrotal bruising. Although these symptoms resolve, a very firm, nontransilluminating mass remains. On exam, the mass typically surrounds the testis, obliterating the epididymis. Surgical intervention is definitely indicated.

Spermatocele is a cystic masses containing sperm. For reasons that are not entirely clear, sperm released from the seminiferous tubules becomes blocked en route to the epididymis, creating a fluid collection. Most spermatoceles are the size of a marble or smaller (1 cm in diameter) and lie above and posterior to, but separate from, the testes. Occasionally, they become quite large and are mistaken for hydroceles. On exam, the mass is firm, uniformly spherical, and nontender. It is also freely movable and transilluminating. Aspirated fluid, which is white and cloudy, reveals sperm (usually dead) under the microscope. No specific therapy is indicated, since most spermatoceles are small and cause no discomfort. However, on occasion some do become large enough to warrant surgical excision.

A pooling of venous blood around the testicle is called ***varicocele.*** It results from incompetent or congenitally absent valves along the spermatic vein. Varicocele is more likely to occur on the left side, where spermatic vein drainage into the vena cava is naturally compromised by a sharp angle. Further compounded by gravity, the problem results in a mass or dilated and tortuous vessels. By interfering with sperm maturation and motility, varicocele may contribute to infertility. Furthermore, its sudden appearance may signal venous obstruction from a retroperitoneal mass, particularly renal. Some patients remain asymptomatic. Others complain of a dull ache or a slight dragging sensation in the groin that may be exacerbated by sexual activity. On examining the standing patient, the varicocele can be palpated posterior to and above the testes (in a recumbent position, the dilated veins collapse and are not palpable). The mass has the consistency of a bundle of worms. The diagnosis is confirmed with ultrasound. Scrotal support or suspension to relieve any discomfort may be the only treatment necessary. However, if these measures fail, surgery to ligate the spermatic vein is indicated. It should also be performed if unwanted infertility is associated.

One of the most important purposes of investigating cystic masses (hydroceles, hematoceles, spermatoceles, and varicoceles) is to rule out ***testicular cancer,*** since malignancy is very frequent in patients with a painless testicular mass. Testicular cancer is relatively rare in blacks. Its onset is almost entirely limited to three age periods: infancy, ages 20–25, and ages over 50. It is the leading cause of male deaths from solid neoplasm in the 21–40 year age group, although its overall incidence is quite low (3 per 100,000). The cause of testicular cancer is not known. A 20- to 40-

fold increase of malignant change in undescended testes suggests degeneration, perhaps from excessive body heat, as a possible cause, while a high incidence in brothers (particularly twins) and family members points to a genetic predisposition. Trauma and infection have been causally linked as well. Tumors arise from either seminiferous tubules (germinal) or interstitial tissue (nongerminal). Germinal tumors, which are more common, include seminomas, embryonal tumors (embryoma, choriocarcinoma, embryonal carcinoma, teratocarcinoma, adult teratoma), and gonadoblastomas. Nongerminal tumors may be interstitial cell, Sertoli cell, or stromal cell tumors. Mixed tumors are not unusual. Patients with testicular cancer present with testicular enlargement and occasionally mild discomfort. In addition, nongerminal tumors tend to produce excessive quantities of androgenizing hormones, which may cause virilism and precocious puberty in young boys and impotence and gynecomastia in adults. Since 30–40% of patients have metastases when they are first seen, the symptoms may be related to other systems as well. For example, there may be abdominal pain or mass (bowel or urinary tract obstruction) and/or supraclavicular nodes, a cough, or weight loss (lung tumor). On exam, important physical findings include testicular enlargement and a firm mass that fails to transilluminate. Laboratory findings may be negative except for increased urinary or serum chorionic gonadotropins and, when metastasis is present, anemia. Alphafetoprotein is a useful marker for embryonal tumors. Ultrasound confirms the solid nature of the tumor and identifies retroperitoneal nodes. If biopsy confirms the diagnosis, the testicle is removed. Iliac and inguinal nodes are examined at the time of surgery and radically resected if there is evidence of involvement. Radiation therapy and chemotherapy are sometimes used as adjuncts. The prognosis for seminomas is good, and with early intervention, 90% of patients achieve 5-year cures. It is more guarded for other tumor types, particularly in the presence of metastases or high gonadotropin secretion. Since early detection is of the utmost importance, all male patients should be instructed on ▶ ***testicular self-exam.***

Sperm Maturation and Storage (Epididymis)

After formation in the seminiferous tubules, sperm travel to the epididymis. Lying on the posterolateral surface of each testis, the epididymis consists of 20 ft of tubing coiled into a sausage-like structure (see Fig. 9.1). It is divided into three portions: the globus major, which communicates with the testes by means of the efferent ductules; the corpus; and the globus minor, which is continuous with the vas deferens. In the globus major, sperm reach their full maturity. From the time of initial germ cell division, the process requires almost 10 weeks. A mature spermatozoon consists of a head, neck, body, and tail. A small structure tipping the sperm head (the acrosome) contains rich supplies of hyaluronidase and proteinases, enzymes that allow penetration through the female cervical mucosa and the protective covering of the ovum. The dense cephaloid body is packed with fertilizing nuclear material. The tail generates considerable amounts of adenosine triphosphate (ATP), which is used as a source of energy for motility. Sperm are stored in the globus minor until ejaculation, when approximately 400 million are eliminated at one time. They remain viable in the genital tract for up to 6 weeks and, if not ejaculated within that time, are reabsorbed. Ejaculated sperm survive for only 1–3 days. The process of ejaculation is discussed in a later section.

Congenital abnormalities of the epididymis are relatively rare. Absence of the epididymis is usually associated with cryptorchidism. Occasionally, the epididymis and testes are not fused properly.

By contrast, inflammation, or ▶ ***epididymitis,*** is quite common, particularly in sexually active men aged 20–40. It is caused by infectious organisms that reach the epididymis through the vas deferens from primary infections in the urine, posterior urethra, prostate, or seminal vesicles. Rarely, infection spreads via the lymphatics or along hematogenous routes. Urethral stricture or trauma may contribute, along with bowel straining in patients who have a prostatic condition. Staphylococci, colon bacilli, and streptococci are typically isolated organisms. In men under age 35, mumps virus and chlamydia are likely to be the causative agents. Epididymitis may also be associated with gonorrhea, which causes an acute inflammation, or with tuberculosis, which causes chronic painless swelling. Concurrent involvement of the testes (epididymo-orchitis) is not unusual.

The onset of acute epididymitis is marked by mild discomfort in the inguinal canal or lower abdomen. Within a few hours to a day or two, the discomfort develops into significant pain located in the testes. On exam, the epididymis (and testes if they are involved) is noted to be exquisitely tender, enlarged, and indurated. Cord structures may be slightly thickened and tender as well. A complete blood count (CBC) may reveal leukocytosis, with a left shift. Urethral discharge may be present and, if so, should be cultured. Urinalysis may or may not reveal evidence of infection. Antibiotic therapy should be instituted if there is evidence of systemic involvement or abscess (fever, leukocytosis). Symptomatic relief can be offered in the form of a scrotal support, ice packs, and analgesia. Sedentary activity or bed rest for 3–5 days is advised. When the patient appears toxic with fever and leukocytosis, hospital admission for administration of parenteral aminoglycosides may be necessary. Complete resolution of epididymitis can be expected in 1–8 weeks. Pure viral infections may take longer. With delayed or inadequate treatment, ***chronic or relapsing epididymitis*** may ensue, a complication that often requires surgical removal of the epididymis (epididymectomy).

Epididymal tumors arise with epithelial or connective tissues. Malignant tumors, spreading via veins, offer a very poor prognosis. Fortunately, epididymal tumors are quite rare, and most are benign. Patients present with mild testicular discomfort but very rarely with frank pain. A hydrocele, if present, should be aspirated so that the testes can be properly palpated. Surgical exploration of the region is required. Treatment consists of epididymectomy, orchiectomy if malignancy is diagnosed, and radiotherapy to regional lymph nodes.

Vas Deferens, Spermatic Cord, and Seminal Vesicles

The tail of the epididymis (globus minor) connects with the vas deferens (also called the "ductus deferens"). A slim, firm, muscular tube approximately 18 in. (47.5 cm) in length, the vas deferens is divided into five portions; epididymal, scrotal, inguinal, retroperitoneal (pelvic), and vesicoprostatic. For protection, the scrotal and inguinal portions are encased in the spermatic cord.

As previously mentioned, the spermatic cord is a tough fibrous sheath that serves as a conduit, not only for the vas deferens but also for spermatic vessels and the cremastic muscle. Any infectious disease affecting the urogenital tract may affect the vas, blood vessels, lymphatics, or connective tissues of the spermatic cord. In the case of orchitis or epididymitis, infectious organisms may cause retrograde inflammation of the vas deferens ***(deferentitis).*** Occasionally, deferentitis develops without an associated infection elsewhere in the genital tract. In either instance, palpation of the spermatic cord reveals the vas deferens to be enlarged, tender, and indurated. It may feel nodular or fibrous if inflammation has been chronic. Acute deferentitis responds readily to systemic antibiotics, while chronic lesions (e.g., tuberculosis) may require surgical removal of the vas.

Inflammation of the cord itself is called ***funiculitis.*** Acute funiculitis is usually caused by bacteria (notably streptococci) that invade the cord through the lymphatics and initiate cellulitis. Patients are quite ill, with fever and scrotal pain. Palpation of the scrotum reveals normal testes and epididymis, but overall cord enlargement that obscures the vas deferens. The cord is tender and indurated. If abscess or necrosis is present, the induration may be several inches in diameter. Aggressive antibiotic therapy is mandatory. Without it, thrombosis of the spermatic vein or toxemia may ensue. Even with antibiotic treatment, ***chronic funiculitis*** may develop. It is characterized by the presence of palpable fibrous nodules along the cord. Relatively asymptomatic infection of the cord is referred to as ***subacute funiculitis.*** Usually associated with lymphogranuloma venereum, syphilis, or parasitic infection, it requires treatment of the underlying disease.

Spermatic cord neoplasms are extremely rare. Presenting as a palpable mass, occasionally accompanied by local pain, cord tumors must be investigated with ultrasound and surgical exploration. Benign cord tumors (adenomatoid tumor, lipoma, fibroma, cysts) may be removed or simply followed clinically. Malignant tumors (rhabdomyosarcoma, fibrosarcoma, or metastatic lesions) require appropriate oncologic treatment. Rapid spread to the lymph nodes, lung, and liver is not uncommon.

The spermatic cord passes through a cleft in the thick muscular layers of the abdominal wall to its point of origin in the peritoneum. Called the "inguinal canal," the 4-cm cleft is defined by two fibrous rings: the superficial inguinal ring at the scrotal opening and the deep inguinal ring at the peritoneal opening. To prevent herniation of the peritoneal viscera, the deep inguinal ring is guarded by a sphincter (musculoaponeurotic apparatus). In addition, the insertion point of the cord within the peritoneum is partially surrounded by a V-shaped fascial sling. Contraction of the abdominal muscles with any kind of straining (e.g., coughing), draws the sling together and closes off the cord. Finally, the floor of the canal is supported by the fascia, abdominal muscle, Cooper's ligament, and musculoskeletal structures of the pelvis. Congenital or acquired variations in any of these structures may result in an ***inguinal hernia.***

Indirect inguinal hernia is the protrusion of peritoneal viscera into the deep inguinal ring. It is classified according to the extent of internal ring dilatation. An infantile or childhood hernia, usually associated with delayed testicular descent, may have a normal or slightly enlarged internal ring, with the major defect being only the protrusion. A simple adult hernia is characterized by ring enlargement that begins to push the inferior epigastric vessels medially. Greater dilatation is more often found in young men in whom herniation has been present for some time. ***Direct inguinal hernia*** is the protrusion of the peritoneal viscera through the floor of the canal rather than through the internal ring. It usually develops in the presence of a structural defect in the pelvic floor, a particularly high position of abdominal muscles, above the superior ramus of the pubis. Both types of hernias are compounded by prostatic hypertrophy, chronic cough, constipation, or some other condition associated with repeated abdominal straining. Once they begin, hernias continue to enlarge in all directions until marginal resistance is great enough to halt their progression. Patients with an inguinal hernia usually seek medical attention after finding a groin mass or protrusion of some type. The mass itself may not be painful, but it is usually associated with varying degrees of groin discomfort. A nagging sensation of pressure suggests direct herniation. Acute pain with straining that has a testicular radiation pattern points to indirect hernia. On examination, herniation is felt (and sometimes seen) as a palpable bulge, swelling, or thickening along the fibrous cord (indirect) or above the ring (direct). It is helpful to have the patient cough or tense his abdominal muscles, preferably while holding a deep breath. In the presence of direct hernia, the lower border of the internal oblique muscle is felt high in the medial triangle by the finger examining through the external ring. The hernial sac can usually be retained by the thumb and compressed against the deep inguinal ring in the case of an indirect hernia. Auscultation over the inguinal region may reveal bowel sounds. Ideally, patients with inguinal hernia should undergo surgical repair before the hernia becomes large enough to risk strangulation of peritoneal tissue.

With ***strangulated hernia,*** the protruding bowel is cut off from its blood supply. In such cases, the hernia mass is exquisitely tender and discolored. If the tissue becomes gangrenous, fever, leukocytosis, tachycardia, and other signs of advanced infection may be present. The problem is a medical emergency necessitating immediate surgical intervention.

Once in the peritoneal cavity, the left vas deferens skirts the bladder, widens into an opening (ampulla), and converges with the duct of the left seminal vesicle (see Fig. 9.1). The same anatomic progression occurs with organs on the right side. Lobulated structures about 5 cm long and 1.5 cm wide, the paired seminal vesicles contain tubular glands and cylindrical secretory epithelial cells that produce ejaculate fluids needed for sperm nutrition and motility. The point of fusion between the vas deferens and the seminal vesicle is called the "ejaculatory duct." Congenital obstruction here is the cause of ***seminal vesicle cyst.*** These cysts are usually discovered in men aged 30–40. They are almost always solitary but may reach immense proportions. On rectal exam, they are palpated lateral and distal to the prostate. Normal seminal vesicles cannot be palpated. Frequently, the ipsilateral epididymis is enlarged. Patients with these findings should be referred to a urologist. The cyst may require aspiration.

Tumors of the seminal vesicles include benign lesions such as fibromas, myomas, and cystic adenomas. ***Vesicle and duct adenocarcinoma*** is the most common type of malignancy. Patients present with hematuria and sometimes mucus passage, especially in the beginning of the urinary stream. Bladder outlet obstruction occurs with advanced disease. An enlarged, irregular mass is usually found on rectal exam. Patients suspected of having any type of vesicle tumor require urologic work-up. In the case of adenocarcinoma, metastases to the urinary bladder or rectum occur early in the disease. Tumor invasion of lung and bone tissue is also common. Radial surgical treatment is necessary to accomplish a cure; however, the prognosis for patients with carcinoma of the seminal vesicles and ejaculatory ducts is poor.

Inflammation of the ejaculatory duct and seminal vesicles is called ***seminal vesiculitis (vasitis).*** Since it is an extension of prostatitis, the diagnosis and treatment are discussed in the next section.

Prostate

The ejaculatory ducts pass into the prostate. A compact organ about the size and shape of a chestnut, the prostate surrounds the bladder neck and urethra. It is encased in a fibromuscular capsule, extensions of which, along with the ejaculatory ducts, divide the prostate into five lobes (posterior, median, anterior, and two lateral). The ejaculatory ducts enter at the posterior lobe and unite with the urethra in the median lobe. Then the posterior urethra exits the anterior lobe of the prostate.

Prostatic tissue is mostly fibromuscular. Some portions also contain branched tubules (the external glands). The external glands open into elongated canals, which in turn converge to form 12–20 ducts (excretory ducts). Emptying into the urethra, the excretory ducts serve as conduits for a colorless, thin, alkaline substance produced by the external glands. As discussed later, this substance is a vital part of the ejaculatory fluid.

A number of infectious processes may affect the prostate, causing an inflammation of the gland referred to as ***prostatitis.*** Organisms gain access to the prostate from an ascending urethral infection, reflux of infected urine through the posterior urethra into the prostatic ducts, and invasion of rectal bacteria either directly or via lymphatic/hematologic spread. Sexual transmission may be possible; this is yet to be proved.

▶***Acute bacterial prostatitis*** is most commonly caused by gram-negative organisms (particularly *Escherichia coli,* pseudomonas, and enterococcus). In attempt to clear the infection, polymorphonuclear leukocytes, lymphocytes, plasma cells, and macrophages invade prostatic tissue, causing hyperemia, edema, and microabscess formation. The onset of disease is marked by sudden fever, chills, myalgia, and low back and perineal pain. Within a few days, urinary frequency, dysuria, urgency, and varying degrees of bladder outlet obstruction develop. Because of the risk of bacteremia, the rectal exam must be conducted carefully, vigorous prostatic massage is contraindicated. On gentle palpation of the prostate, the gland usually feels enlarged, boggy, very tender, and warm. Expressed prostatic fluid (EPS) is typically purulent. Urine samples, especially the first, contain pus and bacteria, while the CBC often shows leukocytosis. Microscopic exam, C&S of urine, and EPS exam should be done. Pending the results, patients should be started on antibiotics. Bed rest, increased fluid intake, analgesics, antipyretics, and stool softeners are also advised. Sexual abstinence is important for recovery as well as to prevent possible transmission of the infection. Antibiotics must be continued for at least 30 days.

Prostatic abscess may develop secondary to acute bacterial prostatitis, particularly in men aged 50–70 who have a history of diabetes mellitus. Prior to the use of penicillin, gonorrhea was the causative organism in most cases; today it is *E. coli.* Patients present with all the signs and symptoms of acute bacterial prostatitis and, in some cases, epididymo-orchitis, as noted above. Rectal exam is significant for prostatic enlargement and tenderness predominating on one side. The affected side may be fluctuant. In addition to the measures for acute bacterial prostatitis, the abscess must be surgically drained. Spontaneous rupture into the urethra is not uncommon.

Inadequate treatment of an acute bacterial infection may lead to ▶***chronic bacterial prostatitis.*** With this condition, patients remain asymptomatic until significant bacteremia develops. Complaints of dysuria, urgency, frequency, nocturia, and/or pain (suprapubic, peripheral, low back, scrotal, penile) are thus intermittent. Hematospermia and painful ejaculation are other less frequent symptoms. Diagnosis on the basis of the physical exam is impossible, since rectal palpation discloses no significant findings. Laboratory results may also be negative except for one important finding: relapsing urinary tract infection due to the same pathogen. Long-term therapy (12 weeks) is required to cure chronic bacterial prostatitis. Trimethoprim/sulfonamide has the best-documented success, although geocillin, minocin, and erythromycin may also be effective. Rarely, patients must be referred for surgical intervention (prostatectomy).

The most common form of prostatitis, ▶ ***nonbacterial prostatitis,*** is of uncertain etiology, cultures being persistently negative. The symptoms and physical findings are similar to those of chronic bacterial prostatitis. Diagnosis is based on the evaluation of EPS showing more than 10 white blood cells (WBCs) per high-power field. Biopsy is sometimes necessary to rule out a specific cause of inflammation. If none can be determined, nonbacterial prostatitis is sometimes treated with a clinical trial of antibiotics despite its classification. Should antibiotics prove unsuccessful, symptomatic relief with anti-inflammatory agents is all that can be offered.

Prostatic calculi are common in middle-aged and elderly men. They are usually discovered as incidental findings on x-ray films or during surgery and are rarely of clinical importance. Sometimes, however, bacteria become deeply embedded in the stone matrix. Since antibacterial agents are unable to sterilize such calculi, bacteria continually reinfect the surrounding prostatic tissue and urine. Transurethral extrusion of the stone may be required.

In addition to its own external glands, the prostate houses the paraurethral glands. Found in the mucosa lining the excretory ducts and roof of the urethra, the paraurethral glands manufacture mucus to lubricate the urethra. Normally, the paraurethral glands, along with other prostatic tissues, begin to atrophy after age 40. Sometimes, however, these tissues begin a rapid and abnormal proliferation that leads to ***benign prostatic hypertrophy (BPH).*** The etiology is poorly understood, though atherosclerotic, inflammatory, metabolic, nutritional, and especially hormonal factors are thought to play a part. The risk seems unrelated to social class, marital status, celibacy, or sexual drive. Although BPH afflicts men of all races, the age of diagnosis in blacks averages 5 years earlier than that of whites. In the beginning, tissue hyperplasia results in a general enlargement of the prostate, which is typically unnoticed by the patient. With progression, it produces a well-defined layer (surgical capsule) that limits outward expansion. Further enlargement may then be directed in various patterns: lateral lobe; posterior commissural or median lobe; lateral and median lobe; subcervical; lateral and subcervical; lateral, median, and subcervical; anterior commissural; or subtrigonal. Symptoms develop from progressive pressure on the urethra and/or bladder. These symptoms remain minimal as long as the detrusor muscle in the bladder can compensate enough to force urine past the obstruction (see Chapter 8). Eventually, however, patients note frequency (nocturia can be quite bothersome), difficulty in starting the urinary stream, continued dribbling after voiding, and stress incontinence. The most significant clinical finding is an enlarged, smooth prostate with an elastic consistency on rectal exam. It should be noted, however, that the degree of urethral obstruction is not reflected by the size of the gland as determined by rectal palpation. There may be little or no obstruction in the presence of significant lateral lobe enlargements, which are readily palpated. By contrast, marked obstruction is likely with middle lobe hypertrophy, which is barely if at all palpable. Patients with severe obstruction may display signs of secondary renal failure and congestive heart failure (CHF) such as pallor, weight loss, hand and facial edema, anemia, or even pulmonary edema.

The work-up for suspected prostatic obstruction begins with urinalysis and urine cultures. Blood urea nitrogen (BUN) and serum creatinine levels are determined to check renal function and serum prostatic acid phosphatase to screen for prostate carcinoma. Because prostatic manipulation causes a transitory elevation, serum prostatic acid phosphatase should not be drawn for several days after a rectal exam. An intravenous pyelogram (IVP) with postvoiding films displays the degree of upper urethral obstruction and/or the presence of residual bladder urine. Cystourethroscopy is essential to evaluate the obstruction of the bladder neck properly. Definitive treatment for BPH is transurethral prostatectomy. However, this is reserved for cases complicated by urinary retention, hydronephrosis, recurrent urinary tract infections, or severe hematuria.

An important reason for the work-up for BPH is that ***cancer of the prostate*** often originates within the surgical capsule in the posterior lobe. Prostatic adenocarcinoma is the second most common form of cancer in the United States, affecting 65,000 men annually. It rarely affects men younger than age 50, and its incidence peaks around age 70. The etiology is not known, although significant familial tendencies suggest a genetic component. Strikingly influenced by hormones, particularly androgen, the tumor may extend via the ejaculatory ducts to the seminal vesicles and via the urethra to the bladder. Early metastasis (to pelvic bone, skin, liver, lung, and bone marrow) is also the rule. Patients present with perianal discomfort and/or symptoms of upper urinary tract obstruction similar to those seen with BPH. Those with tumor extension or metastatic disease may have additional complaints such as hematuria, lumbosacral pain, nausea, vomiting, chronic cough, or weight loss. In the early disease, rectal exam of the prostate may reveal no abnormality, an area of altered texture, or a distinct nodule. In advanced disease, the prostate is stony hard and fixed, and the seminal vesicles are indurated. Significant laboratory tests include urinalysis, urine cultures, SMAC, CBC, and prostatic acid phosphatase. Acid phosphatase levels on SMAC may be elevated in metastatic bone disease. Biopsy confirms the diagnosis. Patients with prostatic cancer are staged and treated with radical surgery, radiation therapy, and/or chemotherapy. The earlier the stage, the better the prognosis. Therefore, primary care providers should do rectal exams with careful palpation of the prostate in all men over age 50 at least annually.

Urethra and Penis

In the man, the urethra serves as a conduit for the urinary tract as well as the genital tract (see Chapter 8). It is an S-shaped tube about 20 cm long divided into three portions. The "prostatic" urethra extends from the neck of the bladder through the prostate. Within the prostate it communicates with both the ejaculatory and prostatic ducts (see the previous section). Perforating the urogenital diaphragm, the "membranous" urethra passes out of the pelvic cavity. Finally, the "cavernous" urethra enters the bulb of the penis, situated just below the prostate. Here it communicates with the ducts from two pea-sized structures (bulbourethral or Cowper's glands) that flank the bulb. These glands secrete a viscoid, alkaline fluid that washes out the urethra in preparation for ejaculation.

The bulk of the penis narrows into a cylindrical mass of erectile (cavernous) tissue called the "corpus spongiosum." Wedging the entire length of the corpus spongiosum from above are two other cylindrical masses of erectile tissue, the corpora cavernosa. The three corpora, each encased in a fibrous covering (tunica albuginea), form the shaft of the penis.

At the end of the shaft, the corpus spongiosum widens to form the glans penis, from which the urethra exits through a small longitudinal slit (external urethral meatus). The skin from the shaft of the penis folds back around the glans to create a protective covering called the "prepuce" or "foreskin" (see Fig. 9.1). In a minor surgical procedure, ***circumcision,*** the prepuce is pulled forward and part of it is cut off, leaving the glans and neck of the penis totally exposed. Circumcision is usually performed for cultural and religious reasons. Currently there are no medical indications for routine circumcision in infancy, and, in fact, the procedure may result in damage to the glans.

In the uncircumcised male, a small amount of urine is always trapped under the foreskin after each voiding. Because a cheesy, odoriferous substance produced by the glans also collects there, the foreskin should be retracted manually and the area carefully cleaned and dried routinely. Poor hygiene predisposes the area to bacterial, fungal, parasitic, or mixed infection. This, in turn, causes inflammation of the glans alone ***(balanitis)*** or of the glans and foreskin together ***(balanoposthitis).*** Regardless of hygiene, balanitis and balanoposthitis may occur secondary to gonorrhea, syphilis, or Reiter's syndrome. It may also be the manifestation of a drug eruption, contact dermatitis, psoriasis, lichen planus, seborrheic dermatitis, and lichen sclerosis. Patients complain of tenderness, redness, and swelling around the glans penis, with or without foreskin involvement. Foreskin constriction due to edema of the glans and prepuce, and erosion and superficial ulceration of both, may be present. Tenderness and enlargement of the inguinal lymph nodes sometimes also occur. Purulent discharge indicates infectious complications. The search for the offending agent should begin with a culture and sensitivity test to isolate any causative pathogen. Use or exposure to local irritants and ingestion of urticariogenic substances should be determined. Depending on the underlying disorder, treatment consists of topical antifungal, antibacterial, and/or steroid ointments. Meticulous personal hygiene is mandatory. Once the inflammatory reaction has subsided, referral for circumcision is advisable.

Chronic balanoposthitis may produce thickening and hardening of the foreskin. ***Phimosis,*** a condition in which the prepuce cannot be retracted over the glans, may follow. Although it usually occurs in uncircumcised men, it may also be seen in circumcised men who underwent an improper procedure. Some patients are bothered only by the inability to retract the foreskin, but most are plagued by ongoing infections. After bringing the inflammation and infection under control as described above, patients should be referred for circumcision.

In rare cases, uncircumcised individuals are also at risk for ***paraphimosis,*** which occurs when a relatively snug foreskin is forcibly retracted (during intercourse) and cannot return to its normal position covering the glans. This is due to chronic inflammation under the foreskin with eventual contracture of the skin. If it remains untreated, edema, vascular insufficiency, and gangrene of the glans penis may result.

Patients with paraphimosis should be sent immediately to a urologist for manual reduction or incision of the constricting tissue and circumcision.

Inflammation of the anterior portion of the urethra, or ***urethritis,*** is the most common manifestation of sexually transmitted infection in the man. Characterized by dysuria and/or urethral discharge and irritation, urethritis is usually associated with gonorrhea and chlamydia infections. For this reason, it is discussed in a later section on sexually transmitted diseases.

Along the penile shaft, progressive fibrosis of the tunica albuginea with plaque formation results in ***Peyronie's disease (acute cavernositis).*** It is found in men aged 50–70. The cause of the condition is not known. Neoplastic changes or irritation (following abscess, extravasation of urine, or trauma) have been suggested as initiating events. Associations with arteriosclerosis, diabetes mellitus, phlebitis, vitamin E deficiency, increased levels of serotonin, and the use of beta blockers are under investigation. Fibrosis usually begins in the septum and spreads linearly, eventually compressing erectile tissue. Many patients seek attention for the presence of a lump in the penis. Others complain of penile pain, curvature, and/or distal flaccidity on erection; any of these conditions may lead to impotence. On examination of the penis, well-demarcated, raised, fibrotic plaques are easily palpated. Myriad medical measures have been employed, including vitamin E, estrogens, oral and intralesional steroids, ultrasonic vibration, irradiation, dimethyl sulfate, and potassium *p*-aminobenzoate. However, surgical intervention is considered the only definitive treatment. Excising the fibrotic area and replacing the defect with a dermal graft is one widely used technique. The Nesbit procedure (an ellipse is excised from the point opposite the plaque to counteract the curvature) is another. For the impotent man, insertion of a penile prosthesis after excision of the plaque is recommended.

FEMALE GENITAL TRACT

Female Sex Hormones and Oogenesis (Ovaries)

The organs of the female genital tract are illustrated in Figure 9.3. Oogenesis (egg formation) and hormone production take place in the ovaries, a composite of which is shown in Figure 9.4. During fetal life, germ cells, contained within the ovaries, divide to create 500,000 oocytes per ovary. A layer of granulosa cells surrounds each oocyte and engulfs it with secretions of a mucoid substance forming a primordial follicle cell, which in turn is surrounded by two layers of theca cells (theca externa and theca interna). After birth, a large number of these follicles (about 20–30%) undergo a degenerative process (atresia), whereby the oocyte dies and the follicle becomes fibrous (corpus albicans). The remaining follicles secrete estrogen and progesterone, the two main female sex hormones, described in Table 9.3. Hormone secretion is largely controlled by the hypothalamic-pituitary-ovarian axis. Low levels of circulating estrogen stimulate hypothalamic secretion of luteinizing hormone releasing factor (LH-RF), causing pituitary release of LH and FSH. This, in turn, results in a subsequent increase in ovarian steroid production.

In the young girl, the immature hypothalamus barely responds to the small amounts of estrogen produced by the ovaries. Just before puberty, it becomes increasingly sensitive to low levels of estrogen. Though it is not known for sure, the

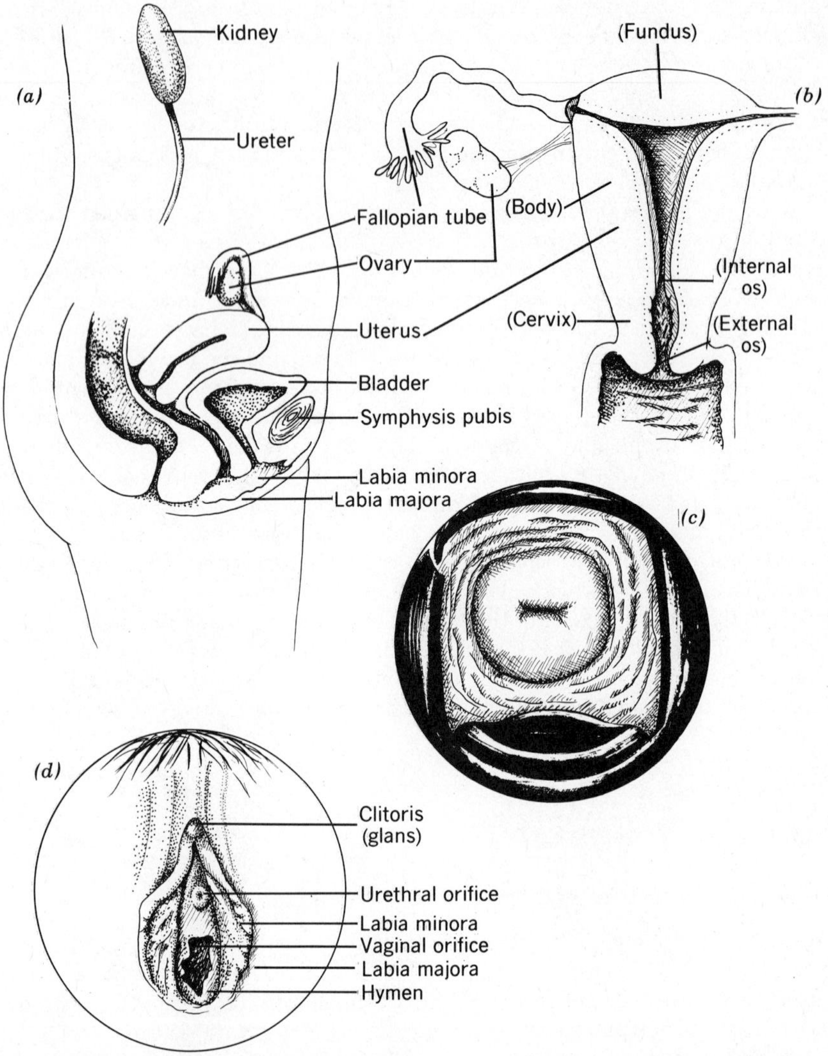

Figure 9.3 Female genital tract: (*a*) lateral view; (*b*) anterior/sagittal section of the uterus; (*c*) view of the cervix through a speculum; (*d*) external genitalia.

altered sensitivity may be related to a change in body fat composition, the prepubescent girl having a 5:1 ratio of muscle to fat and the pubescent girl a ratio of 3:1. In any case, a surge of sex hormone activity follows, along with a number of body changes that mark the onset of puberty. Androgens are released from the adrenal glands, causing a growth spurt and the appearance of pubic hair (andrenarche). Estrogens are secreted from the ovaries, causing breast budding and initiating the first ovulatory cycle and menses (menarche).

The onset of puberty is variable, being influenced by geographic, racial, socioeconomic, nutritional, and emotional factors. In the United States, female pubescence

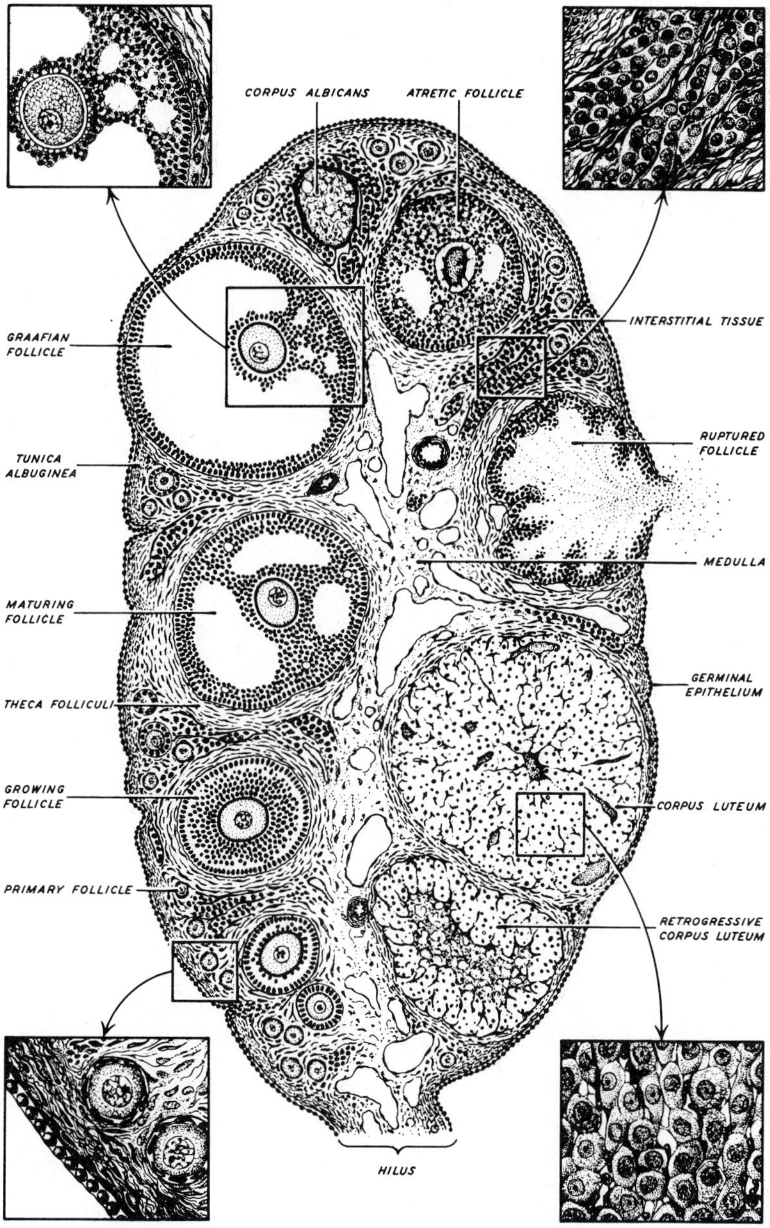

Figure 9.4 Composite of the female ovary. (From Brown, *Medical Physiology*, © 1983, John Wiley and Sons, Inc., New York.)

TABLE 9.3 FEMALE SEX HORMONES

Estrogens (three major types)

Estradiol Secreted by the ovaries in response to ACTH stimulation. Responsible for development of female sex characteristics at time of puberty. Also responsible for adolescent increase in bone formation (growth spurt, epiphyseal closure) and changes in total body configuration (increased deposition of fat in subcutaneous tissue, buttocks, thighs) and breast development (growth of ducts, deposition of fat). Stimulates cyclic growth of uterine lining to regulate menses. Responsible for growth and maintenance of vaginal mucosa. Stimulates cervical glands to produce clear, watery secretions at time of ovulation in order to facilitate sperm passage into the uterus. Increases action of cilia in fallopian tubes at the time of ovulation to enhance movement of ovum toward the uterus. Prepares breast for lactation. Maintains the strength of capillary walls. Helps reduce blood cholesterol levels. Helps maintain bone density.

Estriol Secreted by the placenta during pregnancy.

Estrone Major circulating estrogen after menopause. Derived from peripheral conversion of androstenedione (an androgen) secreted by the adrenal gland.

Progesterone

Secreted by the corpus luteum (cyclically with the menstrual cycle and persistently during pregnancy). Increases body temperature shortly after ovulation. Reduces motility in fallopian tubes. Prepares endometrial lining for implantation. Inhibits uterine contractions so that the implanted ovum will be retained. Stimulates lobular/alveolar growth in breasts. Causes cervical mucus to become viscous, inhibiting further sperm passage through the os. Increases excretion of water and sodium from the kidneys (aldosterone antagonist). Contributes to positive nitrogen balance and overall weight gain. Has a balancing effect on the increased plasma insulin response to glucose loads (retards the hypoglycemic effect). Plays a significant role in fat deposition.

generally occurs between the ages of 9 and 16. Occasionally, sex hormone secretion increases in the absence of pituitary gonadotrophic stimulation. This results in a condition called ***pseudoprecocious puberty.*** It is marked by early breast budding and pubic hair development before age 9 that is not accompanied by menarche. The causes include primary ovarian and adrenal lesions, including neoplasms and nonneoplastic cysts. By contrast, a premature activation of the hypothalamic-pituitary-ovarian axis results in ***true precocious puberty.*** Characterized by the development of both secondary sexual characteristics and menarche at an abnormally early age, the problem may be idiopathic and benign. On the other hand, it may be caused by a central nervous system (CNS) tumor, an adrenal lesion, or a correctable endocrinopathy, particularly hypothyroidism. If menarche occurs late in its course, true precocious puberty may be difficult to distinguish from pseudoprecocious puberty. In either case, endocrinologic work-up is imperative. The treatment depends on the underlying cause.

When growth of breasts, appearance of pubic hair, and menarche have not occurred by age 16, the patient has ***delayed puberty.*** Congenital defects, a hypogonadotrophic state or other endocrinopathy, sclerocystic ovaries, follicles insensitive to gonadotropins, idiopathic delayed puberty, and endometrial synechiae are possible causes. Most cases require endocrinologic work-up and treatment. A few resolve spontaneously.

In 1938, Turner described a syndrome genetically linked to a single X chromosome and characterized by maldevelopment of the ovaries. The ovary of ***Turner's syndrome*** contains no follicles, only rudimentary elongated streaks of spindle-shaped tissue and whorls of connective tissue. It was once believed that the clinical manifestations appeared only at puberty (i.e., failed sexual maturation). However, Turner's syndrome can be recognized as early as infancy and throughout life, according to the signs outlined in Table 9.4. Treatment (estrogen replacement) begins after ages 13–15 to avoid premature epiphyseal closure and continues throughout life.

TABLE 9.4 CHARACTERISTIC FEATURES OF TURNER'S SYNDROME

Feature	Description
Musculoskeletal	Dwarfism (patients usually 4–4.5 ft tall). Increased carrying angle of arms. Webbing of neck. Stocky chest with widely spaced nipples. Short fourth metacarpals. Exostosis of tibia. Osteoporosis.
Sexual development	"Streak" ovaries. Primary amenorrhea. Genital hypoplasia with infantile uterus, vagina, and breasts. Scant axillary and pubic hair. High levels of serum FSH and LH.
Cardiovascular	Coarctation of aorta and congenital valve defects common.
Skin	Multiple nevi. Premature senile appearance.
Metabolic	Increased incidence of diabetes and autoimmune thyroiditis.
Hematologic	Lymphedema of hands and feet seen in infants. Chromatin sex pattern often shows a negative buccal smear and a 45, X chromosomal pattern. Mosaicism is common.

Ovulation occurs in a cyclic fashion due to the waxing and waning of hormones illustrated in Figure 9.5. On day 1 of the cycle, when estrogen levels are lowest, FSH begins to rise. In response, about 20% of the ovarian follicles begin to grow, both granulosa cells and surrounding theca cells proliferating. As the cells proliferate, they secrete large amounts of estrogen, which leads to a feedback fall in FSH beginning at around day 6. In the absence of large amounts of FSH, all but a single follicle begin to regress. Because it is more advanced than the other activated follicles, or because it requires less hormonal support, this "dominant" (graafian) follicle continues to grow. If more than one graafian follicle gains ascendancy, multiple births may occur. The graafian follicle moves toward the outer part of the ovary, where it forms a surface bulge. Then rising estrogen levels suddenly have a positive rather than a negative effect on the feedback loops. For 48 hours, FSH and LH rise sharply (LH rises three to five times faster than FSH), causing the follicle to swell with fluid. Stretched follicular walls begin to leak and then rupture, extruding the ovum. Actual release of the ovum (ovulation) can take a few seconds or as long as 15 minutes. In four out of five women, it occurs exactly 14 days before menstruation begins, regardless of cycle length.

It is surmised that when the follicle bursts, a few drops of blood or follicle fluid are sometimes released into the abdominal cavity, causing local peritoneal irritation. Such irritation produces the typical one-sided lower quadrant pain known as ***mittelschmerz*** (German for "middle pain"). Mittelschmerz lasts for periods ranging from a few hours to a day. Most patients respond to reassurance and mild analgesics.

With collapse of the follicle walls after ovulation, granulosa cells increase in size and accumulate a yellow pigment (lutein). Secreting progesterone, they became known as "luteal cells" and the empty graafian follicle as the "corpus luteum." The corpus luteum reaches its peak of endocrine activity 5–7 days later and then, if fertilization does not occur, begins to regress. Like other follicles undergoing atresia, it becomes fibrotic and is transformed into a corpus albicans. Both the rise and sudden withdrawal of progesterone associated with progression of the corpus luteum play an important role in endometrial development and menstruation, as discussed in a later section.

If a graaffian follicle or corpus luteum fails to regress, an ***ovarian cyst*** may form. A ***follicular ovarian cyst*** develops when a mature ovum is not released and the

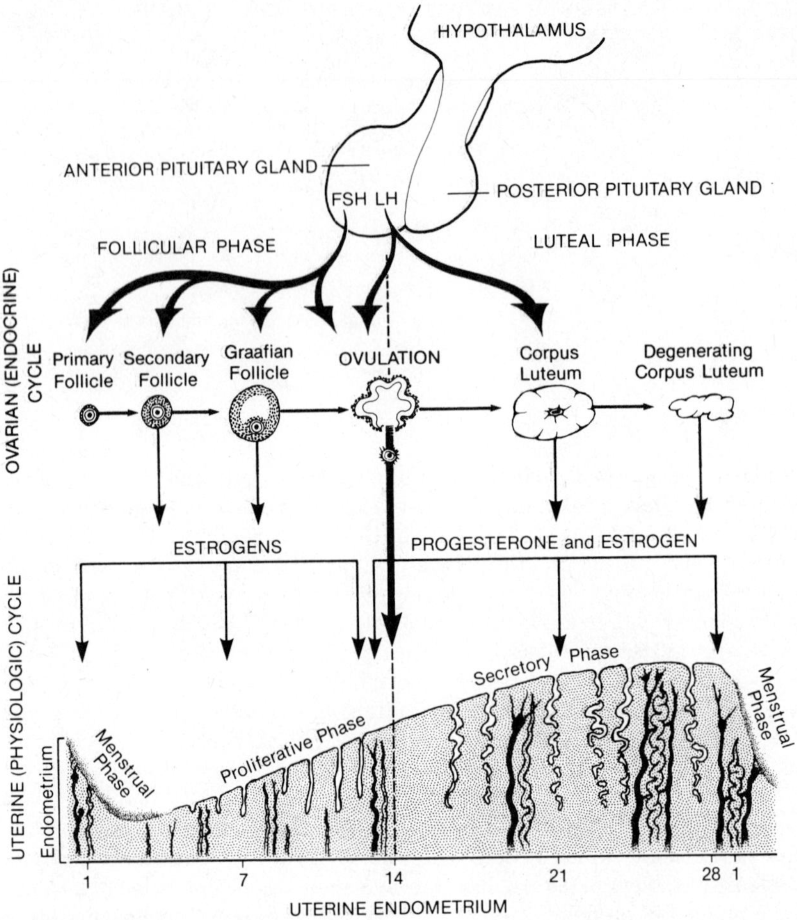

Figure 9.5 Ovulation cycle. (From Butnarescu, *Maternity Nursing: Theory to Practice*, © 1983, John Wiley and Sons, Inc., New York.)

follicle continues to produce fluid and estrogen. ***Corpus luteum cyst*** follows persistent enlargement of luteal cells and progesterone secretion. It may be associated with rupture of a small blood vessel ***(hemorrhagic cyst),*** particularly if the corpus is in a vascularization stage. These cysts often produce no noticeable symptoms. On the other hand, they can be responsible for menstrual irregularities (delayed onset, prolongation, increased frequency) and/or abdominal discomfort (heaviness, ache, or pain). The diagnosis is based on the finding of a soft irregularity on bimanual exam of the ovaries and on ultrasound studies. Most ovarian cysts reabsorb spontaneously and require no treatment. Aspiration or surgical removal may be undertaken for large, painful cysts. Surgical intervention may also be necessary for ruptured hemorrhagic cysts associated with extensive bleeding.

A particular disturbance in the hormonal relationship along the hypothalamic-pituitary-ovarian axis leads to the ***polycystic ovary syndrome (PCO).*** LH is hypersecreted, occasionally in bursts, with absence of the typical LH surge. Concurrently, levels of androgen, testosterone, and estrogen are elevated, while FSH is diminished. The ovary has a cystic texture within a thickened, whitish capsule. Hirsutism and infertility are hallmarks of PCO; however, androgen-producing adrenal tumors may have similar effects. Hirsutism, usually involving the face, may precede menarche. The menstrual history often reveals irregular menses or oligomenorrhea commencing 1–2 years after menarche; eventually amenorrhea may follow. Alternatively, the patient may experience irregular, heavy bleeding. Anovulation is usual, but occasional ovulatory cycles are not uncommon. Obesity is a finding in more than 30% of women with PCO. The ovaries are enlarged in some cases. The diagnosis is based on a hormonal assay as well as on the clinical presentation. However, differential diagnosis is difficult and should be performed by a specialist. A medical regimen of clomiphene can help induce ovulation in women who wish to conceive. If this fails, gonadotropin administration or ovarian wedge resection may be attempted. For the woman who does not wish to conceive, oral contraceptives, if not contraindicated, when used for at least 6 months, may help control hirsutism. Spironolactone, an aldosterone antagonist, is another agent employed to reduce hirsutism.

Ovarian cancer is the fourth leading cause of cancer deaths in U.S. women. Neoplastic changes usually arise from epithelial cells, germ cell tumors being less common. Increased sex steroid secretion (manifested by amenorrhea, erratic or excessive vaginal bleeding, virilization, and/or pseudopuberty) may be associated with ovarian cancers. Several investigators have noted a lower risk among women who use birth control pills and who have had multiple pregnancies. This suggests a protective effect of progesterone. The peak incidence of ovarian cancer occurs in the fifth decade. The early stages are almost always asymptomatic, but may be found on yearly gynecologic exam through the finding of an irregular and/or enlarged ovary (more than 5 cm in diameter in premenopausal women or a palpable ovary in postmenopausal women). Tumors that are not discovered in an early stage tend to reach considerable size before clinical symptoms develop. Women may then develop vague lower abdominal discomfort and mild digestive complaints. Abnormal vaginal bleeding sometimes occurs from hormone secretion by the tumor, but this is uncommon. An abdominal mass, ascites, pelvic pain, anemia, and cachexia are signs of advanced disease. In such cases, Pap smears of the vaginal pool or ascitic fluid may reveal cancerous cells. Ultrasound and pathology reports confirm the diagnosis and aid in staging the disease (Table 9.5). In a young patient with an early unilateral lesion of low-grade malignancy (e.g., mucinous tumor), treatment can be confined to removal of the involved ovary and tube, thereby preserving reproductive function. In more advanced cases or with more malignant tumors (e.g., germ cell tumors), total abdominal hysterectomy, bilateral salpingo-oophorectomy, and omentectomy are undertaken. Chemotherapy and radiation therapy are important adjuncts of treatment. Good responses are being obtained with combination chemotherapy, especially platinum-containing regimens.

Fallopian Tubes

As soon as it is released, the ovum passes into a fallopian tube (see Fig. 9.3). The egg is pulled into the opening of the tube (ostium) via a funnel-shaped structure (infundibulum) that has ciliated, finger-like projections (fimbriae). Activated by the same surge of LH and FSH that initiated ovulation, the fimbriae wave back and forth,

TABLE 9.5 STAGES OF OVARIAN CANCER[a]

Stage	Description
I	Growth limited to ovaries.
A	Growth limited to one ovary; no ascites.
(i)	Ovary capsule intact; no tumor on external surface.
(ii)	Capsule ruptured and/or evidence of tumor on external surface.
B	Growth limited to both ovaries; no ascites.
(i)	Capsules intact, no tumor on external surfaces.
(ii)	Capsules ruptured and/or evidence of tumor on external surfaces.
C	Stage I tumors with ascites or positive cytologic findings on peritoneal washings.
II	Tumor of one or both ovaries plus pelvic extension.
A	Involvement of uterus and/or tubes.
B	Extension to other pelvic tissues.
C	IIa or IIb tumor with ascites present or positive cytologic findings on peritoneal washings.
III	Tumor of one or both ovaries with intraperitoneal metastases (i.e., small bowel, omentum) and/or positive retroperitoneal nodes.
IV	Tumor of one or both ovaries with distant metastases (liver parenchyma, pleural effusion with positive cytologic findings).
Special	Unexplored cases thought to be ovarian carcinoma.

[a]Federation of Gynecology and Obstetrics (FIGO) classification.

pulling the ovum into position. The ovum is pushed along the 10-cm length of the tube by peristaltic waves. After a journey of 3–4 days, it reaches a narrow passageway into the uterus (isthmus) where further progress is delayed for 2–3 days. Unless fertilization has occurred, the egg disintegrates and the debris is eliminated by macrophages.

Infections may ascend from the uterus to the fallopian tubes ***(salpingitis)*** and the peritoneal cavity ***(pelvic inflammatory disease, PID).*** PID has reached epidemic proportions in recent years, affecting 10 women per 1,000 every year. In women below age 25, the problem is even more prevalent (20 cases per 1,000). The causative organisms include chlamydia, gonococcus, bacteroids, streptococcus, staphylococcus, *E. coli, Mycobacterium tuberculosis,* fungi, and parasites. They are usually, but not always, transmitted sexually. A history of vaginal discharge, irregular bleeding, long heavy menses, recent abortion, or dilatation and curettage (D&C) is common. Patients with acute PID complain of a sudden onset of bilateral lower quadrant pain described as sharp or cramping. Classic signs are fever, cervical discharge, and intense pain with cervical manipulation (chandelier sign). An adnexal mass is usually present but may be difficult to assess due to abdominal tenderness with guarding. Abdominal rigidity, nausea, and vomiting suggest peritonitis or tubo-ovarian abscess. Laboratory studies reveal an elevated erythrocyte sedimentation rate (ESR) and WBC count (may be normal or slightly elevated with chlamydial PID). Cervical cultures help identify a lower reproductive tract infection. However, since cervical culture results do not always correlate with the upper reproductive tract infection, transabdominal culture of peritoneal and tubal fluid may also be necessary.

Treatment of PID consists of rest and antibiotics for 10–14 days. The Center of Disease Control (CDC) now recommends that in patients experiencing their first episode of PID, this should be done in a hospital due to the high rate of infertility evolving from inadequate therapy. Hospitalization should also be considered for the following: patients who have signs of peritonitis or abscess, or who are acutely ill; uncertain diagnosis (particularly if associated with GI symptoms or recent gynecologic procedures such as abortion); patients with an intrauterine device (IUD) in place; pregnant or nulliparous patients; and patients who fail to respond to outpatient therapy. In all cases of PID, sexual contacts should receive appropriate treatment. Sexual intercourse should be resumed only after complete recovery.

Unlike other reproductive organs, the fallopian tubes are rarely affected by malignancy. In fact, only 1,100 cases of ***fallopian tube carcinoma*** have been reported. Among these, the highest incidence occurred within the first 5 years following menopause. Many patients have a history of PID. Developing insidiously, symptoms include vaginal discharge, abnormal vaginal bleeding, abdominal pain and distention, and urinary frequency. Exam may reveal an adnexal mass or a poorly defined uterus. The diagnosis is based on pelvic ultrasound and surgical exploration. Treatment is total hysterectomy and bilateral salpingo-oophorectomy followed by radiation therapy and/or chemotherapy. Mortality is highest among women with poorly differentiated and/or advanced tumors.

Uterus

The fallopian tubes enter the uterus, a hollow organ with thick, muscular walls (see Fig. 9.3). Pear-shaped, the uterus has a rounded upper portion (body) and a narrow lower portion (cervix). The size and shape of the uterus are altered with age and childbearing status.

Situated above the bladder and in front of the rectum, the uterus is held by four ligaments (cardinal, broad, round, and uterosacral) in an anterior position, with the cervix at a right angle to the vagina. Though securely supported, the uterus is freely movable, its position varying with distention of the bladder or rectum. ***Uterine displacement*** is also common. ***Retroversion,*** backward tilting of the entire uterus, and ***retroflexion,*** backward bending of the uterine body at the cervix, are the two most common types. In such instances, the cervix points toward either the symphysis or the sacrum, with the fundus felt posteriorly. Displacement may be congenital. However, it may also be secondary to an adnexal mass, neoplasm, or traumatic stretching of the ligaments from pregnancy and childbirth. If acquired pathology is the cause, patients are likely to complain of dysmenorrhea and backache. In such cases, uterine displacement should be evaluated with pelvic ultrasound.

In older women, the pelvic musculature and fascia become lax and flaccid, and may lead to ***uterine prolapse.*** Younger women who have sustained injury to or overstretching of the pelvic floor structures are also at risk. Traction of the uterine ligaments and venous congestion produce lower abdominal heaviness, a "bearing down" feeling, and backache. On exam, a mildly prolapsed uterus is evidenced by displacement of the cervix toward the vaginal opening; this becomes more pronounced with straining. In more severe cases, the cervix may be visible at the vaginal opening or may protrude outside the vagina. Patients should be evaluated for surgical correction, since the problem is not only uncomfortable but can result in cervical ulceration and/or hypertrophy.

Fibroids are uterine fibromyomas—discrete sessile or pedunculated benign tumors composed of smooth muscle and connective tissue. Fibromyomas are very common, especially among black women, with a markedly increased incidence over age 35. They may grow in any of the layers of uterine tissue. Usually multiple, fibroids often cause no symptoms. However, large tumors may exert pressure on the bladder and bowel, causing urinary frequency and constipation. Menometrorrhagia (heavy periods) and dysmenorrhea (painful periods) are common, since the growing fibroid increases the surface area of the endometrium. Anemia may result. Fibroids tend to proliferate in the presence of estrogen. During pregnancy, they grow at an accelerated rate, sometimes leading to spontaneous abortion, malpresentation, failure to engage, premature or ineffectual labor, or postpartum hemorrhage. Infertility due to the presence of fibromyomas is not uncommon.

Fibroids are usually diagnosed on bimanual pelvic exam when an enlarged, irregular uterine outline is discerned. Pelvic ultrasonography confirms the diagnosis and helps differentiate fibroids from an adnexal mass. It can be performed serially to measure fibroid growth or regression. The asymptomatic woman with small fibroids should be monitored at 6-month intervals to assess tumor size. If conception is desired, myomectomy (removal of the tumor only) helps increase fertility. If symptoms are severe or the growth is very large (a large fibroid can mimic advanced pregnancy), hysterectomy without oophorectomy is indicated in premenopausal women. An acute situation arises if the tumor twists on its pedicle or becomes infarcted. In such cases, intense pain results and emergency surgery is indicated. Uterine myomas tend to regress after the menopause.

The uterine cavity is lined by a mucous membrane called the "endometrium." The cellular components of the endometrium (columnar epithelial cells, stromal connective cells, and glandular cells) undergo recurrent changes that constitute the menstrual cycle. These changes correspond to the rise and fall of hormone levels associated with the ovarian cycle (see Fig. 9.5). In the beginning of the cycle, estrogen produced by the ovarian follicles stimulates a rapid multiplication of endometrial cells; this is called the "proliferative stage." Lasting for approximately 14 days (beginning on day 4 of the cycle and ending just after ovulation), this proliferation of cells repairs denuded areas in the uterine lining. With the secretion of progesterone by the corpus luteum after ovulation, endometrial glands dilate and fill with glycogen, fats, and other secretions (progestational or secretory phase). To prepare for implantation of a fertilized egg, increased vascularization also occurs and the endometrium reaches a thickness of 6 mm. Unless the ovum is fertilized, the corpus luteum atrophies and progesterone levels fall suddenly. Without hormone support, the thickened endometrial lining regresses, causing uterine arteries to twist and constrict until the blood supply is cut off. Portions of the endometrium become necrotic, slough off, and disintegrate. Raw bleeding occurs wherever there is sloughing, the blood being discharged through the cervix and into the vagina. Since the entire endometrium does not become necrotic at the same time, and since menstrual blood is uniquely nonclotting, blood flow remains relatively moderate and controlled for 3–7 days.

Although the average characteristics of the menstrual cycle have been determined using samples of women of different nationalities, socioeconomic classes, and ages, much variability in menstrual symptoms, frequency, duration, and amount of menstrual flow exists. The average interval between menses is 27 to 31 days; however, shorter or longer intervals may be normal. Approximately two-thirds of all cycles vary in length by 6 days; one-third vary even more. Irregularity occurs most often during the first few and last several menstrual years. The greatest regularity occurs around age 30. Breast tenderness, bloating, lower abdominal cramping, and back pain may accompany menses but are not normally debilitating. A menstrual

TABLE 9.6 CAUSES OF AMENORRHEA

- Primary amenorrhea
  - Hypothalamic
    - Delayed puberty
    - Debility or serious organic illness
    - Lack of LH-RF
  - Pituitary (low or absent FSH)
    - Supersellar cyst
    - Pituitary tumors
    - Isolated lack of pituitary gonadotropins
  - Ovarian (high FSH)
    - Ovarian agenesis (Turner's syndrome)
    - Ovarian destruction (infectious or autoimmune)
  - Uterine
    - Malformations
    - Congenital Mullerian dysgenesis
    - Imperforate hymen
    - Hermaphroditism
    - Unresponsive or atrophic endometrium
  - Virilizing syndromes
    - Defects in testosterone synthesis or androgen resistance
    - Androgen excess (adrenal or ovarian tumors, polycystic ovaries)
    - Use of alcohol, hormones, certain drugs
- Secondary amenorrhea
  - With positive medical D&C
    - Metropathia hemorrhagica
    - Stein-Leventhal syndrome
    - Estrogen medication
    - Estrogenic tumors (i.e., granulosa cell tumors)
    - Hyperthyroidism
    - Liver disease
    - Psychogenic stress
    - Depletion of body fat (e.g., as seen in dancers)
  - With negative medical D&C
    - Pregnancy
    - Premature menopause
    - Pituitary tumor
    - Pituitary infarction (Sheehan's syndrome)
    - Arrhenoblastoma
    - Cushing's disease
    - Addison's disease
    - Anorexia nervosa
    - Profound myxedema
    - Irradiation of uterine lining
    - Asherman's syndrome (intrauterine adhesions)

flow for as few as 2 days or as long as 8 days is considered normal, but the average duration is 4–6 days. Usually heaviest during the first 2 days, menstrual loss normally ranges from 30 to 100 mL. Up to 200–300 mL is not unusual for some women. Differences in flow are usually noted in women over age 30, who report one day of very heavy flow preceded by a day or two of spotting, and in women in their mid-forties, who experience heavy, lengthy menses known as "flooding."

Amenorrhea is the absence of menstrual periods. The most common causes are pregnancy and menopause, both of which are discussed in later sections. When pregnancy or menopause is not the cause, the problem may be classified as ***primary amenorrhea*** (in which the woman has never menstruated) or ▶***secondary amenorrhea*** (lack of menstruation for 6 months in a woman who has had regular periods in the past or for 12 months in a woman with a history of irregular periods). It may be traced to hypothalamic, pituitary, ovarian, uterine, or other origins, as noted in Table 9.6. Many drugs, particularly psychotropic agents and excessive amounts of alcohol, are known to cause amenorrhea. Pituitary tumors and hormone imbalances are other sources of the problem, along with undue stress and anxiety. Nutrition also has a powerful effect on menstruation, as indicated by the loss of menses following rapid weight loss and crash diets. It is believed that weight loss of 10–15% or a fat:muscle ratio below 3:2 will stop menses, primarily by decreasing the sensitivity of FSH and LH to LH-RF. According to this theory, women athletes, who have exercised away much of their body fat, are candidates for amenorrhea.

Primary amenorrhea should be investigated and treated by a specialist. In cases of secondary amenorrhea, the first step is to rule out pregnancy or menopause. After this, progesterone to induce bleeding (medical D&C) may be used diagnostically. If progesterone fails to produce bleeding (secondary amenorrhea with negative medical D&C), pregnancy should again be investigated, and FSH and LH levels should be measured. High levels of these two gonadotropins suggest an ovarian problem, while low levels point to a hypothalamic-pituitary origin. In the latter instance, prolactin levels and further pituitary work-up may be indicated. If progesterone produces bleeding (secondary amenorrhea with positive medical D&C), the problem may be due to metropathia hemorrhagica, Stein-Leventhal syndrome, or high estrogen levels (due to estrogen medication, liver disease, or, rarely, estrogen-secreting tumors). However, the most likely cause is "psychogenic amenorrhea" related to emotional stress such as going to college, a new job, a new home, or divorce. Secondary amenorrhea with positive medical D&C often requires little more than reassurance, particularly in unmarried women, since menses are often corrected spontaneously after marriage or the first pregnancy. However, it may also be treated with continued administration of progesterone during the last 5–10 days of each month, with clomiphene citrate (Clomid), or with psychotherapy. If amenorrhea persists for many years, a severe estrogen deficiency usually develops; it should be treated as well.

► ***Dysfunctional uterine bleeding (DUB)*** is profuse and prolonged menstrual periods caused by hormone imbalance, usually anovulatory cycles in which high levels of estrogen remain unopposed by progesterone. In the latter case, the endometrium continues to proliferate until ovarian theca and granulosa cells disintegrate and estrogen levels decrease. Subsequent menstruation is prolonged and heavy, and the endometrium is shed irregularly in clots. Bleeding continues until the ovarian follicles secrete enough estrogen to spark new endometrial cell growth. DUB is most common among adolescent girls and premenopausal women, since both groups are prone to anovulatory cycles. However, hormone imbalance cannot be assumed, since abnormal uterine bleeding accompanies early abortion, salpingitis, or, more rarely, thrombocytopenia, clotting factor/platelet disorders, adrenal disorders, polycystic ovarian disease, and hypothyroidism. In the older woman, it may signal uterine cancer.

For these reasons, the diagnostic work-up and treatment of DUB depend on the patient's age. After infection and pregnancy have been ruled out in adolescents and young women, estrogen-progesterone combination pills in high doses (4 pills a day for 5 days) may be used diagnostically and as treatment (unless there are contraindications). In cases of simple hormone imbalance, bleeding subsides in the first couple of days (if not, diagnostic D&C should be performed without delay.) To ensure control, a low-dose oral contraceptive should be started on the fifth day of the next menstrual cycle and continued for 3 months. In women who wish to use the pill as a contraceptive method, it may be continued. Alternatively, medroxyprogesterone acetate (Provera), 10 mg orally, may be given for the last week of the next three cycles. DUB in premenopausal women over age 45 must always be investigated with endometrial or suction biopsy and Pap smears. To halt bleeding, estrogens alone or estrogen-progesterone combinations may be used; to control it over the next few cycles, Provera is usually given. Postmenopausal women with uterine bleeding must be worked up for cancer of the reproductive tract. Hormones should not be used.

► ***Primary dysmenorrhea*** is pain occurring with menstrual periods for which no organic cause can be found. By inducing myometrial spasm and ischemia, estrogens, progestins, and prostaglandins are thought to play important roles in the pathogenesis. Affecting 10–17% of menstruating women, the problem begins 1–2 years after menarche with the onset of ovulatory menses; it continues into adulthood but often subsides after pregnancy and childbirth. Women describe a lower midline, dull abdominal ache or cramp that tends to be spasmodic and cyclic. Beginning 2 days before the onset of menses, the pain often radiates to the back or inner aspects of the thigh. It may be associated with headache, breast tenderness, and gastrointestinal symptoms (nausea, vomiting, diarrhea). In severe cases, syncope may occur. Management begins by ruling out the causes of secondary dysmenorrhea, described below. Relief of symptoms may be achieved with the use of birth control pills or prostaglandin inhibitors, particularly nonsteroidal anti-inflammatory drugs. Several home remedies—intercourse, heating pads, exercise, and yoga—may also be beneficial.

Secondary dysmenorrhea is pain occurring with menses that can be traced to an organic pelvic lesion. The most common cause is PID with or without IUD use. Salpingitis, endometriosis, adenomyosis, and uterine or adnexal tumors are other sources. To help distinguish secondary dysmenorrhea from primary disease, the history is extremely important. Suspicion of an organic problem should always be aroused by the development of dysmenorrhea more than 3–5 years after menarche. Pain that localizes to the right or left side, involves the abdomen generally, is exacerbated by intercourse, or peaks premenstrually and diminishes with the onset of vaginal bleeding is another telling feature. The underlying cause should be determined through physical and pelvic exam, and possibly laparoscopy, and treated accordingly.

Many women experience a constellation of emotional, behavioral, and physical symptoms just before and during the first few days of menstruation referred to as ▶***premenstrual syndrome (PMS).*** The exact cause is unknown. Some investigators believe that ovarian hormones—either estrogen excess or progesterone withdrawal—play a role. This theory is partially supported by the finding that the most severe symptoms accompany irregular or heavy menses. Other theories center on vitamin B_6 deficiency, altered glucose metabolism, imbalance of hypothalamic-pituitary neurotransmitters, and psychosocial factors. Over 150 symptoms have been reported. Among the most frequent physical symptoms are fatigue, abdominal bloating, headache, edema of the extremities, and breast fullness and tenderness. Prominent psychologic symptoms include anxiety, irritability, forgetfulness, depression, panic attacks, mood swings, paranoia, and insecurity. Binge eating, increased alcohol intake, and violence have also marked the syndrome.

Since there are no specific laboratory tests or universal agreement about its definition, PMS is a diagnosis of exclusion. Evaluation begins with a complete history and physical exam to rule out an underlying medical or psychiatric problem. In addition, patients are asked to keep a diary of symptoms throughout their menstrual cycle for several months. If recurrent physical and emotional complaints coincide consistently with the onset of menses, PMS may be considered as a diagnosis. Patients should be informed that though many interventions have been tried, none have been proven effective by controlled studies. Furthermore, the most reliable treatments are safe, simple, and inexpensive. For instance, many patients respond to exercise, stress reduction, multiple vitamins, or hypoglycemic diets. If these measures fail, diuretics, birth control pills, lithium, antidepressants, or prostaglandin inhibitors may prove helpful. As a final resort, progesterone therapy may be initiated.

Endometriosis, the aberrant growth of endometrial tissue, is commonly associated with menstrual cycle disturbances. Ectopic tissue usually establishes itself somewhere in the pelvic cavity, notably along the external uterine surface, ovaries, broad ligaments, or bowel. In rare cases, the vagina, cervix, vulva, perineum, arms, legs, lungs, pleura, or eyes may be involved. Invasion of the uterine walls constitutes a benign subtype of disease called ***adenomyosis.*** Responding to ovarian hormone changes, the endometrial tissue, like normal endometrium, proliferates and then becomes necrotic and sloughs off, causing localized bleeding. The exact pathogenesis of the problem is still uncertain. One theory is that menstrual blood containing endometrial fragments regurgitates through the fallopian tubes into the peritoneal cavity. This risk increases with strong menstrual cramping, douching, or coitus during menstruation. Though still widely accepted, this theory does not explain the occurrence of ectopic endometrium in areas outside the peritoneum. Another theory does. It proposes that embryonic cells differentiate abnormally into endometrial cells, which then begin to function under hormonal or inflammatory stimulation. The presentation of disease is extremely variable. Many patients experience pelvic pain, which starts as a dull ache 2–7 days before the onset of menstruation, and/or coital pain. Bowel involvement may be signaled by painful defecation and rectal bleeding. Both dysmenorrhea and GI symptoms increase in severity until menstrual flow slackens. DUB is not uncommon. It should be noted, however, that the severity of symptoms does not correlate with the extent of disease; women with relatively few complaints can have widespread involvement, and vice versa. Besides significant pain, infertility is the outcome in 75% of cases. In evaluating the problem, colonic involvement can be defined by contrast x-ray films and invasion of the uterine muscle can be defined with hysterography. However, definitive diagnosis rests with laparoscopic visualization and biopsy of suspicious lesions. Treatment depends on the extent of the disease and the age of the patient. In young women with mild disease, symptoms can often be controlled with exogenous hormones such as low-dose oral contraceptive pills or danazole, a synthetic androgen. Analgesics are invariably needed as well. Patients with more extensive disease who desire pregnancy may respond to surgical resection of lesions. However, extensive disease at any age often necessitates the removal of the uterus, ovaries, and tubes by surgery.

Endometrial cancer is the most common invasive cancer of the female reproductive tract, being newly diagnosed in 40,000 women each year. Ninety percent of all cases develop in women over age 40, postmenopausal hormones (androstenedione and estrone) evidently playing a significant role. Obesity is another risk factor, rates of endometrial cancer being three times greater in women 20–50 lb overweight and 10 times greater in women more than 50 lb overweight. This is undoubtedly related to the facts that androstenedione is converted predominantly to estrone in fat tissue and that the rate of conversion increases with excess fat. Hypertension and diabetes are also associated with endometrial cancer. Nulliparity, early menarche, late menopause, menstrual irregularity, liver disease, polycystic ovaries, exogenous estrogen therapy, and estrogen-secreting tumors are other risk factors. Characterized by either excess estrogens and/or lack of cyclic progesterone, such conditions can all cause progressive endometrial changes ranging from benign proliferation to atypical hyperplasia with errors in normal cell division. While levels of endogenous estrogens and cyclic progesterones may be normal in women with early menarche or late menopause, hormone exposure is prolonged. Furthermore, women with early menarche have a higher incidence of anovulatory cycles marked by elevated estrogen levels unopposed by progesterone. In keeping with these associations, combined oral contraceptive pills that provide controlled doses of progesterone throughout the menstrual cycle protect against the eventual development of endometrial cancer. A recent CDC study revealed that the incidence of endometrial cancer among women who used oral contraceptives for at least 6 months was 50% less than that among women who had never used the pill. Persisting for at least 10 years after the pill is discontinued, this protective effect is most notable in nulliparous women.

The cardinal symptom of endometrial cancer is inappropriate uterine bleeding—either postmenopausal bleeding or, in the younger patient, metrorrhagia. There may be no other evidence of disease until the malignancy spreads. Extension occurs (1) down the surface of the uterine cavity into the cervical canal; (2) through the uterine walls into the peritoneal cavity; (3) through the fallopian tube to the ovaries and broad ligaments; and (4) via blood or lymphatics with metastatic spread. Patients with involvement of the cervix or vagina often present with a mucosanguinous discharge. In evaluating a patient with possible endometrial cancer, the Pap smear has limited value, picking up changes in only 60–70% of cases. For this reason, endometrial cell sampling is now being used as a routine screening technique similar to the Pap smear. While endometrial biopsy is even more reliable (yielding accurate results 92% of the time), the diagnostic procedure of choice is fractional curettage. Performed by curetting the endocervix and then sounding the uterus, dilating the cervical canal, and curetting the endometrium, fractional curettage provides specimens that can be used for staging (Table 9.7) as well as diagnosis. Staging may also entail IVP, cystoscopy, barium enema, chest x-ray films, and sometimes mammography, bone and liver scans, and lymphangiography. The treatment is hysterectomy combined with bilateral salpingo-oophorectomy and retroperitoneal lymph node sampling. If the cervix is involved, radical hysterectomy with retroperitoneal lymph node dissection is warranted. In advanced stages, surgery is followed by progesterone therapy.

Cervix

The cervix (see Fig. 9.3) is a spool-like structure through which passes a 2- to 4-cm-long canal (endocervical canal). The canal opens into the vagina through the external os. Round to begin with, the os assumes a "fishmouth" figuration after childbirth.

TABLE 9.7 STAGES OF ENDOMETRIAL CANCER

Stage	Description
O	Carcinoma in situ (histologic findings suggestive of malignancy).
I[a]	Carcinoma confined to the uterine body.
A	Length of uterine cavity 8 cm or less.
B	Length of uterine cavity more than 8 cm.
II	Carcinoma limited to body of uterus and cervix.
III	Carcinoma extends outside the uterus, but not outside the true pelvis.
IV	Extension outside the true pelvis or obvious involvement of bladder or rectum.
A	Spread to adjacent organs.
B	Spread to distant organs.

[a]Stage I cases should be histologically subgrouped as follows:

G1 Highly differentiated adenocarcinoma.
G2 Moderately differentiated adenomatous carcinoma with partly solid area.
G3 Predominantly solid or entirely undifferentiated carcinoma.

The endocervical canal is lined with secretory cells that produce mucus. Under the influence of ovarian hormones, both the os and mucus secretions undergo changes that augment sperm transport into the uterus at around the time of ovulation and hinder it thereafter. During the proliferative stage, the external os widens progressively and the cervical mucus becomes clear, white, profuse, and watery. When placed on a glass slide, preovulation mucus produces a fern-shaped pattern as it dries. After ovulation the os shrinks and cervical mucus becomes scant, viscid, and sticky.

The endocervical glands extend down almost to the cervical mucosal surface. Blockage of the endocervical ducts results in tiny pearly-yellowish ***nabothian cysts*** (retention cysts). Only a few millimeters in diameter, these tiny benign cysts can be observed on the cervix upon speculum exam and are also palpable. Nabothian cysts are often associated with a history of chronic cervicitis but in themselves require no treatment.

Infiltration of the cervical mucosa and underlying tissue by infectious organisms leads to ***acute cervicitis.*** Gonorrhea, chlamydia, trichomonas, gardnerella, herpes, monilia, and condyloma accuminata are common causes. As sexually transmitted diseases, they are discussed in a later section. Patients with acute cervicitis may be asymptomatic but more often complain of a vaginal irritation and discharge. The latter may be variably described as thick and curdy, purulent, and/or malodorous. Speculum exam reveals the cervix to be reddened, irritated, and swollen. Certain organisms (particularly gonococcus and chlamydia) produce a profuse white or yellow exudate that discharges from the os. Herpetic cervicitis is characterized by vesicles and ulcers rather than mucopurulence. In addition to the presenting complaints and appearance of the cervix, wet preparations, KOH smears, Gram stains, and Pap smear help distinguish the causative organism. Treatment consists of the appropriate antimicrobial drugs for both the patient and any sexual contact.

Chronic cervicitis may follow one of the acute infections described above, but a more likely cause is pathologic invasion of vaginal microflora, particularly streptococci or staphylococci. Chronic inflammation leads to cellular infiltration of the mucous membrane as well as deeper cervical layers. Patients complain of a persistence discharge that is thick and viscous, like egg white. Occasionally, the discharge is mucopurulent. Lower abdominal discomfort and coital pain are other symptoms. Two presentations may be noted on speculum exam. In one, most of the cervical surface appears normal, but the endocervix is thickened and a wide reddish area (erosion) sometimes dotted with translucent or opaque retention cysts radiates from the os. In the other, the entire cervix appears large and hypertrophic, with an infected and swollen mucous membrane extending from the os. Given the abnormal appearance of the cervix, patients should be referred for colposcopic exam and biopsy. If biopsy reports are negative, the treatment is long-term antimicrobials guided by cultures and sensitivities. Cervical intraepithelial neoplasm, discussed below, is treated with cryotherapy, cauterization, or conization.

Cervicitis is one of the risk factors for ***cervical carcinoma,*** particularly if the infectious agent is herpes virus type 2 or certain strains of human papilloma virus (HPV) responsible for condyloma acuminata. Most likely to develop in women who have a history of early and frequent coitus and multiple sex partners, cervical carcinoma is the second most common malignancy of the female reproductive tract. The earliest histologic change is abnormal proliferation of epithelial cells, referred to as "dysplasia" or "cervical intraepithelial neoplasm (CIN)." In mild cases (CIN I), dysplastic cells are confined to the lower one-third of the epithelium. They can revert to normal spontaneously. On the other hand, they may extend into deeper layers of the epithelium, severe dysplasia (CIN III) being characterized by abnormal cells in two-thirds of the epithelium. Most cases of CIN III progress to ***carcinoma in situ*** (intraepithelial carcinoma), in which the full thickness of the epithelium consists of abnormal cells. Dysplasia and carcinoma in situ produce few if any warning symptoms. Postcoital bleeding sometimes occurs, but even this does not usually develop until the later stages. In order to detect problems early, ▶ ***Pap smear screening*** is extremely important. Beginning at the age at which she becomes sexually active or by age 18–20, every woman should have a regular Pap smear examination. The American Cancer Society recommends Pap smears every three years after two normal Pap smears have been obtained a year apart, but the American College of Obstetricians and Gynecologists and many individual providers advocate yearly screening. The specimen must be correctly collected and sent to a reliable laboratory. Laboratories should report the smears in descriptive terms, using either traditional or more recent classifications, as noted in Table 9.8. Women whose Pap smear reveals mildly atypical cells should be reexamined for cervicitis or vaginitis and treated accordingly. Following treatment, the Pap smear should be repeated in 3 months. If the repeated smear is still abnormal, the patient should be referred for colposcopic exam. Any woman with signs of an abnormal cervix on exam or dysplasia on the Pap smear should also be referred for colposcopy. Depending on the colposcopic findings, further treatment such as cryotherapy may be indicated. With correct screening and early intervention, complete cures for cervical carcinoma are possible with fairly noninvasive procedures. However, more advanced disease must be staged (Table 9.9) and treated with surgery, radiation therapy, and/or chemotherapy.

Diethylstilbestrol (DES) exposure refers to the synthetic estrogen prescribed from the 1940s through 1971 for pregnant women who were diabetic or had a high risk of miscarriage. It was later found not only that DES probably did not help maintain the pregnancy but also that children of mothers who took this drug were at greater risk for potentially serious health problems. The length of use, dosage, and

TABLE 9.8 PAP SMEAR CLASSIFICATIONS

Class	Traditional Definition	Newer Definition
I	Normal	No premalignant or malignant cells; specific infections identified
II	Inflammation with or without atypia	Mildly atypical squamous cells; specific infections identified
III	Changes suggestive of cancer (dysplasia)	Mild or moderate to severe squamous cell dysplasia (CIN I–II)
IV	Highly suggestive of cancer	Severe squamous cell dysplasia or carcinoma in situ (CIN III)
V	Diagnostic of cancer	Invasive cancer
Unclassified	No such category	Atypical repair; endometrial cells in postmenopausal smear; atrophy versus carcinoma, etc.

Source: Luff MD: Abnormal Pap smears: Newer approaches to class II evaluation, *Consultant,* November, 1984. Used with permission.

TABLE 9.9 STAGES OF CERVICAL CANCER

Stage	Description
O	Preinvasive cancer (CIN). Positive CIN status not included in therapeutic statistics of cervical cancer.
I	Carcinoma limited to cervix.
A	Microinvasive (early stromal invasion).
B	Other than microinvasive.
II	Carcinoma extends beyond the cervix but not to the lower third of the vagina or pelvic wall.
A	No parametrial involvement.
B	Parametrial involvement.
III	Extended pelvic involvement.
A	Involvement of the lower third of the vagina, but no extension to the pelvic wall (cancer-free space noted on rectal exam).
B	Extends to pelvic wall (on rectal exam, no cancer-free space) and/or associated with hydronephrosis or nonfunctioning kidney.
IV	Extension beyond the true pelvis or involvement of bladder/rectal mucosa.
A	Limited to adjacent organs.
B	Spread to distant organs.

time take during pregnancy (adverse effects are most likely to occur in the first 5 months of gestation) all influence the risk of problems. As the DES daughters reached sexual maturity, data began to accumulate that linked drug exposure to an increased risk of clear cell adenocarcinoma, an uncommon malignancy affecting the vagina and cervix. This risk is still small, estimated at approximately 1 case per 8,000 DES daughters. About one-third of DES daughters have vaginal and/or cervical abnormalities, including vaginal adenosis and septa; hooded, hypoplastic, rimmed, or cockscomb cervix; pseudopolyp; and a T-shaped uterine cavity. Women exposed to DES in utero are at greater risk for early abortion, ectopic pregnancy, and premature birth during their childbearing years.

Half of the DES-exposed population is male. Many studies have shown abnormalities of the reproductive tract in a significant number of DES sons. These include varicocele, meatal stenosis, micropenis, epididymal cysts, hypoplastic and undescended testes, abnormal sperm, oligospermia, and infertility. A direct association between DES exposure and malignancy in men has not been established; however, any man with cryptorchidism is at greater risk for testicular cancer and should be promptly referred for evaluation and treatment.

Since DES-exposed men and women have not reached age 50, the long-term multisystemic effects have not been investigated completely. Those born between 1940 and 1971 should attempt to determine if their mothers used DES. A history of diabetes, prior miscarriage, abnormal bleeding, or a pregnancy that was almost lost suggests a DES prescription. If questioning of the parents is unproductive, medical records from the obstetrician or hospital should be obtained if possible. A list of the trade names under which DES was marketed may be found in Table 9.10. There is no treatment for DES exposure. ▶ ***Screening women exposed to DES*** for early detection of malignancy is of prime importance. Specially obtained Pap smears should be instituted near menarche, usually around age 14. Staining of the vaginal vault with Lugol's iodine may reveal abnormal areas that will not pick up stain and should be biopsied. Colposcopy is also recommended initially and possibly intermittently.

TABLE 9.10 TRADE NAMES OF DES

Oral Nonsteroidal Estrogens			
Benzestrol	Domestrol	Mikarol forti	Stilbetin
Chlorotrianisene	Estilben	Milestrol	Stilbinol
Comestrol	Estrobene	Monomestrol	Stilboestroform
Cyren A	Estrobene DP	Neo-Oestranol I	Stilboestrol
Cyren B	Estrosyn	Neo-Oestranol II	Stilboestrol DP
Delvinal	Fonatol	Nulabort	Stilestrate
DES	Gynben	Oestorgenine	Stilpalmitate
DesPlex	Gyneben	Oestromenin	Stilphostrol
Dibestil	Hexestrol	Oestromon	Stilronate
Diestryl	Hexoestrol	Orestol	Stilrone
Dienestrol	Hi-Bestrol	Pabestrol D	Stils
Dienoestrol	Menocrin	Palestrol	Synestrin
Diethylstilbestrol	Meprane	Restrol	Syndestrol
Dipalmitate	Mestilbol	Stil-Rol	Synthoestrin
Diethylstilbestrol	Methallenestril	Stilbal	TACE
Dipropionate	Microest	Stilbestrol	Vallestril
Diethylstilbenediol	Mikarol	Stilbestronate	Willestrol
Digestil			
Oral Nonsteroidal Estrogen-Progesterone Combination			
Progravidium			
Vaginal Preparations with Nonsteroidal Estrogens			
AVC cream with Dienestrol			
Dienestrol cream			

Source: National Institutes of Health, NIH Publication No. 80-1118, Washington, D.C., revised March 1980.

▶ ***DES information/organizations*** offer important education and support for patients.

Vagina

The cervix protrudes into the 9- to 10-cm-long vaginal canal. It is surrounded by the cup-shaped upper end of the canal (fornix). During intercourse, sperm are deposited in the posterior fornix, where they have direct access to the cervical os. The reception and transport of sperm is facilitated by the vagina in other ways as well. Though normally collapsed, the muscular walls of the vagina can distend considerably to allow penetration of an engorged penis. During intercourse, they constrict around the penis, providing tactile stimulation that leads to ejaculation. Finally, a mucous membrane lines the vaginal walls, producing lubricants to facilitate intercourse.

At birth, the vaginal introitus is covered by a delicate membrane with no apparent physiologic function called the hymen. Thin and flexible, the hymen normally perforates and regresses as the child develops. Later, residual hymen tissue may tear when a finger, tampon, or penis is introduced into the vagina for the first time, causing a show of blood. This is normal. However, the persistence of an ***imperforate hymen*** leads to a potentially serious complication. Though it may go unnoticed during childhood, a thick, fibrous hymen that remains intact seals off the vaginal canal, preventing the escape of blood once the girl begins to menstruate. The blood collects in the vagina ***(hematocolpos)*** and eventually backs up through the uterus and into the tubes. Seepage of blood into the peritoneum initiates peritonitis. Patients present with abdominal pain, fever, and rebound tenderness. WBC counts and

TABLE 9.11 SOME ORGANISMS THAT MAY INHABIT THE VAGINA WITHOUT PATHOLOGIC COLONIZATION

Lactobacillus	Gram-negative rods
Gram-positive cocci	*Escherichia coli*
Staphylococcus epidermidis	*Proteus*
Beta-hemolytic streptococcus group B	*Klebsiella*
Alpha-hemolytic streptococcus	*Enterobacter*
Nonhemolytic streptococcus	Anaerobic bacteroids
Group D streptococci	

the ESR may be elevated. The problem is diagnosed by visual inspection of the introitus, which shows the intact, bulging membrane. It is quickly corrected with surgical perforation.

The breakdown of glycogen by vaginal mucosal cells produces lactic acid, which helps to keep the vaginal environment highly acidic (pH 3.5–4.5). Lactobacilli, normally found in great numbers in the vaginal canal, may also be involved in acidogenesis. The acidic environment allows a wide range of flora to survive but prevents their disease-producing colonization. Some of these organisms are listed in Table 9.11.

Infectious invasion of the vaginal mucosa leads to inflammation or ***vaginitis.*** Trichomonas, herpes, condylomata, gardnerella, and monilia are common causes; they are discussed in a later section on sexually transmitted disease. Vaginitis may also follow allergic reactions to soaps, laundry detergents, bath oils, feminine deodorant sprays, douches, and spermicides. Finally, it can be initiated by a forgotten tampon or diaphragm, a retained condom, or excessive intercourse. Almost all patients present with vaginal itching, burning, and/or discharge. Many complain of dysuria and pain with intercourse as well. Exam reveals inflammation, swelling, and edema of vulvar tissue and/or vaginal walls. A vaginal discharge may also be present. A saline wet mount probably provides the most important diagnostic clues but should be substantiated with KOH preparations, cultures, and possibly Gram stains. In cases of sexually transmitted diseases, treatment consists of an appropriate antimicrobial drug for the patient as well as her sexual contacts. Preventive measures should also be discussed. Frequent douching (alters pH) and sitting in wet bathing suits or sweaty gym clothes (traps body heat and moisture) should be avoided, along with deodorized or colored toilet paper, deodorized tampons, vaginal sprays, and bath salts and oils (common allergens). Loose-fitting clothing and underwear with cotton crotches are advisable.

Toxic shock syndrome (TSS) is a rare but serious febrile illness caused by exotoxins produced by certain strains of *Staphylococcus aureus.* It may occur in men and women at any time but most commonly strikes girls between the ages of 15 and 19 during menstruation. The loci of the pathogenic *Staphylococcus* have been traced to wound or surgical infections, boils, osteomyelitis, endocarditis, and, most commonly, to the vagina. In the last case, the organism is probably transferred from the nasal passages or vaginal labia via the hands. Indeed, vaginal *Staphylococcus* is more commonly isolated in women who use diaphragms, IUDs, and tampons, all of which require frequent insertion of fingers into the vagina. Although many women seem to carry vaginal *Staphylococcus,* only 1 in 10,000 ever develop TSS. The reason for this is unclear. Menstruation and tampon use are highly associated with disease.

Bacterial growth is favored by vaginal pH changes associated with menstruation, as well as the blood itself. Tampons, which absorb and retain the blood, create a particularly fertile medium. By creating small abrasions in vaginal epithelia, insertion of tampons may provide the entrance for exotoxins into the bloodstream. Oxygen tension may be another factor, *Staphylococcus* growth being impeded by the normally anaerobic environment of the vaginal canal. Oxygen may be introduced into the vaginal canal with insertion of tampons or with distention of the vaginal opening and walls when tampons are in place. Rely, a superabsorbent brand of tampon associated with a high proportion of TSS cases, has been taken off the market. In addition, all tampons are now mandated by the Food and Drug Administration (FDA) to carry a warning about TSS.

The symptoms of TSS, which are often severe, appear quickly. They include high fever (often greater than 102°F), vomiting, diarrhea, dizziness, fainting, and a sunburn-like rash. Aching muscles, red eyes, and a sore throat are other symptoms. Patients suspected of having TSS should be hospitalized. The criteria for diagnosis are noted in Table 9.12. Developing within 72 hours of onset, hypotension is the most dangerous, sometimes life-threatening, element of the disease. Electrolyte imbalance, thrombocytopenia, and renal and hepatic damage are also possible. Cultures of local infections, blood, urine, throat, and, if appropriate, cerebrospinal fluid (CSF) and vagina should be taken. SMAC, CBC, and platelet counts should also be followed. Treatment consists of cardiovascular support (maintaining blood pressure and fluids) and antibiotics. Abscesses should be drained. Initially, patients should be covered with broad-spectrum agents until sepsis or any other specific infection is ruled out. Although there is no evidence that antistaphylococcal antibiotics affect the acute course of disease, they do reduce the risk of recurrence in menstrually associated TSS. For this reason, a semisynthetic penicillin or first-generation cephalosporin is given for 7–10 days during the next three to four menstrual cycles. Avoidance of tampon use by women who have a history of TSS also reduces the risk

TABLE 9.12 DIAGNOSTIC CRITERIA OF TSS[a]

Fever (>102°F)
Rash (diffuse macular erythroderma) with desquamation (particularly of the palms and soles) 1–2 weeks after onset of illness
Hypotension or orthostatic syncope
Other etiologies ruled out:
Cultures of blood, throat, CSF
Serologic tests for Rocky Mountain spotted fever, leptospirosis, measles
Involvement of organ systems (three or more)
GI tract (vomiting or diarrhea at onset of illness)
Muscles (severe myalgia and/or creatinine phosphokinase elevations[b])
Mucous membranes (hyperemia of vaginal, oropharyngeal, or conjunctival membranes)
Renal (BUN/creatinine elevations[b]; pyuria without evidence of urinary tract infection)
Hepatic (bilirubin, SGOT, or SGPT elevations[b])
Hematologic (thrombocytopenia)
CNS (disorientation or altered consciousness without focal neurologic signs other than those associated with hypotension or fever)

Source: Centers for Disease Control MMWR 1980, 29:441–445

[a]Definite TSS when all criteria are present. Probable TSS in the presence of three or more criteria with desquamation or five or more criteria without desquamation.
[b]Twice the upper limit of normal for the laboratory.

of recurrence. Steroids have been given for 3–4 days at the beginning of acute cases. It is reported that they ameliorate and shorten the course of the illness. However, this practice may favor recurrence and needs further study before being recommended. With immediate intervention, most TSS patients begin to recover within 1–2 weeks. At this time desquamation, particularly of the palms of the hands and soles of the feet, usually occurs; it may result in some loss of hair. Full return to previous feelings of well-being and energy levels takes many months. Death or permanent sequelae are now uncommon. For prevention, primary care providers should educate patients, particularly menstruating women, about ▶***measures to minimize the danger of TSS.***

The muscular vaginal walls support the bladder, urethra, rectum, and bowel. Weakening of the walls from obstetric injury, age, excessive abdominal straining, or spinal cord injury can lead to various types of ***vaginal hernias. Cystocele,*** herniation of the bladder wall, causes anterior vaginal fullness, which can be observed on exam and felt by the patient. Cystocele is often accompanied by ***urethrocele,*** which is not a hernia but the sagging of the urethra following its detachment from the symphysis pubis due to childbirth. In addition to the sensation of fullness, both problems may interfere with complete emptying of the bladder. The presence of residual urine then contributes to frequency (though only small amounts may be voided) and sometimes to cystitis. Stress incontinence (uncontrolled seepage of urine with laughing, sneezing, coughing, or straining) is also common. ***Rectocele*** is herniation of the rectum through the vaginal floor. Often following traumatic delivery of a large infant, it causes constipation or a sense of rectovaginal fullness from the presence of feces in the rectocele pouch. Bowel straining increases rectocele size. ***Enterocele*** is the herniation of a pouch of small bowel through the vaginal floor. It is recognized by a bulging high up on the rectovaginal septum during rectovaginal exam, which is noted most prominently when the patient bears down while in a standing position. Enteroceles produce a sense of weight in the pelvis and contribute to constipation. Symptomatic vaginal hernias can be surgically corrected. Most patients, however, do well with supportive measures alone—a high-fiber diet for constipation, weight reduction, and limitation of lifting or straining. Pessaries provide temporary relief in some cases. The Kegel exercise is an important preventive measure but is of little value once the muscular walls become stretched and damaged.

Vaginal carcinoma is an uncommon malignancy that accounts for approximately 1% of gynecologic cancers. The most common type is squamous cell carcinoma; it develops almost exclusively in postmenopausal women. Other types, including clear cell adenocarcinoma linked with DES exposure, may affect younger women. Squamous cell lesions usually originate in the upper third of the vagina, with metastases likely to affect the rectum and bladder. The tumor ulcerates, and during intercourse or trauma, pain and bleeding can occur. The ulcerated tumor may produce a watery discharge or become secondarily infected. During the pelvic exam, slow extraction of the speculum with careful visualization of the vaginal vault is necessary to identify suspicious lesions. An abnormal cell structure will show up on the Pap smear only if the involved area is sampled. When the vagina is stained with iodine solution, cancerous areas (which do not contain glycogen) will not stain. These areas should be biopsied. Surgical excision of the carcinoma is indicated (hysterectomy and/or upper vaginectomy) and may be combined with radiation therapy. The 5-year survival rate, depending on the existence of metastases, is usually less than 50%.

Vulva

The vulva includes the external opening of the vaginal canal (introitus, vaginal orifice), the labia minora and majora, and the clitoris (see Fig. 9.3). Homologous to the penis, the clitoris is a small erectile organ, the major focus of female sexual stimulation. Richly endowed with blood vessels and nerves, it is covered by the upper folds of the labia minora. Secretions of the sebaceous glands in this area can become trapped under the labial folds, causing ***clitoritis,*** an irritation and inflammation similar to balanitis (see the previous section).

Bartholin's glands are two bean-sized glands situated deep in the perineum on both sides of the vaginal introitus. Bartholin's ducts, the glands' openings located at the base of the labia majora on either side of the vaginal orifice, are generally not visible. In function, Bartholin's glands are believed to parallel the bulbourethral glands in the man. During sexual arousal, they secrete small amounts of mucus to lubricate the vestibule. The area of Bartholin's glands should be felt during the exam of the external genitalia. When enlarged, Bartholin's glands become palpable and frequently visible.

Local inflammation and infections such as gonorrhea can cause ▶ ***acute bartholinitis.*** Patients develop vulvar pain, swelling, and erythema, as well as dyspareunia. A thorough pelvic exam and appropriate laboratory studies (wet mount, gonorrhea culture) should be done to look for pathogenic organisms. Pending the results, patients should be started on broad-spectrum antibiotics and warm soaks.

Chronic bartholinitis may follow the acute inflammation. It is characterized by persistent small nodular swelling of the gland, which is apparent only on careful palpation. Patients are usually asymptomatic and require no treatment.

A common sequela of bartholinitis is stenosis of Bartholin's duct(s). Secretions are unable to drain, leading to a swollen, not necessarily tender, gland referred to as ***Bartholin's cyst.*** Bartholin's cysts may also occur when the ducts become obstructed for no apparent reason. If the patient is asymptomatic, they require no specific treatment and often resolve spontaneously or after application of warm soaks. If the cyst becomes infected, however, ***Bartholin's abscess*** may form. It is marked by fluctuation, redness, and possibly enormous swelling of the entire labium. A purulent exudate can often be expressed from the duct with gentle pressure. Bartholin's abscess requires immediate incision and drainage. An indwelling Word catheter inserted into the affected gland aids drainage and forms a new duct when the natural duct is too stenotic to function. Other important aspects of treatment include antibiotics, bed rest, analgesics, and warm compresses.

Numerous sebaceous glands are found in the labia. Sebum, a mixture of oil, waxes, and triglycerides, cholesterol, and cellular debris, produced by these glands, lubricates the skin and, along with the secretions of sweat glands, forms a waterproof protective barrier against urine, feces, menstrual blood, and bacterial infection. These same protective secretions, however, can lead to vulvular irritation when retained against the skin by tight synthetic underwear, girdles, pantyhose, and slacks. In addition, painful pea-sized ***sebaceous cysts*** are a not uncommon development as glandular ducts are blocked by inflammation or sebum retention. Most of these cysts drain spontaneously and require no treatment, but some become secondarily infected and must be surgically excised. Other ***benign lesions of the vulva*** are described in Table 9.13.

After uterine and ovarian cancer, ***vulvar carcinoma*** is the third most common

TABLE 9.13 BENIGN LESIONS OF THE VULVA

Lesion	Description
Bartholin cyst	Cystic mass felt lateral to the inferior vaginal opening. Caused by obstruction of Bartholin's duct and accumulation of fluid in the gland.
Sebaceous cyst	White, raised, painless lesions on vulva. Caused by obstruction of sebaceous glands with accumulation of sebum. May be locally excised.
Hidradenoma	Small, raised, nodular cystic or solid tumor arising from vulvar sweat glands; overlying skin may be reddened, glandular, or ulcerated.
Fibroma	Firm, pedunculated (sometimes smooth) subcutaneous nodules arising from vulvar fibrous tissue. Caused by proliferation of fibroblasts.
Lipoma	Soft, solid mass usually seen on labia majora. Arises from adipose tissue in vulva.
Condylomata acuminata	Warty growths of various sizes. May appear in clusters. May be sexually transmitted.
Angioma	Solid tumor consisting of blood or lymph vessels. May be congenital.
Granular cell myoblastoma	Irregular clumps of large, pale-staining cells with eosinophilic cytoplasmic granules that arise from myelin sheath of nerves.
Neurofibroma	Small, fleshy, pinkish-tan, polypoid mass that arises from the neural sheath. Usually asymptomatic. No treatment necessary.
Nevus	Pigmented lesion (mole) with malignant potential. Should be surgically excised.
Sebaceous adenoma	Raised, yellow-tan nodule (round or oval). May be pedunculated. Premalignant. Should be surgically excised.
Cystic epidermal inclusion	Round, white, yellow, or orange lesion that constantly drains a thick, purulent exudate. Caused by retention of squamous epithelia beneath skin or mucosa.

type of primary pelvic cancer. Luckily, it involves a less occult area than the others and thus allows earlier detection. Squamous cell carcinoma accounts for most cases. Usually developing in postmenopausal women, it is initially marked by a white or red ulcerated, granulomatous, and/or raised lesion appearing on any part of the vulva. The lesion enlarges steadily, with increased induration, ulceration, and surrounding edema, until there is significant vulvar tissue destruction and atrophy. The cancerous squamous cells may spread to the perineum and rectum or to the urethra and bladder; distant metastases may follow involvement of the inguinal and femoral lymphatics. In contrast are the relatively noninvasive intraepithelial lesions usually seen in young women aged 20–39. They appear as slightly elevated multicentric patches that may be reddish, whitish, or pigmented. Intraepithelial lesions are thought to be causally associated with sexually transmitted diseases (particularly herpes virus type 2, human papilloma virus, and chlamydia).

The suspicion of vulvar cancer should be aroused by a local itch, irritation, or bleeding of an atypical vulvar lesion. Any unusual lesion should be biopsied. The differential diagnosis includes local cysts or lesions of lymphogranuloma venereum or syphilis. Early diagnosis is important, since carcinomas less than 3 cm in diameter without inguinal lymph node enlargement are associated with a 90% 5-year survival rate after excision. Larger lesions and those with metastases require more radical disfiguring surgery (vulvectomy) and are associated with a 5-year survival rate of less than 25%. Full vulvectomy is rarely necessary in cases of intraepithelial lesions. Localized excision of a unifocal lesion with a 1-cm margin around the tumor is usually curative. Skinning vulvectomy, chemotherapy, and laser therapy are also effective.

Menopause

The influence of ovarian hormones has been discussed throughout this chapter. With bilateral oophorectomy for any reason prior to age 50, ▶ ***surgical menopause*** results from the sudden cessation of ovarian hormone production. Surgical menopause encompasses all of the changes occurring with natural menopause (see the subsequent discussion), but at a greatly accelerated rate and at an earlier age than normal. To prevent early tissue changes (particularly osteoporosis) and to alleviate uncomfortable vasomotor symptoms, hormone replacement is usually given.

Depending on the genetic predisposition, ▶ ***natural menopause*** occurs between the ages of 35 and 60 (50 being the average). Defined as the cessation of menses, it develops in three phases, as described in Table 9.14. The menopausal phase includes

TABLE 9.14 PHYSIOLOGIC PHASES OF MENOPAUSE

Phase	Discussion
Premenopausal	After age 40, ovaries begin to decline. This causes variability in the amount of estrogen and progesterone secretions. During some months the ovaries function normally, resulting in regular ovulation and menstruation. During others, they secrete abnormally low amounts of estrogen, resulting in anovulation and scantier periods, or abnormally high amounts of estrogen, resulting in anovulation and longer, heavier periods. During anovulatory cycles, there is no progesterone to block the flow of estrogen. This may lead to rapid growth of fibroid tumors and/or overgrowth of the endometrial lining and abnormal uterine bleeding. The latter frequently requires D&C to stop bleeding and rule out endometrial cancer. Unchecked estrogen flow can produce fluid retention, causing breast tenderness, a bloated feeling in the abdomen, fatigue, and irritability. The premenopausal phase may last as long as 5 years before actual menopause begins.
Menopausal	By age 50 the ovaries have declined significantly. During some months, they fail to produce any estrogen. Estrogen withdrawal may affect the autonomic nervous system, causing vasomotor instability. Heart palpitations may be quickly triggered by fatigue or stress. Capillaries in the skin (particularly in "blush areas") may open suddenly. "Hot flashes" and night sweats then result from the rush of blood. Occurring once a month to 20 times a day, they may last for a few months or up to a year. Cycles marked by lack of estrogen are also marked by anovulation, lack of progesterone, and amenorrhea. After 12 consecutive months without a period, menopause has arrived. Due to the estrogen decline, it may be associated with decreased muscle strength and elasticity (stiffness, tension, or weakness may be noticed); decreased caloric requirement (if caloric intake is not adjusted, weight gain occurs); decreased elasticity of skin (wrinkles appear); slowing of GI motility (gas and constipation may become bothersome); and CNS changes (recent memory may become uncertain or patients may be vulnerable to emotional low periods).
Postmenopausal	After the menopausal transition, the body becomes adjusted to lower estrogen levels. However, some effects of decreased estrogen are cumulative. They cause changes that appear some time after menopause. Within 6 months to 10 years, vaginal atrophy occurs (the vagina becomes shorter, narrower, and less elastic, with a thinner wall and reduced secretions). Loss of muscle, ligament, and connective tissue elasticity may lead to uterine prolapse or vaginal hernias such as cystocele or rectocele (pelvic discomfort, stress incontinence, or constipation may complicate the picture). The growth and tone of hair on the head decrease, while the growth of facial hair increases. With estrogen withdrawal, there is increased rate of bone loss. In over half of the female population, it depletes bone mass below the level needed for mechanical support (osteoporosis).

a period of ovarian decline (climacteric) that may last for 1 or 2 years. The climacteric is initiated by the dwindling ability of follicle cells to produce estradiol. Estradiol withdrawal disrupts the hypothalamic-pituitary-ovarian axis. At first, this leads to increased FSH levels, manifested by shortened menstrual cycles. However, as estradiol withdrawal continues, the follicles fail to develop and anovulation results. Menstrual cycles become lengthened and irregular, and eventually menses stop altogether.

In addition to amenorrhea, climacteric women often experience ***vasomotor instability*** from disturbance of hypothalamic temperature control and compensatory peripheral vasodilatation. Sometimes preceded by a chill, peripheral vasodilatation begins in the lower chest and rises to the head and neck. It is marked by flushing (particularly facial) followed by drenching sweats. Occurring one to two times a day or even every half hour and lasting for periods ranging from a few seconds to an hour, these "hot flashes" may be triggered by a warm environment, exercise, eating, or emotional stress. In some women they disappear in a few weeks; in others, not for years.

When estradiol levels fall during the climacteric, the body turns to estrone as its major source of estrogen. Estrone is converted mainly from androstenedione (which is produced by adrenal glands), and thus androstenedione levels increase. Testosterone production by the declining ovary also increases, rendering the endocrine milieu of the postmenopausal woman androgenic. As a result, many body tissues change with menopause (see Table 9.14).

In the vagina, the tissue lining tends to shrink, rugae disappear, and the mucosal surfaces become dry and thin. Lubrication is scant, causing dyspareunia as well as local tenderness, pruritis, and dysuria. Thinned tissues may fissure and bleed after intercourse. A vaginal discharge, stemming from irritation of the delicate mucosa, may develop as well. This condition is referred to as ***atrophic vaginitis.*** A history of onset after the menopause, characteristic symptoms, and a pelvic exam aid in making the diagnosis. A wet mount reveals mostly parabasal cells, with the absence of specific pathogens unless there is concurrent infection. In any case of abnormal vaginal bleeding in the postmenopausal woman, the suspicion of malignancy must be maintained.

Atrophic vaginitis, severe vasomotor instability, and osteoporosis are indications for estrogen replacement. Due to the risk of gynecologic cancer and cardiovascular disease, estrogen replacements should not be given if the following conditions are present: breast or estrogen-dependent neoplasm, undiagnosed vaginal bleeding, active thrombophlebitis, or a history of thromboembolic disease. They should also be withheld if pregnancy is known or suspected. The drugs should be titrated to the lowest dose required to control symptoms and should be continued for the shortest possible time. They should be discontinued if nausea, vomiting, abdominal cramps, bloating, headaches, dizziness, depression, or breast changes (tenderness, enlargement, secretion) ensue. For the duration of therapy, patients should be followed on a twice-yearly basis; some clinicians advocate routine endometrial washings or biopsy at these visits, even in asymptomatic women.

In addition to physical changes, women are subject to a developmental crisis during the climacteric as their fertility status changes and children leave the home. It is important to note, however, that menopause is not normally associated with depression. On the other hand, an exaggerated response to menopause can be an important clue to underlying depression. These problems are discussed in Chapter 13.

BREASTS

The female breast (Figs. 9.6 and 9.7) belongs functionally to the reproductive system, and the male breast is discussed here as its counterpart. However, the breasts are actually part of the integument.

Male Breast

Each breast consists of 15–20 modified sweat glands separated into lobes by bands of connective tissue. The lobes converge toward the nipple in a spoke-like pattern. Typical of all sweat glands, secretory mammary cells (acini) line sac-like structures called "alveoli." Grouped in grape-like clusters on a stalk, alveoli stem into an enlarging system of collecting ducts (lactiferous ducts). Both the alveoli and the ducts are surrounded by specialized contractile cells (myoepithelial cells). After widening into an ampulla, three to five lacteriferous ducts from each gland open onto the surface of the nipple. A pigmented area around the nipple (areola) contains several large sebaceous glands that open to the surface in small papillae.

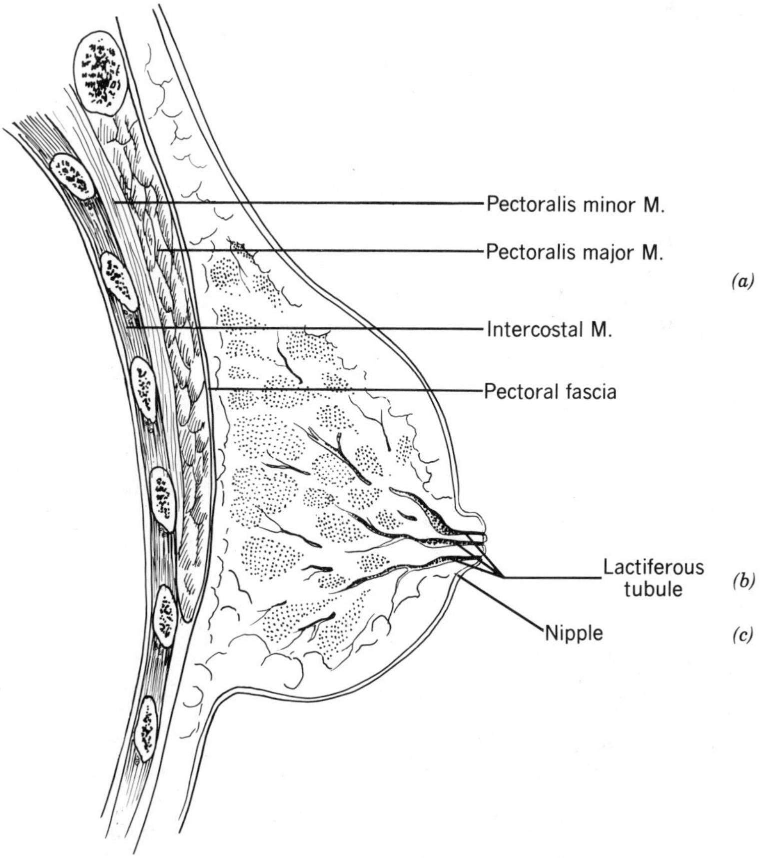

Figure 9.6 Breasts—sagittal section: (*a*) muscles; (*b*) lactiferous tubules; (*c*) nipple.

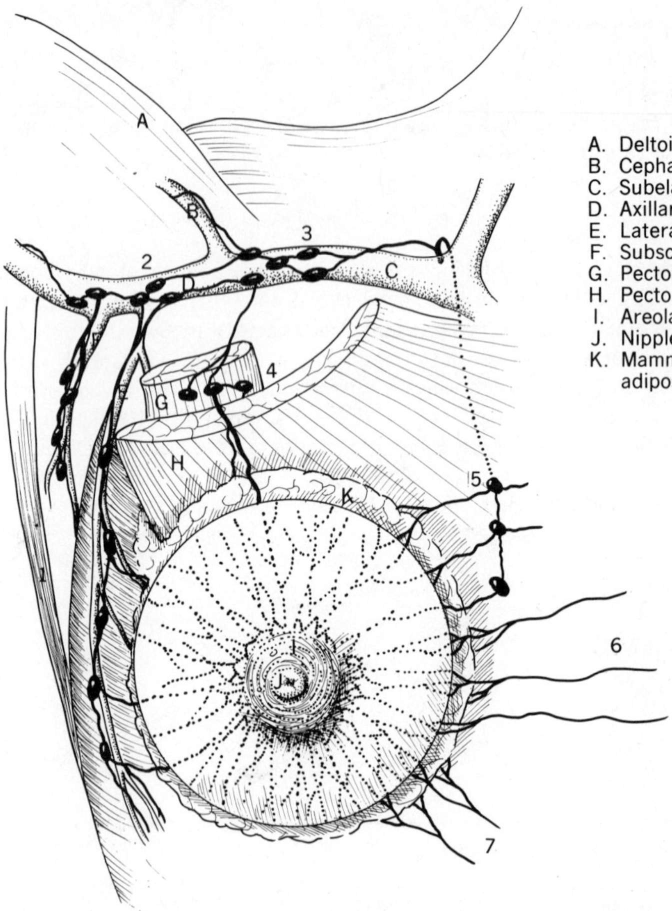

A. Deltoid muscle
B. Cephalic vein
C. Subclavian vein
D. Axillary vein
E. Lateral thoracic vein
F. Subscapular vein
G. Pectoralis minor muscle
H. Pectoralis major muscle
I. Areola
J. Nipple
K. Mammary gland with adipose tissue

(a) Superficial
1. Anterior pectoral group
2. Central axillary
3. Subclavian nodes

(b) Deep
4. Rotter's lymph nodes
5. Internal mammary nodes
6. Cross-mammary pathway
7. Paramammary pathway

Figure 9.7 Lymphatic drainage of the breast: (*a*) superficial; (*b*) deep.

During fetal life, acinar cells may be stimulated by high levels of pregnancy hormones. The newborn then demonstrates some engorgement of breast tissue and may actually secrete small amounts of fluid referred to as ***witch's milk.*** Following withdrawal of the mother's estrogen and progesterone, neonatal breast tissue regresses and secretory activity ceases. Composed of only a few scattered ducts, supported by dense collagenous tissue and loose connective tissue, male breasts remain small throughout life.

Excessive development of one or both breasts in the male is called ***gynecomastia.*** There may be ductal hyperplasia and lobular formation with some secretory activity,

TABLE 9.15 CONDITIONS ASSOCIATED WITH GYNECOMASTIA

Benign hypertrophy With puberty With old age (particularly with weight gain) With sudden weight gain after prolonged illness Organic disease Liver disease (cirrhosis, hepatoma) Hyperthyroidism Adrenal disease (Addison's disease, feminizing adrenal tumors) Testicular disease (tumors, hypogonadism) Breast cancer	Drugs Hormones (estrogens, androgens, HCG) Antihypertensives (reserpine, spironolactone, methyldopa) Antineoplastic agent Digitalis Cimetidine Isoniazid Psychiatric drugs (phenothiazines, tricyclic antidepressants, amphetamines, diazepam)

or an increase in dense connective and adipose tissue. Afflicting 40% of boys between the ages of 14 and 15, ***pubertal gynecomastia*** is related to minor hormonal disruptions that decrease the ratio of testosterone to estradiol. It resolves spontaneously within a few months to 2 years but can be painful and embarrassing.

Adult-onset gynecomastia is related to more severe estrogen-androgen imbalances associated with congenital or acquired endocrine diseases, tumors, or drugs (Table 9.15). Patients seek medical attention for the altered breast appearance. Breast enlargement from excess adipose tissue may also be seen in the obese patient. In such cases, careful palpation of the breast fails to reveal the ridgy glandular changes that occur with true gynecomastia. Any adult who presents with gynecomastia should be worked up for one of the conditions listed in Table 9.15. Treatment aims at curing or removing the causative problem. Androgen replacement can reverse the changes in many cases. However, long-standing hypertrophy causes irreversible tissue changes. In such cases, patients may be offered cosmetic mastectomy.

Male breast cancer is a rare but serious disease. As in women, hormonal influences (high estrogen levels, shift in the androgen:estrogen ratio, or abnormal susceptibility of breast tissue to estrogen concentrations) may play a role in the pathogenesis. The average age of onset is the sixth decade. Patients present with a painless breast lump commonly preceded by gynecomastia. A discharge, retraction, ulceration, or erosion of the nipple may be associated. Examination reveals a hard, ill-defined, nontender mass located under the areola. The work-up and staging are similar to those for female breast cancer (see the later discussion). Unfortunately, blood-borne metastasis of malignant cells has usually occurred by the time the patient seeks medical attention. Leading to immediate tumor growth in distant sites or remaining latent for several years, it is responsible for a poorer prognosis in men with breast cancer than women. In operable patients, treatment consists of modified radical mastectomy. Metastatic disease localized to the skin, lymph nodes, or bone is treated with irradiation. Disseminated disease is managed with chemotherapy and endocrine manipulation (including estrogens and corticosteroids, as well as castration and bilateral adrenalectomy).

Female Breast

Throughout fetal life and childhood, the female breast (see Figs. 9.6 and 9.7) remains histologically and functionally similar to the male breast (see the previous section). However, with activation of the hypothalamic-pituitary-ovarian axis at puberty, the female duct system enlarges, and adipose tissue begins to deposit around the surface of the glands just under the skin. Connective tissue, vascularity, and elasticity increase as well, and breasts begin to develop.

In the United States, 95% of girls experience breast budding by age 12 and full breast maturity by age 15 or 16. Primary amenorrhea or delayed puberty may result in absent development ***(aplasia)*** or underdevelopment ***(hypoplasia),*** respectively. These problems have been previously discussed. Due to the insensitivity of breast tissue to hormone stimulation, the breasts sometimes fail to develop in the girl who has regular menses and no other endocrine abnormalities. Unlike other forms of the problem, hormone therapy is not helpful and is contraindicated due to the risk of thromboembolism and other toxic effects. Breast implants may be considered for cosmetic reasons.

Hormonal hypersecretion (secondary to ovarian, adrenal, or pituitary tumors) or hypersensitivity of the breast to normal levels of circulating hormones can lead to undue enlargement known as ***breast hypertrophy*** (macromastia). Affecting one or both breasts, the problem may also develop in pregnancy from high levels of estrogen and progesterone. It may be of psychologic as well as physical concern. Hypertrophied breast tissue is associated with retracted, ulcerated nipples and intertriginous excoriations. Due to enlarged veins, increased fibrous tissue, and hyperplastic duct epithelium, there may be irregular lobular development and decreased secretory activity during lactation. Pain is common. Macromastia associated with pregnancy reverses with delivery or abortion. However, for the most part, tissue hypertrophy is irreversible unless the underlying cause can be treated before or during pubertal breast development. In such cases, many patients benefit from reduction mammoplasty.

Like cervical, endometrial, and vaginal tissue, breast tissue in the nonpregnant woman undergoes menstrual cyclic changes in response to fluctuations in ovarian hormone levels. As estrogen levels rise in the first half of the cycle, ducts dilate and epithelial cells proliferate. In the second half, rising progesterone levels oppose these estrogen effects, preventing further dilatation or proliferation but resulting in glycogen deposition and secretory activity. This accounts for the breast fullness and tenderness that many women experience just prior to their periods when hormone influence on breast tissue peaks. Hormone influence is lowest about one week after menstruation. This is the ideal time for the monthly ▶ ***breast self-exam (BSE).*** Requiring only a few minutes, this simple practice may be truly lifesaving, since many breast changes subsequently described are first discovered by women themselves.

▶ ***Fibrocystic breast disease (FBD)*** develops in the wake of abnormally low progesterone levels, which may be due to a hyperprolactinic state (prolactin inhibits production of progesterone by the corpus luteum). Without adequate progesterone, estrogen stimulation continues and the mammary ducts undergo undue enlargement. In addition, high aldosterone levels (progesterone is an aldosterone antagonist) causes an influx of water and electrolytes. Fluids collect in the enlarged ducts, forming cysts. FBD is the most common disease of the breast, affecting 20% of premenopausal women. The patient notes swelling and tenderness of breast tissue (unilateral or bilateral) just before her period. On exam, one or more lumps of varying size may be palpated. The lumps are usually sensitive, soft, and freely movable. If tense with fluid, they may feel hard and somewhat fixed. To confirm its benign and cystic nature, any dominant mass should be aspirated and the fluid sent

TABLE 9.16 DIAGNOSTIC TESTS FOR DETECTING BREAST PATHOLOGY

Test	Comment
Xeromammography (mammography)	Beam of radiation (less than 0.4 rad per exposure) is passed through the breast; an image is recorded on a selenium plate, processed, and transferred to film. Detects abnormal masses smaller than 1 cm and dense parenchyma with connective tissue hyperplasia. From 70 to 90% accurate.
Thermography	Special instrument used to take photographic image of infrared emanations from each breast. Normal thermal patterns are symmetric, while most cancerous patterns are increased (due to high metabolic activity of the tumor with increased temperature from venous blood flow). No radiation exposure. However, misses a substantial number of cancers clearly defined on mammography and has a 20% incidence of false positives. Does not offer good localization for biopsy. Good screening method for low-risk groups. Should not be used in high-risk groups.
Ultrasound	Sound waves used to distinguish cystic from solid masses. Only useful for masses greater than 3 cm. No radiation exposure. Not for screening use.
Cytology	Pathologic evaluation of cells (Pap smear of nipple discharge, cytologic exam of fluid from fine needle aspiration) or of tissue taken via excisional biopsy. Excisional biopsy is the most reliable means of ruling out cancer in any questionable case.

for cytologic study. Ultrasound can distinguish between cystic and solid masses only when they are 1 cm or larger in diameter. Mammography is particularly useful for masses characterized by diffuse nodularity with no dominant mass (Table 9.16). A mass that fails to produce fluid on aspiration or persists after aspiration must be removed for biopsy. Once the diagnosis of FBD has been confirmed, patients may receive symptomatic relief by wearing a supportive bra night and day, and by avoiding trauma (e.g., jogging) when the breasts are most sensitive. Danazole, a synthetic androgen, is used for unusually severe cases. The role of caffeine remains controversial. Although double-blind studies have failed to verify an exacerbating effect of caffeine, many patients note improvement of symptoms with curtailed caffeine consumption. Reassurance is also in order; patients should be informed that they are not at higher risk for the development of breast cancer, as was once thought. Several investigations have shown that there is no greater incidence of microscopic fibrocystic disease in cancerous breasts than in noncancerous breasts studied at autopsy. Retrospective and prospective epidemiologic studies have concurred. Nonetheless, all patients should practice monthly BSE and should have careful breast exams by a health care provider at least yearly.

Fibroadenoma (adenofibroma, fibrosis) is the most common solid breast lesion in young women, the peak incidence being the early thirties. Abnormally sensitive to estrogen, focal areas of intralobular connective tissue undergo rapid overgrowth and nearby ducts display haphazard branching. Lesions can grow rapidly, particularly during pregnancy. Patients present with a painless lump that appears most often in the upper outer quadrant. One or both breasts may be involved. On exam, masses are noted to be well defined or encapsulated, with a rubbery consistency. The breasts are otherwise unremarkable and the axillae are negative. Lesions must be surgically removed and sent for pathologic study. The problem requires no other treatment and resolves with menopause. However, since recent studies have found a high association between fibroadenoma and breast cancer, health care providers should arrange breast exams every 6 months and urge the patient to practice BSE monthly.

Cystosarcoma phyllodes is a rare form of fibroadenoma characterized by extremely rapid growth of the lesions. The presentation is the same as that of fibroadenoma except that the masses can reach a very large size and tend to recur if inadequately removed. Though they are considered benign, metastases to regional lymph nodes can occur. Wide excision or sometimes simple mastectomy is the treatment.

Overgrowth of fibroepithelial tissue within terminal nipple ducts leads to ***papillomatosis*** (intraductal papillomas). The cardinal sign is a cloudy or bloody discharge from the nipple that may be spontaneous or expressed. Projecting from the wall of a duct, the raspberry-like lesions are often too small to palpate. Affected ducts must be carefully excised and tissue examined for signs of malignancy. While no other treatment is necessary, women must be carefully followed, since papillomatosis is considered a significant risk factor for future development of breast cancer.

Mammary duct ectasia is the dilatation of subareolar ducts that sometimes occurs in postmenopausal women. Once dilated, the ducts become filled with lipid-containing material that is responsible for most of the symptoms. Patients complain of burning, itching, or a painful drawing sensation around the areola and/or a thick, sticky nipple discharge that varies in color from gray to greenish-black. With time, the duct material becomes infiltrated by plasma cells and lymphocytes. Patients then develop a palpable abscess-like mass under the areola and a bloody discharge from the nipple. The acute inflammatory reaction ***(periductal mastitis)*** resolves spontaneously in 7–10 days. Meanwhile, cultures, Gram stains, and a Pap smear of the discharge help rule out bacterial mastitis and/or malignancy. If fibrosis follows the acute reaction, hardened subareolar lesions and nipple retraction may persist. They must be investigated (along with any continued discharge) with mammography and biopsy. The major mammary ducts, including the mass, are excised, usually by a circumareolar incision that preserves the nipple.

Breast cancer is the most common malignancy in women. Hormone imbalances (notably prolonged exposure to cyclic estrogen unopposed by progesterone, increased aldosterone levels, and hyperprolactinemia) seem to play a role by damaging DNA and thus initiating malignant changes in epithelial stem cells. Such imbalances are associated with early menarche, late menopause, nulliparity, first child after age 30, estrogen therapy, obesity, a high-fat diet, and hypothyroidism—all of which are risk factors in breast cancer. Furthermore, there is a strong genetic tendency; women whose mother or sister suffered from the disease are clearly at increased risk (Table 9.17). Very early tumors can be detected by noting small lesions, areas of thickening, increased vascularity, and/or microcalcifications on screening mammography. However, most cases are uncovered when a painless breast lump is discovered by the woman herself or by a health care provider. Other signs and symptoms include distortion of the areola, retraction of the nipple, enlargement or altered contour of the breast, skin edema (indicated by peau d'orange skin), or the appearance of prominent vascular patterns. There may be enlarged axillary or supraclavicular nodes or signs of metastasis to other organs (notably the lungs, liver, and bone). Skin nodules, which ultimately ulcerate, may be present in far advanced disease.

With one atypical form of breast cancer, ***inflammatory carcinoma,*** the symptoms resemble those of acute mastitis. The skin overlying a rapidly growing tumor is edematous, red, warm, indurated, and painful. In another typical form, ***Paget's disease,*** the only symptom of disease may be a chronic crusting of the nipple causing itching and an eczematoid appearance of surrounding skin. The crusting comes from

TABLE 9.17 FACTORS ASSOCIATED WITH AN INCREASED RISK OF BREAST CANCER

Racial background	Caucasian, particularly Northern European or Northern American descent.
Age	Over 40.
Diet	Postmenopausal obesity. High-fat diet.
Family history	Mother or sister with breast cancer (particularly if cancer is bilateral or developed in premenopausal years).
Medical history	Endometrial cancer. Previous breast cancer. Breast irradiation (greater than 100 rads). Previous biopsy. Cystic disease of the breast associated with proliferative changes, papillomatosis, or atypical epithelial hyperplasia. Cancer of a major salivary gland. Hypothyroidism (slight increase). Estrogen therapy (inconsistent data).
Menstrual history	Early menarche (before age 12). Nulliparity. First full-term pregnancy after age 30. Late menopause (more than 40 menstrual years).

invasion of the nipple epidermis by malignant "Paget's cells" shed from an intraductal lesion deep within the breast. The abnormal cells can be detected by Pap smear, but the primary lesion is usually too small to palpate.

Though the history, physical exam, and/or mammographic findings may strongly suggest its presence, breast cancer is definitively diagnosed only with examination of tissue removed by open surgery or aspiration. After diagnosis, patients are staged (Table 9.18) and treated accordingly. The surgical treatments include excision of the lump (lumpectomy); removal of the lump along with some surrounding tissue and overlying skin (segmental mastectomy); removal of the breast and sample lymph nodes (simple mastectomy); and of the breast and regional lymph nodes (modified radical mastectomy). Radical mastectomy, whereby the breast, lymph tissue, and pectoral muscle are excised, is no longer considered necessary. Furthermore, reconstructive procedures are now being done at the time of mastectomy or several months later. Radiotherapy and chemotherapy (hormones, cytotoxic agents, immunosuppressives) may be employed as adjuncts to surgery. One out of 15 women in the United States develops breast cancer. Every victim suffers physical and psychologic distress, and many die. Primary care providers must educate all women about the importance of low-fat diets, maintaining ideal weight, annual or semiannual breast exams, and monthly BSE. They should also advise screening mammography for high-risk patients and for all women when they reach age 40. For diagnosed patients and their families, ▶ ***organizations for breast cancer*** can offer valuable information and support.

Lactation

During pregnancy, high levels of estrogen, progesterone, human chorionic gonadotropin (HCG), cortisol, and insulin stimulate the activity of breast glands and ducts in readiness for lactation. A dramatic drop in these hormones and a rise in prolactin (PRL) stimulate milk production 3–5 days after delivery. Secretion of milk is preceded by that of colostrum, a thin yellowish fluid containing significant amounts of immunoglobins during the later months of pregnancy and after childbirth. Low circulating levels of PRL and subsequent failure to lactate may be the first symptoms of ***Sheehan's syndrome,*** vascular injury to the pituitary gland incurred during delivery.

TABLE 9.18 STAGES OF BREAST CANCER

Stage	Clinical Assessment
I	Tumor less than 2 cm in diameter. No evidence of lymph node involvement. No evidence of metastases.
II	Tumor more than 2 cm but less than 5 cm in diameter. Axillary nodes may be palpable but not fixed. No evidence of distant metastases.
III	Tumor more than 5 cm or tumor of any size that has invaded the skin or is attached to the chest wall. Supraclavicular nodes. No evidence of distant metastases.
IV	Distant metastases present.

Breast engorgement marks the onset of milk secretion. The result of distended blood and lymph vessels, this painful condition resolves with breast feeding. For women who are not breast feeding, it may persist until circulating PRL levels become normal and menses resume (4–12 weeks). For this reason, estrogen-androgen combinations (e.g., TACE or Diatate) are sometimes given to non-breast-feeding mothers immediately after birth to prevent lactation and avoid the problem. However, there is increasing evidence that such hormones have a carcinogenic effect, and they are being used less and less often. Anti-PRL substances have shown promising results in preliminary studies. Until they are available, many physicians are advising the time-honored practices of ice packs, tight binders, and analgesics.

Breast feeding involves two important components. The first is the let-down reflex. Initiated by infant suckling, it triggers the hypothalamus to release oxytocin from the posterior pituitary. Oxytocin stimulates the myoepithelial cells surrounding the mammary glands to contract, forcing milk into the ducts and toward the nipple. Let-down is also triggered by the baby's cry or the mother's thoughts about breast feeding. Besides affecting breast tissue, oxytocin has a constricting effect on uterine smooth muscle, helping to return the uterus to normal size after delivery. Unfortunately, it also results in painful uterine contractions associated with the first few minutes of breast feeding called ***after pains.*** For an unknown reason, after pains do not occur with the first child but can be extremely uncomfortable immediately after the birth of subsequent children. They disappear spontaneously.

Supply-and-demand response is the second component of breast feeding. By influencing the amount of PRL released by the pituitary, the baby's suckling controls the amount of milk produced from the nutrients and fluids provided by the mother's body. For the health and well-being of both mother and baby, primary care providers must keep a number of ▶ ***breast-feeding considerations*** in mind. They should also be able to offer advice about breast-feeding techniques and problems. They should pay special attention to the dietary requirements, birth control measures, and drug use of all breast-feeding patients. Common drugs that should be avoided or used with extreme caution are listed in Table 9.19. Finally, primary care providers can help new mothers keep in touch with ▶ ***breast-feeding information/support groups.***

A potentially serious problem, almost always associated with breast feeding, is ▶ ***mastitis.*** *Staph. aureus* (66–90% of cases) or streptococci spread from the infant's nose or mouth through nipple fissures into the ducts. Infection is most likely to be established during weaning when milk collects in the ducts after missed feedings, providing a perfect medium for bacterial culture. Occasionally, mastitis develops in the non-breast-feeding woman. In such cases, bacteria gains entrance to breast tis-

TABLE 9.19 DRUG USE DURING BREAST FEEDING

Drug	Comment
Antiarrhythmia drugs	
Quinidine	Absolutely contraindicated. May cause dangerous arrhythmia in infant.
Anticoagulants	
All types except heparin	Contraindicated. May cause bleeding episodes in infant.
Antimicrobials	
Chloramphenicol	Absolutely contraindicated. May cause bone marrow suppression in neonate with anemia, shock, death.
Metronidazole	Should be avoided. If used, nursing may resume 48 hours after last dose.
Penicillin/ampicillin/amoxicillin	Small amounts excreted in milk. Infant may develop allergic sensitization and/or candidal diarrhea.
Sulfonamides	Absolutely contraindicated. May lead to jaundice in neonate. May cause hemolytic anemia in infants with glucose-6-phosphate dehydrogenase (G-6-PD) deficiency.
Tetracycline	May be used if clearly indicated. Amount received by infant too small to cause discoloration of teeth.
Antineoplastics	
All types	Excreted in measurable amounts in breast milk.
Cyclophosphamide	Absolutely contraindicated.
Heavy metals	
Bismuth	Absolutely contraindicated. Toxic to infant. May be contained in some dermatologic preparations (check all skin preparations before using for nipple care).
Mercury	Absolutely contraindicated. Excreted in milk. Toxic to infant.
Hormones	
DES	Absolutely contraindicated. Inhibits milk secretion.
Oral contraceptives	Absolutely contraindicated. Reduces milk supply. May have feminizing effect on male infants.
Progestins	Contraindicated. Can produce feminization in male infants.
Motion sickness agents/antihistamines	
Most types	Not appreciably excreted in the milk except when taken in large doses.
Transderm-Scop	Avoid.
Psychiatric drugs	
Lithium	Absolutely contraindicated. Definitely toxic to infant.
Sedatives/tranquilizers	Avoid. Can have sedating effect on infant.
Recreational drugs	
Alcohol	If taken in excess, amount secreted in milk may be harmful to infant. May interfere with caretaking ability of mother.
Cocaine	No data available.
Lysergic acid diethylamide (LSD)	Absolutely contraindicated. Likely to interfere with caretaking ability of mother.
Marijuana	Absolutely contraindicated. No data on human infants, but known to impair DNA and RNA in animals.
PCP	Absolutely contraindicated. Same as for LSD.

TABLE 9.19 *(Continued)*

Drug	Comment
Testing materials	
Gallium	Insignificant amount excreted in breast milk; nursing should be suspended for 2 weeks after testing.
Iodine-125	Discontinue nursing for 48 hours.
Iodine-131	Discontinue nursing until secretion is no longer significant (24–36 hours after test dose, 2–3 weeks after treatment dose).
Radioactive iodine	Absolutely contraindicated. May affect thyroid function in infant.
Technetium-99	Discontinue nursing for 48 hours.
Thyroid medications	
Methimazole	Absolutely contraindicated. May cause goiter or depression of WBCs.
Thiouracil	Absolutely contraindicated. Same as above.

Source: Based on Sahu MD: Drugs and the nursing mother, *American Family Practice,* (Dec.) 1981, 24(6).

sue through small scratches, scrapes, or abrasions incurred during sexual foreplay or from eczema or bug bites. The signs and symptoms of mastitis appear almost a week after inoculation, since extension of the infection is temporarily contained by Cooper's ligaments. Thereafter, redness, swelling, heat, and tenderness of the breast ensue. Mastitis tends to develop in a diffuse pattern with streptococcal infections and in a nodular pattern with staphylococcal infections. Systemic symptoms include rapid onset of fever, shaking chills, and increased heart rate. A milk sample should be taken for culture and sensitivity testing. Heat, analgesics, and antistaphylococcal antibiotics should be instituted immediately. Continued nursing is a controversial issue. Those opposed assert that continued breast feeding perpetuates the problem, since bacteria are passed through infected milk to the baby and then back to the mother. Advocates feel that antibiotics in the breast milk treat the infant as well as the mother. Further, they note that sudden cessation of breast feeding results in caking and engorgement, which only worsen the situation.

Unless mastitis is treated with antibiotics in an early stage, ***breast abscess*** may form. The patient has continuous fever, chills, and general malaise. The breast becomes erythematous, tender, and swollen with an exquisitely painful mass. In addition to antibiotics, patients should be referred for immediate aspiration and drainage. Hospitalization may be necessary.

Galactorrhea is secretion of breast milk that is not associated with childbirth or that persists for more than 6 months after breast feeding is discontinued. Usually a milk discharge can be distinguished from a serous or purulent discharge by its thin blue-white appearance alone; if necessary, fat stains or tests for specific milk products may be done. Galactorrhea is classified as grade I or II when milk is expressed manually but not otherwise observed and as grade III or IV when copious secretions occur spontaneously. It is usually harmless but may be associated with the conditions noted in Table 9.20, particularly when accompanied by menstrual irregularity or infertility. In the latter instance, work-up and treatment of underlying disorders are indicated.

TABLE 9.20 CONDITIONS ASSOCIATED WITH GALACTORRHEA

Idiopathic	Breast stimulation
	  Sexual foreplay
	  Thoracic trauma (including burns)
	  Inflammation (mastitis, herpes)

Hypothalamic
  Histiocytosis
  Metastatic cancer
  Tumor impingement
  Infarction
  Embolism
	Drugs
	  Morphinergic drugs (including methadone, heroin, marijuana)
	  Psychiatric (butyrophenones, phenothiazines)
	  Oral contraceptives
	  Metoclopramide

Pituitary
  Pituitary adenoma
  Impingement from exogenous tumors (e.g., meningioma)
  Chairi-Frommel syndrome (persistent galactorrhea, amenorrhea after pregnancy)
  Section of pituitary stalk
  Vascular insult
	Decreased prolactin clearance
	  Renal failure
	  Liver failure
	  Hypothyroidism
	  Renal failure

Other endocrine
  Addison's disease
  Feminizing adrenal tumor
  Polycystic ovarian syndrome
	Ectopic prolactin production
	  Renal tumor
	  Bronchogenic tumor

	Unclassified
	  Stress
	  Empty sella turcica syndrome

SEXUAL ACTIVITY

Physiology of the Sex Act

As noted in Table 9.21, four stages of the sex act are described: excitement, plateau, orgasm, and resolution. For each stage, specific physiologic changes occur throughout the body. With the initiation of sexual excitement in the woman through erotic imagery, caressing, and clitoral stimulation, there is a local genital vasocongestive response equivalent to male penile erection. Clitoral stimulation may occur either directly by hand or other objects or indirectly by the thrusting movements of the penis, which put traction on the labia minora pulling the hood of the clitoris back and forth over the sensitive, highly innervated clitoral glans. All of the clitoral structures, the glans, the crura, and the urethral and perineal sponges, are richly supplied with vascular beds and sensory networks from the parasympathetic nervous system. As stimulation continues, swelling and tightening of the perivaginal and clitoral structures take place through the filling and expansion of the vascular supply to those areas. Specifically, the glans of the clitoris swells, hardens, and becomes erect as the shaft of the clitoris shortens pulling the glans up under the hood, thereby increasing tension on the glans. Engorgement of the clitoral legs, or crura, which extend subcutaneously from the glans posteriorly between the labia minora and majora, also occurs, as it does in the clitoral tissue that surrounds the urethra and underlies the perineum in structures referred to as the urethral and perineal sponges, respectively. An "orgasmic platform" develops at the introitus as vasocongestion of the vagina produces swelling, thickening, and heightened color of the labia, vestibular bulbs, and the lower third of the vaginal musculature, narrowing the introitus. The vaginal mucosa produces a transudative fluid that wets the vaginal walls providing lubrication.

TABLE 9.21 PHYSIOLOGIC CHANGES DURING THE FOUR PHASES OF THE SEX ACT

	Excitement	Plateau	Orgasm	Resolution
General	Sexual arousal following psychologic or physical stimulation.	Heightened sexual tension from continued excitement.	Intense culmination of arousal with sudden rhythmic release of tension.	Relaxation following orgasm.
Skin	Measles-like rash appears on upper abdomen, chest, neck ("sex flush").	Flush spreads over shoulders, down inner arms, abdomen, back, thighs, buttocks.	Flush reaches peak intensity	Flush fades.
Breasts	Nipple erection. Areola enlarges by 20–25%.	No further change.	No further change.	Nipple erection fades. Areola size decreases.
Muscles	Increased muscular tension in arms, chest, abdomen, rectum, and legs.	Further tension in buttock and thigh muscle.	Involuntary contraction of multiple muscle groups.	Muscle relaxation.
Cardiopulmonary	Heart rate and blood pressure increase. No change in respiration.	Heart rate reaches 100–175/min. Blood pressure increases (20–60 mm Hg diastolic, 10–20 mm Hg systolic). Respiration increases.	No further change.	Heart rate, blood pressure, respiration rate return to resting levels.
Sweat glands	No change.	No change.	No change.	Overall body sweating by woman. Sweating of palms of hands and soles of feet in man.
Male genital				
Scrotum	Skin contracts and thickens	No further change.	No further change.	Skin resumes normal baggy appearance.
Testes	Draw upward in scrotum as spermatic cord shortens.	Upward drawing continues until testes pressed against body wall. There is a 50% increase in size due to vasocongestion.	No further change.	Return to normal size and position.
Cowper's gland	Produces small amount of fluid to lubricate urethra (drop appears at end of penis).	No further activity.	No further change.	No further change.
Prostate	None.	None.	Release of ejaculate. Rhythmic convulsions.	No further activity.
Penis	Engorges.	Further engorgement.	Rhythmic pumping of cavernous muscles. Bulbous urethra increases in size.	Detumescence.

TABLE 9.21 (*Continued*)

	Excitement	Plateau	Orgasm	Resolution
Female genital				
Vagina	Immediate vasocongestion. Lubrication of vaginal mucosa by vaginal glands ("sweating"). Dilatation of posterior fornix. Color change to deep purple.	As muscles become turgid and swollen, vaginal opening reduces in size by 50% (increases tactile stimulation of the penis).	Rhythmic contraction of outer third of vaginal walls.	Blood rapidly drains from congested vessels. Purple color fades within 10–15 minutes. Walls return to normal size.
Uterus	Engorges. Increases in size. Draws upward.	Further engorgement. Continued elevation (may cause irritability of uterine muscles —myotonia). Uterine contractions in late stage.	Contractions with peristalsis toward fallopian tubes.	External cervical os dilates slightly. Contractions gradually cease.
Clitoris	Vasocongestion and erection. Gland doubles in size.	Gland elevates and retracts. Stimulation must continue for orgasm.	No further change.	Returns to normal position. Engorgement usually dissipates within 5–10 minutes but may last for hours, causing discomfort.
Labia	Swelling of minora with darkening of color. Majora becomes congested.	Changes continue.	No further change.	Return to normal size and color.
Bartholin glands	Secrete small amount of fluid.	Secretions continue.	None.	None.

At the plateau phase vasocongestion is at its fullest in all of the genital structures. In addition, the broad ligaments supporting the uterus shorten pulling the engorged uterus, ovaries, and tubes up out of the pelvis. This change in uterine position elongates the vagina and the distal end of the vagina balloons outward. Pulse, respirations, and blood pressure increase, the areola of the breasts may darken, and vasocongestion of the skin produces a mottling flush, especially on the upper chest.

With sufficient clitoral stimulation orgasm occurs producing reflex, involuntary, rhythmic contractions of the circumvaginal orgasmic platform and the uterus. In addition to these contractions, equivalent to the expulsive phase in the man, the woman also experiences a bodily sensation of pleasure and warmth and breaks into a light sweat. As in the male, orgasm is followed by a resolution phase when the muscular contractions end, vasocongestion resolves, and the clitoris relaxes. However, the woman does not experience the refractory period that in the man prevents him from being able to come to orgasm again immediately; rather, she may have repeated orgasms with continued clitoral stimulation before resolution is complete.

In the male with the onset of sexual excitement, parasympathetic nerve impulses are transmitted from the hypothalamus to the penis, causing the muscular walls of penile arteries to relax (normally, the strong muscular walls of the arteries passing through shaft tissue serve as floodgates to prevent venous blood from filling the cavernous sinuses and thus keep the penis in a flaccid state). As a result, venous blood floods the cavernous sinuses and the penis becomes erect. With this occurrence, Cowper's glands secrete a viscous alkaline fluid into the urethra. The fluid lubricates the urethra in preparation for ejaculation. It also washes out the urethra and neutralizes lingering traces of acid urine, which would kill delicate sperm. If sexual excitement continues, further physiologic changes take place. Rhythmic friction during intercourse or masturbation stimulates nerve endings in the skin of the penis, which send impulses to the thalamus and cerebral cortex. The latter, in turn, creates the urge for intensified stimulation.

Eventually, a second reflex mechanism is set off and impulses from the sympathetic nervous system pass to the genital organs, initiating ejaculation. These same sympathetic impulses cause the internal sphincter at the bladder neck to close, preventing urine from entering the urethra. Layers of smooth muscle in the testes and epididymis milk sperm into the vas deferens, while those of the seminal vesicles and prostate milk the contents of these organs into the urethra. Peristaltic waves move along the vas deferens, ducts, and urethra, mixing all fluids and sperm together into semen, a description of which appears in Table 9.22. This process is called "emission."

Actual ejaculation occurs when pudendal nerves send parasympathetic impulses to skeletal muscles encasing the base of the penis. The muscles contract rhythmically, increasing pressure in the urethra and causing semen to be expelled in spurts. The initial contractions are strong (propelling semen as far as 12–24 inches) but then grow progressively weaker. The "end" ejaculate consists of gel from the seminal vesicles that washes the remaining sperm out of the urethra. The total volume of ejaculated semen normally ranges from 2 to 6 mL. The act of ejaculation and the accompanying feeling of intense pleasure constitute orgasm. Following orgasm, there is a refractory period during which further ejaculation is not possible.

Freshly ejaculated semen is a coagulant within which sperm remain relatively immotile. However, it contains proteolytic enzymes from prostatic fluid that liquefy the semen within 3–25 minutes. After this period, ejaculated sperm become highly motile and remain viable for 24–72 hours at body temperature. Sperm that are not ejaculated remain viable in the male urogenital tract for 6 weeks and are then reabsorbed.

Failure to become sexually aroused and/or to complete satisfactory orgasm leads to ***sexual dysfunction.*** Some causes of sexual dysfunction are listed in Table 9.23. There are several descriptive subclassifications of ***male sexual dysfunction. Erectile failure (impotence)*** is the persistent inability to obtain and/or maintain an erection long enough to achieve coitus. The patient with ***primary impotence*** has never experienced an erection. He often suffers from deep psychic conflicts based on childhood experience. The patient with ***secondary impotence*** develops the problem after a period of normal sexual function. In such cases, hormonal, neurologic, vascular, and particularly medication effects may be the cause 50% of the time. Only after these factors have been investigated should a psychogenic diagnosis be made. Cases with a psychogenic component are often related to performance anxiety. ***Premature***

TABLE 9.22 DESCRIPTION OF SEMEN

Component	Comment
Volume	1–5 mL (3–6% Cowper's fluid, 72% seminal vesicle fluid, 15% prostatic fluid).
Sperm	Form in the testes and "ripen" in the epididymis (takes about 74 days for sperm to reach full maturity). Remain in epididymis until ejaculation, when hundreds of millions are transferred via the vas deferens and empty into the ejaculatory duct at the same time as seminal vesicle fluid and prostatic fluid. Each mature sperm consists of a head (equipped with a small structure containing the enzyme hyaluronidase, which helps break down the protective covering on the ovum), a neck, a body (contains abundant mitochondria, which provide energy for movement), and a powerful tail (flagellating action allows the sperm to swim at a rate of 2–3 mm/min). Normal ejaculate contains 20–200 million sperm/mL, more than 50% of which are motile and more than 60% of which are normal in form. Sperm produce a number of acid metabolic products (urea, creatine, uric acid, ammonia). They can live in the female reproductive tract for up to 72 hours but begin to lose vitality after 24 hours.
Bulbourethral (Cowper's) fluid	Tiny amounts produced by the bulbourethral glands (situated on either side of the urethra below the prostate) during the initial phase of sexual arousal. This thick mucous fluid lubricates and washes out the urethra in preparation for ejaculation. Highly alkaline, it neutralizes any traces of urine, whose acid nature would damage sperm. The fluid may contain small numbers of sperm, which contributes to the failure of coitus interruptus as a contraceptive method.
Seminal fluid	Produced by seminal vesicles. With ejaculation, this slightly alkaloid, mucoid secretion is emptied into the ejaculatory duct at the same time as sperm from the vas deferens. It contains fructose, vitamins (ascorbic acid, inositol), amino acids, phosphorylcholine (a nitrogenous compound), and prostaglandins (PGE, PGA, PGB, PGF). The fluid nourishes and protects sperm (by adding bulk to semen). The prostaglandins provoke uterine contractions, helping to propel sperm on their way to the fallopian tubes.
Prostatic fluid	Produced by the prostate glands. With ejaculation, this milky alkaline fluid is emptied into the ejaculatory duct at the same time as sperm from the vas deferens. It contains electrolytes (calcium, zinc, citric acid), spermine (a nitrogenous compound), and a number of enzymes. The alkalinity of prostate secretions helps neutralize the acid metabolic products of sperm and the acid environment of vaginal secretions. This is crucial, since sperm motility remains suboptimal until the surrounding environment reaches a pH of 6–6.5. Furthermore, within half an hour after ejaculation, enzymes help to dissolve the mucus secretions of the seminal vesicles and bulbourethral glands, which initially make semen so viscous that sperm are immobile.

ejaculation is ejaculation that routinely and readily follows erection. It may be traced to posterior urethritis, prostatitis, degenerative neurologic disease, or, most often, psychologic barriers. Relatively rare by comparison is ***retarded ejaculation,*** the inability to achieve ejaculation through coitus despite a sustained erection and sexual interest. Spinal cord injury or certain medications (particularly monoamine oxidase inhibitors) may contribute to the problem. However, as in the case of premature ejaculation, psychogenic factors are usually at fault. Both men and women may experience loss of sexual desire, which may be a result of individual or relational psychologic problems.

Sexual dysfunction in women has four categories as described by Kaplan: general sexual dysfunction (frigidity), orgastic dysfunction, vaginismus, and sexual anesthesia (conversion). The first three are expressed by physiologic dysfunctions, although they also may have psychologic components, and may occur separately or concurrently with the others. Sexual anesthesia, on the other hand, is felt to be

TABLE 9.23 SOME CAUSES OF SEXUAL DYSFUNCTION

General physical factors: decrease libido, lower sensitivity to stimulation, affect body image, reduce physical stamina, increase pain on coitus
- Fatigue
- Heart disease
- Multiple sclerosis
- Endocrine disorders, particularly diabetes
- Chronic renal failure
- Cirrhosis
- Dialysis
- Vascular disease
- Neuropathy
- Pulmonary insufficiency
- Cancer
- Spinal cord trauma
- Severe headaches
- Arthritis
- Obesity
- Surgery (particularly mastectomy, cardiac bypass, colostomy)

Psychologic causes
- Negative feelings stemming from sexual trauma or exploitation
- Performance anxiety
- Poor self-esteem
- Strict religious or parental upbringing
- Fear of losing control over feelings or behavior
- Marital discord or hostility toward the partner
- Situational stress
- Castration anxiety (men)
- Deep intrapsychic conflicts arising in childhood
- Chronic schizophrenia
- Depression
- Inability to communicate

Female genital causes (coital discomfort)
- Bartholin's cyst
- Bartholinitis
- Clitoral lesions or inflammation
- Cystitis
- Intact hymen
- Endometriosis
- Little or no vaginal lubrication
- PID
- Pregnancy
- Retroverted uterus
- Vaginal atrophy
- Vaginismus
- Varicose veins of the vulva
- Vulvovaginitis
- Vulva or vaginal lesions

Male urogenital causes (coital pain, erection failure)
- Urethritis
- Prostatitis
- Cystitis
- Urethral stricture
- Peyronie's disease
- Epididymitis
- Orchitis
- Hydrocele
- Priapism
- Peripheral neuropathy
- Balanitis
- Phimosis
- Hypospadias

Drugs—decreased libido (l), erectile problems (er), or inability to ejaculate (ej)
- CNS depressants
  - Alcohol (l, er)
  - Heroin (er)
  - Methadone (l, er)
  - Sedative/narcotics (er)
- Anticholinergic/antisecretory
  - Atropine sulfate (er)
  - Cimetidine (er)
  - Clidinium bromide (er)
  - Dicyclomine (er)
  - Isopropamide iodide (er)
  - Methantheline bromide
- Cardiovascular
  - Beta blockers (l, er)
  - Bethanidine (er, ej)
  - Clonidine (er, ej)
  - Digitalis (l)
  - Guanethidine (er, ej)
  - Hydroflumethiazide (er in rare cases)
  - Methyldopa (l, er, ej)
  - Pentolinium (er, ej)
  - Reserpine (l, er, ej)
- Diuretics
  - Chlorthalidone (er in rare cases)
  - Hydrochlorothiazide (er in rare cases)
  - Spironolactone (er)
- Psychiatric agents
  - Antidepressants
    - Amitriptyline (l, er, ej)
    - Cyclobenzaprine (l)
    - Doxepin (l, er)
    - Imipramine (l, er, ej)
    - Phenelzine (er)
  - Anxiolytics
    - Benzodiazepines (l)
  - Antipsychotics
    - Fluphenazine (l, er, ej)
    - Haloperidol (l, er, ej)
    - Lithium (er)
    - Mesoridazine (l, er, ej)
    - Prochlorperazine (l, er, ej)
    - Thioridazine (l, er, ej)
    - Trifluoperazine (l, er, ej)
- Others
  - Amphetamines (l, er)
  - Clofibrate (l, er)
  - Disulfiram (er)
  - Metronidazole (l)
  - Medroxyprogesterone (l)

entirely psychologic in origin. In general sexual dysfunction the woman does not experience erotic feelings and there is an inhibition of the vasocongestive phase of the sexual response. Despite the lack of clitoral and vaginal engorgement, the woman may still experience orgasm with clitoral stimulation, although usually this response is also inhibited secondarily. The most common female sexual dysfunction is orgastic dysfunction, in which the woman has erotic feelings and sexual arousal is intact with vaginal lubrication and vasocongestion, but there is no orgasm with its reflex perivaginal response. Primary orgastic dysfunction occurs in about 10% of sexually active women who have never experienced orgasm under any circumstances; secondary orgastic dysfunction occurs either with all sexual activity or only in selected instances in women who have previously been orgasmic. The woman with orgastic dysfunction may experience intercourse as pleasurable and in general she suffers no adverse effects. However, some women may develop ***chronic pelvic congestion syndrome*** if they never have orgasm with its concomitant full resolution phase. They may also eventually resent sexual activity if their partner is always orgastic, especially if the partner does not attempt to make intercourse mutually pleasurable. Both general sexual and orgastic dysfunctions may be the result of psychologic factors or painful intercourse from causes listed in Table 9.23 or both. Although few studies have been done on the effect of drugs on the female sexual response, it is reasonable to assume that drugs that impair sexual response in men have similar effects on the analogous sexual responses in women. Vaginismus, a relatively rare condition, is the involuntary tightening of the introital muscles preventing vaginal penetration; the sexual responses of vasocongestion and orgasm may remain intact. This condition is often the result of fear based on previous real painful sexual experiences (such as rape or a brutal pelvic examination) or imagined such experiences.

Treatment of sexual dysfunction in either the man or the woman depends on the underlying cause. The primary care provider can help many patients by adjusting medications, treating infections, encouraging communication between couples, teaching normal anatomy and physiology, frankly discussing coital techniques, and/or tracing the origin of anxiety performance/arousal failure. Other patients may require referral to a urologist, psychiatrist, or sex therapist.

During sexual intercourse, organisms from skin and body cavities can be worked into the urethra, vagina, or cervix as a route of entry for infection. By the same token, infectious organisms in the body can be shed in semen and vaginal secretions. Diseases that are sexually transmitted are collectively referred to as ***venereal diseases*** or sexually transmitted diseases (STD). As noted in Table 9.24, the list is long and includes many conditions that, other than the route of transmission, have little to do with the reproductive tract. Such problems (acquired immune deficiency syndrome, hepatitis, parasites, etc.) are discussed in other chapters.

Caused by the spirochete *Treponema pallidum,* ▶***syphilis*** has been clearly described since the fifteenth century. Although it is currently not the most prevalent STD, studies have shown a recent increase in the number of primary infections. The clinical manifestations and chronology of the stages of syphilis are described in Table 9.25 and are also discussed in other chapters (notably Chapter 10). The patient may present with a sore, usually in the genital area, which begins as a dull red macule that subsequently becomes papular and erodes centrally. The eroded area is loaded with *T. pallidum* and thus is highly contagious. This chancre, the characteristic sign of primary syphilis, is usually well circumscribed, painless, and indurated,

TABLE 9.24 SOME STDs

Acquired immune deficiency syndrome (AIDS)	Hepatitis virus
Actinomyces israelii	Herpes simplex virus
Campylobacter jejuni	Lymphogranuloma venereum
Candidiasis	Molluscum contagiosum
Cervical cancer	*Mycoplasma hominis*
Chancroid	*Neisseria gonorrhoeae*
Chlamydia trachomatis	PPNG
Condylomata acuminata	Salmonellosis
Entamoeba histolytica	Shigellosis
Gardnerella vaginitis	Syphilis
Giardia lamblia	Trichomonas vaginitis
Granuloma inguinale	*Ureaplasma urealyticum*

although atypical lesions are not uncommon. Within a week, nontender regional lymphadenopathy occurs. Although common in the inguinal region, lymphadenopathy can be found around other possible chancre sites such as the lips, mouth, nipples, throat, anus, and rectum. Primary syphilis may easily go undetected in the woman or the homosexual man, since chancres may be hidden from view and heal spontaneously within 2–12 weeks. Therefore, thorough case finding and prompt treatment of sexual contacts are necessary to halt further transmission of the disease.

The diagnosis of syphilis may be made by dark field microscopic exam of material from open lesions with *T. pallidum.* A negative dark field exam does not rule out infection. Several serologic tests are also available. Usually used for screening purposes are the nonspecific antibody tests rapid plasma reagin (RPR), venereal disease research laboratory (VDRL), and the automated reagin test (ART). The most widely used specific treponemal antibody test is the FTA-ABS test. False-positive results occur frequently on the nonspecific screening tests; specific treponemal antibody tests must be done if screening tests are positive. False-negative serologic findings are possible in early primary syphilis; repeat testing within 6 weeks is likely to yield

TABLE 9.25 STAGES OF SYPHILIS

Stage	Characteristics	Chronology
Primary	Chancre. Regional lymphadenopathy.	Appearance 10–90 days after exposure. Heal in 2–12 weeks.
Secondary	Skin rash (maculopapular and/or pustular) condylomata. Flu-like symptoms (fever, weight loss, malaise, anorexia, headache). Generalized painless lymphadenopathy. Hepatitis with high alkaline phosphatase levels. Nephropathy with proteinuria. Uveitis.	Begin 6 weeks–6 months after onset of primary infection. Heal in 3 months.
Latent	Positive syphilis serologic findings in the absence of signs of tertiary disease. Normal CSF findings.	Between secondary and tertiary stages. Variable length of progression.
Tertiary	Neurosyphilis (tabes dorsalis, paresis, optic atrophy or asymptomatic). Cardiovascular syphilis (syphilitic aortitis). Iritis. Gummas (granulomatous lesions of any organ, most commonly the skin, skeleton, and respiratory tract).	More than 50% of untreated patients do not develop overt tertiary syphilis.

positive results if disease is present. Pharmacologic therapy differs based upon the stage of the disease, specifically when the duration of illness is greater than 1 year. If the patient has no known history of illness or symptoms and serologic exam reveals a syphilis infection, CSF analysis is indicated to rule out tertiary syphilis, which requires more aggressive treatment. It is important that the history include a prior history of syphilis, since antibody titers may remain elevated after past treated infections.

Neisseria gonorrhoeae, a gram-negative intracellular diplococcus, is the cause of ▶***gonorrhea.*** The gonococcus can directly infect the urethra, endocervix, anal canal, pharynx, and conjunctivae, with possible resultant systemic infections. Various organs including the skin, joints, heart, CNS, liver, and female reproductive tract may be potentially affected. Humans are the only natural hosts for the gonococcus, which is transmitted principally by sexual contact. Gonorrhea is currently the most commonly reported STD in the United States. The incubation period is 2–14 days in the man and 7–21 days in the woman. In the man, the urethra is usually the primary site of infection, although the rectum and pharynx are common areas among homosexuals.

Occurring in 90% of infected men, symptoms of gonococcal urethritis include tingling or burning on urination, local urethral redness, and a milky and later a yellowish or blood-tinged discharge. Pharyngeal gonorrhea may be asymptomatic or may present as a red and/or exudative sore throat associated with regional lymphadenopathy. Pharyngeal infection rarely results from oral contact with the infected female genitalia, hence the greater association with the homosexual population and with women who have had oral-penile contact. Gonococcal infection of the rectum may be asymptomatic or may cause symptoms as severe as proctitis with pain, tenesmus, mucopurulent discharge, and rectal bleeding. Gonococcal proctitis infrequently causes symptoms in the woman, although the organism may be isolated from that area in many cases. Conjunctival infection is almost always confined to infants as they pass through an infected birth canal and is treated by instillation of antibacterial eye drops at birth. The sites of colonization of the female genital tract are the urethra, Skene's ducts, Bartholin's glands, vagina, cervix, and adnexae. Due to the conducive vaginal environment, women are more likely to become infected than men. In fact, after intercourse with an infected partner, 60–80% of women will develop gonorrhea, as opposed to only 20–30% of men. At least half of all infected women have no symptoms. If the urethra is affected, women may experience a urethritis that mimics cystitis without positive urine cultures. Dysuria, frequency, urgency, purulent urethral discharge, and urethral erythema characterize "gonococcal urethral syndrome" in the woman. The endocervix is the most frequently infected area. Manifestations include vaginitis, bartholinitis with abscess formation, and cervicitis with a mucopurulent discharge, friable tissue, and possibly abnormal menstrual bleeding.

Complications of untreated gonorrhea may be disastrous for the woman. In 15% of women with gonococcal cervicitis, infection ascends to the fallopian tubes, causing PID (see the previous section). This often occurs at the time of menses. Women using IUDs have a threefold increased chance of contracting PID. The sequelae are tubal scarring with infertility and a greater risk of ectopic pregnancy. Direct spread of the gonococcus via the peritoneum to the liver may cause perihepatitis ***(Fitz-Hugh-Curtis syndrome).*** Complications in the man are rare, although epididymitis and prostatitis may occur. Approximately 1% of individuals with gonorrhea (mostly women) develop gonococcal bacteremia. Individuals with deficiencies of certain complement factors appear to be particularly susceptible. Manifestations of disseminated infection may include migratory arthralgias, septic arthritis, fever, and skin lesions (papular, pustular, or hemorrhagic). Other complications include endocarditis, myocarditis, and meningitis.

The diagnosis of gonococcal infection in the symptomatic man is usually made by Gram staining a urethral discharge and inspecting the slide for neutrophils containing multiple gram-negative diplococci. Ideally, the specimen should be obtained at least 2 hours after urination. Though this is a sensitive test, it will not rule out the presence of ***penicillinase-producing Neisseria gonorrhoeae (PPNG)***—a penicillin-resistant strain believed to have developed in Southeast Asia with subsequent spread to the United States. Culture on chocolate agar (e.g., modified Thayer-Martin medium) from sites of suspected infection in the man and woman allow positive identification of *N. gonorrhoeae* at the laboratory. The beta-lactamase test, performed on the same specimen, will determine penicillin resistance. Cultures of blood and/or synovial fluid may reveal gonococci in cases of disseminated infection. Treatment consists of appropriate antibiotic therapy. Postgonococcal urethritis (recurrence of symptoms after adequate treatment) is usually caused by a concurrent chlamydial or ureaplasma infection.

Chlamydia trachomatis, a bacteria-like intracellular parasite, is the cause of the most prevalent STD in the United States. In the man, *C. trachomatis* (serotypes D–K) causes ***nongonococcal urethritis,*** with possible complications being acute epididymitis and, in the homosexual man, proctitis. It is estimated that approximately 50% of nongonococcal urethritis and 70% of postgonococcal urethritis are due to ▶***chlamydia infection.*** The remaining cases are probably caused by condylomata acuminata, trichomonas, and mycoplasmas such as *ureaplasma urealyticum.* A feeling of discomfort at the penile tip approximately 7–21 days after exposure may be the initial symptom in the man. Dysuria may follow, along with a discharge scantier and clearer than that associated with gonorrhea. Typically, the discharge is most evident in the early morning, but symptoms may vary. An asymptomatic carrier state has been documented. The woman with chlamydia is usually symptom free; estimates of asymptomatic female carriers are as high as 30%.

Chlamydia is often implicated in the syndrome, which is characterized by frequency, urgency, dysuria, and pyuria in the woman without positive urine cultures for bacteria. Chlamydia may also cause cervicitis, which is associated with a mucopurulent cervical discharge that is often irritating to the vaginal tissues and ectropion. However, the most serious complication for women is the high association between chlamydial infection and PID, which often results in infertility or an increased incidence of ectopic pregnancy. Infants born to mothers with cervical chlamydial infections may develop neonatal inclusion conjunctivitis and chlamydial pneumonitis. Adults with genital chlamydia and poor hygiene practices may self-inoculate and develop inclusion conjunctivitis.

The diagnosis of chlamydia is challenging, since so many infected individuals are without symptoms and since the present laboratory culture methods are expensive and often inaccessible. A man with a Gram-stained urethral discharge devoid of gonococci but with more than five neutrophils per high-power field is likely to have chlamydia. Culture of the urethra in the man (ideally, at least 2 hours after voiding) and the endocervix in the woman should be attempted if possible. In cases where laboratory confirmation is not feasible, the diagnosis may be presumed in men with nongonococcal urethritis, in women with nongonococcal cervicitis, and in their respective partners. A high level of suspicion of chlamydia is warranted in women with PID and their contacts, women with sterile pyuria, and men under 35 years of age with acute epididymitis. Gonorrhea and chlamydia infections are often concurrent; diagnosis of the former thus does not preclude that of the latter. Treatment consists of appropriate antibiotic therapy.

Different strains of *C. trachomatis* (serotypes L1, L2, L3) are pathogens causing ***lymphogranuloma venereum (LGV).*** The illness is transmitted sexually and may affect the urethra, vagina, or rectum. After an incubation period of 2–5 days, a small vesicular lesion or erosion may appear, but frequently lesions are not evident. Several weeks later regional adenopathy occurs, beginning as soft, discrete, tender inguinal nodes that later become larger, matted, and adherent to erythematous overlying skin. There may be associated nonspecific systemic symptoms. Diagnosis is based on this distinctive presentation. The treatment of choice is tetracycline, 500 mg po qid for at least 2 weeks. Without early treatment, complications may develop: draining fistulas, lymphatic obstruction with secondary local swelling (elephantiasis), and rectal or urethral strictures.

Usually referred to as "genital warts," ▶***condylomata acuminata*** are sexually transmitted warts caused by human papilloma virus (HPV), some 20 subtypes of which have been identified. Lesions may be observed on the external genitalia, vagina, cervix, and anorectal area, as well as in the mouth. Condylomata acuminata are usually multiple, pink, moist, raised lesions that may appear as cauliflower-like, elongated, or pedunculated. They may grow large enough to block the introitus or anus. The incubation period is long, lasting for 1–6 months. Patients are often asymptomatic, but women may develop a secondary vulvitis, profuse, irritating vaginal discharge, or dyspareunia. A positive connection has been suggested between CIN progression and certain subtypes of condylomata acuminata (HPV subtypes 16–18 are most strongly implicated). Thus, the annual Pap smear should be encouraged. In the man, warts may be found inside the urethra, hidden from view, possibly causing urethral discharge.

The diagnosis of condylomata acuminata is usually made by observing the characteristic appearance of the warts. Alternatively, typical changes associated with condylomata acuminata may be noted on the Pap smear before lesions are observed. In contacts of documented condylomata patients, all possible infected areas should be examined. Urethroscopy may be necessary in cases of recurrent meatal warts and proctoscopy for patients with extensive or proximal anorectal warts. Biopsy should be considered for atypical or persistent lesions. Traditional treatment consists of wart removal with topical podophyllum (10–25%) in tincture of benzoin followed by bathing to remove the podophyllum 4 hours after application. However, recent studies have raised some concern that podophyllum may be associated with dysplastic changes. Until the issue is clarified, cryosurgery may be a safer form of treatment. Recurrence is common.

▶***Herpes genitalis*** is an acute, recurrent viral infection characterized by the appearance of small, single or grouped, tense vesicles on mucous membranes or skin in the genital region. The responsible virus is herpesvirus hominis, a virus with two subtypes—1 and 2. Subtype 1 is responsible for about 80% of herpes infections in the mouth (fever blisters or cold sores), discussed in Chapters 3 and 10. Herpes genitalis is mostly due to type 2 virus, although both types can occur on any area of the skin. Usually contracted venereally, primary infections may be preceded by general malaise, muscular aches (particularly in the lower back), mild fever, and regional lymphadenopathy. Within a day or two, small vesicles filled with clear fluid appear on a slightly raised, erythematous base. In the man, they usually develop on the penis; in the woman, they may involve the labia, urethra, vagina, or cervix. The anal area is another common site of involvement. Soon rupturing, the vesicles leave painful ulcers that are slow to heal. Although the primary lesions resolve spontaneously within a week or two, many patients suffer from recurrences that can be precipitated by emotional stress, menstruation, local trauma, (intercourse, tight jeans), fever, smoking, or certain foods or drugs. Recurrences are usually preceded by a prodromal period of tingling, burning, stinging, or itching at the site of the eventual vesicle eruption. If pain is severe, patients may have difficulty urinating or defecating. In the woman, repeated infections have been associated with CIN progression. Furthermore, an active infection at the time of childbirth may be contracted by the newborn.

The diagnosis of herpes genitalis can usually be made on the basis of the classic history and typical skin eruptions. It may be confirmed by cultures for the virus and/or a positive Tzanck test of scrapings for vesicles stained with Giemsa stain (which reveals multinucleated giant cells). Treatment consists of topical acyclovir for primary infections and oral acyclovir for severe recurrent infections. Mild analgesics may be indicated for discomfort and antibiotics for secondary skin infection. All patients should be advised that exposing another person to an active lesion can result in transmission of disease. The disease can also be transmitted in the asymptomatic phase. Condoms decrease but do not entirely eliminate the possibility of transmission. Women should be informed about the association with cervical neoplasia and possible transmission of infection to a newborn child. Because of these complications, frequent Pap smears (at least yearly) and vaginal cultures prior to labor are indicated. The presence of herpesvirus at the time of delivery necessitates Caesarean section and temporary isolation of the mother from the baby. Because discomfort, embarrassment, and misinformation about the disease abound, patients may benefit from ▶ ***herpes support groups.***

Trichomonas vaginalis is a pear-shaped protozoan that causes ***trichomonas vaginitis*** in approximately 75% of infected women, but rarely causes symptoms in men. Transmission is usually sexual but may be by moist fomites. Incubation periods range from 3 to 21 days. Women may notice a vaginal discharge that is usually greenish-white, seropurulent, malodorous, and sometimes has a frothy appearance. Accompanying symptoms can include dysuria, dyspareunia, vulvar itch, and intertrigo. The cervix may be hyperemic and friable, with the classic "strawberry" stippling observed in some cases. Inguinal lymphadenopathy may be evident. A wet mount slide (vaginal discharge mixed with 1 drop of normal saline) will often demonstrate the trichomonads propelling themselves with their flagella. The vaginal pH is usually in the range of 5 to 6. *T. vaginalis* may be noted incidentally on the Pap smear. If this is the case the smear should be repeated after treatment, since changes related to a current trichomonas infection can mask other cytologic abnormalities. Flagyl is the drug of choice, with a 1-day treatment regimen being effective in most cases. Trichomonads may be found in the male genitalia for up to 2 weeks in most cases. Treatment of the steady male partner, even if he is asymptomatic, appears to decrease the rate of recurrence in the woman. Alternatively, the use of condoms for 2 weeks (the time needed for the organisms to vacate the male genitals) can prevent reinfection of the woman; however, if recurrence does occur, the man should be treated.

Gardnerella vaginalis, a gram-negative coccobacillus, has been implicated in ***gardnerella vaginitis*** (nonspecific, hemophilus vaginitis). It appears that vaginal anaerobes and *G. vaginalis* in combination cause the clinical syndrome. The predominant symptom is a thin, whitish-gray-green vaginal discharge that may be odorous. Vulvar itch, dysuria, and dyspareunia may also be present. The cervix is usually normal in appearance. Men are generally asymptomatic, but they harbor *G. vaginalis.* The diagnosis is made by ruling out other vaginitis syndromes and identifying "clue cells" on wet mount with normal saline. The latter are epithelial cells that have granular stippling. Addition of 1 drop of 10% potassium hydroxide to the vaginal discharge produces a fishy odor (positive "whiff" or "amine" test). The vaginal pH ranges from 4.5 to 5.5. There is considerable debate regarding the appropriate treatment for gardnerella vaginitis, concerning the pharmacologic agent and whether to treat the male partner. Antibiotic creams are not consistently effective. Flagyl and ampicillin administered orally seem to produce the highest cure rates. There is general agreement that the male partner should be treated if the woman becomes reinfected after a documented cure.

The fungus *Candida albicans,* generally a normal resident of the vagina, can overgrow inhibitory lactobacilli and cause ▶***monilia*** (yeast infection). Factors that predispose to overgrowth include the use of antibiotics (especially broad-spectrum types), hyperglycemia (diabetes, a diet high in refined carbohydrates), and the use of steroids (birth control pills, anti-inflammatory drugs, immunosuppressive agents). Pregnancy, frequent douching, and moisture in the genital areas (garments of synthetic materials, tight jeans, and pantyhose) are also conducive. Just as *Candida* can affect the skin of various parts of the body, it can irritate the glans penis and prepuce, and in rare cases affects the urethra. Thus, the infection can be sexually transmitted. Symptoms in the woman, which can be severe, are vulvar irritation and excoriation, dysuria, and dyspareunia. A white, curd-like, cheesy, musty-smelling, adherent vaginal discharge is typical. In the man, monilial balanitis (balanoposthitis in the uncircumcised individual) is manifested by irritation, itchiness, and soreness of the glans and prepuce, especially after intercourse. There may be local erythema, perhaps accompanied by vesicular eruptions, erosion, and a thick, adherent white discharge. Urethral discharge is uncommon. The appearance and symptoms aid in making the diagnosis, which is confirmed by the observation of hyphae or mycelia on a slide of discharge mixed with 1 drop of 10% potassium hydroxide. Culture on Nickerson medium can reveal cases where yeast were not visualized on wet mount. Treatment consists of the application of clotrimazole or miconazole cream or suppository.

Granuloma inguinale, rare in the United States, is caused by a gram-negative bacterium called *Calymmatobacterium (Donovania) granulomatis.* Transmitted usually but not solely by sexual means, the disease is manifested as a lesion of the penis, scrotum, groin, anus, rectum, thighs, vulva, vagina, or perineum. After an incubation period of 10–80 days, the lesion begins as a subcutaneous nodule that later erodes through the skin surface and contains beefy red, granulomatous tissue within a well-demarcated border. The painless ulcer tends to spread, leading to complications such as scar tissue formation, secondary infection, and, in advanced cases, cachexia, anemia, and death. The presence of Donovan bodies when Wright or Giemsa stains are applied to lesion scrapings confirms the diagnosis. Treatment consists of ampicillin or tetracycline, 500 mg po qid for 2 weeks.

Hemophilus ducreyi is a short, gram-negative coccobacillus that causes a genital lesion called ***chancroid.*** From 3 to 14 days after sexual contact, a tender papule on a nonindurated, erythematous base appears. The papule later becomes pustular and erodes to form a friable lesion with an irregular border. Soft, fluctuant, tender regional lymphadenopathy may be present; the nodes may actually rupture. Chancroids are not commonly seen in women, although they do carry and spread the infection. To diagnose chancroid, a culture may be taken of a lesion exudate or bubo aspirate and grown on chocolate agar containing 3 mg/mL vancomycin. Alternatively, a Gram stain may be done of a lesion exudate to look for gram-negative bacilli with rounded edges. Both partners should be treated with erythromycin, 500 mg po qid, or trimethoprim/sulfamethoxazole DS bid, for at least 10 days.

Conception

Under natural conditions, the sperm ejaculated into the vagina during intercourse swim directly through the cervical os. Their effort is enhanced by the thin, watery consistency of the cervical mucus at the time of ovulation. Aided by the propulsive movements of the uterus that occur with female orgasm, sperm can reach the entrance of the fallopian tubes in about 5 minutes. If conception is to occur, viable sperm must meet a viable ovum. Although sperm can live in the female reproductive tract for 72 hours, they lose vitality after 24 hours. By the same token, an ovum begins to degenerate after 24 hours. Fertilization therefore rarely occurs in the uterus, since it takes about 4 days for an unfertilized egg to reach the uterus. It almost always takes place in the upper third of the fallopian tube within a day or less of the actual moment of ovulation and intercourse. Of the 300–500 million sperm in the ejaculate, only a few reach the ovum. Many are lost before they reach the entrance to the fallopian tubes; of those that remain, one-half enter the tube that contains no ovum. Once in the fallopian tube, about 35 million of the strongest sperm surround the egg and begin to ram its protective covering. With the impact, a structure on each sperm head releases a minute amount of the enzyme hyaluronidase, which eats away at the covering until a breach in the surface is made. The next sperm to ram the weakened surface penetrates the egg and fuses with it. Instantly the outer membrane of the ovum thickens, preventing the entrance of additional sperm. The head of the penetrating sperm swells rapidly, forming the male pronucleus; at the same time, the ovum undergoes meiosis, forming the female pronucleus. The two pronuclei align themselves to form a structure with a full complement of 46 chromosomes (zygote, embryo). Beginning to divide and living on the supply of food provided by the ovum, the embryo normally travels down the fallopian tube and into the uterus a day or two later. On the seventh to ninth day after conception, it implants in the endometrium.

Ectopic pregnancy is implantation of the embryo in an area other than the uterus. It may sometimes occur in the interstitium (2–4% of cases), or, more rarely, in the ovary, cervix, or abdominal cavity. In 95% of cases, the ectopic implantation is in the fallopian tubes (tubal pregnancy). In delaying embryo descent by altering tubal motility, IUD placement contributes to the risk of ectopic pregnancy. The problem is also more likely to develop in a fallopian tube scarred by surgery or PID. In such instances, microscopic sperm continue to pass unimpeded through the narrowed lumen, but a dividing zygote becomes blocked. In rare cases, abdominal pregnancies can go almost completely to term with successful delivery through abdominal section. However, tubal pregnancies eventually cause the fallopian tube and/or ovary to rupture. An ectopic implant within the isthmus (narrow, muscular portion of the tube) is prone to rupture early in the course of gestation; that in the infundibulum or ampulla (wider, less muscular, and more distensible portions) may not rupture until the pregnancy is more advanced. In either case, associated hemorrhage and peritonitis can be life-threatening.

About 50% of patients with ectopic pregnancy report a missed period followed in 1–8 weeks by spotting. Profuse hemorrhagic bleeding is uncommon, and only 10–25% of patients experience symptoms of pregnancy. Eventually, patients develop a crampy, dull abdominal pain that is typically confined to the lower quadrant. Pain radiating to the shoulder and back suggests intraperitoneal bleeding, while severe stabbing pain warns of rupture. Exam may or may not reveal the tender, distended adnexal mass that is presumed to be a classic sign. Uterine enlargement, which often accompanies ectopic pregnancy, should not be misconstrued as diagnostic evidence of intrauterine pregnancy. The WBC count and ESR may be slightly elevated. If severe bleeding is present, hemoglobin and hematocrit may be low. Human chorionic gonadotropin (HCG) levels are typically lower in ectopic than intrauterine pregnancy. For this reason, some older urine tests measuring HCG levels lack the sensitivity to detect the pregnancy. Newer urine antibody tests or blood assays may be needed to make the diagnosis of pregnancy, and emergency ultrasound may be required to determine the location of implantation. If an ectopic pregnancy is found, patients should undergo immediate surgery.

When a fertilized egg implants in the endometrium, a placenta develops to provide continuous transport of materials back and forth between the mother and fetus. The placenta immediately begins to secrete HCG and the ***intrauterine pregnancy (IUP)*** is underway. Peaking at 8–10 weeks and then gradually decreasing, HCG sustains the corpus luteum and prevents endometrial sloughing and vaginal bleeding. Thus, one of the earliest signs of IUP is a missed period. Other symptoms and signs are breast tenderness and enlargement, nausea, urinary frequency, and fatigue. Quickening, or the first perception of fetal movement, occurs at 18–20 weeks. On physical exam at 6 weeks' gestation, the cervix and vagina may have a blue "blush" (Chadwick's sign). The uterine isthmus is thickened and soft (Hegar's sign), and the fundus is softer and slightly enlarged. There should be little if any adnexal tenderness or enlargement. Table 9.26 shows further changes in uterine size according to the number of weeks of gestation. A positive pregnancy test in the presence of clinical signs and symptoms confirms the diagnosis. Previously, urine tests were based on the clearance of HCG by the kidneys when blood levels peaked (10 days to 2 weeks after a missed period to 16–20 weeks' gestation). However, these tests could not be counted on to detect the lower amounts of HCG secreted before or after this time. Furthermore, factors such as proteinuria, dilution, or medication use often interfered with the results, as noted in Table 9.27. Some of these factors are not an issue with newer urine tests, which measure antibodies to HCG. Furthermore, antibody tests can be counted on to detect pregnancy within a few days after conception. Even so, if a urine test is negative and pregnancy seems likely, serum levels of HCG should be measured.

The woman who has any doubts about her pregnancy may seek information regarding her alternatives. ▶ ***Birthright organizations*** provide important services for women whose pregnancy presents a social, moral, and/or financial dilemma. In the first two trimesters, ***pregnancy termination*** may also be undertaken; the various procedures are described in Table 9.28. The method of abortion chosen depends on the duration of the pregnancy and locally available options. Vacuum aspiration is

TABLE 9.26 THE UTERUS IN PREGNANCY

Weeks of Gestation	Uterine Fundus: Size	Uterine Fundus: Position
6	Normal or slightly larger than normal	In pelvis
7 to 9	Tangerine to small orange	In pelvis
10	Large orange	In pelvis
12	Grapefruit	At or just above symphysis pubis
16		Halfway between umbilicus and symphysis pubis
18		2 fingerbreadths below umbilicus
20	Small melon	At umbilicus
20–24		Measurement in centimeters from symphysis pubis to top of fundus roughly equal to number of weeks of gestation

usually performed before the twelfth week of pregnancy (dated from the last menstrual period). It consists of inserting a sterile vacuum tube with a curetting end through the cervical os into the uterine cavity. The products of conception are then removed by suction. D&C may be done up to 14–16 weeks. The cervix is gradually dilated and a surgical curette is used to remove the products of conception. Saline abortions are performed from week 16 to week 24 of pregnancy. The amniotic sac is localized by ultrasound, and a small catheter or needle is inserted into it through the abdominal wall. A small amount of fluid is removed and relaced with hypertonic saline. Uterine contractions begin 5–15 hours after injection, with labor lasting for another 8–15 hours. Prostaglandin abortions are also performed after the sixteenth week and involve prostaglandin injection or cervical absorption from prostaglandin suppositories, which cause the onset of labor. The decision to terminate or continue the pregnancy may be made with or without the involvement of family or friends.

TABLE 9.27 PREGNANCY TEST ERRORS

False negatives
- Error in reading
- Test performed too early or too late in pregnancy
- Urine too dilute
- Urine stored too long at room temperature
- Impending spontaneous abortion
- Missed abortion
- Ectopic pregnancy
- Interfering medication
- Too much antiserum

False positives
- Error in reading
- LH cross-reaction (test at the time of ovulation or in a perimenopausal client)
- Proteinuria
- Hematuria
- Lipemia or turbidity of serum specimen
- Persistent corpus luteum cyst
- Recent pregnancy (less than 10 days after abortion or delivery)
- Detergent residue on glassware
- Premature menopause
- Drug interference (Aldomet, marijuana, methadone, aspirin, phenothiazines, antidepressants, antiparkinsonians, anticonvulsants)
- HCG treatment within the preceding 30 days
- Recent radioisotope diagnostic study or treatment (serum) only
- Tubo-ovarian abscess
- Trophoblastic disease (hydatidiform mole or choriocarcinoma)
- HCG secreted by malignant tumor (of breast, ovary, lung, kidney, GI tract, sarcoma, malignant melanoma)

TABLE 9.28 THERAPEUTIC ABORTION METHODS

Method	Gestation	Anesthesia	Complications
Vacuum curettage	≤12 weeks	Local or none	Vasovagal reactions Allergic reaction to anesthesia Uterine perforation Retained products of conception Infection
Dilation and curettage (D&C)	≤16 weeks	General or local	Same as for vacuum curettage In addition: Hemorrhage Uterine atony
Hypertonic saline	16–24 weeks	Local	Same as for D&C In addition: Myometrial necrosis Emboli Electrolyte imbalance CVA
Prostaglandins	16–24 weeks	Local or none	Same as D&C In addition: Cervical lacerations Delivery of live fetus

For women who decide to undergo abortion, it is important to explain the procedure and follow-up care and to explore subsequent plans for contraception. Patients should also be warned about the possible feelings of sadness and loss that may accompany termination.

▶ ***Prenatal considerations*** are extremely important for any woman who decides to continue the pregnancy. Primary care providers can institute early referral for prenatal care and reinforce special needs for proper nutrition, exercise, and rest. Alcohol and caffeine intake, as well as cigarette smoking, should be avoided. The benefit of any drug use must always be weighed against the potential harm it may cause the fetus (Table 9.29). Occupational hazards should also be considered (Table 9.30). Since the first trimester is the time when the developing fetus is most vulnerable to outside influences, these interventions decrease the chance of complications.

Ideally, ***family planning*** means more than choosing a method of contraception; it means having children when they are wanted and preventing conception when pregnancy is not desired. For this reason, when ▶ ***counseling patients on birth control measures,*** it is important to discuss their plans for child bearing. It may be helpful to review the considerations listed in Table 9.31. Patients should also be informed about various birth control methods being used in the United States today. These methods should be reviewed in terms of how they work, their effectiveness, and their risks and benefits. The health effects of each method should be presented, along with a comparison of the mortality risk and the risk of pregnancy. Figure 9.8 shows that the mortality risk of pregnancy when no method of birth control is being used is much greater than the mortality risk of any method of contraception except for the pill when used by smokers who are more than 40 years old.

When counseling patients, primary care providers should be aware that several factors influence a patient's choice, continuation, and success with a particular method of birth control. Older patients are generally more successful than younger ones because of their greater experience and practice and relative decreased fertility.

TABLE 9.29 DRUG USE DURING PREGNANCY

Drug	Comment
Adrenocorticosteroids	
All types	Low incidence of cleft palate if given during first trimester. Low incidence of placental insufficiency with increased perinatal mortality if given in second and third trimesters. Mild adrenal suppression and hypoglycemia if given at term. Risks considered small enough to justify use in cases of serious illness.
Analgesics	
Aspirin	Conflicting reports about large doses. No evidence that therapeutic doses are harmful but is generally avoided.
Nonnarcotic analgesics	Avoid. Can cause withdrawal syndrome in newborn.
Newer nonsteroidal anti-inflammatory drugs	Little information available. Indomethacin not recommended.
Anticoagulants	
All types except heparin	Contraindicated. May cause bleeding episodes in baby. Warfarin is definitely embryotoxic.
Anticonvulsants	
All types	Embryotoxic. In general, cause two to three times more fetal abnormalities (cleft lip/palate, spontaneous abortion, heart defects, microcephaly) than those occurring in the general population.
Antimicrobials	
Aminoglycosides (amikacin, garamycin, kanamycin, streptomycin, tobramycin vancomycin)	May have toxic effects on the eighth cranial nerve.
Cephalosporins (cefazolin, cephalexin, cephalothin, cephradine)	No adverse effects reported.
Chloramphenicol	Reported effects include gray baby syndrome, failure to feed, hypothermia, death.
Chloroquine	Reports suggest that proper dosages are not contraindicated. Prolonged use in pregnancy may produce fetal damage.
Clindamycin	No adverse effects reported.
Erythromycin	Considered apparently safe.
Ethambutol	Slight increase in fetal malformations if given in first trimester.
Ethionamide	Small increase in fetal malformations if given in first trimester.
Isoniazid	Use with caution. May cause CNS effects.
Metronidazole	Should be avoided, although recent reports suggest that it may be safe.
Methenamine	Appears safe.
Nalidixic acid	May cause chromosomal abnormalities.
Nitrofurantoin	Appears safe in correct doses. May cause hemolysis in G-6-PD–deficient fetuses.
Pencillins (ampicillin, amoxicillin, floxacillin, penicillin)	Appears safe but may cause sensitization in utero.
Primaquine	Reports suggest that proper dosages are not contraindicated. Prolonged use in pregnancy may produce fetal damage.
Rifampin	Some fetal malformations reported from use in first trimester.
Sulfonamides	No adverse effects noted in first trimester. Contraindicated in second and third trimesters due to theoretical risk of jaundice.

TABLE 9.29 *(Continued)*

Drug	Comment
Tetracycline	Contraindicated. Causes discoloration of teeth and interferes with bone growth.
Trimethoprim/sulfamethoxazole	Appears safe in first trimester. Contraindicated in second and third trimesters due to risk of jaundice from sulfonamide component.
Asthma preparations	
Aminophylline/	No increased risks to fetus in studies.
Theophylline	May cause vomiting and tachycardia if given during labor and delivery.
Epinephrine	Use with caution during labor and delivery.
Antineoplastics	
All types, with possible exception of tamoxifen	Reports of embryotoxicity. Use only for treatment of malignant conditions.
Cardiovascular preparations	
Reserpine	No reported effects during pregnancy. May cause bradycardia and temperature fluctuations during labor and delivery.
Methyldopa	Appears safe when used under close medical supervision.
Propranolol	Fetal growth retardation with low birth weight. If taken during labor and delivery, can impair cardiac output, and cause hypoglycemia and respiratory distress.
Digitalis	No adverse effects on fetus reported.
Cold/cough preparations	
Ammonium chloride	May cause acidosis.
Diabetic agents	
Diazoxide	Should not be used in the second and third trimesters or during labor and delivery.
Insulin	Harmless as long as maternal hypoglycemia is avoided. Monocomponent insulins are preferable.
Sulfonylureas (all types)	Not recommended in pregnancy. Increase in fetal mortality and fetal defects suspected. Neonatal hypoglycemia possible.
Diuretics	
Acetazolamide	Use with caution in first trimester.
Chlorthalidone	Avoid. May cause thrombocytopenia and potassium depletion.
Ethacrynic acid	Avoid. Can cause hyponatremia.
Furosemide	Avoid. Can cause hyponatremia.
Hydrochlorothiazide	Avoid. Same as for chlorthalidone.
Spironolactone	No adverse effects reported.
GI preparations	
Antacids	Single study shows a slightly higher incidence of fetal malformations. Avoid in early pregnancy if possible.
Atropine sulfate	No studies. Should be avoided.
Cimetidine	Animal studies only. Crosses placenta. Should be avoided.
Dicyclomine HCL	Conflicting study results.
Metoclopramide HCL	Has not been used widely in pregnancy. Avoid if possible.
Heavy metals	
All types	Contraindicated.

TABLE 9.29 *(Continued)*

Drug	Comment
Hormones	
Clomiphene	Slightly higher level of anencephalic births if taken during first trimester.
DES	Absolutely contraindicated. Definitely embryotoxic.
Estrogens	Prolonged exposure can cause masculinization of female fetus and less aggressive male fetus.
Oral contraceptives	Contraindicated. Both estrogens and progesterones may be embryotoxic.
Oxytocin	Widely used during labor and delivery without many problems.
Progestins	Contraindicated. Can produce feminization of male infants and masculinization of female fetus.
Progestasert IUD	Increased incidence of ectopic pregnancy.
Testosterone	Contraindicated. Can cause masculinization of female fetus with clitoral enlargement and labial fusion.
Motion sickness agents/antihistamines	
Meclizine	Original reports of increased abnormalities not confirmed.
Promethazine	Keep use to minimum. Hip dislocation is suspected.
Diphenhydramine	Suspicion of cleft palate not confirmed.
Transderm-Scop	Avoid.
Nutritional agents	
Nicotinamide	Avoid. Possibly embryotoxic.
Vitamin D	Excess amounts can cause hypercalcemia and aortic stenosis.
Vitamin K	Risk of hyperbilirubinemia if taken in excess at term.
Parkinson's disease agents	
Amantadine	Limited use.
Levodopa	Limited use. No adverse effects reported.
Bromocriptine	Normal infants reported with continuous use throughout pregnancy.
Psychiatric drugs	
Lithium	Absolutely contraindicated. Definitely toxic to infant.
MAO inhibitors	Use with extreme caution at term and during delivery.
Phenothiazines	Avoid if possible. Adverse effects reported in all stages of pregnancy.
Tricyclic antidepressants	Original reports of higher incidence of fetal abnormalities have not been confirmed in British studies.
Sedatives/hypnotics	Avoid. May cause fetal malformations, premature labor, intrauterine death, withdrawal syndrome in neonate.
Tranquilizers	Avoid. All types may be embryotoxic. If given at term, can cause reduced Apgar score. Withdrawal syndrome possible in newborn.
Recreational drugs	
Amphetamines	May cause fetal malformations.
Alcohol	If taken in excess, definitely embryotoxic.
Cocaine	Serious abnormalities, increased rates of stillbirth, miscarriage, and sudden infant death syndrome reported.

TABLE 9.29 *(Continued)*

Drug	Comment
Cigarettes	Associated with low-birth-weight infants.
Heroin	Withdrawal syndrome in newborn.
Marijuana	No data on human infants, but known to impair DNA and RNA in animals.
Methadone	Serious withdrawal syndrome in newborn.
Thyroid medications	
Iodides	Contraindicated in large dosages and for long-term use. Can cause goiter, hypothyroidism, and cretinism in infant.
Methimazole	Absolutely contraindicated. May cause goiter or hypothyroidism.
Propylthiouracil	Appears safe in minimum doses.
Thyrouricil	Contraindicated. Can cause thyroid enlargement, hypothyroidism, and cretinism in infant.
Thyroxine	Appears safe, but thyroid levels in newborn should be monitored if taken by mother during pregnancy.

Source: Based on Balke et al.: Drugs in pregnancy: Weighing the risks, *Patient Care,* (May) 1980.

Couples who desire to prevent further pregnancies are more likely to succeed with whatever method of birth control they choose than are couples who only wish to delay future pregnancies. Women who do not want more children may be more willing to choose a method that poses more risks to future fertility (e.g. IUD, sterilization) than women who have not finished childbearing. Ultimately, it must be the patient who chooses, since it is she who has to live with the consequences. Some of the ***experimental birth control measures*** described in Table 9.32 may make future choices easier.

Abstinence is an important birth control measure that should not be overlooked.

TABLE 9.30 OCCUPATIONAL HAZARDS TO REPRODUCTION[a,b]

Anesthetic gases (halothane, nitrous oxide, cyclopropane, others)
Cadmium
Carbamates
Chromium compounds
Fluorine
Formaldehyde
Mercury
Nickel
Polychlorinated biphenyls
Vinyl chloride
Viruses
*Carbon disulfide
Carbon monoxide
*Chloroprene
*Estrogens (manufacturing of)
*Ionizing radiation
*Kepone
*Lead
*Microwaves

Organic solvents: *toluene, *xylene, benzene, ethylene dibromide, 1,1,1-trichloroethane, chlorinated hydrocarbons (methylene chloride, *trichlorethylene, perchlorethylene, chloroform, carbon tetrachloride)

Pesticides: aldrin, DDT, heptachlor, methoxychlor, endrin, dieldrin, *dibromochloropropane, chlordane, lindane, toxaphene, parathion

Source: Based on Hunt Z: *Work and the Health of Women.* CRC Press, Boca Raton, Fla., 1979.

[a]Unstarred substances or hazards are associated with various adverse pregnancy outcomes with exposure of either partner.
[b]Starred substances are associated with infertility in either men or women.

TABLE 9.31 CHILDBEARING ISSUES

Issues for all future parents Affinity for children Expectations of the child Willingness of both partners to have children Shared values by partners regarding work, religion, family, and childbearing Changes in lifestyle necessitated by the presence of children Finances Commitments to job, elderly parents, or others Personal health Personality characteristics such as patience, emotional control, and communication ability Motivations for childlessness Health risks of pregnancy Political beliefs regarding overpopulation Children by a previous marriage Homosexual preference	Motivations for childbearing Continued growth of a satisfying relationship Creation of a new human being that will grow and develop with the parents' loving guidance Affirmation of religious beliefs regarding procreation as the reason for marriage and intercourse Establishment of adulthood and independence from one's family of origin Resolution of marital problems by obligating partners to each other Replacement of a lost child Substitution for a satisfying adult relationship Proof of sexual adequacy Escape from boredom of work Production of an heir or security in old age Attainment of economic support from a spouse or the state Frustration with birth control methods that may have unpleasant or unacceptable side effects

Sources: Bradshaw BR et al.: *Counseling on Family and Human Sexuality,* Family Service Association of America, New York, 1977; Moore MD, Davis OS: *Realities in Childbearing,* Saunders, Philadelphia, 1978, pp. 110–111.

It is used by teenagers and unmarried couples who view intercourse as appropriate only within a well-defined or sanctified relationship such as marriage. Other couples practice ***periodic abstinence (PA)*** as part of natural family planning techniques or for reasons of medical illness, recent termination of a pregnancy, pelvic pain, or inability to achieve erection. During periods of abstinence, they may continue to have sexual contact that may range from holding hands to mutual masturbation or oral-genital sex. Patients should be encouraged to exercise their right to defer intercourse until the time they deem appropriate. This may be a particularly important consideration for teenagers exposed to peer pressure.

► ***The pill*** (oral contraception, OC) is a widely used birth control method, particularly by women younger than 30. Available preparations are listed in Table 9.33. Containing the hormones estrogen and progesterone in fixed or triphasic combinations, they work by suppressing the hypothalamic-ovarian feedback axis and thus preventing ovulation. The pill also works by causing cervical mucus to become thicker (interfering with sperm passage) and by altering the lining of the uterus (interfering with implantation in the event of ovulation). The effectiveness of the pill is 98–99% depending on user compliance. It is given in one of two ways: (1) a pill every day for 21 days and stopping for 7 days (21-day pack) or (2) a pill every day with no stopping between packs (28-day pack). In the 28-day regimen, only the first 21 pills contain hormones; the last 7 pills are inert reminder pills to encourage the daily habit of pill taking.

Pill use is associated with the benefits and risks described in Table 9.34. Users generally like the convenience of being able to have sex without any special preparation and of having predictable, lighter periods. As studies show, they also have a lower incidence of benign breast disease, ovarian cancer, iron deficiency anemia, dysmenorrhea, and PID than other groups of women. On the other hand, pill use is associated with some adverse health effects, the most serious being an increased

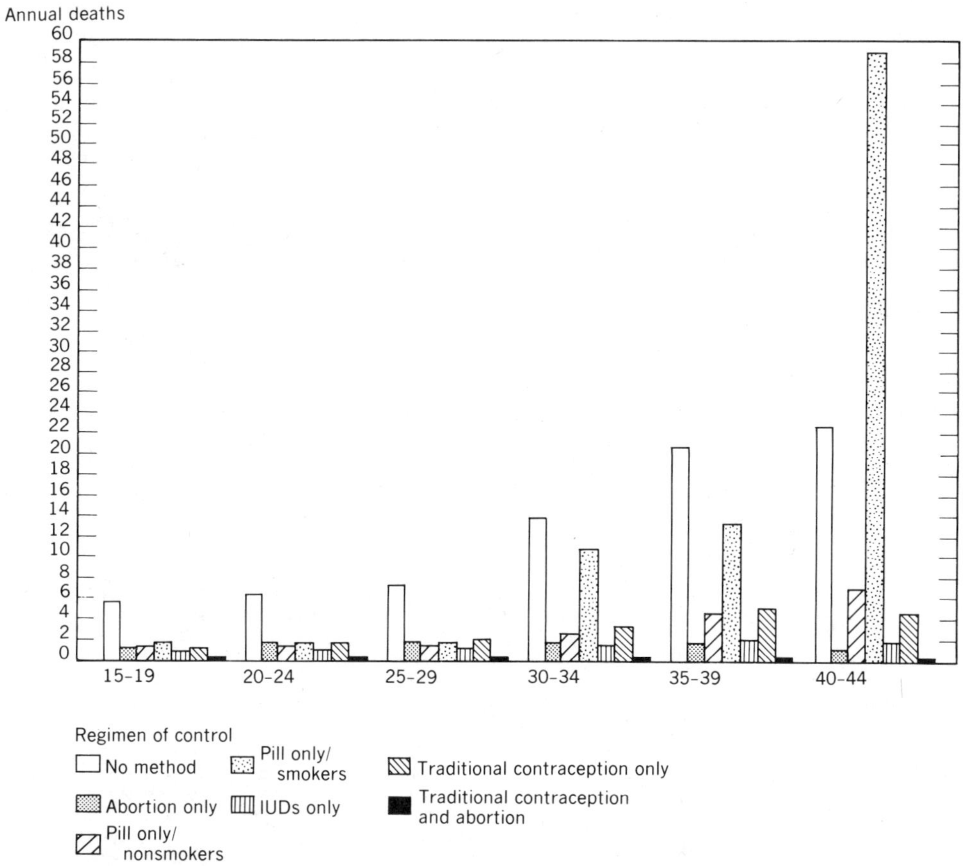

Figure 9.8 Estimates of mortality associated with fertility control. (Reprinted by permission from Tietze, *Family Planning Perspectives,* 9(2):76, © 1977.)

cardiovascular risk of stroke, heart attack, pulmonary emboli, and thrombophlebitis. In addition, some drugs (Table 9.35) reduce the contraceptive effectiveness of the pill, and vice versa. The risks and benefits of the pill should be discussed with prospective users. In addition, before prescribing the pill, a thorough history should be taken and a physical exam performed to rule out the contraindications noted in Table 9.36. Patients receiving a prescription should be instructed on how to take the pill, and advised about warning symptoms of thromboembolic complications and necessary follow-up.

Six types of progestins are used in pill preparations. They differ with regard to their estrogenic, androgenic, and antiestrogenic potency, as noted in Table 9.37. As a result, patients can develop ▶ ***minor side effects of the pill*** such as nausea, breakthrough bleeding, acne, or other conditions described in Table 9.38. Many of these problems resolve spontaneously after 3 months of pill use and are best managed with reassurance. Others require simple interventions such as salt restriction for weight gain or taking the pills at night to prevent nausea. Starting patients on the newer

TABLE 9.32 EXPERIMENTAL BIRTH CONTROL METHODS

Method or Product	Description
Depoprovera	A long-acting form of medroxyprogesterone acetate given by IM injection every 3 months. It has not been approved for use as a contraceptive in the United States but is widely used in other countries. The FDA has denied approval because of controversy regarding its association with breast, uterine, and growth abnormalities in test animals. There have also been reports of fertility problems and congenital abnormalities in humans. Although its use as a contraceptive is not recommended, Deprovera is available by prescription in the United States under the authority of a physician.
Subdermal contraceptive (Norplant)	Silastic rods containing levonorgestrel are planted under the skin of the upper arm. They release gradual amounts of the hormone each day for a period of 5–6 years (although studies demonstrate that optimum effectiveness is reached if the implants are replaced at 3-year intervals). Removal is followed by immediate fertility. This method may soon be available in Europe; however, there is no immediate plan to release it in the United States.
Contraceptive vaginal ring (CVR)	Silastic ring placed in the vagina. Kept in place for 3 weeks, it releases an average of 300 mg levonorgestrel and 180 mg 17-beta-estradiol daily. It is then removed for 1 week, during which time withdrawal bleeding occurs. CVR has been found to be highly effective and convenient in experiments. However, it has been associated with decreased serum HDL-cholesterol levels in some of the women participating in investigations.
Gossypol	A contraceptive pill for men that works by decreasing the motility of sperm and arresting spermatogenesis without suppressing testicular hormone production. The usual gossypol regimen during investigations in China between 1974 and 1978 consisted of 20 mg/day for 3 months followed by 50 mg/week for maintenance. Serious issues have been raised regarding its toxicity and irreversibility. Some Chinese men had reduced plasma protein levels; others experienced lengthy delays in restoration of spermatogenesis.
Experimental IUD	Modified versions of presently available IUDs. Some new designs aim to reduce the chance of expulsion in postpartum women. The modified structure of the Population Council's Copper-T 380A (already FDA approved) gives it a longer life span in the uterus and requires less frequent replacement than present copper-bearing devices. A T-shaped IUD (Nova T) that releases 30 mg levonorgestrel a day over a 3-year period has shown promise in protecting against pelvic infection. Reduced menstrual and intermenstrual bleeding is another advantage of this IUD.
Cervical cap	The cervical cap is a rubber or flexible plastic device that did not withstand FDA testing for effectiveness and user acceptability. The cap is inserted into the vagina and held in place directly over the cervix by suction. It works by blocking entry of sperm into the uterus. Used with or without a spermicide, it can be left in place for 2 days and perhaps longer. Problems included the development of a malodorous discharge within the cap, a somewhat difficult insertion procedure, and possible dislodgement during intercourse.
The contracap	A rubber-like plastic cervical cap with a one-way valve that permits unidirectional flow from the cervix while preventing sperm from reaching the os. An impression of the cervix, using dental impression techniques ensures its exact fit. The contracap may then be worn for long periods of time, perhaps up to 2 years. FDA trials were abandoned in 1985 due to an unacceptable pregnancy rate.

TABLE 9.33 ORAL CONTRACEPTIVE PREPARATIONS

Brand (Packaging)	Estrogen	Estrogen (μg/Tablet)	Progestogen	Progestogen (mg/Tablet)	Total Steroid (mg/Tablet)
More than 50 μg estrogen					
Enovid 5 mg (20)	Mestranol	75	Norethynodrel	5.0	5.075
Enovid-E (21)	Mestranol	100	Norethynodrel	2.5	2.60
Norinyl 2 mg (20)	Mestranol	100	Norethindrone	2.0	2.10
Ortho-Novum 2 mg (21)	Mestranol	100	Norethindrone	2.0	2.10
Ovulen (21, 28)	Mestranol	80	Ethynodiol diacetate	1.0	1.10
Norinyl 1+80 (21, 28)	Mestranol	80	Norethindrone	1.0	1.08
50 μg estrogen					
Norlestrin 2.5/50 (21, Fe)	Ethinyl estradiol	50	Norethindrone acetate	2.5	2.55
Demulen (21, 28)	Ethinyl estradiol	50	Ethynodiol diacetate	1.0	1.05
Norinyl 1+50 (21, 28)	Mestranol	50	Norethindrone	1.0	1.05
Norlestrin 1/50 (21, 28)	Ethinyl estradiol	50	Norethindrone acetate	1.0	1.05
Ortho-Novum 1/50 (21, 28)	Ethinyl estradiol	50	Norethindrone	1.0	1.05
Ovcon-50 (21, 28)	Ethinyl estradiol	50	Norethindrone	1.0	1.05
Ovral (21, 28)	Ethinyl estradiol	50	Norgestrel	0.5	0.55
Less than 50 μg estrogen					
Loestrin 1.5/30 (21, Fe)	Ethinyl estradiol	30	Norethindrone acetate	1.5	1.53
Demulen 1/35 (21, 28)	Ethinyl estradiol	35	Ethynodiol diacetate	1.0	1.035
Norinyl 1+35 (21, 28)	Ethinyl estradiol	35	Norethindrone	1.0	1.035
Ortho-Novum 1/35 (21, 28)	Ethinyl estradiol	35	Norethindrone	1.0	1.035
Ortho-Novum 10/11 (21, 28)	Ethinyl estradiol	35	Norethindrone	0.5	0.535 (10 days)
		35		1.0	1.035 (11 days)
Loestrin 1/20 (21, Fe)	Ethinyl estradiol	20	Norethindrone acetate	1.0	1.02
Ortho-Novum 7/7/7 (21, 28)	Ethinyl estradiol	35	Norethindrone	0.5	0.535 (7 days)
		35		0.75	0.785 (7 days)
		35		1.0	1.035 (7 days)
Tri-Norinyl (21, 28)	Ethinyl estradiol	35	Norethindrone	0.5	0.535 (7 days)
		35		1.0	1.035 (9 days)
		35		0.5	0.535 (5 days)
Modicon (21, 28)	Ethinyl estradiol	35	Norethindrone	0.5	0.535
Brevicon (21, 28)	Ethinyl estradiol	35	Norethindrone	0.5	0.535
Ovcon-35 (21, 28)	Ethinyl estradiol	35	Norethindrone	0.4	0.435
Lo/Ovral (21, 28)	Ethinyl estradiol	30	Norgestrel	0.3	0.33
Nordette (21, 28)	Ethinyl estradiol	30	Levonorgestrel	0.15	0.18
Triphasil (21, 28)	Ethinyl estradiol	30	Levonorgestrel	0.05	0.08 (6 days)
		40		0.075	0.115 (5 days)
		30		0.125	0.155 (10 days)

Source: Based on a chart prepared by Wyeth Laboratories, January 1985. Used with permission.

triphasic pills, which have lower total doses of progestins, or switching patients on fixed combinations to another brand of pill may also be helpful.

There are three available brands of the ▶ ***minipill,*** described in Table 9.39. Each contains progestin only. Nor QD and Micronor have one-third the amount of norethindrone contained in the combined pills, Norinyl 1/50 and Ortho-Novum 1/50. Ovrette has slightly more than one-sixth the amount of Lo-Ovral. Like the combined estrogen-progesterone pills, the minipill works by suppressing hypothalamic-ovarian feedback, changing cervical mucus, and altering the endometrial lining; however, hypothalamic-ovarian suppression is less complete than with combined estrogen-progestin preparations. Women take a pill containing the progestin every day; there are no hormone-free days. If the minipill is used consistently in this manner, effectiveness rates approach 97.5–99%.

A significant problem with minipill use is that ovulation and fertilization are highly variable and transport of the ovum through the fallopian tube may be slowed

TABLE 9.34 RISKS AND BENEFITS OF THE PILL

Cardiovascular

The most serious side effects associated with pill use are cardiovascular complications (angina, heart attacks, thrombophlebitis, pulmonary embolism, and stroke). They are related to hormonal effects that alter blood coagulation and increase triglyceride levels. The danger of stroke while taking the pill is enhanced in patients who are prone to vascular headaches. Vascular spasm in conjunction with hypercoagulation changes from estrogens could precipitate a cerebral clot. Furthermore, persons who have frequent headaches may ignore an important warning symptom. Hypertension occurs as a result of pill use in 1–5% of users; its incidence is increased further by obesity and increasing age and parity. If blood pressure rises higher than 140/90 mm Hg and is sustained over 3 months, pill use should be stopped. Such blood pressure changes are reversible upon discontinuation. Cardiovascular complications are greatest when the pill is used by women with other predisposing risk factors: smoking, diabetes, hypertension, type II hyperlipidemia, and age over 40. Within 1 month of discontinuing the pill, the risk of cardiovascular disease returns to age adjusted pre-pill levels. However, without complications, there seems to be no useful effect or need to initiate periodic pill-free intervals, since side effects are related to timing of use rather than duration.

Hepatobiliary

The incidence of cholelithiasis is higher in women who use oral contraceptives than in nonusers. The incidence of cholestatic jaundice is also increased in pill users. Liver tumors have been reported in 500 out of 10 million users of combined pills. Though they are not malignant, deaths have occurred from spontaneous or surgically induced hemorrhage. The risk of tumor development appears to be related to continuous use of the pill for 4 years or longer. Spontaneous regression of tumors occurs when pill use is stopped.

Breasts and reproductive tract

The pill may provide some protection against the development of benign breast disease. It may also have a protective effect against the development of cancer of the breast, ovaries, and endometrium. Amenorrhea and infertility may follow the use of oral contraceptives. Normal fertility returns by the third month after stopping the pill in 90% of women. However, women who have never become pregnant and who have a history of irregular and lengthy menstrual cycles may well be anovulatory to begin with. These women should consider not using the pill because of further ovulation-suppressing effects. There appears to be a slightly increased risk of congenital defects in children born to mothers who were taking the pill at the time of conception. Therefore, if a woman thinks she is pregnant, she should stop taking the pill. There is no increased incidence of congenital abnormalities in former users of oral contraceptives. The incidence of spontaneous abortion in women who become pregnant after using the pill, is apparently similar to that of other groups of pregnant women. Nonetheless, it is recommended that another method of birth control be used for the first three cycles after the pill has been discontinued before trying to become pregnant. Estrogen suppresses lactation. Both the estrogens and progestins in contraceptive pills appear in breast milk. Although the effect on the infant is unknown, breast-feeding mothers should avoid the combined pill. Women with known or suspected cancer of the breasts, ovaries, uterus, or cervix should not take the pill, since these malignancies may be hormone dependent. Although there are no epidemiologic data to support a causal relationship between cancer of the uterus or cervix and the use of combined oral contraceptives, there is a relationship between the use of estrogens by postmenopausal women and subsequent development of uterine cancer.

Metabolic

Metabolic effects of pill use include decreased glucose tolerance, elevation of serum triglycerides, alteration in amino acid metabolism, and increased thyroid-binding globulin. There may be an increased need for vitamins C, B_2, B_6, and folate but a decreased loss of iron due to lighter periods. Women who are at greatest risk for nutritional problems are those who have previous dietary deficiencies, chronic medical illness, a family history of diabetes mellitus, hyperlipidemia, or recent childbirth. Adolescents are also at risk. Most problems are minimized by using pills with low-dose estrogens or are corrected by diet and vitamin supplements.

TABLE 9.35 DRUG INTERACTIONS WITH COMBINED ORAL CONTRACEPTIVES

Effect	Drug		
Reduced contraceptive effectiveness (known or possible)	Antimicrobials Ampicillin Chloramphenicol Tetracycline Nitrofurantoin Rifampicin Penicillin V	Anticonvulsants Phenytoin Phenobarbital Carbamazepine Primidone Ethosuximide Analgesics Phenacetin Phenylbutazone	Hypnotics Barbiturates Methaqualone Tranquilizers Chlordiazepoxide Chlorpromazine Meprobamate Antihistamines Ergotamines
Potentiation of therapeutic effect or side effects of the other drug	Anti-inflammatories Phenylbutazone Antihypertensives Reserpine Corticosteroids		
Reduced therapeutic response of the other drug	Antidepressants Tricyclics	Antihypertensives Guanethidine Methyldopa	

Source: Based on Beard RJ: Some practical aspects of contraception, *Clinics in Obstetrics and Gynecology,* 1979, 6(1):157–170; Read MD: Managing oral contraception, *The Practitioner,* 1980, 224:179–181.

but not prevented. As a result, ectopic pregnancy is more common. This is a potentially life-threatening complication that requires surgical intervention. Thus, the minipill should not be used in women who have a history of an ectopic pregnancy. Another adverse side effect of progestin-only pills is irregular menses and intermenstrual spotting. Since abnormal bleeding is a crucial indicator of possible gynecologic tumors in older women, use of the minipill may obscure symptoms of underlying pathology, particularly in women over 35. The minipill is assumed to have the same thromboembolic complications as the estrogen-containing pills because epidemiologic studies have not separated estrogen effects from progestin effects. However,

TABLE 9.36 CONTRAINDICATIONS TO PILL USE

Absolute contraindications
- Thromboembolic disorders
- Angina, myocardial infarction
- Delivery of pregnancy within past 2 weeks
- Cerebrovascular accident
- Pregnancy
- Pituitary dysfunction
- Impaired liver function, hepatic adenoma
- Malignancy of the breast or reproductive organs

Strong relative contraindications
- Onset of established, regular menses for less than 6 months
- Vascular headaches or migraines
- Breast feeding
- Age over 40 or age over 35 combined with smoking 1 pack of cigarettes per day
- Hypertension
- Diabetes mellitus or a strong family history of the disease
- Sickle cell anemia
- Cardiac, renal, or hepatic insufficiency
- Type II hyperlipidemia
- Undiagnosed abnormal vaginal bleeding
- Termination of first-trimester pregnancy within 2 weeks
- Gallbladder disease
- Mononucleosis
- Long leg cast or prolonged immobilization

Other relative contraindications
- Renal disease
- Varicose veins
- Uterine fibroids (may contribute to enlargement)
- Mental retardation
- Chloasma
- Depression
- Asthma
- Epilepsy
- Acne
- Potential drug interactions
- Valvular heart disease

TABLE 9.37 POTENCY OF PILL PROGESTINS

	Effect		
Potency	**Androgenic**	**Estrogenic**	**Antiestrogenic**
High	Norgestrel/levonorgestrel	Norethynodrel	Norethindrone acetate
↑	Norethindrone acetate	Ethynodiol diacetate	Norgestrel/levonorgestrel
↕	Norethindrone	Norethindrone acetate	Norethindrone
↓	Ethynodiol diacetate	Norethindrone	Ethynodiol diacetate
Low	Norethynodrel	Norgestrel/levonorgestrel	Norethynodrel

TABLE 9.38 MINOR HORMONE-RELATED SIDE EFFECTS OF THE PILL

Estrogen Excess	Estrogen Deficiency	Progestin Excess	Progestin Deficiency
Nausea	Vasomotor symptoms, especially hot flashes	Increased appetite with secondary weight gain	Late spotting
Cyclic weight gain and edema	Early and midcycle spotting	Fatigue	Heavy menstrual flow[a]
Leukorrhea	Decreased menstrual flow, amenorrhea	Depression	Delayed onset of menses
Chloasma	Decreased libido[a]	Decreased libido[a]	
Breast tenderness[a]	Depression	Oily scalp, acne	
Breast enlargement		Alopecia	
Vascular headaches		Decreased length of menstrual flow	
Hypertension		Vaginitis, especially monilia	
PMS if on the pill[a]		Hirsutism	
Heavy menstrual flow[a]		PMS if between cycles[a]	
		Breast tenderness[a]	

Source: Based on Hatcher et al: *Contraceptive Technology 1980–81,* 10th ed., Irvington, New York, 1980, pp. 36–37.

[a]Effects that may be due to excess or deficiency of both hormones.

TABLE 9.39 MINIPILL PREPARATIONS

Brand	Progestin	Dose (mg/Tablet)
Micronor	Norethindrone	0.35
Nor QD	Norethindrone	0.35
Ovrette	Norgestrel	0.075

physiologic data indicate that estrogens are most likely responsible for the thromboembolic effects. Thus, the minipill, while having the same absolute contraindications as the combined pills, may pose fewer risks for women with cardiovascular risk factors than do the combined pills. In fact, there appears to be less risk of hypertension with progestin-only preparations. A switch from combined pills to the minipill is reasonable for women who become hypertensive on the former. Women with preexisting hypertension may also be candidates for minipill use. In addition, women taking combined pills who have developed other estrogen-related side effects such as chloasma, headaches, cyclic weight gain, and nausea may do well on the minipill. Severe venous varicosities are an indication for choosing the minipill over the combined pill. Side effects such as depression, acne, hirsutism, and vaginitis may be due to progestin use, but the strength of progestins in the minipill is less than that in combined pills; a switch to the minipill from the combined pills may therefore alleviate such problems. Lactation can continue successfully in the woman taking the minipill. However, progestins appear in breast milk, and the effects of the hormones on the infant are unknown. There is no known association between the minipill and cancer of the reproductive tract.

For women interested in using the minipill, a complete history and physical exam are necessary to rule out the contraindications noted in Table 9.40. Patients who are prescribed the minipill should be given complete instructions on use and have routine follow-up. If signs or symptoms arise of thromboembolic disorders or other conditions that contraindicate minipill use, it should be stopped immediately and appropriate medical treatment given. The patient who misses a menstrual period, even if she has taken all of her pills, should have a pregnancy test and, if there are any signs or symptoms of an ectopic pregnancy, a pelvic exam. The occurrence of intermenstrual bleeding is common, and reassurance should be provided. However, if it occurs in women over 35, discontinuance of the pills may be warranted for watchful waiting. With persistent bleeding, a work-up is indicated.

As a postcoital method, the ▶***morning-after pill (MAP)*** is not considered a primary means of birth control. The only hormonal preparation approved by the FDA for postcoital birth control is DES. Equivalent preparations are listed in Table 9.41. MAP is used when intercourse was unexpected and/or unprotected. Ideally, the hormones are prescribed only to women who are willing to have a therapeutic abortion if the method fails because of the possibility of birth defects. These hormones should not be used if more than 72 hours have elapsed since unprotected intercourse or if there has been more than one act of unprotected intercourse since the last menstrual period. Contraindications for the combined pill (Table 9.36) also apply. Prior to giving a prescription, a complete history should be obtained and a physical exam performed. The patient should then be given careful instructions for taking the medication. An antiemetic is usually prescribed along with the estrogen-only preparations.

An ▶***intrauterine device (IUD)*** is a small metal or plastic device that is implanted in the uterus through the cervix. It may be left in place indefinitely, depending on the type of device; those with copper wrappings and hormonal impregnations must be changed at specific intervals. The IUD is thought to prevent conception in

TABLE 9.40 CONTRAINDICATIONS TO MINIPILL USE

Absolute contraindications	Strong relative contraindications
Undiagnosed abnormal vaginal bleeding	Previous ectopic pregnancy
Thromboembolic disorders	Breast feeding
Angina, myocardial infarction	Diabetes mellitus
Cerebrovascular accident	Acute mononucleosis
Pregnancy	
Impaired liver function	Other relative contraindications
Malignancy of the breast or reproductive system	Uterine fibroids
	Mental retardation
	Depression
	Irregular menses

TABLE 9.41 HORMONE DOSES OF THE MORNING-AFTER PILL

Drug	Dose	Frequency
Estrogens		
Diethylstilbestrol	25 mg	bid × 5 days
Ethinyl estradiol	2.5 mg	bid × 5 days
Conjugated estrogen	10 mg	bid × 5 days
Estrogen and progestin		
Ethinyl estradiol/ *d*-Norgestrel (Ovral)	100 μg/1.0 mg	q12h × 2 doses

the following ways: (1) by providing mechanical interference with implantation; (2) by producing a sterile inflammatory reaction in which macrophages engulf sperm or the egg; (3) by causing changes in the endometrial fluid; and/or (4) by causing changes in uterine tubal motility. In addition, the copper-covered devices act by altering the endometrial enzyme system necessary for implantation and by producing a more pronounced inflammatory reaction. The devices impregnated with progesterone add the contraceptive effects of progesterone (cervical mucus changes and local hormonal effects on the endometrium). Effectiveness rates range from 95 to 98.5%. Though the FDA has not withdrawn approval of any of the IUDs noted in Figure 9.9, many drug companies have discontinued the distribution of their IUD products in the United States. To date, the Progestasert remains the only IUD to be actively marketed here. Since many women bear IUD models inserted prior to their discontinuation, and since many others are traveling to Canada for new insertions, discussion of various types is still warranted.

IUD use is associated with some serious complications, most of which are related to the reproductive tract. PID occurs three to five times more frequently in IUD users than in women who use other methods of birth control. Women with a prior history of PID are even more prone to the infection with an IUD in place. In general, the

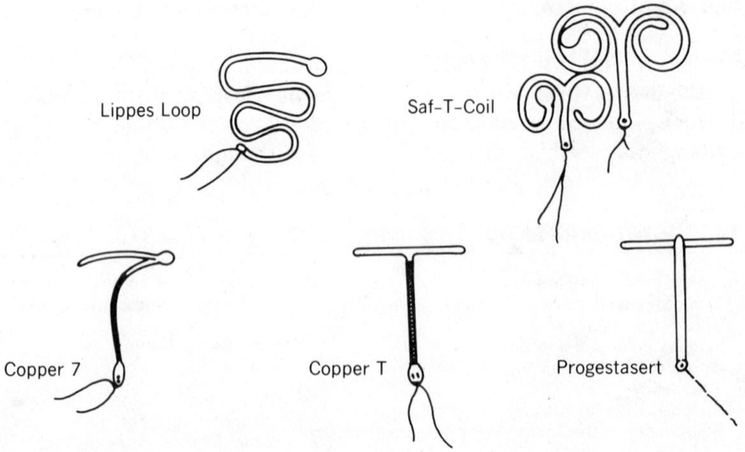

Figure 9.9 Intrauterine devices. (From Butnarescu, *Maternity Nursing: Theory to Practice*, © 1983, John Wiley and Sons, Inc., New York.)

incidence of PID tends to decline with increasing duration of IUD use. The proportion of gonococcal to nongonococcal PID is the same in IUD users as in nonusers. In some cases, PID may lead to tubo-ovarian abscess, peritonitis, or sepsis, or to permanent sterility because of tubal scarring. Complications may necessitate hysterectomy. Furthermore, probably because of its effects on tubal motility, the IUD is associated with a six- to eightfold increase in ectopic pregnancy over that of the non-IUD user. This increase may be apparent rather than actual because the IUD prevents intrauterine pregnancy but not tubal pregnancy. The risk of an ectopic pregnancy increases with duration of use.

When pregnancy occurs with an IUD in place, ectopic pregnancy must be ruled out by physical exam and, if necessary, ultrasound. IUDs must be removed in cases of intrauterine pregnancy. Those left in place have been associated with third-trimester uterine infections and sepsis. This complication has caused several deaths, the majority in women who were using the Dalkon Shield. Although the Dalkon Shield is no longer marketed, any woman who still has one in place should have it removed. IUD removal in the event of pregnancy is associated with a 25% risk of spontaneous abortion. This may be an important moral or religious consideration for a number of women; nonetheless, the risk of sepsis and death during a pregnancy with an IUD in place must be emphasized. There is no increased incidence of fetal malformation when conception occurs with an IUD in place.

If uterine perforation occurs, it usually happens at the time of IUD insertion. It may also happen spontaneously at a later time. Most perforations are asymptomatic, occurring without pain or bleeding. Closed devices that perforate must be removed because of the possibility that they will enclose a loop of bowel and cause obstruction. They are no longer marketed in the United States but may still be in use by some women. If the perforating IUD is a copper-containing device, it must be removed by laparoscopy or surgery because of its harmful interaction with internal organs. Other devices may be left in the abdominal cavity indefinitely. Less serious complications from IUD use are dysmenorrhea, spotting, menorrhagia with resultant iron deficiency anemia, spontaneous complete or partial expulsion, and difficult removal because of a lost string or embedding in the endometrial wall.

Women who wish IUD insertion should have a thorough health history, physical exam, and limited laboratory tests to rule out the contraindications noted in Table 9.42. Insertion should be performed at an appropriate time by a skilled practitioner. Following the procedure, patients should be given written instructions and a follow-up appointment for a string check and pelvic exam. Yearly appointments should be scheduled thereafter. For replacement or discontinuation, IUD removal is easiest to

Table 9.42 CONTRAINDICATIONS TO IUD USE

Absolute contraindications	Strong relative contraindications
Active PID within 3 months of insertion	Concern for future fertility
Recurrent PID	Multiple sexual partners
Pregnancy	Small uterine size
Distorted uterine anatomy, fibroids, congenital anomalies	Endometriosis
Valvular heart disease	Severe dysmenorrhea or menorrhagia
Undiagnosed abnormal vaginal bleeding	Anemia
For the copper devices: copper allergy or Wilson's disease	

accomplish during menses, when the small amount of associated spotting is less noticeable. The IUD should not be removed at midcycle if the woman has had intercourse in the preceding 4–5 days without the use of another method of contraception, since it is possible that a fertilized egg may be present. If ▶ ***IUD problems*** such as infection, pregnancy, expulsion, or missing strings develop, appropriate measures should be taken at once.

The ***morning-after IUD*** is the insertion of a copper-containing IUD within 3–5 days of unprotected intercourse (a lapse of more than 5 days is contraindicated). It prevents implantation of the ovum and provides ongoing birth control. Its use should be limited to women who have had only one act of unprotected intercourse since their last menstrual period in order to avoid interrupting a previously established pregnancy. Because of its association with an increased incidence of PID, this method should not be used for sexual assault victims, who are at greater than normal risk for contracting gonorrhea.

The ▶ ***diaphragm*** is a rubber dome attached to a circular spring. Used with a spermicidal jelly or cream, it is inserted into the vagina to cover the cervix, as shown in Figure 9.10. The diaphragm acts both to block sperm mechanically from reaching the cervical os and to hold spermicide at the os should sperm get past the mechanical barrier. The spermicide is the more important contraceptive protection provided by the diaphragm. According to newer studies, effectiveness rates range from 81–98% depending on correct use and motivation. As special considerations, the user must feel comfortable touching herself for insertion and must be willing to prepare in advance for intercourse. Diaphragm users may develop cystitis from pressure of the diaphragm ring on the urethra, particularly when diaphragms are left in place for more than the 6–8 hours required after intercourse; otherwise, they are not at risk for any adverse health risks. In fact, diaphragm use offers significant protection against the development of STDs. The relatively few contraindications are noted in Table 9.43. Before being fitted, the woman should have a complete health assessment and physical exam, including breast and pelvic exams. During the pelvic exam, the clinician should look specifically for cystocele, rectocele, prolapse, or shallow pubic notch. No laboratory tests are required.

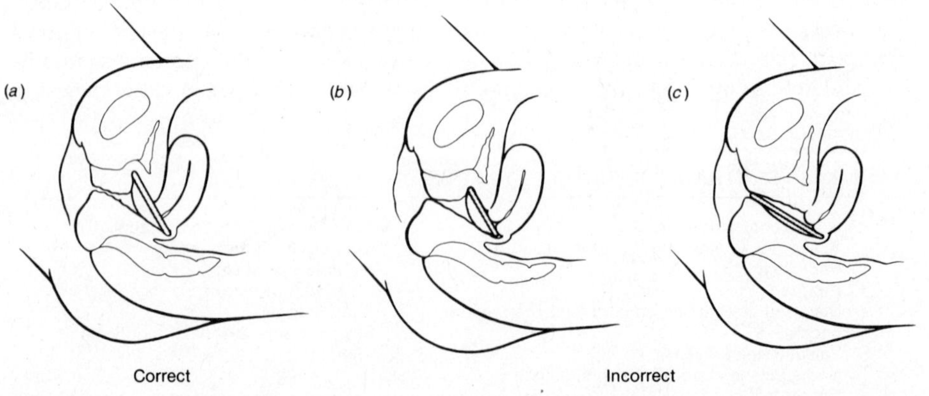

Figure 9.10 Diaphragm placement. (From Butnarescu, *Maternity Nursing: Theory to Practice,* © 1983, John Wiley and Sons, Inc., New York.)

TABLE 9.43 CONTRAINDICATIONS TO DIAPHRAGM USE

Absolute contraindications Medical conditions in which pregnancy would impose undue hazards for the mother	Uterine prolapse or extreme retroversion Small or button cervix Allergy to rubber or spermicide
Strong contraindications Client unable to learn insertion and removal techniques Moderate to severe cystocele Severe rectocele	Relative contraindications Shallow pubic notch Recurrent urinary tract infections Client who is averse to touching her genitals

There are three types of diaphragms: flat spring, coil spring, and arcing spring. Flat and coil spring diaphragms maintain a straight spring line when their sides are pressed together. The spring edge of the arcing spring forms a half circle when compressed. The sizes for all three types are in 5-mm increments and range from 55 to 95 mm in diameter. The most commonly used sizes are 65 to 85 mm. All diaphragms provide equal protection from pregnancy. In fitting the patient, the type and size of the diaphragm chosen depend on the pelvic anatomy and the woman's preference. After the fitting, the clinician should instruct the patient (and her partner) on diaphragm use and care.

The ▶ ***contraceptive sponge*** (Today) is a nonprescription method that was introduced to the American public in 1983. Made from a piece of soft polyurethane about 5.5 cm wide and 2 cm thick, the sponge is impregnated with the spermicide nonoxynol-9. After wetting, it is inserted into the vagina before intercourse, to provide contraception by blocking the cervical os, soaking up sperm, and killing sperm. Because the spermicide is released gradually, the sponge remains effective for 24 hours regardless of how many times the user has intercourse. It must be left in place for at least 6 hours after the last intercourse, even if intercourse occurred during the twenty-fourth hour after sponge insertion. The sponge is removed by pulling it out with the loop sewn to its bottom. Its effectiveness rate is 80–90%. As a special consideration, the user must feel comfortable touching her body in order to insert the sponge and must be willing to plan for intercourse. There are no health risks other than an allergy to spermicide. Isolated cases of TSS have been reported in Today users, but the rate is not statistically higher than that of users of other birth control methods. Patients should be instructed on how the method works, as well as its effectiveness, advantages and disadvantages, and proper use.

▶ ***Condoms*** are disposable sheaths that fit over the penis. They collect semen and prevent sperm from reaching the cervical os. Used alone, they have an effectiveness rate of about 90–98%. As a special consideration, the condom cannot be used until erection is achieved. This requires that the man not be overly modest about physiologic phases of the sex act and be willing to prepare for intercourse. Both the man and the woman may note decreased sexual pleasure, since the condom may reduce transmission of body heat, secretions, and sensation. There are no health risks except for the minor one of contact dermatitis from allergy to latex or the lubricant. In fact, because condoms help prevent transmission of venereal disease, their main effect on health is a beneficial one. Available without a prescription, condoms are made of latex (at a cost of approximately $0.30 to $0.50 each) or from the cecum of lamb intestines (about $1.50 each). Latex condoms come in a variety of colors and textures, either lubricated or unlubricated. They may be tapered, flared at the end, or narrowed, and may have a reservoir tip to hold the sperm. The thinness of the latex varies with the brand. In general, condoms come in only one size but may be available through mail order in different sizes. Condom choice is determined by user preference. Patients should be advised that condom effectiveness is greatly improved with concurrent use of a vaginal spermicide. It is important that both the man and the woman be instructed on use.

► ***Vaginal spermicides*** are creams, jellies, effervescent tablets, suppositories, or foams that contain nonoxynol-9 or some other active spermicide. The preparations available in the United States are listed in Table 9.44. Inserted by a finger or special applicator into the vagina just before each act of intercourse, the inert base blocks entrance to the cervix, trapping the sperm while the spermicide incapacitates them. Depending on the preparation used, effectiveness rates vary from 82–95%. Some creams and jellies are made to be used alone (e.g., Conceptrol, Delfen, Ramses); others contain less spermicide and are to be used only with a diaphragm or cervical cap (e.g., Koromex IIA, OrthoGynol). Because of this difference and because of poorer cervical coverage, the use of creams or jellies alone is not recommended. For spermicides to be properly used, the woman must feel comfortable touching her body and must be willing to prepare for intercourse. Dripping and burning are two com-

TABLE 9.44 SPERMICIDE PREPARATIONS

Brand	Type	Active Ingredient
Encare Oval	Foaming suppository	Nonoxynol-9, 2.27%
Semicide	Suppository	Nonoxynol-9, 6.6%
S'positive	Suppository	Nonoxynol-9, 5.8%
Today	Sponge	Nonoxynol-9, 1 g
Crescent Vaginal Jelly	Jelly	Glyceryl ricinoleate, 1%
Koromex II Jelly[a]	Jelly	Octoxynol, 1%
Koromex II-A Jelly[a]	Jelly	Nonoxynol-9, 2%
Orthogynol[a]	Jelly	*p*-Diisobutylphenoxypolyethoxyethanol
Preceptin	Jelly	*p*-Diisobutylphenoxypolyethoxyethanol
Ramses "10 hour" Vaginal Jelly	Jelly	Nonoxynol-9, 5%
Anvita	Cream	Phenylmercuric borate 1:2,000
Conceptrol	Cream	Nonoxynol-9, 5%
Crescent Cream	Cream	Glyceryl ricinoleate, 0.36%
Milex Cream	Cream	Glyceryl ricinoleate, 0.36%
Delfen Cream	Cream	Nonoxynol-9, 5%
Immolin Cream-Jel	Cream	Nonoxynol-9, 1%
Ortho Cream	Cream	Nonoxynol-9
Because	Foam	Nonoxynol-9, 8%
Delfen Foam	Foam	Nonoxynol-9, 12.5%
Emko	Foam	Nonoxynol-9, 8%
Emko Pre-Fill	Foam	Nonoxynol-9, 8%
Koromex	Foam	Nonoxynol-9, 12.5%

[a]For use only with a diaphragm or cervical cap.

monly cited disadvantages of the method. The major advantages are that prescriptions are not needed and there are no systemic side effects. Its effectiveness is greatest if the condom is used concurrently (approaching that of the combined pill). It is also improved if the clinician provides full instructions and follow-up, encourages use of the preparation with each coital act, and inspires confidence in the method when it is used consistently.

Coitus interruptus (withdrawal) is the practice of removing the penis from the vagina just before ejaculation. If no sperm are deposited in the vagina, conception will not take place. Unfortunately, effectiveness rates are quite low (around 77–84%). There are several reasons for this. First, some sperm may be present in the lubricating fluid that is released from the penis long before ejaculation. Second, control of ejaculation may not be complete and thus withdrawal may not occur soon enough. This risk is increased by the fact that there is a strong desire for deeper penetration just before orgasm. Alcohol use and fatigue tend to decrease the awareness of impending ejaculation. Advantages of the method include (1) lack of cost, (2) no need for a prescription or special equipment, (3) acceptability to those whose religion prohibits artificial contraception, and (4) no systemic side effects. The major disadvantage is the high failure rate. All of these factors should be discussed with the patient and the technique explained. The method is not advised for men who have a history of premature ejaculation or lack of self-control.

Natural family planning involves observation and recording of certain natural symptoms and bodily changes during a woman's menstrual cycle that indicate fertile and infertile phases for the purpose of either preventing or achieving pregnancy. It is based on three scientific facts: (1) for most women, ovulation occurs 14 days before the beginning of menstruation; (2) the egg survives for 24 hours; (3) sperm survive in the female genital tract for 48–72 hours. The major benefits of natural family planning are the lack of adverse health effects and its general acceptability to couples whose religion prohibits artificial means of birth control. Important considerations are that the woman must be diligent about keeping daily records and that both partners must be willing to find means other than vaginal intercourse for sexual expression and gratification during fertile days. Sex on safe days is unencumbered by preparations, but such spontaneity is not permissible on fertile days. Some couples may find this situation frustrating; others may appreciate the intercourse-free days or may find the sense of control and responsibility gratifying. A woman who is not in a stable relationship may not find the support she needs to use this method.

The ► ***basal body temperature (BBT) method*** is based on temperature changes that occur in the woman's body shortly after the time of ovulation. The BBT is the temperature taken in the morning before the woman begins her daily activities. At the beginning of the cycle, in the preovulation period (phase I), the temperature remains at a constant but lower level. Just prior to ovulation it drops momentarily (nadir) and over the next 1–5 days (at the time of ovulation and with progesterone increase) begins a thermal shift upward (phase II). Phase II is the fertile period. It begins on the first day of temperature rise above the preovulation base and lasts until the temperature remains elevated at least 0.4°F for 3 days. There are four different thermal shift patterns: immediate rise in 1–2 days, a slow rise over 3–4 days, a stairstep rise with increases every 2–3 days, or a zigzag rise with increases and decreases over several days. Examples are given in Figure 9.11. In the postovulation period (phase III), temperatures remain at a constantly higher level than those observed in the preovulation period. This period begins on the night of the

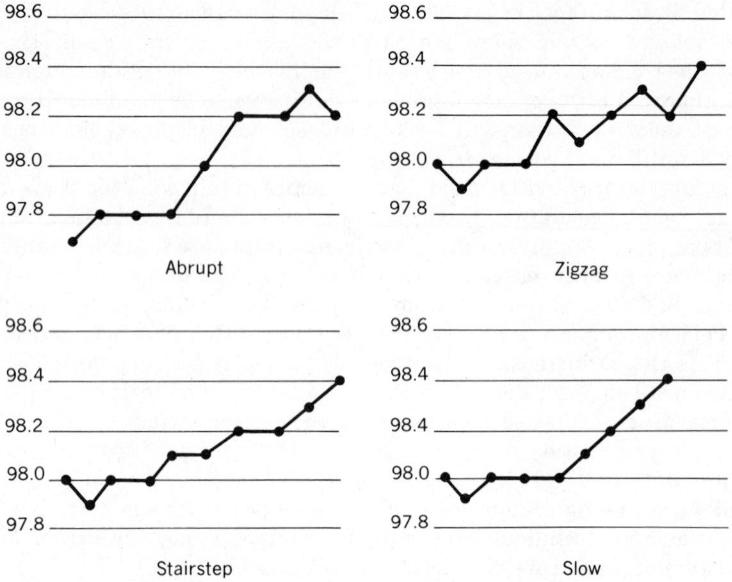

Figure 9.11 Temperature rise patterns.

third or fifth day of the thermal shift (depending on the pattern) and ends with the first day of menses. By keeping a monthly record of BBT such as that illustrated in Figure 9.12, the woman can identify her postovulation infertile time in each cycle.

The strict BBT method confines intercourse to phase III. It has an effectiveness rate of 94–98%. The relaxed BBT method allows for intercourse in phase I as well as in phase III. Its effectiveness rate is somewhat lower: 80–95%. However, neither BBT method is a reliable means of birth control during postpartum, lactation, or menopausal periods. The advantages and disadvantages of the BBT method were mentioned in the discussion of natural family planning. For management, no special health assessment is required. However, extensive counseling is needed to instruct the patient and her partner on equipment (special thermometer, graphs), temperature taking, charting, temperature patterns and interpretations, and determination of safe times.

The ▶ ***cervical mucus (Billings) method*** is based on monitoring the physiologic changes of the cervical mucus to determine ovulation. Influenced by the rise and fall of estrogen and progesterone levels, the uterine cervix continually produces a mucus discharge that changes in amount and consistency. At the beginning and end of the menstrual cycle the mucus is scant, cloudy, thick, and tacky. These days are referred to as "dry." In response to rising estrogen levels at the time of ovulation, the mucus is abundant, clear, thin, and elastic ("wet days"). The elastic quality of midcycle mucus is called "Spinnbarkheit" when it can be stretched into a thread 5–20 cm long. If allowed to dry on a glass slide, it forms a crystalline, fern-like pattern because of its relatively high salt and protein content. This egg white texture enhances the movement and survival of sperm. The last day of abundant wet mucus is referred to as the "peak day." By keeping a monthly record of mucus changes, the woman can identify fertile and infertile periods. As soon as the mucus appears, the

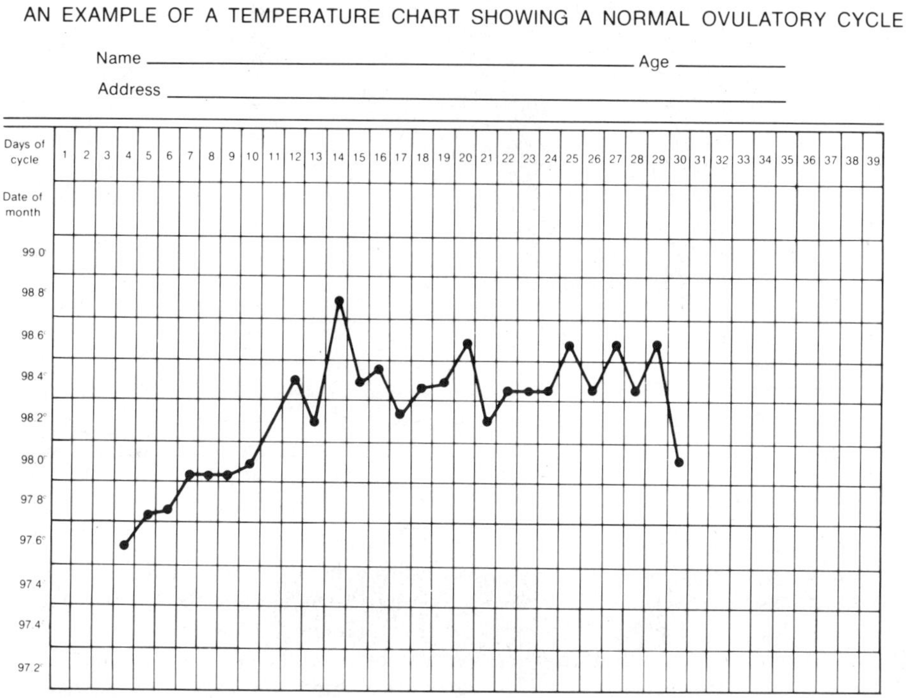

Figure 9.12 BBT chart. (From Butnarescu, *Maternity Nursing: Theory to Practice,* © 1983, John Wiley and Sons, Inc., New York.)

fertile phase of the cycle begins. Four complete days after the peak day marks the beginning of the postovulatory infertile phase. The effectiveness rate of this method ranges from 75 to 98%. Although it can be safely used by lactating, premenopausal, and perimenopausal women, this method is not advised for women who have chronic or recurrent vaginal infections. Its advantages and disadvantages are the same as those of any natural family planning technique. For management, no special health assessment is required. However, extensive counseling is needed to instruct the patient and her partner on mucus changes, charting, interpretations, and determination of safe times.

The ▶***symptothermal method*** combines the principles of BBT and cervical mucus changes with the observation of other physiologic indicators of ovulation. The latter may include Mittelschmerz (midcycle unilateral pelvic pain), breast changes (swelling, tenderness), abdominal bloating, a slightly bloody discharge, increased libido, vulvar swelling, and/or palpable changes of the cervix (it becomes softer, flatter, and more slippery, and the os opens slightly). All indicators are recorded on a calendar. The fertile period begins with the first symptom of cervical mucus and lasts through phase II of temperature rise and the fourth morning after peak mucus. As with the ovulation method, effectiveness rate ranges from 75 to 98%. Although it can be safely used by lactating, premenopausal, and perimenopausal women, this method is not advised for women who have chronic or recurrent vaginal infections. Its advantages and disadvantages are the same as those of any natural family

TABLE 9.45 CALENDAR METHOD: CALCULATIONS OF FERTILITY

Shortest Cycle	First Unsafe (Fertile) Day	Longest Cycle	Last Unsafe (Fertile) Day
21	3rd	21	10th
22	4th	22	11th
23	5th	23	12th
24	6th	24	13th
25	7th	25	14th
26	8th	26	15th
27	9th	27	16th
28	10th	28	17th
29	11th	29	18th
30	12th	30	19th
31	13th	31	20th
32	14th	32	21st
33	15th	33	22nd
34	16th	34	23rd
35	17th	35	24th

Day 1 = first day of bleeding.

planning technique. For management, no special health assessment is required. However, extensive counseling is needed to instruct the patient and her partner on BBT and ovulation methods as well as other symptoms of ovulation.

The ► ***calendar (rhythm) method*** has also been used as a natural family planning technique. However, since failure rates are as high as 14–35%, its use alone is no longer recommended by experts in the field. The calendar method is based on the premise that for the majority of women, ovulation occurs 14 ± 1 days before the onset of menses. Fertile (unsafe) days are computed by counting forward and backward from this time to account for both sperm and ovum survival times. Thus, there are a total of 11 unsafe days in an average 28-day cycle (Table 9.45). Some couples do not like to have intercourse during menstruation, which further decreases the number of days free for intercourse. The problem is that cycles vary in length from month to month. Thus the menstrual history must be recorded for at least 6–8 months prior to relying on the method and then in an ongoing fashion (Figure 9.13). At the onset of each menses, cycle lengths of the previous 6–8 cycles are used to determine safe and unsafe days which are then suitably marked on the calendar for the upcoming month.

Sterilization procedures are available for both sexes. They may be chosen for a number of reasons: attainment of desired family size, side effects of other contraceptives, personal political beliefs, or medical or genetic conditions. These procedures should be considered permanent, although some are surgically reversible. Counseling is therefore recommended for couples or individuals seeking sterilization to emphasize its consequences, to explore the reasons for making this choice, and to discuss alternatives. Counseling should address a number of factors, particularly the reasons for choosing to end all future childbearing. Sterilization should not be performed immediately after a stressful event such as the birth of a child with a genetic disease or after therapeutic abortion. A decision at that time may be a reaction to the stress rather than a well-thought-out choice. Also, sterilization should not be presented as a choice to women while they are in labor or shortly after delivery; rather, the decision should always be made well in advance of the procedure. Single persons

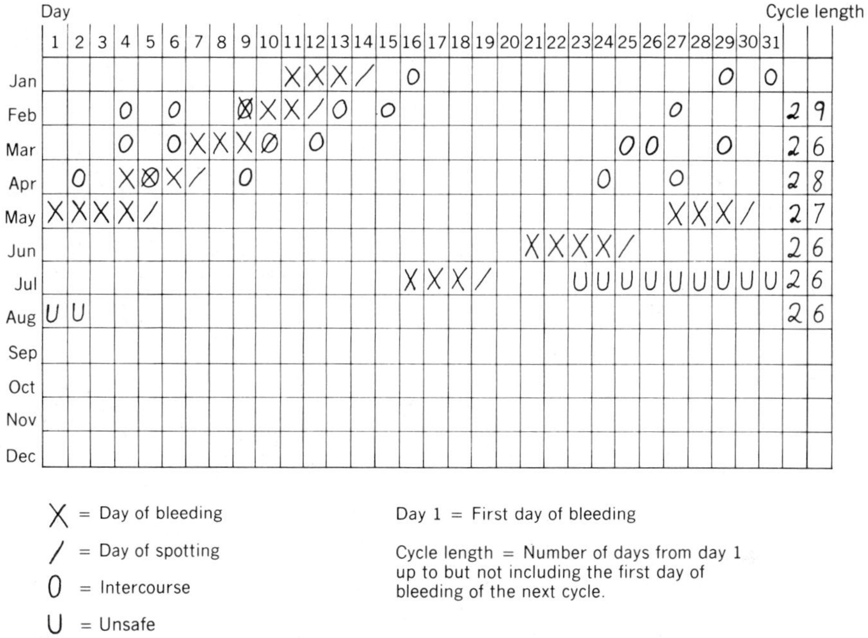

Figure 9.13 Ovulation calendar.

and those without children can generally be legally sterilized at their request; however, women who have tubal ligations when they are younger than 25 are among the majority of those few who later request reanastomosis. When sterilization is requested by a couple because of genetic disease, the partner with the disability or trait should usually be the one to undergo the procedure.

Male sterilization for contraceptive purposes is achieved by a surgical procedure, vasectomy, performed by a qualified surgeon or urologist. Through one or two small scrotal incisions made under local anesthesia, the vas deferens leading from each epididymis is surgically cut and tied, preventing the transport of sperm from the testes to the ejaculate. Sperm are still manufactured by the testes but are reabsorbed by the body. Directly after the surgery, there is usually some scrotal swelling and pain. Complications such as bleeding and infection may also occur. Until sperm-free semen has been demonstrated, usually within 6–8 weeks after the procedure, another method of birth control must be used. After three aspermic semen analyses, the vasectomy has a failure rate of only 0.15%. Long-term complications are rare, since hormonal function and ejaculatory ability are unaffected. Some men find that the psychologic impact of sterilization weakens their libido. The body may produce antibodies to the unconducted sperm, but these have not been found to be dangerous. Rare instances of spontaneous reanastomosis or incomplete ligation do occur, resulting in pregnancy. The possibility of this event is highest in the first 6 months following the procedure. Therefore, some surgeons recommend monthly sperm checks up to that time. Surgical reanastomosis is possible, but its success is limited.

Female sterilization for birth control alone is accomplished by tubal ligation.

TABLE 9.46 METHODS OF FEMALE TUBAL LIGATION

Procedure	Surgical Approach	Anesthesia	Procedure
Laparotomy	Abdomen near pubic hair-line	General	Exposure of uterus and tubes with ligation
Minilaparotomy	Abdomen through smaller incision than laparotomy	General or local	Uterus stabilized through the vagina; tubes exposed and ligated
Laparoscopy	Abdomen through very small incision just below the umbilicus	General	Carbon dioxide inflation of abdomen with ligation done entirely within the abdomen
Culpotomy	Posterior vagina	General	Vaginal exposure of tubes with ligation

One of the several surgical approaches presented in Table 9.46 may be used. Tubal ligation is usually done under general anesthesia by tying and cutting the fallopian tubes through an abdominal or vaginal incision. This prevents sperm from reaching the ovum and prevents ovum transport from the ovary to the uterus. Ova continue to mature in the ovaries, however, and ovarian hormonal function continues. Immediate complications from the surgery include the risks of general anesthesia, bleeding, embolism, intestinal burns or perforation, and infection. Unlike vasectomy, tubal ligation is immediately effective. Long-term effects are rare, though some women may have difficulty adjusting to the psychologic change that may accompany loss of fertility. Rarely (in 4 out of 10,000 women), postligation intra- or extrauterine pregnancy does occur, so any missed period is an indication for a pregnancy test. Tubal ligation is considered permanent, since reanastomosis has very

TABLE 9.47 POSSIBLE CAUSES OF INFERTILITY

Male	Female
Hypothalamic/pituitary	Hypothalamic/pituitary
Pituitary insufficiency	Pituitary insufficiency
Hyperprolactinemia	Hyperprolactinemia
Occupational toxins	Occupational toxins
Testicular	Ovarian
Mumps orchitis	Polycystic ovary syndrome
Undescended testicle(s)	Endometriosis
Chronic renal failure	Cancer chemotherapy
Lead and other occupational toxins	Radiation therapy
Sperm antibodies	Genetic disorders
Varicocele (excess heat)	Tubal
Radiation	Infection
Genetic disorders	Adhesions
Spermatogenesis deficit or failure	Sperm antibodies
Ejaculatory	Uterine
Obstruction of ducts	Malformations
Cystic fibrosis	Fibroids
Hypospadias	Adhesions
Impotence	
Prostatitis	Cervical/vaginal
Diabetes mellitus	Inadequate cervical mucus
	Vaginitis/cervicitis

limited success. After discussing with the woman her reasons for choosing sterilization, its permanence, and alternative methods of birth control, she should be referred to a qualified gynecologist.

Infertility is a common problem, striking one out of every eight couples. Some possible etiologies of male and female infertility are listed in Table 9.47. Most of them are complicated problems requiring special investigation and intervention. However, simple interventions by primary care providers can sometimes help couples achieve a wanted pregnancy. Any pelvic and/or urethral infection should be identified and treated. Counseling, particularly a review of reproductive anatomy, can also be important. Patients can be taught to use BBT, ovulation, and symptothermic methods and use of home urine testing kits (e.g., First Response) to identify fertile times for intercourse. Other simple measures can be suggested such as a change in coital position (man on top), avoidance of immediate withdrawal by the man, and maintenance of a supine position by the woman for at least 20 minutes following intercourse. Douching should be avoided. A semen analysis may be necessary, particularly in men who have not fathered children before or who are exposed to reproductive toxins at work (see Table 9.30). If fertility is still not achieved, referral should be made to a qualified gynecologist or infertility specialist.

Details of Management

▸ *Testicular Self-Exam*

Laboratory Tests: None.

Therapeutic Measures: None.

Patient Education: Provide men with written information such as the following:

HOW TO EXAMINE YOUR TESTICLES. Develop the habit of examining your testicles once a month. This simple self-exam takes only 3 minutes and provides the best chance for early detection of testicular cancer. It should be performed after a warm bath or shower when the scrotal skin is most relaxed. Using the fingers of both hands, gently roll the left testicle (which normally hangs slightly lower than the right) between the thumbs and forefingers. Check the right testicle in the same manner. Normal testes are equal in size, smooth in contour, and have a rubbery consistency. If you note any pain, enlargement, lumps, or bulges on the outside surface of the testes, check with your doctor. These changes may not represent a malignancy, but if one is present, early treatment can be lifesaving.

Follow-up: None.

▸ *Epididymitis*

Laboratory Tests: CBC. Urinalysis. Culture and sensitivity tests and gonorrhea culture of available discharge.

Therapeutic Measures: Start patients on antibiotics as follows: tetracycline 500 mg, 1 tablet qid for 10 days, or amoxicillin 500 mg, 1 tablet qid for 10 days. For pain relief, have patients use an athletic supporter (even during sleep) and give an anti-inflammatory/analgesic such as Indocin 25 mg, 1 tablet q8h prn or Naprosyn 375 mg, 1 tablet bid prn or extra-strength Tylenol, 1 or 2 tablets q4h prn. Advise patients to remain sedentary for several days. Bed rest for 3–5 days is required in severe cases. Patients with signs of toxemia must be hospitalized.

Patient Education: Use an anatomic drawing to point out the area of infection. Review the proper use of medication. Stress the importance of completing the prescribed course of antibiotics, of following instructions to remain sedentary, and of reporting any worsening or change of symptoms.

Follow-up: Patients should return weekly until normal testes, epididymis, and spermatic cord are clearly palpable. If abnormal findings persist after 4 weeks, patients should be referred to a urologist.

▶ *Acute Bacterial Prostatitis*

Laboratory Tests: CBC. Culture and sensitivity of available discharge. Gonorrhea culture of urethra. Two-glass urinalysis (the patient should void small amounts both before and after prostatic massage) with microscopic evaluation of both specimens, culture and sensitivity of the second urine specimen.

Therapeutic Measures: Start antibiotics as follows: Septra or Bactrim DS, 1 tablet bid for 14 days (usually effective against pathogens causing prostatitis). If the patient is allergic to sulfur, Geocillin 100 or 200 mg, 2 tablets qid for 14 days can be substituted. Analgesics are rarely necessary, but if requested, give acetylsalicylic acid (ASA) or acetaminophen, 2 tablets q4h prn. Severe cases may require hospitalization.

Patient Education: Use an anatomic drawing to point out the area of infection. Stress the importance of completing the course of antibiotics. Instruct patients to report any worsening or changes in symptoms.

Follow-up: Schedule weekly visits until all signs of the infection have resolved (negative prostate exam and cultures). If immediate improvement is not apparent or if complete resolution is not achieved in 4 weeks, refer the patient to a urologist.

▶ *Chronic Bacterial Prostatitis*

Laboratory Tests: CBC. Culture and sensitivity of available discharge. Gonorrhea culture of urethra. Two-glass urinalysis, as for acute bacterial prostatitis, with culture and sensitivity testing of the second urine specimen.

Therapeutic Measures: Prescribe long-term antibiotic therapy as follows: Septra or Bactrim DS, 1 tablet bid for 12 weeks, or Geocillin 100 or 200 mg, 1 tablet qid for 4 weeks, or Minocyn 100 mg, 1 tablet bid for 4 weeks, or erythromycin 500 mg, 1 tablet qid for 2 to 4 weeks. Although not usually necessary, ASA or acetaminophen, 2 tablets q4h, may be given for discomfort.

Patient Education: Use an anatomic drawing to point out the area of infection. Stress the importance of long-term antibiotic use to clear a chronic condition (frequent reinforcement is advisable). Review the proper use of medication. Patients should also be reminded to report any worsening or changes in symptoms.

Follow-up: Patients should be followed every 7–10 days until the condition resolves. Treatment failure mandates referral to a urologist.

▸ Nonbacterial Prostatitis

Laboratory Tests: CBC. Culture and sensitivity of available discharge. Gonorrhea culture of the urethra. Two-glass urinalysis, for chronic bacterial prostatitis, as described with culture and sensitivity of the second urine specimen.

Therapeutic Measures: Antibiotic therapy should be started until bacterial prostatitis is ruled out and then discontinued unless symptoms improve. Have patients avoid alcohol, caffeine, and spicy foods, since these substances may aggravate the condition. To relieve inflammation, give Indocin 25 mg, 1 tablet q8h prn, or Naprosyn 375 mg, 1 tablet bid prn. Tylenol, 1 or 2 tablets q4h prn, helps to relieve discomfort in patients who cannot tolerate anti-inflammatory drugs. Pyridium 100 mg, 1 tablet tid for short-term use, alleviates dysuria. Hot sitz baths are also soothing.

Patient Education: Stress the nonbacterial nature of the problem and the ineffectiveness of antibiotics. Reassure patients that the condition resolves spontaneously, but warn that recurrence is possible. Review the use and side effects of anti-inflammatory agents and Pyridium. Review diet modifications.

Follow-up: Patients should be followed for 7–10 days until the condition has resolved. Referral to a urologist is recommended if symptoms persist for more than a month.

▸ Secondary Amenorrhea

Laboratory Tests: Pregnancy test in all cases. FSH, LH, prolactin levels in cases of a negative response to progesterone challenge (see below).

Therapeutic Measures. Once pregnancy has been ruled out, patients may be challenged with progesterone (medical D&C). Give 20 mg norethindrone or 10 mg medroxyprogesterone orally every day for 4–5 days.

Positive medical D&C: If menstrual bleeding occurs within 2–3 days, it may be assumed that endogenous estrogen production is adequate but that progesterone is lacking. Treatment is then aimed at the underlying disorder (see Table 9.6). In cases of psychogenic stress, watchful waiting is advisable, since menses usually return spontaneously without any treatment. Alternatively, administration of medroxyprogesterone acetate (Provera) 10 mg daily on the last 5–10 days of the month may be used to produce withdrawal bleeding.

Negative medical D&C: If menstrual bleeding does not occur within 2–3 days of progesterone administration, further testing is advised. Pregnancy should be again be ruled out. FSH, LH, and prolactin levels should be drawn (high FSH and LH levels point to an ovarian problem, while low levels suggest a hypothalamic-pituitary origin). Treatment is aimed at the underlying cause (see Table 9.6). In cases associated with low FSH and LH, the endometrium usually suffers from hypoestrin effects (confirmed by vaginal smears and endometrial biopsy). In such cases, menses may return after several cycles induced with conjugated estrogen (e.g., Premarin) 1.2 mg, daily from days 1 to 20, and medroxyprogesterone (e.g., Provera) 10 mg, from days 21 to 25. As an alternative, clomiphene citrate (Clomid) 50 mg daily may be given for 5 days. Bleeding should follow within 30 days; if it does not, a second course of 100 mg daily may be given for 5 days. In underweight women, menses may return with appropriate weight gain, negating the need for drugs.

Patient Education: Explain the cyclic changes that normally occur to produce the menstrual cycle. Give careful instructions for taking medication.

Follow-up: While the patient is taking medication, schedule visits every 1–3 months. Patients with other than stress-related amenorrhea should be referred to an endocrinologist or gynecologist.

▸ *Dysfunctional Uterine Bleeding (DUB)*

Laboratory Tests: Hematocrit. Pap smear. Cervical biopsy and endometrial biopsy in women over age 35. Pregnancy test, pelvic ultrasound, cervical stains/cultures, WBC, ESR, thyroid function, and/or clotting work-up if indicated by the history and physical exam.

Therapeutic Measures

Spontaneous abortion, ectopic pregnancy, PID, polyps, fibroids, pelvic neoplasia, IUD complication, acute blood loss: immediate referral to an obstetrician or emergency room.

Endogenous hormone imbalance (estrogen stimulation without adequate progesterone): Give medroxyprogesterone acetate, 10 mg daily, or norethindrone acetate, 5 mg daily for 10–14 days starting on day 15 and repeat three or more cycles. Young women may be treated with a fixed combination oral contraceptive (e.g., Ovral), one pill qid until bleeding stops (usually 5–7 days) followed by three cycles of the same pill taken in the usual manner (one daily beginning with withdrawal bleeding). Also, give a nonsteroidal anti-inflammatory drug (e.g., Motrin, Indocin) in the usual dose to reduce uterine cramping and blood loss. Give iron therapy as needed. Investigate the underlying causes of anovulation, particularly psychogenic stress.

Exogenous hormone imbalance (prolonged use of progestins in the form of a minipill, injectable contraceptives, endometriosis therapy): treat with conjugated estrogens (e.g., Premarin), 1.25 mg daily for 7 days. Refer patients with severe bleeding to an emergency room (intravenous conjugated estrogens may be required).

Patient Education: In cases of hormone imbalance, explain the cyclic changes that normally occur to produce the menstrual cycle. Give careful instructions for taking medication. Have patients report continued bleeding or pain.

Follow-up: Schedule an exam in 3 days. Refer patients with persistent bleeding to an endocrinologist or gynecologist.

▸ *Primary Dysmenorrhea*

Laboratory Tests: None.

Therapeutic Measures: Prescribe a prostaglandin inhibitor such as ibuprofen (Motrin), 400 mg, or naproxen (Naprosyn), 275 mg, at the onset of bleeding (minimizes inadvertent drug use during pregnancy), repeated every 6 hours as needed. Oral contraceptives may be given to young women who are good candidates and have no objection to using the pill. Acupuncture, orgasm, the knee-chest position, and a hot water bottle applied to the lower abdomen are other effective interventions for pain relief.

Patient Education: Review the normal physiology of endometrial shedding with menses and excessive vascular spasm as a source of pain in some women. Explain the theoretical role of prostaglandin inhibitors. Review drug use and side effects.

Follow-up: As needed.

▸ *Premenstrual Syndrome (PMS)*

Laboratory Tests: Pap smear. Fasting blood sugar. CBC. If ovarian-hypothalamic imbalance is suspected, FSH, LH, estradiol, progesterone, and prolactin levels may be obtained within 7 days prior to the onset of menses.

Therapeutic Measures: Pharmacologic therapy for PMS remains controversial. Vitamin B_6, 50–800 mg po daily, has proven to be somewhat effective. PMS associated with luteal phase progesterone deficiency may respond to natural progesterone, 400 mg intravaginally on a daily basis from day 14 to day 28 of the menstrual cycle. Treat dysmenorrhea as outlined above. For water retention (evidenced by breast and abdominal enlargement and bloating) consider a diuretic (e.g., Dyazide, 1 capsule daily, or Hydrodiuril 25 mg, 1 tablet daily) given 2 days before and the first day or two of menses. Heating pads and exercise may be of limited help.

Patient Education: Warn patients taking vitamin B_6 not to exceed a daily dose of 800 mg because large doses (over 2 g/day) have been associated with neurologic symptoms. Stress the fact that prescribed medication should not be continued after symptoms abate. Explain to patients that other factors such as stress reduction, exercise, alcohol intake reduction, smoking withdrawal, and diet modifications (low-sodium, high-protein, low-sugar diet, weight management) can reduce PMS symptoms.

Follow-up: As needed.

▶ *Pap Smear Screening*

Laboratory Tests: An optimum Pap smear sampling depends on the following:

Patient considerations: Try to time sampling at the patient's midcycle. Instruct the patient not to douche or use intravaginal medication for at least 24 hours prior to the exam.

Clinician technique: For all sampling, use a speculum lubricated with plain water only (jelly will interfere with the smear). *To obtain a routine smear,* take a sample from the squamocolumnar junction of the cervix, including the distal 2–3 mm of the endocervical canal and the ectocervix. Cotton swab smears are unacceptable because of the high percentage of poor-quality smears and the extensive damage to cells. If a swab is used, Dacron swabs moistened with normal saline provide a more acceptable smear. The best samples are obtained by cervical scrape or cervical aspiration. *To obtain a cervical scrape,* use either the Ayer or the modified Ayer spatula (elongated tip). Other spatulas also reach into the cervical canal but tend to have acute angles that miss the squamocolumnar junction. Gently introduce the tip into the os and rotate it 360 degrees (remember, only the distal 2–3 mm of cervical canal bear the majority of dysplasias, and it is not necessary to scrape deeply into the canal). It should be noted that the upper portions of epithelial lesions are removed by cervical scraping and must be permitted to regrow before an accurate biopsy can be taken. Thus, the recommended interval between cervical scrape and biopsy is 8 weeks. A biopsy can be performed earlier after aspirate smears. *For cervical aspiration,* use a disposable pipette and a nondisposable bulb (firm bulbs such as the strong-suction 1-oz Asepto rubber bulb offer the strongest suction). Fit the bulb to the pipette and compress it completely. Position the tip of the pipette firmly against the external os without forcing it into the canal. Slowly release the bulb a bit to aspirate secretions from the endocervix. Continue the slow release of bulb pressure and rotate the tip of the pipette around the ectocervix, concentrating on the area around the external os. *To transfer the sample to a slide,* spread the secretions from the spatula once, using even pressure, beginning at the labeled end of the slide. When transferring from a pipette, rest the tip of the pipette perpendicular to the label end of the slide and with a quick squeeze blow the secretions onto the slide and use the pipette lengthwise to spread them. Do not rearrange the secretions. *To fix a smear,* hold the slide 1–2 ft from a well-shaken can of fixative and spray the slide evenly with a fine mist of fixative (do not drench the slide; a single pass is usually sufficient). Secretions must be fixed while they are still wet (within 3–5 seconds). Taking additional samples (vaginal pool samples, endocervical swabs) delays fixation and reduces screening reliability rather than enhancing it. A single cervical sample that covers the entire slide provides the optimum amount of critical material to examine. *To label the test properly,* write the patient's name and date on the frosted end of the slide in pencil (best done prior to the exam). Include in the Pap smear requisition (1) the patient's age, (2) the date of the last menstrual period, (3) the birth control method used, (4) exogenous hormone therapy, (5) previous cytologic or biopsy findings, (6) significant medical history, and (7) pertinent physical findings.

Laboratory expertise: Use a reputable laboratory with qualified cytopathologists. To be acceptable, laboratory reports must include a specific definition along with a classification such as that given in Table 9.8.

Therapeutic Measures: Refer the following for immediate colposcopy and/or treatment: any patient with a Pap smear of class III or above or with a Pap smear showing evidence of herpes or papilloma virus. Treat patients with class I or II Pap smears showing infection accordingly. After treatment, such patients with a class II Pap smear should have a repeated Pap smear in 3 months. If atypia persists, they should be referred for colposcopy.

Patient Education: Explain the purpose of Pap smear screening and its importance in detecting pelvic cancers. Note the fact that progression of cervical cancer can be prevented with early intervention.

Follow-up: Advise routine Pap smears on a yearly basis. Follow up abnormalities as noted above.

► *Screening Women Exposed to DES*

Laboratory Tests: Pap smears of the cervix (see the previous section) and vaginal mucosa every 3–12 months. It must not be done during the menses or if an inflammatory discharge is present. Obtain smears after wiping all secretions from the cervix and upper vagina. On four separate labeled vaginal slides, take smears of the upper vaginal vault: anterior, posterior, and two lateral (this is in the order of the most common sites of adenosis). Fix slides promptly.

Therapeutic Measures: Any patient with a visual abnormality or abnormal Pap test must be referred to a qualified colposcopist. Suspicious areas should be biopsied.

Patient Education: Explain the risks of DES exposure and the rationale for continuous and regular follow-up. Explain the nature of the screening tests and what to expect. Avoid making the parents feel guilty (if one's mother took DES it was because she wanted her child). Advise the patient to inform all other health care providers of her DES exposure. Note that fertility is usually normal in women but that there is a greater incidence of spontaneous abortion, premature birth, and ectopic pregnancy.

Follow-up: Every 3–12 months for Pap smears as described above (if initial exams reveal no abnormality, annual exams and Pap smears may be sufficient).

▸ DES Information/Organizations

Laboratory Tests: None.

Therapeutic Measures: None.

Patient Education: Provide patients with the pamphlet "Questions and Answers About DES Exposure during Pregnancy and Before Birth." It can be obtained by writing to the U.S. Department of Health and Human Services and requesting NIH Publication No. 80-1118. Information can be obtained from:

DES Action USA
2845 24th Street
San Francisco, CA 94110
Tel: (415) 826-4403

DES Action USA
Long Island Jewish Medical Center
New Hyde Park, NY 11040
Tel: (516) 775-3450

This group provides referral information for support groups. It also publishes "Fertility and Pregnancy Guide for DES Daughters and Sons" and the newsletter, "DES Action Voices."

Department DES
National Cancer Institute
Office of Cancer Communications
Bethesda, Maryland 20205

or

Cancer Information Centers
Toll-free number: (800) 638–6694

Encourage both DES sons and daughters to participate in voluntary DES registries run by state deparments of health. Information obtained for the registry promotes the ongoing effort to understand DES and the problems associated with its use. It is kept strictly confidential. Persons who are listed receive periodic information on DES-related developments.

Follow-up: As needed.

▸ Measures to Minimize the Danger of TSS

Laboratory Tests: None.

Therapeutic Measures: None.

Patient Education: Explain the nature of the illness. Note that although TSS is a rare problem and can strike women at any age, the incidence is highest among menstruating women who use tampons. Advise women that the risk of TSS can be lowered by using sanitary pads rather than tampons during menses. This is particularly important for patients with a history of TSS, since tampon use greatly increases the risk of recurrence. If tampons are used, those of the lowest absorbency and size to meet menstrual flow needs should be chosen. At the present time there is no standard measure of absorbency; "regular" in one brand can be more or less absorbent than "regular" or "super" in another brand. If the tampon causes irritation, "sticks," or is difficult to remove, another brand/absorbency/size should be tried. Alternating tampons and pads (particularly at night) and switching to lower-absorbency or smaller tampons at the end of the period are also helpful. Avoid leaving tampons, vaginal sponges, or diaphragms in any longer than necessary. On the other hand, excessive tampon changes (more often than every 3–4 hours) may also increase the risk of TSS (perhaps by introducing extra oxygen into the vaginal canal and/or irritating the vaginal mucosa). Store tampons in a clean, dry place. Wash hands with soap and water before and after inserting and removing tampons. Always insert or remove tampons carefully. In addition to giving information on tampons, teach patients to recognize the symptoms of TSS (sudden high fever, vomiting, diarrhea, dizziness, rash) and to take the following steps if symptoms develop: (1) remove the tampon if one is being used, (2) seek medical attention immediately, and (3) tell the medical practitioner that TSS is suspected.

Follow-up: None.

▸ *Acute Bartholinitis*

Laboratory Tests: Vaginal wet preparation. Gonorrhea culture. Culture and sensitivity of any drainage.

Therapeutic Measures: Start tetracycline 500 mg, 1 tablet qid for 7 days, or erythromycin 500 mg, 1 tablet qid for 7 days, or doxycycline 100 mg, 1 tablet bid for 7 days. If the gonorrhea culture is positive, treat accordingly (see the later section on gonorrhea). Prescribe frequent warm soaks. Give ASA, 2 tablets q4h for pain and to reduce inflammation.

Patient Education: Point out the area of inflammation on an anatomic drawing. Note that sexually transmitted organisms are the usual source of the problem. Stress that all sexual contact should be avoided until after treatment. Review the specifics of medication. Advise the use of loose-fitting clothing as long as swelling and pain persist. Have patients report signs of abscess formation (fever, increased swelling/pain, drainage). Warn that cyst formation and/or recurrence are common.

Follow-up: If an abscess develops, provide immediate referral for incision and drainage. Otherwise, schedule a return visit in 7–14 days for reexamination.

▸ *Surgical Menopause*

Laboratory Tests: Pap smear, SMAC (repeated yearly) while the patient is on hormone replacement. Other tests as needed for health maintenance according to age.

Therapeutic Measures: To prevent vasomotor symptoms and abrupt onset of osteoporosis/atrophic vaginitis, which occurs with bilateral oophorectomy, estrogen replacement* is usually started soon after surgical recovery. The usual choice is conjugated estrogen (e.g., Premarin) 1.25 mg, or ethinyl estradiol (e.g., Estinyl) 0.5 mg, or estrone sulfate (e.g., Ogen) 1.25 mg given for days 1–25, days 26–30 off hormones. Many providers are now giving estrogens in the above doses for days 1–15 and progesterone† for days 16–25 to reduce the risk of breast cancer. The usual prescription is medroxyprogesterone acetate (e.g, Provera) 10 mg or norethindrone acetate (e.g., Norlutin) 5 mg (whole or half tablet) on days 16–25. Most oophorectomized patients have a concurrent hysterectomy so that endometrial cancer is not a risk. After age 45–50, taper the hormone doses to half. Hormones may be discontinued after age 50–55.

Patient Education: Explain the role of the ovaries in the production of hormones. Note the importance of estrogens in maintaining bone mass and other tissue function. Review the use of medication. Advise the use of calcium, vitamin D, and exercise for prevention of osteoporosis (see Chapter 11).

Follow-up: Schedule appointments every 6 months for blood pressure, weight check, and medication review. Do a thorough gynecologic exam and check blood chemistries annually.

▶ *Natural Menopause*

Laboratory Tests: As needed for health maintenance in this age group. FSH and LH levels (show elevations) and a vaginal Pap smear (shows low estrogen effect with predominantly parabasal cells) may be useful, particularly in cases of premature menopause. Pap smear, SMAC (repeated yearly) for patients on hormone replacement.

Therapeutic Measures

Minimal symptoms: None needed other than education and support.

Vasomotor symptoms: Consider giving conjugated estrogens* (e.g., Premarin) 0.625 mg, or ethinyl estradiol (e.g., Estinyl) 0.02 mg, or estrone sulfate (e.g., Ogen) 0.625 mg on days 1–15 with medroxyprogesterone acetate (e.g., Provera) 10 mg, or norethindrone acetate (e.g., Norlutin) 5 mg (whole or half tablet) on days 16–25. The addition of progesterone† reduces the risk of endometrial cancer (and possibly of breast and ovarian cancer as well). For patients with hysterectomy, estrogens may be given on days 1–25.

Atrophic vaginitis: For patients with atrophic vaginitis and vasomotor symptoms, consider oral hormone therapy as noted above. For patients whose main complaint is atrophic vaginitis, topical hormone creams in small doses relieve

*Estrogens should not be given to women with cancer of the breast or uterus, estrogen-dependent ovarian cancer, thromboembolic disease, hypertension, diabetes, significant hepatobiliary disease, or large uterine myomas.

†Progestin should not be given to women with thromboembolic disease, cancer of the breast, or undiagnosed vaginal bleeding.

symptoms with minimal systemic absorption. Give conjugated estrogen cream (e.g., Premarin vaginal cream) 0.625 mg/g, ⅛th applicatorful (0.3 mg) at bedtime for 7–10 nights to start and twice weekly thereafter. If estrogen is contraindicated,* testosterone propionate 1-25 in vanishing cream may be given in the above manner.

Osteoporosis: Treatment as outlined in Chapter 11.

Patient Education: Explain hormone changes and their influence on body systems (see Tables 9.3 and 9.14). Suggest simple measures such as layers of natural fiber clothing that absorbs perspiration and "breathes" and that can be put on and taken off quickly with rapid body temperature changes. Obtain pamphlets for handout use such as the following:

"The Menopausal Years"
Patient Information Library
Physician's Art Service, Inc.
Daly City, California

or

"Your Menopause" by Ruth Carson
Public Affairs Pamphlet No. 447
381 Park Ave. South
New York, New York 10016

Encourage participation in midlife discussion groups, daily exercise, healthy diet.

Follow-up: For patients on hormone replacement, schedule appointments every 3–6 months for blood pressure, weight check, and medication review, as well as a thorough gynecologic exam, Pap smear, and blood chemistries annually.

▸ *Breast Self-Exam (BSE)*

Laboratory Tests: None.

Therapeutic Measures: None.

Patient Education: From menarche to menopause, women should be encouraged to perform BSE monthly as soon as menstruation is over. At this time, hormonal levels are low and the breasts are less likely to be painful, swollen, or nodular. Women with amenorrhea (e.g., due to hysterectomy, oophorectomy, or menopause) should choose a particular date on which to perform monthly BSE. Women should be instructed on the three-step breast examination procedure illustrated in Figure 9.14 and described as follows:

Step I. Examining the breast while wet: During a bath or shower, while the hands and breasts are soapy, examine every part of the breast, beginning at the

*Estrogens should not be given to women with cancer of the breast or uterus, estrogen-dependent ovarian cancer, thromboembolic disease, hypertension, diabetes, significant hepatobiliary disease, or large uterine myomas.

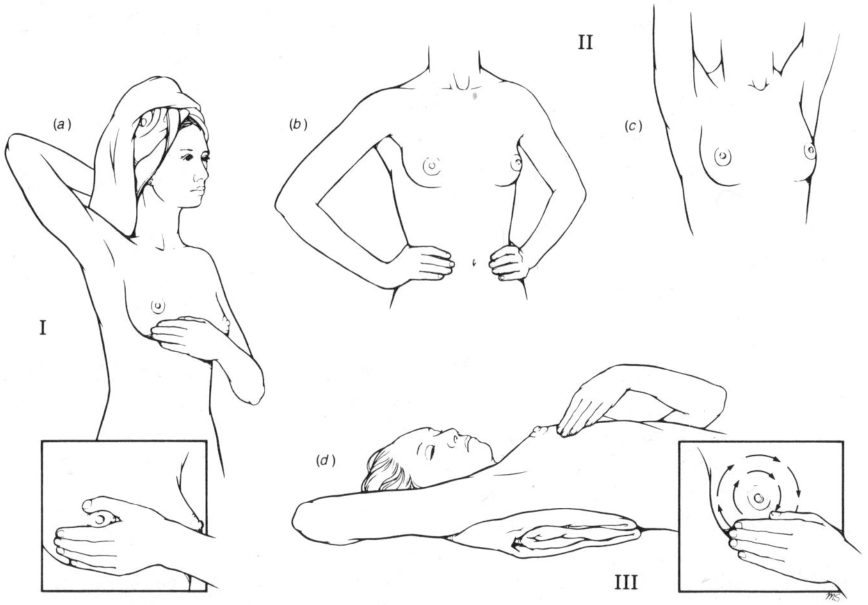

Figure 9.14 Breast self-exam. (From Butnarescu, *Maternity Nursing: Theory to Practice*, © 1983, John Wiley and Sons, Inc., New York.)

outermost top, moving in decreasing concentric circles to the nipple. Be sure to check the armpits. With the left arm raised above the head, use the right hand to check the left breast, and vice versa. If any lump, hard knot, or thickening is felt, seek medical advice immediately.

Step II. Inspection before a mirror: With arms at your sides, turning slowly from side to side, inspect the breasts for any bulges, asymmetry, or areas of surface flattening. It is normal for the breasts to be of unequal size. Check for skin redness, ulceration, edema (causes breast skin to look like the skin of an orange), and nipple/areola displacement or retraction. Next, with the arms raised overhead to reveal the sides and undersurfaces of the breast, repeat the inspection. Finally, place the palms of the hands on the hips, pressing down in order to contract the pectoral muscles and repeat the inspection. If any changes are noted, seek medical advice immediately.

Step III. Inspection while lying down: To examine the breast in this position, place a pillow or folded towel under the corresponding shoulder and place the corresponding arm under your head to distribute breast tissue more evenly. With the finger pads of the opposite hand, press gently in small circular motions, beginning at the outermost top of the breast (12:00) and moving clockwise around the breast back to 12:00. Each time you reach the top of the breast, move inward and continue in this manner until you reach the nipple. At least three or four circles are necessary for a complete exam. When this exam is completed, follow the procedure for the opposite breast. Finally, squeeze the nipple of each breast gently between the thumb and index finger of the opposite hand, noting any discharge (clear, bloody or purulent). Any lump, hard knot, thickening, or discharge should be brought to a practitioner's attention immediately.

Pamphlets with similar information in Spanish and English can be obtained by requesting:

"Breast Exams, What You Should Know"
NIH Publication No. 83-2000
Office of Cancer Communications
National Cancer Institute
Bethesda, Maryland 20205

"How to Examine Your Breasts"
Publication No. 2088-LE
American Cancer Society
90 Park Ave.
New York, New York 10016

Regular inspection of the breasts helps each woman to establish what is normal for her and gives her confidence in the practitioner's exam. Women should also be assured that most abnormalities are not breast cancer, but if they are, early detection and treatment can be lifesaving.

Follow-up: Reinforcement and review of BSE with annual gynecologic exams.

▸ *Fibrocystic Breast Disease (FBD)*

Laboratory Tests: In the presence of a single mass, diagnosis should always be confirmed by mammography and/or aspiration.

Therapeutic Measures

Mild disease (i.e., pain and tenderness do not limit activity or sleep): Reassurance and mild analgesics in the form of ASA or Tylenol, 1 or 2 tablets q4h prn may be sufficient. Also, recommend that the patient wear a properly fitting, supportive bra, particularly when engaged in sports and exercise. Start overweight patients on a weight loss program. Advise premenstrual restriction of fluid and sodium intake. Although not yet scientifically proven, reduced use of substances containing methylxanthine and nicotine may alleviate symptoms of fluid retention. Alternatively, diuretics may prove beneficial: Dyazide, 1 capsule daily or Hydrodiuril 25 mg, 1 tablet daily when symptoms occur.

Moderate to severe disease (i.e., activity is restricted, the patient cannot sleep on the stomach, a strong analgesic is needed): Danazol may be considered but is associated with serious side effects such as amenorrhea, loss of normal body fat distribution, deepening of voice, decreased fertility, and hirsutism. It is also very expensive. The usual prescription is 200 mg/day for 6 months and 400 mg/day for 6 months. In patients who do not show 75–100% improvement after the initial 6 months, danazol should be stopped and not reused. High doses of vitamin E (not to exceed 400 U/day) have also been shown to be effective.

Patient Education: Describe the cyclic changes that occur in FBD. Provide patients with a list such as the following

SUBSTANCES CONTAINING METHYLXANTHINE AND NICOTINE

(avoid or limit, particularly 1–2 weeks before period)

Caffeine beverages (coffee, soda, tea)	
Chocolate	Caffeine capsules
No-Doz	Cigarettes
Anacin	Excedrin
Midol	Aqua Ban
Dristan	Triaminicin
Dietac	Dexatrim
Theophylline	

Patients on danazol should be able to recognize its side effects:

Acne	Headache
Hot flashes	Hair growth
Nausea	Weight gain
Menstrual disorders	Muscle cramps
Skin oiliness	

Warn patients using vitamin E not to exceed the recommended dosage, since too much vitamin E causes cardiovascular and coagulation problems. Instruct patients in BSE techniques as described in the previous section, stressing the need for immediate medical attention if any changes are noted.

Follow-up: Careful breast exam every 6–12 months. After age 40, an annual mammogram is advised. Patients on danazol should be seen every 1–2 months for medication review.

▸ *Organizations for Breast Cancer*

Laboratory Tests: None.

Therapeutic Measures: None.

Patient Education: Information and support can be obtained from local chapters of the American Cancer Society and from:

Reach to Recovery
90 Park Ave.
New York, New York 10016
Tel.: (212) 599-8200

Cancer Care
One Park Avenue
New York, New York 10016
Tel.: (212) 679-5700

Cancer Information Service
Toll-free number: (1-800) 4-CANCER

Follow-up: As needed.

▸ *Breast-Feeding Considerations*

Laboratory Tests: None.

Therapeutic Measures: (Throughout this section, masculine nouns and pronouns are used to refer to the baby and feminine nouns and pronouns to the mother in order to eliminate confusion. The information, of course, applies to both male and female infants.)

Nutrition: Have the mother increase fluid intake and prescribe additional nutrients (particularly calcium) to meet the Recommended Daily Allowance during lactation (see Chapter 5).

Engorgement: Before nursing, have the mother massage her breasts in a warm shower, standing with her back to the shower head while water runs over her shoulders and down her breasts. Advise frequent, short nursing sessions.

Sore nipples: Soreness usually results from improper positioning. Review the correct nursing technique with the mother as described below (it is especially important that the baby suck not only on the nipple but on the areola as well, and that he is properly removed from the breast). Soreness can also result from repeated stroking by the baby's tongue in one spot. For example, if the baby is always nursed in the sitting position, his tongue always strokes the nipple at about 7:00. Soreness developing in this area can be relieved by having the mother nurse in a lying position with the baby's head pointing toward her feet (the tongue would stroke the top of the nipple) or by sitting with the baby tucked under her arm in a "football hold" (tongue would stroke at 5:00). Review proper nipple care.

Mastitis: Treat immediately as outlined in the section on "Mastitis."

Drugs: Be familiar with medication/substance indications as outlined in Table 9.19.

Patient Education: Provide patients with the following information:

Nipple preparation: Preparing the nipples before the baby is born helps to toughen the skin and may lessen the risk of soreness later on. Starting during the seventh or eighth month of pregnancy, the nipples may be periodically rubbed, rolled, or exposed to sunlight, air, or rough clothing. Specific techniques are outlined in the pamphlet "Prenatal Breast Care, Preparing for Breastfeeding," available from Health Education Associates, 520 School House Lane, Willow Grove, Pennsylvania 19090.

Nipple care: Colostrum may begin to ooze from the nipple at around the fourth or fifth month of pregnancy or later. It should be gently washed away with plain water each day but never expressed (expression may reduce the amount of this fluid, which supplies the baby with valuable immunoglobins). Soap or alcohol weakens nipple skin and should not be used. After the baby is born, the breasts should be washed daily with clean water, but it is not necessary to clean the nipples before or after feeding in any special way. A correctly fitted nursing bra provides breast support and may add to your comfort at night as well as during the day. To prevent milk from leaking on your clothes, tuck a clean cotton handkerchief or breast shield into your bra or casually press your arm against the nipple for a minute when you feel the milk starting to flow. Never use a shield with plastic liners, since moist milk trapped against the nipples can irritate the skin. In fact, it is helpful to leave the flaps of your nursing bra open from time to time, exposing the nipples to air. Air drying can be accomplished under clothing by using the Hobbitt Shield for Sore Nipples (HSS). A Hobbitt Shield for Inverted Nipples (HSI) may be used by the small percentage of women who have very flat, inverted nipples. It is placed inside the bra over the nipples half an hour prior to nursing to help draw the nipples out. Both HSI and HSS can be obtained from Health Education Associates, Inc., 211 South Easton Road, Glenside, Pennsylvania 19038.

Nursing technique: The hands should be washed before breast feeding. Settle in a comfortable lying or sitting position. In the beginning, hold the baby on his side so that his whole body is facing you (later, you can use various positions so that the baby's tongue does not always stroke one area of the nipple). A pillow can be placed on your lap or behind the baby to bring him closer to the breast without straining your arm muscles. Supporting the breast with one hand, draw the baby close to your body and stroke his cheek or corner of his mouth with your nipple. This causes the baby to turn and open his mouth ("rooting reflex"). As he does so, pull the baby closer so that your nipple and part of the areola extend far back into his mouth. Pressing the area behind the nipple also helps position the nipple and at the same time keeps breast tissue away from the baby's nose so that he can breathe freely. After several minutes of nursing, it is not uncommon to feel a slight tingling sensation and to notice a strong surge of milk ("let-down" reflex). You may still have plenty of milk even without experiencing this sensation. Allow the baby to nurse for about 10 minutes. Then remove the baby by pressing the breast away from the corner of his mouth to break the suction. Diapers can be changed and the baby burped if necessary. The baby can then nurse on the other breast as long as he wants. At the next nursing, start the baby on the breast he finished with the previous feeding.

Feeding schedule: Breast-fed babies usually prefer about 2-hour spans between feedings, though some babies nurse more or less frequently. If your baby sleeps a great deal during the day, wake him after 3 hours to nurse. The more you nurse, the more milk there will be. Indications that your baby is getting enough milk are as follows: (1) he has six or more wet diapers a day (completely breast-fed babies do not become constipated and may normally have several quite loose stools of varying color per day; (2) he gains 1 lb or more per month; (3) he nurses 8–10 times in 24 hours. Giving too many bottles or food can cause the baby to go longer between nursings, and this lowers the production of breast milk. In general, it is advisable to wait until the baby is 2 weeks old before giving a bottle. An occasional bottle containing water, formula, or expressed breast milk may then be given. The bottle can be given by someone else if you need some time to get away.

Breast massage and milk expression: To store milk in a bottle or to relieve full or engorged breasts, milk may be hand expressed or pumped* from the breast.

*The Kaneson Expressing Unit is available from Health Education Associates, Inc., 211 South Easton Road, Glenside, Pennsylvania 19038.
The Loyd-B-Pump can be ordered from Lopuco, Ltd., 1615 Old Annapolis Rd., Woodbine, Maryland 21797.

Before pumping or expressing milk, wash your hands with soap and water and then perform breast massage to stimulate milk let-down. Move the milk from the back of the breast forward to the nipple to increase the amount of milk expressed. Breast massage can be done through clothing or, if breasts are engorged, in a warm shower, standing with the back to the shower head while water runs over the shoulders and down the breasts. Place the palms of your hands on the periphery of the breast and stroke gently toward the nipple. Massage from several starting points (shoulder, under the arm, waist, center of the chest), always working toward the nipple. Massage around each breast several times. After massaging, open your clothing so that the entire breast is exposed. Express the milk into a wide-mouthed container (plastic or glass jar or cup). A sterilized container* must be used for any milk that is to be fed to the baby. To express milk by hand, cup the breast in your hand with the thumb above and fingers below. Push back toward the chest wall and squeeze the breast rhythmically between your fingers and thumb. Do not slide your hand along the skin. Rotate your hand slightly and repeat. Do this until you have covered the entire breast, reaching all the milk ducts that radiate from the nipple. Repeat the process (it should take about 3–5 minutes) on the other breast and then on each breast a second time. Changing back and forth allows time for milk to come down the ducts. If you are using a breast pump, follow the manufacturer's directions. Discontinue expression when milk no longer squirts out but appears only as an occasional drop. The amount that can be expressed varies and helps keep up the milk supply when nursing sessions are missed. However, it is always less than the amount the baby can suckle out.

Storing breast milk: Milk that has been expressed or pumped into a sterilized collecting container can be transferred to a sterilized baby bottle or another sterilized container for storage in the refrigerator or for freezing. Collected milk must be chilled immediately in the refrigerator. Chilled milk can be used within 24–48 hours or frozen. Small amounts of new chilled milk can be added to previously frozen milk, up to $3\frac{1}{2}$–4 oz in a 6-oz bottle for a young baby, more in a 12-oz bottle for older babies. Never fill a freezer container to the top, since space is needed for expansion. Frozen milk can be kept for months but should be defrosted just before use as follows: hold the frozen container under cold, then warmer water, shaking gently. As soon as it is thawed, heat the milk to body temperature in a pan of water and give it to the baby immediately. Always discard any unused defrosted milk.

Nutrition and general health: Drink extra fluids and eat prescribed foods and vitamin supplements. Get plenty of sleep and exercise. Both smoking and drinking of alcoholic beverages affect breast milk; avoid or reduce these practices. Check with your medical provider before taking any medications, since these, too, may affect milk production or content.

Follow-up: As needed.

*For easy sterilization, wash and rinse all containers, place them in a pan, and cover them with cold water. Bring the water to a boil, boil for 5 minutes, turn off the heat, and drain off water using the lid of the pan. Leave the jars in the covered pan until they are ready for use. Do not touch the inside parts of the containers.

▸ *Breast-Feeding Information/Support Groups*

Laboratory Tests: None.

Therapeutic Measures: None.

Patient Education: In addition to the organizations and suppliers mentioned in the preceding section, information and support for breast-feeding mothers can be obtained from:

La Leche League International
9616 Minneapolis Ave.
P.O. Box 1209
Franklin Park, Illinois 60131
Tel.: (312) 455-7730

Women, Infants, and Children (WIC) and Food Stamp Programs

The Womanly Art of Breastfeeding, 166-page softcover booklet available for approximately $3.50 from La Leche League at the above address.

The Complete Book of Breastfeeding by Eiger and Olds (210-page paperback available for approximately $1.95 from Bantam Books, New York, New York 10022).

Nursing Your Baby by Pryor (290-page paperback available for approximately $1.95 from Pocket Books, New York, New York 10020).

Follow-up: As needed.

▸ *Mastitis*

Laboratory Tests: For lactating women, culture and sensitivity and Gram stain of milk and the baby's nasopharynx. For nonlactating women, culture and sensitivity and Gram stain of any discharge, skin scrapings, or biopsied tissue.

Therapeutic Measures: Treatment should begin even before cultures results are available. Start penicillin VK 500 mg, 1 tablet qid for 10 days or erythromycin 500 mg, 1 tablet qid for 10 days (the treatments of choice, since they cover the widest range of the usual pathogens). If staphylococcal infection is definite, nafcillin 500 mg, 1 tablet qid is recommended. After the organism has been identified, antibiotic therapy should be changed or continued as appropriate. Lactating women should be encouraged to continue nursing unless frank pus is evident. If pus occurs, the patient should nurse from the other breast and pump milk from the affected one.

Patient Education: Explain the etiology of infection. Review the correct usage and side effects of medication. If needed, teach patients how to express milk. To prevent mastitis, nonlactating women should be told about the importance of keeping skin eruptions, cuts, and abrasions clean and of seeking immediate medical care if any unusual discharge or pain develops.

Follow-up: If symptoms persist, patients should be referred for surgical evaluation of possible breast abscess. Symptoms should abate within 36–48 hours with proper treatment.

▶ *Syphilis*

Laboratory Tests: VDRL, ART, or RPR. If they are positive, use FTA-ABS, TPI, or MHA-TP (even these specific antibody tests yield approximately 1% false-positive results). Dark-field exam of chancre material (no longer done by many laboratories). If indicated, do CSF exam for protein, VDRL, pleocytosis to stage infection.

Therapeutic Measures

Early syphilis (primary, secondary, or latent of less than 1 year's duration): Benzathine penicillin G 2.4 million units IM at once (1.2 million units in each buttock), or (if the patient is allergic to penicillin) tetracycline HCL, 500 mg po qid for 15 days, or (if the patient is allergic to penicillin and pregnant or allergic to penicillin and unable to tolerate tetracycline) erythromycin 500 mg po qid for 15 days (not always effective).

Syphilis of more than 1 year's duration without neurosyphilis (negative CSF): Benzathine penicillin G 2.4 million units once a week for 3 weeks (total of 7.2 million units), or (if penicillin allergic) tetracycline HCL 500 mg po qid for 30 days, or (if penicillin allergic and pregnant or penicillin allergic and unable to tolerate tetracycline) erythromycin 500 mg po qid for 30 days (not always effective).

Neurosyphilis (positive CSF): Refer the patient to an infectious disease specialist; intravenous therapy may be required.

All cases: Evaluation and treatment of sexual partners.

Patient Education: Discuss the nature and progression of the illness in order to motivate patients to complete the therapeutic regimen. Stress the importance of finding and treating contacts. Review the correct usage and potential side effects of prescribed medication. Review STD prevention such as condom use, prompt medical evaluation if illness is suspected, and the increased risk of multiple partners.

Follow-up

Nonneurosyphilis: Quantitative VDRL titer at 1, 3, 6, and 12 months after treatment. The titer should progressively decline.

Neurosyphilis: After treatment, lumbar puncture to examine CSF every 3–6 months for 3 years.

▸ *Gonorrhea*

Laboratory Tests: Gram stain of urethral discharge and chocolate agar culture in men. Chocolate agar culture from endocervix or urethra in women. In both men and women, additional pharyngeal, rectal, blood, or synovial cultures as indicated by the history or symptoms.

Therapeutic Measures (uncomplicated infections): Treat the patient and all sexual contacts with the most appropriate regimen as follows:

Treatment A: Aqueous penicillin G 4.8 million units IM in divided doses after administration of 1 g probenicid po. Advantages: it is effective against concurrent syphilis infection and involves no compliance problem. Disadvantages: it is ineffective against concurrent chlamydia infection and may cause anaphylaxis.

Treatment B: Tetracycline hydrochloride 500 mg po qid for 7 days. Advantage: it is effective against chlamydia, the drug of choice for penicillin-allergic patients. Disadvantages: it is ineffective against syphilis, and the need for a longer dosage period increases compliance problems. It must be taken on an empty stomach (1 hour before or 3 hours after meals).

Treatment C: Amoxicillin 3 g or ampicillin 3.5 g po at once; then tetracycline 500 mg qid for 7 days (effective against gonococcus and chlamydia).

For PPNG: Spectinomycin 2 g IM preceded by 1 gm probenicid po (ineffective against pharyngeal infections). As an alternative, oral amoxicillin, ampicillin, or tetracycline as outlined above (ineffective against anorectal infections in men).

Patient Education: Discuss the nature and progression of gonorrhea in order to motivate patients to complete the therapeutic regimen. Stress the importance of finding and treating contacts. Review the correct usage and potential side effects of prescribed medication. Review STD prevention.

Follow-up: Reculture infected sites in men 4–7 days after treatment and in women approximately 7–14 days after treatment. Always obtain a rectal culture in women on follow-up exam (rectal cultures in women indicate treatment failures quite accurately). Unless IM penicillin is used, do syphilis serology in 1–3 months.

▸ *Chlamydia Infection*

Laboratory Tests: Chlamydia culture or direct specimen test (e.g., Microtrak) of urethra or endocervix. Follow laboratory instructions for special collection and transport. Wet preparation of urethral or cervical discharge under a microscope (look for increase in WBCs and absence of visible organisms). Evaluation for concurrent gonorrhea by Gram stain and chocolate agar.

Therapeutic Measures: For uncomplicated infections, treat the patient and sexual contacts with one of the following regimens:

Treatment A: Tetracycline HCL 500 mg po qid for at least 7 days or doxycycline 100 mg po bid for at least 7 days.

Treatment B: Erythromycin 500 mg po qid for at least 7 days (use in pregnancy or for other contraindication to tetracycline).

Patient Education: Discuss the nature, progression, and prevalence of chlamydia infections in order to motivate patients to complete the therapeutic regimen. Stress the importance of finding and treating contacts. Review the correct usage, potential side effects of prescribed medication. Explain the risk of self-inoculation to other sites and teach appropriate hygiene practices. Review STD prevention methods such as barrier contraceptives (notably condoms), prompt medical evaluation if illness is suspected, and increased risk of multiple partners.

Follow-up: Reculture after 3–6 weeks following treatment. Reassess if treatment fails to relieve symptoms.

▸ *Condylomata Acuminata*

Laboratory Tests: Syphilis serology to rule out condylomata lata (contagious lesions of secondary-stage syphilis that resemble condylomata acuminata). Pap smear of the cervix to rule out cervical warts.

Therapeutic Measures: Preferably, refer patients and sexual contacts with symptoms for colposcopy and treatment with cryotherapy, electrosurgery, or surgical removal by scissors or curette. Podophyllum 10–25% in tincture of benzoin is being used, but recent reports raise the question of an association with neoplastic changes. If it is used, apply podophyllum to external warts less than 1 cm in diameter. When possible, coat the area around the lesion with petroleum jelly or zinc oxide to avoid damaging healthy tissue. Allow podophyllum to dry completely before the treated area contacts normal tissue. Treat weekly for up to 4 weeks until lesions disappear (contraindicated in pregnancy and in patients with oral, intraurethral, or cervical lesions and large lesions). Have patients keep the affected area clean and dry, if possible, since moisture encourages growth.

Patient Education: Describe the nature, transmission, and incubation period of the disease. Advise patients with lesions to use condoms to prevent spread. If podophyllum used, instruct patients to wash the treated area thoroughly about 4 hours after application. Note the likelihood of recurrence and teach patients to inspect the genitals for new lesions. Discuss the importance of colposcopy and annual Pap tests due to the association of condylomata acuminata with neoplastic changes. Home remedies should be avoided.

Follow-up: If podophyllum is used, schedule weekly visits for treatments until lesions disappear or as recommended after surgical removal. Obtain annual Pap smears in women.

▸ *Herpes Genitalis*

Laboratory Tests: The diagnosis of herpes infection may be proven or supported by the following:

1. Viral culture if laboratory facilities are available (can be costly).
2. Pap smear of a freshly opened lesion taken with a saline-moistened swab and fixed promptly. Instruct the laboratory to look for herpes.
3. Tzanck smear of a freshly opened lesion with a saline-moistened swab, spread on a slide, fixed with methanol or ethanol, stained with Giemsa or Wright's stain, and examined for multinucleated giant cells.
4. Serology to detect a primary infection if there has been no previous exposure to herpes types I or II.

Syphilis serology should be done if the lesion is suspicious.

Therapeutic Measures

Topical antiviral medication (for primary infection): Acyclovir ointment (5%) applied to the lesion with a gloved finger q3h for 1 week.

Oral antiviral medication (to reduce the frequency and severity of recurrent infections): For an initial infection, give acyclovir capsules 200 mg po q4h while awake (5/day) for 10 days. For recurrences thereafter, give acyclovir capsules 200 mg po q4h while awake (5/day) for 5 days, starting with the earliest symptoms. For chronic suppressive therapy, give acyclovir capsules 200 mg po tid for up to 6 months.

Symptomatic treatment: Cool sitz baths or cool moist soaks to lesions (heat may spread the virus and exacerbate the inflammation). If dysuria is present, force fluids to keep urine dilute; suggest urinating into the bath for urinary retention secondary to pain. Suggest Tylenol or ASA for discomfort.

Patient Education: Discuss the nature and transmission of the disease and the importance of informing contacts. Advise condom use, since the virus may be shed even when symptoms are absent (sheep gut condoms may not be as protective as latex, since the virus may cross the natural membrane). Note that stress, menses, and intercurrent illness can all trigger illness; counsel patients regarding stress reduction strategies and self-care techniques to prevent illness. Note also that the virus can be transmitted to other sites (e.g., eyes) by self-inoculation and stress that proper hand-washing techniques are imperative. Advise women to tell their obstetrician about their history of herpes genitalis in the event of pregnancy. Review the correct usage and side effects of prescribed medication. If appropriate, explain that the risk of STD increases with the number of sexual partners.

Follow-up: Annual Pap smears for women.

▸ *Herpes Support Groups*

Laboratory Tests: None.

Therapeutic Measures: None.

Patient Education
HELP (Herpetics Engaged in Living Productively)
Call 1-800-227-8922 or write:
HELP/ASHA
260 Sheridan Ave., Suite 307
Palo Alto, California 94306

Follow-up: As needed.

▸ *Trichomonas Vaginitis*

Laboratory Tests: Wet mount with normal saline (look for mobile trichomonads). Vaginal pH (5.0–6.0 is consistent with disease). The organism may be identified incidentally on Pap smear. Cultures for *T. vaginalis* are available but rarely necessary since the organism is easily identifiable on wet mount. The amine test may be positive (add 1 drop of 10% KOH to the discharge; production of a fishy odor indicates a positive test). Tests as indicated for concurrent STDs (the gonorrhea culture may be falsely negative in the presence of trichomonas infection and should be repeated after treatment if there is any question).

Therapeutic Measures: Treat both the woman and her sexual partners by giving with milk after eating, metronidazole (Flagyl) 2 g at once or in the case of relapse 500 mg bid for 7 days. Flagyl is contraindicated in pregnancy, lactation, previous intolerance, and in patients with a history of blood dyscrasias, active neurologic disease, or gastric ulcers. Always inform patients to avoid alcohol use for 24–48 hours before and after Flagyl intake due to its Antabuse effect. If the patient cannot take Flagyl and is not pregnant, try betadine douches hs for 10 days and the use of condoms. If both partners are being treated with Flagyl, advise condom use for at least the first 2 days after treatment. If the man is not being treated, advise condom use for 2 weeks after diagnosis (unless reinfection occurs, trichomonads often resolve spontaneously in men). Advise the use of a warm or cool sitz bath to help reduce vulvovaginal swelling and itching.

Patient Education: Discuss the nature of the disease and methods of transmission (not always sexual). Explain the use and side effects of Flagyl: alcohol use should be avoided for 1 or 2 days before and after medication; urine may turn brownish; the effectiveness of oral contraceptives may be decreased; and a backup method for the balance of the current pill cycle is advised. Stress the importance of condom use to prevent transmitting disease or becoming reinfected.

Follow-up: As needed if symptoms do not respond to treatment. Repeat the Pap test in 3 months after treatment if trichomonads and inflammation are noted on the report.

▸ *Gardnerella Vaginitis*

Laboratory Tests: Wet mount with normal saline (look for the absence of WBCs and the presence of "clue cells"—epithelial cells with intracellular organisms producing a ground-glass appearance in the matrix). Amine test (add 1 drop of 10% KOH to the discharge; production of a fishy odor indicates a positive test). Vaginal pH (4.5–5.5 is consistent with disease). Cultures for *G. vaginalis* may be done. Additional tests as indicated for concurrent STDs.

Therapeutic Measures: Metronidazole 500 mg po bid for 7 days with milk after eating (contraindicated in pregnancy, lactation, previous Flagyl intolerance, and in patients with a history of blood dyscrasias, active neurologic disease, or a history of gastric ulcers). Always inform patients to avoid alcohol intake while taking Flagyl due to its Antabuse effect. As an alternative to Flagyl, ampicillin 500 mg po qid for 7 days or Sultrin cream bid for 14 days may be used (treatment failures are higher with both). Automatic treatment of sexual partners is a controversial issue. When both partners are being treated, advise condom use during and for at least the first 2 days after completion of medication. If the man is not being treated, advise condom use for at least 2 weeks after diagnosis (unless reinfection occurs, many organisms do not survive in the male urethra and disappear spontaneously). Advise the use of a warm or cool sitz bath to help reduce vulvovaginal swelling and itching.

Patient Education: Discuss the nature of the disease and methods of transmission (not always sexual). If Flagyl is being used, explain its use and side effects: alcohol intake should be avoided for 1 or 2 days before and after medication; urine may transiently turn brownish; the effectiveness of oral contraceptives may be decreased; and a backup method for the balance of the current pill cycle is advised. If Sultrin is prescribed, review the use of intravaginal application of medication. Stress the importance of condom use to prevent transmitting disease or becoming reinfected.

Follow-up: As needed if symptoms do not respond to treatment. Repeat the Pap test in 3 months after treatment if inflammation is noted on the report.

▸ *Monilia*

Laboratory Tests: Wet mount slide of discharge mixed with 1 drop 10% KOH (look for budding yeast or branch-like forms). Culture may be done (using Nickerson's medium). In women, infection may also show up incidentally on a Pap smear. For frequent recurrences, check blood sugar levels to rule out diabetes.

Therapeutic Measures: For women, give miconazole, butaconazole, or clotrimazole cream or suppositories as directed (there are 7-, 3-, and 1-day regimens on the market; longer or intermittent courses may be needed in recurrent infection). Plain yogurt applied intravaginally may help mild infections or prevent recurrence in the individual at high risk. A vinegar or liquid acidophilus douche (2–4 tbsp in 1 qt of warm water) may also be used prophylactically or at symptom onset in mild cases. In men, give miconazole cream applied topically for 7–14 days. Advise condom use until both partners have been treated. Advise patients to keep the genitals clean and dry and to allow air flow to the area as much as possible by wearing loose clothing made of natural fibers.

Patient Education: Discuss the factors that predispose to yeast infections and counsel patients to avoid them if possible. Demonstrate the use of intravaginal creams or suppositories and advise their continued use even if menses begin. Women should avoid bubble baths and excessive douching. Uncircumcised men should be told to retract the foreskin of the penis, exposing the glans for thorough cleaning at least once daily, and to wipe the area dry after voiding and intercourse.

Follow-up: If symptoms recur or do not resolve.

▸ *Birthright Organizations*

Laboratory Tests: None.

Therapeutic Measures: None.

Patient Education: Birthright (headquarters)
Toronto, Canada
Tel.: (416) 469-1111
Birthright (regional organizations)
Check your local telephone directory

Follow-up: As needed.

▸ *Prenatal Considerations*

Laboratory Tests: None.

Therapeutic Measures

Early referral: Since the first trimester is the time when the developing fetus is most vulnerable to outside influences, early referral for prenatal care greatly decreases the chance of complications. Include a careful summary of the patient's pertinent medical history.

Nutrition: Have the mother increase fluid intake and prescribe additional nutrients (particularly calcium) to meet the Recommended Daily Allowance during lactation (see Chapter 5). The minimum daily prenatal diet should include 2 eggs, 1 quart of milk, two 3-oz servings of meat, fish, or poultry, three servings of vegetables with one dark green or yellow vegetable, three servings of fruit with one citrus fruit, and five servings of whole grain breads or cereals. Snacks should be nutritious foods such as cheese, peanut butter, granola, or fruit. Salt may be added to taste. Most women should take supplementary B vitamins, folic acid, and iron. Even if a woman is overweight, pregnancy is not the time to begin or continue weight-loss dieting. Refer eligible patients to Women, Infants, Children (WIC) and food stamp programs.

Exercise: In general, a pregnant woman can continue any exercise that she did routinely before becoming pregnant. For those who are relatively inactive, a daily walk for 15–30 minutes will provide needed fresh air and circulatory stimulation.

Drugs: Be familiar with the medication/substance indications as outlined in Table 9.29. Note that alcohol and caffeine intake and cigarette smoking should be avoided. Warn pregnant women not to take any medications without checking with their obstetrician. Advise women to ask their employers about hazardous chemical or physical substances on the job and then to avoid those substances.

Nausea: For the nausea that often accompanies the first trimester of pregnancy, recommend smaller, more frequent meals. Eating foods high in carbohydrates, such as crackers, before getting up in the morning may prevent morning sickness. Elimination of fatty foods and strong spices may also help. Vitamin B_6 (pyridoxine) decreases nausea. Good sources of this nutrient are brewer's yeast, whole grain breads, meat and poultry, or pill supplements.

Patient Education: In addition to the above information, give patients written information for on-hand reference. Some available pamphlets are as follows:

"Be Good to Your Baby Before It Is Born"
March of Dimes Birth Defects Foundation
1275 Mamaroneck Ave.
White Plains, New York 10605

"How to Have a Healthy Pregnancy"
A Scriptographic Booklet by the Channing L. Bete Co., Inc.
South Deerfield, Massachusetts 01373

Follow-up: As needed.

▸ *Counseling Patients on Birth Control Measures*

Laboratory Tests: None.

Therapeutic Measures: None.

Patient Education: Review the considerations listed in Table 9.31. Discuss patients' feelings about an unplanned pregnancy. If the woman becomes pregnant despite contraception, she will have to decide whether or not to continue the pregnancy or terminate it with a therapeutic abortion. This decision will be determined not only by the various factors regarding the choice of parenthood but also by religious or personal convictions regarding family and lifestyle. The effectiveness of the contraceptive method may be the major determinant of contraceptive choice if an unplanned pregnancy is highly undesirable for the patient. Another determinant is the patient's past success or failure with various methods of birth control. There may also be methods that she or her partner find unacceptable because of religious convictions or the experience of relatives or friends.

Explain or review available methods of contraception in terms of how they work, as well as their effectiveness, risks, and benefits. Explain that effectiveness rates account not only for the physiologic effectiveness of the methods but also for the human error introduced with actual use. Methods that require more action on the part of the user generally leave more room for error and therefore are less effective. Such methods, however, are often the ones with the fewest medical side effects. When discussing risks and benefits, note that methods such as the pill and the IUD involve serious medical risks, as well as other less serious but nonetheless bothersome effects. Life-threatening complications such as thromboembolism or sepsis can result from hormonal and intrauterine methods, respectively. Permanent effects on future fertility may result from an ectopic pregnancy secondary to minipill or IUD use or from IUD-associated PID. It is difficult to compare the significant side effects of oral contraceptives and the IUD in order to advise the client on which are "preferable"; neither a stroke related to use of the pill nor an ectopic pregnancy related to use of the IUD is desirable.

Some women may prefer to have less contraceptive effectiveness from a mechanical or natural method than to assume the small but serious medical risks associated with the pill or the IUD. Women over 40 face several factors that add to the difficulty of choosing contraception. Sympto-thermic methods are less reliable for women who do not restrict intercourse to Phase III of their cycles and for older women who may have anovulatory, irregular cycles. There is a higher incidence of genital cancer in this age group, and use of the IUD with its associated intermenstrual spotting may obscure the need for a D&C. The pill triples the risk of mortality for a woman of 40 or over compared to that of a woman of 30. Smoking and the pill in women over 40 push the mortality risk even higher: a 10-fold increase compared to the complications of pregnancy. Women who do not want more children may be more willing to choose a method that poses more risks to future fertility (e.g., IUD) than will women who have not finished childbearing. The health effects of each method should be presented, along with a comparison of the mortality risks of pregnancy. Note that the mortality risks of pregnancy, when no method of birth control is being used, are much greater than those of any method of contraception except for use of the pill by smokers who are more than 40 years old.

Discuss the relationship between sexual practices and various types of birth control methods. Note that many couples find that the initiation and enjoyment of intercourse are increased when their fear of pregnancy is diminished by effective contraception. However, certain methods of birth control such as the diaphragm, condoms, and foam require advance planning, and this planning is thought by some to interfere with sexual spontaneity. Discuss the fact that women often fear that the preparation needed for some methods will be interpreted as "looseness" by a partner and that men may hesitate to use condoms for the same reason. Emphasize that natural methods—calendar rhythm, BBT, and cervical mucus—require a great deal of advanced planning and a commitment to periodic abstinence from intercourse. These methods may be most suitable for couples who have a strong relationship and an understanding of the need for a certain amount of sexual self-control or for means of sexual expression other than intercourse.

The frequency of intercourse and the number of sexual partners have a bearing on the acceptability of any method of contraception. Women who have intercourse infrequently may not feel the need to have the continuous protection provided by oral contraceptives or the IUD. For women with several sexual partners, the risk of PID is increased by the use of an IUD. By contrast, condoms and diaphragms provide some protection against venereal disease and PID.

Convenience is a major factor in contraceptive success. Oral contraceptives are very convenient, since their use is daily and therefore habitual and not related to the act of intercourse itself. The IUD requires no planning or action on the part of the user other than periodic checking of its placement; this does not have to be coitus related, however. Although the diaphragm and the vaginal sponge can be inserted at the time of intercourse, they can also be inserted several hours beforehand and thus are not necessarily coitus related. Condoms can only be used once the man has achieved erection. Most spermicides must be used 30 minutes to 2 hours before intercourse. Natural methods require several months of record keeping for accuracy and demand abstinence from intercourse during certain times during the menstrual cycle.

In reviewing the methods of contraception, it is helpful to use a written handout with comparative information. Some available printed pamphlets are as follows:

"Family Planning Methods of Contraception"
DHEW Publication No. (HSA) 80-5646 (English or Spanish)
For sale by the Superintendent of Documents
U.S. Government Printing Office
Washington, D.C. 20402

"What Everyone Should Know About Contraception"
A Scriptographic Booklet by the Channing L. Bete Co., Inc.
South Greenfield, Massachusetts 01373

"Contraception: Comparing the Options"
DHEW Publication No. (FDA) 78-3069
U.S. Department of Health, Education, and Welfare
Office of Public Affairs
5600 Fisher Lane
Rockville, Maryland 20857

Pamphlets can be mailed before or given at the time of the visit.

In addition, make up a tray containing the following items for demonstration:

- Birth control pills (fixed combinations, triphasic, 21-day cycle, 28-day cycle, minipill)
- IUD (those used in your clinic or office)
- Diaphragm (various types)
- Spermicidal cream and jelly
- Vaginal sponge
- Condom
- Foam
- Menstrual calendar
- Basal body thermometer
- Billings method kit (optional)
- Other optional items: penis model (to demonstrate condom use) and pelvic model (to demonstrate foam and diaphragm use)

Drug companies that specialize in contraceptive products often supply prepackaged kits containing these items or other teaching material. With addresses listed in the *Physician's Desk Reference,* they include:

Eaton-Merz Laboratories
Holland-Rantos
Lederle
Meade-Johnson
Ortho Pharmaceutical Corporation
Parke-Davis
Schering Corporation
Schmid Laboratories
Searle
Syntex
Wyeth

Follow-up: As needed.

▸ *The Pill*

Laboratory Tests: Pap smear. Urinalysis. Hematocrit. Fasting levels of serum triglycerides and cholesterol, GTT if indicated by personal or family history.

Therapeutic Measures: To establish that there are no contraindications to pill use (Table 9.36), a complete history and physical exam should be obtained prior to giving a prescription. Blood pressure, pulse, weight, and height should be measured. Special attention should be given to the ocular fundi, breasts, lungs, heart, abdomen, skin, extremities, and pelvis. For patients with no contraindications, prescribe a brand of combined oral contraceptives (see Table 9.33) with a low dose of estrogen, generally 30–35 μg. Pills with less than 30 μg of estrogen (e.g., LoEstrin 1/20) do not reliably prevent contraception and therefore should not be used. Most women may be started on the pill at the time of menses. In the postabortion patient, the pill may be started immediately after the procedure if the gestation period was less than 12 weeks or 2 weeks after the procedure if it was more than 12 weeks. The postpartum woman may be started on the pill at the time of her 6-week checkup. This delay decreases the risk of thromboembolism.

Patient Education: Each patient (and her partner) should be instructed on how the pill works, its risks and benefits, and how to take it. Use a calendar and the due date of her next period to explain the correct pill start. Use a pack of the pill brand being prescribed to show patients how to read day labeling, how to extract pills from the foil, and how to take pills in order. In addition to verbal counseling, give each patient a written handout with information such as the following:

INSTRUCTIONS FOR PILL USE

Education: Each pill manufacturer distributes a small pamphlet on the contraindications, risks, and benefits of the pill. Read it thoroughly and carefully, and ask your clinician to explain anything you do not understand.

Triphasil start: Take the first pill on the first day of your period. Continue to take it at the same time every day. If you have a 21-day pack, stop for 1 week at the end of the pack and then begin your next pack. If you have a 28-day pack, begin a new pack the day after finishing the first one. Start each new pack on the same day of the week.

Sunday start: Start your first pill pack on the first Sunday after your period begins. If your period starts on a Sunday, start the pill that day. Continue to take the pill at the same time every day. If you have a 21-day pack, stop for 1 week at the end of the pack, and then begin your next pack on the Sunday at the end of that week. If you have a 28-day pack, begin a new pack the day after finishing the first one.

Fifth-day start: Start the first pill on day 5 of your next period. Continue to take the pill at the same time every day until all pills are gone. Stop for 1 week at the end of the pack and then begin your next pack. Start each new pack on the same day of the week.

First-month backup: Unless you start the first pill of your first pack on day 1 of your period, use a backup method (e.g., foam, condoms, diaphragm, sponge) until you have taken the first 7 pills. This extra precaution against pregnancy is necessary only with the first pack.

Missed pills: If you miss one pill, take it as soon as you remember it even if this is the next day. Take today's pill at the regular time. You probably will not get pregnant, but to be sure, use another method such as foam or condoms. If you miss 2 pills, double up for 2 days. You may have some spotting and you are definitely at risk for pregnancy, so use another method of birth control while you finish the pack. If you miss more than 2 pills, stop the pills and use another method. Consider a permanent change of method if you are having this much trouble remembering to take the pill. Start a new pack of pills with your next normal period.

Spotting: Bleeding between periods for the first several cycles is not unusual. If the bleeding is very heavy or persists beyond the first three cycles, call your clinician.

Missed period: Call your clinician.

Pregnancy: If you become pregnant while taking the pill, stop taking it and consult your clinician. If you plan to become pregnant, discontinue taking the pill 3 months beforehand. Use another method of birth control until you have had three normal periods off the pill.

Side effects: See your clinician or go to the emergency room immediately for any of the following: severe headache, loss of vision, blurred vision, flashing lights, severe chest pain or sudden shortness of breath, severe abdominal pain, severe leg or calf pain. These may indicate the occurrence of one of the following very serious problems: migraine headache; stroke; blood clot in the legs, lungs, or other blood vessel; heart attack; or gallbladder or liver disease.

Health care: If you consult another physician or nurse or are hospitalized, be sure to tell them that you are taking the pill.

Clinician's name, phone number, and address.

Before the patient leaves, be sure that she understands the importance of stopping the pill and seeking immediate attention for warning signs of thromboembolic complications: severe headache; chest pain; shortness of breath; pain, redness, or swelling of the leg; or visual disturbance. Patients should also know that to prevent the development of thromboembolic complications, the pill should be stopped and another birth control method used within 4 weeks of planned surgery, during prolonged bed rest, or when the lower extremities have been immobilized for long periods in casts or splints.

Follow-up: A visit should be planned after three cycles on the pill for symptom and health information review and blood pressure check. If there are no contraindications, 6-month refills may be provided. At yearly intervals, the woman should have a physical exam including blood pressure check and breast, abdominal, and pelvic exams. Yearly laboratory studies should include a Pap smear, cervical gonorrhea culture for high-risk women, urinalysis, and hematocrit. Blood pressure checks only may need to be done every 3–6 months; adolescents should be seen that often as well to reinforce earlier instructions.

▸ *Minor Side Effects of the Pill*

Laboratory Tests: None.

Therapeutic Measures: Use Table 9.38 to determine if the side effect is likely to be caused by an estrogen or progestin excess or deficiency. Adjust the brand of pill according to the potency of the progestin first, the estrogen second (see Table 9.37) and/or advise the following:

Nausea: Advise the client to take her pill at bedtime or with a meal. The lower the estrogen dose, the less often this symptom occurs.

Breakthrough bleeding: Intermenstrual spotting is common when pill use begins and usually resolves by the third cycle. If spotting continues beyond the third month, ascertain if it occurs early (days 1–14) or late (days 15–21). Early bleeding is a side effect of estrogen deficiency and may be remedied by choosing a pill with a progestin that has a higher estrogenic effect. If this is not successful, then a 50-μg pill such as Demulen or Norlestrin 2.5 should be used for 3–6 months. After such a trial, the 30- to 35-μg pills should be reintroduced. If spotting recurs, the patient may need to be maintained on the 50-μg pill. Late spotting and breakthrough bleeding are due to progestin deficiency. A pill with a stronger androgenic progestin such as LoOvral, Ovral, or Norlestrin can be tried. Triphasil, a brand that adjusts both estrogen and progesterone throughout the cycle, may also prove helpful.

Weight gain: For women who gain weight cyclically while on the pill, lower doses of estrogen and avoidance of sodium-containing foods for the last half of the cycle may be helpful. If the weight gain is from increased appetite, choose a pill that has a low androgenic effect, such as Demulen.

Acne and hirsutism: Acne may increase with any pill. Low-progestin, low-androgen pills are preferable for this condition (e.g., Demulen, Norinyl, or OrthoNovum). The high estrogenic effect of Enovid may be helpful. Hirsutism can also be avoided with a similar choice of pill.

No withdrawal bleeding: If a woman has no bleeding at the end of the cycle and has missed no pills, she should continue with the pills. If at the end of the next (second) cycle she still has no withdrawal bleeding, she should have a pregnancy test. If she has missed any pills, she should have a pregnancy test after the first missed period. If pregnancy is ruled out, then several months on a 50-μg estrogen pill or a higher-progestin pill such as Ovral, Demulen, or Norlestrin 2.5 is recommended. Reassurance that she is not pregnant may be the most helpful intervention.

Patient Education: Explain the hormonal effects responsible for various side effects.

Follow-up: As needed.

▸ *The Minipill*

Laboratory Tests: Pap smear. Urinalysis. Hematocrit.

Therapeutic Measures: Women interested in using the minipill should give a complete history and receive a thorough physical exam. Blood pressure, pulse, height, and weight should be recorded. The examiner should concentrate on the ocular fundi, heart, lungs, abdomen, pelvis, skin, and extremities. If there are no contraindications (Table 9.40), the patient can be started on one of the three available brands of the minipill described in Table 9.39. Nor QD and Micronor have one-third the amount of norethindrone contained in the combined pills, Norinyl 1/50 and Ortho-Novum 1/50. Ovrette has slightly more than one-sixth the amount in Lo-Ovral.

Patient Education: Explain how the minipill works, as well as its risks and benefits. Give the patient written instructions such as the following:

INSTRUCTIONS FOR MINIPILL USE

Education: Read carefully and thoroughly the manufacturer's warnings enclosed with your pills. Ask your clinician to explain anything you do not understand.

How to take the minipill: Start your first pill on the first Sunday after your period begins. If your period starts on a Sunday, take your first pill that day. Then take one pill at the same time every day. Begin a new package of pills immediately upon finishing each package; there is no waiting time between packages. The chance of pregnancy on the minipill is most likely during the first 6 months of use; therefore, you may want to use another method such as foam and condoms together with the minipill during this time to increase its effectiveness. After the first 6 months, continued use of a backup method at midcycle will also decrease the chance of pregnancy.

Missed pills: It is important not to miss pills because of the greatly increased chance of pregnancy if you do. If you miss a pill, take it as soon as you remember it or with the next day's pill. You will need to use another method of birth control, such as foam and condoms or abstinence, while taking the remainder of the package.

Spotting: Spotting between periods is common while taking the minipill.

Missed period: If your period is 2 weeks late, see your clinician to determine if you are pregnant. The risk of pregnancy in the fallopian tubes rather than in the womb (ectopic pregnancy) is increased while taking the minipill. If you have severe abdominal pain, you should also contact your clinician, especially if you miss a period, to determine if you have an ectopic pregnancy.

Pregnancy: If you become pregnant while taking the minipill, stop using it and consult your clinician. If you plan to become pregnant, discontinue minipill use 3 months beforehand. Use another method of birth control until you have had three normal periods off the minipill.

Side effects: See your clinician or go to the emergency room for any of the following: severe abdominal pain, severe headache, loss of vision, blurred vision, flashing lights, severe chest pain or shortness of breath, severe leg or calf pain. These may indicate an ectopic pregnancy, blood clot, or stroke.

Health care: If you consult another physician or nurse or are hospitalized, be sure to tell them that you are taking the minipill.

Clinician name, address, telephone number.

Follow-up: Each patient should be seen after her first six cycles on the minipill for symptom and information review. A 6-month refill may then be given provided there are no contraindications. If signs or symptoms arise of thromboembolic disorders or other conditions that are contraindications for beginning the minipill, it should be stopped immediately and appropriate medical treatment instituted. The patient who misses a menstrual period, even if she has taken all of her pills, should have a pregnancy test and, if there are any signs or symptoms of ectopic pregnancy, a pelvic exam. Although intermenstrual bleeding is common, if it occurs in women over 35, discontinuance of the pill may be warranted for watchful waiting. Persistent bleeding should be worked up. Patients with no problems should be seen annually for a complete exam.

▸ *The Morning-After Pill*

Laboratory Tests: Pap smear. Urinalysis. Hematocrit. A serum pregnancy test is essential to rule out preexisting pregnancy. Microscopic exam of cervical mucus for ferning helps to establish whether the woman is presently ovulating. STD testing is mandatory in all rape cases.

Therapeutic Measures: High-dose female hormones (morning-after pill) should be given only when intercourse was unexpected and/or unprotected. Ideally, the hormones are prescribed only to women who are willing to have a therapeutic abortion if the method fails because of the possibility of birth defects. These hormones should not be given if more than 72 hours have elapsed since unprotected intercourse or if there has been more than one act of unprotected intercourse since the last menstrual period. To ensure that there are no contraindications (same as for birth control pills; see Table 9.36), a complete history and physical exam should be obtained. Blood pressure, pulse, weight, and height should be measured. Special attention should be given to the optic fundi, breasts, lungs, heart, abdomen, skin, extremities, and pelvic exam. The only hormonal preparation approved by the FDA for postcoital birth control is DES, 25 mg bid for 5 days. Other equivalent preparations are listed in Table 9.41; Ovral 2 tablets q 12 h for 2 doses is also commonly used. With DES, an antiemetic is prescribed one-half hour before each dose and as needed afterward (Tigan tablets 250 mg or suppositories 200 mg up to qid, or Compazine tablets, 5–10 mg up to qid, or suppositories, 25 mg bid).

Patient Education: Describe how the hormones work, as well as their risks and benefits. Stress the possibility of teratogenic effects if pregnancy occurs in spite of hormone use. If DES is used, give the patient an introduction sheet with information such as the following:

INSTRUCTIONS FOR MORNING-AFTER PILL USE (DES)

How to take the pills: Take the pills twice a day for 5 days until they are all gone. You must start taking them within 72 hours of the time of intercourse. They will not work if you wait beyond this period.

Nausea: Many women find that these pills cause nausea and vomiting. You may be able to avoid these problems by taking the other pills or suppositories prescribed at least one-half hour before taking the hormones. If you do vomit after taking a dose, call your clinician to determine whether to repeat the dose.

Bleeding: Your next period may be early, late, or on time.

Pregnancy: If your next period is 2 weeks late, see your clinician for a pregnancy test. If you become pregnant even though you took the pills, you should strongly consider having a therapeutic abortion, since the child may develop a birth defect.

Side effects: See your clinician or go to the emergency room immediately for any of the following: severe headache, loss of vision, blurred vision, flashing lights, severe chest pain or sudden shortness of breath, severe abdominal pain, severe leg or calf pain.

Clinician name, address, phone number.

Follow-up: As needed.

▸ *Intrauterine Device (IUD)*

Laboratory Tests: Hematocrit. Pap smear. Gonorrhea culture. Serum pregnancy test to rule out antecedent pregnancy and slide tests for cervical mucus ferning to evaluate the patient's ovulation status should be done before insertion of a morning-after IUD.

Therapeutic Measures

Exam: Women who wish IUD insertion should have a thorough health history, heart, abdominal and pelvic exam to rule out contraindications (see Table 9.42).

Timing of insertion: Recommendations depend on the parturition status of the patient:

Parturition Status	Time of Insertion
Not pregnant	During menses Immediately after menses Between menses providing no unprotected intercourse occurred since last menses
After first-trimester abortion	Immediately after procedure or 2 weeks after procedure
After second-trimester abortion	2 weeks after procedure
After full-term pregnancy	6 weeks after delivery
After unprotected intercourse (morning-after IUD)	Within 72 hours of intercourse providing no other unprotected intercourse occurred since last menses

Choosing the correct device: Selection of the IUD should be made according to the patient's history and pelvic exam and availability of devices (many drug companies are phasing out IUD products in the U.S.). The Lippes Loop is available in four sizes (A–D). The large Lippes Loop is particularly suited to parous women. The Copper-7 and Copper-Ts are smaller than the inert plastic devices and are therefore well suited for nulliparous women. They may also produce less dysmenorrhea than the larger Loop. The Copper-7, however, has its string looped over the outside of the insertion barrel, which may increase the incidence of uterine infection or cause problems with interpretation of expulsion or with ease of removal. Expulsion rates are lowest with the Copper-7 and Copper-T. For the woman with a history of a previously expelled IUD, the more rigid Loop or the Progestasert should be tried. Impregnated with progesterone, the Progestasert T is least associated with cramping and bleeding. The pregnancy rate is lowest with the Copper T-380 and highest with the Lippes Loop. However, the rates for both pregnancy and expulsion are dependent on the skill and experience of the clinician who inserts the device. The Copper-7 and the T-shaped devices have the highest continuation rates after 1 year, the Loop the lowest. The inert devices are the least expensive. The Lippes Loop may be left in place indefinitely. The Copper-7 is FDA approved for 3 years use while the Copper-Ts are approved for 4. The Progestasert must be replaced yearly.

Inserting the IUD: Clinicians must be prepared for the possible occurrence of perforation and vasovagal reaction, which may lead to syncope, arrhythmias, or cardiac arrest during insertion. Appropriate treatment procedures for any of these complications should be available. The insertion procedure should be carried out according to the manufacturer's instruction. The following steps offer general guidelines for the insertion procedure:

1. Explain the procedure to the woman and choose a suitable device.
2. Perform a bimanual exam to ascertain uterine size, shape, and position (perforation is most common in the retroflexed uterus). Check for signs of preexisting PID.
3. Insert a warm speculum and perform a Pap smear and cervical culture.
4. Swab the whole cervix with antiseptic solution at least three times. If the solution contains iodine, be sure to inquire whether the patient has an iodine allergy.
5. Attach a sterile tenaculum to the anterior lip of the cervix to provide traction for IUD insertion and to straighten the cervico-uterine angle.
6. Insert a sterile sound into the uterine cavity to determine further its position and depth. Place a cotton swab next to the sound at the cervix; remove the sound and the swab at the same time, using the swab to mark the depth at which the sound is inserted. If the cavity sounds less than 4.5 cm, no IUD can be inserted.
7. Load the IUD into the inserter barrel, using sterile technique.
8. Insert the IUD according to package instructions, using the tenaculum for traction. If possible, use withdrawal technique, since it is associated with fewer perforations and IUD displacements.
9. Remove instruments.
10. Trim the IUD tail strings to 5 cm. They can be trimmed shorter later if necessary.

Patient Education: Following the insertion procedure, patients should be given written instructions such as the following:

INSTRUCTIONS FOR IUD USE

Your IUD: You have a __________ intrauterine device (IUD). It should be changed every __________ year(s), but an examination is recommended yearly for an IUD check, breast and pelvic exam, Pap smear, and blood count. If you go through the menopause (change of life), have your IUD removed.

Bleeding: It is not unusual to have spotting and mild cramping between periods for the first several months after getting your IUD, as well as heavier periods with more cramps. If bleeding is very heavy or spotting continues, contact your clinician. You may have the IUD removed at any time.

Strings: Check for your IUD strings at least after every menstrual period, when the chance of expelling the device is highest. If you check for the string each time you have intercourse, you can be more sure of having protection. If you feel hard plastic or if your partner feels pain on penetration, you may be losing your IUD. You are not protected from pregnancy if you cannot feel the IUD strings. Use another method of birth control such as foam and condoms until you can see your clinician.

Backup: A second method of birth control such as foam and condoms, used for the first 3 months and then at midcycle (days 10–18 of a 28-day cycle), will provide added protection against pregnancy.

Missed periods: If you miss a period or are late for a period, call your clinician immediately.

Pregnancy: If you become pregnant with an IUD in place, it should be removed as soon as possible. During and after removal, there is an increased chance of miscarriage. If the IUD is not removed, there is a chance that serious infection may occur, which may even lead to death.

Warning signs: Signs of serious problems that require immediate medical attention include pain in the lower abdomen and with intercourse, late period or no period, foul discharge, clots, heavy bleeding, new spotting or bleeding, and fever and chills, especially if associated with any of the other signs.

Clinician's name, address, and telephone number.

Follow-up: An appointment should be arranged in 6 weeks for string check and pelvic exam. All instructions should be reinforced at that time. Yearly appointments should be scheduled for breast and pelvic exams, Pap smear, and hematocrit.

▸ *IUD Problems*

Laboratory Tests: Cervical cultures, CBC, ESR in the event of infection. Hematocrit if heavy periods occur. Pregnancy test for a missed period or any possibility of ectopic pregnancy. Pelvic ultrasound for suspected ectopic pregnancy or if IUD placement is in question.

Therapeutic Measures

Infection: Cramping, pain, or a vaginal discharge must first and foremost be considered as indicators of PID in the IUD user. If a pelvic exam confirms the presence of PID, the IUD should be removed and the appropriate treatment instituted. If the cramping and pain are instead determined to be due to a uterine reaction to the device, the device may be left in place. Measures that are useful for dysmenorrhea may be helpful. If there is any doubt about the possibility of an infection, the IUD should be removed.

Pregnancy: If a woman is late for her period, she should have a urine or blood pregnancy test and a pelvic exam to rule out an ectopic pregnancy. If the pregnancy test is positive and the pregnancy is intrauterine, the device must be removed. The risk of subsequent spontaneous abortion is approximately 25%. The risk of spontaneous abortion with the IUD in place is 50%. The risk of sepsis is greatly increased in the IUD user who is pregnant. Any pregnant IUD user should be medically evaluated immediately should she develop flu-like symptoms of fever, chills, headache, and myalgia. If the pregnancy is ectopic, refer the patient to a gynecologist or emergency room.

Expulsion: If an IUD is partially expelled, it should be removed and a new one inserted or a new method of birth control chosen. Pregnancy should be ruled out with both complete and partial expulsions.

Missing strings: Strings that cannot be felt or visualized may be coiled in the uterine cavity. Missing strings may also indicate that the device has been expelled unnoticed or that perforation has occurred. Diagnostic procedures are as follows:

1. Exclude pregnancy first.
2. Sound the uterus, feeling for the IUD. If it is felt, the strings may be retrieved with careful probing. A specially designed sterile plastic helix or a hook may be used in place of a sterile sound.
3. If the device is not felt, refer the patient for pelvic ultrasound.
4. Alternatively, if the device is not felt, insert another IUD and refer the client for posteroanterior and lateral x-ray films of the abdomen, using the new IUD as the known landmark for locating the missing IUD. If the old device is not seen, the new one can be left in place for continuing contraception with the assumption that the previous device was expelled unnoticed.
5. If the device is located outside the uterus, refer the patient for removal.

Removal: Removal is easiest to accomplish during the menses, with the small amount of associated spotting going unnoticed at that time. The IUD should not be removed at midcycle if the woman has had intercourse in the preceding 4–5 days without using another method of contraception, since it is possible that a fertilized egg may be present. To remove the IUD, supply steady, firm, but gentle traction on the string. If the strings are not visible, use the procedure for finding missing strings, discussed above. If removal is difficult, refer the patient to a gynecologist.

Patient Education: Teach patients the warning symptoms of problems and stress the importance of immediate attention for symptoms of pelvic infection or pregnancy.

Follow-up: As needed.

▸ *Diaphragm*

Laboratory Tests: As needed for women's health care. No specific tests are required.

Therapeutic Measures

Exam: To rule out the relatively few contraindications to diaphragm use (see Table 9.43), the woman should have a health assessment and pelvic exam before being fitted. During the pelvic exam, the clinician should look specifically for cystocele, rectocele, prolapse, or a shallow pubic notch.

Diaphragm selection: There are three types of diaphragms: flat spring, coil spring, and arcing spring. Flat and coil spring diaphragms maintain a straight spring line when their sides are pressed together. The spring edge of the arcing spring forms a half circle when compressed. The sizes for all three are in 5-mm increments and range from 55 to 95 mm in diameter. The most commonly used sizes are 65–85 mm. All diaphragms provide equal protection from pregnancy. The type chosen depends on the pelvic anatomy and the woman's preference. The coil spring diaphragm is the most commonly used and is suitable for women with good vaginal tone, an anterior cervix position, and an adequate pubic notch. The flat spring has a thinner rim than the coil spring and is best suited for women with a shallow pubic notch. The flat spring also may be better for women with recurrent urinary tract infection because it exerts less pressure on the urethra. The arcing spring is well suited for the woman with a posterior or midline cervical position, some laxity of vaginal tone, a deep vaginal vault, and, in some cases, a shallow pubic notch. The Koroflex arcing spring is the best choice for women with poor vaginal tone or a slight cystocele because the rim spring is stronger than that of the other diaphragms and compensates for the poor tone.

Fitting instructions: It is best to use a set of fitting diaphragms, not fitting rings, and to have sets with all three spring types. This permits the patient to practice insertion and removal with the same equipment that she will be using at home. The following steps are taken to fit a diaphragm:

1. Perform a pelvic exam and assess vaginal tone, cervix position, and depth of the pubic notch. Based on this assessment, choose the appropriate diaphragm type.
2. Measure the depth of the vaginal vault for diaphragm sizing by inserting the first two fingers into the vagina behind the cervix and the thumb of the same hand just to the depth of the pubic notch. Hold the thumb in that position, remove the examining hand, and select a diaphragm that is the length of the distance from the tip of the examining finger to the tip of the thumb. If there is any doubt, choose a larger rather than a smaller size.
3. Insert the fitting diaphragm. It should fit behind the cervix and sit securely in the pubic notch, with no more than a fingertip breadth between the rim and the pubic bone.
4. Once a diaphragm is chosen that seems to be the correct size, do two things: have the woman bear down (Valsalva maneuver) with the diaphragm in place to see if the rim dislodges from the pubic notch, and then have her do the same with the next larger size. The largest comfortable diaphragm that does not gap with the Valsalva maneuver is the correct size.
5. After teaching the patient how to feel for her cervix, teach her how to feel the proper placement of the diaphragm: the cervix is covered by the rubber, the posterior rim is behind the cervix, and the anterior rim is securely lodged in the pubic notch (see Fig. 9.10).
6. Have the patient remove the diaphragm by putting a finger between the rim and the anterior vaginal wall, gently pulling it down and out.
7. Have the patient practice diaphragm insertion. This may be easiest in a supported, semisitting position or standing with one leg on a chair. Squatting may be easier for some women, particularly those who are obese. The patient should have at least one successful insertion and removal before leaving.
8. When prescribing a coil or flat spring type, a demonstration of the use of a diaphragm introducer may be helpful. The diaphragm is stretched across the notches of the introducer; the device is inserted into the vagina, and then

twisted and removed. Proper placement must then be checked as outlined in step 5.

Patient Education: Explain how the diaphragm works, as well as its effectiveness rates, risks, and benefits. After the fitting, instruct the patient (and her partner) on diaphragm use and care. These instructions can be reinforced with a written handout such as the following:

INSTRUCTIONS FOR DIAPHRAGM USE

Your diaphragm: You have a __________ spring diaphragm, size __________ mm.

Holes and tears: Before each use, check the diaphragm for holes by holding it up to the light or filling it with water. Check carefully for tears under the rim. You may want to have an extra diaphragm on hand in case you do find a tear.

Spermicide: Rinse the diaphragm and dry it. Put a teaspoon of spermicidal cream or jelly (not foam) in the diaphragm cup; spread it in the cup and under the rim with your finger. Jelly and cream are equally effective in killing sperm, but jelly is more lubricating. Do not use Vaseline with your diaphragm, since it can corrode the rubber.

Insertion: You may try inserting the diaphragm standing with one leg on a stool, squatting, or lying down with your knees up and apart. With the dome side down, looking into the cup, squeeze the rims of the diaphragm together and insert it into your vagina at the same angle as you would insert a tampon: up and in toward the small of your back.

Placement: Check the diaphragm for proper placement. The front rim nearest the opening of your vagina should be firmly in the pubic notch behind the pubic bone. Follow the front rim of the diaphragm back behind the cervix to make sure that the rubber cup covers the cervix. The cervix is at the back of the vagina and feels firm, like the tip of your nose.

Misplacement: Your partner may feel the diaphragm, but if it is uncomfortable for him or for you, it is probably not in the proper position. The diaphragm is more likely to become dislodged in sexual positions with the woman on top; guiding the penis in slowly may avoid this problem.

Timing: You may insert the diaphragm up to 6 hours before intercourse. You must leave it in place in the vagina for at least 6 hours after intercourse so that all sperm in the vagina are dead before diaphragm removal. If you have intercourse more than once after insertion, add an extra applicator of cream or jelly to the back of the vagina without removing the diaphragm. Do not douche with the diaphragm in place.

Removal: Put your finger between the rim and the pubic bone. Pull the diaphragm down and out.

When to use: For maximum effectiveness, use the diaphragm every time you have intercourse. If used during the menstrual period, the diaphragm will trap the menstrual flow. You may find it convenient to insert the diaphragm habitually every night before bedtime or before you usually have intercourse so that you do not need to interrupt lovemaking for its insertion.

Care of the diaphragm: After removal, wash the diaphragm with a mild soap and warm water. Dry it carefully and dust it with cornstarch (not perfumed powders). Store it in its case.

Replacement: Your diaphragm should last for about 2 years. If you gain or lose 15–20 lb or if the diaphragm is uncomfortable after wearing it for several hours, it should be refitted. If you have not had intercourse before, you should return for refitting after 6–8 weeks of use. Refitting should also be scheduled 6 weeks after having a baby.

Clinician's name, address, and telephone number.

Follow-up: One week after fitting, the woman should return with the diaphragm in place. Fitting and placement can be checked and problems discussed. Thereafter, the patient should return yearly or when she has a weight change of more than 15 lb, has a baby, or has problems with the device.

▸ *Contraceptive Sponge*

Laboratory Tests: None.

Therapeutic Measures: The contraceptive sponge (Today, 1983) has no major side effects on health. For this reason, there are no recommendations for assessment. Prescriptions are not needed.

Patient Education: Explain how the sponge works, as well as its effectiveness rates, risks, and benefits. Discuss the use of the sponge with the patient and demonstrate its use on a pelvic model or on the patient herself. Provide the patient with a written handout containing information such as the following:

INSTRUCTIONS FOR VAGINAL SPONGE USE

Education: A pamphlet insert containing consumer information and colored illustrations can be found in each box of vaginal sponges. Study them carefully.

Preparation: To be effective, the sponge must be available. Be sure to plan ahead and have it on hand.

Insertion: Briefly wet the sponge to activate the spermicide and gently squeeze it out so that it is damp, not dripping wet. Fold the sponge between two fingers and insert it into the vagina so that the indentation is on top and the removal loop underneath. Push the sponge deep into the vagina, firmly against the cervix.

Timing: The sponge is effective as soon as it is in place and remains so for 24 hours regardless of how many times you have intercourse. You must leave it in place in the vagina for at least 6 hours after intercourse so that all sperm will be dead before removal. If you have intercourse during the 24th hour after insertion, the sponge must still remain in the vagina for 6 hours.

Removal: Reach into the vagina and pull the sponge out by taking hold of the removal loop and pulling downward and out. Throw away the used sponge; it cannot be used again.

When to use: The sponge must be in place before intercourse. You may use it during menses, but you will need to wear a pad or a tampon too. When using it during menses, do not leave it in place for a full 24 hours; instead, remove it 6 hours after intercourse.

Douching: Douching is not recommended at any time. If you do douche, do not do so with the sponge in place or within 6 hours after intercourse.

Hotline number: A 24-hour hotline service has been established by the Today manufacturer to answer any questions and give advice about problems. It can be reached by dialing (800) 223-2329.

Follow-up: None necessary.

▸ *Condoms*

Laboratory Tests: None.

Therapeutic Measures: There are no contraindications to the use of condoms and therefore no recommendations for assessment. Prescriptions are not needed.

Patient Education: Explain how condoms work, as well as their effectiveness rate, risks, and benefits. Specifically, note that because condoms help prevent transmission of venereal disease, their main effect on health is a beneficial one. Note that condoms are made of latex (at a cost of \$0.30–0.50 each) or from the cecum of lamb intestines (\$1.50 each). Latex condoms come in a variety of colors and textures, lubricated or unlubricated. They may be tapered, flared at the end, or narrowed and may have a reservoir tip to hold the sperm. The thinness of the latex varies according to the brand. In general, condoms come in only one size but may be available through mail order in different sizes. Condom choice is determined by user preference.

Advise patients that condom effectiveness is greatly improved with concurrent use of a vaginal spermicide. It is important that both the man and woman be instructed on condom use and given an instruction sheet with information such as the following:

INSTRUCTIONS FOR CONDOM USE

Preparation: Condoms do not work unless you use them. Therefore, be prepared. Condoms have a shelf life of about 5 years but will not last that long if exposed to high temperatures.

Use: Unwrap the condom and place it on the tip of the erect penis before making any contact with the vagina. Unroll it over the shaft of the penis, leaving a $\frac{1}{2}$-in. space free of air at the tip to collect sperm if there is no built-in reservoir tip. Immediately after ejaculation, hold the base of the condom firmly on the penis and withdraw the penis and condom together. Remove the condom and discard. There will still be sperm on the penis, so contact with the vagina should continue to be avoided.

Backup: Contraceptive foam used before each act of intercourse will greatly increase the effectiveness of condoms as a method of birth control. If the condom breaks or slips off in the vagina, foam should be inserted immediately.

Lubrication: Although some condoms are lubricated, you may lubricate dry ones with K-Y Jelly, saliva, or spermicidal foam. Do not use Vaseline or other oils, since they may corrode the rubber.

Availability: You can buy condoms without a prescription in drugstores. Condoms vary in the thickness of the rubber; try several brands until you find one that is suitable for you. Brand name condoms are usually of higher quality, allow greater transmission of body heat and tactile sensation, and are less likely to break or tear.

Follow-Up: None necessary.

▸ *Vaginal Spermicides*

Laboratory Tests: None.

Therapeutic Measures: Vaginal spermicides have no major adverse effects on health. There are no recommendations for assessment, and the only contraindication to their use is a known allergy to the spermicide.

Creams and jellies: Although no prescription is necessary for any of the vaginal spermicides, it is helpful to review the various preparations available in the United States (see Table 9.44) and provide information that can help patients make the best choice. Creams and jellies, when used alone rather than with a diaphragm or cervical cap, are probably the least effective spermicidal preparations because they provide less surface coverage per dose and because placement in the vagina is more prone to error. They are inserted into the vagina with the use of a plunger-type applicator up to half an hour before vaginal penetration, providing the woman remains lying down after insertion. Although some creams and jellies are made to be used alone (e.g., Conceptrol, Delfen, Ramses), others contain less spermicide and are to be used only with a diaphragm or cervical cap (e.g., Koromex IIA, OrthoGynol). Because of this difference and because of poorer cervical coverage, the use of creams or jellies alone is not recommended.

Aerosolized foams: Aerosolized foams are considered more effective than creams or jellies. They can be inserted deep into the vagina up to half an hour before penetration with a plunger-type applicator. A new application of foam must be used with each act of intercourse. Common errors with foam application include not shaking the can long enough to ensure mixing of the base and spermicide; inserting too little spermicide; inserting spermicide more than half an hour before intercourse; inserting spermicide too shallow or deep into the vagina; douching sooner than 6 hours after intercourse; maintaining an upright position after spermicide insertion, which may allow spermicide to leak out; and not having spermicide available at the time of intercourse. Because of variations in applicator size, some brands of foam require two doses, rather than one, per act of intercourse if used as the only method of birth control. If foam is being used as a backup method, one application of any brand is sufficient. Purse or pocket-size container-applicators are available (e.g., Because).

Suppositories: Both regular and foaming suppositories are available. They require at least a 10- to 15-minute waiting period after insertion before penetration to allow for the suppositories to melt, and in the latter case, to foam. The foaming suppositories release heat as a by-product of the foaming action; some women and men find this disturbing or irritating, while others find it pleasurable. In addition, because of the added coverage of the foaming suppository, it is preferable to suppositories that are essentially creams or jellies in a wax base. Care must be taken with storage of the suppositories. If they become too warm, either from storage on a sunlit shelf or from body heat when carried in a pocket, they will melt and will no longer be insertable. To solve this problem, the unopened package should be held in cold water as soon as warming occurs, before the suppository has fully melted. Common errors with suppository use are the same as with foam, with the addition of these factors: inadequate waiting time to allow suppository melting and dispersal; rectal, rather than vaginal, insertion; and lack of wrapper removal before insertion.

Patient Education: Spermicidal preparations may be the only acceptable method of birth control for some clients; under such circumstances, they are better than no method at all. Their effectiveness is greater if the clinician provides full instructions and follow-up, encourages the use of the preparation with each coital act, and inspires confidence in the method when used consistently. Explain how spermicides work, as well as their effectiveness rates, risks, and benefits. When discussing the use of vaginal spermicides with patients, it is most helpful to demonstrate how to fill and insert the product using a pelvic model. The demonstration can also be incorporated into the pelvic exam. Written instructions such as the following should also be given:

INSTRUCTIONS FOR VAGINAL SPERMICIDE USE

Education: A pamphlet insert containing consumer information and illustrations can be found in each package of vaginal spermicide. It is often offered in both English and Spanish. Be sure to follow the specific instructions carefully.

Preparation: To be effective, spermicides must be available. Be sure to plan ahead and have the product handy. To increase its effectiveness, use the foam or suppositories with another method of birth control such as condoms, IUDs, or rhythm.

Use of foam: Before filling the applicator, shake the can 20–30 times to build up bubbles. Fill the applicator by putting it on the top of the can nozzle and either pushing straight down or tilting the applicator to one side while pushing, depending on the brand. Fill to the line marked on the applicator. Then insert the applicator into the vagina as far as it will go. Next, pull it out half an inch; the applicator is now pointing at your cervix. Push the plunger, depositing the foam into your vagina. Remove the inserter. It is best to use the foam with another method such as condoms. If you are using only foam, insert one or two applicatorfuls according to manufacturer's instructions. If you do not have intercourse within half an hour of using the foam, insert another application. Once the foam is inserted, you should remain in a lying position as much as possible to prevent the foam from running out. Each time you have intercourse, you must insert more foam in the vagina.

Use of suppositories: Make sure that the suppository you buy says "contraception" on the box; some are for vaginal hygiene and will not prevent pregnancy. Insert the suppository deep into the vagina, about 3–4 in. Wait 10 minutes before having intercourse to allow the suppository to melt. If you are using Encare Ovals, you may feel a warm or burning sensation as the tablet begins to foam. As with the foam, you should remain in a lying position as much as possible after inserting the suppository so that the spermicide does not run out. If you do not have intercourse within 1 hour, insert another suppository. Each time you have intercourse, you must use another suppository. If the suppositories become warm in their wrapper, either from being carried in your pocket or from being stored in another warm place, put them immediately into cold water still in their wrapper. If they are foaming suppositories and have already begun to foam, they may no longer be effective.

Hygiene: There may be dripping from the vagina after spermicide use. Minipads are useful to soak up the discharge. Most people do not like the taste of spermicides. If you plan to have oral sex, do so before inserting the spermicide and having vaginal sex.

Douching: In general, douching is not recommended. If you do douche, wait at least 8 hours after intercourse before doing so. It is all right to bathe or shower at any time.

Follow-up: None needed.

▶ *Basal Body Temperature (BBT) Method*

Laboratory Tests: None.

Therapeutic Measures: BBT combines the calculation of menstrual cycle lengths and the changes in body temperature caused by hormonal variation to predict ovulation and infertile days of the menstrual cycle. Since ovulation varies during the postpartum period, lactation, and menopause, the BBT method may be less reliable at those times. Understanding the body's thermal response to ovulation is essential to proper use of BBT. Although there are minor daily variations, there are three general temperature phase shifts during the menstrual cycle. Phase I is the relatively infertile time before ovulation, when the base temperature is the lowest and is calculated by subtracting 21 days (rather than 18 days, as with the calendar method) from the shortest length of the preceding six to eight cycles. It extends from day 1 of the menstrual cycle to the first possible fertile day, as determined by such calculation. The preovulation base temperature is the highest temperature recorded during phase I. Phase II is the fertile period when a thermal shift takes place at the time of progesterone increase with ovulation. Over 1–5 days, basal temperature rises 0.4–0.6°F above the preovulation base. Phase II begins on the first day of temperature rise above the preovulation base and lasts until the temperature remains elevated at least 0.4°F for 3 days. There are four different thermal shift patterns during phase II: an immediate rise in 1–2 days, a slow rise over 3–4 days, a stairstep rise with increases every 2–3 days, or a zigzag rise with increases and decreases over several days (see Fig. 9.11 for examples). When the pattern is the immediate one, the first safe time for coitus is the night of the third day of the shift. When the pattern is slow, stairstep, or zigzag, the first safe time is the night of the fifth day of progressive elevation. These conservative waiting periods allow for a second ovulation and its following 24-hour ovum survival time (a second ovulation may occur within 24 hours of the first before progesterone levels are high enough to inhibit another ovulation). Phase III begins on the night of the third or fifth day of the thermal shift, as described above, and ends with the first day of menses. It is the absolutely infertile time. The strict BBT method confines intercourse to phase III; the relaxed BBT method allows for intercourse in phases I and III. BBT kits are available at pharmacies and many family planning clinics. They include a Fahrenheit thermometer marked in 0.1° increments from 96° to 100°, rather than the standard fever thermometer, which has a higher range and 0.2° increments. There are also sample temperature graphs, as in Figure 9.12, some of which allow for concurrent recording of menstruation and coitus. If prepared charts are not available, they can be made using a piece of graph paper. Body temperature can be measured orally, vaginally, or rectally, but the same site must be used consistently. Vaginal and rectal temperatures are less subject to environmental variation. The temperature should be taken on awakening in the morning after 5–6 hours of sleep and before any activity occurs. Getting up during the night for a few minutes or even for an hour or so will not have a significant effect on the early morning temperature. Restriction of activity before temperature taking should be studiously maintained while patterns are being determined. After that time, some experimentation is possible.

Patient Education: Explain how the BBT method works, as well as its risks and benefits. Instruct the patient and her partner on temperature taking, charting, temperature patterns and interpretations, and the determination of safe times. Give them an instruction sheet such as the following:

INSTRUCTIONS FOR THE BBT METHOD

Equipment: Use either a special basal body Fahrenheit thermometer, sold at pharmacies or family planning clinics, that is marked in tenths of a degree or a standard fever thermometer. The BBT thermometer is easier to read. Use a copy of the accompanying graph or the graphs that come with the BBT kit to keep a record of your daily temperature and menstrual periods.

Taking your temperature: You may use oral, rectal, or vaginal temperatures, but once you have decided which site to use, always use the same site. Insert the thermometer as soon as you wake up in the morning, preferably at the same time every day, and leave it in place for 5 minutes. Then record the temperature on the graph, shake down the thermometer, and store it in a safe, convenient place for the next day's use. Factors that interfere with an accurate reading are kissing, eating or drinking, cigarette smoking, illness, using an electric blanket, immunizations, getting less than 5–6 hours of sleep, drinking alcohol the night before, climate extremes, and sleeping pills. Getting up during the night will not affect your morning temperature significantly. If you are ill with an elevated temperature, record the temperature but note the illness on your graph. These days cannot be used to help in your determination of safe and unsafe days.

Cycle pattern: Before using your BBT records and interpretations as a dependable method of birth control, you should have kept temperature records for three cycles and discussed them with a trained natural family planning counselor. Note: Do not attempt to use this method without detailed instructions first. If you are unsure about how to interpret any of your cycle patterns, contact your clinician or family planning counselor.

Safe days: About 2 weeks before your next menstrual period, your body temperature will begin to rise above the preovulation baseline established in the first 2 weeks. The rise of 0.4–0.6°F, or thermal shift, occurs just after ovulation and may take place in 1 day or over several days. When the temperature has been elevated more than 0.4°F above baseline for 3 days, the safe period begins: intercourse is safely allowed on the night of the third day of the thermal shift. The safe period begins that night and lasts until your next period begins.

21-day rule: Some persons practice a more relaxed BBT method by having intercourse not only after the third day of postovulation temperature rise but also in the relatively infertile time before ovulation. This time is determined by subtracting 21 from the number of days in the shortest cycle in the preceding six months. The result is the number of preovulation days starting with the first day of menses that are relatively safe for intercourse. For example, if your shortest cycle has been 26 days long, 26 − 21 = 5. Days 1–5 are relatively safe for intercourse in addition to the days after the thermal shift.

Combining BBT with other methods: The BBT method, when combined with other natural methods such as cervical mucus determination or with barrier spermicide methods such as condoms, foam, diaphragm, or sponge, will have increased effectiveness.

Clinician's name, address, phone number.

Follow-up: The patient should return at the end of her first cycle to review her temperature chart and to ask questions. At the end of her third cycle, she should return for detailed review of her temperature charts and discussion of their interpretation. Clinicians who are not experienced with temperature chart interpretations should refer their patients to someone who has such experience if possible. Thereafter, follow-up is needed only for problems or regular health maintenance.

▸ *Cervical Mucus (Billings) Method*

Laboratory Tests: None.

Therapeutic Measures: The cervical mucus method is based on monitoring the physiologic changes of the cervical mucus to determine ovulation. Although it can be safely used by lactating, premenopausal, and perimenopausal women, this method is not advised for women who have chronic or recurrent vaginal infections. Understanding the cervical responses to ovulation is necessary for proper use of the cervical mucus method. Influenced by the rise and fall of estrogen and progesterone levels, the uterine cervix continually produces a mucus discharge that changes in amount and consistency. At the beginning and end of the menstrual cycle the mucus is scant, cloudy, thick, and tacky. These days are referred to as "dry days." Around the time of ovulation the mucus is abundant, clear, thin, and elastic. Its slippery, egg white texture enhances the movement and survival of sperm. The elastic quality of midcycle mucus is called "Spinnbarkheit" when the mucus can be stretched into a thread 5–20 cm long. If allowed to dry on a glass slide, it will form a crystalline, fern-like pattern because of its relatively high salt and protein content. These days are referred to as "wet days." The last wet day (the "peak day") corresponds to ovulation. The first safe or infertile day begins the morning of the fourth day after the peak day. A calendar is used to record the type of mucus observed, the day of the cycle, days of intercourse, and menses. The following abbreviations can be used: M = menses, D = dry days, W = wet days, P = peak day, I = intercourse. As an alternative, the Billings kit is a system of colored stamps designed by the developers of the cervical mucus method: red for menses, white with a baby outline for wet and peak days, light green with a baby outline for the three days after the peak, and green for safe, dry days.

Patient Education: Explain how the method works, as well as its risks and benefits. Advise the patient that combining this method with other methods such as BBT or foam and condoms will increase its effectiveness. Instruct the patient and her partner on the different kinds of cervical mucus and how to keep a calendar. Give the couple an instruction sheet with information such as the following:

INSTRUCTIONS FOR CERVICAL MUCUS METHOD USE

Checking your mucus: Every morning upon awakening, feel your vaginal opening with your fingers for wetness or dryness. If there is wetness, decide if it is infertile wetness: white or yellow, sticky or tacky, very scant; or fertile wetness: slippery, like egg white, clear or cloudy, stretchy, abundant.

Calendar: Note on your calendar the day of your cycle, with day 1 being the first day of your period, and the kind of mucus wetness or dryness you felt that morning, using the following abbreviations: M = menses, D = dry or sticky, infertile mucus, W = wet, P = peak day, I = intercourse since yesterday morning. The peak day is the day that you feel the most wetness with slippery, stretchy mucus, usually halfway between one period and the next. Calculate the estimated first unsafe day according to the calendar method (shortest cycle length − 18).

Intercourse: The times when intercourse is unsafe are (1) during menses, because the bleeding covers up the mucus and some women may ovulate during menses; (2) the day after intercourse in the period before ovulation, because the semen from the day before will make the mucus "wet," covering up the normal mucus; (3) the first safe day as calculated by the calendar method and all of the days that follow, through ovulation, even if no mucus wetness is felt; (4) during any wet days, the peak day, and 3 days after the peak day, because this is the time of ovulation; and (5) on days when there is spot bleeding, because this may be a sign of ovulation. The times when intercourse is safe are (1) only at night on dry days before ovulation; morning intercourse is all right if you check your mucus beforehand, and (2) anytime after the peak + 3 days.

Pregnancy: If you strongly desire not to get pregnant, do not have intercourse in the time between the start of your period and the third day after the peak day, or use another method of birth control in addition to checking your mucus.

Vaginal discharge: Days when you have an abnormal discharge, such as one with a bad smell or itching or burning, should be considered unsafe days. Medical treatment may be necessary.

Special conditions: If you have not had a regular period and thus cannot anticipate ovulation based on the calendar, either because you recently stopped using birth control pills, had a baby, are breast feeding, or are nearing menopause, you must be sure not to have intercourse 2 days in a row. The semen from the first day's intercourse will make the next day a wet day and will cover up your own mucus.

For more information see:

Billings, E. and Westmore, A. *The Billings Method: Controlling Fertility without Drugs or Devices*. New York: Random House, 1980.

Follow-up: The patient should return at the end of her first cycle to review her chart and to ask questions. At the end of her third cycle, she should return for detailed review of the charts and discussion of their interpretation. Thereafter, follow-up is needed only for problems or regular health maintenance.

▸ *Symptothermal Method*

Laboratory Tests: None.

Therapeutic Measures: The symptothermic method combines the principles of the calendar, BBT, and cervical mucus methods with an assessment of ovulation signs and symptoms. Although it can be safely used by lactating, premenopausal, and perimenopausal women, the symptothermic method is not advised for women who have chronic or recurrent vaginal infections. Proper use of the symptothermic method depends on an understanding of the physiologic responses to ovulation. The cervical mucus and BBT changes were described in the previous sections. At midcycle the cervix becomes softer, flatter, and more slippery and the os opens slightly. Mittelschmerz, or midcycle, unilateral pelvic pain may be felt by some women. Other changes with ovulation may be swollen, tender breasts, abdominal bloating, a slightly bloody discharge, increased libido, and vulvar swelling.

Patient Education: The patient and her partner should be instructed on keeping a menstrual cycle calendar and chartng BBT and cervical mucus changes as previously described. In addition, midcycle symptoms should be discussed. Give a handout with information such as the following:

SYMPTOMS AND SIGNS OF OVULATION

Cervix	Softening, flattening, opening up
Cervical mucus	Abundant, slippery, clear and stretchy, like egg white
Breasts	Enlargement, tenderness
Other	Abdominal bloating
	Lower abdominal pain on one side
	Slightly bloody discharge
	Increased sex drive

For more detailed information on natural family planning see:

Nofziger, M. *A Cooperative Method of Natural Birth Control.* Summertown, TN: The Book Publishing Co., 1979.

Follow-up: The patient should return at the end of her first cycle to review her charting and observed symptoms and to ask questions. At the end of her third cycle, she should return for detailed chart and symptom review and discussion of their interpretation. Thereafter, follow-up is needed only for problems or regular health maintenance.

▸ *Calendar (Rhythm) Method**

Laboratory Tests: None.

Therapeutic Measures: Because many women have variable cycle lengths from month to month, it is important to have an initial baseline menstrual calendar for 6–8 months to check cycle variation. Figure 9.13 shows a menstrual calendar with several sample cycles filled in. Whether ovulation can be reliably predicted should be established before attempting to use the calendar method of birth control alone. The method is inadvisable in the following cases: menstrual cycle variability more than or equal to 8 days, menstrual cycle shorter than 25 days, and in postpartum, lactation, or menopausal periods. Women who have little or no variation in cycle length will be most successful with this method. Effectiveness can be increased by combining this method with other natural family planning methods such as BBT, cervical mucus, or withdrawal.

Patient Education: Stress the fact that the calendar method is no longer recommended by experts in natural family planning, since it has an estimated failure rate of 14–35%. For patients using this method, a basic understanding of the fertilization process is imperative. Explain that ovulation occurs 14 $\pm$ 1 days before the onset of menses. The ovum survives for up to 24 hours, and sperm can remain viable in the female reproductive tract for up to 2 and perhaps even 3 days. If intercourse occurs 19 days before menses, fertilization can therefore theoretically occur when the egg is released 4 or 5 days later. Adding the survival times for sperm and ovum together, this makes a total of 11 unsafe days out of an average 28-day cycle. Some couples do not like to have intercourse during menstruation, and this further decreases the number of days free for intercourse.

Instruct couples on how to keep a menstrual calendar and how to calculate safe and unsafe days. A sample menstrual calendar should be given, along with the list for calculating safe and unsafe days (Table 9.45). In addition, give a written handout such as the following:

INSTRUCTIONS FOR CALENDAR METHOD USE

Recording: Keep a monthly record of the first day of your menstrual period to determine the length of your menstrual cycle. Day 1 of your menstrual cycle is the first day of menses; the last day of your cycle is the day before your next

*Due to its high failure rate (14–35 pregnancies per 100 women using the method for 1 year), use of the calendar method alone is no longer recommended by experts in natural family planning.

menses. A total of 6 consecutive cycles, if regular, and 12 if irregular, should be recorded before depending on the method.

Fertile, unsafe days: From the previous six cycles, determine your shortest and longest cycles. Use a fertility calculation table to find your unsafe days. If no such table is available, you can calculate the unsafe period by subtracting 18 from your shortest cycle and 11 from your longest cycle. An example follows:

Shortest cycle	= 25 days	−	18	=	day 7 first unsafe day
Longest cycle	= 29 days	−	11	=	day 18 last unsafe day
Menses this month started			Oct 3		Oct 3
			+7		+18
First unsafe day			Oct. 10		
Last unsafe day					Oct. 21

Calculations: Every month on the first day of your period, recalculate your fertile days based on the cycles from the most recent 6–8 months.

Backup: You can increase the effectiveness of the calendar method, and possibly identify a shorter unsafe period, by combining this method with other natural methods such as cervical mucus awareness and BBT recording.

Checkup: If your cycles vary by more than 8 days or if your shortest cycle is less than 25 days, consult your clinician. You may need to choose another method of birth control. Bring your calendar to every visit, even if you have no problems with the method.

Clinician's name, address, phone number.

Follow-up: The woman should be seen after she has recorded for several months to review the calculation of cycle length and the fertile period. If she has already done this and has brought her calendar to the first visit, she need return only for problems or her annual visit.

BIBLIOGRAPHY

Albertsen PC, et al. A critical method of evaluating tests for male infertility. *The Journal of Urology,* (Sept.) 1983, 130(3):467–75.

Alexander B. Sexual problems: Now that they're out of the closet: How can you help? *Consultant,* (June) 1984, 217–223.

American Cancer Society. *How to Examine Your Breasts.* Pamphlet No. 2088-LE. Tuckahoe, N.Y., May 1975.

American Cancer Society. *Facts on Testicular Cancer.* Pamphlet No. 2645-LE. Tuckahoe, N.Y., February 1978.

American Council for Healthful Living. *Nine Common Sexually Transmitted Diseases.* Orange, N.J., 1983.

American Social Health Association. *Some Questions and Answers About Herpes.* Palo Alto, Calif., 1983.

Arndt K. *Manual of Dermatologic Therapeutics,* 2nd ed. Little, Brown, Boston, 1978.

Ban Y, Murphy GP. Antigen marker assays in prostate cancer. *Laboratory Management,* (Apr.) 1983, 19–24.

Barrier methods. *Population Reports,* series 11, no. 4, 1976.

Bartosch JC. Oral contraception: Selection and management. *Nurse Practitioner,* (May) 1983, 56–63.

Barwin JJ, et al. The intrauterine contraception device. *Canadian Medical Association Journal,* 1978, 118.

Bates B. *A Guide to Physical Examination,* 3rd ed., Lippincott, Philadelphia, 1983.

Begley B. Amenorrhea: A primary care approach. *Physician Assistant,* (Apr.) 1985, 13–28.

Benson RC, Patterson DE. The Nesbit procedure for Peyronie's disease. *Journal of Urology,* (Oct.) 1983, 130:692–693.

Berkow RB (ed.). *The Merck Manual of Diagnosis and Therapy,* 14th ed. Merck Sharp & Dohme Research Laboratories, Rahway, N.J., 1982.

Berman RL. Current perspectives in gynecology. (KJ Bean, ed.). *Clinical Symposia,* 1985, 37(1):2–32.

Bettoli EJ. Herpes: Facts and fallacies. *American Journal of Nursing,* (June) 1982, 924–929.

Blake JP, et al. Drugs in pregnancy: Weighing the risks. *Patient Care,* (May) 1980, 22–37.

Boston Collaborative Drug Surveillance Program. Oral contraceptives and venous thromboembolic disease, surgically confirmed gallbladder disease, and breast tumors. *Lancet,* 1973, 1.

Bradshaw BR, et al. *Counseling on Family and Human Sexuality.* Family Service Association of America, New York, 1977.

Brown AM, Stubbs DW (eds.). *Medical Physiology.* Wiley, New York, 1983.

Burke L, et al. Observations on the psychological impact of diethylstilbestrol exposure and suggestions on management. *Journal of Reproductive Medicine,* 24(3):99–102.

Burroughs Wellcome Co. *Sexually Transmitted Disease Bulletin,* (Oct.) 1984, 4(5).

Burroughs Wellcome Co. *Sexually Transmitted Disease Bulletin,* (June) (1985), 5(3).

Caine VA, Spence MR. Treating sexually transmitted infections. *Therapeutics,* 1982.

Carson R. *Your Menopause.* Public Affairs Pamphlet No. 447. New York, May 1981.

Cherniak D. *A Book About Birth Control,* 2nd ed. Montreal Health Press, Montreal, 1980.

Comstock B. Dysfunctional uterine bleeding. *PA Outlook,* (Mar.–Apr.) 1984, 4–16.

Conn HF, Conn RB Jr (eds.). *Current Diagnosis.* Saunders, Philadelphia, 1980.

Coordinated Human Services of Westchester, Inc. *What Everyone Should Know About Contraception.* Channing L. Bete Co., Greenfield, Mass., 1977.

Coughlin PWF, Carson CC, Paulson DF. Surgical correction of Peyronie's disease: The Nesbit procedure. *The Journal of Urology,* (Feb.) 1984, 131:282–285.

Coustan DR, Carpenter MW. The use of medications in pregnancy. *Medical Times,* (June) 1984, 45–51.

Crafts RC. *A Textbook of Human Anatomy,* 3rd ed. Wiley, New York, 1985.

Crouch J. *Functional Human Anatomy.* Lea & Febiger, Philadelphia, 1972.

Crouch JE, McClintic JR. *Human Anatomy and Physiology,* 2nd ed. Wiley, New York, 1976.

Cutick R. Special needs of perimenopausal and menopausal women. JOGN *Nursing* (suppl.), (Mar.–Apr.) 1984, 68s–73s.

Demarest CB. Advising women on sterilization options. *Patient Care,* (May) 1983, 128–172.

Dicken RP. *Managing Contraceptive Pill Patients,* 2nd ed. Creative Infomatics, Aspen, Colo., 1980.

Dosey MA, Dosey MF. The climacteric woman. *Patient Counseling and Health Education,* 1980, 2(1):14–21.

Duncan SL. Ethical problems in advising contraception and sterilization. *The Practitioner,* 1979, 223.

Elegbe I, Modupe C. A preliminary study on dressing patterns and incidence of candidiasis. *American Journal of Health,* (Feb.) 1982, 72(2):176–177.

Elias H, Pauly JE, Burns ER. *Histology and Human Microanatomy,* 4th ed. Wiley, New York, 1978.

Eschenbach D, et al. Polymicrobial etiology of acute PID. *New England Journal of Medicine,* (July) 1975, 295(4):166–171.

Fayez JA. Dysfunctional uterine bleeding. *American Family Physician,* (Mar.) 1982, 25(3):109–115.

Federation of Feminist Woman's Health Centers. *A New View of a Woman's Body.* Simon & Schuster, New York, 1981.

Fogel C, Woods N. *Health Care of Women.* Mosby, St. Louis, 1981.

Foster RS Jr. New approaches to breast cancer management: Part I, management of local and regional disease. *Continuing Education,* (Dec.) 1982, 56–68.

Friedman D. Premenstrual syndrome. *The Journal of Family Practice,* 1984, 19(5):669–678.

Fuchs F. Primary dysmenorrhea: New theories promote "rational" therapy. *PA Practice,* 1985, 4(2):15–16.

Fuller E. Herpesvirus: Agent of many ills. *Patient Care,* (Nov.) 1981, 200–227.

Gambrell RD, et al. Breast cancer and oral contraceptive therapy in premenopausal women. *The Journal of Reproductive Medicine,* 1979, 23(6).

Gibbs RS. Management of pelvic inflammatory disease. *Sexual Medicine Today,* (Jan.) 1985, 9(1):21–25.

Gorline LL, Stegbauer CC. What every nurse should know about vaginitis. *American Journal of Nursing,* (Dec.) 1982, 1851–1855.

Goroll AH, May LA, Mulley AG. *Primary Care Medicine: Office Evaluation and Management of the Adult Patient.* Lippincott, Philadelphia, 1981.

Graham SD Jr. Male infertility: Treatment options. *PA Drug Update,* (Oct.) 1983, 45–55.

Gray, H. *Anatomy of the Human Body,* 29th American ed. (CM Goss, ed.). Lea & Febiger, Philadelphia, 1973.

Green T. *Gynecology: Essentials of Clinical Practice,* 3rd ed. Little, Brown, Boston, 1977.

Greenblatt RB, Gambrell RD Jr. Primary dysmenorrhea: Mechanisms and management. *The Female Patient,* (Oct.) 1984, 9:63–79.

Greenblatt RB, Vasquez J, Samaras C. Fibrocystic breast disease: Current status of diagnosis and treatment. *Postgraduate Medicine,* (Mar.) 1982, 71(3):159–167.

Grey H. *Anatomy, Descriptive and Surgical.* Running Press, Philadelphia, 1974.

Gump FE. Common errors in the treatment of benign breast lesions. *Drug Therapy,* (Mar.) 1982, 209–217.

Guyton AC. *Textbook of Medical Physiology,* 6th ed. Saunders, Philadelphia, 1981.

Haddock DA. Pelvic inflammatory disease. *Diagnostic Challenges,* (Jan.) 1983, 2(5):1–5.

Handsfield HH. PPNG infections: Current status and guidelines for therapy. *PA Drug Update,* (Jan.) 1983, 68–75.

Harry JD (ed.). *Rhoads Textbook of Surgery: Principles and Practice,* 2 vols., 5th ed. Lippincott, Philadelphia, 1977.

Hatcher RA, et al. *Contraceptive Technology 1986–1987,* 13th rev. ed. Irvington, New York, 1986.

Health Education Associates. *Breast Massage and Hand Expression of Breast Milk: Collection and Storage of Breast Milk.* Willow Grove, Pa., 1977.

Health Education Associates. *Breast Feeding: Those First Weeks at Home.* Willow Grove, Pa., 1978.

Health Education Associates. *Prenatal Breast Care: Preparing for Breastfeeding.* Willow Grove, Pa., 1978.

Health Education Associates. *Have You Thought About Breastfeeding?* Willow Grove, Pa., 1980.

Health Education Associates. *Breastfeeding Problems Can Be Avoided.* Willow Grove, Pa., 1984.

Health Education Associates. *Nursing Is Easy When You Know How.* Willow Grove, Pa., 1984.

Health Education Associates. *Time Out for Breastfeeding Mothers.* Willow Grove, Pa., 1984.

Helzer M. Differential diagnosis of scrotal swellings. *Physician Assistant,* (July) 1983, 94–108.

Henzl MR. Dysmenorrhea: Achievements and challenges. *Sexual Medicine Today,* (Jan.) 1985, 9(1):7–10.

High rates of pregnancy and dissatisfaction mark first cervical cap trial. *Family Planning Perspectives,* 1981, 13(1).

Hoole AJ, Greenberg RA, Pickard CG Jr. *Patient Care Guidelines for Nurse Practitioners.* Little, Brown, Boston, 1982.

Hull MGR, et al. Normal fertility in women with post-pill amenorrhea. *Lancet,* 1981, 1.

Impotence: Mostly medical and curable. *Acute Care Medicine,* (July–Aug.) 1984, 15–23.

Jacob S, Francone C, Lossow W. *Structure and Function in Man,* 4th ed. Saunders, Philadelphia, 1978.

Jaffe HW. Nongonococcal urethritis: Treatment of men and their sexual partners. *Reviews of Infectious Diseases* (suppl.), (Nov.–Dec.) 1982, 4:s772–s776.

Jay MS, Taylor W. Primary dysmenorrhea: Current concepts. *American Family Physician,* (Nov.) 1981, 24(5):129–134.

Johnson NE. Nutritional needs of middle-aged women. *Midpoint: Counseling Women Through Menopause,* (Dec.) 1984, 1(2):7–13.

Jones EF, Paul L, Westoff CF. Contraceptive efficacy: The significance of method and motivation. *Studies in Family Planning,* 1980, 11(2).

Kaplan H. *Disorders of Sexual Desire.* Simon & Schuster, New York, 1979.

Kaplan HS. *The New Sex Therapy.* Brunner/Mazel, New York, 1974.

Katzenstein DA. Chlamydial infections. *Continuing Education,* (Aug.) 1982, 34–45.

Kaufman SA. Diagnosis and management of infertility. *Physician Assistant and Health Practitioner,* (Mar.) 1981, 16–27.

Kaye CI. Genetic counseling. *Medical Aspects of Human Sexuality,* (Mar.) 1981, 15(3):164–180.

Kelaghan J, et al. Barrier-method contraceptives and pelvic inflammatory disease. *Journal of the American Medical Association,* 1982, 248(2).

Kellum MD, Loucks A. Genital herpes infections. *Nurse Practitioner,* (Feb.) 1982, 14–21.

Kemmann E, Jones JR. The female climacteric. *American Family Physician,* (Nov.) 1979, 20(5):140–151.

Keye WR Jr, Strong T. Premenstrual syndrome: An enigma. *Continuing Education,* (Oct.) 1983, 913–918.

King J. Vaginitis. JOGN *Nursing* (suppl.), (Mar.–Apr.) 1984, 41s–48s.

Kistner RW. Endometriosis as a cause of infertility. *Sexual Medicine Today,* (Jan.) 1985, 9(1):12–14.

Klaus H, et al. Use-effectiveness and analysis of satisfaction levels with the Billings ovulation method: Two year pilot study. *Fertility and Sterility,* 1977, 28(10):

Kradjian RM. Breast Lumps. PAS, Daly City, Calif., 1981.

Krupp MA, Chatton MJ, Werdegar D (eds.). *Current Medical Diagnosis and Treatment 1985.* Lange, Los Altos, Calif., 1985.

La Leche League International. *When You Breastfeed Your Baby: Helpful Hints for the Early Weeks.* Pamphlet No. 124. Franklin Park, Ill., October 1983.

Lee LM, Wright JE, McLaughlin MG. Testicular torsion in the adult. *The Journal of Urology,* (July) 1983, 130:93–94.

Lipman AG. Oral contraceptives: Eight interactions you should remember. *Modern Medicine,* (Nov.) 1981, 227–228.

Lossick JG. Treatment of *Trichomonas vaginalis* infections. *Reviews of Infectious Diseases* (suppl.), (Nov.–Dec.) 1982, 4:s801–s814.

Luckmann J, Sorensen KC. *Medical Surgical Nursing: A Psychophysiologic Approach,* 2nd ed. Saunders, Philadelphia, 1980.

Luff RD. Newer approaches to class II evaluation. *Consultant,* (Nov.) 1984, 24(11):177.

Macaluso JN Jr. Priapism: Update for the non-urologist. *Sexual Medicine Today,* (Feb.) 1985, 11–15.

Martin LL. *Health Care of Women.* Lippincott, New York, 1978.

Massey LK, Davidson MA. Effects of oral contraceptives on nutritional status. *American Family Physician,* 1979, 19(1).

Masters W, Johnson V. *Human Sexual Response.* Little, Brown, Boston, 1966.

Mattox JH. The infertile couple: Evaluating the woman. *Diagnosis,* (Mar.) 1985, 69–76.

McCormack MK. Screening for genetic traits and diseases. *American Family Physician,* (Oct.) 1981, 24(4):153–166.

Mead Johnson & Co. *Weaning Your Baby: A Helpful Guidebook About Weaning for the Breast-Feeding Mother.* Pamphlet No. L-F58-10-81. Evansville, Ind., 1981.

Meyer JK. The treatment of sexual disorders. *Medical Clinics of North America,* (July) 1977, 61(4):811–823.

Micha JP. Genital warts: Treatable warning of cancer? *The Female Patient,* (Oct.) 1984, 9:31–36.

Moore MD, Davis OS. *Realities in Childbearing.* Saunders, Philadelphia, 1978.

Morgan S. *Coping with Hysterectomy.* Dial Press, New York, 1982.

Morgan S. Sex after hysterectomy. *MS,* (Mar.) 1982, 82–85.

Mostofi FK. Testes tumors: Epidemiologic, etiologic, and pathologic features. *Cancer,* 1983, 32:1186–1205.

Murphy CA. Abnormal vaginal bleeding. *Physician Assistant and Health Practitioner,* (Oct.) 1982, 69–76.

National Women's Health Network. *Menopause.* Resource Guide No. 3. Washington, D.C., 1980.

Nelson JH Jr, Averette HE, Richart RM. Dysplasia, carcinoma in situ, and early invasive cervical carcinoma. *Ca—A Cancer Journal for Clinicians,* (Nov.–Dec.) 1984, 34(6):306–325.

Neuwirth RS. New approaches to female sterilization. *Physician Assistant and Health Practitioner,* (Dec.) 1980, 52–58.

New York State Department of Health. *DES: The Wonder Drug Women Should Wonder About.* Albany, N.Y., May 1981.

New York State Department of Health. *DES Sons.* Albany, N.Y., March 1981.

Notelovitz M. Menopause: When to treat. *Hospital Medicine,* (Oct.) 1980, 9–21.

Novak E, Jones G, Jones H. *Gynecology.* Williams & Wilkins, Baltimore, 1975.

On making the best of antibiotics in pregnancy. *Emergency Medicine,* (May) 1980, 67–77.

Ortho Pharmaceutical Corporation. *A Guide to the Methods of Postponing or Preventing Pregnancy.* Pamphlet No. 3-6. Raritan, N.J., rev. October 1974.

Ortho Pharmaceutical Corporation. *For Your Information . . . Vaginitis.* Pamphlet No. 3-95. Raritan, N.J., rev. May 1979.

Ory HW. Ectopic pregnancy and intrauterine contraceptive devices: New perspectives. *Obstetrics and Gynecology,* (Feb.) 1981, 57:137–144.

Patrick JK. Congenital absence of the vas deferens. *American Family Physician,* 26(3):147–149.

Pelosi MA. Diagnosis: Ectopic pregnancy. *Hospital Medicine,* (Mar.) 1982, 37–64.

Petersdorf, RG. *Harrison's Principles of Internal Medicine,* 10th ed. McGraw Hill, New York, 1983.

Pfizer Laboratories Division. *Sexually Transmitted Diseases: What You Should Know.* Pamphlet No. X-011-X-83. Pfizer, New York, 1983.

Pheifer P, et al. Nonspecific vaginitis. *New England Journal of Medicine,* (June) 1978, 298(26):1429–1434.

Portnoi V. Urinary incontinence in the elderly. *American Family Physician,* (June) 1981, 23(6):151–154.

Potter S. Menopausal attitudes and symptoms: A psychosexual duality. Master's thesis. Yale School of Nursing, 1977.

Prout GR. Testicular symptoms that may mean cancer. *Diagnosis,* (June) 1984, 125–129.

Prout GR, Griffin PP. Testicular tumors: Delay in diagnosis and influence on survival. *American Family Physician,* (May) 1984, 29(5):205–209.

Quinn PA. Mycoplasmas: What kind of association with non-gonococcal urethritis? *Sexually Transmitted Diseases Bulletin,* (Oct.) 1984, 4(5):2–9.

Reid RL. Premenstrual syndrome: A therapeutic enigma. *PA Drug Update,* (July) 1982, 14–22.

Reimer BL. *The Menopausal Years.* Physicians Art Service, Daly City, Calif., 1980.

Renshaw DC. Sexual dysfunction in the elderly couple. *The Female Patient,* (Oct.) 1984, 9:59–62.

Riddick DH. Hormonal management of the climacteric. *Physician Assistant,* (Apr.) 1983, 37–46.

Romanowski B, Harris JRW (D. Shephard, ed.). Sexually transmitted diseases. *Clinical Symposia,* 1984, 36(1):2–32.

Rosenfield AG. Contraception: Where are we in 1985? *Contemporary OB/GYN,* (Feb.) 1985, 79–81.

Rosenwaks Z. New approach to dysmenorrhea. *PA Drug Update,* (Jan.) 1983, 38–49.

Ross LS. Diagnosis and treatment of infertile men: A clinical perspective. *The Journal of Urology,* (Nov.) 1983, 130(5):847–854.

Sabiston DC (ed.). *Davis-Christopher Textbook of Surgery: The Biological Basis of Modern Surgical Practice,* 2 vols. Saunders, Philadelphia, 1981.

Sandberg E. Benign cervical and vaginal changes associated with exposure to stilbestrol in utero. *American Journal of Gynecology,* 1976, 125(6):777–789.

Sex Information and Education Council of the U.S. *Characteristics of Male and Female Sexual Responses.* SIECUS Study Guide No. 4. Behavioral Publications, New York, 1974.

Shapero GH. Mastitis and breast abscess during lactation. *Physician Assistant,* (July) 1984, 45–50.

Siever A, Tolins P. *Be Good to Your Baby Before It Is Born.* National Foundation—March of Dimes, 1979.

Silverstein A. *Human Anatomy and Physiology.* Wiley, New York, 1980.

Slag, MF, Morley JE, Elson MK, et al. Impotence in medical clinic outpatients. *Journal of the American Medical Association,* 1983, 249:1736–1748.

Sloan E. *Biology of Women.* Wiley, New York, 1980.

Smith EL. The role of exercise in the prevention of osteoporosis. *Midpoint: Counseling Women Through Menopause,* (Dec.) 1984, 1(2):3–6.

Soloway HB, Peter JB (eds.). Interpretation of tests. *Diagnostic Medicine,* (Oct.) 1983, 17.

Spark RF. Neuroendocrinology and impotence. *Annals of Internal Medicine,* 1983, 98:103–104.

Speroff L, Glass R, Kase N. *Clinical Gynecologic Endocrinology and Infertility,* 3rd ed. Williams & Wilkins, Baltimore, 1983.

Stadel BV. Oral contraceptives and cardiovascular disease, part II. *New England Journal of Medicine,* 1981, 305(12).

Tallent DD. Cytologic examination of the breast: A safe, simple, and accurate technique. *Postgraduate Medicine,* (Feb.) 1981), 69(2):91–98.

Tetirick JE. Nipple discharge. *American Family Physician,* (Nov.) 1980, 22(5):101–103.

Thorp VJ. Effect of oral contraceptive agents on vitamin and mineral requirements. *Journal of the American Dietetic Association,* 1980, 76.

Townsend CM Jr. Breast lumps. *Clinical Symposia,* 1980, 32(2):3–32.

U.S. Department of Health, Education, and Welfare. *Family Planning for Completed Families.* Pamphlet No. 75-16015. Washington, D.C., 1975.

U.S. Department of Health, Education, and Welfare. *Contraception: Comparing the Options.* Pamphlet No. 78-3069. Washington, D.C., 1978.

U.S. Department of Health, Education, and Welfare. *Family Planning Methods of Contraception.* Pamphlet No. 80-5646. Washington, D.C., 1978.

U.S. Department of Health and Human Services. *Breast Feeding.* Pamphlet No. 80-5109. Washington, D.C., 1980.

U.S. Department of Health and Human Services. *Natural Family Planning.* Pamphlet No. 80-5621. Washington, D.C., 1980.

U.S. Department of Health and Human Services. *Questions and Answers About DES Exposure During Pregnancy and Before Birth.* Pamphlet No. 80-1118. Washington, D.C., National Institutes of Health, March 1980.

U.S. Department of Health and Human Services. *Were You or Your Daughter or Son Born After 1940?* Pamphlet No. 80-1226. National Institutes of Health, Washington, D.C., May 1980.

U.S. Department of Health and Human Services. *Breast Self-Examination.* Pamphlet No. 80-649. National Institutes of Health, Washington, D.C., August 1980.

U.S. Department of Health and Human Services. *Sexually Transmitted Diseases Treatment Guidelines 1982.* Pamphlet No. 82-8017. Washington, D.C., 1982.

Utian W. *Menopause in Modern Perspective: A Guide to Clinical Practice.* Appleton-Century-Crofts, New York, 1981.

Vana J, et al. Primary liver tumors and oral contraceptives: Results of a survey. *Journal of the American Medical Association,* 1977, 238.

Varney H. *Nurse-Midwifery.* Blackwell Scientific Publications, Boston, 1980.

Vaughn TC. Benign breast lesions: New therapy for a common but worrisome disorder. *Consultant,* (Jun.) 1983, 129–138.

Vessey M, Lawless M, Yeates D. Efficacy of different contraceptive methods. *Lancet,* (Apr.) 1982, 841–842.

VLI Corporation. *Use Instruction Booklet* (for the Today vaginal contraceptive sponge). 1983.

Walbroehl GS. Sex and pregnancy: Advising the patient. *Sexual Medicine Today,* (Jan.) 1985, 9(1):18–20.

When to think ectopic pregnancy. *Patient Care,* (Nov.) 1984, 18(19).

Wiesenthal AM. Toxic shock syndrome: An update. *PA Drug Update,* (Apr.) 1983, 32–221.

Wilson EA. Infertility: Methods of evaluation and treatment. *PA Practice,* 1985, 4(2):7–14.

Wyngaarden JB, Smith LH Jr (eds.). *Cecil Textbook of Medicine,* Vols. 1 and 2, 16th ed. Saunders, Philadelphia, 1982.

Yuzpe AA. Postcoital contraception. *International Journal of Gynecology and Obstetrics,* 1979, 16.

Zuna RE. The Pap smear revisited. *Postgraduate Medicine,* (Nov.) 1984, 76(6):37.

10

Skin

Connie Main

Outline

DERMIS

Blood Vessels and Lymphatics

Heat disruptions (syncope, cramps, exhaustion, stroke)
Fever
Burns (epidermal, partial-thickness, full-thickness)
▶ Minor burns

Cold Injuries

Cold urticaria
▶ Localized cold injuries (frostnip, chilblains, frostbite)
Hypothermia
Contact dermatitis (irritant, allergic)
▶ Toxicodendron (plant) dermatitis
Seborrheic dermatitis
▶ Atopic dermatitis
Nummular dermatitis
Dyshidrosis
Dermatophytids
Generalized exfoliative dermatitis
Stasis dermatitis
Pityriasis rosea
Lichen planus
Hypertrophic lichen planus
Secondary form of early (infectious) syphilis
Urticaria
Angioedema
Erythema multiforme
Erythema multiforme bullosum
Stevens-Johnson syndrome
Toxic epidermal necrolysis (TEN)
Erythema nodosum
Cutaneous drug reactions
Granuloma annulare
Bullous disorders
Bullous pemphigoid
Cicatricial pemphigoid
Pemphigus vulgaris
Dermatitis herpetiformis
Herpes gestationis
Porphyria cutanea tarda
Bacterial infections
Impetigo (ecthyma, bullous)
Folliculitis

Sycosis
Furuncles
Carbuncle
Cellulitis
Erysipelas
Wound infections
Hidradenitis suppurativa
Scalded skin syndrome
Scarlet fever
Leprosy (lepromatous, tuberculoid)
Viral infections
Herpes simplex
▶ Herpes zoster
▶ Chickenpox
Measles
Measles vaccination
Atypical measles syndrome (AMS)
Rubella
▶ Rubella virus vaccine
▶ Insect bites
Insect stings (ordinary response, generalized systemic reaction, anaphylaxis, delayed hypersensitivity responses)
Tick bites
Rickettsial diseases
Rocky Mountain spotted fever
Erythema chronicum migrans (ECM)
▶ Pediculosis (capitis, corporis, pubis)
▶ Scabies
Chronic discoid lupus erythematosus

Sensation

Pruritis

EPIDERMIS

Ichthyosis
Xeroderma (dry skin)
Keratosis pilaris
Calluses and corns
Warts (common, periungual, plantar, filiform, flat)
Molluscum contagiosum
▶ Psoriasis
Pustular psoriasis
Guttate psoriasis
Fungal infections
▶ Tinea (capitis, corporis, cruris, manuum, pedis, unguium)
Candidal onychomycosis
Intertrigo
Cutaneous candidiasis
Tinea versicolor

Pigmentation

Sunburn (mild, severe)
Photosensitivity reactions
Ephelides
Lentigines
Seborrheic keratoses
Skin tags
Acanthosis nigricans
Stucco keratosis
Nevi (melanoma, junctional nevus, compound nevus, intradermal nevus)
▶ Actinic keratoses
Squamous cell carcinoma
Keratoacanthoma
Lentigo maligna
Lentigo-maligna melanoma
Basal cell carcinoma
Keloids
Albinism (congenital, partial)
Vitiligo
Secondary hypopigmentation
Hyperpigmentation
Melasma

ACCESSORY ORGANS OF THE SKIN

Hair

Alopecia (male and female pattern loss)
Alopecia areata
Trichotillomania
Hirsutism
Pseudofolliculitis barbae
Folliculitis keloidalis

Nails

Onycholysis
Onychomycosis (distal ungual, white superficial, proximal ungual, candidal)
Paronychia
"Green nails"
Dystrophic nail changes

Sebaceous Glands

Sebaceous nevus
Sebaceous hyperplasia
▶ Acne
Rosacea

Sweat Glands

Hyperhidrosis
Miliaria

SKIN

The integument, which includes not only the skin but also its accessory organs (hair, nails, sebaceous and sweat glands, sensory receptors), is a complex organ system covering a surface area of about 2 m^2 and representing about 6–16% of total body weight. Its functions include protection of underlying structures, excretion, secretion, thermoregulation, sensation, and production and storage of various products.

There are two distinct skin layers. The inner, thicker layer, the dermis (or corium), is made up of dense areolar connective tissue. All of the accessory organs of the skin are located in this layer, although some are actually products of the outer layer, the epidermis. This layer, composed of stratified squamous epithelium, is thinner than the dermis and has four or five layers or zones, each containing cells in varying stages of metamorphosis (Fig. 10.1).

Lying beneath the skin, but inseparable from it, is the subcutaneous fascia (also called the "hypodermis" or "superficial fascia"), a layer of loose connective tissue that varies from areolar to adipose. It is not considered part of the skin, but one of its functions is to bind the skin loosely to the underlying structures, attaching directly to the fascia around the muscles, or, in some cases, to the periosteum. Varying numbers of fat cells occur in this layer, depending upon the body region and the organism's state of nutrition. In addition to enabling storage of fat, this layer provides insulation and cushioning for the structures beneath it. Wherever continuous lobules of fat occur, they form a pad called the "panniculus adiposus," which on the abdomen may be as thick as 3 cm or more. No fat is present in the subcutaneous tissue of the eyelids, scrotum, and penis.

The subcutaneous layer varies in thickness throughout the body, but is generally thicker than the dermis and contains large arteries, veins, lymphatics, and nerve trunks. Parts of the hair follicles and sweat glands are also located in the uppermost region of this layer.

DERMIS

The dermis, sometimes called the "corium" or "true skin," is a thick layer of vascular, dense connective tissue containing primarily white collagenous fibers with some reticular and yellow elastic fibers embedded in a ground substance of glycosaminoglycans. There are numerous capillaries, lymphatics, nerves, and nerve endings in the dermis, as well as hair follicles, sebaceous glands, sweat glands and their ducts, and smooth muscle fibers. Extending from the fatty, areolar subcutaneous tissue to the epidermis, it varies in thickness from less than 1 mm to over 3 mm and can be subdivided into two strata (see Fig. 10.1): the inner reticular layer (closest to the subcutaneous fascia) and the outer papillary layer (next to the epidermis).

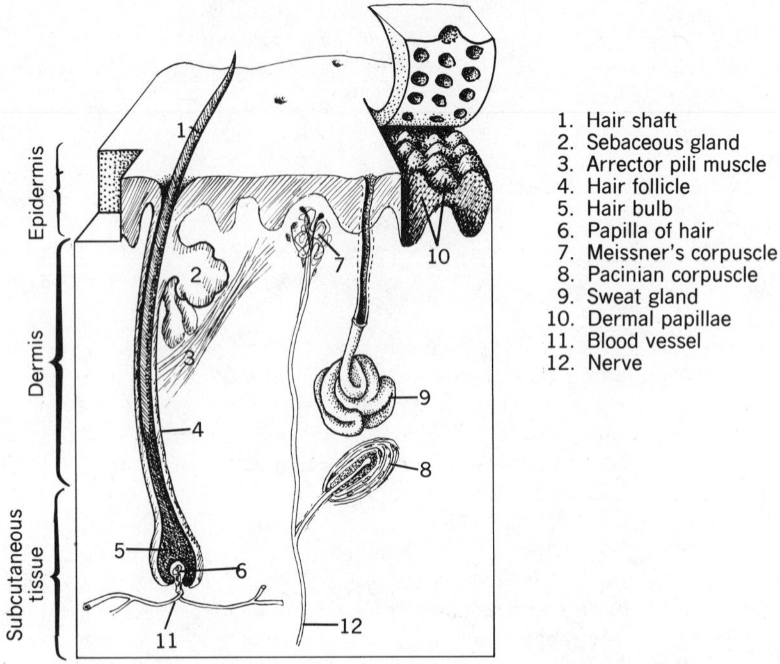

(*a*)

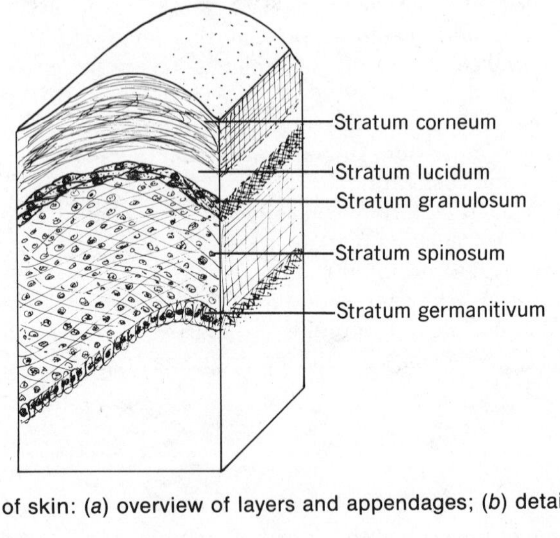

(*b*)

Figure 10.1 Layers of skin: (*a*) overview of layers and appendages; (*b*) detail of epidermal layers.

The deeper reticular layer is a dense mesh network of coarse fibers (mainly white collagenous) that provides most of the skin's reinforcement. The fibers are arranged predominantly parallel to the skin surface, and their directional orientation in a particular site results in lines of skin tension called "Langer's lines." These lines are of surgical importance, since incisions made parallel to them gape less and heal with a fine linear scar, but those made perpendicularly or obliquely across the lines of tension may result in unsightly scarring. Bundles of fibers also extend downward from the dermis into the subcutaneous fascia, thereby anchoring the skin. Except in local areas such as the soles of the feet and palms of the hands, the loose structure of the subcutaneous tissue permits a great deal of mobility for the skin.

Above the deeper reticular layer is the papillary layer, so called because its surface has numerous projections, called "papillae," which extend into the overlying layers of the epidermis. Papillae are composed of cellular connective tissue and vary in size and number throughout the body surface. On the palms and soles, where they are often branched, they are tallest and most numerous. Within each papilla is a small bundle of reticular fibers arranged parallel to its long axis, which extend perpendicularly from the dermis to insert into the basal lamina of the epidermis as anchoring fibrils. Some papillae contain a terminal knot of capillary blood vessels (a capillary loop) that provides a blood supply to the epidermis, the sebaceous glands, and the intermediate portion of hair follicles. Others (sensory or nervous papillae) contain specialized nerve endings that respond to touch.

Papillae are often arranged in double rows that run in various directions along the surface of the dermis. The conformity of the overlying epidermis to these dermal ridges, particularly on the soles and palmar surfaces, results in noticeable patterns consisting of whorls, loops, and arches. The fact that the arrangements of ridges and creases are unique to each individual and never change (apart from enlargement) after they form in fetal life forms the basis for the use of fingerprinting as a means of personal identification. These surface ridges also improve the frictional characteristics of the palms and soles. The degree of development of the ridges varies across the body surface; the papillae of facial skin are poorly developed, and the skin of the forehead, external ear, scrotum, and perineum lacks ridges altogether.

The bundles of connective tissue of the papillary layer are finer and more closely interwoven than those of the reticular layer. Dispersed throughout both layers of the dermis are yellow elastic fibers that give some resilience to the skin. With increasing age there is a noticeable decrease in skin elasticity, and wrinkles form. Even in young skin, large tumors, pregnancy, or extremely rapid weight gain may stretch the skin beyond the limits of its elasticity. The skin will not return to normal but will display silver-white "stretch marks" (striae albicans, s. distensae, s. gravidarum), which are actually tiny tears.

The main muscle fibers of the dermis are the arrectores pilorum, small bundles of smooth muscle fibers attached to the hair follicles. Smooth muscle fibers are also distributed throughout the skin of the nipple, scrotum, penis, and parts of the perineum, forming a layer permeated with elastic tissue known as the "tunica dartos." The skin of these regions appears wrinkled when these muscle fibers contract. Only on the neck and face does the skin possess striated muscle fibers (platysma myoides); these terminate in fine elastic fiber networks of the dermal layer.

Fibroblasts and macrophages (lymphocytes and polymorphonuclear leukocytes) are the predominant cellular components of the dermis, and fat cells may occur singly or in groups. In addition to the usual connective tissue cells, chromatophores, branched, pigmented connective tissue cells, may also be present, particularly in areas where the overlying epidermis is heavily pigmented, such as the perineal region and the areola of the nipple. These cells apparently are not involved in the elaboration of pigment, but obtain it from melanocytes. Melanocytes (pigment cells) are not common in the dermis, but when they accumulate in the sacral region, they form the mongolian spot. They may also occur in certain tumors of the dermis such as blue nevi.

Blood Vessels and Lymphatics

The dermal layer of the skin is replete with blood vessels and lymphatics. Arteries that proceed from networks in and just above the subcutaneous connective tissue branch as they ascend toward the skin surface. In the lower portion (reticular layer) of the dermis they anastomose to form a horizontally oriented plexus (rete cutaneum), and just below the superficial (papillary) layer of the dermis branches again anastomose to form the rete subpapillare. Branches from the deeper cutaneous plexus feed into the fat lobules in the adipose tissue of the underlying hypodermis, supply deeper portions of hair follicles, and also form "baskets" of capillaries around the coils of the sweat glands that are situated deep in the dermis or the hypodermis. Branches from the superficial subpapillary plexus furnish blood to the sebaceous glands and intermediate portions of the hair sheaths, and terminal arteries extend into the papillae as "capillary loops." There are no blood vessels in the overlying epidermis.

Veins receiving blood from the areas supplied by the subpapillary plexus form a plexus immediately beneath the papillae and sometimes a second one just below that and connected with it. Veins from these plexuses go into the deep reticular layer of the dermis, branching and receiving veins from the fat lobules and sweat glands; joining with larger veins, they continue into the subcutaneous tissue. Only when they become larger veins and arteries in the hypodermis do vessels receive specific names.

The blood in the vessels of the dermis gives a pinkish tint to less pigmented skin. Dilation of these blood vessels due to emotional or physiologic factors produces a "flush," which is more noticeable in fair-skinned persons than in darker-skinned ones; likewise, constriction of these vessels results in pallor. This dilation and constriction of peripheral vessels plays an important role in thermoregulation. Exposure to excessive heat results in prompt dilation of superficial cutaneous blood vessels, increased cardiac output, and sweating. With peripheral vasodilation, more blood is brought closer to the body surface, where heat can be lost by radiation to the environment. Conversely, constriction of these superficial vessels helps to preserve body heat by keeping more blood deep within the body core so that less surface heat is lost. Constriction of cutaneous blood vessels is also brought on in situations of stress as part of the body's "fight-or-flight" mechanism. Diversion of blood from surface vessels results in additional blood being supplied to the brain, vital organs, and muscles. All of these peripheral responses are controlled and mediated by the central nervous system (CNS).

There are four major disorders resulting from excess environmental heat. In order of increasing severity, they are heat syncope, heat cramps, heat exhaustion, and heat stroke.

Heat syncope is the term for fainting that occurs suddenly after exertion in the heat. The skin becomes pale, cool, and clammy, the pulse is weak and either slightly rapid (100–120 beats per minute) or slow (vasovagal syncope), and there is a transient decrease in blood pressure. The response to treatment, which includes rest in a recumbent position, cooling, and oral fluid administration, is usually prompt.

Heat cramps are painful spasms of the skeletal muscles of the abdomen and extremities that are caused primarily by salt depletion from excessive sweating (the salt content of sweat increases to 0.2–0.5% with increased environmental temperatures). Cool, moist skin, possible muscle twitching, and normal or only slightly increased body temperature are present. Hemoconcentration and low serum sodium levels are shown in laboratory studies. Treatment includes administration of sodium chloride, 1 g every 30–60 minutes, with large amounts of water or saline solution orally or IV. In addition, gentle massage of the affected muscles and rest in a cool place for 1–3 days are indicated.

Fatigue and collapse following prolonged (hours to days) or unaccustomed exposure to heat is termed ***heat exhaustion.*** This systemic response is due primarily to the low blood pressure and low blood volume that result from loss of body fluids and salts through excessive sweating. If the heat exhaustion is due primarily to fluid loss (heavy work at high temperatures may result in loss of up to 3–4 L/h from sweating), symptoms include intense thirst, weakness, muscular incoordination, hyperthermia, delirium, psychosis, and coma. This condition may progress rapidly to heat stroke if major seizures or circulatory failure occur. In heat exhaustion that is due predominantly to salt depletion (e.g., occurring when adequate fluids are taken following sweating but salts are not replaced), symptoms include muscle cramps, weakness, nausea, vomiting, and diarrhea. Pallor, tachycardia, hypotension, and low serum levels of sodium also occur, and body temperature is usually near normal. Measures to replace lost fluid and salt should be instituted immediately, including cool water, salted fruit drinks, or salt tablets, depending upon the primary cause of the condition (i.e., salt depletion or fluid loss). If the patient is unable to take these orally, IV normal saline or isotonic glucose solutions should be administered, depending on what the clinical appearance and laboratory findings reveal as the need. Marked sodium depletion with excess water intake (water intoxication) may require intravenous hypertonic saline solution.

Heat stroke occurs when the rectal temperature exceeds 40°C (104°F), and death is common if this condition remains untreated. This is a true medical emergency, characterized by a sudden loss of consciousness and high fever without sweating (caused by failure of the thermoregulatory mechanism). This condition most often results from excessive exposure to heat or strenuous physical exertion under hot conditions. However, very old, obese, or ill [from infection or gastrointestinal (GI) upset] persons and persons with alcoholism or cardiovascular disease are also susceptible to the development of heat stroke in the absence of unusual heat exposure. Diuretics, sedatives, and anticholinergic and antipsychotic drugs may be contributing factors.

Heat stroke related to exertion results from normal responses for diminishing the heat load (high cardiac output and low systemic vascular resistance), but in elderly patients there is an unexplainable decrease in cardiac output and increased peripheral resistance. Prodromal symptoms include headache, dizziness, faintness, staggering, and nausea, which progress to various signs of CNS involvement (confusion, lethargy, agitation, visual disturbances, convulsions, and coma). The body temperature is usually greater than 40°C (it may be as high as 43°C) but may be lower if even simple measures to relieve heat stress have been initiated prior to examination. The skin is hot and flushed, and usually dry; the pulse is strong and its rate high (140 beats per minute or more); systolic blood pressure may be normal or elevated, but the diastolic presure is usually lowered; however, in the late stages, the blood pressure may be lowered due to circulatory failure. Hyperventilation may result initially in respiratory alkalosis, but this is often followed by metabolic acidosis. Sweating may be present, or it may be reduced or absent (an ominous sign). Other findings include a high hematocrit, decreased coagulation, low serum levels of potassium, calcium, and phosphorus and increased serum transaminase, and scanty urine with proteinuria, tubular casts, and myoglobin.

Treatment of heat stroke aimed at the reduction of body temperature and support of the circulation should be instituted immediately, including physical cooling measures such as application of ice, alcohol, or wet towels, using a strong fan in a cool, dry room, or a cold tub bath (placing the patient in a cool, shady place and removing all clothing may be used as a preliminary first aid measure); aggressive cooling measures may be necessary for extremely high body temperatures, and sedation may be required if the patient struggles or begins to convulse (chlorpromazine, 25–50 mg IM, will help to control shivering and delirium and make the process of cooling more tolerable for a conscious patient). Cooling measures should be continued until the rectal temperature drops below 38°C and should be reinstituted if the patient shows a later rise in temperature (continued monitoring of temperature is necessary). Other measures include maintenance of an adequate airway (endotracheal intubation may be required if arterial oxygen pressure drops below 65 mm Hg) and administration of a high concentration of oxygen, IV fluid replacement, continuous monitoring of arterial blood gases and pH and central venous or pulmonary artery wedge pressure, maintenance of blood pressure and urinary output (with IV crystalloids and inotropic agents such as dopamine as necessary), and careful observation for complications (renal failure, cardiac arrhythmias, rhabdomyolysis, disseminated intravascular coagulation, hepatic failure).

Peripheral vasoconstriction is also employed by the body, in conjunction with shivering, in the production of pyrexia or ***fever*** in response to stimulation of the thermoregulatory center in the hypothalamus by circulating endogenous pyrogens. This is a valuable physiologic response, since it has been observed that the host defense response may be enhanced in the presence of a fever. However, a prolonged elevation of body temperature (e.g., rectal temperature over 41°C or 105.8°F) is a dangerous condition that can damage brain tissue, disturb metabolic processes, and distort the pharmacokinetics of drugs used for treatment of an associated disease. Birth defects apparently unrelated to the cause or treatment of fever may result from maternal fever during the first trimester of pregnancy, and extreme fevers in children 6 months to 5 years of age may result in seizures. Table 10.1 lists the causes of fever and hyperthermia. Symptomatic treatment of fever is not always recommended. It may be a benign and transient phenomenon, especially in children, and, as mentioned above, it has been shown to play a role in the body's defense against infection. Symptomatic treatment of fever may mask or eliminate important diagnostic information about an illness as well.

However, there are some justifiable instances in which fever should be treated: when it causes such discomfort that the patient is unable to get adequate rest; or when there is a preexisting cardiovascular, pulmonary, neurologic, renal, or metabolic condition, since the increase in fluid loss and metabolic rate that accompany a

TABLE 10.1 CAUSES OF FEVER AND HYPERTHERMIA

Cause	Examples
Infection	Viral, bacterial, rickettsial (e.g., Rocky Mountain spotted fever), fungal, and parasitic infectious causes are all common. Infections may be: 1. Localized (e.g., pyelonephritis). 2. Generalized, with localizing signs (e.g., scarlet fever). 3. Generalized, without localizing signs (e.g., septicemia).
Cardiovascular disease	Bacterial endocarditis, myocardial infarction, paroxysmal tachycardias, pulmonary embolism, thromboembolic diseases.
CNS disease	Cerebral hemorrhage, degenerative CNS disease (e.g., mutiple sclerosis), injuries to the head and spinal cord, tumors of the brain and spine.
Collagen diseases	Dermatomyositis, polyarteritis nodosa, rheumatic fever, rheumatoid arthritis, SLE.
Endocrine disease	Hyperthyroidism, pheochromocytoma.
GI disease	Inflammatory bowel disease, cirrhosis (necrotic phase), liver abscess.
Hematologic disease	Hemolytic anemias, hemorrhagic disease (e.g., hemophilia), leukemias, lymphomas, pernicious anemia.
Malignant neoplastic disease	Primary neoplasms (genitourinary tract, liver, lung, pancreas, thyroid), secondary neoplasms, carcinoid.
Environmental causes	Heat stroke, radiation sickness, trauma (e.g., surgery).
Chemical causes	Anaphylactic reactions, chemical poisoning, drug reactions, malignant hyperpyrexia from anesthesia (succinylcholine, potent inhalation anesthetics), pyrogen reactions following IV fluids.
Others	Fluid imbalance (dehydration, acidosis), sarcoidosis, amyloidosis.

fever may place considerable stress on an already weakened body system. In addition, fever in an epileptic or brain-damaged child may result in convulsions, and in a normal child it may trigger seizures. Fever should also be treated in patients who are known or suspected of being in bacterial shock. In general, if a fever is a hypothalamic response to exogenous (e.g., toxins, radiation, CNS lesions) or endogenous pyrogenic stimulation (e.g., infection, allergies, collagen disease), the treatment should include antipyretic medication (e.g., aspirin or acetaminophen, 300–600 mg qid) that will restore the hypothalamic set point to normal; oral or parenteral fluid replacement; and avoidance of physical measures for heat removal (e.g., ice application, sponge baths). However, in significant hyperthermia (greater than 40°C), physical measures to reduce the body temperature may be used in combination with antipyretic medications to reduce the fever and hypothalamic set point, since high body temperatures carry a significant risk of brain and metabolic disturbances. Hyperthermia resulting from heat production or an environmental heat load that exceeds normal heat loss mechanisms (examples of the former are malignant neoplastic diseases and thyroid storm; examples of the latter are overexposure to heat in the work environment or a sauna) or from defective heat loss mechanisms (e.g., heat stroke, sweat gland disorders, burns) should be treated by removal of excess clothing, elimination of any excess external heat source, and physical heat removal measures (sponging, application of ice), but should not include antipyretic drugs.

Burns are another common type of thermal injury. Every year they cause a significant number of deaths, particularly in children. Scalds, a minor form of burn, may be prevented to some extent by regulation of the water heater temperature. Burns are classified according to the extent of body surface involvement, depth of the burn, age of the patient, and association with other illnesses or injuries. To make an accurate assessment of the extent of a burn injury, it is necessary to view the patient's entire body after any soot has been cleaned off. In general, each of the following body surface areas is estimated to be equivalent to about 9% of the total body surface of an adult: the entire head and neck, the posterior surface of the upper trunk (above the level of the diaphragm), the anterior surface of the upper trunk, the posterior surface of the lower trunk, the anterior surface of the lower trunk (excluding the genital region, which is estimated to be 1% of the total body surface), the posterior surface of each leg, the anterior surface of each leg, and the entire surface of each arm.

Determination of the depth of a burn injury can be difficult, but ***epidermal*** (first-degree) ***burns*** appear red (due to dermal vasodilation) or gray and demonstrate excellent capillary refill. There is generally extreme tenderness and pain, increased warmth, erythema, and edema. No blisters are present initially in first-degree burns, and they do not present a significant danger of fluid loss. These burns heal without treatment and do not result in scarring. The epithelium sloughs in about a week (similar to the peeling following a sunburn). The presence of a blistered burn injury is representative of partial-thickness involvement of the dermis (second-degree burn). ***Partial-thickness burns*** may be distinguished clinically as superficial or deep. Although the damage in this burn extends through the epidermis and into the dermis, in the superficial partial-thickness burn this does not interfere with rapid epithelial regeneration (these burns heal in less than 3 weeks and rarely scar or cause functional impairment). Superficial partial-thickness burns are extremely painful, and the dermis at the base beneath the blisters (after debridement) appears wet and uniformly pink, blanches with pressure, and is usually raised above the surrounding skin. A deep partial-thickness burn may have lost its blister and appear reddened like an epidermal burn, but capillary refill is not good. This burn lacks the extreme sensitivity of the more superficial (epidermal and partial-thickness) burns, and unlike the superficial partial-thickness burn is uncomfortable, rather than painful, to debridement (in fact, pricking the skin beneath this burn will often produce only a sense of pressure). The base beneath the blisters is dry and white or bright red, and does not blanch with pressure. The skin after debridement appears white, with multiple red dots that represent the deep dermal vascular plexus.

Full-thickness (third-degree) ***burns,*** which destroy the entire dermal layer, often have a charred, coagulated surface (or, in scalds, white and lifeless), but no pain after the initial acute pain at the time of the injury because of the destruction of nerve endings. Blisters are often absent. The skin surface after debridement is depressed and may appear white or red, like that of a deep partial-thickness burn, or it may resemble dry, inelastic tanned leather. The division between deep partial-thickness and full-thickness burns is somewhat indistinct, but this is of little consequence since treatment is essentially the same for both types. The healing potential of both of these burns varies according to the location. Areas with a rich blood supply and a large number of appendages (hair follicles, sweat glands, etc.) have a better prognosis for reepithelialization, but burns in other areas, even if the dermis is quite healthy, tend to result in slower healing and more scarring. In both of these types, there may be some limitation of function. Since no epithelial tissue remains in deep partial-thickness and full-thickness burns, they must heal by contraction from the wound periphery or must be closed with skin grafts. The age of the burn patient is a critical factor in the chance for healing, and even fairly small burns in infants or elderly persons may be fatal. Likewise, the association of other injuries, such as smoke inhalation (a common complication of burn injuries); cardiac arrhythmias (from electrical injuries); preexisting cardiovascular, renal, or pulmonary disease; alcoholism; drug abuse; or psychiatric illness tend to complicate the recovery from a burn injury.

All patients with major burn injuries and many with moderate, uncomplicated burn injuries should be treated in specialized burn care facilities; moderate injuries may be treated in other facilities that have personnel with expertise in burn care. The American Burn Association (ABA) may be contacted for a list of known burn care facilities in particular states (contact the secretary of the ABA, Thomas Wachtel, M.D., at Good Samaritan Medical Center, 1130 East McDowell Road, Suite B-2, Phoenix, Arizona 85006). The criteria for classification of major, moderate, and mild burn injuries are given in Table 10.2. The vast majority of burns that are serious enough to require medical treatment may be managed by the primary care provider and do not require hospitalization. Most of these burns, if kept clean, will heal within 3 weeks with a minimum of scarring or functional impairment. However,

TABLE 10.2 CRITERIA FOR CLASSIFICATION OF BURN INJURIES

Classification	Thickness	Surface Area in Adults	Surface Area in Children	Other Variables
Major burn injuries	Partial-thickness	More than 25%	More than 20%	—
	Full-thickness	More than 10%	More than 10%	—
	Any thickness	—	—	Involving the face, eyes, ears, hands, feet, perineum or Complicated by inhalation injury (suspected if any of the following exist: a history of burn sustained in a closed or confined space, facial burns, singed nasal hairs, cough or hoarseness, or sooty sputum) or The cause of injury was chemical or electrical or Complicated by fractures or other trauma or Possible suicide attempt, child abuse, or neglect or Patient in a high-risk category 1. Under 2 or over 60 years of age. 2. Associated with a preexisting systemic condition (e.g., cardiovascular, renal, or pulmonary disorders), alcoholism or drug abuse, autoimmune disorder, or immunosuppressive therapy.
Moderate uncomplicated burn injuries	Partial-thickness	15–25%	10–20%	And without the above-mentioned complications
	Full-thickness	Less than 10%	Less than 10%	
Minor burn injuries	Partial-thickness	Less than 15%	Less than 10%	Usually candidates for outpatient management
	Full-thickness	Less than 2%	Less than 2%	

improper management of a more complex burn injury may result in unnecessary hospitalization or a number of serious consequences, including joint dysfunction, hypertrophic scarring, and considerable loss of time from work or school. Therefore, the initial assessment of the severity of a burn injury (based on its depth, extent, cause, and location) and consideration of other factors, such as the patient's age and the presence of other injuries or illness (e.g., smoke inhalation, preexisting cardiovascular, pulmonary, or renal disease, psychiatric illness, drug abuse, or alcoholism) are important for determining whether outpatient treatment will be adequate for a particular patient.

Adult patients with superficial burns covering more than 15% of the total body surface (10% of the body surface in children) or deep burns covering more than 2% of the total body surface should be hospitalized. Also, as already mentioned, the age of the burn patient influences the healing potential. Children less than 2 years of age have thin skin and tend to have poorly developed immune systems, making conversion of superficial burns to full-thickness injuries and infection more likely. Also, children are apt to refuse food when they do not feel well. Elderly patients who have poor psychosocial support or a concomitant disease are also more likely to develop complications than patients of other ages. Therefore, very young and very old patients should be hospitalized unless it is certain that a burn injury is very minor and that a strong family support system is available to the patient. Any condition that predisposes a patient to infection (e.g., diabetes, immunosuppressive or corticosteroid therapy, immunodeficiency diseases) or a concomitant injury to the viscera or extremities should be an indication for inpatient care. So should a significant smoke inhalation injury (suggested by facial burns, debris in the throat, stridor, respiratory distress, or a history of a burn occurring in a closed space), a suspicion of patterns of drug or alcohol abuse, circumstances that may indicate child abuse or neglect, or burns of the face, hand, foot, or perineum (unless the burn is very superficial).

The initial treatment for ▶***minor burns*** (after applying the immediate cooling measures) is gentle cleansing with a saline solution or water and removal of all loose skin and debris. This is followed by the application of a nonadherent gauze dressing (impregnated with sterile petrolatum to facilitate future dressing changes) and several additional layers of gauze for protection and pain control, since exposure to air may be extremely painful for many burn injuries. Topical antibacterial ointments are not only not necessary for very small burns but may even interfere with the natural process of healing. However, they may be helpful for larger burns to prevent early streptococcal invasion. A 3- to 5-day course of systemic antibiotics after the injury may also be beneficial. Silver sulfadiazine, 1% cream (may be impregnated into the innermost gauze instead of petrolatum) or povidone-iodine are the preferred topical antibacterial agents for outpatient use, since they are painless, easy to use, and have a very low incidence of associated side effects. A prophylactic tetanus booster should be administered for even relatively minor burns. The dressings should be changed every day and checked every 2 or 3 days until healing has occurred. An appropriate topical lubricant (with a base of lanolin or cocoa butter) may be used as follow-up treatment once the burn is healed, and the area should be protected from exposure to sunlight by avoidance or by application of a sunscreen or sunblock. Some physicians advise using these precautions for at least a year after the injury and thereafter increasing exposure to sunlight only very gradually.

Exposure to low temperatures can cause a variety of ***cold injuries.*** The extent of the injury is influenced by such factors as temperature and wind velocity (wind chill factor), humidity, and the nature and duration of the exposure. High wind velocity and/or wetness may significantly increase the severity of a cold injury, since they accelerate the chilling of exposed skin. Other contributing factors include fatigue, nonacclimatization, smoking, the use of alcohol or sedative drugs, hunger, emotional stress, very young or old age, systemic illness, the presence of wounds or fractures, and anoxia.

Cold urticaria is a familial or acquired hypersensitivity to cold that may result in the development of pruritus and sometimes burning urticaria in body parts that have had even limited exposure to cold. In some extremely sensitive individuals, the response can be generalized. Immersion in cold water can cause a massive release of histamine and other mediators, which may result in severe systemic symptoms such as hypotension and shock. Drowning may result if the reaction occurs during a swim. The familial variety, which results in a burning sensation in the skin about 30 minutes after exposure to cold, may not be a true urticarial reaction. However, acquired cold urticaria may be due to an underlying disease that is associated with cryoglobulinemia, Raynaud's phenomenon and leg ulceration. Lymphoma, multiple myeloma, and collagen diseases are examples of diseases associated with these signs. Acquired cold urticaria may also be associated with cold hemoglobinuria from syphilis, but most often the cause is not known. The diagnosis of cold urticaria can usually be made by producing the reaction by the application of an ice cube to the skin or by immersing part of an extremity in cold water. Avoidance of the cold is obviously the treatment of choice for this disorder, but when this is not feasible (as in the winter months), pretreatment with cyproheptadine, 4–8 mg four times daily, will prevent the urticarial reaction for most patients. However, the side effects of this drug include an increase in appetite, weight gain, and sedation (these are more pronounced when this drug is combined with the antihistamine hydroxazine). A less effective treatment is the use of H-1 and H-2 antihistamines such as diphenhydramine or hydroxazine and cimetidine (Tagamet) or ranitidine (Zantac). Also, since there is evidence to suggest that this reaction may be IgE mediated, desensitization by slowly increased periods of exposure to the cold may be helpful.

►***Localized cold injuries*** may occur from prolonged exposure to low temperatures. When an extremity is exposed to low temperatures, there is an immediate localized vasoconstriction followed by a generalized vasoconstriction. The skin's response to cold exposure includes a progressive decrease in tissue metabolism with a simultaneous increased demand for oxygen to the tissue, resulting in localized cyanosis followed by redness that results from a decreased dissociation of oxyhemoglobin. When the skin temperature reaches about 15°C (59°F), tissue damage occurs, with ischemia and thromboses in small vessels or the actual formation of ice crystals in or between cells (frostbite). ***Frostnip,*** a milder superficial injury due to dampness and cold, results in firm, whitened, cold skin areas, usually on the face, ears, or extremities. There may be peeling or blistering (such as occurs in sunburns) in 24 to 72 hours and, occasionally, long-term mild sensitivity to the cold. Red or pale, itching, numb, and inflamed lesions caused by cold exposure are known as ***chilblains*** (pernio). Edema or blistering may be present, but there is no actual freezing of tissues. Chilblains are aggravated by warmth, and with continued exposure may progress to ulcerative or hemorrhagic lesions, scarring, fibrosis, and atrophy. ***Frostbite,*** a superficial tissue injury due to actual freezing of the tissues, may vary from a very mild form with numbness or mild prickling sensations and itching to paresthesia and joint stiffness. The frostbitten area is cold, hard, glossy, white or grayish-yellow, and anesthetic, and with rewarming becomes blotchy red and edematous and exhibits tenderness or a burning pain. Blisters, necrosis, and gangrene may develop.

The initial treatment of all cold tissue injuries is rapid rewarming, preferably by immersion in water just warmer than body temperature (38–42°C but no warmer than 43°C) unless there is any possibility of refreezing (i.e., if the person must walk for a considerable distance to receive care). In this case, the frostbitten part should not be thawed until the patient is able to be protected from the cold, since refreezing results in increased tissue necrosis. All patients with frostbite should be hospitalized.

Hypothermia, severe exposure to cold, is a medical emergency. It may result from exposure to prolonged or extremely cold temperatures (atmospheric or water immersion). It may affect healthy individuals through recreational or occupational exposure, or it may occur in accident victims. Any of the above-mentioned factors predisposing to cold injury may contribute to the development of hypothermia (e.g., the use of alcohol or sedative drugs, fatigue, hunger, stress). Acute alcoholism, illness, cardiovascular or cerebrovascular disease, myxedema, hypopituitarism, and mental retardation are among the conditions that may make an individual more vulnerable to systemic hypothermia at relatively normal temperatures. A wide range of early signs and symptoms may signal the development of hypothermia, including irritability, confusion, weakness, drowsiness, and impaired coordination. A slightly lowered body core temperature (rectal temperature of 33–35°C) may be the only sign of mild hypothermia (oral temperatures should not be relied on), but a slowed pulse and delirium may also occur, and shivering is common. Moderate (core temperature of 30–33°C) to severe (core temperature below 30°C and even as low as 25°C) hypothermia may involve more serious signs, including a pale, grayish skin color, absent peripheral pulses, extremely shallow respirations, extremely slow or absent pupillary reflexes, and coma. The patient's skin is cold to the touch, joints may resist bending, and the thermoregulatory shivering mechanism is absent. Metabolic acidosis, hypo- or hyperglycemia, pneumonia, ventricular fibrillation, renal failure, and respiratory arrest may occur. As in localized cold injuries, rewarming is the initial concern in the treatment of hypothermia.

Patients with mild hypothermia and some degree of consciousness in the absence of other injuries or illness should be removed from the cold environment, undressed if their clothing is wet, and placed in a sleeping bag or warm bed with blankets (passive rewarming). Active rewarming (application of an external heat source) may be used as an alternative to restore normal body temperature more quickly. It may be provided in the form of a warm bath, warm packs, or an electric blanket kept near normal body temperature. Rapid, active rewarming and appropriate supportive treatment measures are necessary for moderate to severe hypothermia. A core body temperature below 32.2°C (90°F) is a true medical emergency. In a remote area where no other suitable heat sources are available, the patient may be put into a sleeping bag, unclothed, with one or two other persons to provide body warmth through skin-to-skin contact as an emergency measure. There is considerable controversy about the optimal methods, temperature, and rate to be used in rapid, aggressive rewarming of hypothermic patients in the hospital. It should be attempted only by persons who are experienced in these methods and prepared to deal with any consequences that may result from this hazardous treatment. Respiratory support and cardiopulmonary resuscitation may be necessary.

The abundant supply of lymphatics in the skin takes the form of a deep horizontal plexus of larger vessels in the reticular layer of the dermis and a more superficial fine capillary plexus in the papillary layer. These two plexuses communicate with each other and drain alongside the blood vessels into the subcutaneous tissue. The superficial plexus in the papillary layer sends branches up into the papillae, where they end blindly, or into pariendothelial lymph spaces around the capillary loops. Hair follicles and sebaceous and sweat glands possess their own lymphatics, which also drain into the subcutaneous plexus of larger lymph vessels.

The skin may be affected by a number of disorders, all of which may result in changes in the skin, only one of which is the appearance of lesions. Since the character of an eruption often provides information about the underlying cause, it is imperative that the practitioner use an organized approach in examining the skin in order to proceed toward a diagnosis. Examination of the entire body, and not just the portion of the skin that the patient presents, should be done in good light, preferably daylight. Note both the distribution (location and pattern) of the eruption and the arrangement of the lesions (e.g., linear, concentric). Although skin diseases do sometimes depart from the norm, they tend to follow a customary pattern of distribution and arrangement of lesions, both of which can provide important information in helping to establish a diagnosis.

Next, the practitioner should try to locate the primary lesion, which is the earliest form in which the disorder appears. Note the color of the lesion, whether it is flat or raised, or filled with fluid (serum, pus). Table 10.3 gives a list of skin lesions and arrangements and their descriptions. Note also whether individual lesions are discrete or blend into one another, whether they are localized or spread over extensive areas of skin, and whether there is evidence of excoriation or crusting.

The sequence given in Table 10.4 organizes a number of common skin disorders according to the appearance of the primary lesion. If the lesions are fluid filled, the vesicular, bullous, or pustular diseases should be considered. If these are not present, the color of the lesions should be checked. If they are red, the underlying cause may be a vascular reaction, one of the disorders characterized by inflammatory lesions, or one of the papulosquamous diseases. The presence of flesh-colored, white, brownish, or yellow lesions signifies certain disorders, many of which are also listed in Table 10.4. The examiner should keep in mind that the appearance of an eruption may be modified by a secondary infection, by excoriation, or by a sensitivity reaction to a primary disorder (such as a fungal infection).

After the physical exam, a history should be obtained from the patient, focusing particularly on aspects that are relevant in terms of what was observed in the physical exam and the subjective complaints of the patient. For instance, if the eruption only involves areas of the body normally not covered by clothing, one should ask what type of work, sports, or other activities the patient participates in, because these may help to determine what substances he is usually or has recently been exposed to. If the lesions involve the genitals, it is necessary to find out whether a sexual partner or family members have a similar problem.

Finally, unless the clinical picture is straightforward, laboratory tests may be employed to make a diagnosis. Referral to a specialist may be necessary for such procedures as biopsy, cultures, scrapings, patch tests, immunofluorescence tests, and examination by Wood's light (black light), unless the primary care provider has received training in them. A number of common diagnostic procedures are described in Table 10.5. Referral is also warranted whenever generalized peeling of the skin is the first manifestation of a disorder, since this occurrence may signify a potentially

TABLE 10.3 DEFINITIONS OF SKIN LESIONS AND OTHER TERMS

Term	Definition
	Lesions
Macule	Circumscribed region of skin color change (e.g., brown, red, tan, white, blue) that is neither raised nor depressed and is less than 1 cm in diameter
Patch	Similar to a macule but larger than 1 cm in diameter
Papule	Raised, circumscribed, solid lesion 1 cm or less in diameter; may or may not be flesh colored, with a rounded, flat, angular, smooth, or verrucous (warty) surface
Nodule	Palpable, circumscribed, solid lesion similar to a papule but with deeper penetration into the dermis; usually 0.5–1 cm or more in diameter (nodules larger than 2 cm are called "tumors") and may or may not be raised
Urticarial lesions	Wheals or hives; raised, rounded or flat-topped, edematous, erythematous, evanescent lesions; a common allergic skin reaction
Vesicle	Raised, fluid-filled lesion (blister) less than 0.5 cm in diameter
Bulla	Fluid-filled blister larger than 0.5 cm in diameter; may be tense or flaccid
Pustule	Superficial, raised lesion filled with neutrophils (pus)
	Arrangement of Lesions
Linear	Lesions arranged along a line
Serpiginous	Wavy arrangement of lesions resembling a snake
Annular	Ring-shaped arrangement of lesions; also used to describe primary lesions that tend to have or develop a central clearing ("iris" or "target" lesions), such as those seen in granuloma annulare, erythema multiforme, dermatophyte (ringworm) infections, and secondary syphilis
Zosteriform	Lesions that occur within a dermatome, as in herpes zoster
Koebner phenomenon	"Isomorphic response"; the lesion mimics the shape of a skin trauma (e.g., along the line of a scratch in *Toxicodendron* dermatitis)
	Other Terms
Umbilicated	Lesion has a central depression
Plaque	Relatively large, circumscribed area of raised, abnormal skin (group of confluent lesions)
Erosion	Relatively superficial area of skin surface denudation (all or part of the epidermis is lost)
Ulceration	Denuded area of skin surface in which the defect penetrates the level of the dermis
Scales	Fragments of the stratum corneum; may be scant and adherent (e.g., in lichen planus), profuse, flaking, and silver to white (e.g., psoriasis), or greasy and yellowish (e.g., in seborrheic dermatitis)
Crust (scab)	Coagulated blood elements (blood, serum, pus); appearance may be altered by local medications
Excoriations	Marks where the skin has been scratched, rubbed, or picked by the patient, usually indicating pruritus as a subjective symptom
Lichenification	Thickening of skin and accentuation of normal epidermal markings; seen commonly in atopic dermatitis
Telangiectasia	Superficial dilated blood vessels; may be wispy (e.g., as a consequence of solar damage) or coarse
Morbilliform	Describes an eruption that resembles the rash of measles (rubeola)
Nikolsky's sign	Epidermis is easily detached from the underlying skin by slight friction (e.g., rubbing with a finger)
Atrophy	Thinning and wrinkling of the skin (resembling cigarette paper); seen in discoid lupus erythematosus and as a consequence of long-term topical fluorinated corticosteroid use
Scar	Results from healing when there has been some destruction of the dermis; may be pink and vascular at first, and then white, depressed, and avascular (atrophic)

TABLE 10.4 A SEQUENCE FOR IDENTIFICATION OF SKIN DISEASES BY THE APPEARANCE OF LESIONS

Blistering Conditions

Blisters Filled with Clear Fluid	**Blisters Filled with Pus**
Vesicular diseases Dermatitis herpetiformis Dyshidrosis Herpes simplex Herpes zoster (shingles) Scabies Varicella (chicken pox) Vesicular tinea pedis Bullous diseases Bullous impetigo Bullous lupus erythematosus Bullous urticaria pigmentosa Cold or thermal injury Dermatitis herpetiformis Epidermolysis bullosa Erythema multiforme bullosum Herpes gestationis Lichen planus Pemphigold (bullous and cicatricial) Pemphigus Pompholyx Porphyria cutanea tarda Stevens–Johnson syndrome Toxicodendron dermatitis	Pustular diseases Acne Bacterial folliculitis Candidiasis or intertriginous skin Fungal folliculitis Rosacea Pseudopustules Keratosis pilaris Milia

Nonblistering Conditions with Red Lesions

Scaling Red Lesions with No Epithelial Disruption (Papulosquamous Diseases)	**Scaling Red Lesions with Epithelial Disruption (Eczematous Diseases)**	**Nonscaling Dome-Shaped Lesions (Inflammatory Papules and Nodules)**	**Nonscaling Flat-Topped Lesions (Vascular Reactions)**
With prominent plaque formation Lupus erythematosus Mycosis fungoides Parapsoriasis Psoriasis Tinea corporis Predominantly papular Guttate psoriasis Lichen planus Pityriasis rosea Rubella Rubeola Secondary syphilis	With prominent excoriation Atopic dermatitis Candidiasis Dyshidrotic eczema Fungal eczema Scabetic eczema Stasis dermatitis Without prominent excoriation Contact dermatitis Perioral dermatitis Seborrheic dermatitis Xerotic eczema	Inflammatory papules Cherry angiomas Granuloma annulare Insect bites Pityriasis rosea Pyogenic granulomas Secondary syphilis Inflammatory nodules Cellulitis Cystic acne Erythema nodosum Furuncles Hidradenitis suppurativa Inflamed epidermoid cysts	Nonpurpuric (blanchable) lesions Cellulitis Erythema multiforme Erythema nodosum Fixed-drug eruption Gyrate erythemas Macular and diffuse erythemas Urticaria Purpuric lesions Palpable purpura (vasculitis) Petechial and ecchymotic diseases

TABLE 10.4 (*Continued*)

Nonblistering Conditions with Nonred Lesions			
Flesh-Colored Lesions	**White Lesions**	**Yellow Lesions**	**Brown Lesions**
Keratotic (rough-surfaced) Actinic keratoses Callouses Corns Paronychial warts Plantar warts Verruca vulgaris warts Nonkeratotic (smooth-surfaced) Basal cell carcinomas Condyloma acuminata Epidermoid (sebaceous) cysts Flat warts Lipomas Molluscum contagiosum Nonpigmented dermal nevi Skin tags Squamous cell carcinomas	White patches, plaques Pityriasis alba Pityriasis versicolor (tinea versicolor) Postinflammatory hypopigmentation Morphea Vitiligo White papules Kertosis pilaris Milia Molluscum contagiosum	Smooth-surfaced Necrobiosis lipoidica diabeticorum Xanthelasma Xanthomas Yellow-crusted lesions Actinic keratosis Impetigo Seborrheic dermatitis	Brown macules Freckles Junctional nevi Lentigines Brown papules, nodules Compound nevi Dermatofibromas Intradermal nevi Melanomas Seborrheic keratosis Skin tags Brown patches, plaques Cafe-au-lait patches Chloasma Giant hairy pigmented nevus Pityriasis versicolor (tinea versicolor) Postinflammatory hyperpigmentation

Source: Adapted from tables and figure in "A Problem-Oriented Approach to Clinical Dermatology," by W. Mitchell Sams, Jr., *Continuing Education,* August 1982, pp. 73–78.

fatal response to a staphylococcal infection that requires immediate hospitalization (e.g., scalded skin syndrome) or toxic epidermal necrolysis (TEN), which is usually caused by a drug reaction and is also potentially life-threatening. Toxic shock syndrome (TSS) is another extremely serious disorder associated with cutaneous or subcutaneous staphylococcal infections; its symptoms may include a bright red tongue ("strawberry tongue") and desquamation of the skin on the hands. Any skin disorder that does not improve within a week should be referred to a specialist. In addition, any suspicious tumor, particularly pigmented tumors that have undergone a change in color, size, or shape, or that have an irregular border or show signs of inflammation, should be referred for evaluation and possible biopsy or excision.

The occurrence of a skin eruption in areas normally uncovered by clothing or otherwise exposed to particular substances is suggestive of an environmental cause. ***Contact dermatitis*** is an acute or chronic dermatitis that may affect a localized area such as that portion of the wrist or finger in contact with a piece of jewelry, or it may involve whole patches of skin that have come into direct contact with irritants or allergens or indirect contact by fomites (e.g., contaminated hands, tools, athletic equipment, clothing, pets). Most of such reactions fall under the category of ***irritant contact dermatitis,*** which is due to excessive contact or additive effects of an irritant such as a soap, detergent, or organic solvent that interferes with the integrity of the skin surface and makes it less resistant to the drying effects of the environment and penetration by foreign substances. Others are actual sensitivity reactions to

TABLE 10.5 COMMON DIAGNOSTIC PROCEDURES FOR SKIN DISORDERS

Procedure	Purpose
Biopsy	Essential for the diagnosis of any lesion suggestive of malignancy or for any obscure skin disorder, particularly if chronic. May be a shave or punch biopsy, curettage, or (for large tumors) removal of a portion (e.g., wedge) of the lesion. An excisional biopsy is sometimes preferred for small lesions when malignancy is suspected, with obvious financial and time savings, but for large lesions or those in obvious locations, a definitive diagnosis is generally obtained before deciding upon excision.
Examination of scrapings of lesions	For suspected superficial fungal infections; scrapings are fixed with 15% potassium hydroxide (KOH) solution and examined microscopically.
Culture of fluid from lesion	For suspected viral infection, fluid is taken from an early lesion (e.g., vesicle, bulla, or pustule).
Culture of swab sample from lesion	For diagnosis of bacterial infections, culture and tests for antibacterial sensitivity are advised for any acute bacterial infection, but treatment should be initiated immediately without waiting for test results.
Examination by Wood's light (black light)	Skin is examined in a dark room under long-wave UV light filtered through "Wood's glass," providing important diagnostic clues: 1. The skin in tinea versicolor fluoresces golden. 2. The scalp hairs in tinea capitis fluoresce light bright green (if due to *Microsporum canis* or *M. audouini*). 3. Pseudomonas infection causes involved tissues to fluoresce green. 4. Depigmented lesions of vitiligo fluoresce ivory-white (helping to differentiate these from areas of hypopigmentation due to other causes). 5. Large amounts of uroporphyrin in urine specimens (in porphyria cutanea tarda) fluoresce red.
Diascopy	Observation of a reddened macule under firm pressure of a clear glass or plastic slide will help to differentiate erythema due to dilated capillaries from purpura due to extravascular blood (erythema will blanch with pressure, whereas purpura will not), as well as a raised hemangioma (which exhibits a delayed blanching reaction) from a melanoma, which will not blanch.
Tzanck test (Tzanck smear)	For cytologic exam when the primary lesion is a vesicle or bulla, smears of scrapings taken from the base of lesions are stained with Wright's or Giemsa stain and then examined microscopically. 1. Multinucleated epidermal giant cells may be seen in certain viral infections (herpes simplex, herpes zoster, and varicella). 2. Acantholytic cells are seen in pemphigus.
Immunofluorescence (IF) tests	Direct IF microscopy of skin biopsy sections reveals characteristic findings in bullous disorders (pemphigus, bullous and cicatricial pemphigoid, dermatitis herpetiformis, herpes gestationis, porphyria cutanea tarda), SLE, and discoid lupus erythematosus. Indirect IF microscopy of patients' serum reveals the presence of specific antibodies to certain regions of the epidermis in bullous disorders (pemphigus, bullous pemphigoid) and other circulating antibodies in scleroderma, SLE, and occasionally dermatitis herpetiformis.
Electron microscopy	Examination of a glass slide smear of fluid from vesicles may be used to identify a causative virus.
Patch tests	May be useful in diagnosing allergic contact dermatitis, but should be performed by persons trained and experienced in performing the procedure and interpreting the results, since application and occlusion of irritating substances may result in severe bullous reactions (which are actually chemical burns) and scarring, and false-positive reactions are common (from simple irritation caused by occluding a mildly or highly irritating substance).
Photopatch test	When a photosensitivity contact reaction is suspected, the patch test site should be exposed to sunlight after 24 hours.

skin contact with an allergen ***(allergic contact dermatitis).*** Plant dermatitides, such as those occurring with poison ivy, oak, or sumac, are common examples of allergic contact reactions. Other common substances causing allergic contact dermatitis include dermatologic agents such as topical anesthetics (e.g., benzocaine), some minerals (nickel is a common example), ethylenediamine, turpentine, and formalin (see Table 10.6).

Often the location of the eruption is sufficient for identification of a possible irritant or allergen, but a patch test with a suspected agent may elicit a reaction (if the response is an allergic one) and confirm the suspicion (see Table 10.5). There are limitations to this diagnostic procedure, however; if the reaction is positive, it may still not confirm an allergic response, and a control test on another individual may be necessary to rule out primary irritation. If a photosensitivity contact reaction is suspected, exposure of the patch test site to sunlight after 24 hours (photopatch test) is called for.

The eruption of a contact dermatitis usually takes the form of localized swelling and erythema initially, followed by the appearance of lesions (macules, papules, vesicles, bullae), which may eventually weep and crust and are vulnerable to secondary infection. The lesions are usually accompanied by pruritus, burning, and stinging pain. The arrangement of the lesions may also be diagnostic. For example, transfer of the cross-reacting oleoresin, urishiol, from members of the *Toxicodendron* genus (poison ivy, oak, and sumac) usually occurs as the plant brushes the skin, and results in a contact dermatitis ▶ ***(Toxicodendron*** or ***plant dermatitis)*** characterized by a typical linear streaked arrangement of vesicles on the extremities. Indirect contact via contaminated fomites may result in a nonlinear arrangement, however, and systemic absorption of the antigen may produce an eruption pattern quite different from the usual contact dermatitis, with an eruption that is morbilliform, scarlatiniform, or urticarial. Usually an asymmetric distribution helps to rule out systemic causes, but differentiation from other skin disorders may be difficult if the area of involvement is consistent with patterns seen in those disorders, such as atopic dermatitis and other eczemas, dermatophytid, and scabies.

Treatment of acute severe contact dermatitis (involving more than one-third of the patient's body, especially if the hands, face, or genitalia are involved) should include oral administraton of prednisone. For most cases, one should begin with an initial daily dose of 40–50 mg for the first 4 days; this dose should then be decreased by 10 mg every 4 days until the total daily dosage is 20 mg, at which time it is changed to 20 mg every other day for a week and then discontinued. Other systemic corticosteroids are listed in Table 10.7. Systemic therapy may be supplemented by local treatments aimed at providing symptomatic relief (Table 10.8). For moderate (affecting 10–30% of the body and excluding the hands, face, and genitalia) and mild contact dermatitis, treatment should be restricted to local measures, which include wet dressings for localized areas of involvement, soaks for lesions on the extremities, and lukewarm baths (15 minutes two or three times daily) for generalized involvement. If the eruption results in drying of the skin, application of petrolatum following the soaks or bath will assist in hydrating the keratin, or a small amount of oil may be added to the bath water. If the lesions are wet, however, drying agents such as starch or calamine lotions and powders may be beneficial. These are also indicated for involvement of intertriginous areas. Topical corticosteroids in ointment or cream form may help to suppress acute lesions and relieve pruritus. Table 10.9 lists some

TABLE 10.6 COMMON CAUSES OF CONTACT DERMATITIS

Cause	Where Found
	Irritant Type
Hexachlorophene	Topical antiseptic.
Formalin/formaldehyde	Wash-and-wear clothing, antiseptics, disinfectants, fixing agents for histologic specimens, ingredients in fingernail polishes.
Phenol	
Alkalis and acids	
Acetone	
Plants	Cactus spines, stinging nettles, buttercups, Compositae family members (chrysanthemum, brown-eyed Susan, feverfew, gaillardia, Shasta daisy).
	Allergic Type
Hexachlorophene	Topical antiseptic.
Antibiotics	Topical medications: penicillin, sulfonamides, neomycin are common causes.
Antihistamines	Contact may occur in medical personnel who handle chlorpromazine and other phenothiazines such as prochlorperazine, promazine HCl, promethazine HCl, and diphenhydramine.
Topical and locally injected anesthetics	Ingredients in some topical medications; medical personnel may come into contact through handling and injecting anesthetics. Benzocaine, procaine, butethamine, tetracaine, cyclomethycaine sulfate, dibucaine, and butacaine are common examples; there may also be an associated hypersensitivity to paraphenylenediamine (used in hair dyes), sulfonamides, hydrochlorothiazide, and sunscreens containing *p*-aminobenzoic acid (PABA) esters.
Benzalkonium chloride (BAK)	Preoperative skin disinfectant, surgical instrument disinfectant, ingredient in many cosmetics, deodorants, and mouthwashes.
Thimerosal (Merthiolate)	Topical antiseptic.
Ethylenediamine HCl and derivatives	Stabilizer in medications; cross-reactions with aminophylline and antihistamines derived from ethylenediamine may occur.
Topical vitamin E	Soaps.
Mercaptobenzothiazole and tetramethylthiuram disulfide	Ingredients in rubber products (e.g., surgical gloves, shoes, undergarments).
Nickel sulfate	In some metal jewelry.
Potassium dichromate	Trace ingredient in cement; leather-tanning agent.
Paraben	Ingredient (preservative) in some topical medications.
Paraphenylenediamine	Found in hair and fur dyes, industrial chemicals.
Oil of turpentine	Found in cleaning agents, paint thinners, polishes, waxes.
Wood wax alcohol	Ingredient in lanolin.
Ammoniated mercury	Ingredient in topical medications.
Ethyl alcohol	Hypersensitivity may extend to butyl, isopropyl, amyl, and methyl alcohol.
Plant oils	Toxicodendron (poison ivy, oak, and sumac) urishiol, primrose, ragweed.

TABLE 10.7 ANTI-INFLAMMATORY ACTIVITY OF CERTAIN SYSTEMIC CORTICOSTEROIDS

Corticosteroid	Anti-inflammatory Activity (Relative to Hydrocortisone)
Cortisone acetate	0.8
Hydrocortisone	1
Prednisone	3–5
Prednisolone	3–5
Triamcinolone	3–5
Methylprednisolone	4–6
Fluprednisolone	8–10
Fludrocortisone	10
Dexamethasone	20–30
Betamethasone	20–30
Triamcinolone acetonide (parenteral)	4–5

TABLE 10.8 SOME LOCAL AND SYSTEMIC TREATMENTS FOR SKIN DISORDERS

Compresses and Soaks

Aluminum chloride hexahydrate (AluWets Wet Dressing Crystals)

Aluminum subacetate (Burow's solution)

Aluminum sulfate and calcium acetate (modified Burow's solution)

Boric acid solution

Cold skim milk

Milk of bismuth

Saline

Sodium bicarbonate

Water

Bath Preparations

Bath oils (Alpha-Keri, Lubath, Domol), 5–25 mg/tubful (50 gal) warm water

Colloidal oatmeal (Aveeno Colloidal Oatmeal, Aveeno Oilated Bath)

Oatmeal and baking soda (sodium bicarbonate)

Starch bath (Linit starch)

Starch and baking soda

Tar bath (coal tar solution USP), 50–100 mL/tubful (50 gal) warm water

Antipruritic Agents

Oral antihistamines and "antiserotonin" drugs
- H-1 receptor blockers (hydroxyzine, tripelennamine, diphenhydramine)
- H-2 receptor blockers (cimetidine, ranitidine) may be used with H-1 antihistamines for unresponsive cases
- Beta agonists (albuterol)
- Cyproheptadine (Periactin) for urticaria

TABLE 10.8 *(Continued)*

Corticosteroids

Systemic corticosteroids

Topical corticosteroids (lotion, cream, ointment)

Corticosteroid suspension for intralesional injections

Oral Antifungals

Griseofulvin (Fulvicin P/G, Fulvicin-U/F, Grifulvin V, Grisactin, Grisactin Ultra, Gris-PEG tablets) for tinea

Ketoconazole (Nizoral) for candidiasis, tinea, and tinea versicolor

Nystatin (Mycostatin, Nilstat, Tetrastatin) for candidiasis

Topical Antifungals

Specific
- Ciclopirox
- Clotrimazole (Lotrimin or Mycelex) cream or lotion
- Haloprogin (Halotex) cream or solution
- Miconazole (Monistat-Derm, MicaTin) cream
- Nystatin (Mycolog, Mycostatin, Nilstat) cream, powder, or ointment for candidiasis
- Sulconazole cream
- Tolnaftate (Tinactin) cream or solution

Nonspecific
- Carbol-fuchsin solution (Castellani's paint)
- Coal tar in lotion or paste
- Compound undecylenic acid ointment
- Gentian violet for candidiasis
- Iodine solution (dilute)
- Potassium permanganate or aluminum acetate for wet compresses
- Selenium sulfide (adjunct to oral griseofulvin)
- Sodium thiosulfate (Tinver lotion)
- Sulfur-salicylic acid ointment or cream
- Whitfield's ointment, alcoholic Whitfield's solution

Nonsteroidal Anti-inflammatory Drugs

Diflunisal (Dolobid)

Fenoprofen (Nalfon)

Ibuprofen (Motrin, Rufen, Advil, Nuprin)

Meclofenamate sodium (Meclomen)

Naproxen (Naprosyn)

Naproxyn sodium (Anaprox)

Piroxicam (Feldene)

Sulindac (Clinoril)

Tolmetin sodium (Tolectin)

Miscellaneous

Acyclovir for herpesvirus and herpes zoster infections

Anthralin (topical) for psoriasis

Antibiotics, systemic and topical, for prevention and treatment of bacterial infections

Antiparasitics (for lice, mites)

Oral retinoids (lichen planus, acne, pseudofolliculitis barbae)

Papain (Adolph's Meat Tenderizer) for insect stings

PUVA therapy (psoralens plus UV radiation) for psoriasis and repigmentation in vitiligo

Sedatives for stress-related disorders (e.g., lichen planus, psoriasis)

Topical tar preparations for eczema, psoriasis, seborrheic dermatitis

TABLE 10.9 POTENCIES OF SOME COMMONLY USED TOPICAL CORTICOSTEROIDS

Brand Name	Generic Name
High Potency	
Aristocort cream 0.5%	Triamcinolone acetonide
Benisone gel 0.025%	Betamethasone benzoate
Diprosone cream 0.05%	Betamethasone dipropionate
Diprosone ointment 0.05%	Betamethasone dipropionate
Florone ointment 0.05%	Diflorasone diacetate
Halciderm cream 0.1%	Halcinonide
Halog cream 0.1%	Halcinonide
Lidex cream 0.05%	Fluocinonide
Lidex ointment 0.05%	Fluocinonide
Maxiflor cream 0.05%	Diflorasone diacetate
Maxiflor ointment 0.05%	Diflorasone diacetate
Topicort cream 0.25%	Desoximetasone
Topsyn gel 0.05%	Fluocinonide
Valisone ointment 0.1%	Betamethasone valerate
Medium Potency	
Aristocort ointment 0.1%	Triamcinolone acetonide
Cordran cream 0.05%	Flurandrenolide
Cordran ointment 0.05%	Flurandrenolide
Fluonid cream 0.01%	Fluocinolone acetonide
Kenalog cream 0.1%	Triamcinolone acetonide
Kenalog lotion 0.025%	Triamcinolone acetonide
Kenalog ointment 0.1%	Triamcinolone acetonide
Synalar cream 0.025%	Fluocinolone acetonide
Synalar ointment 0.025%	Fluocinolone acetonide
Synalar-HP cream 0.2%	Fluocinolone acetonide
Synemol cream 0.025%	Fluocinolone acetonide
Valisone cream 0.1%	Betamethasone valerate
Valisone lotion 0.1%	Betamethasone valerate
Westcort cream 0.2%	Hydrocortisone valerate
Low Potency	
Alphaderm cream 1%	Hydrocortisone (urea 10%)
Cort-Dome cream 1% or 0.5%	Hydrocortisone
Hytone cream 2.5% or 1%	Hydrocortisone
Hyetone lotion 2.5% or 1%	Hydrocortisone
Hytone ointment 2.5% or 1%	Hydrocortisone
Locorten cream 0.03%	Flumethasone pivalate
Meti-Derm cream 0.5%	Prednisone
Synacort cream 2.5% or 1%	Hydrocortisone
Tridesilon cream 0.05%	Desonide
Lowest Potency	
Hexadrol cream 0.1% or 0.04%	Dexamethasone
Medrol Acetate ointment 0.25% or 0.1%	Methylprednisolone acetate

available topical corticosteroid products. Oral antihistamines may also be given for pruritus.

Seborrheic dermatitis is an acute or chronic eczematous disease that is genetically based, although a variety of factors such as nutrition, emotional stress, hormones, and infection contribute to outbreaks. This condition, which most commonly affects the scalp, is characterized by redness and microscopic exudative vesicles in severe cases and, in milder forms, by dry, yellowish scales on the skin that may be reddened. "Dandruff," which is heavier than normal physiologic scaling of the scalp, is one example, although seborrheic dermatitis may occur in areas of the neck, eyebrows, ear canals, and posterior pinna, face (particularly the "butterfly area" over the nose and cheeks), intertriginous areas (axillae, umbilicus, groin, gluteal cleft), and central anterior and posterior chest. The skin may also be fissured, and pruritus is often but not always present. The moisture and warmth of intertriginous areas tend to foster the development of a secondary infection as a complication. *Candida albicans* is the most common organism in these sites, and *Staphylococcus aureus* or gram-negative bacteria are often responsible for infections superimposed on the dermatitis in other areas. Therefore, tests for these organisms should be performed in order to rule out their occurrence as a differential diagnosis or as a secondary involvement. A scraping of lesions on the chest (which includes the roof of vesicles) should be prepared with 15% potassium hydroxide and examined microscopically to rule out fungal infections such as tinea corporis and tinea versicolor. For scalp involvement, selenium sulfide (Selsun) suspension or Exsel may be applied once a week after shampooing the hair. Sebulex or Fostex cream may be used once a week as a shampoo for patients with oily hair. The patient should be instructed to shampoo the hair vigorously twice with the product, leaving the shampoo on the hair for 5–10 minutes the second time before rinsing. Other shampoos for seborrheic dermatitis of the scalp include Sebutone (with tar) and those that contain zinc pyrithione (Zincon, Head & Shoulders). A medium-potency corticosteroid lotion (e.g., 0.1% betamethasone valerate) may also be applied after shampooing the hair. For nonhairy affected areas, an ointment containing 3–5% sulfur or one that combines sulfur and 1% salicylic acid (to aid in removal of scales) is helpful. Topical corticosteroid preparations may also be used, and a combination of 0.5% hydrocortisone with 10% sodium sulfacetamide in an emulsion base is particularly helpful. Patients should be warned that steroid rosacea may result from regular use of high-potency fluorinated corticosteroids on the face. Aluminum subacetate (Burow's solution) may be used as soothing astringent wet dressings for affected intertriginous areas, followed by the application of an emulsion base containing 3% iodochlorhydroxyquin and 1% hydrocortisone. Since seborrheic dermatitis tends to recur throughout life, with each outbreak lasting for weeks to years, patients should be instructed that good nutrition, regular work and sleep habits, and measures to manage emotional stress are important as preventive factors. Systemic infections should also be treated quickly whenever they occur, since they also tend to initiate outbreaks.

▶ ***Atopic dermatitis*** (eczema, neurodermatitis) is a common inherited condition that is associated with respiratory allergy (asthma, allergic rhinitis) and a family history of the condition. Skin involvement generally begins at an early age, as early as the first few months of life, with erythema, weeping lesions (papules, vesicles, pustules), and eventually dry, lichenified scales on the face, scalp, neck, and upper trunk, and, less often, on the extremities. With age, the distribution becomes more widespread, but in older children and adults eruptions tend to be more localized, most often to the extremities (antecubital and popliteal fossae and wrists) and on the eyelids and neck. In all cases, marked pruritus may be present. A secondary bacterial infection and lymphadenitis or cellulitis or very extensive eruptions are potential complicating factors. Since the tendency is for lifelong recurrence of this disease, topical corticosteroids and other medications are greatly preferred to systemic steroid therapy, except in cases where the severity of the attacks interferes with the patient's normal functioning or patient compliance is very poor because of dissatisfaction with the use of topical therapies. In prescribing systemic corticosteroids, keep in mind the recurrent nature of this condition and the fact that the patient may rely on their use for flareups, which occur throughout life.

Another common form of intrinsic or idiopathic dermatitis is ***nummular dermatitis*** (nummular eczema), which has discrete coin-shaped, inflamed, and pruritic lesions with irregular surfaces. The widespread lesions begin as patches of confluent vesicles and papules, which later become exudative and form crusts and scales. They appear most commonly on extensor surfaces and buttocks but may also affect the trunk. These lesions frequently become secondarily infected by bacteria and produce significant amounts of dark yellowish crusting. The treatment is the same as for atopic dermatitis, and oral antibiotics should be administered as well for secondary bacterial infection (cloxacillin or erythromycin 250 mg, four times a day for extremely infected lesions, or tetracycline 250 mg, four times a day for less infected lesions). Topical corticosteroids should be applied three times daily after the lesions have dried. As with atopic dermatitis, long-term corticosteroid treatment should be avoided, but in severe cases a short-term course (e.g., 40 mg prednisone given in one dose every other day) may lessen the severity of the symptoms. Patients should be instructed that temperature or humidity changes, emotional stress, and infections may trigger recurrences, and should be avoided or dealt with promptly.

Dyshidrosis (pompholyx) is a chronic dermatitis with deep pruritic vesicles on the palms of the hands, between the fingers, and on the soles of the feet, which are often followed by erythematous swelling and oozing. Very often the primary cause is an allergen or fungus, so patch tests and microscopic exam of scrapings (including the roofs of vesicles for a fungus) will help to locate these causes. Fungal infections on the feet are quite common and may produce a strong immunologic reaction to the fungus resulting in a dermatitis elsewhere on the body ***(dermatophytids*** or "id" eruptions). Whenever a fungal, irritant, or allergic cause is involved in a dermatitis of the hands or feet, treatment should be aimed at its removal: avoidance of irritants and allergens, and, in the case of fungal infections, griseofulvin (micronized form), 250 mg orally two to four times a day until the infection is cleared, which may take months. Topical corticosteroid lotions, ointments, and creams may provide symptomatic relief but are not helpful if the dermatitis is superimposed on an underlying fungal infection (in the same location). Id eruption sites, however, may benefit from topical corticosteroid preparations.

A ***generalized exfoliative dermatitis*** (erythroderma) with widespread erythema and scaling (involving 70% of the body surface) is secondary to a number of conditions, including any dermatitis that has become generalized, a hereditary or acquired disease, a manifestation of a systemic disease (including lymphoma, mycosis fungoides, leukemia, carcinoma, and others), or a drug reaction. Cutaneous diseases that may become generalized to take this form include seborrheic, atopic, contact, and stasis dermatitis, psoriasis, dermatophytosis, pityriasis rubra pilaris, pemphigus foliaceus, and ichthyoses. Drugs that have provoked this response include penicillin, sulfonamides, isoniazid, phenylbutazone, phenytoin, *p*-aminosalicylic acid, gold, carbamazepine, barbiturates, and a number of irritating topical agents. The incidence in men is about two to three times greater than that in women, and although it can occur at any age, about 75% of the cases of erythroderma occur in persons over 45 years of age. Exfoliative dermatitis may have an insidious or rapid onset, with widespread erythema and slight to generalized scaling. The skin is initially thin and dry, but as the condition progresses, it thickens. The rate of cell turnover in the epidermis increases and the time of transit toward the surface decreases, resulting in an increased loss of protein, a major cellular constituent, and possibly a negative nitrogen balance in the body. The patient's temperature may be elevated (most patients have at least a temperature of 38°C at some point), but patients may report feeling chilled, since there is an increase in blood flow in the skin and excessive sweating, and occasionally tachycardia and edema may result. Prompt hospitalization is often necessary, since the disease is potentially life-threatening, and determination of the cause should be the immediate concern. If the patients history or physical exam strongly suggests a primary dermatitis, the condition can be expected to lessen in severity within a few weeks from the onset of the exfoliative process and then take on the usual features of the underlying disorder. All possible systemic and topical medications should be discontinued immediately, since drug reactions and contact dermatitis may be the cause, and any necessary systemic medications should be replaced by ones that are chemically dissimilar whenever possible. Drug reactions usually improve within a week or two after discontinuation of the causative agent. However, the course of an exfoliative dermatitis secondary to a malignant process is characteristically more protracted. A generalized superficial lymphadenopathy is usually present, but unless leukemia or lymphoma is suspected, biopsy is generally not helpful; however, in the former, a bone marrow biopsy, and in the latter, a lymph node biopsy, may be diagnostic. Topical measures for symptomatic relief should be employed, including baths followed by the application of petrolatum and cool, wet dressings or warm compresses, depending on the symptoms. Oral fluid replacement is critical because of the tendency for dehydration from the excessive perspiration. Topical low-potency steroid preparations (see Table 10.9) are most effective if they are given in an ointment base during the initial phase of the disease, since lotions and creams are less resistant to removal by sweating, and oral antihistamines help to relieve pruritus. When topical measures are unsuccessful, a short (2- to 3-week) course of an oral corticosteroid (e.g., prednisone, 40–60 mg given in a single daily dose for about 10 days and then tapered to every other day) is often highly beneficial. However, if the underlying cause is not determined and eliminated, the symptoms may recur whenever an attempt is made to discontinue the steroid, and a longer course may be necessary.

A persistent eruption of the skin of the lower legs with erythema, mild scaling, and a brownish discoloration (due to erythrocyte diapedesis) may be indicative of ***stasis dermatitis,*** a condition frequently associated with deep venous incompetence. Neglect of the condition may result in increasing edema, subcutaneous induration, and eventually painful ulceration and secondary bacterial infection. Treatment should include elevation of the leg above heart level to promote venous return, as well as topical therapy selected according to the stage of the disease. For acute nonulcerative dermatitis, wet dressings (plain water) may be applied and then allowed to dry somewhat before removal so that some of the crust is removed with them. A topical corticosteroid preparation (cream or ointment) or one that is incorporated into plain zinc oxide paste may be applied to the lesion three times daily as the condition becomes less acute. Lesions that are ulcerated may be treated similarly with wet compresses followed by petrolatum or zinc oxide paste. If a bacterial cellulitis is present, a course of oral antibiotics should be given, but topical antibiotics should never be used, since they are useless and may cause a contact dermatitis as well.

Pityriasis rosea is a common, self-limiting skin disease characterized by the appearance of an initial "herald" or "mother patch" (most often on the trunk) followed in 1 or 2 weeks by a generalized eruption of smaller lesions (0.5–2 cm in diameter) parallel to the lines of cleavage on the trunk, typically in a "Christmas tree" pattern, radiating from the spinal column diagonally downward and outward. The arms and face may also be involved. The individual lesions are slightly erythematous, round or oval, fawn- or rose-colored macules with a scaly, slightly elevated border. Pruritus is a common symptom; in rare cases, malaise and headache occur. The etiology of the disorder is unknown, but it occurs most frequently in the spring or fall, does not appear contagious, and generally resolves without complication about 6 weeks after the appearance of the herald patch, conferring "immunity" (recurrences are rare). There is no specific treatment, but topical measures may be required for itching and inflammation, such as 0.25% menthol in a cream base or a low-potency topical corticosteroid cream for severe lesions. Wet dressings may also be helpful, and ultraviolet light seems to hasten resolution. Since the lesions of pityriasis rosea may resemble those of secondary syphilis, serologic tests for the latter should be performed if the clinical appearance is suspicious (e.g., if there is involvement of mucous membranes, fever, or weeping of lesions).

The occurrence of a spreading pruritic eruption consisting of numerous flat-topped, violaceous papules that may be discrete or coalesce to form rough, scaling plaques on an otherwise healthy individual may be indicative of ***lichen planus,*** a common benign papulosquamous disease. There is a predilection for the flexor surfaces of the wrists and forearms, sides of the neck, sacral region, genitalia, and legs, especially around the ankles. In about 30–70% of cases there is involvement of the tongue, buccal mucosa, or other mucous membranes, and in some patients the mucosa may be the first or the only site of eruption. Cutaneous lesions are 1–4 mm in diameter and have lacy white streaks (Wickham's striae) on the surface. They are best observed with a hand magnifying lens when mineral oil is placed on the surface of a lesion. A positive Koebner reaction may occur during the acute phase, with new papules appearing along the site of a skin trauma; a common example is a linear configuration of lesions resulting from a superficial scratch. Hyperpigmentation and atrophy may result from persistent lesions. Approximately 10% of patients also have nail involvement, with such changes as longitudinal grooving, nail bed atrophy, pterygium, and subungual hyperkeratosis. ***Hypertrophic lichen planus,*** a variant that may accompany the common form, has lesions that may become large, verrucous, scaly, and extremely pruritic. The lesions occur most commonly on the shins and ankles, and may persist after the other areas of involvement have resolved. Referral for possible biopsy is indicated whenever mucosae are involved, since although lichen planus of the oral or vaginal mucosa generally has a distinctive clinical appearance, biopsy is warranted to rule out dysplastic changes and to differentiate lichen planus from other mucosal lesions. Biopsy of cutaneous lesions may be done and will reveal characteristic histiopathic features. As with all papulosquamous disorders, serologic tests for secondary syphilis must be ordered to rule out this possibility.

Since emotional stress is believed to play a causative role in both the initial outbreak and recurrences, a mild sedative may be helpful in the treatment of lichen planus. For pruritus, an antihistamine such as diphenhydramine 50 mg or chlorpheniramine 4 mg, four times a day may be beneficial, and other nonspecific local therapies such as topical tar preparations and bath oils may provide relief. However, topical and occasionally systemic (in severe cases) corticosteroid therapy is most helpful for extensive involvement and severe pruritus. For small, recalcitrant, highly pruritic or hypertrophic plaques, intralesional injections of triamcinolone acetonide suspension, diluted with saline to 2.5 to 5 mg/mL, is generally the preferred treatment. One should inject only enough to elevate the lesion slightly and should not repeat the treatment more often than once every 3 weeks. An occlusive covering such as an ordinary plastic wrap may also be secured over a site where a topical steroid preparation has been applied for severe localized plaques. A 0.05 or 0.1% tretinoin solution (Retin-A) applied with a cotton-tipped applicator at night and supplemented with an application of a corticosteroid cream or ointment (see Table 10.9) three times daily is beneficial for cutaneous lichen planus. Oral griseofulvin (microsize) therapy, 500 mg daily, has also been used with some success. Oral lesions may be treated with triamcinolone acetonide in an emollient dental paste (Kenalog in Orabase), but since this product contains a corticosteroid, it is contraindicated in cases of fungal, bacterial, or viral infections of the mouth or throat. A small amount should be applied directly to lesions to form a thin film at bedtime; for severe lesions, the preparation may be applied two to three times a day, preferably after meals. Lichen planus is a benign disease and treatment usually shortens the course and lessens the severity of symptoms, but in about 50% of patients active lesions may still be present 1 year after the onset. Oral lesions and hypertrophic lichen planus tend to be the most persistent, with as many as 20% of patients having at least one relapse. Recurrences, however, tend to be less severe than the initial eruption. The lesions eventually flatten and become asymptomatic, but there may be residual hyperpigmentation for years. Prolonged lichen planus, especially the mucosal and hypertrophic forms, is susceptible to malignant degeneration.

The ***secondary form of early (infectious) syphilis*** is characterized by a generalized nonpruritic eruption that can mimic a number of disorders. The most common manifestation is a maculopapular rash, but macules, papules, pustules, follicular lesions, or any combination of these can occur. Mucosal lesions and involvement of the palms and soles are common. Mucous membrane involvement varies from ulcers and papules to a diffuse pharyngeal redness. Condylomata lata are fused papules that develop at the mucocutaneous junctions and in moist skin areas and may become hypertrophic, flattened, and dull pink or gray. All lesions are highly infectious in the early stages (primary and secondary) of syphilis. A generalized, nontender lymphadenopathy, fever, and meningeal, hepatic, renal, bone, joint, and ocular involvement may occur, with resulting cranial nerve palsies, jaundice, nephrotic syndrome, periostitis, iritis, and iridocyclitis. Serologic testing and treatment for syphilis are discussed in Chapter 9.

Urticaria is a common acute or chronic vascular reaction of the skin that is characterized by an eruption of local, pale, evanescent wheals ("hives") and erythema in the dermal layer. Acute urticaria is most often an allergic reaction, but chronic urticaria is rarely allergen induced. ***Angioedema*** is a similar reaction but covers larger edematous areas, involves the deeper dermis and subcutaneous tissue, and tends to be asymmetric. Urticaria is frequently, though not always, accompanied by severe pruritus, while angioedema is usually not. The disorders may occur simultaneously or individually. There are a number of possible causes of urticaria and angioedema (see Table 10.10), and the first step of treatment is to try to locate the specific underlying cause and, if possible, to eliminate it. A good history and physical exam may point to a particular etiology, but should they provide no clues, a battery of tests to rule out underlying disease should be performed including a

TABLE 10.10 CAUSES AND TREATMENT OF URTICARIA AND ANGIOEDEMA

Type	Mediators	Causes	Treatment
Direct activation of mast cells	Histamines, kinins	Nonspecific histamine liberators 1. Drugs, including tubocurarine chloride, morphine, meperidine, codeine, polymyxin, thiamine, dextran, pilocarpine 2. Food additives, including benzoates, metabisulfites 3. Insect bites and stings	H-1 antihistamines, such as hydroxyzine, tripelennamine, or diphenhydramine, 75–200 mg/day (divided into three or four doses) to begin H-2 antihistamines (cimetidine, ranitidine) may be used in combination with H-1 antihistamines for cases unresponsive to H-1 antihistamines alone, but this type of regimen has given inconsistent results Beta agonists (e.g., albuterol, 2 mg four times a day) may occasionally be added For severe symptoms, corticosteroids may be given (e.g., oral prednisone, 40–60 mg/day for 7–10 days); a few minums of epinephrine 1 : 1,000 sc given sequentially may also be beneficial
Interference in cyclooxygenase pathway of arachidonic acid metabolism	Prostaglandins plus subsequent mediator	Aspirin Nonsteroidal anti-inflammatory drugs (naproxen, ibuprofen, aminopyrine, indomethacin, mefenamic acid, etc.) Tartrazine (yellow dye No. 5) and other azodyes Benzoic acid derivatives Naturally occurring salicylates	Avoidance of the responsible agent H-1 and H-2 antihistamines, as noted above
Allergen-induced	IgE, histamine	Drug allergies: penicillin and sulfonamides are common Inhaled (rare) or contact allergens: ragweed, animal dander, etc. Food allergies: shellfish, peanuts, chocolate, fresh fruits, milk products, and eggs are common	Avoidance of the implicated allergen H-1 antihistamine; add H-2 antihistamine Beta agonists may be tried Steroids may be used (rarely) for severe reactions unresponsive to the above treatments
Induced by physical stimuli	IgE, histamine	Pressure Light (solar urticaria) Vibration (familial vibratory urticaria) Skin trauma (dermographia occurs in about 4% of the normal population, with light stroking or scratching resulting in an urticarial reaction Water (aquagenic urticaria)	Avoidance of the causative stimulus Sunscreens for solar urticaria H-1 antihistamines if the condition is severe enough to require treatment H-2 antihistamines (rarely) Steroids (rarely) Beta agonists (rarely)
Cold-induced	IgE, kinins, histamine, serotonin	Exposure to cold	Avoidance of the cold (weather, water immersion, etc.) Pretreatment with cyproheptadine, 4–8 mg, four times a day H-1 and H-2 antihistamines Desensitization through slowly increased exposure may be helpful, since this appears to be an IgE-mediated disorder

TABLE 10.10 (*Continued*)

Type	Mediators	Causes	Treatment
Cholinergic (heat-induced)	Histamine	Heat Emotional stress Exercise Sweating	H-1 antihistamines, alone or in combination with cyproheptadine (25 mg hydroxyzine plus 4 mg cyproheptadine taken four times daily), are usually effective; severe or frequent outbreaks may require up to 50 mg hydroxyzine plus 8 mg cyproheptadine four times daily H-2 antihistamines may be added
Immune-complex-mediated	Activation of complement system, kinins, many inflammatory mediators	Viral infections: rubella, hepatitis B, mononucleosis Parasitic infestations: *Ascaria, Ancylostoma, Echinococcus, Fasciola*, filaria, *Schistosoma, Strongyloides. Toxocara, Trichinella* Serum sickness Nephritis Transfusion reaction Collagen vascular disease: SLE, rheumatoid arthritis, vasculitis, Sjögren's syndrome, polycythemia vera	Treatment of the underlying infection or infestation H-1 and H-2 antihistamines Steroids may be used to treat the primary disease condition (not for viral infections)
Complement abnormalities	Activation of complement system (excess activation of C4 and C2), kinins, inflammatory mediators	Decreased levels or functional inactivity of C1-esterase inhibitor (C1INH), which may be hereditary (hereditary angioedema) or acquired (secondary to neoplasms, such as carcinoma of the lung, colon, or rectum)	In an acute attack, C1-inhibitor concentrate (lyophilized and partially purified) in 5% dextrose may be given IV in 10–45 minutes Aminocaproic acid or tranexamic acid (plasmin inactivators) may also be used to control an acute attack Methyltestosterone buccal tablets, danazol, or stanozolol may be used for long-term therapy to reduce episodes
Metabolic disease	Heat	Hyperthyroidism Generalized hyperpyrexic states	Treat primary disorder
Idiopathic	Questionable	Unknown	H-1 antihistamine (e.g., hydroxyzine), alone or in combination with an H-2 antihistamine Beta agonists may be added in cases unresponsive to antihistamines Corticosteroids may be used (as a last resort only) in severe cases unresponsive to H-1 and H-2 antihistamines; administer 40–60 mg prednisone per day for 1 week to 10 days

complete blood count (CBC), determination of the erythrocyte sedimentation rate (ESR), serum C3, C4, and CH-50 levels, liver function tests, T_4, and antinuclear antibody (ANA) testing and urinalysis. The treatment for urticaria and angioedema is outlined in Table 10.10.

Erythema multiforme is an acute cutaneous inflammatory disease that may range from a mild, localized skin eruption to a severe, widespread bullous form with multiple system involvement (erythema multiforme bullosum). It may occur as a primary disorder or as a manifestation of any number of systemic causes, including systemic infection (herpes simplex and atypical mycoplasma infections are common), a chronic or malignant internal disease process (including chronic ulcerative colitis, lupus erythematosus, dermatomyositis, and rheumatoid state), or as a reaction to a drug or injected serum [vaccinia, bacille Calmette-Guérin (BCG), and poliomyelitis vaccines]. Characteristically, there is a sudden onset, without prodromal symptoms, of isolated or clustered groups of violaceous, edematous macules and/or papules. However, as the name implies, the lesions of this disorder are variable; in addition, there may be vesicles, bullae, pustules, wheals, and dome-shaped nodules. With time the lesions enlarge, and varying amounts of hemorrhage within some of them may give a purpuric appearance. The "erythema iris," an erythematous papule with a clear center giving a "bull's-eye" appearance, is a characteristic lesion. Lesions occur most frequently on extensor surfaces but may also be found on the soles or palms. Hemorrhagic ulcerative lesions (aphthae) can also occur on the lips and oral mucosa. Constitutional symptoms are common and variable, including malaise, arthralgia, and fever. The disease itself tends to be self-limiting but may occasionally be recurrent (as in erythema multiforme associated with herpetic infection). A rare form, erythema perstans, may persist for months or years. Another variant, ***erythema multiforme bullosum*** tends to have a sudden onset of large bullae that are often surrounded by wide, erythematous halos. Pruritus, malaise, and fever often accompany the eruption. The trunk is less frequently affected than the extremities, and the most common sites of involvement are the palms and soles. The occurrence of large vesicobullous lesions not only on the skin but also on the mucosal surfaces, including the eyes, nostrils, and oral and anogenital regions, constitutes ***Stevens-Johnson syndrome*** (erythema exudativum), a serious and sometimes even fatal variant. With this severe form there may also be involvement of the tracheobronchial mucosa, with bronchitis and atelectasis. Permanent eye damage from residual corneal scarring is a common complication, so obviously an ophthalmologic consultation is always essential. Renal and pulmonary involvement may also necessitate consultations with a specialist for related complications.

Toxic epidermal necrolysis (TEN) is another severe manifestation of erythema multiforme that is almost always due to a drug reaction. (It should be differentiated from staphylococcal scalded skin syndrome, which most often occurs in children; see Table 10.11 and the section on scalded skin syndrome.) This disease is characterized by generalized erythema with large, flaccid blisters occurring anywhere on the body, followed by separation of the entire epidermal layer (cleavage is at or just above the basal layer, the stratum germinativum, as a result of disintegration of cells of that layer) in sheets. A positive Nikosky's sign (slight friction can rub off the epidermis) is seen in the uninvolved skin at the edges of blisters. There is frequent mucosal involvement and sometimes large areas of the body are affected, making fluid and heat loss a serious concern. Exam of frozen sections of the skin, which is readily detached, reveals the full epidermal thickness. Inflammatory cells, basal cells (i.e., of

TABLE 10.11 DIAGNOSTIC FEATURES OF TOXIC EPIDERMAL NECROLYSIS (TEN) AND STAPHYLOCOCCAL SCALDED SKIN SYNDROME (SSS)

	TEN	Staphylococcal SSS
Histologic distinction	Necrosis of entire epidermal layer with separation near the basement membrane level (just above or within the stratum germinativum from disintegration of basal cells).	Epidermal separation occurs in the stratum granulosum (induced by staphylococcal toxins).
Laboratory tests	1. Biopsy (frozen section of skin peeled from fresh wound) shows full thickness of epithelium. 2. Tzanck preparation from denuded base of lesions shows inflammatory cells and cells with a high nucleus-to-cytoplasm ratio (i.e., basal cells). 3. Eosinophil counts (usually elevated when due to a drug reaction).	1. Biopsy (as for TEN) shows the stratum corneum with foci of adherent granular cells. 2. Tzanck smear of cells from denuded base of lesions shows broad cells with low nucleus-to-cytoplasm ratio (granular cells). 3. Eosinophil counts usually reduced.
Other findings	Frequent mucosal involvement; some reports of associated membranoproliferative glomerulonephritis.	Mucous membranes rarely involved.
Age predilection	Over 10 years of age.	Most common in children, especially newborns.
Prognosis	Serum loss may be significant (since the entire thickness of the epidermis is separated), so the prognosis is guarded.	Good.
Therapeutic measures	Discontinue all possible medications or replace necessary ones with chemically dissimilar drugs. Provide supportive therapy, with careful attention to fluid balance (steroids or possibly renal dialysis may be required).	Prompt, specific antibiotic therapy is indicated for this staphylococcal infection (e.g., dicloxacillin); aspirin may be given, and topical lubricating (but not anitmicrobial) agents may be useful during the period of desquamation.
Etiology	Drugs are common precipitating agents (especially penicillin, sulfonamides, tetracycline, mithramycin, aspirin, phenylbutazone, hexametaphosphate, barbiturates, amidopyrine, procaine, phenolphthalein, allopurinol, gold salts, hydantoin, dapsone); less common causes are immunizations, vaccinations, and nonstaphylococcal infections.	Staphylococcus, phage type 71.

the stratum germinativum), and a high nucleus-to-cytoplasm ratio (which is characteristic of cells of the deeper levels of the epidermis) are seen in a Tzanck test of scrapings from the denuded base of lesions. Eosinophil counts provide further help in differentiating this condition from staphylococcal scalded skin syndrome; eosinophilia is a common finding when the disorder is due to a drug reaction, but eosinophil counts are reduced when the cause is staphylococcal. With any of the forms of erythema multiforme, drug eruptions, secondary syphilis, and urticaria should be ruled out, and the more severe bullous form of erythema multiforme should be differentiated from other bullous disorders such as pemphigoid, pemphigus, and dermatitis herpetiformis.

The primary concern in treating various forms of erythema multiforme should be the location and elimination or treatment of the causative factor. All unnecessary medications should be discontinued. The patient's history may suggest an infectious cause (e.g., a recent upper respiratory tract infection or herpetic cold sores weeks prior to the skin eruption) and should be followed up. Systemic antibiotics (e.g., tetracycline, 250 mg, four times daily for several days) may be helpful for some infections. Mild erythema multiforme generally requires no treatment or plain wet dressings, but systemic corticosteroids may be beneficial for severe cases. One should begin with a daily dose equivalent to 60 mg prednisone or more, continue or increase it until a response is seen, and then taper off over a 2- or 3-week period. If there is no improvement within 5 days, however, it is probably best to discontinue the steroid, since the small chance of achieving a significant benefit after that point does not seem to outweigh the risk of steroid-related complications. Systemic corticosteroid treatment also seems to render some patients, particularly those with severe oral and pharyngeal involvement, more susceptible to fatal respiratory infections, so the decision to use them must be made with great caution. Oral antihistamines may provide some relief, and local measures used in other skin disorders may be helpful. Severe forms (Stevens-Johnson syndrome and TEN) require IV fluid and electrolyte replacement and reverse isolation (as for severe burns) to prevent suprainfection. Oral lesions may be treated with zinc sulfate solution, 0.01–0.025%, used as a mouth rinse several times a day.

Erythema nodosum is an inflammatory disease of the skin and subcutaneous tissue that is often a manifestation of internal disease but may also be associated with various infections, pregnancy, or a drug reaction. It occurs as an eruption of painful red nodules of variable size (1–10 cm in diameter) scattered predominantly on the anterior aspects of the legs and joints and, rarely, on the arms, trunks, and face. The nodules are pink or red at first, but over several weeks become bluish to brown, resembling contusions. Fever, malaise, and arthralgia commonly precede the eruption, and hilar adenopathy is a less frequent accompaniment. The condition is more common in young adults, and women are predominantly affected. The disease usually lasts for about 6 weeks and then resolves, but recurrences may continue for months or years. Leukemia, sarcoidosis, regional ileitis, and ulcerative colitis are disease processes associated with erythema nodosum. Infectious causes include streptococcosis (the most common cause in the United States), primary coccidioidomycosis, histoplasmosis, leprosy, primary tuberculosis, psittacosis, lymphogranuloma venereum, rheumatic fever, North American blastomycosis, and syphilis. Drugs that may cause the reaction include sulfonamides, iodides, bromides, penicillin, phenacetin, and progestins. Laboratory findings may include an elevated ESR and leukocytosis. Determination of the specific cause (systemic disease or infection or a drug) and elimination or treatment of that cause whenever possible is primary.

The treatment for erythema nodosum is essentially the same as for erythema multiforme, with systemic antibiotics for infections and/or corticosteroid therapy, unless it is contraindicated, as in suspected tuberculosis. Intralesional injections of a corticosteroid suspension (directly into each nodule) seem to be particularly helpful. Alternatively (where corticosteroids are contraindicated), prompt involution may be obtained with 5–15 drops of a saturated solution of potassium iodide three times daily. Other local treatment measures are usually not necessary, but hot or cold compresses may be beneficial.

Table 10.12 lists a number of ***cutaneous drug reactions*** and the drugs most often associated with them. Some reactions are due to allergic responses, which result from an initial prior exposure in which sensitization occurs and then from a

TABLE 10.12 CUTANEOUS DRUG REACTIONS

Type of Reaction	Description	Agents Often Responsible
Toxic erythema	Most common skin reaction to drugs; often the trunk is more severely affected than the extremities; appears on about the ninth day of treatment in primary use and in 2–3 days with subsequent administrations.	Antibiotics (especially ampicillin), barbiturates, *p*-aminosalicylic acid, phenylbutazone, and sulfonamides and related compounds (e.g., furosemide, thiazide diuretics, sulfonylurea hypoglycemics).
Fixed drug eruptions	Round, erythematous, circumscribed patches occurring in the same site whenever a drug is readministered.	Barbiturates, glutethimide, methaqualone, phenolphthalein, quinine, sulfonamides, tetracycline.
Eczematous eruptions	Resembles a contact dermatitis; occurs with systemic administration of the same (or a related) substance that caused sensitization in prior (external) contact.	Local anesthetics, neomycin, penicillin, phenothiazines.
Lichenoid or lichen planus–like eruptions	Flat-topped papules that coalesce to form scaling plaques.	Arsenic, chloroquine, chlorpromazine, gold, *p*-aminosalicylic acid, phenothiazines, quinacrine.
Urticaria	Erythematous wheals.	Aspirin, codeine, dextran, meperidine, morphine, nonsteroidal anti-inflammatory drugs (ibuprofen, naproxen, etc.), penicillins, pilocarpine, polymyxin, sulfonamides, thiamine, tubocurarine chloride.
Allergic vasculitis	Inflammatory changes that are most severe around veins and venules.	Ibuprofen, indomethacin, phenylbutazone, phenytoin, sulfonamides.
Exfoliative dermatitis/erythroderma	Scaling and erythema (redness) over the entire skin surface.	Barbiturates, carbamazepine, gold, isoniazid, *p*-aminosalicylic acid, penicillin, phenytoin, phenylbutazone, sulfonamides.
Erythema multiforme	Characteristic "iris" or "target" lesions appear mostly on extensor surfaces; bullae may also occur.	Barbiturates, fenoprofen, phenylbutazone, sulfonamides, sulindac.
Toxic epidermal necrolysis (rare)	Generalized regions of erythema followed by separation of the epidermis in sheets (resembles wet tissue paper).	Barbiturates, methotrexate, oxyphenbutazone, penicillin, phenylbutazone, phenytoin, tetracycline, sulfonamides, sulindac, mithramycin, aspirin, amidopyrine, procaine, phenolphthalein, allopurinol, dapsone, hydantoin, gold salts.
Erythema nodosum	Characteristic tender red nodules occurring predominantly on the anterior aspect of the lower legs and occasionally on the arms or other areas.	Bromides, iodides, oral contraceptives, penicillin, phenacetin, sulfonamides.
Drug-related lupus erythematosus	Lupus-like rash exacerbated by sun exposure and accompanied by other characteristic symptoms (fever, myalgia, pleural and pericardial serositis, polyarthritis).	Hydralazine, isoniazid, phenytoin, procainamide.
Photosensitivity	Exaggerated response to sunlight (UV radiation) on exposed skin surfaces.	Chloroquine, nalidixic acid, phenothiazines, sulfonamides and related compounds, tetracyclines (especially demeclocycline), thiazides, artificial sweeteners, and a number of other agents.

TABLE 10.12 (*Continued*)

Type of Reaction	Description	Agents Often Responsible
Purpura	Nonblanching purple or brownish macules of variable size (usually minute) on dependent body areas (e.g., legs); pruritus is common.	Anticoagulants, apronalide, barbiturates, carbromal, chlorothiazide, meprobamate, phenylbutazone, quinine, sulfonamides, sulfonylureas, sulindac.
Pigmentary upsets	Ranging from chloasma to discoloration of light-exposed areas to generalized discoloration.	Oral contraceptives (in chloasma), chlorpromazine and other phenothiazines, heavy metals (arsenic, bismuth, gold, silver), and quinacrine are common causes of pigmentary upsets.
Pruritus	Due to overgrowth of *Candida*. Due to biliary stasis.	Following systemic antibiotic treatment. Oral contraceptives, phenothiazines, rifampin.
Toxic alopecia	Hair loss.	Anticoagulants (coumarin, heparin, phenindione), antithyroid drugs (carbimazole, thiouracil), cytotoxic agents, oral contraceptives, vitamin A (excessive amounts).

later exposure to the drug that results in an eruption within minutes or as late as hours or days afterward. True allergic drug reactions occur in response to even very low levels of the drug (below the therapeutic range), manifestations that differ from the usual drug effects, restriction to certain types of reactions (e.g., urticarial, anaphylactic), and reproducibility of the reaction. The onset of this type of reaction is usually sudden, but may be delayed, and is marked by bright erythema and often pruritus, which may be severe. Other symptoms that may be present include headache, fever, malaise, and arthralgia. Other drug reactions may result from accumulation of a drug, its normal pharmacologic action (e.g., purpura from excessive anticoagulants), or interaction of genetic factors. Treatment of a drug reaction centers on the determination of the specific causative agent. A detailed history with inquiry about all prescription and nonprescription drugs, keeping in mind that some drug eruptions may continue for weeks or months after discontinuation of the drug, is often necessary. Topical measures for treatment of the cutaneous eruption should first be tested by application of a small amount of the agent to a localized area; if it is effective, it may then be applied to the entire eruption. Acute allergic reactions may require injection of 0.2–0.5 mL of a 1:1,000 solution of epinephrine (adrenaline) SC or IM, once or repeated after 5 minutes if necessary. An antihistamine may also be administered (e.g., chlorpheniramine maleate, 20 mg) parenterally, and an IM injection of 100–300 mg hydrocortisone hemisuccinate may be beneficial.

Granuloma annulare is a chronic skin disorder characterized by the development of asymptomatic yellowish or flesh-colored papules or nodules that in time spread peripherally, appearing as a slightly elevated ring with a center that is normal or slightly depressed. This benign lesion may occur in persons of all ages and is not associated with any systemic conditions, except that there is a statistically significant incidence of diabetes mellitus in adults who have a number of lesions. One or more lesions may be present, and the arms, legs, hands, and fingers are the sites most commonly affected. High-potency corticosteroid creams used in conjunction with occlusive covering (e.g., plain plastic wrap) at bedtime or direct intralesional injection of a corticosteroid suspension (e.g., triamcinolone acetonide suspension diluted with saline to 2.5–5 mg/mL) may hasten involution of the lesion. It should be explained to patients that the condition may be chronic but is benign. Spontaneous resolution of lesions is common.

A number of conditions are characterized by the appearance of blisters (bullae). These often have distinct clinical, histologic, and immunologic features. Table 10.13 lists some of these ***bullous disorders*** with their associated diagnostic features. Since nearly all of these conditions are treated differently, an exact, prompt diagnosis is an essential first step. Consultation with a physician familiar with the diagnosis and treatment of these disorders may be advisable, since a number of factors (severity of the disease, the patient's general health status, etc.) may have to be taken into account in selecting the exact therapeutic regimen to be followed.

Bullous pemphigoid is a chronic, benign disease characterized by a localized (particularly on the abdomen and flexor surfaces) or generalized eruption of subepidermal bullae or multiple vesicles. The blisters may be preceded by erythematous, eczematous, or pruritic urticarial eruptions or may appear suddenly on normal skin. Lesions may occur on the oral mucosa, but these are infrequent and heal rapidly. The disease is most common in persons over age 60. The bullae are initially tense and resist rupture, and may be accompanied by dusky red, edematous, annular lesions with or without vesicles at their peripheries. This disorder is considered an autoimmune disease because direct immunofluorescence of biopsy sections reveals immunoglobin G (IgG) and complement (C3) at the dermal–epidermal junction (basement membrane level). Histopathologic exam also reveals subepidermal bullae, and autoantibodies are demonstrated in the patient's serum by indirect immunofluorescent tests. In fact, the presence of IgG antibodies against the basement membrane zone in the serum of a patient with a chronic blistering disease is always strongly suggestive of bullous pemphigoid.

Low to moderate doses of systemic corticosteroids are the treatment of choice for bullous pemphigoid (e.g., prednisone, 40–60 mg orally every morning for several weeks and then gradually tapered to a maintenance level). However, if large doses are required over a long period of time for management, immunosuppressives such as methotrexate, azathioprine, or cyclophosphamide may be used to reduce or replace the amount of corticosteroids needed for control. The use of medium-potency topical corticosteroids (see Table 10.9) may also allow lower doses of oral corticosteroids. Some cases may respond to dapsone (Avlosulfon), 100–300 mg initially and then reduced to a maintenance dose. This disorder may be self-limited but usually persists for several years. In the elderly patient, additional new lesions do not warrant increasing the oral corticosteroid dosage because the benefits do not generally outweigh the significant side effects.

In ***cicatricial pemphigoid*** (benign mucosal pemphigoid), subepidermal bullae form on the mucous membranes but rarely on the skin. These bullae frequently ulcerate, and residual scarring is common. Oral, pharyngeal, laryngeal, esophageal, anogenital, and conjunctival involvement are all possible. Hoarseness, dysphagia, and stenotic anogenital orifices may result from secondary fibrous bands, and scarring of the palpebral conjunctiva may result in blindness. In this disorder, which is twice as frequent in women as in men, linear deposition of IgG and complement (C3) is seen with direct immunofluorescent microscopy (as in bullous pemphigoid), but indirect immunofluorescence tests fail to reveal circulating antibodies to basement

TABLE 10.13 DIAGNOSTIC FEATURES OF CERTAIN BULLOUS DISORDERS

Disorder	Indirect IF Test	Direct IF Test
Bullous pemphigoid	Serum IgG to basement membrane (titer does not correlate with severity or extent of clinical involvement).	Linear deposition of IgG and C3 at basement membrane level seen on biopsy of perilesional or normal skin.
Cicatricial pemphigoid	Circulating antibodies generally not found.	Linear deposition of IgG and C3 at dermal–epidermal junction, as in bullous pemphigoid.
Pemphigus vulgaris	Anti-intercellular antibody. Antibody titer may correlate with severity of disease.	IgG on epidermal or epithelial cell surfaces invariably seen on biopsies of perilesional skin or mucous membranes.
Dermatitis herpetiformis	Circulating antibodies usually not found, but IgA antibody to normal basement membrane tissue or IgG antibody to reticulin found in some patients.	Biopsies of perilesional or healthy skin show granular deposits of IgA and C3 at junction of dermis and epidermis, especially in upper zone of dermal papillae; IgG or IgM also seen occasionally, and sometimes linear IgA deposition along entire dermal–epidermal junction.
Herpes gestationis	Circulating antibodies not ordinarily found, but complement to normal basement membrane tissue may be demonstrated using special techniques.	Linear deposits of C3 at junction of dermis and epidermis in perilesional or normal skin.
Porphyria cutanea tarda		Deposits of IgG and IgM seen ar dermal–epidermal junction and in blood vessels, but these are not diagnostic (urinary uroporphyrin levels must be determined).

membrane in the serum of most patients. Local treatment measures are sometimes all that is required (e.g., Kenalog in Orabase for oral lesions, Decadron Phosphate or Hydrocortone Acetate ophthalmic ointments and solutions), but systemic corticosteroids or immunosuppressives are frequently also necessary.

The term "pemphigus" refers to a number of blistering disorders characterized by intraepidermal bullae, disruption of epidermal intercellular connections (acantholysis) seen on a smear taken from the base of a lesion and stained with Giemsa's stain (Tzanck test), and the presence of autoantibodies in the serum and skin to an intercellular antigen in the epidermis. The disorder is seen throughout the world, with no apparent sexual or racial predilection, although it seems to occur more commonly in adults, particularly between the ages of 40 and 60. ***Pemphigus vulgaris*** has an

Histologic Features	Other Features	Treatment
Subepidermal bullae without acantholysis (negative Tzanck test)	Numerous eosinophils, especially in papillary dermis; chronic form is most common in the elderly; lesions favor the abdomen, groin, and flexor surfaces.	Systemic and topical corticosteroids; immunosuppressives (methotrexate, azathioprine, or cyclophosphamide) for severe, unresponsive cases.
Subepidermal bullae and ulceration (no acantholysis) involving mucous membranes and sometimes skin	Twice as common in women as in men; may involve the conjunctiva, mouth, esophagus, pharynx, larynx, and anogenital region; residual scarring may be severe.	Local (oral, ophthalmic, etc.) treatments may be sufficient, but systemic steroids are sometimes necessary.
Intraepidermal bullae and erosions; acantholysis seen with Tzanck smear from lesions (diagnostic)	Possibly leukocytosis and eosinophilia; positive Nikolsky's sign on involved and uninvolved skin; most common between 40 and 60 years of age; mucosal involvement common.	Hospitalization and systemic corticosteroids; immunosuppressives (methotrexate, azathioprine, cyclophosphamide) or IM gold sodium thiomalate may limit steroid requirements for maintenance.
Subepidermal bullae, acantholytic cells not seen in Tzanck smear	Neutrophils seen in upper region of dermal papillae; severe pruritus and excoriation are common.	Dapsone or sulfapyridine and gluten-free diet.
Subepidermal bullae indistinguishable from those of bullous pemphigoid	Marked eosinophilia, intense pruritus, asymmetric distribution; oral contraceptives, estrogens, and subsequent pregnancies may induce recurrences.	Corticosteroids (topical and systemic).
	Autosomal dominant inheritance, but a secondary factor (e.g., alcoholism, chronic liver disease) is necessary for the expression of the condition. Bruising, photosensitivity, blisters, and erosions occur.	Elimination of possible aggravating factors (e.g., administered iron, estrogen, alcohol, noxious chemicals); phlebotomy, low-dose chloroquine, urine alkalinization (with sodium carbonate), avoidance of sun (sunscreens are usually not helpful to prevent sun-induced damage).

acute onset and is potentially fatal unless aggressive treatment with steroids is instituted. It is characterized by the appearance of relapsing crops of flaccid, easily ruptured bullae on apparently normal skin, and often by a positive Nikolsky's sign on both lesioned and unlesioned skin. Very extensive erosions may result, and mucosal involvement (particularly in the mouth) is common and may be the initial manifestation; oral lesions are associated with a poorer prognosis. Toxemia and a foul (mousy) odor may occur. The eruption is often localized at first and then becomes generalized within about a year.

If the Tzanck and immunofluorescence tests confirm the diagnosis of pemphigus vulgaris (direct immunofluorescence tests of perilesional skin or mucosa show IgG on epidermal or epithelial cell surfaces, and indirect immunofluorescence tests demonstrate circulating antiintercellular antibody), treatment should include hospitalization and large doses of systemic corticosteroids to halt the eruption of new lesions. An initial dose may be the equivalent of prednisone, 40–80 mg orally two times daily, but it should be doubled after 1 week if new lesions continue to appear. When no new lesions have appeared for 7–10 days, the dosage may be tapered slowly by giving the total daily dose in the morning initially, then every other morning, and then gradually decreasing this to a maintenance level (the minimum level necessary to control local or systemic manifestations). Concomitant therapy with an immunosuppressive drug (methotrexate, azathioprine, cyclophosphamide) and IM gold salt (given as for rheumatoid arthritis after initial corticosteroid therapy) has been used successfully as an alternative in cases where high-dose or prolonged corticosteroid therapy would have been necessary, thereby limiting the potential side effects of the steroid use. However, these drugs have their own serious risks. Dapsone (Avlosulfon), 100 mg or less daily, may control some cases of pemphigus. Additionally, appropriate systemic antibiotic therapy should be administered for secondary infections, and silver sulfadiazine cream (Silvadene Cream) may be used to prevent secondary infection of erosions. Other local measures appropriate to the severity of the lesions may be used as well, including baths, protective ointments, and intralesional injection of corticosteroid suspension (e.g., triamcinolone acetonide) when there is a small number of lesions. Blood transfusions and IV feedings may be necessary, and anesthetic lozenges may be used before eating for painful oral lesions.

Dermatitis herpetiformis is a chronic, intensely pruritic disease characterized by groups of tense papules, vesicles, bullae, or urticarial lesions distributed in a classic, usually symmetric, pattern over extensor surfaces (elbows, knees, shoulders, sacrum, buttocks, scalp), and sometimes also over the face, ears, and neck. Mucosal involvement may also occur. Due to the highly pruritic nature of the disorder, the lesions are often obscured by excoriation. There is generally a gradual onset. The disorder is most common in persons between the ages of 15 and 60 and is twice as common in men as in women. The term "herpetiformis" refers to the typical grouping pattern of small vesicles, which resembles that seen in herpes simplex and herpes zoster; it is not meant to suggest a viral cause. Histopathologic exam of lesions often reveals subepidermal vesicles with aggregates of neutrophils within the dermal papillae, numerous eosinophils, and widespread destruction of the basement membrane. Direct immunofluorescent microscopy done on biopsy specimens of perilesional or normal skin reveals granular deposits of IgA and usually C3 at the dermal–epidermal junction, especially in the upper regions of dermal papillae, and is an important aid to diagnosis. IgG and IgM are also sometimes seen, and a linear deposition of IgA along the dermal–epidermal junction may be seen in some patients. Indirect immunofluorescence tests generaly fail to reveal circulating autoantibodies or significant serum complement levels, although circulating IgA antibody to normal basement membrane and IgG antibody to reticulin may be seen in the sera of some patients. In 70–90% of patients with dermatitis herpetiformis (and in many of their relatives), there is an associated asymptomatic gluten-sensitive malabsorptive enteropathy, with decreased disaccharidase and dipeptidase activities and villous atrophy of the small intestine apparent on biopsy of the small bowel. Aggravation of the disease has been known to occur from halogens, and a skin patch test with 20% potassium iodide is often positive and may produce typical lesions with IgA deposition.

The symptoms of dermatitis herpetiformis usually respond readily to dapsone or sulfapyridine. Both of these drugs inhibit neutrophil function (other sulfonamides are not effective in this manner), but both are also likely to produce side effects including hemolytic anemia, agranulocytosis, thrombocytopenia, peripheral neuropathies, and drug reactions such as erythema multiforme and toxic epidermal necrolysis. Therefore, patients receiving these medications should have a weekly CBC for the first 4 weeks, then every 2 or 3 weeks for 12–18 weeks, and then every 8–10 weeks thereafter. Consultation with a physician familiar with the use of these drugs is also advisable. Adherence to a gluten-free diet for a prolonged period will often help to reduce the symptoms and may eventually induce a remission, but it is often months before the skin response becomes evident (the bowel reverts within days to a normal state), and convincing the patients, who rarely have symptomatic enteropathy, to adhere to the diet is usually difficult.

The occurrence of an extremely pruritic vesiculobullous disease during pregnancy is most likely indicative of ***herpes gestationis,*** a chronic disorder that, like dermatitis herpetiformis, is not caused by a herpes virus. The name refers to the characteristic arrangement of lesions and its occurrence during pregnancy. In an early, unsuspected pregnancy, the intense pruritus and unique clustering of lesions may suggest dermatitis herpetiforme, but in this disorder the distribution lacks symmetry and the lesions are frequently bullous and occasionally urticarial. The first episode usually occurs in the first trimester but can take place any time during pregnancy. The condition often becomes worse within a day or two after delivery, but within several months it usually remits and finally disappears. Some women have recurrences associated with menses for a year or more after delivery, and oral estrogens or contraceptives and subsequent pregnancies are likely to reinduce active disease. In the mother, the major problem is the symptomatic discomfort of the condition, but fetal death is a possibility. In addition, the newborn may be affected by the condition through passive transference of antibodies against skin from the mother in utero, but the eruption in the infant is transient. Direct immunofluorescence of biopsy specimens of perilesional or normal skin reveals linear deposition of C3 and occasionally IgG at the dermal–epidermal junction. Indirect immunofluorescence tests are ordinarily negative, but complement may be induced to bind to the basement membrane zone in normal skin that has previously been incubated with serum from patients with herpes gestationis. Topical corticosteroids may be sufficient, but systemic corticosteroid therapy is often necessary during gestation for this disorder, and early delivery may be recommended because of the increased risk of fetal death. Because oral contraceptives and estrogen will induce recurrences, these are often contraindicated in women with herpes gestationis.

Porphyria cutanea tarda is an autosomal recessive disease associated with partial deficiency of the enzyme uroporphyrinogen decarboxylase, which results in an accumulation of large amounts of photosensitizing uroporphyrin that are excreted in the urine. The incidence is equal in both sexes, and symptoms are generally limited to the skin. However, liver dysfunction also occurs; it may be due both to concomitant diseases (alcoholic cirrhosis, tuberculosis, intestinal disease) and to the excessive uroporphyrin, which is thought to be toxic to the liver. The onset of the disorder, as the name implies, is commonly late (in middle age rather than childhood), because the expression of the genetic disorder requires a secondary factor; the most common of these is alcoholism, although excessive iron intake, estrogen or oral contraceptives, busulfan, barbiturates, phenytoin, and tolbutamide may also activate the disease. Photosensitivity and a tendency to bruise easily are the major clinical findings, and cutaneous involvement takes the form of areas of erythema, with vesicles or bullae occurring on exposed portions of the body, usually preceded by sun exposure and followed by crusting and scabs and then scarring. Erosions in which the epidermis may shear off following minor trauma may also occur. Hypertrichosis (increased numbers of coarse, dark hairs on areas of the face where terminal hairs are not normally found, such as the zygoma and forehead), areas of hyper- and hypopigmentation, milia, and sclerodermoid changes may be evident in areas of chronic lesions.

In porphyria cutanea tarda, since urinary uroporphyrin is considerably increased, a random acidified urine specimen will fluoresce red when examined under Wood's light. However, the diagnosis is usually made by determining the quantitative 24-hour urinary uroporphyrin level. Other laboratory findings include an increased urinary coproporphyrin and aminolevulinic acid (ALA) levels and increased levels of other porphyrins with 7-, 6-, and 5-carboxyl groups. There are also variable amounts of fecal porphyrins (isocoproporphyrins). There may be an increased serum iron level and abnormal liver function tests. Direct immunofluorescence tests demonstrate IgG and IgM deposition at the dermal–epidermal junction as well as in blood vessels of the dermis.

The initial step in the treatment of porphyria cutanea tarda is to identify the factor(s) that cause expression of the disease. If it is alcohol, for instance, discontinuation of alcohol intake may induce an asymptomatic state. Phlebotomy will usually induce remission by the removal of iron, which functions as a cofactor in the buildup of uroporphyrin levels. If there are no contraindications, 300–500 mL blood can be removed about every 3 weeks. Hemoglobin and urinary porphyrin levels should be monitored, and if the hemoglobin level drops to below 11 g/dL, phlebotomy should be discontinued until the level increases. The procedure is continued until the daily rate of urine uroporphyrin excretion is less than 500–600 μg. Remissions induced by this method often last for years, and recurrences can be treated similarly. Therapeutic alkalinization of the urine will also cause increased uroporphyrin excretion. Very low doses of chloroquine (125 mg twice a week) over a long period (8–18 months) will also aid mobilization of tissue porphyrins, but an acute reaction that includes toxic hepatitis and systemic illness (fever, headache, malaise, abdominal pain, vomiting, and red urine) results from larger doses of chloroquine, so these are always contraindicated. Occasionally the dosage must be increased (to 250 mg twice a week) after about a year of this therapy in order to obtain a remission. Phlebotomy is a much quicker method of achieving remission and is therefore the preferred treatment. In addition, patients should be instructed to avoid the precipitating factors mentioned above, and a sunscreen should be used during the active phase of the disease for protection from photosensitivity reactions.

A number of skin infections may be caused by bacteria, and the determination of the specific bacterial cause is of primary importance. In general, primary ***bacterial infections*** of the skin (e.g., impetigo, erysipelas) usually respond readily to treatment with an appropriate systemic antibiotic, but secondary infections (e.g., of wounds or burns) tend to clear more slowly. Topical antibiotic preparations are generally useless and may actually produce an allergic contact dermatitis. Therefore, these preparations are not recommended, except as preventive treatments against an initial infection in abrasions or surgical wounds, or, in some cases, in the treatment of acne. Recurrent infections should alert the primary care provider to the possibility of an underlying systemic disease (e.g., diabetes mellitus).

Impetigo (impetigo contagiosa) is a common superficial infection of the skin that is usually due to group A beta-hemolytic streptococci (*Streptococcus pyogenes*) but may also be caused by staphylococcal (especially *Staphylococcus aureus*) organisms or both. ***Ecthyma*** is a deeply ulcerated form that often causes scarring. The causative organisms can be introduced in a number of ways; purulent nostrils or ears are a common source of staphylococci. The term "pyoderma" is used collectively in reference to localized purulent streptococcal skin infections, but it is sometimes used synonymously with "impetigo." Impetigo initially appears as a transient eruption of pustules, vesicles, and macules that range from less than 1 cm in diameter to large ringworm-like lesions. The lesions are surrounded by erythema and after 4–6 days become exudative and develop into sticky, yellow-brown crusts that heal slowly, leaving areas of depigmentation. The ulcerated lesions of ecthyma are small, shallow, purulent, and punched-out, with thick, dark brownish crusts and a surrounding area of erythema. When these crusts are removed, a denuded red area of skin is seen beneath. Impetigo is generally a primary infection affecting exposed areas of skin, while the legs and covered areas are more frequently involved in ecthyma. Pruritus is a frequent symptom, and scratching may spread the infection. ***Bullous impetigo*** (impetigo neonatorum), a more severe form seen frequently in children, is highly contagious, associated with systemic toxicity, and potentially fatal. The lesions, as the name suggests, are initially massive bullae and later form thin, varnish-like crusts. Bullous impetigo is invariably staphylococcal.

Folliculitis is a superficial or deep staphylococcal infection of hair follicles usually caused by *Staph. aureus*. The lesion in the acute phase is a superficial pustule or inflamed nodule within the hair follicle. A chronic form, ***sycosis,*** occurs where hair follicles are deep, as in the bearded region. It is usually spread by the trauma and autoinoculation of shaving, and the surrounding skin resembles eczema, with redness and crusting. Tests should also be performed to differentiate bacterial folliculitis from a fungal infection (tinea barbae), and acne vulgaris and impetigo should also be ruled out.

Furuncles (boils) are acute perifollicular swellings due to *Staph. aureus* and, less commonly, to *Staph. epidermis* (*albus*) infections that result in a deep-seated infection (abscess). The lesions are extremely tender and occur most frequently on hairy areas (face, neck, axillae, breasts, perineum, buttocks, thighs) exposed to irritation, friction, pressure, moisture, or blocking of the follicle by products containing petroleum. Pruritus may be an early symptom, but pain and tenderness (due to pressure on nerve endings) always accompany the acute phase, particularly on the nose, ears, or fingers, where the skin is closely attached to underlying structures and there is little room for swelling. Fever and malaise may also be present, and laboratory tests may reveal slight leukocytosis. The primary lesion is a rounded or conical papule that gradually enlarges, becomes fluctuant and necrotic, softens, and then drains spontaneously after a few days to a couple of weeks. Relief of pain and the onset of healing occur soon after drainage of necrotic tissue and pus occurs, but a furuncle that regresses without drainage may form a "blind boil," which is indolent and susceptible to exacerbation with minor trauma. Lesions may be multiple since they are autoinoculable, but multiple lesions should also prompt a search for a predisposing cause, such as diabetes mellitus or nephritis. A debilitating disease may not be present but should always be ruled out or treated if found.

A large furuncle or a conglomerate of several furuncles that have developed in adjoining hair follicles and coalesced is called a ***carbuncle.*** This deep-seated mass will often drain through multiple skin openings. It is most common on thick skin (e.g., the back of the neck) and represents an acute suppurative inflammation of the subcutaneous (fibrous and adipose) tissues. Carbuncles may reach a diameter of several centimeters and may be accompanied by more severe pain, fever, and malaise than are present with furuncles, as well as chills, prostration, leukocytosis, and bacteremia, and may be fatal in weakened or elderly persons. Both furuncles and carbuncles should be differentiated from other bacterial infections (e.g., anthrax and tularemia), from deep fungal infections (e.g., sporotrichosis, blastomycosis), and from various cysts (acne, epidermal, pilar).

Cellulitis is a diffuse, spreading bacterial infection of the skin characterized by acute inflammation, hot, red, edematous skin, and an infiltrated surface that resembles the skin of an orange (peau d'orange) or "solid edema" (a permanent swelling due to recurrent attacks that have affected the lymph vessels). A break in the skin usually precedes the infection, and therefore cellulitis is often preceded by a burn or other wound. Petechiae, vesicobullous lesions (which may rupture), and occasionally necrosis may occur on the involved skin. It is most commonly due to *Strep. pyogenes* (group A beta-hemolytic) or *Staph. aureus,* but may also be caused by *Staph. epidermis* (*albus*). Streptococcal skin infections are associated with the subsequent development of an acute glomerulonephritis based on an antigen–antibody reaction in the glomerulus (see the section on renal disease in Chapter 8). Systemic symptoms of cellulitis, which include fever, chills, headache, malaise, tachycardia, lymphangitis (tender, red, linear streaks directed toward enlarged, tender lymph nodes), hypotension, and delirium, may occur, but sometimes the patient may not appear ill. Leukocytosis is a common but variable finding.

A superficial form of cellulitis is ***erysipelas,*** which is distinguishable from the former by sharply demarcated, slightly elevated borders. It is caused by a group A streptococcal infection. Rapidly progressing bilateral involvement most commonly occurs on the face (especially the cheek), an arm, or a leg. When the trunk or extremities are involved, it is often at the site of a surgical or traumatic wound. The lesion is a well-circumscribed patch that is shiny, red, edematous, hot, and tender. The lesion may show evidence of resolution in the center while continuing to spread peripherally. Vesicles and bullae may also be present, and significant swelling occurs when the infection involves the eyelids. Erysipelas of the face may resolve spontaneously in 4–10 days, but lesions of the trunk or extremities may be very extensive and even fatal. Constitutional symptoms include high fever, chills, and malaise. Areas of peripheral redness and regional lymphadenopathy may also be present, and recurrent erysipelas may result in lymphedema. Laboratory findings include an elevated ESR and leukocytosis. Erysipelas should be differentiated from contact dermatitis, angioneurotic edema, cellulitis, and erysipeloid (*Erysipelothrix rhusiopathiae* infection), a benign bacterial infection commonly seen on the skin of fingers or the backs of hands of fishermen and meat handlers and characterized by an area of reddened skin that gradually enlarges over a period of several days. (Treatment of this condition with penicillin or a broad-spectrum antibiotic is promptly curative.)

Wound infections may result from a number of factors, including the person's own nasal discharge, another local infection, or external sources (e.g., other persons or objects). Newborns, elderly persons, persons receiving immunosuppressive therapy, and those with debilitating conditions (diabetes mellitus, obstructive jaundice, severe extensive burns) are particularly susceptible to secondary infection of wounds, including surgical ones (drainage equipment, orthopedic hardware, and sutures greatly increase the potential for bacterial invasion of tissue).

In all acute bacterial skin infections, antibiotic treatment should be instituted immediately, but cultures of the organism and tests for antibacterial sensitivity should be performed as well, because it is impossible to distinguish between a staphylococcal and a streptococcal skin infection simply by inspection. For cultures, it is essential that an adequate sample be obtained from an involved site (in wounds or lesions, under crusts). A swab sample is usually sufficient for frankly pustular lesions. The swab should be placed in a broth culture immediately without allowing it to dry. However, obtaining an adequate sample in the case of chronic infections may require scraping or even a biopsy specimen. Also, although there are some distinguishing features that help to suggest a bacterial as opposed to a viral or fungal origin (e.g., cellulitis with fever and swollen lymph nodes is most likely due to a bacterial cause, but herpes zoster, which is viral, can cause the same signs, and although fungal infections are notorious for occurring in intertriginous areas, bacterial infections may also arise), if there is doubt about the diagnosis, it is a good idea to sample some of the blister fluid in order to rule out a viral cause or a scraping from the roof of a blister in order to examine it for fungus.

Cultures from streptococcal infections usually yield large numbers of group A hemolytic streptococci, of which more than 95% are inhibited by low-potency bacitracin disks, but species from other serogroups (e.g., C and G) may be responsible for pyodermal lesions. Until recently, cutaneous infections were due predominantly to beta-hemolytic streptococci or to a mixture of staphylococcus and streptococcus. However, in recent years, studies have shown that an overwhelming majority of skin infections are caused by staphylococci (some estimate about three-fourths), less are due to mixed infections (staphylococcal and streptococcal), and a very small percentage are purely streptococcal. This is of particular importance when one considers that the majority of staphylococcal infections are resistant to penicillin G or V, ampicillin, and amoxicillin.

Early laboratory findings for cutaneous streptococcal infections include leukocytosis, with an increase in polymorphonuclear neutrophils, and possibly an elevated ESR. Urine tests often reveal proteinuria and a few red blood cells. Within 1–3 weeks of the onset of a streptococcal infection, there is a rise in serum antibodies, particularly to hyaluronidase (AH), streptolysin O (ASO), streptokinase, deoxyribonuclease (anti-DNAse B), and other streptococcal antigenic products. In pyoderma, antihyaluronidase and anti-DNAse B are the most commonly elevated antibodies, but modest ASO responses may be observed when a cutaneous streptococcal infection is accompanied by streptococcal pharyngitis. Elevated antibody levels may persist for months after the infection. Microscopic exam of material taken from skin lesions due to staphylococcal infections will reveal polymorphonuclear neutrophils and staphylococci.

The treatment of staphylococcal and streptococcal skin infections is basically the same, with adequate doses of systemic antibiotics, except that the choice for most strains of staphylococcus must be restricted to the penicillinase-resistant antibiotics. Antibiotic treatment of a streptococcal pyoderma may include a single IM injection of 1.2 million units of long-acting benzathine penicillin G for adults (600,000 units for children) for acute cases or an oral regimen such as penicillin V, 250 mg four times a day for adults (125 mg four times a day for children) for 10 days. Persons who are penicillin sensitive may be given oral erythromycin or a cephalosporin instead.

All of these give cure rates of 97% or greater for streptococcal pyoderma, but if the response to the antibiotic is not rapid, the presence of a penicillin-resistant staphylococcus should be assumed.

For a staphylococcal infection, a penicillinase-resistant penicillin (e.g., oral dicloxacillin, cloxacillin, oxacillin, or nafcillin) may be given in doses of 250 mg four times daily (125 mg qid for children) for 10 days. Alternatively, for penicillin-sensitive adults, a 10-day course of erythromycin, clindamycin, or one of the cephalosporins (cephalexin or cephradine) is effective. Dicloxacillin and cloxacillin are probably the most reliable of the semisynthetic penicillin derivatives, since they are absorbed well even when taken with food and cost the least. Minocycline may be successful with some staphylococcal strains that are resistant to other antibiotics. If the responsible organism is unknown, the infection should always be treated as if it is staphylococcal, since the treatment for staphylococcus will clear up a streptococcal infection, but the reverse is not true.

Local treatments include gentle cleansing with a mild soap solution and soaks or wet compresses (Burow's solution, saline, or plain water) for acute lesions (impetigo, folliculitis, infected wounds). Local measures for furunculitis may be attempted in less severe cases prior to instituting systemic therapy, but if furuncles are large, involve the face or neck or are accompanied by systemic reactions (fever, lymphadenitis), or if the patient has diabetes, a valvular or congenital heart disease, or any other condition prone to complications, systemic therapy is necessary. Local measures include soaks and warm moist compresses to help "draw out" furuncles, followed by applications of a topical anti-infective agent such as iodochlorhydroxyquin, 3% cream or ointment (apply bid after soaking) or a topical antibiotic ointment (e.g., polymyxin B with bacitracin or oxytetracycline in combination with erythromycin). A surgical incision may be performed on mature lesions, but this must not be deep and must be supplemented with systemic antibiotics.

Hidradenitis suppurativa is a chronic, suppurative, cicatricial disease of the apocrine glands that may involve the axillae, anogenital area, or both. The lesions, which resemble furuncles, block the ducts of apocrine glands and result in rupture with painful local inflammation or sometimes discharge. The infection commonly spreads to other local follicles and glands, producing interconnecting draining sinuses and palpable extensive scar formation. When the condition becomes extensive, it may be disabling, particularly if the genital areas are involved (walking may become difficult). Treatment with rest, moist heat, surgical drainage, and prolonged systemic antibiotic therapy may resolve early cases, but extensive involvement may require excision of the involved tissues and skin grafting. Early surgery may therefore be advisable to abort the disease and decrease the number of glands at risk. Susceptible persons should be advised to avoid using substances that may produce irritation, such as antiperspirants.

The occurrence of an intense, diffuse, painful erythema of the skin of the face and body, followed within several hours to 2 or 3 days by the appearance of Nikolsky's sign (gently rubbing the skin surface will cause the superficial epidermis to peel off in sheets resembling wet tissue paper) and a profuse desquamation, may be indicative of ***scalded skin syndrome,*** a potentially fatal complication of a group II staphylococcal infection (particularly type 71, but types 3A, 3C, and 55 are also common). Fever, vomiting, diarrhea, anorexia, hypotension, irritability, and severe malaise are also common. The disease usually begins with a superficial crusted lesion near the nose or ear that becomes surrounded by bright redness within 24 hours and generalizes within 36–48 hours. Unlike TEN from which this should be differentiated (see Table 10.11), mucosal involvement is rare. The cause of scalded skin syndrome is an exfoliative or epidermolytic toxin produced by the straphylococci, which causes an intraepidermal split within the stratum granulosum. Edema in skin areas where hair is scarce gives a fine, stippled appearance that resembles a nutmeg grater pattern. Localized bullae may also be present. Characteristic facies develop as the disease progresses, with red, crusting fissures superimposed on the edema in the folds between the nose and mouth and at the corners of the mouth. When the skin sloughs, the resultant raw, red, moist areas resemble those of a second-degree burn, which gives the disease its name. "Scalded skin syndrome" was once used interchangeably with "toxic epidermal necrolysis" to refer to any staphylococcal or drug reaction producing widespread erythema and epidermal desquamation. Now, however, "scalded skin syndrome" refers to the staphylococcus-induced disorder, which is most common in childhood but occurs in adults as well. "Toxic epidermal necrolysis" is the designation used when the etiology is nonstaphylococcal (e.g., a drug reaction, nonstaphylococcal infection, vaccination, or immunization).

The organism responsible for scalded skin syndrome may often be recovered from the patient's skin, throat, or nares, as well as from cultures of the patient's conjunctivae, stool, and occasionally blood. If additional confirmation is required, frozen section exams of skin peeled from the lesions reveal the stratum corneum with focally adherent patches of granular cells, demonstrating that the separation is confined to the stratum granulosum (unlike TEN, which produces cleavage at the deeper level of the stratum germinativum and shows full epidermal thickness in peeled skin sections). Tzanck preparation of smears taken from the denuded base of lesions shows broad cells with a low ratio of nucleus to cytoplasm (characteristic of cells from upper epidermal levels). Scalded skin syndrome must be differentiated from Kawasaki's disease or mucocutaneous lymph node syndrome (a childhood illness characterized by fever, lymphadenopathy, a polymorphous mucocutaneous eruption, and a "strawberry tongue"), pemphigus, and toxic shock syndrome (see Chapter 9), which is more often associated with diarrhea, desquamation of the skin on the hands, and refractory shock. Because the disease may progress rapidly, prompt, vigorous antibiotic therapy is indicated even prior to obtaining culture results. Since most of the responsible organisms are resistant to penicillin, a pencillinase-resistant drug such as dicloxacillin is the best choice. Aspirin may be given for the fever, and lubricating (not antimicrobial) ointments may be beneficial for the skin during the period of desquamation. However, steroids (oral or topical) are always contraindicated because they can depress the body's immune response.

Scarlet fever (scarlatina) was a once common complication of a streptococcal pharyngitis that is relatively uncommon today with the availability of antibiotics. It is associated with beta-hemolytic group A streptococci that may produce an erythrogenic toxin. In susceptible persons, this toxin causes a rash characterized by a diffuse erythematous flush that blanches on pressure and fine red papules superimposed on the flushed skin surface. The punctate rash is most prominent in the regions of the neck, groin, and axillae, as well as in skin folds, and may become petechial. Other common manifestations include whiteness around the mouth (circumoral pallor) that contrasts vividly with the flushed face, a strawberry tongue (protrusion of inflamed red papillae on a white-coated tongue surface), dark red lines in the cutaneous folds (Pastia's lines), and desquamation of the upper layer of previously reddened skin when the fever begins to subside, particularly on the hands and feet. The onset is sudden, and early systemic signs and symptoms include an elevated temperature (38.3–40.6°C), convulsions in very young patients, and frequent vomiting, chills, malaise, and headache. Cervical lymphadenopathy and a rapid pulse may also be present. Leukocytosis (with counts ranging from 10,000 to 20,000 leukocytes with 75 to 90% neutrophils) and an elevated ESR are common, and proteinuria (related to fever) may develop. The rash of scarlet fever must be distinguished from a sunburn rash, drug reactions, rubella, meningococcemia, toxic shock syndrome, and echovirus infections. A positive throat culture for erythrogenic-toxin producing beta-hemolytic streptococcus will help to establish the diagnosis. There is also an associated rise in serum levels of ASO 1–3 weeks after the onset of the infection. The treatment of scarlet fever is the same as for other group A streptococcal infections, including a 10-day course of penicillin G or V or erythromycin. Aspirin and gargling with warm salt water may relieve the discomfort of the sore throat, and bed rest and adequate fluid intake are important during the febrile period.

Leprosy (Hansen's disease) is a chronic infectious disease caused by the acid-fast bacillus *Mycobacterium leprae,* which has a high incidence of infectivity but a low tendency toward pathogenicity. The mode of transmission is uncertain, but contact with nasal discharges and skin lesions (and possibly indirect contact via fomites and arthropods) is most likely. The incubation period may be as short as 1 year but tends to be quite long (as long as 30 years), and the disease progresses slowly. Since only about 5% of contacts appear to contract the infection, it is believed that an immunity may be developed. The disease is endemic in equatorial regions including Southeast Asia, Africa, South and Central America, the Pacific regions (including Hawaii), and the southern United States (Texas, Louisiana, Florida). Endemic foci in the continental United States seems to be associated with immigrants who have a history of childhood residence in another endemic area.

There are two distinct types of leprosy, which may be distinguished clinically and by laboratory findings: lepromatous and tuberculoid. ***Lepromatous leprosy,*** the more contagious variety, is a generalized, progressive, and malignant infection involving the skin, mucous membranes (oral, nasal, upper respiratory), anterior eye, cutaneous and peripheral nerve trunks, adrenal glands, and testes. Skin involvement is characterized by nodular, erythematous, infiltrated lesions, 1–5 cm in diameter, or by a diffuse skin infiltration lacking any distinct, identifiable lesions. Macules, papules, and plaques may also occur. Nerve involvement is symmetric, and numerous acid-fast bacilli may be easily found in tissue specimens. A lepromin skin test (intradermal injection of autoclaved bacilli taken from lepromatous nodules) is negative for this type, signifying impaired cellular immunity. If untreated, this form is extremely progressive and generally fatal in 10–20 years.

Tuberculoid leprosy has a more benign and nonprogressive course with few asymmetric, localized skin lesions, peripheral nerve involvement, a sudden onset, and a less contagious nature than the lepromatous type. The lesions of tuberculoid leprosy are typically pale, anesthetic macules ranging from 1 to 10 cm in diameter. Few bacilli can be found in the lesions (except during acute reactive periods), but there is an intense inflammatory response, with a swelling that contains epithelioid and Langerhans cells and is surrounded by a large number of lymphocytes. The response to the lepromin skin test is positive, indicating a high resistance to the infection, and spontaneous recovery may occur within 1–3 years. However, there may be eye involvement (keratitis, iridocyclitis), nasal ulcers, epistaxis, anemia, and lymphadenopathy. Peripheral nerve involvement (with caseation necrosis) may result in permanent destruction of peripheral nerves, paralysis of one or more extremities, anesthesia, and crippling deformities. Laboratory confirmation of the diagnosis of leprosy is dependent on the demonstration of the acid-fast bacilli in lesions or nasal discharge and on biopsy of a suspected skin lesion. The lepromin test, usually negative in the lepromatous type and positive in the tuberculoid type, helps to distinguish between the two types. A large amount of disfigurement may result unless treatment is instituted; however, immediate active treatment of a lesion discovered early can be expected to produce a cure, and patients receiving therapy are not considered to be a serious public health problem. However, since children are less resistant to the infection, they should be removed from contact with patients. BCG vaccination and/or dapsone may have prophylactic value for family contacts of patients with the more contagious lepromatous type.

The treatment for tuberculoid leprosy includes oral administration of dapsone (DDS, Avlosulfon), continued for 2 years after the disease becomes inactive. The treatment for lepromatous leprosy is a combination therapy of dapsone plus rifampin or dapsone plus clofazimine, continued indefinitely (sulfoxone may be given instead of dapsone if a gastric intolerance to dapsone occurs). Leprosy caused by dapsone-resistant strains (evidenced by progression or relapses of disease or the presence of bacilli in new lesions during treatment) should be treated with a combined therapy regimen of rifampin plus clofazimine, rifampin plus ethionamide, or ethionamide plus clofazimine. Secondary bacterial infection of skin lesions and traumatic amputation of anesthetic fingers are possible complications. Management of leprosy patients is complex. Physicians at the U.S. Public Health Service Hospital in Carville, Louisiana are available for expert consultation on matters pertaining to the disease.

A number of skin diseases are due to ***viral infections.*** When an eruption is thought to be viral in origin, a glass-slide smear of fluid taken from a vesicle or some of the crusted tissue may be sent for examination. Swabbing for cultures necessitates a special viral transport media.

Herpes simplex is an acute, recurrent viral infection characterized by small, single or grouped, tense vesicles on the skin or mucous membranes, especially the oral ("fever blisters" or "cold sores") or genital regions. The responsible virus is herpesvirus hominis, a double-stranded DNA virus with two subtypes—1 and 2—that are biochemically, immunologically, and serologically distinguishable. About 80% of herpes infections in the mouth region are caused by the more common type 1 herpesvirus, and lesions in the genital region (see Chapter 9) are mostly due to type 2 infections, although both types can occur on any area of the skin. Primary infections, which are usually asymptomatic or very mild, can occur through direct or indirect contact with lesions of an infected individual. By 4 years of age, about half of all children will have had a primary infection with type 1 herpesvirus and will have developed antibodies to it. If it is symptomatic, the disease may resemble an upper respiratory tract infection or part of the teething syndrome, with a mild fever, drooling, some discomfort, or disinterest in food. Recovery occurs within several days. In adults, a sore throat, general malaise, muscular aches, mild fever, and regional or generalized lymphadenopathy may initially accompany the primary infection, followed within a day or two by the appearance of small vesicles anywhere on the body, but most commonly on the oral mucosa (gingiva, hard or soft palate, or buccal mucosa). The vesicles are filled with clear fluid and occur on slightly raised, erythematous bases. They soon rupture, leaving painful ulcers that are slow to heal. Primary infections with type 2 herpesvirus occur more commonly on the genitalia and are usually contracted venereally. In men, clusters of vesicles may occur on the penis, and in women the labia majora and minora, urethra, vagina, or cervix may be involved. These primary infections are usually painful but tend to resolve spontaneously within a week or two. Although not all persons infected with the virus have recurrent lesions, a number do suffer from recurrences that can be precipitated by emotional stress, menstruation, local trauma (rubbing, kissing, dental procedures, shaving, intercourse), minor infections (mostly of the upper respiratory tract), fever, sun exposure, smoking, or certain foods or drugs. Recurrences are usually preceded by a prodromal period of tingling, burning, stinging, or itching at the site of the eventual eruption of single vesicles or clusters of vesicles within a day or two and lasting for 2–4 days. The vesicles may change into pustules and become flaccid or rupture, leaving a shallow ulcer that soon dries and forms a thin yellowish crust before healing. Neuralgia may also occur during the prodromal period or during the eruption, and lymphadenopathy is common. Although pain or discomfort and embarrassment are usually the extent of the problems associated with recurrences, repeated infection or an infection contracted by a newborn from delivery through an infected birth canal can result in encephalitis. A number of other complications may result from recurrences, including erythema multiforme, eczema herpeticum (a very extensive, generalized eruption that may be hemorrhagic), Bell's palsy, aseptic meningitis, temporary bladder and bowel paralysis, and dissemination of the virus through the bloodstream. Blindness may result when the eye is involved.

Cultures for the virus, a positive Tzanck test of scrapings from vesicles stained with Giemsa's stain (revealing multinucleated giant cells), and a progressive increase in serum titers of antibodies to the virus (in primary infections) are diagnostic of herpes. Symptomatic treatment of primary infections and mild recurrences includes aspirin (10 grains every 4–6 hours as needed) and rinses mouth with an elixir containing diphenhydramine hydrochloride or viscous lidocaine or a milk of magnesia and water mouthwash. An antibiotic ointment (e.g., a neomycin-bacitracin ointment) for nonoral lesions may be used to minimize the potential for secondary bacterial infection and painful crusting and cracking; if a secondary bacterial infection does occur, systemic antibiotic therapy may be necessary. However, keeping lesions moist may aggravate the condition and delay healing, so a drying agent may be more effective (e.g., camphor spirit, 70% alcohol). Application of a moistened styptic pencil several times daily will also help to abort cutaneous lesions. Topical corticosteroid preparations are never indicated in herpesvirus infections. Topical acyclovir may be used in primary genital herpes infections, and oral acyclovir may be indicated for severe, recurrent infections (see Chapter 9). Patients should be advised that they are infectious during the primary or recurrent eruptions and should avoid contacting other persons with infected parts. Also, avoidance of the sun or application of a sunscreen (particularly a lip sunscreen product) will help prevent recurrences in those persons who find that sun exposure initiates an outbreak. Using a shaving cream may help to minimize the potential of shaving trauma, and additional lubrication prior to intercourse may help to prevent precipitating skin trauma. Avoidance of foods or other agents that tend to cause eruptions and sometimes oral contraceptive therapy may be beneficial. Frequent gynecologic exams are advisable for female patients with recurrent genital herpes infections, since studies have suggested a strong association between the virus and cervical cancer.

▶ ***Herpes zoster*** (shingles) is an acute infection of the central nervous system (CNS) (primarily involving the dorsal root ganglia) that is characterized by a unilateral vesicular eruption, involving predominantly the trunk and face, and neuralgic pain or other sensations (itching, tingling). The rash and neuralgia tend to be limited to the areas corresponding to the region of cutaneous innervation. The varicella-zoster virus (which also causes chickenpox) is the causative agent. The infection most often occurs in persons who are over age 50, who are receiving immunosuppressive therapy, or who have a systemic disease such as Hodgkin's disease; the first attack almost always confers lifelong immunity. The eruption is usually preceded by malaise, fever, and segmental dysesthesia lasting for about 4 or 5 days; the pain may persist or increase in intensity even weeks after the lesions have disappeared. Other systemic symptoms (chills, GI disturbances) may also precede the eruption by days. The lesions begin as grouped, reddish papules on an erythematous base, changing to patches of tense, deeply set vesicles that may also be confluent. (In rare cases, the lesions are erythematous plaques without vesicles.) Within about 5–10 days the vesicles become dry and crusted, but in severe cases they may develop a gangrenous appearance. Regional lymphadenopathy may accompany the eruption. The prodromal symptoms may be confused with those of a number of other disorders, but once the eruption occurs, the characteristic distribution of the lesions helps to establish the diagnosis of herpes zoster. Exam and direct immunofluorescent tests of scrapings from the base of vesicles will help to establish a viral origin and to determine that the varicella-zoster virus is responsible. Cultures of the virus from vesicle fluid and determination of serum levels of antibodies will also confirm the diagnosis. Herpes zoster should be differentiated from zosteriform herpes simplex, contact dermatitis, dermatitis herpetiformis, cellulitis, other viral infections (e.g., chickenpox), and temporal arteritis. Hodgkin's disease and other lymphomas should also be ruled out by a CBC with white blood cell (WBC) differential.

Most herpes zoster infections are benign and self-limited, but an elderly or immunocompromised patient, or one who is receiving radiation therapy or has an underlying malignancy, is more susceptible to complications such as cranial and peripheral nerve palsies, meningitis, encephalitis, pneumonitis, localized motor weakness, ophthalmic zoster, neuralgia, or dissemination. A secondary bacterial infection of vesicles may occur with intensified erythema, induration, and a fever; scarring may result. Bacterial cultures of the vesicles and treatment with the appropriate systemic antibiotics will help abort this bacterial involvment. There is no specific treatment for herpes zoster, but treatments aimed at relief of symptoms (e.g., wet soaks, topical creams or ointments, an oral analgesic) may be quite helpful, and early institution of a course of systemic corticosteroids may relieve the pain and decrease the incidence of postherpetic neuralgia in severe cases. However, these measures will not influence the rate of healing or shorten the acute phase of the infection. Ophthalmic herpes zoster must always be differentiated from ophthalmic herpes simplex, particularly before prescribing corticosteroids, since these are always contraindicated in acute ocular herpes simplex. Consultation with an ophthalmologist is in line if there is any evidence of eye or nasociliary nerve involvement. Oral acyclovir has shown promise in both shortening the course of the infection and decreasing postherpetic neuralgia, but it is not approved for this use by the Food and Drug Administration (FDA). The rare complication of cutaneous dissemination (lesions outside the original dermatome) may occur with immunocompromised persons. Since this may progress to involvement of the CNS, lungs, liver, or myocardium, antiviral chemotherapy should be instituted (human leukocyte interferon or IV acyclovir), preferably by a physician experienced in the use of these drugs.

▶ ***Chickenpox*** (varicella) is the more common disease caused by the varicella-zoster virus. It is usually seen in children and is highly communicable. Epidemic outbreaks occur most frequently in the winter and early spring. There is an incubation period of 10–20 days following exposure, and then a short (1- or 2-day) prodromal period of mild constitutional symptoms (headache, moderate fever, anorexia, malaise, and sore throat) followed by a morbilliform eruption that may initially be accompanied by an evanescent flush. The prodromal period is mild in children but more severe in adults. The early macular lesions, which are associated with severe pruritus, progress rapidly to papules and vesicles (within 6–8 hours) and then quickly rupture to form ulcers. Successive crops of macules appear just as the lesions of a previous crop begin to crust, resulting in the simultaneous presence of all stages of lesions in the same patient. The trunk is generally the first site (and may be the only site) of the eruption, but lesions can occur on the face, neck, and extremities, and occasionally on the mucous membranes. When the lesions appear on the scalp, the suboccipital and posterior cervical lymph nodes are frequently enlarged and tender. The acute phase lasts about 4–7 days, and most crusts will have disappeared within 20 days from the onset of the first lesions. The infectious period for this disease persists from a few days prior to the onset of symptoms until all of the vesicles have crusted over, and isolation for 6 days after the appearance of the first vesicles can usually control transmission. A single attack will confer lifelong immunity, and a partial immunity in newborns (probably acquired transplacentally) seems to exist until about 6 months of age.

In childhood, chickenpox is generally quite benign, but a rare, but serious, complication (Reye's syndrome) may occur 3–8 days from the onset of the eruption, with acute encephalopathy and some degree of mental disturbance (ranging from mild amnesia and lethargy to episodes of agitation and disorientation), along with a number of other respiratory, hepatic, and other findings. This occurrence is potentially fatal. It requires hospitalization and monitoring, as well as treatment of individual complications as they occur. Since Reye's syndrome seems to be associated with aspirin use during a varicella infection in children, the use of aspirin is contraindicated in any disorder in children that is associated with flu-like symptoms. Other potential complications include secondary bacterial (streptococcal or staphylococcal) infection of lesions that produces a pitted scar, pneumonia (more common in adults and infants than in young children), myocarditis, transient arthritis, hemorrhagic complications, and postinfection encephalitis (uncommon) with CNS complications. The fingernails should be kept trimmed and clean to prevent secondary bacterial infection through excoriation, and if a few lesions do become infected, a bacitracin-neomycin ointment may be applied twice daily. However, penicillin may be given IM for extensive infection of lesions. Other complications (e.g., encephalitis, pneumonia) should be treated symptomatically, and corticosteroids may be helpful for varicella pneumonia. Leukopenia is a common finding. The virus may be isolated from vesicle fluid, and scrapings of the base of vesicles reveal multinucleated giant cells. However, the characteristic clinical appearance and a large number of reported cases in an area are usually sufficient to establish a diagnosis.

Measles (rubeola or morbilli) is another formerly common acute, systemic viral infection that is more common in children than in adults and is highly contagious. Transmission occurs through inhalation of infected droplets from the nose, mouth, and throat of persons in the prodromal or early acute phase of the disease. Following a 7- to 14-day incubation period, there is a prodromal phase with fever, hacking cough, coryza, periorbital edema, conjunctivitis, and photophobia; 2–4 days later, the pathognomonic Koplik's spots (tiny white spots that, in contrast to the dull redness of the mucosa, resemble tiny grains of table salt) appear on the buccal mucosa and occasionally on the mucosa of the labia, vagina, or conjunctival folds as well, and persist for 1–4 days. Other features of the prodromal period include pharyngeal redness, tonsillar edema (sometimes with a yellowish exudate), a central coating and marginal redness of the tongue, moderate generalized lymphadenopathy, and occasionally splenomegaly. A characteristic spreading cutaneous rash (accompanied by mild pruritus) appears 3–5 days after the onset of the symptoms (1–2 days after Koplik's spots appear), beginning on the face, around the ears, and on the sides of the neck. The initial lesions are tiny (the size of a pinhead), irregular macules that soon become maculopapular and spread within 24–48 hours to the trunk and then the extremities, by which time the earlier lesions (on the face and neck) have coalesced and begun to fade. With particularly severe eruptions, petechiae or ecchymoses may be present. The fever may reach as high as 40–40.6°C, and leukopenia is common (with relative lymphocytosis) unless there is a secondary bacterial complication. Proteinuria (from the fever) is also present. The fever subsides within 3–5 days, making the patient more comfortable, and the eruption fades soon afterward, revealing a yellowish-brown discoloration followed by slight desquamation. Hyperpigmentation tends to be more persistent in severe cases or in fair-skinned individuals.

Patients with measles are highly susceptible to secondary bacterial infections (particularly streptococcal), and a number of bacterial complications including pneumonia (especially in infants), otitis media, and cervical adenitis may occasionally follow the measles infection immediately (in about 15% of cases). A switch in the WBC from leukopenia to leukocytosis, exacerbation of the fever, and the development of malaise, pain, or prostration are all possible indicators of a bacterial infection as a complication. General treatment measures include isolation of infected persons for 1 week following the onset of the rash and bed rest during the febrile period. Tylenol (see the preceding discussion of Reye's syndrome), wet (saline) eye compresses, vasoconstrictive nose drops, and sedative cough medicines may provide symptomatic relief. Complicating bacterial infections should receive prompt, appropriate antibiotic therapy whenever they occur.

Encephalitis is an occasional complication of measles. Its onset occurs 3–7 days after the eruption, with vomiting, convulsions, and a number of severe neurologic signs and symptoms, a normal or elevated lymphocyte count, elevated protein levels in the cerebrospinal fluid, and coma. Symptomatic and supportive measures are the only treatments available; there may be a brief course with recovery in about a week, or a prolonged course with a number of permanent CNS sequelae and a significant (15%) mortality. Another complicating condition associated with measles infection is subacute sclerosing panencephalitis (SSPE), a chronic and usually fatal brain disease occurring in children and adolescents months to years after an attack of measles. Convulsive seizures, motor abnormalities, intellectual deterioration, and death may all occur.

Measles vaccination (with attenuated live measles virus) has greatly reduced the incidence of the disease and is an important preventive measure for all children; multiple-virus vaccines (e.g., measles-mumps-rubella) are equally effective. If vaccination is performed after 15 months of age, immunity is lasting (vaccination prior to the age of 12 months is associated with atypical measles syndrome, which is due to an acquired hypersensitivity to the virus as opposed to an immunity), with negligible complications; however, it is not recommended for severely immunodeficient children. The attenuated vaccine, administered to susceptible persons who have been exposed to measles (within 24–48 hours of exposure) may prevent the disease. After 24 hours, or as an alternative in persons whose condition either contraindicates the use of a live measles vaccine or provides reason to defer immunization (e.g., pregnant women, children under 3 years of age, and patients with active untreated tuberculosis, any acute febrile illness, generalized malignancies, an immunologic deficiency disease, or who are receiving immunosuppressive therapy), gamma globulin may be administered IM to prevent clinical manifestations of the illness. This should be followed by immunization 3 months later with the live virus vaccine unless a contraindicating condition is still present at that time (e.g., leukemia, immunosuppressive therapy).

An ***atypical measles syndrome (AMS)*** may result from infection of persons who have previously been immunized against the disease with a killed measles vaccine, or occasionally with live, attenuated measles vaccine (possibly due to inadvertent inactivation of the vaccine by improper storage or to being given before 12 months of age, resulting in hypersensitivity rather than immunity to the virus). This variable infection may begin abruptly with a brief prodrome of numerous symptoms (high fever, headache, toxicity, cough, abdominal pains, and/or arthralgia), followed by the appearance within 1 or 2 days of an unusual rash (maculopapular, vesicular, urticarial, or hemorrhagic), often beginning on the extremities. There is often severe illness, edema of the hands and feet; pneumonitis, and nodular densities in the lungs (which may persist for as long as 12 weeks or more) may occur; and, unlike ordinary measles infection, there is an associated high mortality. As with ordinary measles infection, treatment is limited to whatever symptomatic and supportive measures are indicated by the developing symptoms and complications, including wet compresses, antipyretic and cough medications (e.g., Tylenol, cough syrups and lozenges), and protection from secondary bacterial infection (e.g., cleansing of lesions, topical antibiotic ointments). If a bacterial infection does occur, it should be treated with appropriate systemic antimicrobial medication.

Rubella (German measles) is a contagious systemic viral infection associated with mild constitutional symptoms and a mild maculopapular eruption lasting for about 3 days. The disease is transmitted through inhaled infected droplets or close contact; the communicable period lasts from 1 week prior to the onset of the rash to 1 week after it fades. One attack will usually confer permanent immunity, but rubella is only moderately communicable; consequently, a number of persons are not infected during childhood and are still susceptible during adulthood. This is a significant concern, since abortion, stillbirth, and a number of congenital birth defects (including retarded growth, thrombocytopenia, cataracts, deafness, congenital heart defects, and organomegaly) may occur in infants whose mothers were infected during the early months of pregnancy.

The 14- to 21-day incubation period of rubella may be followed by a 1-week prodrome of mild fever, malaise, and tender occipital lymphadenopathy, but usually there are no prodromal symptoms. The rash is very similar to the eruption of measles, but is more evanescent and less extensive. A flush may appear at the onset of the eruption, particularly on the face. Discrete, rose-colored spots may appear on the palate and later coalesce into a red blush; erythema may also be present on the pharynx in the absence of any complaint of throat pain. Mild coryza and polyarthritis (in about 25% of adult cases) may also be present. The skin eruption, a fine, pink, maculopapular rash, appears first on the face and neck, spreads rapidly to the trunk and then the extremities, and finally fades after having lasted for about 1 day in each area. The total duration of the rash is about 2–3 days. Rubella infection may also occur without the eruption, and if suspected, may be confirmed by laboratory tests. Other findings include postauricular and posterior cervical lymphadenopathy and arthralgia. Encephalitis, a rare complication, may be fatal. Adult men may complain of transient testicular pain. Leukopenia may be present early, but the WBC may be normal (differentiating it from scarlet fever, which has leukopenia as a common finding, as well as a sore throat and more constitutional symptoms. It may be differentiated from measles by the absence of Koplik's spots, a cough, and photophobia, as well as by the milder, more evanescent rash. The eruption of syphilis is more bronze-like and the lymphadenopathy is not tender (quantitative serologic tests for syphilis may be done if there is doubt). The diagnosis of rubella may be confirmed by isolation of the virus, fluorescent antibody tests, and serologic tests of immunity. Treatment is usually not necessary in rubella, but a complication of otitis media (rare) requires appropriate therapy.

Vaccination with live attenuated ▶***rubella virus vaccine*** is an important measure in the prevention of rubella infection and transmission of the disease. Routine vaccination of all children between 15 months of age and puberty is suggested as a means of eliminating the reservoir of infection and thereby reducing the potential for adult exposure, but all girls should certainly be immunized before menarche and immunization of adult women in whom the absence of virus antibodies is established must be done when there is no possibility of pregnancy. Birth control should be used to avoid pregnancy for at least 3 months after vaccination.

▶***Insect bites*** are common causes of skin lesions, particularly during the summer months. A number of biting insects possess salivary secretions that can result in a variety of reactions and skin lesions. The more common of these arthropods include mites, ticks, fleas, lice, biting flies (sand, deer, and horse flies), mosquitoes, bedbugs, certain waterbugs, and kissing bugs. All of these may produce reactions ranging from a small papule to a large ulceration with considerable swelling, pruritus, pain, and sometimes a dermatitis. Severe attacks may cause insomnia (from intense pruritus), fever, faintness, or even collapse, and a secondary infection may follow excoriation, with possible serious consequences.

Identification of the offending insect and localization of the injury are the initial steps in the treatment of insect bites; identification is particularly important if a hypersensitivity reaction ensues and future avoidance is to be accomplished. If the insect is still present on the skin (e.g., ticks), it should be quickly removed. A petroleum product or an irritant (e.g., alcohol) should be applied directly to the insect and then carefully removed with tweezers (it is advisable never to remove ticks with fingers because of the risk of infection, particularly in endemic regions of Rocky Mountain spotted fever), taking care not to leave the head in the wound, since chronic inflammation or deeper migration (resulting in a granuloma) may result. The site should be cleansed thoroughly with soap and water to prevent a bacterial infection of the bite area. Cold compresses or application of an ice cube may control swelling and relieve pain. Oral antihistamines may be given for pruritus, and topical corticosteroid lotions or creams may control inflammation and lessen pruritus. For mites, a crotamiton cream or lotion (Eurax) may be used instead, since it is miticidal as well as antipruritic (see the section on scabies), and for lice another antiparasitic (e.g., Kwell or Rid) may be applied (see the section on pediculosis). Calamine lotion may also be used, and an antibiotic product (cream, lotion, or powder) may be used when there is a possibility of a secondary infection, but local overtreatment should be avoided. For localized persistent lesions, intralesional injection of a corticosteroid suspension may be beneficial. Exercise and excessive warmth may produce an exacerbation of symptoms and should be avoided. Codeine may be given for severe pain, but the use of creams or sprays containing local anesthetics is not advisable, since their use carries a substantial risk of sensitization, making later use of related local anesthetics a problem.

Most ***insect stings*** are caused by members of the order Hymenoptera: the honeybee and bumblebee (both of which tend to sting only if provoked) in one subgroup and wasps, hornets, and yellow jackets in a second subgroup. Of the stinging insects, the honeybee is the only one that loses its stinger and venom sac when they penetrate the skin, so finding an embedded stinger in the skin of a patient is a good means of identifying the sting of that insect. The amount of venom injected in a single sting is so small that it is estimated that about 100 stings would be necessary to inflict a fatal dose in most adults, but in hypersensitive individuals, an anaphylactic reaction to a single hymenoptera sting may be fatal. The chemical composition of the venoms produced by these various insects differs significantly, but there is a strong potential for cross-reaction between different members of a certain subgroup, so a person who is allergic to yellow jacket venom is more apt to have a hypersensitivity reaction to a wasp or hornet sting than to a bumblebee or honeybee sting. The ***ordinary response*** to a hymenoptera sting is an initial sharp pain followed by the development of a small, localized, erythematous wheal that enlarges and becomes edematous and indurated. Pain and pruritus accompany the lesion. The reaction generally subsides within 24 hours unless it occurs on an extremity, in which case there is more extensive edema and a course of several days. Most localized reactions resolve within a day or so without the need for treatment, but if there are severe symptoms, treatment of the ordinary local reaction is the same as for other insect bites and stings: thorough washing with soap and water, ice application to reduce edema, local creams or lotions (e.g., calamine lotion) for itching, and oral antihistamines (for stings measuring more than 5 or 6 cm in diameter) to relieve pruritus and produce a sedative effect. A mild topical antibiotic ointment may be applied to prevent a secondary infection (of course, not in conjunction with other topical lotions or creams). Application of a paste or papain powder (Adolph's meat tenderizer) and water or Panafil ointment to the site of an insect sting may also alleviate the symptoms, and for extensive edema of an extremity, rest and elevation of the affected extremity will help.

A ***generalized systemic reaction*** to the toxin (occurring in persons who have been repeatedly stung within a short time period) may produce systemic symptoms ranging from mild (pruritus of the eyes, mouth, or ears, dry cough, flushing of skin, urticaria) to moderate (abdominal pain, headache, nausea, vomiting, dizziness, fainting, diarrhea, constriction of the throat and chest, wheezing) to severe (hoarseness, confusion, anxiety, weakness, dyspnea). The etiologic factor in such reactions is probably the release of an extreme amount of histamine. This is not a hypesensitivity reaction, however, because its occurrence in a nonallergic person does not indicate that a future sting by the same type of insect will produce a similar generalized response. However, an immediate or delayed (less common) systemic allergic reaction to insect stings occurs in an estimated 0.5% of the population in this country.

Anaphylaxis, the immediate response, typically occurs within 15 minutes of the sting and may involve a number of organ systems. Skin involvement may include widespread urticaria, angioedema, and pruritus, and systemic symptoms include nausea, vomiting, abdominal or uterine cramping, urinary urgency, dyspnea, cyanosis, hypotension, shock, and cardiac arrhythmias. ***Delayed hypersensitivity responses*** may be localized or systemic and may occur hours or days (up to 2 weeks) after a sting. Symptoms include headache, fever, malaise, arthralgia, urticaria, purpura, allergic vasculitis, polyarthritis, lymphadenopathy, secondary infections, and neurologic defects (encephalopathy, peripheral neuritis).

All systemic reactions to stings should be treated as medical emergencies, including the nonallergic generalized systemic variety, since potentially fatal developments (e.g., laryngeal edema or vascular collapse) can occur at any point once systemic involvement has taken place. If the stinger is present, it should be removed at once, since the sac of venom will still be attached and may continue to exude venom into the wound. Epinephrine, 1:1,000 should then be injected SC (0.3–0.4 mL for adults, 0.2 mL for children over 2 years old, and 0.1 mL for younger children and infants). Once the patient is stabilized, this should be followed with administration of an antihistamine orally or IM (e.g., diphenhydramine hydrochloric acid). Systemic corticosteroids are not indicated in the management of acute allergic reactions because an anti-inflammatory effect may take up to 48 hours to occur. If shock occurs, IV saline may be necessary to support the circulation, and pressor agents (e.g., levarterenol bitartrate) may be administered if necessary. If dyspnea and/or hypoxia occur, oxygen should be administered by mask or positive pressure, and endotracheal intubation or tracheostomy may be necessary for maintenance of an adequate airway if laryngeal edema occurs.

Hyposensitization may be induced by the administration of gradually increasing amounts of antigen derived from venom sacs, causing the patient to produce IgG antibodies that block the effect of IgE antibodies and thus prevent the release of histamine and other mast cell–derived mediators. Immunotherapy must be continued indefinitely to maintain a state of hyposensitivity to the insect venom, and since the venoms may induce an anaphylactic reaction in hypersensitive persons, they must be administered with care.

Tick bites are responsible for the transmission of a number of infectious diseases, including rickettsial and spirochetal diseases. The category of ***rickettsial diseases*** includes a variety of illnesses in which transmission involves an insect vector (usually an arthropod) that is known to infect humans. Common features of the rickettsias are a sudden onset, fever lasting for 1 or more weeks, headache, malaise, peripheral vasculitis, prostration, and often a characteristic eruption. The rickettsias penetrate the skin or mucosa when the insect vector bites the host and multiply within the cells of the endothelial lining of small blood vessels. A number of tick-borne rickettsial infections may result in spotted fevers, and probably all are transmitted by ixodid (hard) ticks.

The most common of these infections is ***Rocky Mountain spotted fever,*** an acute disease due to *Rickettsia rickettsii.* About 70% of patients report a history of a tick bite (most common in the western United States is the wood tick, *Dermacentor andersoni,* and in the eastern United States it is the dog tick, *D. variabilis*). After a 3- to 12-day period of incubation (average, 7 days) following the bite by an infected tick, there is a sudden onset of systemic symptoms, including sore throat, severe headache, chills, anorexia, malaise, nausea, prostration, and conjunctival injection.

Within several days, the temperature may be elevated (as high as 39.5–40.0°C) and in severe cases it will remain high for 15–20 days. The fever may be accompanied by progression of the early symptoms, as well as muscular and abdominal pain, nausea and vomiting, restlessness, irritability, and insomnia. As the condition progresses, splenomegaly, hepatomegaly, jaundice, myocarditis, gangrene, uremia, delirium, lethargy, stupor, and coma may also occur. At the time of the onset of the fever, a local lesion (eschar) appears, which is a small (2- to 5-mm) ulcer with a black center, often accompanied by nearby lymphadenopathy. Between the second and sixth day (average, fourth day) of the fever, a red maculopapular eruption appears, first on the wrists, forearms, and ankles, spreading centrally, with individual lesions becoming larger and petechial. The rash spreads for about 2–3 days, extending to most areas of the body, including the palms and soles. The fever subsides by the end of the second week in most mild, untreated cases, and death is uncommon except in very old or debilitated persons (the mortality for untreated elderly persons is about 70%). Leukocytosis and protein and blood cells in the urine are common findings.

Rickettsiae can sometimes be isolated from the blood in the first few days of the illness, but a rise in antibody titer is evident during the second week of illness before antimicrobial drug therapy is begun. Specific complement fixation, immunofluorescence, microagglutination, and a Weil-Felix reaction test with *Proteus* OX19 and OX2 are the methods used to detect the increased number of antibodies. If oral chloramphenicol (50 mg per kilogram of body weight every 6–8 hours) or tetracycline (25 mg/kg every 6–8 hours) therapy is instituted early (when the rash first appears), prompt alleviation of the signs and symptoms will occur. The antibiotic treatment should produce obvious clinical improvement within 36–48 hours, with a reduction in the fever in 48–72 hours, and should be continued until such improvement occurs and for 24 hours after the fever is gone. Antibiotics may also be given IV if the patient is too ill to take oral medication, and in late severe cases, large doses of oral corticosteroids may be given in combination with the antibiotics for about 3 days.

Erythema chronicum migrans (ECM) is the skin lesion of another disease probably transmitted by an *Ixodes* (*dammini*) tick. Lyme disease (or Lyme arthritis) is an illness characterized by an early skin lesion (ECM), a red macule or papule usually occurring on the proximal portion of an extremity (particularly the thigh) or on the trunk (especially the buttocks or axillae). The initial lesion grows as large as 50 cm in diameter, often with a central clearing, giving a characteristic bull's-eye appearance, and is often hot to the touch. About 25% of patients have a history of tick bite 3 days to 3 weeks prior to the onset of the lesion. The patient may not have noticed the lesion, but it may have been brought to his or her attention by a family member. About half of the patients develop additional multiple lesions (usually smaller and without central indurations). ECM generally lasts for a few weeks, but in the course of resolution faint evanescent lesions may appear, and lesions that have previously resolved may reappear faintly afterward, sometimes preceding recurrent bouts of arthritis. Among the symptoms that accompany (or precede) ECM are fever, headache, chills, stiff neck, malaise, and fatigue, and, less commonly, nausea, vomiting, sore throat, lymphadenopathy, backache, myalgias, and splenomegaly. Most of these occur briefly (for a few days) or intermittently, but malaise and fatigue may persist for weeks. *Borrelia burgdorferi,* a spirochete, is the causative organism. The response to early treatment with penicillin G or tetracycline is usually prompt, resulting in the disappearance of the lesion (ECM) and prevention or attenuation of the subsequent complication of arthritis, which occurs within weeks or months of the onset of ECM in about half these patients (see the discussion of Lyme arthritis in Chapter 11).

▶ ***Pediculosis*** (infestation by lice) may occur on the scalp (pediculosis capitis, caused by *Pediculus humanus capitis*), the trunk (pediculosis corporis, caused by *P. humanus corporis*), or the genital region (pediculosis pubis, due to *Phthirus pubis*). Head and body lice are about 3–4 mm long and similar in appearance. Pubic lice are larger. Transmission of ***pediculosis capitis*** occurs through close personal contact and shared use of combs and hats. It is common among school children, spreading rapidly throughout classrooms, camp groups, or other situations of close contact. Infestation is primarily localized to the scalp, but the eyebrows, eyelashes, and beard may also be involved. Severe pruritus and excoriation are common, sometimes with secondary bacterial infection, and moderate swelling of posterior cervical lymph nodes frequently occurs. Once infestation is considered, diagnosis is fairly simple. Examination of the scalp (preferably with a hand lens) reveals numerous small, grayish-white, ovoid specks ("nits") that represent ova, attached to the shaft of scalp hairs close to the base. These are best seen near the ears and at the nape of the neck. The ova cannot be removed and mature in 3–4 days. Lice are more difficult to find but may be seen most easily behind the ears and around the occiput.

The less common ***pediculosis corporis*** involves intense pruritus and excoriation. Inspection commonly reveals small red punctate lesions (due to bites) on the shoulders, buttocks, and abdomen, often associated with linear scratch marks, urticaria, or pyoderma. Nits may be seen on body hairs, but exam of the undergarments and seams of clothing in contact with skin reveals both nits and lice, since the body louse inhabits the clothing and comes onto the skin only to feed. Furunculosis may occasionally occur as a complication.

Pediculosis pubis ("crabs") is usually transmitted venereally but may be acquired by sitting on an infested toilet seat. Pruritus is common, and a careful search for these parasites must be performed for all complaints of anogenital itching. Although these lice are large, a diligent search is often required, since they may be few in number and may resemble the crusts of scratch dermatitis. A scattering of tiny dark brown specks on undergarments (louse excreta), ova attached to the skin at the base of pubic hairs, or small bluish or slate-colored macules (which do not blanch on pressure) on the skin of the pubic region and trunk are all signs of the infestation. Excoriation and a secondary dermatitis (often from self-medication) are common.

Treatment for pediculosis is curative, and relief of symptoms by treatment of uncertain cases may serve to confirm the tentative diagnosis of louse infestation. Application of 1% lindane (Kwell, Scabene) or pyrethrins in lotion form (Rid, Pyrinate 200) once daily for 2 days and then repeated after 10 days to destroy any nits that may have matured in the interim is sufficient in most cases, but simultaneous treatment of infested family members and other close contacts (particularly sexual contacts in the case of pediculosis pubis), as well as decontamination of sources of infection (combs, hats, clothing, bedding), are necessary to prevent recurrences. Recurrences are common, but prolonged parasitide use should be avoided because it may produce a persistent genital dermatitis, particularly in men. Persistent pruritus following treatment is not an indication for retreatment unless living mites are demonstrated after about 7 days.

▶ ***Scabies*** ("the itch") is another common parasitic skin infection caused by the itch mite (*Sarcoptes scabiei*) and characterized by superficial burrows ("runs" or "galleries"), vesicular and pustular lesions, intense (nocturnal) pruritus, and secondary infection from excoriation. Transmission occurs through close contact with an infested person, during which time an impregnated female mite burrows into the stratum corneum, depositing eggs along the tunnel she creates. When the eggs hatch (within a few days), the larvae congregate along hair follicles. The mite may appear to the naked eye as a minuscule white dot. Lesions, which are thought to be due to a hypersensitivity reaction to the parasites, consist of small pruritic vesicles and pustules associated with a generalized excoriation; the head and neck are usually spared (except in infants). Runs or galleries appear as short (2- to 3-mm-long), wavy dark lines resembling pencil marks on the palms, heels, and sides of fingers, and, less commonly, on the axillae, flexor surfaces of wrists and elbows, belt area, lower buttocks, about the areolae of the breasts in women and on the genitals in men. These burrows typically have a single minute lesion (papule) at their open ends. By probing the fresh end of a run with a pointed scalpel, it is possible to demonstrate the female mite, which tends to cling to the tip of the blade. Shaving of an entire run will reveal not only the mite but her eggs and feces (small black dots) as well. If the disease has persisted for a number of weeks, the burrows may be difficult to find, because the severe pruritus soon results in excoriation and possibly a secondary bacterial infection. Secondary lesions (urticarial, eczematous, etc.) may result from a severe hypersensitivity reaction to the mites.

The diagnosis of scabies must be confirmed by examination of a mounted specimen in mineral oil or glycerin, revealing the mite, ova, and/or feces. Treatment of scabies consists primarily of disinfestation with 1% lindane (Kwell or Scabene) or crotamiton (Eurax). All infested family members or other close contacts should be treated simultaneously to prevent reinfestation. Pyoderma should be treated with appropriate systemic antibiotics unless the infection is minimal and localized, in which case a topical antibiotic ointment may be sufficient.

Chronic discoid lupus erythematosus is a variable disorder of unknown etiology, although exposure to sunlight precedes the initial eruption in many cases. An asymmetric distribution of raised, sharply circumscribed, dusky red to purple lesions (macules, papules, and plaques) frequently appears on the face in the typical butterfly arrangement (over the nose and cheeks), but may also appear on the trunk and extensor surfaces without facial involvement. Individual lesions may be single or multiple round, scaling papules 5–20 mm in diameter. As the disease progresses, the lesions become covered with dry, adherent scales that invaginate into dilated follicles, giving a "carpet tack" appearance. The edges of untreated lesions gradually extend to the surrounding skin as the centers atrophy. Telangiectasia, hyperpigmentation and/or hypopigmentation, and scarring are common, and when the scalp is involved, there may be permanent hair loss. Leukopenia, proteinuria, and the appearance of the disorder in a person younger than age 30 are suggestive of the more severe connective tissue disorder systemic lupus erythematosus (SLE). Laboratory tests should always be performed to rule out this possibility. Biopsy of the active margin of the lesion, complete blood count (CBC), ESR, urinalysis, and anti-DNA CH_{50} and C3 tests should be obtained. The antinuclear antibody test is the most helpful one for ruling out the systemic form of the disease, since direct immunofluorescence tests of "uninvolved" skin adjacent to a lesion are negative for the basement membrane antibody in discoid lupus erythematosus but positive in SLE.

Although there are usually no symptoms, early treatment of discoid lupus erythematosus is important before scarring becomes permanent. Sunlight and other forms of strong radiation should be avoided. General measures should include adequate nutrition, supplementary vitamins (vitamin E in oral doses of 400–2,000 IU daily may be particularly helpful) and iron as required, and treatment of chronic infections. Antimalarial drugs may be used for chronic discoid lupus erythematosus, but whenever possible, it is preferable to consider the disorder as a cosmetic defect only and to treat it as such, with topical measures or camouflaging agents. Local measures include injections of a corticosteroid suspension directly into the lesions (e.g., triamcinolone acetonide, 2.5 mg/mL, may be used once a week or once a month), or topical corticosteroid creams may be applied at night and covered with a thin plastic film. If local measures are not helpful, systemic chloroquine phosphate (.025 g/day every day for 1 week, and then 0.25 g twice a week), hydroxychloroquine sulfate (0.2 g/day and then twice a week), or quinacrine (100 mg/day) may be administered (for the discoid form only). An ophthalmic exam should be performed every 3 months if these medications are continued, since they have been known to cause serious eye changes. Quinacrine causes yellowing of the skin, but it may be the safest of the antimalarials, since it has not been reported to cause eye damage.

Sensation

A variety of sensations are perceived through the skin, providing information about both environmental and bodily conditions. Interpretation and discrimination of stimuli received from the external environment (perceived as varying degrees of pain, temperature, touch, and pressure) is dependent on different types of receptors located in the skin, as well as differing patterns of stimulation presented to the cerebral cortex. For example, the sensations of pain, pressure, touch, and itching may be transmitted by the same neurons, but each of these is mediated and perceived differently. Bundles of large nerves in the subcutaneous layer send branches to nerve plexuses in the reticular and papillary dermis, which in turn send branches to the numerous nerve endings and receptors located in different levels of the subcutaneous tissue, dermis, and epidermis. In addition to sensory nerves, sympathetic (afferent) nerve fibers supply blood vessels, secretory cells of sweat glands, and the arrectores pilorum.

Free nerve endings are terminations of sensory nerve fibers that occur everywhere in the skin (and in many other tissues). They are located in and just below the epidermis, in hair papillae and root sheaths, and around the sweat glands. The myelinated nerve fibers that lead to these endings lose their myelin sheath as they near their termination, leaving only the axon with its surrounding neurilemma, which also disappears at the fiber's termination, leaving just the axon, which splits into fine nerve fibrils that, in turn, penetrate the basement membrane (basal lamina) to terminate between epidermal cells. These endings interpret environmental stimulation as varying degrees of touch, pressure, pain (including itching), and temperature.

Meissner's corpuscles are small, encapsulated sensory receptors of touch located within the dermal papillae in the superficial papillary layer of the dermis just beneath the basement membrane. They are most numerous in the highly sensitive regions of skin, such as the palms, soles, fronts of the forearms, lips, nipples of the breasts, and certain mucosal surfaces. These end organs appear as small oval structures surrounded by a connective tissue capsule and filled with layers of tiny "plates" stacked upon one another. When the unmyelinated end of a large sensory nerve fiber penetrates the end organ's capsule, it branches into whorls of terminal nerve filaments that spiral within the corpuscle between the plates and terminate near the top edge. The ability to recognize the exact point on the body that is being touched, as well as the texture of an object that is touched, is thought to be dependent on these receptors, which are characterized by a rapid adaptation to stimulation (probably within about a second after being stimulated). This means that they transmit information about an initial stimulation but cease to respond to that stimulus if it continues much beyond a period of about a second. The tips of the fingers and other highly sensitive areas where large numbers of Meissner's corpuscles are present also contain expanded tip tactile receptors, including Ruffini's end organs, Merkel's disks, and other variants. Merkel's disks are slower at adapting to stimulation than Meissner's corpuscles, enabling them to transmit continuous signals about sustained touch. A few of these expanded tip endings occur on hairy body surfaces, but these regions have almost no Meissner's corpuscles.

The combination of a hair and the nerve fiber that entwines its base is called a "hair end organ," another touch receptor that adapts very soon after stimulation. Therefore, like Meissner's corpuscles, it responds primarily to the initial sensation of touch and movement of an object along the body surface but is unable to transmit continuous information about sustained pressure.

Ruffini's end organs (corpuscles of Ruffini) are oval, encapsulated end organs that occur in the deep subcutaneous skin layers as well as in deeper body tissues. They are most numerous in the subcutaneous tissue of the fingertips very close to the junction of the subcutaneous tissue and the dermis. Within the strong connective tissue sheath of this receptor, nerve fibers branch extensively and end in small knobs. These nerve endings do not adapt rapidly and are therefore capable of signaling continuous touch and pressure sensations, as well as heavy touch (since they also occur in deeper tissues).

Pacinian corpuscles are rapidly adapting spherical receptors sensitive to vibration and other extremely rapid tissue state changes. They are located in the subcutaneous tissue or deep reticular layer of the dermis, and are most numerous in the skin of the palms, soles, and genitalia. Each Pacinian corpuscle is attached to the end of a single nerve fiber and in cross-section appears as a white oval bulb 2–4 mm in diameter with onion-like laminations. As with the nerves terminating in free nerve endings, the nerve fiber traversing the axis of this receptor loses its myelin sheath first and then its neurilemma, until it ends in a tuberculated enlargement within the corpuscle's central cavity. This receptor adapts to incoming sensory information within a fraction of a second and is therefore able to transmit information about tissue changes only at the onset of the stimulus.

Pain may be categorized into a variety of types, including sharp, stinging, burning, aching, throbbing, or cramping. However, most classifications describe three basic types of pain: pricking, burning, and aching. Pricking pain refers to the type of sensation that occurs when the skin is stuck by a needle, cut with a knife, or receives diffuse but strong irritation. Burning pain is typically excruciating, and is the type of sensation felt when the skin is burned. Aching pain is a deeper sensation that may vary from low to high in intensity. The sensation of ***pruritus*** (itching), which originates exclusively in the skin and provokes an urge to scratch, is sometimes considered a mild variation of the pain sensation. Other theories suggest that the nerve fibers that transmit the sensation perceived as itching are different from those that transmit pain sensations. However, certain chemicals have been isolated that have been demonstrated to cause pruritus, including histamine, proteolytic agents, and vasoactive polypeptides.

The list of causes of pruritus is extensive and includes environmental conditions (climate, irritants and allergens, insect bites), parasites, skin diseases (atopic dermatitis, blistering diseases, fungal and bacterial infections, seborrhea, psoriasis, and others), and systemic conditions such as endocrine conditions (including pregnancy and diabetes), hepatobiliary disorders, renal disorders, hematologic disorders, infectious diseases (e.g., herpes zoster, herpes simplex), malignancies, and psychogenic disorders. Some of the factors that influence the perception of pruritus are heat, moisture, level of consciousness of body sensations, and stress. Therefore, pruritus of practically any cause may be reduced by maintenance of a constant temperature, mental or physical occupation, and sometimes cooling measures (e.g., cool compresses). Oral antihistamines may also be useful, particularly if they are supplemented with lubricating agents or cool compresses. Medium-potency topical corticosteroid preparations or other local treatments (e.g., menthol, crotamiton) may also provide symptomatic relief, but the cause of pruritus should always be ascertained as well and treated or eliminated whenever possible.

EPIDERMIS

Above the dermis and firmly adherent to it is the epidermis, a specialized epithelium primarily of ectodermal origin. These two layers together vary in thickness from about 0.5 to over 4.0 mm throughout the body surface, and although it is the thickness of the dermis that primarily determines these variations, it is the thickness of the epidermis that is the basis of the classification of skin as thick or thin. The glabrous skin (smooth, hairless) of the palms and soles, where the epidermis may be as thick as 0.8–1.4 mm, is referred to as "thick skin." The epidermis of this type of skin contains a layer, the stratum lucidum, which is absent in thin skin. The remainder of the body surface is covered by thin skin, the epidermis of which is usually 0.07–0.12 mm thick. The epidermis is thinnest on the eyelids and scalp.

Most of the cells of the epidermis arise from mitotic divisions in the deepest layers of the epidermis. They are gradually displaced through the overlying layers toward the surface, and as they move upward, undergo a process called "keratinization" in which they elaborate a relatively insoluble waxy protein called "keratin." It is partly this substance, which eventually replaces most of the cytoplasm of the cells, that makes the skin surface somewhat waterproof and thereby affords the body some protection against dehydration. As the cells progress toward the surface, they also become flattened, lose their nuclei, and are eventually desquamated (shed).

The epidermis contains no blood vessels, and the cells of the deepest layer depend on diffusion of nutrients and fluid from the vessels in the underlying dermis. As a result, the cells that move toward the surface and away from the blood supply of the dermis gradually dehydrate and die.

The second component of the epidermis is the melanocytes, which are specialized cells derived from the neural crest. These cells produce a pigment called "melanin" and do not undergo keratinization. (These are discussed in the section on pigmentation.)

There are four distinct layers of epidermis throughout the body surface, except on the palms and soles, where there are five (see Fig. 10.1). In order, from the deepest layer to the most superficial, they are the stratum germinativum (or basal layer), stratum spinosum (or prickle cell layer), stratum granulosum, stratum lucidum (present only on the palms and soles), and the outermost stratum corneum (or horny layer).

The deepest layer, the stratum germinativum, is composed of a single row of cuboidal or columnar epithelium resting on a thin basement membrane (or basal lamina), which in turn conforms to the irregular surface of the dermal papillary layer. The nuclei of its cells are elongated and the cell walls are indistinct. The basal surface of each cell possesses thin, short cytoplasmic processes that fit into corresponding indentations in the basal lamina, apparently anchoring the epithelium to the dermis below. Several hemidesmosomes occur on the plasma membrane next to the basal lamina, and desmosomes that appear to bind the cells together occur on the lateral and upper surfaces of the cells of this layer. Mitosis, limited to this layer and possibly to the cells immediately above it, produces cells at the rate at which they are desquamated from the surface of the skin. The epidermis will regenerate without scar formation as long as this layer of cells remains undamaged. Interspersed among the cells of this stratum are melanocytes, which specialize in the production of the pigment melanin.

The cells of the stratum spinosum, several layers thick, are irregular and polygonal, and possess well-defined intercellular bridges that appear as spine-like projections. The bridges consist of short cytoplasmic projections of two neighboring cells that meet at a desmosome. Tonofibrils, bundles of filaments that are present in the cytoplasm of these cells, are thought to be the principal precursor of keratin. As the cells (keratocytes or prickle cells) move toward the surface, they become flattened.

The cells of the stratum germinativum and the stratum spinosum (together termed the "Malpighian layer" or "stratum Malpighii") are responsible for proliferation and initiation of keratinization. Dispersed among the cells of this layer are melanocytes, Merkel cells, and Langerhans cells. The last have been shown to have surface properties similar to those of macrophages, and are believed to play a role in determining susceptibility to the development of allergic contact dermatitis.

The two to three layers of flattened cells of the stratum granulosum are named for the granules of a histidine-rich substance (keratohyalin) present in their cytoplasm that are believed to play a role in the formation of soft keratin. Cells begin to die in this layer of the epidermis.

Present only in the skin of the palms and the soles, the stratum lucidum is a thin layer, three to five cells deep, of flattened cells that in stained sections appear translucent. The cells of this layer are dead, have no nuclei, and contain a diffuse translucent compound called "eleidin," which is presumed to arise from the keratohyalin in the granules of the infra-adjacent layer and to be a precursor of keratin.

Several rows of clear, dry, scale-like, and highly keratinized cells make up the outermost layer of the skin, the stratum corneum, which serves as the body's first line of defense against the external environment. Living cells require a fluid environment with a pH and other variables that are controlled. The high content of keratin in the dead cells of the stratum corneum makes this layer an effective waterproof barrier against dehydration. In addition, the outermost cells have an acid pH that kills some microorganisms and are poor conductors of heat, providing some protection against heat loss or gain. The most superficial cells of this stratum are flattened and continually flake off (desquamate), to be replaced by cells migrating outward from the deeper layers of the epidermis. The thickness of this epidermal layer varies over the body surface, being thickest where the greatest stimulation is received (from weight bearing or abrasion), as on the soles of the feet.

Ichthyosis refers to rough, dry scaling of the skin without erythema. Close exam may reveal a fine scaling with plugged follicles or large, loosely adherent polyhedral scales. There may be an exaggeration of normal creases on the palms and soles. It may be a mild condition due to an enviornmental cause (frequent bathing, cold weather), irritation (e.g., from detergents), or part of the normal aging process (senile dry skin), or it may be a symptom of an underlying systemic disorder. There are also a number of ichthyosiform dermatoses (ichthyoses) that are inherited and have their onset in infancy or childhood. These are characterized by generalized or characteristically distributed dryness and scaling of the skin that is caused by the retention of excessive amounts of keratin on the skin surface. ***Xeroderma (dry skin)*** is the mildest form of ichthyosis, being more common in middle-aged or older persons (because of the decreased amount of lipids in the skin) or in persons who bathe often. It is characterized by fine, dry scaling of the skin and often by mild to moderate itching. It may involve the general body surface or may be confined to one area, particularly the lower legs and feet. Cold weather may aggravate the condition, and the superimposition of an irritation dermatitis (e.g., from detergents or other irritants) is common.

Treatment for this minor condition includes application of an emollient such as petrolatum two or three times a day, preferably after hydration of the skin by soaking, while the skin is still moist. Covering the area with an occlusive dressing at bedtime will increase the amount absorbed by the skin. Lubricants that contain 15–30% urea or a preparation containing 6% salicylic acid in a gel base of propylene glycol, ethyl alcohol, hydroxypropylene cellulose, and water may be helpful in freeing retained keratin on the skin surface. The latter can also be applied two or three times a day and covered with an occlusive dressing at night (it should not be occluded with children). When the scaling has lessened, it may be applied only occasionally. Other lubricants include cold cream, equal parts of hydrophilic petrolatum and water, and 50% propylene glycol in water. Patients should be instructed that too frequent bathing and exposure to cold weather may be etiologic factors. Measures to increase the environmental moisture content (indoor humidifiers) may also be beneficial. Asymptomatic ichthyosis may be associated with a number of systemic diseases, including leprosy, hypothyroidism (yellowish, due to carotenemia), Hodgkin's disease and other lymphomas, multiple myeloma, sarcoidosis, and carcinoma of the breast. It may range from a localized fine, dry scaling on the trunk and legs to a widespread thick scaling. Refsum's syndrome is an inherited metabolic disorder characterized by ichthyosis. Butyrophenones and triparanol are among the drugs that may cause ichthyosis by a similar inhibition of lipid synthesis. Lubrication may be helpful for ichthyosis due to one of these causes, but treatment of the underlying condition is the most helpful. Ichthyosis that is caused by a drug will respond to discontinuation of the responsible agent.

Keratosis pilaris is a common condition in which plugs of keratin block the openings of hair follicles, resulting in numerous small, pointed papules on the outer aspects of the upper arms, buttocks, and thighs. Treatment is usually unnecessary, but the same agents described for use in ichthyosis may help to flatten the papules, making them less noticeable.

Calluses and corns are localized areas of overgrowth of the stratum corneum (hyperkeratosis) due to repeated trauma (pressure and friction) from a number of causes, such as faulty weight bearing, poorly fitting shoes, and deformities. Tenderness to pressure may be the only symptom of a callus, but corns tend to be painful. Corns, which are conical, occur most frequently over toe joints and between toes. Paring away the overlying stratum corneum of a callus or corn will help to differentiate it from a plantar wart, revealing a glassy core (a wart has multiple bleeding points from thrombosed capillaries when pared) and skin lines that go straight through the lesion, rather than circling it. Also, pressing straight down on the lesion will elicit pain in a callus or corn, while lateral squeezing pressure will elicit pain in a wart. Both soft corns and warts may itch, especially if they occur in moist skin areas such as interdigital spaces.

Treatment of corns and calluses consists primarily of correcting the causes of the mechanical pressure on the site. Soft, properly fitted shoes and orthopedic devices (e.g., arch inserts, metatarsal plates or bars) to correct deformities, and foam rubber or moleskin pads or rings may help prevent recurrences by redistributing pressure form weight bearing. The use of protective gloves can often help to prevent calluses of the hands occurring from such activities as driving, sailing, gardening, and racket sports. A callus may be removed by soaking in warm water for several minutes and then rubbing it with a rough towel, pumice stone, or emery board to remove loosened tissue or carefully paring it away. A keratolytic agent (Keralyt gel with 6% salicylic acid) may also be applied locally to the callus or corn each night and covered with an occlusive wrapping. More potent keratolytic agents (e.g., containing 20% or more salicylic acid) are available as well, but great care must be taken to avoid getting any of these products on normal surrounding skin. Persons who tend to form corns or calluses frequently should be referred to a podiatrist for regular care. Patients with diabetes mellitus or other conditions involving impaired peripheral circulation or insensitive extremities also require special foot care.

Warts (verrucae) are common, benign epithelial tumors occurring anywhere on the skin or mucous membranes (hands and fingers are common sites), caused by papillomaviruses (papovaviruses). They may appear at any age, but are most common in children and young adults and least common in elderly persons. They are usually less than 0.5 cm in diameter, but their size and appearance may vary according to their location and the amount of irritation and trauma they receive. Warts may occur singly or in clusters, are contagious, and may be spread by autoinoculation. About one-half to two-thirds of them resolve spontaneously in months, although some may persist for years and new ones may recur at the site of an old one. Most warts are unresponsive to intervention. During resolution the warts may become reddened, painful, and bleed.

Common warts (verrucae vulgaris), which account for about 75% of all such lesions, appear most frequently on the fingers, elbows, knees, scalp, and face. Local trauma is believed to play a role. They are usually well circumscribed, round or irregular, firm, and have a verrucous surface. They range from light gray to yellow to brown to gray-black and from 2 to 10 mm in diameter. ***Periungual warts*** are common warts occurring near the nail plate. Nail biting seems to contribute to their occurrence and spread to other nails. When they disturb the underlying nail matrix, the nail plate may be distorted. ***Plantar warts*** are flattened common warts that occur on the sole of the foot. They are surrounded by thickened cornified epithelium and are often extremely tender. Paring away the surface will differentiate them from corns and calluses, because there will be multiple pinpoint sites of bleeding from thrombosed capillaries. Plaques of multiple, small, closely situated plantar warts are called "mosaic warts." The most common appearance is of a single large lesion surrounded by a cluster of satellite warts. Small, long, narrow, flesh-colored growths occurring on the eyelids, face, neck, or lips are called ***filiform warts.*** They occur more frequently in men than in women and may be clustered or have several finger-like projections radiating from a single base. They are asymptomatic but persist if untreated.

Flat warts (plane warts) are smooth, flat-topped, flesh-colored or yellow-brown lesions that occur mainly in children and young adults, most commonly on the face, hands, and along scratch marks from autoinoculation. Since they lack the rough verrucous texture of common warts, it is sometimes difficult to differentiate them from lichen planus, but the latter have lesions that are often pruritic and violaceous, and tend to occur on the flexor surfaces and oral mucosa. A biopsy of skin lesions will confirm the diagnosis when there is doubt. Moist warts (anogenital or "venereal" warts, condylomata acuminata) are discussed in Chapter 9. Warts, which represent a proliferation and elongation of the stratum corneum by the papillomavirus (as opposed to a simple packing of layers of stratum corneum in corns and calluses), may be differentiated from these other lesions by examination of the surface (a rough appearance is more likely in a wart, and smooth surfaces are typical of calluses and corns) and a careful paring of the stratum corneum of the lesion, which will reveal "seeds" (multiple dark pinpoint sites of bleeding from thrombosed, elongated capillary ends) and skin lines that circle the lesion and form a distinct border. Pressure elicited by lateral squeezing is also characteristic of warts.

Although most warts are self-limited, the development of immunity may require years, and autoinoculation is common with persistent lesions. Therefore, removal is desirable in many cases. Common warts may be removed by cryotherapy, freezing with liquid nitrogen or solid carbon dioxide (most dermatologists or podiatrists can perform this procedure). The freezing agent is applied intermittently (for 20–30 seconds) to the wart until the area of frost that develops extends just beyond the border of the lesion. A blister appears at the site within 2 or 3 days, and healing often occurs in 3–4 weeks, but many warts require multiple treatments, which should be done every 3 weeks. As an alternative for small warts, especially if there are several, cantharidin (Cantharone) may be applied to each wart every 2–3 weeks until the warts resolve. Other agents containing salicylic acid in collodion (e.g., Duofilm) and nonprescription preparations (Compound W, Vergo, and Wart-off) may be applied once daily to the wart after soaking it in hot water for 5 minutes. However, this treatment may take 6–8 weeks, and since the patient will be applying the agent, he or she should be warned to avoid getting it on healthy skin. An application of petrolatum around each wart may help prevent this occurrence. Both the light, repeated freezing and the application of salicylic acid preparations produce a low-grade irritation that disturbs the cell wall of the wart, allowing the papillomavirus to be absorbed into the circulation and thereby promoting the immune response to the virus (through the production of IgG antibodies). Also, a specialist (or properly trained primary care provider) may excise warts surgically with quick and relatively atraumatic results, but scarring may result from this technique (or even from freezing or electrodesiccation with curettage). Experience with each of these methods is important to minimize this potential.

Molluscum contagiosum is characterized by flesh-colored, smooth, shiny, umbilicated papules occurring anywhere on the skin and frequently in the pubic and genital regions. The lesions range in diameter from 2 to 10 mm, but a single "giant" molluscum may grow as large as 2 to 3 cm. They are due to an infection caused by a poxvirus and are spread by direct contact, particularly venereal. There are generally no symptoms unless the lesions become secondarily infected. The characteristic central depression, which is filled with a semisolid material, makes diagnosis easy, and exam of the expressed material from the lesion, stained with Giemsa stain, reveals numerous large cells with inclusion bodies. Autoinoculation may spread the disease, but it may also resolve spontaneously within months. Successful treatment includes removal by cryotherapy or excision.

► ***Psoriasis,*** a common, acute or chronic, recurrent skin disease characterized by one or more sharply demarcated, pink or red elevated patches of skin covered by dry, silvery scales often presents with a dominant inheritance pattern. The disorder may be limited to a small area with one or two lesions, or it may occur as a generalized, life-threatening dermatosis with widespread, intractable exfoliation and, in about 10–15% of patients, an associated arthritis (psoriatic arthritis).

An early primary lesion is usually round and less than 2–4 cm in diameter, but individual plaques may be large enough to cover a major portion of a limb or trunk. Irregularly shaped lesions may also occur, especially on the trunk ("geographic plaques," deriving their name from their map-like appearance). Any area of the body may be affected, but the extensor surfaces of the limbs (e.g., elbows and knees) are characteristically the first sites of involvement. Psoriasis is also common on the scalp, back, and buttocks. On the scalp it may range from a diffuse, fine scaling (resembling dandruff or seborrheic dermatitis) to an adherent crust that may extend to the forehead and temples. When the external ears are involved, there is typically diffuse erythema, scaling, and sometimes crusting that may also affect the region behind the ears. Psoriasis of the body folds and anogenital areas tends to be associated with severe pruritus, some scaling, and a particularly bright erythema. Annular (ring-shaped) plaques with central clear areas are another variation. A Koebner phenomenon is also a common finding, with an eruption within 1–2 weeks at the site of a skin trauma that mimics the shape of the original injury (isomorphic response). Nail involvement occurs in approximately 30% of patients and may be the only manifestation. It may produce a number of changes, including fine stippling, ridging, fraying, pitting, or discoloration of the plate, distal plate separation (onycholysis) and flaring, increased nail plate thickness, and subungual hyperkeratosis (build-up of psoriatic scales beneath the nail). Studies have indicated that psoriasis is most likely rooted in an abnormally rapid proliferation of cells in the epidermis. There is also evidence that suggests an immunologic factor in the disorder, and direct and indirect immunofluorescent tests have revealed a number of antibodies within the skin of persons with psoriasis. The incidence in men and women is equal, and although onset can occur at any age, it is most common prior to age 30.

Pustular psoriasis is characterized by small, discrete, sterile pustules that may be localized to the palms and soles or generalized to include any part of the body. These pustules may be associated with erythema, scaling, and leukocytosis, and there may be common psoriatic lesions in other body regions at the same time. ***Guttate*** (or "spotty") ***psoriasis*** is a variant that is more common in children. It tends to follow acute streptococcal or other upper respiratory tract infections. Lesions are typically 2–3 mm in diameter, discrete, and occur all over the body surface. Treatment for psoriasis may range from topical lubricating, keratolytic, and steroid formulations, exposure to sunlight, and psoralens and ultraviolet radiation (PUVA) therapy to systemic antimetabolites (e.g., methotrexate) for severe skin and joint involvement. The latter has a potential for hematologic, renal, and hepatic toxicity. It requires careful monitoring and should be administered only by persons experienced in its use in the treatment of psoriasis.

Fungal (mycotic) ***infections*** may occur anywhere on the skin or mucous membranes, but cutaneous infections are most common on the scalp, beneath the breasts, and on the legs (especially the upper thighs) and the feet, and the appearance of a dermatosis in a characteristic location (e.g., intertriginous) may be an important clue to the diagnosis. Superficial infections are most frequently caused by dermatophytes, fungi that grow in or on the nonliving tissues of the integument (stratum corneum of the epidermis, hair, nails) and rarely penetrate deeper, but *Candida albicans* and *Pityrosporon orbiculare* (causes tinea versicolor) may also be responsible. Since the treatment for all of these infections is quite different, it is extremely important that the appropriate laboratory procedures be employed to identify the responsible organism as well as to rule out other causes, such as a bacterial infection or allergic contact dermatitis. *Corynebacterium erythrasmae* infection in particular produce skin lesions resembling those of a fungal infection. Laboratory tests for a suspected fungus include exam of scrapings of lesions prepared with 15% potassium hydroxide (KOH), cultures of the organisms, exam with Wood's light (see Table 10.5), and biopsy sections stained with periodic acid-Schiff technique. There are no useful serologic tests at present for detecting fungal causes of infections.

► ***Tinea*** (ringworm) is the name given to any cutaneous fungus infection, and infections occurring at particular body locations are named according to the area of involvement. ***Tinea capitis*** is a fungal infection of the skin of the scalp, once caused predominantly by *Microsporum* infection (*M. gypseum, M. canis,* or *M. audouini*) but now caused almost exclusively by *Trichophyton tonsurans.* It is more common in children than adults and is contagious, spreading quickly through families and other groups with close contact (camps, school classrooms). The condition may be accompanied by slight itching but is generally asymptomatic. Tinea capitis due to *T. tonsurans* infection has a subtle onset with a mild, persistent inflammation and characteristic "black dots" that represent broken hairs. The organism, which is an endothrix (i.e., produces chains or arthrospores within the hairs, as opposed to those that produce spores arranged in a sheath on the outside of hairs and are designated ectothrix), as well as its spores, can be seen on microscopic exam. Affected hairs do not fluoresce under Wood's light. Tinea capitis due to *Microsporum audouini* has lesions that are small, scaly, grayish patches with hair loss (the "bald" spots are due to breaking off of hairs, not to disruption of hair growth). Affected hairs are dry, brittle, lusterless, and break easily. Involvement may be localized to a small area, or there may be extensive involvement with patches that coalesce until the entire scalp is affected. *M. canis* and *M. gypseum* produce a more inflammatory reaction with hair loss as well. Raised, red, and tender granulomas (kerions) commonly occur, followed soon afterward by healing. These kerions look very much like bacterial abscesses, however, so a definitive diagnosis (utilizing laboratory tests) is essential to avoid misdiagnosis and mistreatment. Direct microscopic exam of scrapings of lesions with a 15% KOH preparation reveals the organism, an ectothrix, with the spores it produces forming a sheath around individual affected hairs. In addition, exam of the scalp that is infected with *Microsporum* under Wood's light reveals infected hairs that fluoresce a light bright green. Tinea capitis must be differentiated from other conditions that may result in scalp hair loss, such as trichtillomania (voluntary pulling of one's own hair), alopecia areata, and so on.

Tinea corporis is a fungal infection of the body, particularly of exposed body surfaces (e.g., the face and arms), characterized by severely pruritic, scaling, annular (rings with raised borders and central clearing) lesions and small vesicles that surround the periphery. The lesions tend toward peripheral expansion and central resolution, and the disease is therefore often called "ringworm." All of the genera of dermatophytes have been known to cause this disorder, but *Trichophyton* is the most common. Often there is a history of exposure to an infected animal such as a cat. The rings of vesicles occur generally in clusters and in an asymmetric distribution on exposed body surfaces. The intense pruritus is a significant feature that distinguishes it from other annular lesions such as those of erythema multiforme, pityriasis rosea, and psoriasis. The infection may spread to the hair or nails or may become secondarily infected with bacteria. Also, a sensitivity reaction to the fungus may result in an allergic dermatitis elsewhere on the body (see the discussion of dermatophytids).

Tinea cruris ("jock itch" or "dhobie itch") is characterized by severe pruritus and annular erythematous macular lesions in intertriginous areas, particularly the groin and gluteal cleft. As in tinea corporis, the lesions tend to spread peripherally while the center slowly clears, but these are more indolent than the lesions of tinea corporis, since they are more subject to the effects of maceration and moisture from perspiration. Tinea cruris is more common in athletes and obese persons or those who perspire excessively. Individual lesions are sharply demarcated and may have vesicles at the borders of the erythematous lesions as well as satellite vesicles. Tinea cruris should be differentiated from other conditions that tend to affect intertriginous regions, including candidiasis, intertrigo, "inverse" psoriasis (psoriasis of body folds), seborrheic dermatitis, and erythrasma.

Tinea manuum and ***tinea pedis*** ("dermatophytosis" of the hands and feet, "athlete's foot") are characterized by pruritus, burning, and stinging, which accompany a vesicular eruption in the acute stage, and exfoliation, fissuring, scaling, and maceration and denudation in the subacute or chronic stages. Tinea pedis (dermatophytosis of the feet) is particularly common and is most frequently due to a *Trichophyton mentagrophytes* infection, but can also be due to *T. rubrum* or representatives of the species *Epidermophyton*. Tinea pedis most commonly involves the third and fourth interdigital spaces and is subject to acute flareups, with the formation of vesicles and bullae, in warm weather. There may be a thickening of the skin of the affected soles and palms, and the infection may spread to involve the nails, resulting in ***tinea unguium*** (onychomycosis), a destructive dermatophyte infection of one or more fingernails or toenails. *Trichophyton* (especially *T. mentagrophytes* and *T. rubrum*) and *Epidermophyton* (especially *E. floccosum*) are the most common causes of fungal infections of the nails (onychomycosis), but *Candida* may also cause it ***(candidal onychomycosis).*** In onychomycosis (tinea or candidal), the nail plate may become thickened, brittle, dull, and hypertrophic. Debris may accumulate under the free edge of the nail, and onycholysis (separation of the nail plate) may result in breaking off of irregular portions of the nail plate or loss of the entire nail.

Nail changes may result from a number of causes, and the treatments of each cause are quite specific. Since even the appropriate course of treatment may be prolonged, it is mandatory that cultures and other tests be used to confirm the specific etiologic factor(s) involved. Psoriatic involvement of the nail bed, in particular, may produce changes that resemble those of a fungal infection. Oral griseofulvin is an effective treatment for skin infections caused by *Trichophyton* and *Microsporum* species and *E. floccosum.* Also, topical application of miconazole 2% cream (Monistat-Derm) or clotrimazole 1% cream or lotion (Lotrimin or Mycelex) is effective for certain types of dermatophyte skin infections (not tinea capitis or onychomycosis, except with special measures to aid absorption), as is tolnaftate (Tinactin) solution or cream. Haloprogin (Halotex) 1% solution or cream or ciclopirox 1% cream may also be used topically. These are all strong irritants, and care should be taken to avoid overtreatment. The skin should be kept dry and open to the air as much as possible, and talc or other drying powders or drying soaks may be used. Tinea capitis may be treated with a combination of oral griseofulvin and selenium sulfide (Selsun, Exsel) shampoos. Athlete's foot that is actually ***intertrigo*** (caused by maceration from heat, moisture, and friction) in the absence of tinea infection may be treated by the application of a keratolytic agent (Keralyt gel), 30% aqueous aluminum chloride, or carbol-fuchsin paint. Tinea infections of the nails may require long-term oral griseofulvin therapy (daily for 3–8 months or more) until the nail has been completely replaced and all infected debris has been cast off. There may be risks involved in long-term use of this drug (GI distress, skin rashes, and leukopenia have occurred, and long-term administration of dosages comparable to those used in humans has caused cancer in laboratory rats), and this treatment is useless for candidal infections. Oral ketoconazole, 200 mg daily, is a useful treatment for both dermatophyte and candidal nail infections, but the potential side effects from long-term use (liver abnormalities and decreased adrenal steroid synthesis) should be considered. Either of these may be supplemented with local measures, including filing or sanding down the nails daily (if necessary, to the nail bed) and application of 1% ciclopirox cream (Loprox), 2% miconazole cream, or 1% clotrimazole cream or lotion three to four times daily.

Cutaneous candidiasis (moniliasis) is a yeast infection that may resemble dermatophytid skin infections in intertriginous regions, particularly the groin. Typically, the erythema in candidiasis is brighter ("beefy red"), there is more often maceration and denudation, and there may be satellite vesicopustular lesions at the periphery of the scaling erythematous patches. Severe pruritus, tenderness, or pain are common symptoms, and a whitish, curd-like exudate may be seen on the surface of denuded areas. Paronychial infections and erosion of the skin of the interdigital webs may occur. Microscopic exam of the curds or skin scales prepared with 15% KOH reveals the organism and hyphae, which are most commonly of the species *C. albicans,* but others of the same genus may be responsible (e.g., *C. tropicalis*). The organism may also be cultured in Sabouraud's medium. Pregnant women, obese persons, and immunocompromised or debilitated individuals (e.g., diabetics) are most susceptible to candidal skin infections, as well as to generalized (systemic) candidiasis. Antibiotics, oral contraceptives, steroids, and hyperhidrosis may be contributory factors in other persons. Baseline and yearly follow-up tests to screen for the development of endocrinopathy (diabetes, thyroid, parathyroid, or adrenal dysfunction) should be performed on a patient who presents with chronic mucocutaneous candidiasis.

Treatment of cutaneous candidiasis includes general measures to keep involved areas dry and exposed to the air and local treatments. Nystatin cream (Mycostatin), 100,000 units/g, miconazole or clotrimazole cream or lotion (Monistat-Derm, Mycelex, Lotrimin), or ciclopirox, 1% cream (Loprox), applied three to four times daily, are all effective for candidiasis of the skin. Equal amounts of an antifungal cream and a corticosteroid cream may be mixed to obtain anti-inflammatory and antipruritic actions in addition to the antifungal activity. (See Chapter 9 for a discussion of vaginal candidiasis.) Candidiasis of the diaper area requires frequent diaper changes, as well as measures to keep the area dry and exposed to the air. Gentian violet, 1%, or carbol-fuchsin paint (Castellani's paint) may be used as an alternative treatment for small localized areas one to two times weekly. For resistant or recurrent cases of candidiasis, nystatin may be given orally (500,000 units four times daily). Oral ketoconazole, 200 mg daily, will also eliminate skin lesions, but liver function should be monitored throughout this treatment, since hepatic toxicity has occurred during its use. Ketoconazole treatment should be continued for a minimum of 1 or 2 weeks, and recurrences often follow discontinuation of therapy, so patients with chronic mucocutaneous candidiasis generally require maintenance therapy. Systemic antibiotics should be discontinued if possible, but if it is not possible, oral nystatin should be given concomitantly (500,000 units three to four times daily).

Tinea versicolor (pityriasis versicolor) is a mild, superficial fungal infection of the skin caused by *Pityrosporon orbiculare* (formerly *Malassezia furfur*). The infection is characterized by multiple patches of macules that range in color from white to brown and from 4 to 5 mm in diameter to very large, confluent areas. The lesions are velvety, scale very slightly (when scratched), tend to coalesce, and do not tan with the surrounding skin when exposed to sunlight, so they are noticeable as "sun spots." The trunk (especially the chest and abdomen) is the most frequent site, but lesions may appear on the upper arms, neck, and face. These lesions are usually asymptomatic, but mild pruritus may occur when the patient becomes overheated. Microscopic exam of scrapings taken from the lesions and prepared with 15% KOH reveals yeast and hyphae. Lesions fluoresce golden under Wood's light, thereby demonstrating the extent of the involvement. The organisms are difficult to culture. These tests help to differentiate the disorder from vitiligo (which appears white under Wood's light) and seborrheic dermatitis.

In treating tinea versicolor, good hygiene is particularly important, and local preparations containing selenium sulfide may be helpful. One of these preparations in a shampoo base (Selsun Blue) may be applied to all involved areas at bedtime and washed off in the morning (continued for 3–4 days), taking care to avoid the scrotum. If irritation occurs from this treatment, it may be washed off in 0.5 to 1 hour, or treatment may be stopped altogether for a few days and then resumed. If irritation continues with this preparation, a lotion containing selenium sulfide (Selsun, Exsel) may be applied once daily, left on for 5 minutes, and then washed off. Clotrimazole and miconazole creams or lotions (Mycelex, Lotrimin, Monistat-Derm) are also effective topically applied treatments for tinea versicolor, applied twice daily. Alternative treatments include the application of equal parts of propylene glycol and water (diluted with more water if irritation develops), a 3% salicylic acid and rubbing alcohol preparation or 2% salicylic acid with 2% micropulverized sulfur in a shampoo base (Sebulex), or a lotion containing 25% sodium thiosulfate (Komed or Tinver) may be applied at bedtime for 2 weeks. Regular use of a soap containing sulfur and salicylic acid may also be effective, but with all of these treatments, repigmentation of the lesions may not occur for several months, and the disease may recur in 6 months to a year. Ketoconazole given orally (200 mg daily for 2 weeks) has about a 90% cure rate, but there is a risk of hepatotoxicity with this treatment.

Pigmentation

Skin color is determined primarily by two factors: the amount and nature of blood in the superficial capillaries of the dermal layer, and the presence of pigment in the dermal and epidermal layers of the skin. Blood within the vessels of the dermis accounts for reddish and pink tones, and constriction of superficial capillaries in the skin results in pallor. In skin that contains relatively little pigment, as little as 5 g of unoxygenated hemoglobin per 100 ml of blood will produce the bluish cast known as "cyanosis." In skin that is more darkly pigmented, a greater amount of unoxygenated hemoglobin must be present for these changes to become noticeable.

The second major determinant of skin color is pigmentation. The pigments of the human body are both endogenous and exogenous. In the skin, melanin is endogenous and carotene is exogenous. Other exogenous pigments that may be deposited in the skin and other tissues include carbon, silver, and some dyes. Carotene is a yellowish pigment found in the stratum corneum of the epidermis and in the fatty regions of the dermis, and is responsible for the yellowish tones seen most prominently in the skin of persons of the lighter races, especially Asiatic races. It is derived from foods such as yams, squash, tomatoes, green vegetables (kale, chard, spinach, lettuce), apricots, cantaloupe, citrus fruits, and especially carrots. Prolonged excessive intake of carotenoids through such sources results in carotenemia (hypercarotenemia, hypercarotenosis). It may also be the result of a disturbance of carotenoid metabolism, which may occur in hypothyroidism, hyperlipemia, diabetes mellitus, and anorexia nervosa. When the total serum carotenoid concentration exceeds 250 μg/dL (the normal serum range is 80–120 μg/dL), a yellow or orange discoloration of the skin (but not the sclera, unlike jaundice) may occur. This pigmentation is the result of excretion of carotenoids in the sweat and sebum and subsequent reabsorption into the stratum corneum. It is therefore most obvious in body regions where sweat and sebaceous glands are most abundant and/or where the stratum corneum is thickest (palms, soles, forehead, nasolabial fold, axillae, and groin). There is also a corresponding yellowing of the serum. Although vitamin A may be synthesized in the body from dietary carotenoids, carotenemia is not associated with hypervitaminosis A. Although any associated metabolic disorder must be treated, carotenemia appears not to affect general health, and the skin changes respond promptly to removal of the cause of carotenemia (low-carotene diet if excess dietary intake is the cause). Lycopenia, a harmless condition similar to carotenemia, results from excessive dietary intake of lycopene, a carotenoid that is not converted to vitamin A. Yellow or orange skin discoloration also occurs in this condition. Carotenemia and lycopenia may be differentiated from jaundice (excess bile pigments) by the lack of discoloration of the sclera and buccal mucosa, as well as by the absence of pruritus.

Avitaminosis A and hypervitaminosis A also cause skin changes. The vitamin is essential to the integrity of the epithelium of the skin and its appendages, as well as to other epithelia. Deficiency of the vitamin leads to epithelial keratinization: the epidermis becomes hyperkeratotic, metaplastic keratinizing squamous epithelium replaces the glandular epithelium of sweat glands, and various other mucosal epithelia (e.g., of the eye, nose, salivary glands) display similar changes with a number of associated clinical abnormalities. Dryness of the skin and phrynoderma (follicular hyperkeratosis) are common clinical signs. Hypervitaminosis A also induces disturbances of epithelial function, the most frequent being epidermal hyperplasia, parakeratosis, and a greatly increased epidermal transit time and increased mitotic activity. Common signs include hair loss, patchy erythema, purpura, and dry, fissured lips; a delayed sign of acute toxicity is a generalized desquamation of the skin.

Other nutritional conditions associated with skin changes include protein deficiency (marasmus with dry, thin, wrinkled, inelastic skin and kwashiorkor with circumoral pallor; erosive desquamation and exfoliation; reddish-brown discoloration of skin; dry, brittle, thinning hair, which may become light reddish-brown and then gray or develop bands of light and dark pigmentation—the "flag sign"—which reflect periods of relative improvement or worsening of nutritional status; and transverse nail lines), deficiencies of riboflavin or pyridoxine (seborrhea-like dermatitis), of vitamin B_{12} (occasionally hyperpigmentation), of niacin (erythema, dermatitis, hyperpigmentation, photosensitivity), of biotin (desquamation), of vitamin C (delayed wound healing, exacerbation of acne, hair loss), of calcium (patchy hair loss on the scalp, axillae, and pubic region, cutaneous candidiasis), of zinc (photophobia, delayed wound healing, hyperkeratosis, greasy, scaling dermatitis), and of iron (hair loss). Prolonged ingestion of high doses of niacin (e.g., 500 mg or more daily) may result in drying and thickening of the skin.

Melanin, a dark brownish pigment formed by stellate melanocytes scattered among the cells of the deepest layer of the epidermis, is the factor that accounts for the wide variations in skin color among persons of different races. The amount of melanin elaborated by the melanocytes and distributed to the surrounding epidermal cells is determined primarily by heredity, but other factors that influence melanin production include hormonal changes (primarily melanocyte-stimulating hormone, adrenocorticotropic hormone, estrogen, and progesterone), exposure to sunlight, heat, trauma, ionizing radiation, and inflammation. Either hyperpigementation or hypopigmentation (or both) may result from these influences.

The production of melanin within the melanocytes, specialized connective tissue cells occurring among the cells of the stratum germinativum, is the result of a series of chemical transformations that begins with the conversion of the amino acid tyrosine by tyrosinase to 3,4-dihydroxyphenylalanine (or dopa) and ends with the ultimate formation of the pigment. Melanin is stored in the melanocytes in the form of small cytoplasmic granules (melanosomes), which are "injected" into the cytoplasm of surrounding epidermal cells and become finer and eventually dust-like and better dispersed throughout the cytoplasm as the cells they occupy move outward toward the skin surface.

There may also be fine granules of pigment in some cells of the dermis, but these are generally confined to the deeply pigmented tissue of the eyelids, the axillae, the areolae of the nipples, and the anogenital area.

As already mentioned, melanocyte activity is primarily genetically controlled, but it is also stimulated as a protective response by exposure of the skin to ultraviolet (UV) radiation such as occurs in sunlight. The "suntan" that is caused by an increase in the production of melanin serves to screen out potentially harmful UV rays and protect the underlying tissue from solar damage.

When unprotected skin is first exposed to UV rays, there is an initial acute reaction with hyperemia and redness, followed by venous stagnation in the skin that may last for months. In about 2 days after the exposure, an increase in melanin is apparent; after it reaches a maximum (which is different for each individual), it begins to degenerate and gradually disappears. Exposure to x-rays also increases the enzymatic activity of the melanocytes and results in similar pigmentation.

Depending on the length of the exposure and the amount of skin involved, an acute ***sunburn*** reaction, or dermheliosis, can vary from a mild erythema, which is asymptomatic or accompanied by some tenderness, to a severe debilitating condition with pronounced edema, pain, and even vesiculation. A mild sunburn exhibits erythema within about 6–12 hours following initial exposure, reaches its peak within about 24 hours, and declines over a period of 3–5 days. The skin begins to peel after about a week, and maximal tanning occurs after 2 or 3 weeks. Topical therapy, which includes measures to hydrate the skin, is usually sufficient for ***mild sunburn,*** including cold water dressings applied for 30 minutes four times a day or cool compresses soaked in Burow's solution (aluminum acetate solution). For a generalized sunburn, colloidal sponge or tub baths are soothing (Aveeno Colloidal Oatmeal, Aveeno Oilated Bath). Topical aerosol sprays, such as betamethasone dipropionate (Diprosone) or betamethasone valerate (Valisone) provide further relief, but some experts feel that the major benefit of these corticosteroid aerosols is the cooling effect of the spray's propellant, and that the risks of corticosteroids do not justify their use for mild sunburns. Creams that contain benzocaine or other anesthetics, however, may provide some relief, but there is a slight risk of allergic contact dermatitis or sensitization preventing the later use of related anesthetics. Aspirin or a nonsteroidal anti-inflammatory agent such as ibuprofen, naproxen, or indomethacin, administered regularly, may also help alleviate the discomfort, particularly if taken promptly after sun exposure, since they inhibit the production of prostaglandins, which figure centrally in the skin's inflammatory response to sunburn.

The signs and symptoms of a ***severe sunburn*** from a more prolonged exposure may continue to progress for about 48 hours, accompanied by the development of vesicles and bullae, edema, and pain. Systemic responses suggestive of toxicity, such as fever, chills, nausea, and delirium, may also develop. The topical therapies outlined for mild sunburn should also be administered for severe sunburns. For the vesicular and bullous reactions, early treatment with a short (1-week) course of systemic steroids, such as prednisone (Deltasone, Meticorten), 40 mg/day in a single morning dose, will often halt the development of the signs and symptoms. Codeine or a stronger narcotic may be necessary for pain relief for the first 2 or 3 days. Persons with very severe, generalized sunburns should be treated as second- or third-degree burn patients. Depending on the skin thickness and total body surface involved, as well as other factors such as age and psychosocial variables, hospitalization may be necessary for IV fluid replacement and prevention of infection, particularly if large areas are blistered or denuded, increasing the potential for infection, or if other diseases are present that complicate the condition.

In persons with lighter skin pigmentation, and especially those whose skin burns prior to or without eventually tanning, a sunscreen preparation is an important preventive measure against solar radiation damage. Table 10.14 lists available sunscreen products and their Sun Protection Factor (SPF) values, which may range from 2 to 15 and may be used as a guide in selecting an appropriate sunscreen for a particular skin type. The SPF value is defined as the ratio of the length of exposure required to produce skin erythema with the sunscreen to the time required to produce the same degree of redness without the product. Therefore, if a product has an

TABLE 10.14 SOME SUNSCREEN PRODUCTS AND THEIR SPF RATINGS

Brand Name	SPF Rating	Recommended For:
Clinique 19	15	Maximum sunburn protection for persons who burn easily and tan minimally or not at all; permits little or no sun tanning. Also recommended for any person using drugs or other agents known to cause photosensitivity reactions.
M M M What-A-Tan	15	
Original Eclipse	10	
Pabanol	15	
PreSun 15	15	
Sunbrella	15	
Sundown 15	15	
Total Eclipse 15	15	
Aztec	6	Extra sunburn protection that permits limited sun tanning; recommended for persons who burn moderately, but want to develop a tan.
Blockout	6	
Piz Buin[a]	6	
Solbar[a]	7	
Sundown	6	
Sun Guard	6	
Super Shade Sun-Blocking Lotion	6–9	
Uval[a]	6	
A-Fil Cream	4–8	Minimal to moderate protection from sunburn for persons who rarely burn and tan easily; permits sun tanning.
Coppertone Lite Oil	2	
Maxafil Cream[a]	4–6	
Pabafilm	4–6	
Reflecta	4–8	
RVPaque	4–8	
Sea & Ski Dark Tanning Oil	2	
Sea & Ski Lotion	4–6	

[a]For persons unable to use PABA-based sunscreen products, these products are effective substitutes, but they must be reapplied after swimming or if they are diluted by sweating.

SPF of 6, and it normally takes 10 minutes of exposure to the sun to produce redness, use of the sunscreen would allow six times the length of exposure (six times 10 minutes, or 1 hour) without producing erythema.

Other acute adverse reactions to sun exposure include exacerbation of preexisting disease processes and ***photosensitivity reactions.*** A number of drugs and other substances may induce photosensitivity, which is generally not a true allergic reaction but a sunburn-like sensitivity reaction that is dose related and promoted by exposure to sunlight. Table 10.15 lists some common photosensitizing agents. Any person using a substance known to cause phototoxic reactions should be advised to use a sunscreen with a high SPF rating (applied at least 1 hour prior to exposure to sun) and to take other precautions, such as avoiding sunlight exposure between 10 A.M. and 2 P.M. during the summer months and wearing protective clothing and hats.

Chronic adverse effects of solar radiation include premature aging of the skin, freckling, and premalignant and locally malignant skin tumors. Basal cell and squamous cell carcinomas, the two most common forms of skin cancer, are clearly linked to UV solar radiation, and recent evidence has implicated sunlight as the cause of a third type, the life-threatening malignant melanomas.

Melanin, which is capable of absorbing UV light energy, is quite effective in protecting the skin against the damaging effect of UV radiation in sunlight. In persons who have naturally darker (i.e., more densely pigemented) skin, there is greater natural protection. As a result, the incidence of solar-induced carcinogenesis

TABLE 10.15 DRUGS AND OTHER AGENTS THAT MAY INDUCE PHOTOSENSITIVITY

Systemic substances	Topical Substances
Chloroquine (Aralen)	Aminobenzoic acid esters (in some sunscreen preparations)
Chlorpromazine HCl (Chloramead, Promapar, Thorazine, etc.)	Coal, wood tars
Gold salts	Furocoumarin (in parsley, celery, carrots, limes, and oil of bergamot in perfumes and after-shave lotions)
Griseofulvin (Fulvicin, Grifulvin V, Grisactin, etc.)	Plants, grasses
Methoxsalen (Oxsoralen)	Topical corticosteroids
Nalidixic acid (NegGram)	
Oral contraceptives	
Phenothiazines	
Pyrazinamide (PZA)	
Quinidine gluconate (Quinaglute Duratabs)	
Sulfonamides	
Sulfonylureas (oral antidiabetic agents)	
Tetracyclines	
Demeclocycline HCl (Declomycin)[a]	
Doxycycline (Doxy-C, Doxychel, Vibramycin, etc.)	
Oxytetracycline (Oxlopar, Terramycin, Tet-ramine, etc.)	
Thiazides	

[a]Photosensitivity reaction can occur with all tetracyclines but is most common with this form.

of the skin is significantly less in blacks than in persons of other races, except in body areas that are lightly pigmented (e.g., palms, soles, and mucous membranes).

Another function of the skin is the conversion of the endogenous substance 7-dehydrocholesterol (provitamin D_3) into cholecalciferol (vitamin D_3) upon exposure to UV radiation. This vitamin is then transformed by the liver and kidneys to 25-hydroxyvitamin D_3 and 1,25-dihydroxyvitamin D_3 (or 25-hydroxycholecalciferol and 1,25-dihydroxycholecalciferol, respectively), which, together with the parathyroid hormone and calcitonin, are essential in maintaining homeostasis of calcium in the body. Vitamin D helps maintain normal blood levels of calcium and phosphorus by initiating normal intestinal calcium transport, enabling mobilization of calcium to and from the bones, and controlling the excretion of phosphorus in the urine.

Since UV radiation is required to activate the provitamin D_3 and transform it into the vitamin, the screening effect of melanin in black skin that affords protection against solar skin damage also limits the amount of vitamin D that this skin can produce. Therefore, there is often an increased need for dietary sources of this vitamin in dark-skinned persons. One good source is milk, since regulations in most countries require that it be fortified with vitamins A and D. One quart of vitamin D–fortified milk contains 400 IU of the vitamin. Hypovitaminosis D, which may lead to osteomalacia in children (rickets) or adults or to infantile tetany, is most often due to a combination of factors, including inadequate exposure to sunlight, poor dietary intake, and/or a defect in intestinal absorption or hepatic or renal disease. This deficiency is discussed in Chapter 11.

Freckles are extremely common, small, flat, brownish or yellowish macules due to accumulation of excess amounts of pigment (melanin) in the melanocytes in the basal layer (stratum germinativum) of the epidermis. They are benign, and in children are called ***ephelides,*** which tend to disappear with age. Another form, the benign "senile" or "solar" freckles, are called ***lentigines*** ("age spots" or "liver spots"). They tend to appear later in life on exposed surfaces of the body, particularly the dorsal surfaces of hands and arms or on the face, and often represent a response to sun and weather exposure. These round or oval macules tend to be larger than juvenile ephelides (as large as 1 or 2 cm at times) and, unlike the juvenile freckles, do not darken with sun exposure. They are absolutely benign but may sometimes develop into ***seborrheic keratoses,*** another fairly common benign neoplasm that tends to occur in middle age or later. The superficial, sharply circumscribed, warty or velvety brownish, yellow, or gray lesions are actually epidermal papillomas (composed of immature epithelial cells) that can be easily removed with slight friction. They generally have a greasy, fissured surface that often contains keratin plugs, but on the hands and face they may have rougher and drier surfaces. They tend to increase in number with time, but they are not believed to have any potential for malignancy. Treatment is not necessary but curettage is effective, leaving a flat surface that is covered with normal skin in about a week. Surgical removal is more effective for pedunculated lesions. The development of a black discoloration may occur on a seborrheic keratosis and evoke suspicion about its malignant potential (e.g., melanoma). In this case, although it is often possible to differentiate the two lesions on the basis of their clinical appearance, an excisional biopsy will dispel any doubt about which tumor is present.

Pregnant women may occasionally develop seborrheic keratoses and ***skin tags,*** small, pedunculated, flesh-colored to brown outgrowths of skin occurring predominantly on the neck, axillae, and groin. The keratoses tend to recede after delivery; skin tags require removal only if they are subject to irritation from the friction of movement or clothing. The sudden appearance of large numbers of seborrheic keratoses in a middle-aged or elderly person may signal an underlying internal malignancy (the Leser-Trelat sign). This may also be associated with ***acanthosis nigricans,*** a rare inflammatory condition characterized by a symmetric eruption of blackish hard and soft growths (papillomas), hyperpigmentation, and hyperkeratosis on the axillae, groin, lips, and other regions. ***Stucco keratosis*** is a variant of seborrheic keratosis that features multiple, scaling, whitish lesions on the extremities that appear "stuck on" and are easily removed with a slight scraping.

Nevi (moles) are probably the most common of all skin tumors. A nevus that is present at birth (congenital nevus) is considerably less common than the acquired nevus, which may develop at any age from 6 months on. It also has a greater potential for malignant changes than the acquired nevus. Table 10.16 lists a number of benign, premalignant, and malignant skin tumors and the characteristics of each, as well as the necessity for biopsy or removal of each type. There is a great deal of concern among primary care providers about when to suspect that a pigmented tumor may be a malignant lesion (i.e., melanoma) and not a mole. In general, whenever such a lesion has an irregular margin (it may be scalloped or notched or may have an angular indentation), an uneven, irregular surface (to exam and palpation), an irregularity of pigmentation or coloring (black, brown, blue, gray, red, white), or bleeding, a ***melanoma*** should be suspected. Red, white, or blue coloring within a tumor is particularly suspicious, since red coloring suggests inflammation within the tumor, areas of regression where the body's defense mechanisms have attacked portions of the tumor may appear grayish or whitish, and an irregular bluish discoloration is suggestive of deeper invasion. An admixture of these colors in a skin tumor is a classic feature of the most common type of melanoma, superficial spreading melanoma, which constitutes about 65–70% of melanomas. While a number of nevi appear bluish when they are deep in the skin, irregular blue coloration is

TABLE 10.16 TUMORS OF THE SKIN

Tumor	Features	Potentially Malignant?	Necessary for Removal?
	Flesh-Colored to Pink		
Benign juvenile melanoma	Occurs in children; rapidly growing, flesh-colored, pink, or red; smooth or verrucous surface.	No	Yes, to differentiate it from malignant melanoma
Warts (verrucae)	Caused by papillomavirus; papillated, rough surface is typical; usually less than 0.5 cm in diameter.	No	No, but may be desirable if painful or to prevent spread
Molluscum contagiosum	Flesh-colored, smooth, shiny, umbilicated papules 2–10 mm in diameter (can be 2–3 cm); caused by poxvirus infection.	No	No, but may be desirable to prevent spread
Epidermoid cyst	Well-circumscribed, flesh-colored nodule; more common in men than in women; histologically resembles normal epidermis; multiple cysts may mark genetic syndromes (e.g., Gardner's syndrome).	No	No
Pilar or follicular cyst	Flesh-colored papule commonly occurring on the scalp and face; resembles epidermoid cyst, but a hair-like mode of differentiation is seen histologically.	No	No
Myxoid cyst	Pseudocyst (lacks epithelial lining); occurs on dorsum of finger's terminal digit.	No	No
Milia	White or yellow epidermal inclusion cysts 2–4 mm in diameter occurring on face or skin surfaces that have sustained trauma, burns, or a scarring dermatosis (e.g., bullous disorders).	No	No
Syringoma	Flesh-colored papule (tumor of eccrine sweat glands) occurring on lower eyelid or medial portion of cheeks.	No	No, but biopsy will rule out basal cell carcinoma
Adnexal neoplasms	Well-circumscribed, flesh-colored nodules associated with adnexal structures of skin (hair, eccrine and apocrine glands); resemble intradermal trichoepithelioma, nevi. Examples are syringoma (above), cylindroma, and hidrocystoma.	No	No, but biopsy will differentiate it from basal cell carcinoma
Neurofibroma	Solitary or multiple soft, flesh-colored nodules; may be solitary or multiple (in Recklinghausen's disease) and may be painful.	Yes if part of Recklinghausen's disease (neurofibromatosis)	Possibly

TABLE 10.16 (*Continued*)

Tumor	Features	Potentially Malignant?	Necessary for Removal?
Dermatofibroma (sclerosing hemangioma)	Small, flesh-colored, pink or dark brown, smooth papule that is firm, nontender, and well defined. Histologically represents a collection of histiocytes, fibrous tissue, blood vessels, and iron pigment (hemosiderin) in the dermis.	No	No
Sebaceous hyperplasia	Small, multilobulated, flesh-colored or yellow papules with central punctum; occur in middle age or later.	No	No
Lipoma	Smooth, well-circumscribed, flesh-colored subcutaneous nodule with rubbery consistency.	No	No
Skin tag (acrochordon)	Soft, flesh-colored to brown, 2–4 mm in diameter, pedunculated papilloma occurring commonly at sites of friction (side of neck, axillae, beneath breasts, groin).	No	No, unless irritated
Keloid	Hyperplastic overgrowth in response to injury (even minor trauma).	No	No
Fibrous papule of face	Common, smooth, small, flesh-colored nodule resembling intradermal nevus.	No	No, but biopsy will differentiate it from basal cell carcinoma
Intradermal nevus	Well-circumscribed, small (less than 1 cm in diameter), usually flesh-colored nodule; more common in adults than in children.	No	No
Prurigo nodularis	Extremely pruritic flesh-colored to dark nodule.	No	No
Sarcoidosis	Flesh-colored facial papule.	No	No
Keratoacanthoma	Rapidly-growing, flesh-colored, verrucous tumor with central punctum or keratin plug; usually occurs on sun-damaged skin.	No	No, but biopsy will differentiate it from squamous cell carcinoma
Actinic (solar) keratosis	Rough, irregular, scaly red patch on sun-damaged skin; telangiectasias are common.	Yes (into squamous cell carcinoma)	Yes
Squamous cell carcinoma	Reddish, irregular tumors with rough surface usually occurring on sun- or radiation-damaged skin; may ulcerate or bleed; tendency for early metastasis.	Malignant	Yes

TABLE 10.16 *(Continued)*

Tumor	Features	Potentially Malignant?	Necessary for Removal?
Basal cell carcinoma	Most common form has waxy appearance, central crater-like depression with "pearly" borders (of tiny papules) and telangiectasias; tendency for erosion, ulceration, and bleeding. Usually reddish, but may be brown or black (pigmented basal cell carcinoma).	Malignant	Yes
	Red to Purple (Vascular Tumors)		
Hemangioma	Common red or bluish red macules or papules that blanch with pressure; these represent dilation of blood vessels (may also be pale pink or nearly black).	No	No (rule out melanoma)
Nevus araneus (spider angioma)	Superficial dilation of arterioles that blanches with pressure; often occurs during pregnancy or in association with estrogen therapy or liver disease.	No	No
Senile hemangioma (venous lake)	Smooth, bluish-red papule with well-defined edges; usually less than 5 mm in diameter.	No	No
Pyogenic granuloma (granuloma telangiectaticum)	Deep red or purple pedunculated papule (0.5–2.0 cm in diameter) with a regular border; consists of a proliferation of capillaries and a hyperplastic response of connective tissue usually occurring at the site of an earlier trauma; bleeding and crusting may occur.	No	No
Lymphoma	Blue-red, smooth nodule.	Malignant	Yes
Pseudolymphoma	Red or bluish-red, smooth, well-defined tumor; resembles lymphoma.	No	No, but should be biopsied to rule out malignant lymphoma
Kaposi's sarcoma	Deep berry-red to purple macules, papules, patches, plaques, or nodules; at one time, predominantly affected men of Mediterranean or Jewish descent in sixth or seventh decade (on legs), but now is seen commonly in victims of acquired immune deficiency syndrome (AIDS), with a worse prognosis.	Malignant	Yes
Angiosarcoma	Red, irregular patch with ill-defined border; rare.	Malignant	Yes
Metastatic tumor	Usually firm, flesh-colored or red nodules.	Malignant	Yes

TABLE 10.16 (*Continued*)

Tumor	Features	Potentially Malignant?	Necessary for Removal?
	Brown-Black (Tumors of the Melanocytes)		
Nevus (mole)	Flesh-colored, brown, black, or blue macule or papule; may be congenital or acquired and smooth or rough; may also be congenital or acquired (congenital nevi may be any size and may be hairy, but acquired nevi are typically smaller).	Congenital nevi may occasionally demonstrate change, but malignant development in acquired nevi is rare	No; biopsy if changes take place
Ephelides (juvenile freckles)	Small, flat, brownish or yellowish macules due to excess accumulations of melanin in the melanocytes of the epidermis; darken with sun exposure and tend to fade with age.	No	No
Solar lentigines (senile freckles, age spots)	Ill-defined brownish or yellowish macules that commonly occur in middle-aged or older persons on sun-damaged skin; do not darken with sun exposure and tend to be larger than ephelides (may be as large as 1–2 cm)	No	No
Seborrheic keratosis	Brown, yellow, tan, or gray superficial lesions with a warty or velvety, greasy or dry, and fissured surface; may be easily removed with slight friction. These are actually epidermal papillomas.	No	No, unless bothersome
Lentigo maligna (Hutchinson's freckle)	Large (2–6 cm in diameter) brown or tan macule with an irregular scattering of darker brown or black spots on the surface; the border is frequently irregular with notching.	Yes, into lentigo-maligna melanoma	Yes
Malignant melanoma	Irregular border and surface; may be one color or an admixture of colors (brown, red, blue, gray, white); may occasionally be amelanotic, and may ulcerate and bleed.	Malignant	Yes
	Yellow		
Sebaceous nevus	Yellowish or tan verrucous plaque; congenital lesion of sebaceous glands that becomes most apparent at puberty when adrenal stimulation causes proliferation and enlargement of the sebaceous glands; surface is verrucous.	Rare (may occasionally develop into a basal cell carcinoma)	Controversial; certainly remove if changes suggestive of basal cell carcinoma develop; some experts recommend prophylactic excision
Xanthoma	Soft yellow lump occurring most often around eyelids (xanthelasma); sometimes associated with hyperlipidemia.	No	No
Sebaceous gland carcinoma	Rare yellow tumor.	Malignant	Yes

suspicious. Another type of melanoma, nodular malignant melanoma (constituting about 10% of all melanomas), tends to have a more uniform coloration, however. This type is usually black but occasionally may be amelanotic, presenting as a red, scaling, or crusting papule. A melanoma in the early stages may be flat or barely palpable, but a raised surface with nodule formation and ulceration is characteristic of later stages. A surrounding "halo" of depigmentation is also a suspicious sign, although not a reliable one. In addition to these signs, any sensation, such as itching or burning, may signal a malignant tumor. However, the warning that any change in a wart or mole is potentially indicative of cancer is a bit misleading, since every nevus goes through a series of changes that are normal and harmless.

An acquired nevus typically arises as a ***junctional nevus,*** a flat brownish accumulation of clear nevus cells and melanin situated at the level of the dermal–epidermal junction, with some nevus cells on both sides of the basement membrane. In time, the cells move downward from the basement membrane level, just into the dermis, acquiring a dermal component. The lesion is now called a ***compound nevus,*** which has clear nevus cells within the dermal layer, as well as some junctional elements, and a slightly raised surface. Finally, the entire cluster of cells settles deeper into the dermis to form a prominent lesion, the ***intradermal nevus.*** Of all of these stages of development, the lesion of the earliest (the junctional nevus) has the greatest potential for changing into a malignant melanoma; the compound nevus is next in potential, and intradermal nevi are considered quite benign. Malignant melanomas have the worse prognosis of any of the skin cancers, so any lesion that seems suspicious or about which the diagnosis is unclear should be referred to a specialist for possible biopsy or excision. When a melanoma on the skin of the palm is suspected, fungal infection should be ruled out.

Estimates by the American Cancer Society suggest that skin cancer is the most prevalent form of cancer in the United States. However, it is also one of the most successfully treated forms. A number of nonmalignant skin lesions may be potentially cancerous. The most common of these are actinic keratosis and lentigo maligna (which may be a form of actinic keratosis). Other common premalignant lesions are leukoplakia and radiation dermatitis. Chronic suppurative ulcers, some sebaceous nevi of Jadassohn, and giant congenital nevi may also become malignant.

►***Actinic keratoses*** are a frequent consequence of long-term (years), chronic, excessive exposure to sunlight. Most fair-skinned persons develop at least two or three actinic keratoses in their later years. They tend to occur on areas of the body that receive the most exposure to the sun, such as the forehead, malar areas, the rims of the ears, and sometimes the extremities (dorsal surfaces of the hands and forearms). They occur most frequently on fair-skinned, blue-eyed persons (blacks are rarely affected) and in geographic regions of greatest exposure to ultraviolet radiation. Their development may be signaled initially by a slight localized scaliness or thickness or occasionally erythema. Burning or stinging may also occur, and these symptoms and erythema are heightened by sun exposure. The lesions are red, gray, tan, or flesh-colored, and have a surface that feels rough to the touch (like sandpaper) and ill-defined edges. The roughened surface will sometimes fall off but will re-form a few weeks later. A clue that is helpful in making the diagnosis of actinic keratosis is that the lesion does not respond to treatment for seborrheic dermatitis, and the ill-defined borders and location (i.e., the face and other sun-exposed areas versus the trunk) help to differentiate it from a seborrheic keratosis. A punch biopsy (unless the primary care provider is trained in this procedure, a dermatologist can usually perform it) can be used to differentiate actinic keratosis from solar lentigines, lentigo maligna, and a flat seborrheic keratosis.

Actinic keratoses may either be excised, curetted, electrodesiccated, or treated with a topical fluorouracil (Efudex, Fluoroplex) cream or solution (in the winter, if possible) for 2–3 weeks. With this therapy a small area should be treated initially, and the patient should be advised that temporary crusting, oozing, redness, soreness, burning, stinging, and photosensitivity will occur. Topical 0.5% hydrocortisone lotion in the morning (the fluorouracil cream should be used at night) may help control the inflammatory reaction and photosensitivity. About 3 weeks after this therapy, when the inflammatory reaction subsides (the hydrocortisone lotion may be continued during this period), any lesions that are left should be biopsied, and the patient should be followed for 5 years. Multiple actinic keratoses or heavy, thick lesions may be treated more effectively by dermabrasion or chemosurgical exfoliation (e.g., using trichloroacetic acid or phenolic acid). Both of these treatments remove most of the epidermis and upper papillary dermis, but they should be performed by persons trained and experienced in their use; slightly more trichloroacetic acid than is necessary for successful treatment may cause scarring. Cryotherapy is also effective for these lesions (with a cure rate of about 90–95% in most areas except the scalp) but may result in a permanent area of relative hypopigmentation.

The atypical cells of actinic keratosis are similar to those seen in the malignant tumor ***squamous cell carcinoma*** (squamous cell epithelioma), and when actinic keratoses degenerate, they develop into this lesion. The changes in actinic keratoses are confined to the epidermal layer (the basement membrane is intact), whereas squamous cell carcinomas show invasion into the dermal layer. The appearance of a wart-like growth on the surface (inside or at the edge) of an actinic keratosis should alert the examiner to the possibility of an early squamous cell carcinoma. These tumors may also arise out of a preexisting patch of leukoplakia, or they may develop de novo (the latter have a higher incidence of metastases, which may occur early). Squamous cell carcinomas tend to develop quite rapidly and may reach 1 cm in diameter within 2 weeks. The lesion begins as a small red papule or plaque with a crusted or scaly surface and later becomes a hard, conical, red nodule that may have a warty surface and quickly ulcerates.

If squamous cell carcinoma is suspected, referral to a specialist for evaluation, biopsy, and possible excision is recommended. If the primary care provider is able to do a simple and expedient biopsy, he or she may do so before referring, particularly if the process of referral may take a while. A biopsy will confirm the diagnosis of squamous cell carcinoma (2- to 4-mm punch that continues into the subcutaneous tissue to reveal the depth of invasion). If the results of the histologic exam confirm the diagnosis, the tumor can be excised. For very small lesions, specialists may often prefer to do an excisional biopsy in order to accomplish both diagnosis and removal of the lesion in one visit (microscopic exam is necessary to establish that the entire lesion has been removed). However, it is not always advised for large lesions that may leave a scar, because other lesions that are included in the differential diagnosis (e.g., seborrheic keratosis, actinic keratosis) may be treated with some other treatment that would not result in scarring (e.g., electrodesiccation and curettage, cryosurgery).

A benign growth, ***keratoacanthoma,*** may be clinically indistinguishable from squamous cell carcinoma. Unless a definitive diagnosis of keratoacanthoma can be provided, it should, for all practical purposes, be treated as if it were the cancerous lesion. Keratoacanthoma typically begins as a dome-shaped red papule that evolves very rapidly within a couple of weeks, forming a scale on the surface and then developing a crater-like appearance. This lesion may be dismissed by nonspecialists as a common wart, which can be a serious mistake, since it is potentially malignant. The potential for malignant transformation depends largely upon the duration of the lesion. It may also be misdiagnosed as squamous cell carcinoma when a biopsy is taken from the center of the lesion alone. Keratoacanthomas may disappear spontaneously in months and then reappear, and they may be extremely mutilating and destructive. Treatment for this lesion (by a specialist) may involve excision, irradiation, or cryotherapy. Also, in about 95% of cases, keratocanthomas disappear within 2 weeks following intralesional injection of fluorouracil, often making this the preferred therapy where surgery would be mutilating. Sometimes, however, the surgery is necessary, and both the decision about using fluorouracil therapy versus surgery and the actual procedure should be done by a specialist experienced in the use of local fluorouracil injections.

Lentigo maligna (Hutchinson's freckle) is a premalignant lesion very similar to actinic keratoses appearing on sun-exposed skin areas (e.g., the face) of elderly patients. It is a large (2 to 6 cm), asymptomatic, flat macule that may be brown or tan, with an irregular scattering of darker brown or black spots on its surface. The lesion frequently has an irregular border with some notching; this measure helps to differentiate it from a senile lentigo (liver spot) and is an indication for biopsy. Lentigo maligna has both normal and malignant melanocytes confined to the level of the epidermis and has the potential to develop into a ***lentigo-maligna melanoma,*** a malignant tumor with a dermal component; about one-third of lentigo-malignas will invade the dermis after 10 years or so. This tumor constitutes about 20% of all melanomas. Both the premalignant lesion and its malignant counterpart are usually treated with wide local excision and (when necessary) skin grafting, giving a 90–100% 5-year cure rate.

Basal cell carcinoma also appears more frequently on exposed parts of the body. Unlike squamous cell carcinoma, this tumor grows slowly, taking about a year to reach a diameter of 1–2 cm. The early lesion appears as one or two small, shiny papules with telangiectasias around them. As they enlarge, they develop (in 1 or 2 months) a classic pearly appearance that causes light to be reflected from the surface. This pearly quality is due to the presence of immature cells (basal cells) that have not matured or keratinized. The smaller lesions tend to be firmer nodules, but when a basal cell carcinoma is large, it tends to feel "mushy" and develops a central depression with telangiectasias leading into and over the lesion and into the crater in its center. The central depression, which may begin as a small (2 mm) punctum, may grow to 3–4 mm and turn into a crust, a scale, or a slight ulceration and may begin to bleed. Less often, a basal cell carcinoma may appear as a flat, indurated, scar-like plaque (morphea form) with nodulation and telangiectasias at the edge, or as a lesion that resembles psoriasis or a localized dermatitis. The telangiectasias represent fine papillary vessels that are compressed against the basement membrane. Since the immature basal cell does not form surface skin layers normally, this lesion is often brought to the physician's attention because it received a minor trauma months (or a year) earlier that does not appear to heal, but keeps forming a scab. This is a good indication for biopsy. Metastases rarely occur with this tumor, but when it invades or impinges on an underlying structure or orifice (eye, ear, mouth, bone, dura mater), it may cause complications and even death (rare). The treatment of choice depends on the clinical appearance, site, size, and histologic findings. Electrodesiccation and curettage, surgical excision, or x-ray treatment is possible. Recurrences occur in about 5% of cases. These may be treated with chemical fixation of the tissue followed by microscopically controlled excision (Moh's chemosurgery) or by surgical excision. Topical fluorouracil treatment has been used, but the recurrence rate is high.

Keloids are tumors consisting of an overgrowth of fibrous tissue arising in the area of cuts, burns, or infections, or sometimes arising spontaneously in predisposed persons, especially blacks. The lesions are smooth, shiny, and dome-shaped, and may be pinkish; itching and burning sensations are common. The most common sites are the ears, neck, sternal region, back, and proximal portions of the extremities. Keloids are not malignant, but they behave like neoplasms. They may develop spontaneous finger-like projections from the central growth, and may reach large proportions and be disfiguring. The mechanism involved in the formation of keloids is believed to be an abnormality of the cross-banding of collagen fibers (a normal part of the process of wound repair). Treatment is surgical excision (possibly followed by intralesional injection of triamcinolone acetonide suspension, 40 mg/mL) or cryotherapy, but the results are often unsatisfactory, and they are likely to regrow following excision. Carbon dioxide laser therapy is also being tried, with promising results. It is important to question patients about a personal or family history of keloid formation prior to performing any surgical procedure, since great care should be taken to limit the amount of hyperplasia that will result, and perhaps elective procedures (even ear piercing) should be avoided.

Primary hypopigmentation occurring in otherwise normal skin has a very limited number of etiologic possibilities. ***Congenital albinism*** is a rare inherited condition in which melanocytes are present throughout the skin surface, hair, and irides of the eyes, but to varying degrees fail to produce melanin. If the extent of the defect is minimal, the hair may be yellowish or yellow-brown, the skin may tan somewhat on sun exposure, and the irides may also have some pigment, with minimal eye symptoms. However, if the defect is severe, the skin will be pale, the hair white, and the irides pink. Nystagmus and errors of refraction are common, and there is an associated high risk of malignant skin changes because of the inability of the skin to protect itself by producing melanin to screen out UV radiation. Whereas albinism is inherited as a recessive trait, ***partial albinism*** (or piebaldism) is an autosomal dominant trait. Areas of the skin that lack melanin are present at birth and persist unchanged throughout life. There is often a white lock of hair as well. This disorder may be associated with perceptual deafness in Woolf's syndrome. In Waardenburg's syndrome there is also a lateral displacement of the lacrimal puncta and inner canthi, a prominent nasal root, prominent medial eyebrows, and multicolored irides. Persons with congenital or partial albinism should be advised to make a habit of using a sunscreen product with a high SPF (see Table 10.14) whenever they are in the sun.

Vitiligo, a disorder affecting approximately 1% of the population, may be present at birth, but more often it appears afterward; most cases are manifested by age 20 but may appear at any age. The disorder, which may be localized or universal in effect, is differentiated from partial or complete albinism by a decreased number of melanocytes in the affected areas of skin. A family history of the disorder is present in about one-third of patients, but the cause is unknown. A number of persons with vitiligo also have other disorders such as Addison's disease, diabetes mellitus, pernicious anemia, thyroid dysfunction (Hashimoto's thyroiditis), Graves' disease, halo nevi, mucocutaneous candidiasis, myasthenia gravis, rheumatic arthritis, and hypoparathyroidism. Therefore, a battery of tests to screen for such abnormalities should be ordered, including thyroid function tests, serum glucose, electrolyte assays, and CBC (including morphologic indices). The depigmented areas, which appear chalk white under Wood's light, may range from one or two sharply demarcated, oval or round macules and patches with convex borders to extensive (symmetric) involvement of the skin surface.

In vitiligo there is no associated scaling, and since the hypopigmented areas are asymptomatic, except for advising the patient of the benign nature of the disorder and instructing him or her that the depigmented areas are prone to sun damage and therefore require a protective sunscreen whenever exposure cannot be avoided, there may be no need for treatment. Cosmetic cover-ups may help to disguise the patches. The patient should be advised that there may be a number of exacerbations with interspersed periods of no change, and occasionally some spontaneous repigmentation, although this rarely occurs and is more likely in children than adults. Older patients (over 40 years of age) who have more than 40% of body surface involvement may be candidates for depigmentation of the remainder of the skin surface (with monobenzyl ether of hydroquinone), but the irreversibility of the procedure should be explained. Some new, fairly localized lesions may respond to application of a medium-potency topical corticosteroid product (see Table 10.9), but complications (atrophy, telangiectasias, and striae) must be watched for. PUVA therapy (long-wave UV light and systemic or topical psoralens) may produce perifollicular pigmentation (macules observed after about the 15th or 25th treatment) that eventually coalesces. If full pigmentation occurs, no maintenance therapy is required. This may require 100 or more treatments (given three times weekly). However, some patients do not respond well, and there are also risks associated with the therapy, such as cataract formation, skin cancer, and a phototoxic or blistering reaction to the psoralens. Both depigmentation and PUVA therapy should be performed by physicians experienced in these procedures.

Secondary hypopigmentation (or leukoderma) may occur as a postinflammatory response following bullous dermatoses, burns, skin infections, and other skin conditions such as atopic dermatitis, lichen planus, psoriasis, alopecia areata, and lichen simplex chronicus. In some of these conditions there may also be surrounding hyperpigmentation. Some systemic conditions may also produce hypopigmentation, including syphilis, myxedema, thyrotoxicosis, and toxemias. Monobenzyl ether of hydroquinone, an antioxidant in some rubber products (bra pads, gauntlet gloves) may produce depigmentation, particularly in blacks, as may an aresenic or gold dermatitis or local skin trauma.

Hyperpigmentation due to an increased deposition of melanin may occur as a manifestation of hormonal changes in conditions such as Addison's disease (due to an increased plasma level of immunoreactive beta–melanocyte-stimulating hormone from the pituitary as a result of a lack of inhibitory influence of hydrocortisone) and pregnancy, and from the use of anovulatory hormones. A patterned dark brown pigmentation of the face occurring in pregnancy and in about 30–50% of women taking oral contraceptives is called ***melasma*** (chloasma, melasma gravidarum, the "mask of pregnancy"). The patches of pigmentation are sharply demarcated, roughly symmetric, and occur most frequently on the forehead, temples, and malar areas. The condition is accentuated by sun exposure and in rare cases may occur as an idiopathic finding in some dark-skinned men. In women, it fades somewhat following delivery or cessation of oral contraceptive use. Melasma may be treated with an application of 2 or 4% hydroquinone cream applied two times daily and a sunscreen with an SPF of 15 (see Table 10.14). The hydroquinone cream should be patch tested for a week on a spot behind the ear, since it may lighten the skin excessively or produce a dermatitis. Topical 0.01% tretinoin cream may be used to enhance the effect of the hydroquinone. If melanin deposition is mainly superficial (i.e., epidermal), it will respond well to this treatment, but if it is predominantly dermal, the prognosis is poor.

Increased melanogenesis (e.g., in hemochromatosis) or deposition of exogenous pigment, such as silver (argyria) or other metals, will also produce skin darkening. Metabolic substances that may produce pigmentation include hemosiderin (iron) in hemochromatosis and purpuric processes, mercaptans, homogentisic acid (ochronosis), bile pigments (jaundice), and carotene (carotenemia).

ACCESSORY ORGANS OF THE SKIN

Hair

Hair, which is a modification of the epidermal layer of skin, is well distributed over the surfaces of the body with the exception of the palms, soles, distal phalanges of the fingers and toes, regions of the anogenital openings, and flexor surfaces of the joints. Individual hairs may vary in length from 1 mm or less to 1.5 m and in thickness from 0.05 to 0.5 mm. Surrounding each hair is a tube of epithelial (epidermal component) and connective tissue (dermal component) cells called the "hair follicle," which was formed in utero by invagination of the epidermis into the underlying dermis. In the lowermost portion of the hair follicle is an involution of loose connective tissue derived from the dermis called the "hair papilla," which contains a loop of capillaries to nourish the hair. It is from this papilla that the individual hair, or pili, arises as a thin, flexible shaft of tightly compacted, keratinized cells. The portion of the hair embedded within the follicle is called the "root" and the free portion extending from the opening of the follicle is called the "shaft." The lower portion of the root is enlarged to form an onion-shaped area called the "bulb," which fits like a cap over the papilla (Fig. 10.2). Most hair is associated with two or more sebaceous glands that secrete varying amounts of an oily substance called "sebum" into the follicle near the surface of this skin to coat the hair and skin surface. The combination of hair and sebaceous glands is referred to as the "pilosebaceous unit."

The follicle has three layers: an outer fibrous connective tissue sheath (dermal root sheath) derived from the dermis, and, within that, the internal and external root sheaths derived from the epidermis and covering the hair root. The connective tissue sheath serves as the insertion of the arrector pili muscle, a small bundle of smooth muscle fibers that extends diagonally to connect at its other end with the elastic and fibrous elements in the papillary layer of the dermis and, by contraction, causes the hair to stand on end. The arrector pili is always inserted below the sebaceous gland on the lower surface of the hair. Contraction of these fibers from stimuli such as fear or cold also causes characteristic elevations on the skin surface referred to as "goose flesh" or "goose bumps" (cutis anserina). Lanugo, the fine, lightly pigmented hairs that cover the embryo's body and persist after birth in some

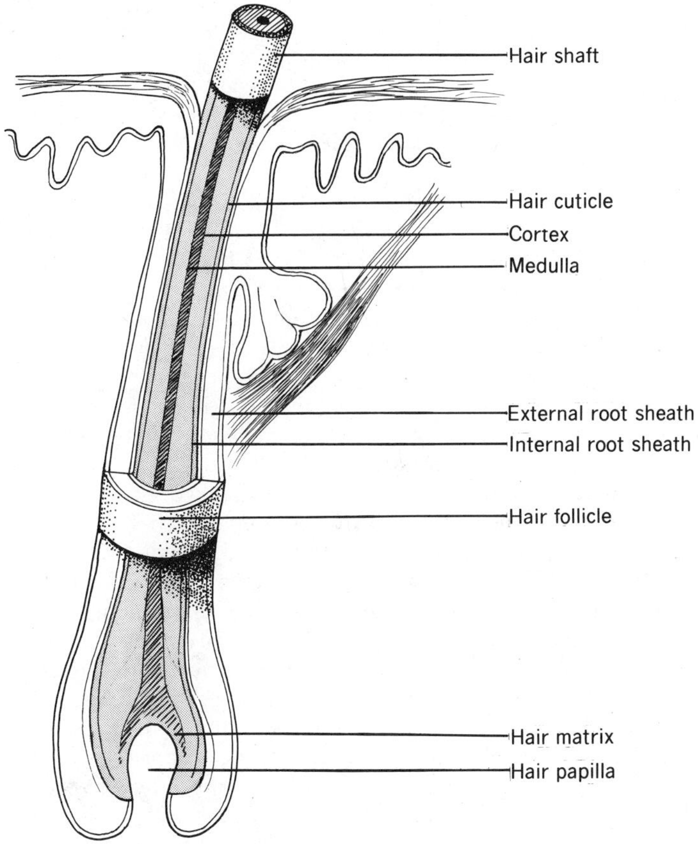

Figure 10.2 Hair shaft and associated structures.

areas (e.g., nose, eyelids, cheeks, lips) lack connective tissue sheaths and arrectores pilorum. Arrector muscles are also absent from the eyelashes and nasal hairs.

The external root sheath is continuous with the stratum germinativum and stratum spinosum of the epidermis and extends only to the level of the sebaceous gland. The internal root sheath covers the growing hair root extending from the sebaceous gland to the bulb, and toward the bulb is divisible into two layers: the outer one or two rows of mostly nonnucleated cells called "Henle's layer" and the inner row (closest to the hair) of nucleated cells called "Huxley's layer." The cuticle of the internal root sheath, a membrane composed of nonnucleated keratinized scales, lines the inner surface of Huxley's layer.

The shaft of the hair is composed entirely of keratinized epithelial cells. In cross-section it has three layers: an outermost cuticle, a cortex, and a central medulla. The surface cuticle is a thin layer of transparent scales that are directed from the center of the hair outward and upward, overlapping in a manner that resembles inverted shingles. These cells are nonnucleated, except for those at the base.

The main portion of the hair is the cortex, which toward the bulb consists of round, soft cells and distally of elongated, compacted, and keratinized cells with linear nuclei. Keratin in the cells of this layer is termed "hard" because it is high in sulfur content. The pigment (melanin) responsible for hair color is found both in solution and in the form of granules in and between the cells of this layer. Melanocytes present in the bulb contribute this pigment, and the presence of air in the intercellular spaces of cortical cells modifies hair color. White hair contains little or no melanin.

The central medulla, consisting of cuboidal cells that contain keratohyalin and degenerating nuclei, is lacking in many hairs, and where it is present, it may not extend the entire length of the hair shaft. Hairs that lack the medullary portion include lanugo, blond hair, and some scalp hair. The keratin of medullary cells is termed "soft" because of its low sulfur content. The hair, like the epidermis from which it originates, has no blood or nerve supply of its own.

Growth of the hair and the internal root sheath and cuticle results from continual mitotic division of the undifferentiated epithelial cells of the lower portion of the bulb, the matrix. Hair goes through phases of growth, atrophy, and rest; during the growth (anagen) phase, the hair root is elongated and new cells from the matrix move upward, increase in size, become keratinized, and are added from below to the cells previously keratinized. Melanocytes present within the matrix contribute melanin in a manner similar to that occurring in the epidermis.

After a period of time, there is a thickening of the inner portion of the connective tissue sheath. The matrix cells stop producing the internal root sheath first, and then the sheath's cuticle and the hair shaft (catagen phase). The hollow bulb becomes a solid keratinized "club" that becomes detached from the matrix; the dead hair is called a "club hair." Once again, the matrix cells increase, but now without differentiating into hair and sheath cells, and the clubbed hair and inner sheath are forced outward to the level of the sebaceous gland, where they may remain for a period of time (rest or telogen phase). After some time, a new hair develops within the old connective tissue sheath and upon the same papilla, and grows toward the surface, forcing the old hair out in the process, if it still remains at the opening. Hair regeneration thus continues even if a hair is cut, shaved, plucked, or otherwise removed, as long as the matrix cells remain alive.

Hairs occurring in different body regions have different periods of growth; the growth period of scalp hair lasts about 2–4 years, whereas that of eyelashes is only about 3–4 months. The hair growth rate also varies in different regions of the body, being most rapid on the chin (about 2.66 mm/week) and scalp (2.45 mm/week) and least rapid on the eyebrow (1.12 mm/week). Hair growth is more rapid in summer than in winter, and overall declines slightly after the third decade. The rate of hair growth and its composition may be altered by stress and by altered nutritional or physiologic states.

Hair on the scalp, eyebrows, and eyelashes is not under the control of sex hormones, but hair in the ears and nose, as well as beard and mustache growth, are androgen dependent, as is the growth of body hair on the chest, shoulders, back, and abdomen. Pubic and axillary hair, as well as other hair under the control of sex hormones, normally occurs only in adults. Pubic hair growth occurs with the onset of puberty and is followed 1 or 2 years afterward by the growth of axillary hair.

Other hormonal changes affect hair growth. After pregnancy, for example, there is a shortening of the growth cycle of hair, which results in temporary hair thinning on the scalp. Oral contraceptives and some medications, including thallium, antimitotic agents, anticoagulants, antithyroid drugs, trimethadione, allopurinol, amphetamines, salicylates, levadopa, gentamicin, clofibrate (rare), and prolonged and excessive ingestion of vitamin A, may also produce hair thinning (drug-induced alopecia). ***Alopecia*** (hair loss) may also result from aging, genetic factors, trauma, and local or systemic disease. Among the systemic conditions that may be associated with alopecia are disseminated lupus erythematosus, lymphomas, cachexia, uncontrolled diabetes, secondary syphilis, dermatomyositis, and severe hypothyroidism or hypopituitarism. Intense emotional stress may also cause alopecia. Traumatic alopecia may occur from traction of tight "ponytails" or from the trauma of hair-curling or straightening methods, and may result in bulb damage and scarring.

Scalp hair loss or balding in the typical ***male distribution pattern*** (affecting primarily the crown and lateral frontal regions) is a sex-linked dominant trait. In rare cases, the pattern may involve the temporal regions as well. This type of hair loss (which may also occur in women with bilateral frontal recession) results from a shortening of the growth cycle. Hair removed from the affected areas by combing are typically short, tapered (indicating that they have not been cut), and clubbed (telogen hairs). ***Female pattern loss,*** which may also appear in men, consists of a diffuse thinning on the scalp that spares the occipital region and a normal hairline. The temporal region is the most severely affected, with as little as one-third of the normal hair density. It usually appears in women after the age of 40 but may occur as early as age 20. The onset is usually gradual but may be abrupt.

Alopecia areata can occur suddenly at any age in individuals who have no obvious skin disorder or systemic disease. There are circumscribed patches of hair loss (most frequently on the scalp or beard area), which may be smooth or have a few hairs remaining. Examination of hairs around the involved area shows numerous small anagen (growing) hairs with abnormally tapered ends (not clubs). Biopsy reveals lymphocytic infiltration of the hair bulbs and follicles that are smaller than normal and set high in the dermis. Other findings include serum antibodies to thyroglobulin, adrenal cells, parietal cells, and thyroid. The cause of the condition is unknown, but it is usually self-limited, with complete regrowth of hair. However, recurrences may take place and some cases, particularly the more extensive forms (alopecia totalis and alopecia universalis) or alopecia that begins in childhood, may be permanent. Severe forms of alopecia areata may be treated with systemic corticosteroids (to suppress adrenal androgen production), in the equivalent of 2.5–7.5 mg prednisone daily plus oral antiandrogens, but the long-term therapy required is usually not justified in light of the serious risks accompanying long-term corticosteroid use. Daily application of anthralin, 0.5% ointment, may provoke hair growth (caution is advised in using this drug with renal patients), and intralesional injections of triamcinolone acetonide suspension are sometimes effective.

Trichotillomania refers to voluntary pulling of one's own hair, a neurotic habit occurring most commonly in children. It may be difficult to distinguish from alopecia areata because of the presence of twisted and broken hairs. However, the hairs around affected areas are not readily plucked and anagen (growing) hairs are always present in the affected patches, since they must reach a certain length before they can be plucked. Biopsy reveals follicular plugging, hemorrhage within the bulb, and pigment casts in the follicular lumen. Covering the biopsy site with a gauze pad held down with collodion for several weeks (under the pretense of wound protection) will help to determine that hairs are growing normally.

Hirsutism, abnormal or excessive growth of hair, may occur in women as a manifestation of an endocrine disorder. The most frequent causes are adrenal virilism, basophilic adenoma of the pituitary, masculinizing ovarian tumors, and the Stein-Leventhal syndrome. It may also occur at menopause, with systemic androgen steroid therapy, systemic corticosteroid therapy, or in porphyria cutanea tarda. A modest amount of excess hair may occur in some women as a family trait. If an underlying disorder exists, it should be treated. Temporary local measures may include plucking, shaving, or waxing. Chemical depilatories may also be used but may cause skin irritation. If the hair is fine, a hair bleach may help to mask the condition. Electrolysis, which destroys individual hair follicles, is the only safe, permanent local treatment. Oral spironolactone, which suppresses androgenic skin activity, is an effective treatment with relatively minor side effects when administered cyclically (100 mg twice daily from day 4 to day 22 of each menstrual cycle). This drug not only decreases hair density but causes hair texture to become finer and softer, with noticeable improvement within 3–5 months of therapy (the lower abdomen and back are the least affected), as well as producing an improvement in acne and regularizing menstrual cycles that were previously disturbed. The side effects generally last for only the first few weeks of treatment.

Pseudofolliculitis barbae (ingrown beard hairs) occurs almost exclusively in black men. The stiff tips of beard hairs may either penetrate the skin before they leave the hair follicle or leave the follicle and then curve back to reenter the nearby skin surface, provoking a foreign body reaction. Pruritus is common. Having the patient grow a beard is the most effective treatment, but if this is not feasible, shaving should be avoided for several weeks until spontaneous resolution of the papules occurs. Then, when shaving is resumed, the hairs should not be cut so short as to encourage recurrence of the condition (a mechanical barber's trimmer may be used for this purpose). As an alternative, thioglycolate depilatory may be used every 2 or 3 days, but skin irritation is common, and growing a beard may be the only successful treatment for many patients. Mild or moderate cases may respond to topical application of 0.05% tretinoin (vitamin A acid, retinoic acid) liquid or cream every day. If irritation develops, it may be used every other day at first and then every day.

Folliculitis, a superficial or deep bacterial infection (usually staphylococcal) and irritation of the hair follicles, was discussed with other bacterial skin infections earlier in the discussion of dermis.

In persons with a predisposition for keloid formation, folliculitis barbae or chronic bacterial folliculitis may result in scarring, a condition known as ***folliculitis keloidalis*** (or acne keloid or dermatitis papillaris capillitii), which occurs most frequently on the nape of the neck and adjacent scalp; black men may develop it in the beard area. The major precipitating factor is the ingrowing of coarse, tightly curved scalp or beard hairs (sometimes related to close razor edging of the hairline or beard area), which results in a foreign body reaction (and possibly a secondary bacterial infection) followed by the development of small, round, firm, pigmented follicular papules. Moderate to severe pruritus and purulent exudation may occur. The treatment is similar to that for folliculitis (see the earlier section on bacterial skin infections) but also includes plucking or debriding with a polyester cleansing sponge (e.g., Buf-Puf Cleansing Sponge) to remove ingrown hairs. The area should be cleansed two or three times daily with an antibacterial soap (the scalp may be shampooed once or twice daily), followed by the application of a topical antibiotic or combination antibiotic-corticosteroid cream or ointment. A course of a culture-directed systemic antibiotic in adequate therapeutic doses will clear up the bacterial involvement. Intralesional injection of triamcinolone acetonide suspension (10 mg/mL) may also be used, and persistent papules may require a shave excision (flush with the skin surface) prior to the intralesional injection.

Fungal (tinea) infections are also discussed earlier in this chapter (see the discussion of epidermis).

Nails

Nails, like hair, are modifications of the epidermis, composed entirely of dead, keratinized epithelial cells. They function as stiff backings to protect the soft tissue at the tips of the fingers and toes. Beneath the nail is the nail bed, which is modified skin derived from the dermis and the deepest layers of the epidermis (Fig. 10.3). Its dermal component is composed of fibrous and elastic tissue. There are no papillae in this dermal layer; instead, there are narrow longitudinal ridges that are lower near the proximal end and increase in height toward its free distal border, abruptly giving way to papillae in the dermis of the skin there. The nail bed also lacks sweat glands and pilosebaceous units. The uppermost portion of the nail bed (closest to the nail) is the matrix, a thin epidermal layer that adheres to the nail plate and is continuous distally with the epidermis of the tip of the finger or toe. The area where these epidermal tissues join (just under the free edge of the nail) is called the "hyponychium," and has a thickened stratum corneum.

The majority of nail growth occurs in the matrix beneath the nail root, the proximal portion of the nail plate that is mostly hidden by a fold of epidermal skin (the nail fold) that is deeper at the nail's root and shallower where it extends forward along the sides of the nail. Mitotic division in the stratum germinativum of the matrix at the end of the root results in an increase in both the length and thickness of the nail plate as the newly formed cells become keratinized and join with the rest of the nail plate. The nail slides forward upon the underlying nail bed, along with the thin epidermal layer to which it adheres; if the nail is surgically or traumatically removed, this epidermal layer will be removed along with the nail. The entire nail may be stripped off and can still be replaced as long as the cells of the stratum germinativum that produce it are intact.

The keratin of nails is high in sulfur content and is therefore termed "hard." The nail root is more opaque than the rest (the body) of the nail plate, due to incomplete keratinization and drying and the presence of air spaces within the keratin matrix of that portion. As a result, the portion of the root that may be visible distal to the nail fold as the crescent-shaped laluna appears whitish. The body of the nail is translucent, and the normally pink color of this portion is due to the highly vascular nature of the underlying nail bed.

Where the epidermis of the skin at the proximal edge of the nail extends distally onto the nail plate, it is called the "cuticle." This structure functions to protect the space between the roof of the nail fold and the nail plate from the introduction of foreign substances from the environment. Cutting or pushing the cuticle back too roughly may destroy it, opening the space to infection. Beneath the cuticle is the eponychium, another solely epidermal structure, which is an extension of the nail fold anteriorly onto the nail plate.

Unlike hair growth, nail growth is normally continuous, but it varies according to

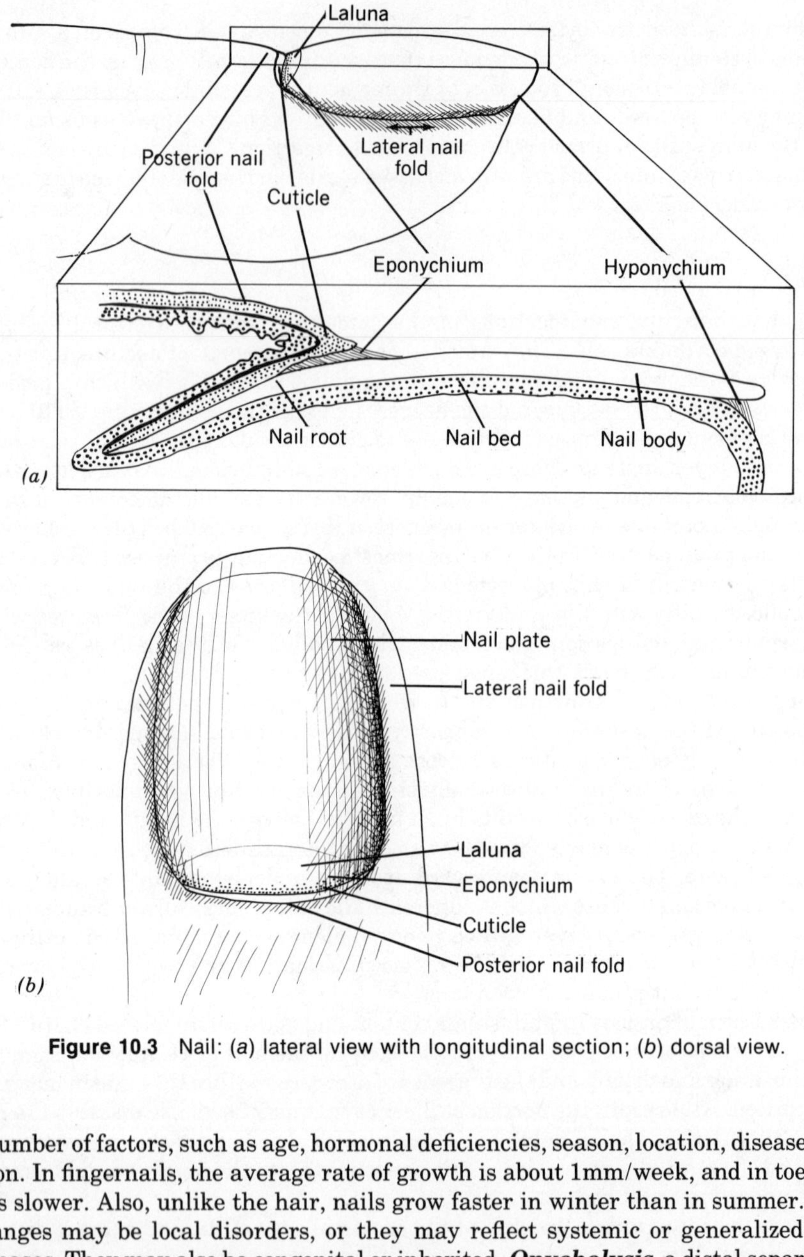

Figure 10.3 Nail: (*a*) lateral view with longitudinal section; (*b*) dorsal view.

a number of factors, such as age, hormonal deficiencies, season, location, disease, and so on. In fingernails, the average rate of growth is about 1mm/week, and in toenails it is slower. Also, unlike the hair, nails grow faster in winter than in summer. Nail changes may be local disorders, or they may reflect systemic or generalized skin diseases. They may also be congenital or inherited. ***Onycholysis,*** a distal separation of the nails from the nail bed (usually fingernail), may be caused by excessive exposure to water, detergents, soap, alkalis, and keratolytic agents. It has also been known to occur with the use of commercial nail hardeners and demeclocycline (an antibiotic), and may be secondary to trauma, onychomycosis (fungal nail infection), psoriasis, contact dermatitis, yellow nail syndrome, and Darier's disease. It may also be indicative of hypo- or hyperthyroidism.

Chronic inflammation of the nail matrix (beneath the eponychium) may result in nail plate distortions. Bacterial (paronychia) and fungal infections (***onychomycosis***) are common causes. The most common type of onychomycosis is ***distal ungual onychomycosis,*** which is frequently caused by *Trichophyton rubrum* infection and primarily involves the stratum corneum of the nail bed, causing a brownish discoloration at the edge of the nail that later spreads and results in thickening and irregularity of the nail plate and possibly onycholysis. Debris accumulates beneath the nail, and the site may be secondarily colonized by other opportunistic organisms. ***White superficial onychomycosis*** is a relatively common toenail infection (usually due to *Trichophyton mentagrophytes*) that is manifested as soft white islands on the nail surface that may spread to become large patches. The stratum corneum of the proximal nail fold is the primary site of ***proximal ungual onychomycosis,*** the least common type of nail fungus. This condition, usually caused by *T. rubrum,* begins as a small white spot near the proximal edge of the nail plate and later develops into larger plaques on the ventral surface of the nail. ***Candidal onychomycosis*** occurs in persons with a chronic mucocutaneous candidal infection. It begins at the distal end (free edge) of the plate and spreads proximally to involve the entire nail plate in both length and thickness, causing white or yellow discoloration of the subungual area, considerable disfiguration, and distal separation of the nail plate (onycholysis). Light microscopy of scrapings of the nail fixed with potassium hydroxide should be performed to verify the presence of a fungal infection. A culture in an appropriate medium will also help to establish the diagnosis.

Onychomycosis due to a member of the *Trichophyton* species or *Epidermophyton floccosum* (but not *Candida*) should be treated with systemic griseofulvin, 1.0 g/day of microsize, or 0.5 g/day of ultramicrosize for 3–8 months (even up to a year for toenails) until the nail has been completely replaced and all infected debris has been cast off. This long-term therapy entails a considerable risk of side effects (renal, hepatic, and hematopoietic, particularly leukopenia). Oral ketoconazole, 200 mg daily, may be used alternatively and is also indicated for candidal infections. It is usually well tolerated, but rare instances of liver toxicity with its use have been reported. It should be stopped immediately when nausea, indigestion, dark urine, clay-colored stools, or jaundice occurs. Decreased adrenal steroid synthesis may also occur, but giving the total daily amount in a single dose will help to prevent this reaction. Either of these systemic therapies should be supplemented by the following local measures: filing or sanding down the nails daily (if necessary, even to the nail bed), followed by the application (three to four times daily) of 1% ciclopirox cream (Loprox), 2% miconazole cream, 1% clotrimazole cream or lotion, or nystatin cream, 100,000 units/g. Carbol-fuchsin paint (Castellani's paint) or 1% gentian violet applied one to two times weekly may be used instead.

Paronychia, an acute or chronic inflammation of the soft tissue surrounding the nail (periungual tissues), is most common in persons whose hands are continuously exposed to water and/or other irritants such as detergents or sterilizing solutions (e.g., laundry workers, housekeepers, medical personnel) and diabetics. The infection usually begins as a red, tender swelling of the proximal nail fold that may extend around the nail margin ("run-around" paronychia) and may lead to eventual loss of the cuticle. Pus may somtimes be expressed from the space between the nail plate and the proximal nail fold. If untreated, the infection can go deeper to form an intradermal or subdermal abscess with throbbing pain and point tenderness, or it may extend beneath the nail plate with suppuration. Rarely, a persistent, untreated infection that penetrates into deeper tissues may involve the tendons, with necrosis and further extension along the sheaths. Chronic infection may cause discoloration (black or brown) of the nail and nail plate dystrophy. An acute paronychia is usually due to staphylococci, but *Streptococcus, Escherichia coli,* and *Pseudomonas* have all been known to cause paronychia.

Treatment of acute paronychia includes hot, wet compresses or soaks, drainage, and elevation of the extremity. If it is treated early (within the first 2 or 3 days), drainage may usually be accomplished by inserting a blunt instrument (a flat metal spatula or the edge of a hardwood stick) under the nail fold and gently but firmly prying the skin away from the nail. If no pus appears, it may be that none is present, but a fluctuant swelling that is not drained by this technique should be incised and drained (the expressed pus should be cultured). If there is subungual extension, a portion of the proximal nail plate should be removed. The fingertip or toe should then be soaked (for 15–20 minutes) in very hot water four times daily for a few days. Between soaks, an antibiotic ointment should be applied, and the nail should be covered with a loose dressing (to allow continued drainage) and the extremity should be elevated. Systemic antibiotics (chosen according to culture and sensitivity test results, if possible) may be administered for 3–5 days as well, particularly for deep infections with subungual extension.

"***Green nails***" is a condition caused by a *Pseudomonas* infection of the nail plate itself. It is characterized by green-black discoloration of the nail plate due to the presence of pyocyanin, a blue-green pigment produced by the bacteria. The coloring and onycholysis usually appear first in the lateral nail fold, but extend to involve the entire plate. Topical application of 15% sulfacetamide (Sebizon) and soaking in a dilute chlorine bleach and water solution (1 part bleach with 4 parts water) have been used to treat this resistant infection.

A number of systemic and local conditions may result in ***dystrophic nail changes.*** Single or multiple longitudinal grooves may occur as a genetic defect or may be a result of trauma or the impingement of warts, nevi, or other growths on the nail matrix. Beau's lines (transverse depressions in the nail plate) often involve all of the nails and may be caused by any serious illness that temporarily interferes with nail growth (e.g., measles, mumps, myocardial infarction, carpal tunnel syndrome); they may also result from faulty manicuring. Hippocratic nails (club fingers) may be congenital or related to prolonged hypoxemia in cardiopulmonary conditions. Splinter hemorrhages may occur in subacute bacterial endocarditis, mitral stenosis, hypertension, malignancy, psoriasis, peptic ulcer disease, trauma, and rheumatoid arthritis. Hemorrhagic streaking may also occur as an allergic reaction to ingredients in commercial nail polishes or hardeners.

Sebaceous Glands

Sebaceous glands, simple, branched or unbranched alveolar glands that are classified as holocrine glands (the secretion contains the cells of the gland), arise from the walls of the hair follicle. In the fetus, these glands develop by invagination of the epidermal layer in the same manner as the hair follicles, and their short duct is actually an extension of the follicle's outer epithelial sheath. Sebaceous glands are found everywhere on the skin surface where hair grows and generally occur in quantities of two or more per hair. They vary in size from 0.2 to 2.2 mm and are largest on the skin of the nose. The size and production of sebaceous glands are controlled entirely by hormonal conditions. The activity of these glands is increased by androgens and suppressed by estrogens.

The secretion of these glands, sebum, is a fatty substance that is formed in cells at the periphery of the gland and contains fats, cholesterol, soaps, inorganic salts, albuminous material, and cell remains. As the cells containing the fluid move slowly toward the centers of the gland's lobules, they degenerate and the sebum is released. This moves continuously through the short duct and alongside the hair shaft toward the skin surface, picking up by-products of epidermal keratinization, bits of bacteria, debris, and sloughed epidermal cell lipids and protein along the way. Joined with the fatty surface epidermal by-products, it forms a film at a pH between 4.2 and 5.6 on the skin's surface. In addition to assisting in waterproofing and insulating the skin surface, this film is somewhat resistant to bacterial and fungal action. It also makes the hair and skin soft and pliable.

Although sebaceous glands generally open into hair follicles, in some regions of the body, such as the anogenital region and the face, certain glands seem to open directly onto the skin surface. In some cases, as at the lip margin or on the labia minora, sebaceous glands may occur independently of hairs. In general, however, these are large glands associated with disproportionately small hair follicles and hairs that fail to be expelled to the outside; they may play a role in the development of acne.

Modifications of sebaceous glands exist on the eyelids (ciliary glands), in the ear canals (ceruminous glands), and on the prepuce and glans of the penis (preputial glands). No such sebaceous glands exist on the glans and prepuce of the clitoris.

Normal changes in the activity of these glands occur throughout the life cycle. At birth the sebaceous glands are small (the vernix caseosa, present at birth, is a sebaceous gland secretion). They increase in size and output by puberty, especially on the face, chest, and back, as a result of androgenic hormones of the testes, ovaries, and adrenals. After puberty the secretion of sebum remains at a high level until menopause and old age, when production returns to preadolescent levels, sometimes resulting in problems with dry skin (see the discussion of xeroderma) and hair.

A ***sebaceous nevus*** is a congenital lesion of the sebaceous glands that often does not become apparent until adolescence, when adrenal stimulation causes proliferation and enlargement of sebaceous glands. The lesion is a tan or yellowish verrucous (warty) plaque, usually on the scalp or face, that is devoid of hair. Although the lesion itself is benign, about 15–20% develop additional lumps within the lesion, some of which turn out to be basal cell carcinoma. Therefore, prophylactic excision is advisable.

Sebaceous hyperplasia (hyperplastic sebaceous glands), more common in middle-aged and older persons than in younger ones, is a disorder characterized by the appearance of small, yellow, multilobulated papules with a central punctum, usually on the face. A "cheesy" sebaceous material may be expressed from the lesions. Although these lesions are little more than a cosmetic nuisance, they should be carefully watched, since they often resemble basal cell carcinoma. Cryotherapy (with liquid nitrogen), light electrodesiccation, or shave excision may be used effectively to treat individual lesions, but systemic isotretinoin therapy may be more effective for multiple diffuse lesions.

►***Acne*** (acne vulgaris) is a common inflammatory disease affecting the pilosebaceous units (hair follicles and sebaceous glands) that usually begins at puberty, when increased androgen production in genetically predisposed individuals causes enlargement and increased production of the sebaceous glands. The disease, which is more common and more severe in boys, may be exacerbated just prior to or during menstruation in girls. Cosmetics and topical corticosteroids may sometimes cause eruptions. The complex pathogenesis of acne involves an interaction of several variables, including hormonal activity, keratinization, sebaceous activity, and bacteria. Hyperkeratosis within the follicles leads to blockage of the follicular infundibulum and sebum retention, which results in overgrowth of *Propionibacterium* (the acne bacillus) within the retained sebaceous material. An accumulation of free fatty acids (from a breakdown of sebum triglycerides by the bacterial lipases) that are irritating to the walls of the follicle and a foreign body reaction to extrafollicular sebum also occur. The lesions, which may affect the face, neck, shoulders, upper back, and chest, consist of inflamed "pimples" (papules or pustules) and open ("blackheads") or closed ("whiteheads") comedones. Cyst formation, slow resolution, and scarring may also occur.

Treatment of acne should include thorough patient education and supportive counseling, as well as scrupulous hygiene. Systemic antibiotic therapy (minocycline or erythromycin), high-estrogen oral contraceptive therapy, and oral isotretinoin (for severe cystic acne), as well as a number of local measures, including keratoplastic and keratolytic agents, dermabrasion, natural and artificial UV radiation therapy, cryotherapy, intralesional corticosteroid injections, topical antibiotic preparations, and a number of commercial cleansers and lotions (most contain benzoyl peroxide) are among those measures commonly used in the treatment of acne.

Rosacea is a chronic inflammatory skin disorder of middle-aged or older persons characterized by rosy erythema and telangiectasia (vascular component), papules, pustules, and seborrhea (acneiform component), and soft tissue hyperplasia, particularly of the nose (rhinophyma). A genetic factor is likely, and seborrheic diathesis, GI dysfunction, and emotional disturbances are often associated. There is a statistically significant incidence of migraine headaches associated with rosacea. Treatment includes a combination of broad-spectrum oral antibiotics (preferably tetracycline, which has few side effects associated with long-term use) and local measures. Clinician should begin by administering 250 mg tetracycline on an empty stomach (i.e., between meals) four times daily until a beneficial response is obtained, and should then switch to a maintenance dose of 250 mg/day every day or every other day to control the disease. Topical 5 or 10% benzoyl peroxide will often eliminate the lesions (but not the telangiectasia) if it is used for 5–8 weeks. Hydrocortisone cream, 0.5–1%, is also effective, but fluorinated cortisones are contraindicated, since they aggravate rosacea. Demodicidosis ("demodex acne") is a variant of rosacea in which a large number of *Demodex folliculorum* (a mite) may be seen on microscopic exam of squeezings taken from the pores and mounted in glycerin on a covered slide. This condition should be treated with a miticidal preparation (see the discussion of scabies). Rosacea should also be differentiated from discoid lupus erythematosus, cutaneous granulomas, and drug eruptions (bromoderma and iododerma).

Sweat Glands

There are two types of sweat or sudoriferous glands in the skin; classified by their method of secretion, they are apocrine glands and eccrine sweat glands. Apocrine glands are found in the axillae, on the nipple and areola, scrotum, prepuce, and labia majora and around the umbilicus, vagina, and anus, but are hormone dependent and do not develop fully until puberty. When mature, they are large (3–5 mm), branched sweat glands whose ducts open onto the surface of the skin and are generally associated with hair follicles. Their secretion, a thick whitish, gray, or yellowish fluid, is stored in the cells of the periphery of the gland, which fill with the fluid, bulge, become stalked, and cast off, losing the edge of their cytoplasm, which enclosed the fluid along with the secretion, into the associated hair follicle. The secretion of this gland is rich in organic matter and contains various chemicals that of themselves are odorous but may take on a stronger and more unpleasant odor when trapped in body hairs and subjected to bacterial action.

Smaller (0.3–0.4 mm in diameter) eccrine sweat glands are important primarily in thermoregulation and maintenance of homeostasis of fluid and electrolytes. They are distributed over the entire body surface (with the exception of the nail beds and the skin of the lips and glans and the inner layer of the prepuce penis) and are most abundant in the axillae, the palms and soles, and the forehead. It is estimated that 1 $in.^2$ on the skin of the palms contains about 3,000 sweat glands.

These structures are long, unbranched tubes that originate in a simple coil located in the deep reticular layer of the dermis and occasionally in the subcutaneous tissue. The duct pursues a straight or winding course toward the epidermis, which it enters between the papillae of the superficial dermal layer, continuing to spiral through the layers of the epidermis and ending independently of hair follicles in a tiny surface pore. The deep, coiled, secretory portion, which comprises about three-fourths of the gland, is surrounded by a mesh of lymphatics, secretory capillaries, and nerves. The secretion, which is eliminated in and between the cells of the gland through these capillaries, is ordinarily an oily fluid that lubricates the skin but, under the influence of the nerves, becomes watery sweat (or sudor), a hypotonic salt solution with a pH ordinarily ranging from 4 to 6 and containing about 99% water with sodium chloride, ammonia, urea, uric acid, creatinine, glucose, lactic acid, amino acids, fatty acids, and traces of the water-soluble vitamins B and C. Since sweat contains nitrogenous wastes similar to those found in urine, the skin is considered to be an excretory organ.

The sequence of activation of these eccrine sweat glands depends on whether the stimulus of activation is thermal or emotional. In thermal activation, whenever the environmental temperature reaches 88–90°F, the sweat glands on the forehead begin first to pour perspiration reflexively over the skin surface. This is followed by activation of the sweat glands over the remainder of the facial skin and then over the general body surface; the last to be activated are the glands on the palms and soles. Interestingly, nervous activation of the sweat glands produces an opposite pattern, beginning with the palms and soles, followed by the general body surface, then the face, and lastly the forehead. Unlike the apocrine glands, the eccrine sweat glands are active throughout life.

Hyperhidrosis (excessive perspiration) may be generalized or localized to the palms, soles, axillae, groin, or under the breasts. The skin is often pink or blue-white in the affected areas, and in severe cases there may be maceration, fissuring, and scaling. The excessive wetness increases the potential for the development of skin diseases, including contact dermatitis and bacterial or fungal infections. Increased perspiration may be a normal physiologic response to increased environmental heat or may accompany fever, but generalized sweating may also be a manifestation of an underlying endocrinopathy or CNS disorder. The cause of localized hyperhidrosis is not known, but if it occurs on the palms, it may be psychogenic. Any underlying systemic disorder that is associated with generalized hyperhidrosis should be treated. Preparations containing an aluminum chlorhydroxy complex (Breezee Mist or Pedi-Dri foot powders) are often effective topical treatments for localized hyperhidrosis of the feet. For axillary hyperhidrosis, a 20% aluminum chloride hexahydrate solution in anhydrous ethyl alcohol (Drysol) may be used. It should be applied to clean, dry skin (not to broken, irritated, or recently shaven skin) at bedtime, tightly covered with an occlusive film (e.g., polyethylene), and removed with soap and water in the morning. Two consecutive applications will often provide 1 week of protection, and it may be used once or twice weekly (or as needed) thereafter. A more dilute solution (Xerac AC is 6.25% aluminum chloride hexahydrate) may be used daily as an antiperspirant instead. Axillary bromhidrosis should be treated by shaving the axillary hair, daily bathing, and daily use of a preparation containing an aluminum chlorhydroxy compound (e.g., Xerac or Drysol), as described above.

Miliaria (heat rash, prickly heat) is an acute inflammatory eruption characterized by aggregates of minute, discrete lesions on covered skin surfaces (usually the arms, trunk, or intertriginous regions) accompanied by burning, itching, and stinging. The lesions are caused by obstruction and inflammation of the ostia of sweat ducts, which results in ballooning and eventually rupture of the ducts. The sweat seeps into the surrounding tissues, causing irritation and, frequently, severe pruritus. If the obstruction is in the deeper dermal layer, the characteristic lesions are red papules (miliaria rubra); if it is epidermal, they are vesicular (miliaria crystallina). If untreated, the condition may progress to fever, heat exhaustion, heat stroke, or death. Symptomatic treatment includes measures to cool and dry the affected area and application of an antipruritic powder or cooling lotion such as menthol, phenol, 0.1% triamcinolone acetonide, or unscented Lubriderm lotion two to four times a day. Preventive measures include avoidance of hot, moist environments and control of environmental temperatures, ventilation, and humidity. Overbathing and the use of irritating soaps should be avoided. An increase in skin aerobes (especially cocci) seems to play a role in the development of this condition, and superficial pyoderma should be treated with systemic therapy (erythromycin, cloxacillin). Oral anticholinergic drugs (e.g., glycopyrrolate, 1 mg two times a day) may help in severe cases.

Details of Management

▸ *Minor Burns*

Laboraotry Tests: None.

Therapeutic Measures: After removing the clothing from the entire wound area, cooling it with a saline solution or water, and establishing that the depth, extent, and site of the injury do not necessitate hospitalization, analgesics may be administered for pain (e.g., aspirin or codeine or, for severe pain, a more potent narcotic for 2 or 3 days). For some burns, prompt and gentle application of a cool compress may provide sufficient relief. Gently cleanse and debride the wound by sponging it with water or saline (no soaps or vigorous washings). Very small blisters may be left intact, as well as those of minor burns on the palms or soles, which should be protected beneath a bulky dressing for 7–10 days after the injury. Although minor burn wounds pose a very low risk for tetanus infection, it is still recommended that tetanus toxoid prophylaxis be administered to patients who have not been immunized within the previous 5 years or whose immunization status is uncertain. Dressings are usually not necessary for epidermal burns, but one of the available products containing aloe vera extracts (at least 60%) may be the best topical medication for this type of burn, since it possesses analgesic and antimicrobial properties and has been said to decrease subsequent pruritus and peeling. Topical sprays containing benzocaine or other anesthetics are never recommended, since their use carries a significant risk of sensitization, preventing later use of related anesthetics. For deeper partial- and full-thickness minor burns, the first (innermost) layer of the wound dressing should be a nonadherent fine-mesh gauze impregnated with petrolatum or, preferably, silver sulfadiazine cream (200 g per 5-yard roll of gauze), which is then covered with several layers of absorbent gauze and loosely wrapped with rolled gauze dressing to make a bulky, occlusive protective covering (the loose dressing accommodates any swelling or drainage and protects against further injury). Secure it with a tape if necessary. Small full-thickness minor burns may be treated initially on an outpatient basis, but they generally require surgical excision of the eschar and grafting for proper healing and reepithelialization to occur.

Patient Education: Instruct the patient or a responsible party in the appropriate use of prescribed medications for pain and the technique of dressing changes. Dressings should be changed every 24 hours, and the wound should be cleansed at the time of the dressing change by rinsing or showering. The injured part (if it is an extremity) should be elevated as much as possible between dressing changes, and the patient should be advised to seek medical help if signs of infection (increased pain or redness around the wound, a persistent temperature above 38.5°C, or chills) develop.

Follow-up: See patients in 48–72 hours and every 2–3 days thereafter until healing has occurred. Examine for the development of cellulitis around the site of the injury, and since endogenous beta-hemolytic streptococcus is the usual infective organism, prescribe oral penicillin (erythromycin for penicillin-allergic persons) if this occurs. A lubricating agent is often necessary to prevent scaling and flaking once the wound has healed, since the destruction of sebaceous glands results in diminished natural skin lubrication. Many products are available, ranging from simple vegetable shortening to vitamin E oil (which may cause contact dermatitis) to a cream with cocoa butter or lanolin base. Since the healed injury site is especially susceptible to solar damage, the patient should be advised to use a sunscreen with a high SPF for as long as 1 year after healing has occurred.

▸ *Localized Cold Injuries (Frostnip, Chilblains, Frostbite)*

Laboratory Tests: None.

Therapeutic Measures: Rapid rewarming is the initial step in treating all cold injuries; it may be passive (bundling the patient in blankets) or active (applying external heat sources). In remote areas, even applying firm, steady pressure with a warm hand or placing the hands in the armpits or groin may be sufficient for very superficial cold injuries, but the preferred method of active rewarming is immersing the affected body part(s) in warm water (38–41°C), since rapid thawing using temperatures slightly above body temperature will decrease the chances of tissue necrosis. Water in this temperature range feels warm but not hot to the normal hand; the temperature should never be warmer than 43°C. Hot water bottles or heating pads may also be used, but immersion is preferable. The area should not be rubbed or massaged, since these actions may cause breakdown of the damaged cellular tissue and increase the chance of gangrene. If the patient is conscious, hot drinks may be given to help warm the body from within. External heat should be discontinued when thawing has occurred and the part has returned to body temperature (usually in about 30 minutes). Patients with frostbite should be hospitalized. The injured areas must be protected from infection after rewarming until healing has occurred. If infection does occur, it should be treated with soaks in mild soapy water or with local application of povidone-iodine for local infections or systemic antibiotics for deep infections. Treatments twice daily for 15–20 minutes in a whirlpool bath (the water should be slightly below body temperature) may be used for 3 weeks or more to aid in cleansing and debridement of superficial sloughing tissue.

Patient Education: The patient should be instructed that the affected body part may be easily injured and should be protected from any trauma, including pressure or friction. Bed rest and elevation of uncovered affected parts (casts, dressings, and bandages are not to be used) at room temperature should be continued throughout the early stage of the healing period. Physical therapy is contraindicated during this stage. Instruct the patient that after the injury heals, the injured areas may be especially sensitive to subsequent cold exposure.

Follow-up: As healing progresses, physical therapy becomes important for promoting circulation to injured body parts.

▸ *Toxicodendron (Plant) Dermatitis (Poison Ivy, Oak, Sumac)*

Laboratory Tests: None.

Therapeutic Measures

Mild dermatitis: Limited involvement (less than 10% of the total body surface) of mild dermatitis requires only local measures for control of pruritus, including cool compresses or soaks (water, saline, Burow's solution, cold skim milk) or baths (with colloidal oatmeal, starch, oatmeal and baking soda, or starch and baking soda) for 20 minutes four to six times daily, followed by application of a bland lotion such as calamine. Protective bandaging between soaks may be used for moist, exudative lesions and may be soaked off at the time of the next treatment. In some instances, topical corticosteroid creams or gels may be used to clear the symptoms and hasten resolution (do not bandage over topical steroids, however, since occlusive dressings increase systemic absorption). Topical agents containing such ingredients as benzocaine, neomycin, zirconium, or diphenhydramine should not be used because of the risk of sensitization. If pruritus is severe and is not manageable with local measures, oral antihistamines may be helpful.

Moderate dermatitis: Dermatitis affecting 10–30% of the body and excluding the hands, face, and genitalia may be managed in much the same manner, with Burow's soaks for drying vesicular lesions followed by a steroid gel. Moderate dermatitis with vesicle formation has an increased potential for secondary infection, and systemic antibiotics should be given whenever bacterial involvement develops.

Severe dermatitis: A severe eruption with bullae and edema (affecting more than 30% of the body surface or involving the hands, face, or genitalia) requires a 2- to 3-week course of systemic corticosteroids, unless it is contraindicated. The equivalent of prednisone, 40–60 mg/day, should be given initially until a clinical response is obtained; then it should be tapered gradually and discontinued by about the 14th or 21st day. Local symptomatic measures may be used to supplement the systemic steroids, as described above. If systemic steroids are contraindicated, a high-potency topical steroid preparation (e.g., betamethasone dipropionate) may be used under occlusion for 24 hours, followed by 24 hours with no treatment, and then used again for 24 hours. Rest is important, since overheating and sweating may intensify the dermatitis. Hospitalization is sometimes required for a severe, incapacitating dermatitis. Secondary bacterial infections should be treated with appropriate systemic antibiotics.

Patient Education

Recognition: Patients should be taught to recognize plants of the *Toxicodendron* genus so that they may avoid them. The following features are common among the toxicodendrons:

1. The stem holding the terminal leaflet is longer than the stems holding lateral leaflets.
2. Poison oak and ivy have 3 leaflets per leaf, and poison sumac has 7–13 leaflets.
3. Leaves are green in the spring and early summer but turn orange or red in late summer and fall.
4. U- or V-shaped scars mark the branches at sites where leaves were attached previously.
5. Flowers and fruit grow at angles between the leaf and branch, and are green initially and cream-colored later (mature fruit of benign sumacs is reddish and occurs at the end of branches).
6. Aerial rootlets occur on larger vines.
7. Oleoresin characteristically turns black when exposed to air, and crushing a suspicious leaflet in a piece of white paper (avoiding skin contact with the plant) will result in black spots on the paper within about 5 minutes if the plant is a toxicodendron.

Prevention: Patients should be instructed that clothing can be an effective barrier (unless it becomes saturated with the oleoresin) and, even in warm summer months, wearing protective attire is an important preventive measure when time is to be spent in woods or other areas where toxicodendrons proliferate. Explain that the dermatitis is not spread by vesicle fluid but that the antigen may remain under fingernails or on clothing, pet fur, or other objects and contact with these fomites may continue to cause a dermatitis in sensitive individuals weeks or months after the initial contamination. The oleoresin remains quite stable at cool, dry temperatures, but water and high temperatures will inactivate it, so routine washing of exposed skin surfaces and nails in hot soapy water (or even plain water) and laundering of clothing immediately after wearing whenever contamination is likely to have occurred is advised. Washing the skin within 10 minutes of contact will usually prevent the dermatitis, but this should be done even if the eruption has developed, since removal of any unbound oleoresin will prevent its subsequent spread. Premoistened alcohol or acetone wipes may be carried to wash the hands and face after working or hiking in a wooded area or field.

Follow-up: As needed.

▶ *Atopic Dermatitis*

Laboratory Tests: Scratch tests with specific allergens produce immediate skin reactivity. There is a delayed blanch reaction to methacholine, abnormal cyclic adenosine monophosphate (cAMP)-phosphodiesterase activity, elevated levels of serum IgE, and possibly eosinophilia.

Therapeutic Measures: Systemic corticosteroid therapy may produce significant improvement but should be avoided in favor of local measures whenever possible, since this is a lifelong problem associated with numerous relapses and chronic steroid use is associated with a number of serious complications. Treat limited sites of cutaneous inflammation with high-potency topical corticosteroids applied in a thin film and rubbed in thoroughly (twice daily). Tachyphylaxis (rapid onset of tolerance to the product) can be avoided when using high-potency steroids by alternating 2-day periods of treatment (applied twice daily) with 2-day periods of no treatment. Warn patients that extensive use can result in high blood levels of steroid and adrenal suppression. For long-term use (more than 3 months) or extensive involvement, use less potent preparations (e.g., containing hydrocortisone) in the same manner. Acute exudative lesions are best treated with wet dressings or soaks (saline, sodium bicarbonate, or aluminum subacetate solution) for 30 mintues three or four times daily or a drying lotion (e.g., calamine or a starch lotion) when soaks are not feasible. If lesions are dry and lichenified (as in chronic lesions), choose agents that are lubricating, keratolytic, antipruritic, or mildly keratoplastic as required. Corticosteroids or tar preparations incorporated in an ointment or paste are the usual treatments for chronic lesions. Persons unable to use tar preparations may benefit from iodochlorhydroxyquin, 3% ointment or cream. High doses of oral antihistamines such as hydroxyzine, diphenhydramine, or chlorpheniramine can be given for their antipruritic and sedative effects (increasing the dosage gradually to avoid extreme drowsiness), and tricyclic antidepressants (e.g., doxepin or amitriptyline) are potent H-1 receptor blockers, making them highly effective for pruritus. Systemic antibiotics (e.g., erythromycin or dicloxacillin) may be indicated when the condition is aggravated by large numbers of *Staph. aureus* colonizing the involved skin. Highly pruritic pustules and painful fissures are signs of a staphylococcal infection. Certain highly allergenic foods, such as shellfish, nuts, chocolate, citrus fruits, milk products, eggs, and tomatoes, may be associated with atopic dermatitis. For severe, recalcitrant cases, these foods should be eliminated from the patient's diet for a week and, if improvement is observed, gradually reintroduced singly to determine if any of them is causing an allergic reaction.

Patient Education: Any of the following may trigger a reaction or exacerbate an existing dermatitis: emotional stress, physical exertion, sweating, skin irritants (e.g., wool, soaps), allergens, environmental temperature or humidity changes, and bacterial infections. Baths or showers should be brief and not too frequent or hot. Soap use should be limited to intertriginous areas, and an emollient should be applied within 3 minutes of bathing to skin that is still moist in order to maintain hydration. Patients with atopic dermatitis tend to have abnormalities in the delivery of sweat to the skin surface and chronic problems with miliaria (prickly heat). They should therefore avoid warm environments and limit activities that cause perspiration. If there is an associated cholinergic urticaria, it should be treated with appropriate anticholinergic agents (e.g., hydroxyzine and possibly cyproheptadine). Most patients may be aware of the role that emotional stress plays in this condition, but they should be encouraged to discuss it with family members and to develop effective strategies for discussing and working through problems in order to keep stress at a minimum.

Follow-up: As needed.

▸ *Herpes Zoster and Chickenpox*

Laboratory Tests: Staining with Wright's stain and performing a Tzanck test of scrapings from the base of vesicles will prove a viral origin, but direct immunofluorescent staining of the scrapings is necessary to differentiate the virus from herpes simplex. The presence of varicella-zoster virus in cultures obtained from vesicle fluid is diagnostic, and determination of serum levels of antibodies also confirm the diagnosis. WBCs often reveal leukopenia as an associated finding. Bacterial cultures of vesicles should be performed if secondary infection is suspected.

Therapeutic Measures

Herpes zoster: Use wet compresses (Burow's solution) and calamine lotion or a topical corticosteroid preparation for fluid-filled blisters and cool wet compresses followed by application of an antibiotic cream or ointment for crusted lesions. A drying agent (e.g., flexible collodion applied to lesions q12h) or a preparation containing glycerin and menthol may provide limited symptomatic relief. In the acute phase, a mild analgesic such as aspirin, 600 mg orally every 4–6 hours, or a combination of acetaminophen and 15–60 mg codeine may be helpful. In severe cases, a course of systemic corticosteroids given early (within 5–10 days of the onset of symptoms) may relieve pain and decrease the incidence of postherpetic neuralgia, but it will not influence the rate of healing or shorten the acute phase of the infection. An initially large steroid dose such as oral prednisone, 60 mg/day in the morning for adults, should be continued for 7 days, followed by 30 mg/day for the next 7 days and 15 mg/day for 1 more week. There is a small risk of dissemination with this treatment, though, so it should certainly not be used for all cases and never in conditions when corticosteroids are contraindicated (e.g., untreated tuberculosis, persons receiving immunosuppressive therapy). Acycylovir has been used for immunosuppressed persons both to shorten the course of herpes zoster and to decrease the incidence of postherpetic neuralgia (oral doses are 200 mg five times daily). Also, fluphenazine hyrochloride (Permitil, Prolixin), 1 mg bid or tid, and amitriptyline hydrochloride, 25–75 mg/day at bedtime, often help to minimize postherpetic neuralgia. Secondarily infected lesions should be treated with appropriate systemic antibiotics.

Chickenpox: In uncomplicated chickenpox, treatment is usually unnecessary. However, wet compresses or lotions may be helpful for pruritus and thus prevent scratching, which may result in widespread infection or secondary bacterial infection of lesions. Severe cases may require antihistamines for pruritus. Secondary bacterial infection of a few local lesions may be treated with an antibacterial ointment (e.g., bacitracin-neomycin), but extensive lesions require appropriate systemic antibiotic therapy. Other complications (e.g., encephalitis, pneumonia) should be treated symptomatically, and corticosteroids may be helpful for varicella pneumonia. Zoster immune globulin (ZIG) or varicella-zoster immune globulin (VZIG) given IM within 72 hours after exposure may be beneficial for exposed immunosuppressed persons (including newborns whose mothers developed chickenpox within 4 days prior to or 2 days after delivery). These globulins may be obtained by contacting the Center for Disease Control, Atlanta, Georgia, at 404-329-3311 or the nearest regional Red Cross Blood Center.

Patient Education: Proper hygiene is particularly important to prevent secondary bacterial infection of chickenpox vesicles; nails should be kept short, and hands and nails very clean. Isolation during the communicable period of an infection (generally about 6 days until all vesicles have crusted over) is important to prevent spread of the infection. Chickenpox in susceptible immunosuppressed children (e.g., those with leukemia receiving antileukemic chemotherapy or those with kidney transplants) can be very serious and even fatal, and herpes zoster in immunosuppressed persons may become disseminated, with a generalized eruption (beyond the dermatome), visceral involvement, encephalitis, and even death as sequelae.

Follow-up: As needed for complications.

▶ *Rubella Vaccination*

Laboratory Tests: Serum levels of rubella hemagglutination inhibition (HI) antibodies should be determined to establish lack of immunity.

Therapeutic Measures: Live attenuated rubella virus vaccine is given routinely to most infants in the United States at about 15–19 months of age. Because of the devastating effect of maternal rubella infection upon the unborn fetus, women of childbearing age should be routinely screened for rubella HI antibodies. Those who are seronegative should be immunized while they are not pregnant, and contraception should be practiced for at least 3 months after immunization. Contraindications for vaccination include pregnancy and a defective or altered immune mechanism (e.g., as in lymphoma, leukemia, other malignancies, febrile illnesses, prolonged corticosteroid therapy, radiation therapy). Persons with an allergy to eggs should not receive vaccines prepared in duck embryo (alternative methods of preparation include the use of rabbit kidney and human diploid fibroblast tissue cultures).

Patient Education: Adult women who are immunized should be advised that pregnancy must be avoided for at least 3 months after receiving the vaccine. Solid immunity persists for more than 7 years in children vaccinated with live virus vaccine, but it may not be permanent.

Follow-up: Not necessary.

▶ *Insect Bites*

Laboratory Tests: None needed (see the subsequent discussions of pediculosis and scabies for specific diagnostic methods and treatments).

Therapeutic Measures: A tick that is still present on the skin should be removed at once. A petroleum product, nail polish, or an irritant such as alcohol should be applied directly to the insect. It may then be carefully removed with tweezers or a tissue, being careful not to leave the head embedded in the skin, since deeper migration, chronic inflammation, and possibly a granuloma may develop. Do not jerk or twist the tick, and avoid using the fingers to remove ticks because of the risk of infection (particularly in regions endemic for Rocky Mountain spotted fever). The tick may be killed by placing it in alcohol or gasoline. Thoroughly clean the site with soap and water to prevent infection of the wound, and apply cold compresses (or an ice cube) to relieve pain and control swelling. Oral antihistamines and topical corticosteroid creams or lotions may be given for symptoms (pruritus and inflammation). The patient should be watched for signs of any infection (rickettsial or spirochetal) that might have been transmitted by the tick, including chills, fever, malaise, headache, disseminated aches and pains, nausea, lymphadenopathy, restlessness, fatigue, a localized eschar, or a rash. A rise in serum antibodies will confirm a suspected infection, which should be treated with appropriate antimicrobial drugs (see the discussions of specific tick-borne infections). The sites of other types of insect bites should also be cleansed thoroughly. Cold compresses, topical corticosteroids, and oral antihistamines may be used, as mentioned above. Other symptomatic treatments include soaks in Burow's solution or application of calamine lotion for pruritus and analgesics (aspirin, Tylenol, codeine) for pain. A topical antibiotic ointment or cream may be applied if there is a possibility of bacterial infection, but creams or sprays containing benzocaine or other anesthetics should not be used, since they carry a risk of sensitization.

Patient Education: Ticks are commonly found in woody or grassy areas and along paths and trails, and are picked up by persons or animals brushing against them. Patients should be advised to wear protective clothing (hats, long-sleeved tops, and long pants tucked into socks) and should use insect repellants whenever entering areas likely to be infested. White, tan, or green colors and clothing made of tightly woven materials or containing a slick finish are best. Each person should thoroughly check his or her own body (and that of any pet) at least twice daily whenever any time is spent in a wood, field, or any area known to be infested with ticks. Pets should be treated with tick-repellant shampoos, powders, sprays, and collars. Perfumes, colognes, and other scented products (hair sprays, cosmetics, after-shave lotions) tend to attract insects and should be avoided when spending any time outdoors where insects might be found. Walking barefoot is also to be avoided.

Follow-up: None needed.

▸ *Pediculosis (Capitis, Corporis, Pubis)*

Laboratory Tests: None needed. Direct examination of the scalp, pubic region, body surfaces, and clothing (particularly undergarments in the case of pediculosis corporis and pediculosis pubis) will usually reveal lice, nits, louse excreta, and/or bites.

Therapeutic Measures: Applying 1% lindane (Kwell, Scabene) shampoo or lotion once daily after bathing (leaving it in place for 8–12 hours and then washing it off entirely) for 2 days and then repeating it after 10 days to destroy any nits that may have matured in the interim is promptly curative. Over-the-counter products containing pyrethrins in lotion form (Rid, Pyrinyl, A-200 Pyrinate, R&C Shampoo) may be applied undiluted to infested areas until they are wet and then washed off after 10 minutes and dried. (Do not exceed two applications in 24 hours.) After either of these treatments, hair should be combed with a fine-toothed comb to remove any remaining nits. Demonstration of living parasites after 7 days indicates that retreatment is necessary.

Patient Education: Recurrences are common, and simultaneous disinfestation of all close contacts (family members, sexual partners, etc.) who demonstrate lice, as well as decontamination of all sources of infestation (e.g., combs, hats, clothing, bedding), are necessary to decrease the potential for reinfestation. Decontamination should be accomplished by boiling, thorough laundering and steam pressing, or dry cleaning. Rugs, carpeting, and upholstery should be vacuumed frequently, and toilet seats should be scrubbed. Patients should be instructed that a single application of the parasitide as directed will kill the lice, and that prolonged use is not only unnecessary but has the potential to induce a persistent dermatitis, as well as CNS toxicity (for lindane), particularly in very young or pregnant patients.

Follow-up: As needed.

▸ *Scabies*

Laboratory Tests: Exam of a mounted specimen (obtained by shaving a tunnel with a scalpel or probing the end of a fresh tunnel with a needle or blade tip) in mineral oil or glycerin reveals the mite, ova, and/or feces, confirming the diagnosis.

Therapeutic Measures: Disinfestation may be achieved with 1% lidane (Kwell, Scabene) in a cream or lotion base applied in a thin layer after bathing once daily from the neck down, paying special attention to hands, feet, and intertriginous areas, left on for 12 hours (or overnight), and then thoroughly removed by showering or bathing. This treatment is not recommended in infants, young children, or pregnant women because of its potential for inducing CNS toxicity. Crotamiton (Eurax) cream or lotion may be used alternatively, massaging the medication into the skin for 2 consecutive nights after bathing. The medication should be thoroughly removed with soap and water 24 hours after the second application. Undergarments, nightwear, and bed linens should be changed and laundered after treatment. A second treatment 4–7 days after the first is occasionally necessary. Sometimes treatment of long-standing infestation will not provide rapid relief of signs and symptoms of the infestation, although the mites are successfully killed. Persistent pruritus after treatment is probably due to dead mites that are retained for a few weeks within the epidermis until the layers they occupy are shed, but patients may overuse the scabicide or overbathe in an attempt to stop the itching, and instead cause even more irritation and pruritus. Colloid baths or a topical corticosteroid product may help, and pruritic papules may be painted with undiluted crude tar oil or Estargel. An oral antihistamine may also be prescribed for severe pruritus that persists after therapy is completed, but if there is no improvement after several days, the miticide should be used again. If itching still persists, a short course of oral prednisone (e.g., for 7–10 days in tapered doses starting with 40 mg/day) will often provide relief. Because of the potential for overuse, nonrefillable prescriptions should be made out only for the amount needed (about 30 g or 1 oz for adults and less for children). A secondary pyoderma should be treated with appropriate systemic or topical (for localized involvement) antibiotics.

Patient Education: Patients should be advised that reinfestation is likely to occur from close contact with other infested persons, so simultaneous treatment of infested family members or sexual partners is an important measure for prevention of recurrences. Bedding and clothing are not common sources of infestation, but these should be laundered or cleaned. Patients should be instructed that a single treatment with an appropriate miticide is usually curative and that prolonged or prophylactic use (i.e., shampooing regularly with Kwell) is not only unnecessary but carries a significant risk of causing a dermatitis or sensitization, as well as absorption of large amounts of the active ingredients and CNS toxicity. Explain that pruritus that persists after treatment with a scabicide is not usually an indication of therapy failure and does not warrant repeated treatment.

Follow-up: As needed.

▶ *Psoriasis*

Laboratory Tests: The clinical appearance is usually sufficient to distinguish psoriasis from seborrheic dermatitis or other conditions. A skin biopsy may help to establish the diagnosis, but chronic eczematous conditions and seborrheic dermatitis may resemble psoriasis histologically. There may be an elevated uric acid level, reflecting an increased cellular turnover in the skin from the psoriasis.

Therapeutic Measures: For acute psoriasis, it is best to avoid irritating or keratolytic agents; a mild lotion such as calamine may be helpful during this stage. As the lesions become less acute, warm baths may be given daily and the lesions scrubbed with soap and water and a brush. Topical steroids are helpful for small new spots as well as older, tougher plaques, particularly on the scalp, face, and hands, but tachyphylaxis is a common occurrence with the long-term corticosteroid use common in psoriasis. To avoid this problem, always begin with weaker preparations and build up to stronger ones as required, applying them sparingly (in a thin film) by massaging gently into the skin. Steroids in an ointment base are more potent and preferable to creams, except for use in intertriginous areas. Because psoriasis is a lifelong condition, there is an increased potential for development of the complications of long-term steroid use (thinning of the skin, dermal atrophy, acneiform eruptions, superimposed fungal infections, and a high level of systemic absorption). Therefore, patients should be advised to keep track of the amount used and to limit their use of steroids whenever possible. It is advisable to prescribe no more than 60 g/week of the more potent steroid ointments (far less in children) for psoriasis patients, and patients should avoid using them for more than 3 weeks. Intralesional steroid injections (e.g., triamcinolone acetonide, 5 mg/mL) are extremely effective for discrete, resistant plaques, but the amount given at any one time should not exceed 2–3 mL and injections should not be repeated more than once every 3 weeks. Topical tars (in water-soluble or oil-soluble bases) are also commonly used in psoriasis. They are less expensive, give longer remissions, and have fewer side effects than steroids. However, they are greasy, so patients should be warned not to wear good clothing after applying them (tars in an alcohol base are not greasy and do not stain). They may be used on the general body surface, but not the face or intertriginous areas (e.g., groin, armpits, beneath breasts). Using downward strokes to apply the tars will help to prevent folliculitis. Whenever the hair is washed, a medicated shampoo (e.g., Sebutone, Ionil T, Polytar, Zetar) should be used. It is helpful to leave the shampoo on the scalp for at least 10 minutes (preferably 30 minutes) before rinsing it out. Tar and topical corticosteroid lotions may also be used on the scalp, and a nightly application of 0.5% anthralin (a coal tar distillate) cream or ointment followed by an oil (Neutrogena T/Derm oil) may be used for recalcitrant scalp lesions. Because of the irritating potential of anthralin, it is best to use a weaker strength (e.g., 0.1%) initially and then to progress to a higher concentration. This treatment also stains skin, light hair, and clothing and should not be used near eyes or in intertriginous areas. Both topical steroids and tar preparations may be used in combination with a keratolytic agent (e.g., 6% salicylic acid in a propylene glycol base) for thick psoriatic plaques. For psoriasis that is not manageable by the above treatments, patients should be referred to a specialist experienced in PUVA therapy, in which oral 8-methoxypsoralen is given and followed in 2 hours by exposure to long-wave UV light (330–360 nm). This is a highly effective method, usually clearing lesions after 10–25 treatments (given two to three times weekly) over a period of about 4–8 weeks. Maintenance treatments twice a month thereafter will generally prevent recurrences, but PUVA therapy is associated with serious side effects, such as an increased risk of skin cancer, cataract formation, and alteration of lymphocyte function.

Patient Education: The chronic but noncontagious nature of psoriasis should be explained fully to patients and the advantage of a healthy lifestyle emphasized. A balanced diet, regular exercise, adequate rest, and avoidance of excessive alcohol intake and smoking, as well as early management of coexisting illnesses (especially upper respiratory tract infections), are all important measures to keep the disease in remission or prevent exacerbations. Breaks in the skin (cuts or other traumas) are particularly susceptible to development of lesions and should be avoided. Also, since emotional stress is a factor in outbreaks, patients should be encouraged to work on managing the stress in their lives. Stress reduction and affirmation techniques may be very helpful and are described in a number of books. Helping the patient come up with ways to explain psoriasis to others is very important, and role playing of everyday situations may be helpful. Patients may find support and additional information and resources by contacting:

National Psoriasis Foundation
Dept. N81, Suite 110, 6415 S.W. Canyon Court
Portland, Oregon 97221
(503) 297-1545

Follow-up: As needed.

▸ *Tinea (Capitis, Corporis, Cruris, Manuum, Pedis, and Unguium)*

Laboratory Tests: Exam of scrapings of lesions prepared in 15% potassium hydroxide, cultures of the organisms, and exam of biopsy sections stained with periodic acid-Schiff technique are all used to diagnose dermatophyte infections. To obtain a culture of a superficial infection, brush the affected area with a sterile toothbrush and implant the brush on an appropriate medium. Tinea due to *Microsporum* fluoresces a light brown green under Wood's light, but affected hairs of *Trichophyton tonsurans* infection (the most common cause of tinea capitis) do not fluoresce at all.

Therapeutic Measures: Small, localized skin lesions usually respond to topical antifungal preparations used twice daily for about 2–3 weeks (tinea pedis and tinea manuum may require 4 weeks). A number of effective local treatments (cream, lotion, solution) are available for tinea of the body surface, including miconazole, clotrimazole, ciclopirox, haloprogin, tolnaftate, and sulconazole nitrate. All of these are strong irritants, and overtreatment should be avoided. The skin should be kept dry and open to the air as much as possible, and drying powders or soaks may be helpful, especially for tinea cruris and foot and hand infections. Loose-fitting underwear and nonirritating clothing are advised for tinea cruris, and wads of cotton may be placed between the toes at night for tinea pedis. Oral griseofulvin may be indicated for severe or unresistant infections (250–500 mg one or two times daily for about 2 weeks). Oral ketoconazole, 200 mg/day, is also effective for griseofulvin-resistant dermatophytosis, but relapse may occur when therapy is discontinued (there is some risk of hepatotoxicity with this treatment). Tinea capitis (scalp infection) is more difficult to treat, but a 2-week course of microsize oral griseofulvin (as described above) will cure most infections (occasionally a 4- to 6-week course is required). This systemic treatment can be supplemented by a shampoo containing selenium sulfide (Selsun, Exsel) used twice weekly. Kerion (raised, red, tender granuloma) may be treated with a saturated solution of potassium iodide taken orally. Tinea unguium (dermatophyte infections of the nail plate) are particularly difficult to treat. Griseofulvin should be given orally, 0.5–1.0 g/day (usually in 2 doses), until the entire nail has been replaced and the infected debris has been shed, which may take 3–8 months (or even a year for toenails). Oral ketoconazole, 200 mg/day, may be used as an alternative. To supplement the systemic therapy, the nail plate may be sandpapered or filed down daily (to the nailbed, if necessary) and a topical antifungal agent may be applied. Ciclopirox olamine (Loprox) cream is effective against dermatophyte infections and appears to penetrate better than any of the other available topical agents.

Patient Education: Discuss general hygienic measures to be observed for controlling sources of infection and reinfection (e.g., for tinea pedis, changing socks frequently, drying carefully between the toes after showering or bathing, and wearing rubber sandals in community showers and bathing areas). Emphasize the need to use topical agents as directed, since with localized tinea corporis there is often a tendency to discontinue treatment once a response is obtained (sometimes it is recommended to continue using the agent for 2 weeks after symptoms have disappeared). With more resistant infections requiring long-term treatment, patients may fail to use medications regularly. Caution patients against using occlusive dressings or wrappings and instruct them to report any signs of unusual irritation from topical antifungal agents. Also, explain that these are specific treatments for fungal infections and are not to be used for other types of dermatoses.

Follow-up: For less resistant infections (tinea corporis), reconsider the diagnosis if no response is seen after 4 weeks of therapy. For other infections requiring long-term systemic therapy with griseofulvin, monitor renal, hepatic, and hematopoietic function; for long-term ketoconazole therapy, hepatic function should be monitored.

▸ *Actinic Keratoses*

Laboratory Tests: The clinical appearance, location, and a history of sun exposure are usually sufficient to identify actinic keratoses, but biopsy of the lesion will confirm the diagnosis.

Therapeutic Measures: Excision, curettage, electrodesiccation, and cryotherapy are all effective treatments of actinic keratoses. However, when scarring or hypopigmentation would be a problem (cryotherapy has a cure rate of about 90–95% in most places on the body but may result in an area of relative hypopigmentation) or lesions are extensive, topical fluorouracil may be the best theapy. Fluorouracil, 1% cream or liquid (Efudex, Fluoroplex), should be applied sparingly every night (in the winter if possible) for 2–3 weeks. For patients using this therapy for the first time, a small area should be treated initially, and the patient should be advised that temporary crusting, oozing, redness, soreness, burning, stinging, and photosensitivity will occur. Topical 0.5% hydrocortisone lotion applied in the morning throughout the 3 weeks of treatment will help control the inflammatory reaction and photosensitivity; it may be continued after the fluorouracil therapy until the healing is complete (generally about 3 more weeks). Any lesions remaining after this point should be biopsied and the patient referred to a specialist to decide on further treatment. Multiple actinic keratoses or heavy, thick lesions may be treated more effectively by dermabrasion or chemosurgical exfoliation (e.g., trichloroacetic acid or phenolic acid). Both of these treatments remove most of the epidermis and upper papillary dermis, but they should be performed by persons trained and experienced in their use. Slightly more trichloroacetic acid than is necessary for successful treatment may cause scarring.

Patient Education: Explain to patients that actinic keratoses are a result of solar damage and must be treated, since they are precancerous. Patients receiving fluorouracil therapy should be carefully advised about how to use it, to wash their hands after each application in order to prevent accidentally getting it into the eyes (where it can cause conjunctivitis), and to avoid sun exposure while using it. Also, explain fully the skin reaction to expect with this treatment after about the third or fourth day of therapy (oozing, crusting, redness, soreness, stinging, burning) and emphasize compliance with the therapy in spite of discomfort, urging patients to contact you if they become concerned about severe reactions. Explain also that any lesions that do not respond to this treatment will have to be biopsied and may have to be removed surgically by a specialist, but that this does not necessarily mean that they are malignant. Stress the importance of regular use of sunscreen products whenever any time is spent in the sun, particularly in the summer and between 10 A.M. and 2 P.M.

Follow-up: Check on patients weekly. About 3 weeks after the end of fluorouracil therapy the inflammatory reaction usually subsides (the hydrocortisone lotion may be continued during this period), and any lesions that are left should be biopsied. The patient should be referred to a specialist for any remaining lesions and should be followed up for 5 years.

▸ *Acne*

Laboratory Tests: None needed.

Therapeutic Measures

General measures: Good hygiene is an important aspect of acne treatment and prevention. A mild soap (e.g., Neutrogena, Aveeno Bar, or Dove) and water should be used for skin cleansing (no more than two or three times daily), and the face should be rinsed thoroughly to remove any remaining soap. A number of prescription and nonprescription cleansers specific for acne are available (containing sulfur, salicylic acid, or benzoyl peroxide). However, acne is a follicular disease, and in order for any of these agents to be of help, they must remain on the skin long enough to penetrate the follicle, which does not occur with most face-cleansing agents.

Topical measures: Very mild acne (an occasional pimple) may often be treated sufficiently and least expensively with an over-the-counter product containing salicylic acid, sulfur, or benzoyl peroxide (Fostex, Listerex, Oxy 5, Oxy 10, pHisoAc BP). Since one factor in the pathogenesis of acne is an altered keratinization of the follicular canal due to excess sebum, the use of a keratolytic agent such as salicylic acid or sulfur helps to correct the defect in keratinization and to unplug comedones. Benzoyl peroxide also affects keratinization to a lesser extent, causing peeling within the follicle, but in addition it is bacteriostatic for *Propionibacterium* acnes because it releases oxygen into the follicle, which oxidizes the bacterium's proteins and inhibits the full development of new lesions. However, all of these agents are somewhat irritating and should be used initially in low concentrations on alternate days until tolerance develops. Then they can be used in higher concentrations once or twice daily to obtain the desired therapeutic effect. For mild acne with comedones, low-strength (0.05 or 0.1% cream or 0.01 or 0.025% gel) topical tretinoin (Retin-A) may be used. Initially, it should be applied sparingly (30 minutes after washing) every 2 or 3 nights, and after 1 or 2 weeks the potency or frequency of application may be increased as tolerated. Tretinoin is highly effective for comedonal acne, helping to unplug comedones by penetrating the follicle and stimulating epithelial production of nonadherent cells. This increased cellular turnover helps to dislodge and discharge comedo contents. The patient's condition may appear to worsen in the initial period of treatment with tretinoin, but substantial improvement can be expected in 2–3 months. Advise patients that tretinoin increases photosensitivity, so they should limit sun exposure and use a noncomedogenic sunscreen (Coppertone for Faces Only). A combined therapy using tretinoin and benzoyl peroxide is very effective for moderate acne (with inflammatory pustules, papules, and comedones), and some studies have shown that it may be as effective as a therapy using oral tetracycline in conjunction with topical agents. Since benzoyl peroxide may oxidize tretinoin if they are applied together, benzoyl peroxide should be applied at night and tretinoin in the morning. If excessive irradiation or drying develops, the topical agents should be discontinued and a moisturizer used for a while; therapy can then be resumed gradually. A number of topical antibiotic agents (containing erythromycin, tetracycline, minocycline, meclocycline) are available for the treatment of inflammatory acne that is not responsive to a combination therapy of tretinoin and benzoyl peroxide. They can also be used as an alternative therapy for patients unable to use benzoyl peroxide (because of sensitivity or allergy) and have a lower incidence of side effects than systemic antibiotic therapy. Meclocycline sulfosalicylate (Meclan) cream seems to be the least irritating. The topical antibiotic should be applied twice daily (e.g., in the morning and early evening), and tretinoin and/or benzoyl peroxide may be applied at other times (e.g., at bedtime).

Systemic: Systemic antibiotic therapy is usually effective for severe inflammatory acne that is unresponsive to topical therapy alone. Some patients with long-standing acne who have been discouraged by previous topical treatment failures may also benefit from systemic therapy combined with topical measures. Tetracycline is the preferred antibiotic for acne, since it is associated with the fewest side effects, can be used for long periods, and is inexpensive. For less severe cases, give 250 mg two to four times daily; for severe cystic acne, give a higher dosage (1–2 g two to four times daily). Instruct patients to take antibiotics on an empty stomach (1 hour before meals or 2 hours after) to ensure maximum absorption, and advise them about the risks of photosensitivity with tetracycline. Discontinue antibiotic therapy when there is clinical improvement, and have patients continue with topical medications. Erythromycin (250 mg qid) or minocycline HCl (50–100 mg bid) may be used if there is an allergy, if side effects develop (GI irritation), or if a response is not obtained with tetracycline. Penicillin and sulfa drugs are not effective in the treatment of acne, since they are not fat soluble and are therefore not concentrated in sebum. Isotretinoin (Accutane), a synthetic derivative of vitamin A, may be effective for severe cystic acne that is unresponsive to other forms of therapy. A response is obtained in about 4 months with maximum amounts of 0.5–1 mg/kg given twice daily, and remissions may last for several years. However, it is associated with significant side effects (mostly affecting the skin and mucosa).

Other measures: For selected patients when immediate improvement is necessary, specialists are able to perform comedo extraction (does not influence the course of acne but provides immediate improvement in the patient's appearance), intralesional steroid injection (induces involution of nodules and cysts within hours, speeds healing, and lessens the chance of scarring), and cryotherapy (accelerates resolution of inflammatory cysts and pustules). Topical application of trichloroacetic acid at monthly intervals and dermabrasion may also be used for disfiguring scars, but complications (hyper- and hypopigmentation, infection, further scarring) may result. Atrophic scars are sometimes treated with collagen injections and punch grafts. All of these procedures must be performed by specialists experienced in their use.

Diet: Although a number of foods are often believed to cause or worsen acne breakouts, research does not support the theory that diet plays any role in the pathogenesis of acne. However, emotional stress, heredity, hormonal changes (menstruation, oral contraceptive use), exposure to cooking oils or petroleum derivatives in the workplace, and long-term use of oil-based cosmetics may all be contributory factors.

Patient Education: Thoroughly discuss the pathogenesis of acne and be sure that the patient understands his or her role in controlling the condition. Advise patients that frequent or vigorous washing or the use of harsh soaps or abrasive cleansers or pads may produce irritation and worsen acne. If cosmetics are used, water-based products should be used instead of oil-based ones and should be thoroughly removed as soon as possible. Patients should be instructed that touching, squeezing, or picking at acne lesions can perpetuate the condition (crusting and scabs are suggestive of manipulation of lesions) and should be avoided. They should also be reminded that, in reduced concentrations, the topical medications are prophylactic and should be incorporated into the daily routine (not used only when an outbreak occurs) until the patient is beyond the acne-prone years of adolescence.

Follow-up: It is important to see patients on a regular basis until the condition is controlled, evaluating their progress and adapting therapy as required. It may be important to discuss with them periodically the role that they play in managing their disease, but keep in mind that patients with acne are often very self-conscious about their condition and need support and encouragement. Patients who require long-term systemic antibiotic therapy should have a baseline CBC and blood tests to check liver and renal function; these should be repeated annually.

BIBLIOGRAPHY

Adams RM. Contact dermatitis: Taking the confusion out of the Dx. *Modern Medicine*, (June) 1984, 128–142.

Bates B. *A Guide to Physical Examination,* 3rd ed. Lippincott, Philadelphia, 1983.

Berkow RB (ed.). *The Merck Manual of Diagnosis and Therapy*, 14th ed. Merck Sharp & Dohme Research Laboratories, Rahway, N.J., 1982.

Bickers DR. Treating skin disorders: Topical versus systemic therapy. *Drug Therapy*, (Mar.) 1982, 196–208.

Blank H. Skin in distress: A guide for generalists. *Acute Care Medicine*, (June) 1984, 20–28.

Brown AM, Stubbs DW (eds.). *Medical Physiology*. Wiley, New York, 1983.

Callen JP. Cutaneous manifestations of collagen-vascular disorders. *Continuing Education*, (Apr.) 1981, 31–39.

Chapman J, Rosen T. Cutaneous hemangiomas: Which ones to treat, and how to do it. *Consultant*, (Oct.) 1983, 289–303.

Conn HF, Conn RB Jr (eds.). *Current Diagnosis*. Saunders, Philadelphia, 1980.

Connolly SM. Allergic contact dermatitis: When to suspect it and what to do. *Postgraduate Medicine*, 1983, 74(3):227–235.

Cornell RC. Getting the most out of topical steroids. *Modern Medicine*, (Feb.–Mar.) 1981, 20–27.

Crafts RC. *A Textbook of Human Anatomy*, 3rd ed. Wiley, New York, 1985.

Crouch JE, McClintic JR. *Human Anatomy and Physiology*, 2nd ed. Wiley, New York, 1976.

Dahl MV. The blistering diseases: What to do when the skin bubbles. *Modern Medicine*, (May–June) 1980, 52–59.

Ecker RI. Dermatology for the primary care physician: Contact dermatitis. *Hospital Medicine*, (Jan.) 1984, 41–65.

Elias H, Pauly JE, Burns ER. *Histology and Human Microanatomy*, 4th ed. Wiley, New York, 1978.

Epstein WI. Poison ivy and oak: How to handle the severe reaction. *Modern Medicine*, (July) 1984, 92–103.

Fekety R. Office treatment of infection: Nonrespiratory bacterial infections, antibiotic prophylaxis, fungal and viral infections. *Postgraduate Medicine,* 1980, 67(2):87–96.

Fenske NA, Greenberg SS. Solar-induced skin changes. *American Family Physician,* (June) 1982, 109–117.

Fisher AA. Preventing and treating contact dermatitis. *Consultant,* (Mar.) 1980, 45–48.

Fitzpatrick KT, et al. Outpatient management of minor burns. *Physician Assistant,* (May) 1985, 16–28.

Frazier CA. Axioms on insect bites and stings. *Hospital Medicine,* (Aug.) 1984, 13–26.

Goldberg GN. The "hellfire" of shingles: How to help your patient cope. *Modern Medicine,* (May) 1984, 94–103.

Goroll AH, May LA, Mulley AG. *Primary Care Medicine: Office Evaluation and Management of the Adult Patient.* Lippincott, Philadelphia, 1981.

Gray H. *Anatomy of the Human Body,* 29th American ed. (CM Goss, ed.). Lea & Febiger, Philadelphia, 1973.

Greer KE. Acne. *Physician and Patient,* 1984, 3(11):37–40.

Grekin RC, Swanson NA. Cutaneous tumors: A pictorial guide with suggestions for treatment. *Consultant,* (June) 1984, 69–90.

Griffin DE. Shingles: Dealing with the recurrent virus. Consultant, (Oct.) 1983, 231–238.

Guin JD, Beaman JH. Toxicodendrons and toxicodendron dermatitis. *Continuing Education for the Family Physician,* 14(6):23–32.

Guyton AC. *Textbook of Medical Physiology,* 6th ed. Saunders, Philadelphia, 1981.

Hanifin JM. Atopic dermatitis: Special clinical complications. *Postgraduate Medicine,* 1983, 74(3):188–199.

Heckel P. Teaching patients to cope with psoriasis: The unshared disease. *Nursing 81* (June):49–51.

Heimbach DM, Engrav LH, Marvin J. Minor burns: Guidelines for successful outpatient management. *Postgraduate Medicine,* 1981, 69(5):22–32.

Hoole AJ, Greenberg RA, Pickard CG Jr. *Patient Care Guidelines for Nurse Practitioners.* Little, Brown, Boston, 1982.

Hurwitz S. Signals from the skin. *Emergency Medicine,* (July) 1979, 91–115.

Inkeles B. A rational approach to treating urticaria and angioedema. *Drug Therapy,* (Sept.) 1983, 105–112.

Isselbacher KJ, et al. *Harrison's Principles of Internal Medicine,* 9th ed. McGraw-Hill, New York, 1980.

Jacobs AH. The skin in childhood. *Hospital Practice,* (Aug.) 1977, 91–112.

Johnson RT. Shingles: What you should and shouldn't do. *Modern Medicine,* (July) 1981, 68–82.

Kaplan AP. Chronic urticaria: Possible causes, suggested treatment alternatives. *Postgraduate Medicine,* 1983, 74(3):209–221.

Krupp MA, Chatton MJ, Werdegar D (eds.). *Current Medical Diagnosis and Treatment 1985.* Lange, Los Altos, Calif., 1984.

Labson LH (ed.). Unraveling clues to the cause of itching. *Patient Care,* (Aug.) 1984, 18–60.

Lamb C (ed.). Skin cancer: Assessing suspicious skin lesions. *Patient Care,* (Nov.) 1979, 20–61.

Lamb C (ed.). Skin cancer: Explaining causative factors and risks. *Patient Care,* (Nov.) 1979, 62–70.

Lamb C (ed.). Skin cancer: Exploring biopsy and treatment options. *Patient Care,* (Nov.) 1979, 72–115.

Leeson SL, Leeson CR. *Histology,* 4th ed. Saunders, Philadelphia, 1981.

Levine N. Sunburn: How to stop the pain, how to prevent the damage. *Modern Medicine*, (July) 1984, 76–91.

Levine N. Insect stings: Acute care for the office emergency. *Modern Medicine*, (July) 1984, 108–121.

Levinson AI. Urticaria and angioedema: Current approach to common problems. *Postgraduate Medicine*, 1984, 76(1):183–190.

Litt JZ. Lupus erythematosus. *Cross Section*, 1982, 10(2):4–9.

Lloyd JR. Burn care: Early assessment and treatment. *PA Practice*, 1984, 3(2):3–7.

Lorin MI. Elevated body temperature: Symptomatic treatment. Consultant, (Jan.) 1980, 130–137.

Luterman A, Curreri PW. Guidelines for early management of burn injuries. *Drug Therapy Hospital*, (Dec.) 1980, 15–26.

Maull KI. Current concepts of wound management. *Continuing Education*, (Oct.) 1983, 950–958.

McDonald CJ. Cutaneous manifestations of systemic disease. *Postgraduate Medicine*, 1981, 69(5):132–149.

Menter A. Dermatology for the primary care physician: Psoriasis. *Hospital Medicine*, (Apr.) 1984, 43–72.

Millikan LE. Atopic dermatitis: Clinical spectrum and approach to treatment. *Postgraduate Medicine*, 76(1):139–146.

Millikan LE. Systemic steroid therapy for skin disorders: Common mistakes. *Consultant*, (Nov.) 1979, 158–170.

Millikan LE. Axioms on summer plant dermatitis. *Hospital Medicine*, (July) 1984, 43–69.

Morgan RF, Nichter LS, Edlich RF. Coping with accidental hypothermia and frostbite. *Geriatric Consultant*, (Jan.–Feb.) 1984, 11–13.

Morman MR. Possible side effects of topical steroids. *American Family Physician*, (Feb.) 1981, 171–174.

Neelon FA. Nail changes in thyroid disease. *Drug Therapy*, (Nov.) 1980, 153–155.

Orkin M, Maibach HI. Scabies, a current pandemic. *Postgraduate Medicine*, 1979, 66(1):52–62.

Parish LC, Witkowski JA, Schwartzman RM. Getting rid of scabies once and for all. *Current Prescribing*, (Sept.) 1977, 94–101.

Parish LC, Witkowski JA. Herpes zoster: How to spot it, how to treat it. *Drug Therapy*, (Mar.) 1982, 122–126.

Ragaz A. Skin growths: Differentiating the benign from the malignant. *Consultant*, (May) 1984, 128–142.

Riley WB Jr. Wound healing. *American Family Physician*, 1981, 24(5):107–113.

Rosenfield RL. Hirsutism in women: Its diagnosis and treatment. *Consultant*, (Feb.) 1980, 239–242.

Rottenberg R (ed.). Common problems: How to individualize acne therapy. *Patient Care*, (Aug.) 1983, 133–157.

Sams WM Jr. A problem-oriented approach to clinical dermatology. *Continuing Education*, (Aug.) 1982, 73–78.

Silverstein A. *Human Anatomy and Physiology*. Wiley, New York, 1980.

Vance JC. Skin cancer: Making a difference with early Dx. *Modern Medicine*, (Aug.) 1983, 60–84.

Whiting D. Recognizing skin tumors: Moles, melanomas, and miscellaneous lesions: Which are malignant? *Modern Medicine*, (June) 1981, 86–100.

Wilkerson MG, Goldberg LH, Rapini RP. Actinic keratoses. *American Family Physician*, (July) 1984, 103–108.

Witkowski JA, Parish LC. Summer dermatoses. *Drug Therapy*, (Aug.) 1983, 167–181.

Witkowski JA, Parish LC. Summer hazards: Stings and blisters. *Drug Therapy*, (June) 1984, 58–71.

Witkowski JA, Parish LC. Summer hazards: Poison ivy, poison oak, and poison sumac. *Drug Therapy*, (June) 1984, 81–88.

Wyngaarden JB, Smith LH Jr (eds.). *Textbook of Medicine*, Vols. 1 and 2, 16th ed. Saunders, Philadelphia, 1982.

Yardley DE, Schwartz RA, Adams HG. Herpes zoster. *American Family Physician*, 1983, 28(6):138–144.

11

Musculoskeletal System

Carla Greene

Outline

Torn rotator cuff
Ruptured biceps
Mallet finger deformity
Ruptured Achilles tendon
▶ General measures for mild to moderate strains
▶ Use of NSAI agents
▶ Cervical strain
▶ Correct posture
▶ Acute lumbar strain
Low back syndrome
Subluxation of a facet joint
Tendinitis
▶ General measures for tendinitis
Calcific tendinitis
▶ Tennis elbow

BURSA

▶ Acute bursitis
Septic bursitis
Chronic bursitis
Calcific bursitis
Adhesive capsulitis or frozen joint
Bunion
Hallux valgus
Hallus rigidus

TENDON SHEATH

Synovial cyst
Ganglion
Tenosynovitis
▶ Tendinitis/bursitis/tenosynovitis of the shoulder
Rotator cuff tendinitis
Tendinitis/tenosynovitis of the biceps insertion
Frozen shoulder
Stenosing tenosynovitis
Trigger finger

FASCIA

Felon
Fasciitis
Bone spurs
Fibromyalgia

FORMATION AND GROWTH OF BONE TISSUE

Osteomalacia
Rickets
Scurvy

MATURE BONE

Osteomyelitis
Skin splints

BONE TURNOVER

Osteomalacia
Osteopenia
Secondary osteoporosis
Compression fractures
Kyphosis
Postmenopausal osteoporosis
▶ Preventive measures for postmenopausal osteoporosis
▶ Established postmenopausal osteoporosis
Paget's disease
Bone tumors
Osteogenic sarcoma
Bone metastases

BONE REGENERATION

Fractures
Fibrous unions
Delayed unions
Nonunions
▶ First aid for fractures
Casts
Cast-related complications
Fat embolism

JOINTS AND CONNECTING STRUCTURES

Costochondritis
Tietze's syndrome
Sprain
Severe sprains
▶ General measures for mild/moderate sprains

Knee sprains
Cruciate ligament damage
Torn cartilage
Ankle sprains
▶ Mild/moderate ankle sprain
Dislocations
Subluxations
Chondromalacia

JOINT CAVITY AND SYNOVIUM

Synovial effusion
Noninflammatory effusion
Hemarthrosis
Inflammatory effusion
▶ Gout
Tophi
Pseudogout
Chondrocalcinosis
Arthritis associated with autoimmune disease
Rheumatoid arthritis (RA)
Felty's syndrome
▶ General measures for RA
▶ Arthritis organizations
Ankylosing spondylitis
Reiter's syndrome
Systemic lupus erythematosus (SLE)
▶ SLE organizations
Lupus-like syndrome
Scleroderma
CREST syndrome
▶ Scleroderma organizations
Mixed connective tissue disease (MCTD)
Septic arthritis
Gonococcal septic arthritis
Nongonococcal septic arthritis
Tubercular joints
Viral arthritis
▶ Lyme disease
Erythema chronicum migrans (ECM)

ARTICULAR CARTILAGE

Degenerative joint disease (DJD)
Secondary osteoarthritis
Primary osteoarthritis
Subchondral cysts
Bone spurs
▶ General measures for osteoarthritis

ANATOMIC SPACES FOR SPINAL CORD AND NERVE PASSAGE

Cord injury
Complete cord injury
Concussive shock
Incomplete spinal cord injury
Nerve root entrapment syndrome
Sciatica
Slipped disc
Ruptured disc
Thoracic outlet syndrome
Peripheral nerve entrapment syndromes
▶ Carpal tunnel syndrome
Compartment syndromes

ACTIVITY

Prolonged confinement
Endurance training
Isometrics
Body building
Weight lifter's blackout
▶ Exercise prescribing
Accidental falls
▶ Preventing fall injuries
Motor vehicle accidents
Seat belt use
▶ Seat belt use and motor vehicle safety

NEUROMUSCULAR TRANSMISSION

Motor neurons in the cerebral cortex initiate impulses for contraction of skeletal muscles. Cell bodies from these "upper motor neurons" form the motor strip, an area in the frontal lobe of the cerebrum (see Chapter 12). Portions of the motor strip are responsible for movement in specific regions of the body. The larger the portion, such as that allotted hands and feet, the more skilled the functions carried out by the body part.

Axons from upper motor neurons extend to the medulla, where a large percentage (75–95%) cross over and then pass down the spinal cord along the corticospinal (pyramidal) spinal tract. Individual axons eventually meet a lower motor neuron, the cell bodies of which make up the anterior horns in the spinal cord and the axons of which form peripheral nerves. Impulses initiated by the upper motor neurons synapse to lower motor neurons and travel out through peripheral nerves across branching axons. To enhance the speed of transmission, axons of peripheral nerves are encased in a layer of fat (myelin sheath). For protection, the myelin sheath is surrounded by an outer covering, the neurilemma, containing specialized cells (Schwann cells). Capable of mitosis, Schwann cells are responsible for some regenerative properties of peripheral neurons not shared by central nervous system (CNS) neurons that lack a neurilemma.

From the branching axons, impulses travel to an individual muscle cell. Surrounded by a flexible membrane, the sarcolemma, an individual muscle cell contains numerous contractile organelles called "myofibrils" (Fig. 11.1). Myofibrils are made up of protein chains, the myofilaments, some of which are thin (actin) and others thick (myosin). Because they alternate, segments of actin and myosin appear under the electron microscope as two distinct optical bands. The A-band is a dark region containing both actin and myosin, with a pale strip of myosin only (the H-zone) at its center. I-bands are lightly shaded regions containing only actin. The end of one actin myofilament overlaps the beginning of another to form Z-lines. The area between Z-lines, the sarcomere, shortens under the influence of calcium to contract the cell.

Branching nerve axons have button-like endings (motor end plates) that contain vesicles filled with the chemical acetylcholine. The end plates fit into grooves along the sarcolemma, forming the neuromuscular junction (Fig. 11.2). The small gap between the nerve ending and muscle membrane is called the "synaptic cleft." As also seen in the figure, a resting muscle fiber is electrically polarized, with the interior of the cell slightly more negative than its exterior environment. This gradient is maintained by the low permeability of the sarcolemma to sodium ions. Furthermore, any leakage of sodium into the cell is balanced by the outward diffusion of an equal amount of potassium. A nervous impulse sent to the neuromuscular junction triggers the release of acetylcholine into the sarcolemma. Acetylcholine makes the membrane suddenly permeable to sodium so that the positive ions rush into the cell, upsetting the usual separation of charges (depolarization). However, diffusion and sodium pumps quickly restore the ions to their original positions (repolarization). Rapid depolarization and repolarization create a capacitor-like force referred to as the "action potential." Following the all-or-nothing principle, the action potential spreads along the sarcolemma, causing the release of calcium ions. As it travels along invaginations of the sarcolemma (transverse tubules or t-tubules), calcium is channeled to the myofibrils. It is theorized that strongly positive calcium ions neutralize the negative chains of actin and myosin, thereby disrupting the tendency of negative charges to repel one another. Actin and myosin slide together, the sarcomere shortens, and as discussed later, the cell contracts.

In the ***muscular dystrophies,*** muscle cells fail to respond normally to nervous stimulation due to a genetic defect of cellular metabolism. As a result, they remain

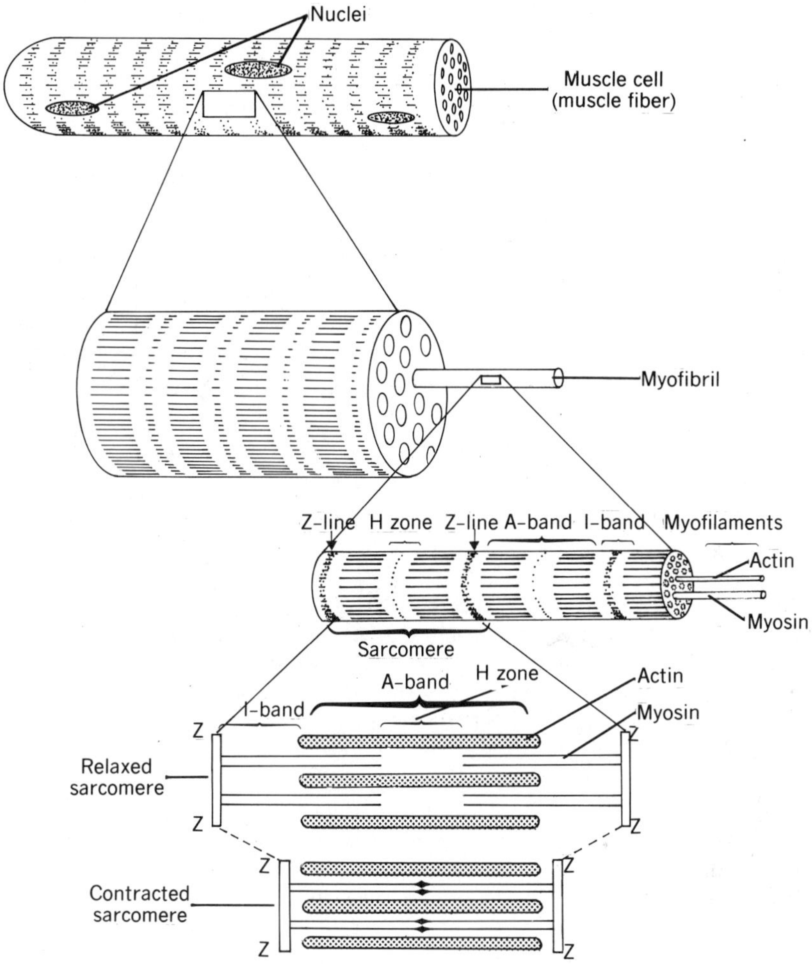

Figure 11.1 Individual muscle cell.

in a state of continual contraction or fail to contract at all. In either case, cells decline progressively and eventually die. Several forms of muscular dystrophy exist, and it may be that the primary abnormality, such as an absent enzyme system, is different for each. A brief description of the dystrophies is given in Table 11.1. Most cases are diagnosed in youth when an apparently healthy child begins to display clumsy behavior. He or she may fall frequently, be unable to run, and have trouble climbing stairs. Interstitial deposits of fat cause arm and leg muscles to become unusually large and firm, even though the muscle fibers are atrophied and weak. Because several of the dystrophies are manifested in adulthood, the possibility should be explored in anyone with progressive loss of motor function in the absence of metabolic or thyroid imbalance. Such patients should be referred to a myologist for muscle biopsy, electromyography, and nerve conduction tests, as well as special endocrine and enzyme studies. No specific treatment for muscular dystrophy exists,

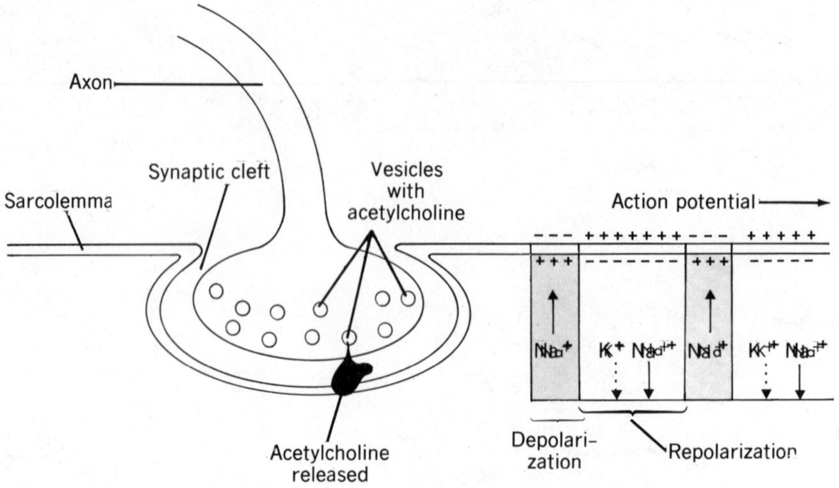

Figure 11.2 Neuromuscular transmission.

though certain drugs (quinine, procainamide, and diphenylhydantoin) relieve the prolonged contractions (myotonia) seen in some forms of the disease. Physical therapy, orthotic devices, pulmonary hygiene, and orthopedic surgery allow patients to lead as full and active a life as possible, but the long-term prognosis is very poor. Genetic counseling is important. ▶ ***Muscular dystrophy organizations*** supply up-to-date information about the disease, trends in treatment, and local support groups.

Sodium, potassium and calcium play key roles in neuromuscular activity. Other electrolytes and certain hormones are also important. For instance, phosphates make up structural portions of the sarcolemma and, as part of the adenosine triphosphate (ATP) molecule, generate energy within the cell. Magnesium is necessary for the operation of the sodium-potassium pump as well as all enzyme systems. Thyroid hormone somehow influences the contractile process of the myofibrils without disrupting neuromuscular transmission. Muscle disturbances resulting from electrolyte and/or hormone imbalance are referred to as ***metabolic myopathies.*** They are outlined in Table 11.2.

The amount of acetylcholine released by the motor endplate is potent enough to perpetuate several muscle cell contractions in a row without further stimulation from the motor nerves. If this were to happen, muscle action would be uncontrollable. Therefore, as soon as acetylcholine comes in contact with the sarcolemma, it is attacked and inactivated by the enzyme cholinesterase. Drugs and poisons that interfere with cholinesterase activity produce severe muscle spasm. The opposite effect occurs with curare-like substances. They block transmission of impulses and paralyze muscles.

Some of the most potent neuromuscular poisons are the exotoxins (types A, B, C, D, E, and F) that cause ***botulism.*** Produced during the anaerobic growth of *Clostridium botulinum* (a spore-forming, gram-negative rod), the exotoxins interfere with the activity of acetylcholine and thus block neuromuscular transmission. The usual source is a canned product that has been inadequately heated during processing. Exposure at 100°C for 10 minutes is necessary to destroy toxins and at 120°C for

TABLE 11.1 MUSCULAR DYSTROPHIES

Type, Incidence, and Onset	Clinical Course
Pseudohypertrophic (Duchenne) Usually X-linked recessive. Rare in women. Onset of symptoms occurs during first 3 years of life.	Main involvement of pelvic, shoulder, and girdle muscles. Pseudohypertrophy of calf muscles, quadriceps and deltoids in 80% of cases. Progressive immobility and weakness. Death occurs from respiratory infection or cardiac failure in third decade.
Facioscapulohumeral (Landouzy-Déjerine) Usually autosomal dominant. Incidence same in men and women. Symptoms begin early in life.	Shoulder girdle and facial muscles major sites of involvement (winging of scapula, drooping of eyelids, overhanging of lips) common. Slowly progressive, with prolonged periods of apparent remission. Survival and activity not significantly affected.
Lamb-girdle (Erb) Usually autosomal recessive. Incidence same in men and women. Onset of symptoms is variable (late childhood to middle age).	Spares facial muscles. Unilateral involvement of shoulder, pelvic, and girdle muscles, later becoming bilateral. Pseudohypertrophy uncommon. Progresses over 20 years to severe disability.

30 minutes to destroy spores. Because acids tend to inhibit spore germination, some foods (such as citrus fruits and tomatoes) are relatively safe from contamination. On the other hand, canned fish, peppers, and vichyssoise have been implicated in outbreaks of the disease. Muscle weakness is first manifested by visual disturbances (diplopia, blurred vision, photophobia) and difficulty in talking or swallowing. Other signs of neuromuscular blockade include nausea, vomiting, constipation, abdominal cramping, and urinary retention. Any of these signs can develop 12–36 hours after the patient has ingested foods contaminated with preformed toxin. Patients with symptoms of botulism of known exposure should be hospitalized for observation and supportive therapy. The first step is to eliminate toxins in the gastrointestinal (GI) tract with gastric lavage, laxatives, and emesis. Barring hypersensitivity to horse serum, trivalent (types A, B, and E) antitoxin should be given as soon as possible. Guanidine hydrochloride, a drug that enhances the release of acetylcholine, may be helpful except in patients who develop severe respiratory problems. For them, death is nearly certain, and they account for the 10% mortality.

Like botulism, ***tetanus*** is caused by the exotoxin of a spore-forming, gram-negative rod. The organism, *Clostridium tetani,* abounds in superficial layers of the soil and easily enters the body through lacerations, punctures, burns, infections, or surgical sites. The toxin, however, is produced only when oxygen levels in the tissues are lower than normal. This is likely to occur in the presence of necrotic tissue, foreign bodies, or calcium salts. Toxins forming around a wound enter the bloodstream and travel to muscle cells, where they cause contractions that are dissociated from action potentials. Toxins are also carried to the CNS, where they interfere with synaptic functions. As a consequence, nervous stimuli overload the peripheral system, throwing muscle groups into severe spasm. Patients who develop tetanus poisoning first note pain and stiffness in the jaw, abdomen, or back. Low-grade fever, profuse sweating, and tachycardia may be present. As the disease progresses, they may experience rigidity of facial muscles (risus sardonicus) and difficulty in opening the mouth (lockjaw). If the rigidity becomes generalized, painful contractions of antagonistic muscle groups (trismus) or respiratory distress occurs. Hospital admission for supportive treatment is imperative. Wounds should be carefully debrided to

TABLE 11.2 METABOLIC MYOPATHIES

Cause	Characteristics
Electrolyte imbalance	
Hypernatremia and hyponatremia	Muscle weakness and cramps.
Hypercalcemia	Decreased neuromuscular irritability, resulting in muscular hypotonicity, weakness, fatigue, aches and pains.
Hypocalcemia	Increased neuromuscular irritability, resulting in tetany (characterized by paresthesias and spasms of both skeletal and smooth muscles). Initial symptoms include numbness of fingers and tingling/burning of hands, feet, circumoral region, and tongue. Progression signaled by skeletal muscle cramps and spasms (carpopedal muscles typically affected first). Spasm of laryngeal muscles produces hoarseness, breathing difficulty, and possibly asphyxia. Convulsive seizures may occur, particularly in infants and children.
Hyperkalemia	Increased neuromuscular irritability, producing muscular weakness and paralysis in severe conditions. Affects first the legs, then the trunk and arms, and lastly the respiratory muscles.
Hypokalemia	Decreased neuromuscular irritability results in muscle weakness and fatigue, usually occurring first in the legs (particularly the quadriceps muscles). Muscle tenderness, cramps, and paresthesias may also be present. Severe conditions affect arm and trunk muscles, as well as respiratory muscles (paralysis with respiratory failure may occur). Chronic potassium depletion may lead to atrophy.
Hyperphosphatemia	Enhanced deposition of calcium and phosphate in bone and precipitation of calcium phosphate in the soft tissues results in hypocalcemia. Signs and symptoms are thus due to hypocalcemia (described above).
Hypophosphatemia	General malaise. Profound muscle weakness, functional paralysis in severe cases. Acute respiratory failure may occur, especially in persons with pulmonary disease. Seizures and other neurologic abnormalities may also result.
Hypermagnesemia	Impairs acetylcholine release at neuromuscular junctions, suppressing reflex activity. Decreased neuromuscular irritability. Possible respiratory arrest.
Hypomagnesemia	Symptoms (if they occur) are similar to those of hypocalcemia: weakness, tremor, sometimes tetany and convulsions.
Endocrine disturbance	
Hyperthyroid	Weakness and atrophy of shoulder and pelvic girdle muscles.
Hypothyroid	Generalized reduction in contractility. Notable weakness of proximal limb muscles.
Cushing's syndrome	General weakness and fatigue. Wasting of quadriceps and pelvic girdle muscles.
Long-term steroids ("steroid myopathy")	Reversible weakness and atrophy of limb girdle muscles.
Severe diabetes	Asymmetric weakness of pelvic girdle and thigh muscles. Diffuse pain and reduced reflexes.
Acromegaly ("growth hormone myopathy")	Pseudohypertrophy of proximal limb muscles; mild weakness.
Hyperparathyroid	Weakness, atrophy (particularly of quadriceps muscles). Normal tendon reflexes. Generalized skeletal pain and easy fatigability.
Hypoparathyroid	Marked elevation of CPK, but no myopathies described.

remove foreign bodies or necrotic tissue. Antiserum, though it does nothing to neutralize toxins already found in the CNS, reduces circulating toxins and greatly improves the overall chances for survival. Therefore, human tetanus immune globulin (TIG) should be administered as soon as possible. In order to control muscle spasms, combinations of sedatives, muscle relaxants, and sometimes neuromuscular blocking agents are used. If the patient survives, the spasms begin to recede after 10 days and disappear entirely in 2 weeks. The 40–60% mortality reflects the severity of the disease as well as its tendency to strike persons older than age 60.

The potential for tetanus is everywhere, but in recent years fewer than 100 cases annually have been reported in the United States. The reason for this low incidence is the mandatory childhood vaccination program. Absorbed tetanus toxoid is given in combination with pertussis vaccine and diphtheria toxoid (DPT) in three doses by age 6. After that, DPT is contraindicated because the pertussis component carries an increased risk of CNS effects and the relatively high dose of diphtheria toxoid may cause severe reactions in older children and adults. Therefore, anyone over the age of 6 should receive the adult type of vaccine, which combines tetanus toxoid with reduced levels of diphtheria toxoid (Td). Adults who have never been vaccinated should receive ▶ ***primary tetanus immunization*** with three initial doses of Td and boosters every 10 years. ▶ ***Tetanus prevention in wound management*** is another issue, and it must be addressed whenever a patient seeks attention for punctures, lacerations, burns, bites, or open skin infections. Other indications include some surgical operations such as GI and orthopedic surgery, any operation on the foot, and septic abortion or delivery (pregnancy is not a contraindication). Persons who have had primary immunization (two or more doses) will need a booster shot if more than 10 years have passed since the last vaccination. When the wound is dirty, deep, or contains a foreign object, boosters are given if more than 5 years have elapsed since the last vaccination. TIG is also recommended in the event of a tetanus-prone wound when prior immunization is incomplete or was obtained more than 10 years previously.

A toxin secreted by female ticks may affect neuromuscular transmission, leading to ***tick paralysis.*** Carried by two species of ticks (Rocky Mountain wood tick and American dog tick), the toxin is released only after the tick has been attached and feeding for more than 24 hours. Patients initially develop restlessness and irritability. They may also experience numbness and tingling of the face and extremities followed by difficulty in swallowing. Within a day or two, speech, vision, and gait become impaired as bulbar, trunk, and limb paralysis progresses. There is usually mild fever. However, the erythrocyte sedimentation rate (ESR), complete blood count (CBC), and urine and spinal fluids typically remain normal. Removal of the tick leads to full recovery within a few hours to days as long as the paralysis is not too far advanced. However, failure to find the tick (which is often embedded in scalp hair) may result in death from respiratory failure or aspiration pneumonia. Fortunately, the condition is extremely rare.

In ***myasthenia gravis,*** which occurs twice as often in women as in men, abnormally thin motor endplates display bizarre branching patterns; subsequently, many neuromuscular junctions fail to function. The pathologic changes are thought to be the consequence of an autoimmune reaction against acetylcholine receptors in the endplates of skeletal muscles. Thymic abnormalities (tumors or hyperplasia) are found in 80% of patients with myasthenia gravis, and remission of the disease often follows thymectomy. Diplopia, due to episodic weakening of extraocular muscles, is usually the presenting symptom. Even though palsy may eventually evolve, the pupils of the eyes remain normal. Facial and laryngeal muscles can also be affected, leading to varying complications: an immobile expression with a hanging jaw, a furrowed "trident tongue," unintelligible speech, and choking. Weakness of skeletal muscles occurs only in advanced disease. Easy fatigability, however, which improves promptly with rest, is an early clue and can be easily elicited by having the patient look up at the ceiling for 2–3 minutes. If the eyelids droop progressively but elevate normally once the exercise is over, the patient should be sent to a neurologist for further evaluation. The diagnosis is confirmed by observing muscle function before and after controlled injections of edrophonium (Tensilon) or neostigmine. Treatment with combinations of cholinesterase inhibitors, corticosteroids, immunosuppressive drugs, and thymectomy has been quite successful. Nonetheless, a small number of patients have fulminant attacks and die of respiratory complications. Patient education materials, information about current research issues, and referrals to local support groups are available from ▶ ***myasthenia gravis organizations.***

CELL CONTRACTION AND MOTOR UNITS

Contraction of the individual muscle cell is referred to as a "muscle twitch." It occurs in three phases (latent, contraction, and relaxation). The muscle twitch lasts for longer than the action potential, which makes it possible for successive electrical waves to initiate new contractions while the cell is still partially contracted. When one contraction occurs on top of another, the cell shortens more than it would in an isolated twitch (summation effect). As the frequency of stimulation increases, the cell has less time to relax between contractions. Rates of 10–12 stimuli per second preclude relaxation and produce a smooth, sustained contraction called "tetany" (Fig. 11.3). Tetany is a maximal response. Faster rates cannot be accommodated because each action potential has to complete its course before another can begin. While the action potential is spreading along the sarcolemma, the membrane remains impervious to further stimulation, no matter how strong. The few milliseconds during which this occurs have been designated the "absolute refractory period."

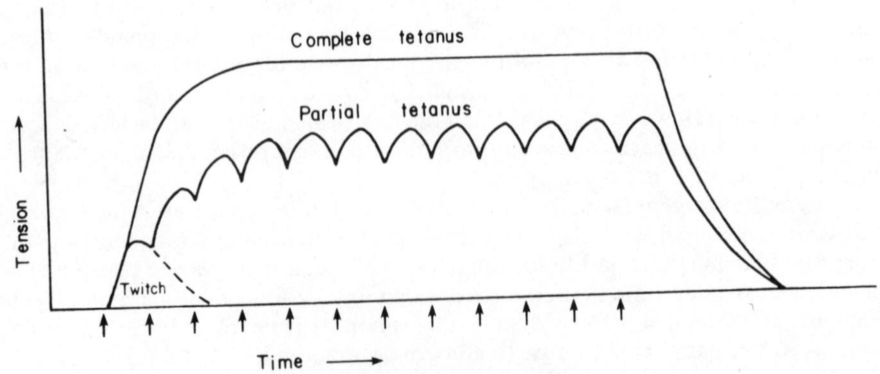

Figure 11.3 Muscle twitch.

Some muscle cells contract longer and with greater force than others. This is because they contain varying amounts of myoglobin, a pigment that transports oxygen. Muscle cells rich in myoglobin (known as "red fibers") are small cells with a vast blood supply, numerous mitochondria, but few myofilaments. Red fibers predominate in muscle groups requiring slow, powerful contractions such as the paravertebral, masseter, and diaphragm muscles. In contrast, myoglobin-deficient cells (white fibers) are large and contain few mitochondria but numerous myofibrils. Because they are able to sustain long periods of rapid contractions, white fibers abound wherever skilled movements are required, such as in the extraocular muscles.

Myoglobin is released with toxic results in ***rhabdomyolysis,*** the acute breakdown of muscle cells. This can occur in chronic alcoholism, viral illness, barbiturate or carbon monoxide poisoning, crush injuries, and some forms of dystrophy. It may also be seen in chronic potassium depletion and narcotic-induced coma, as well as in idiosyncratic reactions to heroin, clofibrate, and phencyclidine (PCP, angel dust). Finally, cases have been reported in marathon runners. After entering the blood, myoglobin is cleared by the kidneys. As a water-insoluble substance, it poses a significant risk of renal damage. Therefore, patients who present with signs of rhabdomyolysis (muscle pain, rapidly progressing weakness, elevated creatinine phosphokinase, and myoglobinuria) require immediate hospitalization. Myoglobinuria is easily recognized as dark red urine that contains neither bile nor red blood cells but tests heme positive on dip stick. Until it clears, urine output and serum electrolytes must be closely monitored. Corticosteroids are given to reduce the inflammatory aftermath of muscle cell destruction. If patients are dehydrated, they should be rehydrated.

The motor neuron, together with the cells it feeds, is referred to as a "motor unit" (Fig. 11.4). The number of cells controlled by a nerve helps determine the functional level of activity for each group of muscles. For example, the motor units found in extraocular muscles contain 6–10 cells per nerve, making rapid, highly refined eye movements possible. Those in calf muscles that require strength more than fine coordination have 2,000 cells per nerve.

In normal muscles, the cells of one motor unit are interspersed with those of adjacent motor units. The units fire asynchronously. Even during sleep, when muscle activity is at a minimum, some cells are found in the smooth, sustained contractions of tetany, while neighboring fibers relax before taking up the load. This "round robin" effect prevents muscle cell fatigue while keeping muscle groups ready for action. The residual degree of contraction is referred to as "muscle tone." It is partially maintained by receptors (muscle spindles) that send reflex signals to the brain whenever muscles are stretched. Kept thus informed, the brain adjusts the level of stimulation necessary to maintain muscle tone.

A mixup of spindle signals may be the initiating factor in ▶***muscle cramps,*** since these painful, hard contractions yield to massage and stretching. Muscle cramps usually develop after strenuous activity or long periods without a change in position. For some unknown reason, they also occur with annoying frequency during pregnancy. However, for the most part, muscle cramps are considered benign. Those related to strenuous activity can be avoided by replacing fluids and salt. ***Nocturnal cramps*** can be relieved by prescribing diphenhydramine (Benadryl) or quinine at bedtime. In cases of severe or recurrent cramps, chronic metabolic or electrolyte disorders should be ruled out (see Table 11.2).

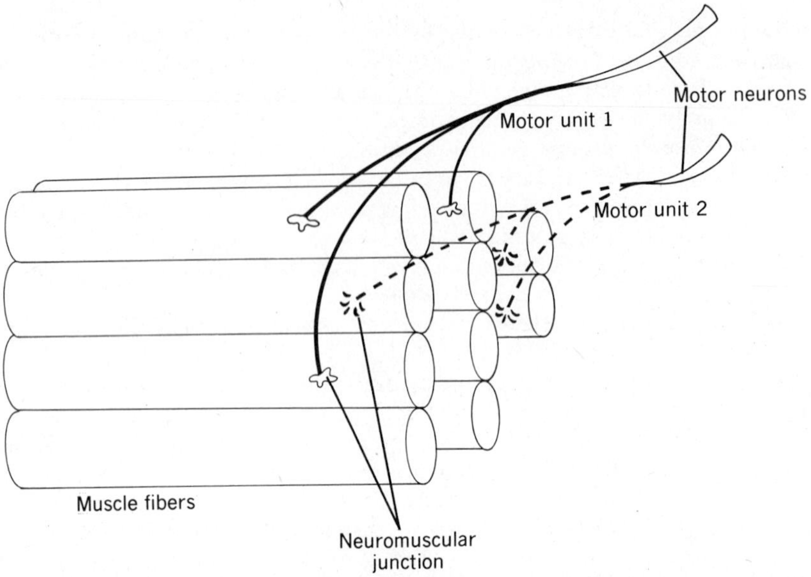

Figure 11.4 Motor unit.

Sustained contractions of scalp and neck muscles cause ***tension headaches.*** Accounting for four out of five headaches, they result from the stress of concentration and are usually relieved by over-the-counter analgesics. When sustained muscle contractions become a continuous reaction to stress, tension headaches lasting for weeks or months may result. Such chronic tension headaches are described as a steady, nonpulsatile pressure occurring at various sites. Spasm of scalp and neck muscles is apparent on physical exam, and electromyography (EMG) changes can always be demonstrated. Studies indicate that drugs seldom reduce their frequency, intensity, or duration and can cause side effects, dependency, or withdrawal symptoms. Relaxation techniques, including massage, application of heat, and biofeedback, give greater benefits (see also the discussion of chronic muscle contraction headaches in Chapter 12).

Damage anywhere along the motor neuron tract affects muscle contraction; disorders of muscle cells and of neuromuscular transmission were previously discussed; cord injuries and nerve entrapment are covered in a later section. Loss of lower motor neurons (in the anterior horns of the spinal cord) and/or upper motor neurons (in the motor cranial nuclei) characterizes the ***motor neuron diseases*** described in Table 11.3. The most widely known of these is ***amyotrophic lateral sclerosis (ALS).*** This progressive disease of unknown cause occurs mainly between ages 50–70. Fasciculations following widespread denervation of motor units are likely to be the first signs. They may be accompaned by muscle cramps and mild paresthesia. Over time, muscles in the hands, forearms, and shoulder girdle atrophy in symmetric or asymmetric patterns. This is eventually followed by signs of upper motor neuron involvement (spasticity, hyperreflexia, clonus, and extensor plantar responses). Characteristically, the superficial abdominal and cremasteric reflexes remain normal and there are no sensory changes. The disease spares extraocular,

TABLE 11.3 MOTOR NEURON DISEASES

Disease	Description
Progressive spinal muscular atrophy	Muscle wasting in the limbs follows degeneration of anterior horn cells in the spinal cord.
Primary lateral sclerosis	Neuromuscular deficit in limbs secondary to upper motor neuron involvement.
Pseudobulbar palsy	Upper motor neuron dysfunction due to bilateral corticobulbar disease. Bulbar involvement predominates.
Progressive bulbar palsy	Bulbar involvement secondary to disease process that affects motor nuclei of cranial nerves.
Amyotrophic lateral sclerosis	Limb and bulbar involvement following mixed upper and lower motor neuron degeneration. May be associated with dementia, Parkinson's disease, and other neurologic diseases.

bladder, and anal sphincter muscles, though in the bulbar form of ALS, musculature controlled by cranial nerves V, VII, X, XI, and XII may be predominantly affected. Intellectual function is preserved except in cases associated with dementia, Parkinson's disease, and other neurologic disorders. Diagnosis is based on an EMG showing chronic partial denervation, fasciculations, and reduction of motor units under voluntary control. Motor conduction velocity and sensory conduction are usually normal. Biopsy shows histologic changes of denervated muscle. Cerebrospinal fluid (CSF) is normal, CPK normal to mildly elevated. There is no proven treatment for ALS or any of the motor neuron diseases, though a number of experimental drugs are under clinical investigation. Progression of the disease to the terminal stages is variable (18 months to more than 7 years). Severe dysphagia or respiratory paralysis is the usual cause of death. The poor prognosis makes the work offered by ►***ALS organizations*** extremely important.

In ***poliomyelitis,*** polio viruses types 1, 2, and 3 spread from person to person by oral and/or fecal transmission. Although the viruses have also been isolated from flies, cockroaches, food, sewage water, and shellfish, disease attributed to these sources has not been demonstrated. Paralytic disease occurs in 0.1% of infected patients. The first symptoms include listlessness, fever, headache, sore throat, vomiting, and achiness. This "minor illness" resolves in 1–3 days. From 2 to 5 days later, the patient displays signs of the "major illness": headache, fever, vomiting, stiff neck, and acute muscle pain. During this time the virus destroys neurons in the anterior horn of the spinal cord and/or motor nuclei of the pons and medulla. If the damage is severe, muscles become permanently paralyzed without sensory loss. If it is less severe, portions of nerve fibers remain viable, sprouting new endings that then attach to denervated muscle cells. The reconstructed motor units contain many times the normal number of fibers, so some impairment is likely. The muscle group becomes either flaccid (less tone than usual) or spastic (more tone than usual). Epidemics of paralytic polio reached a peak in the late 1940s and early 1950s, when 15,000 to 21,000 cases were reported annually. Mortality rates approached 10%. Although long-term rehabilitation improved the degree of recovery from muscle wasting, one-third of the survivors were left with permanent damage.

With the introduction of ***inactivated polio vaccine (IPV)*** in 1955, there has been a dramatic reduction in the disease. Since 1969 an ***oral vaccine*** combining all three strains of polio (trivalent OPV) has been used almost exclusively in the United

States. As a live virus vaccine, OPV has the potential to cause genetic mutations that fail to elicit secretory immunity in the gut. The shed mutant is associated with a rare paralytic disease called ***OPV-associated paralysis.*** The paralysis can develop in vaccine recipients who are immunodeficient or in vaccine recipient contacts who lack antibody protection to the polio viruses. An example of the latter is the young mother who contracts the virus shed from her recently vaccinated infant. However, the risk of disease far outweighs the unlikely risk of OVP paralysis, and outbreaks of polio are certain to recur if the nation falls behind in the administration of childhood vaccinations (four primary doses starting in infancy and a booster at age 12).

▶ ***Adult polio vaccination*** is given only to individuals living in or traveling to endemic areas and to certain health care workers. IPV is recommended for initial vaccination to minimize the chance of OPV-associated paralysis. However, OPV can be given to adults who have been previously vaccinated or when the time constraints of imminent travel do not permit the full series of IPV.

Guillain-Barré syndrome results from an inflammatory cell attack on the myelin sheath, which in severe cases leads to axon damage. The peripheral nervous system (including the cranial, motor and sensory, and autonomic nervous systems) may be affected at any level from nerve roots to distal endings. The cause of the inflammation is not known. A viral illness precedes the syndrome in about 50% of patients. Immunization, animal bites, surgical procedures, lymphoma, and systemic lupus erythematosus (SLE) also seem to have some connection. The first signs are tingling of the hands and feet and motor difficulty. Patients have difficulty getting out of chairs, walking, and performing hand maneuvers. This is generally followed by the development of progressive symmetric paralysis, Bell's palsy, respiratory distress, and/or pure autonomic dysfunction. The last is marked by supraventricular tachycardia or bradycardia, swings in blood pressure, and postural hypotension. Areflexia is bilateral and universal. A glove and stocking anesthesia may be noted, along with altered proprioception, unsteady gait, and ataxia. Severe segmental pain is not uncommon. Patients suspected of having Guillain-Barré syndrome are best hospitalized for monitoring and testing. Supportive care for respiratory and autonomic dysfunction has greatly reduced the mortality. A number of laboratory tests are significant. CSF reveals elevated protein levels but a normal blood cell count. This "albuminocytologic dissociation" is a classic finding. It may not be seen in the first week of the illness, though serial determinations eventually demonstrate the protein elevation in almost all patients. Nerve conduction studies prove myelin damage when nerve stimulation immediately above or below the lesion reveals significantly decreased motor and sometimes sensory conduction velocity. Conduction velocity may be less than 60% of normal. During the acute illness, patients may be treated with steroids, immunosuppressants, and/or plasmapheresis, even though the efficacy of these regimens has yet to be proven. The syndrome is self-limiting, with deficits peaking in 2–4 weeks. If axonal damage is severe, improvement can be slow and recovery incomplete. In rare cases, the syndrome recurs. Patients with a history of Guillain-Barré should never receive influenza vaccines.

GROSS FORMATION OF SKELETAL MUSCLES

Figure 11.5 illustrates the gross formation of a skeletal muscle. Individual cells are packed in a capillary-rich layer of connective tissue called the "endomysium." The endomysium supplies nourishment and binds vast numbers of cells into bundles

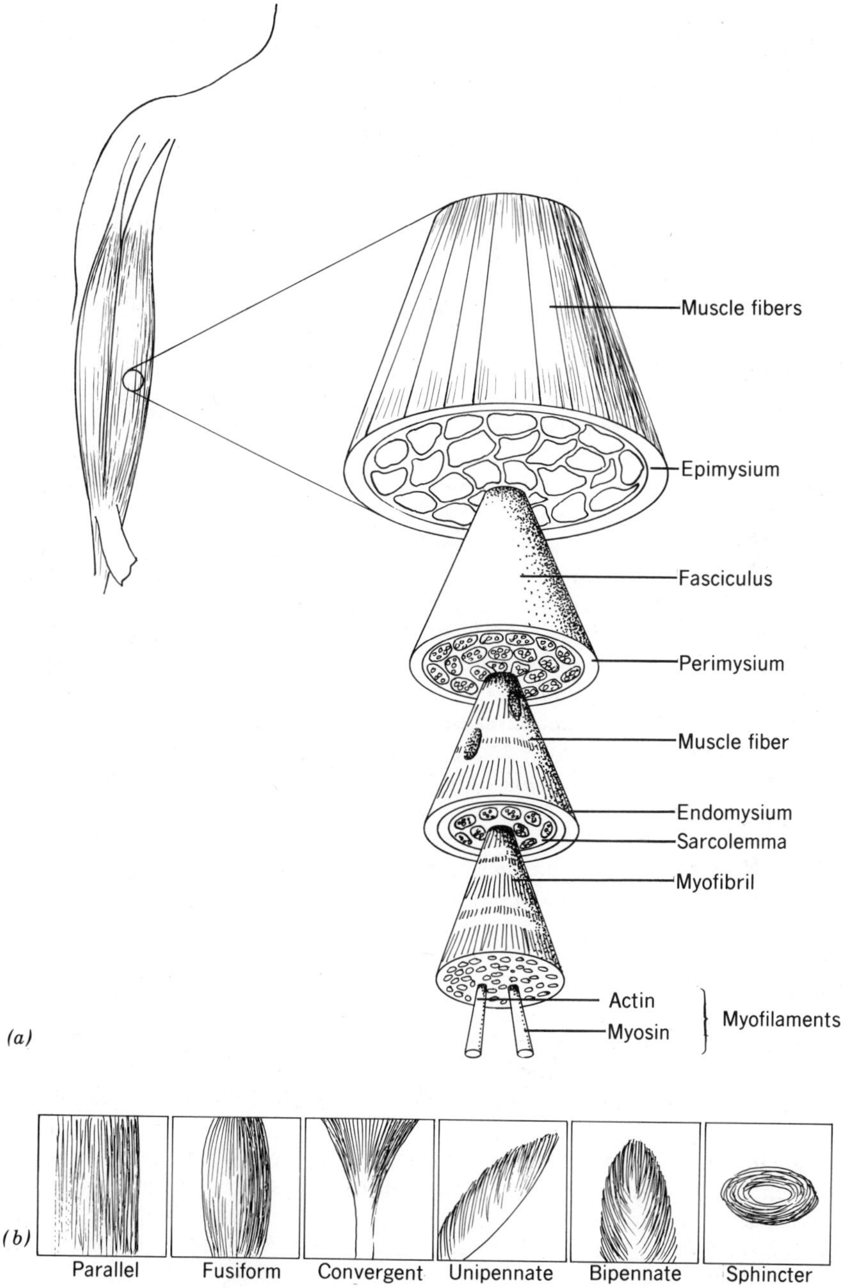

Figure 11.5 Skeletal muscle: (*a*) gross formation; (*b*) types of muscles.

called "fascicles." Surrounded by a thicker layer of connective tissue (the perimysium), fascicles are grouped into fasciculi. Fasciculi are then arranged into one of six specific structural patterns by which the 605 skeletal muscles are classified.

Widespread inflammation of skeletal muscles occurs in ***polymyositis/dermatomyositis.*** There are five classifications of the disorder: type I (adult polymyositis), type II (dermatomyositis), type III (myositis with malignancy), type IV (childhood polymyositis), and type V (myositis associated with other connective tissue diseases). In all cases, the principal changes include inflammatory infiltrates and phagocytic reactions, suggesting an autoimmune mechanism as the etiology. These diseases have a bimodal tendency to appear between the ages of 5 to 15 and 45 to 60. They are twice as common in women as in men. The onset of polymyositis is insidious, with symptoms progressing slowly over weeks or even years. Most complaints can be traced to weakness of the proximal muscle groups. Patients have difficulty rising from chairs, climbing stairs, or combing their hair. Weaknesses of laryngeal, esophageal, and neck muscles are also common, causing problems in speaking, swallowing, and holding the head erect. Ocular muscles are spared, and patients have no pain. Those who describe eye changes and aching sensations in the buttocks, joints, and calves, are likely to have mixed connective tissue disorders. Cardiac abnormalities may present as conduction defects seen on electrocardiogram or as symptoms of myocarditis. Diffuse interstitial fibrosis is the most common pulmonary manifestation. The form of polymyositis affecting the skin is called ***dermatomyositis.*** As similar muscle degeneration occurs, skin changes including maculopapular rash, erythema, eczematoid eruptions, or exfoliative dermatitis develop. Characteristic lilac-colored bands (heliotrope) appear over the face and around fingernails. The diagnosis is based on clinical findings, interpretation of enzyme studies [elevated CPK, serum glutamate oxaloacetic transaminase (SGOT), lactic dehydrogenase (LDH)], EMG, nerve conduction testing, and muscle biopsy. Steroids, aspirin, and physiotherapy are employed, with most patients making a full recovery from acute episodes. Chronic disease is treated with long-term steroids. Ongoing cancer screening is an important aspect of management. Ten percent of patients have type III disease and harbor some form of tumor, usually of the lungs, breast, colon, or prostate.

Rhabdomyosarcoma is a highly malignant tumor of the skeletal muscle. It is typically seen in infancy through young adulthood and in adults older than 50. The malignancy has a high incidence of rapid growth with early hematogenous metastases. Mortality rates, once greater than 50%, have improved significantly with multimodal use of surgery, radiation therapy, and chemotherapy. Since early detection is important, any patient who has a mass arising from muscle tissue should be referred for biopsy.

Although an outer layer of connective tissue, the epimysium, protects fasiculi, ***muscle injury*** is easily sustained. ***Crush injuries*** (e.g., a hand mangled in machinery or a thigh run over by an automobile) result in extensive hemorrhaging, edema, and breakdown of muscle tissue. They require emergency hospitalization. ***Complex laceration*** describes any deep wound that damages not only muscle but also tendons, blood vessels, and nerves. Automobile accidents, broken glass, kitchen and workshop mishaps, and stabbings are common causes. Before closing a complex laceration, wounds must be surgically explored to locate and repair damaged vessels or nerves. They must also be debrided, since nonviable tissue is invariably complicated by infection, particularly with clostridium (gas gangrene). Because muscle fibers do not hold sutures, wound closure involves meticulous reapproximation of all fascial planes.

Contusions result from any blunt trauma that causes bleeding within muscle tissue. Mild, diffuse bleeding produces a ***bruise,*** which may be unsightly and tender but which disappears within several days without serious consequences. Extensive bleeding may result in ***hematoma*** (collection of blood). This is most likely to happen when a muscle in active contraction receives a direct blow. At the line of scrimmage in football, for example, one player may use his padded shoulder to ram an opponent's highly developed and straining quadriceps muscle. The hurt player experiences dysfunction of thigh muscles as swelling and discoloration increase visibly within minutes. The problem is not the contusion itself but the potential for intramuscular blood clots to be replaced by bone tissue. This is an unfortunate complication known as ***myositis ossificans.*** Bone deposition may be noted on x-ray films as early as 2–3 weeks after the injury. It causes painful dysfunction that takes months or even years of intensive rehabilitation to overcome. In some cases, the disability is permanent. To avoid myositis ossificans, it is extremely important to manage contusions with ice packs, elevation, and ace bandages. These measures are usually sufficient to limit interstitial bleeding and tissue damage. However, patients with evidence of large blood collections or whose range of motion is less than 80% of normal should be referred to an orthopedic specialist.

Snakebite by any of the venomous species noted in Table 11.4 is sustained by more than 45,000 people and accounts for approximately 12 deaths per year in the United States. Chiefly made up of proteins, the venoms are complex mixtures with a number of enzymatic activities. They cause severe muscle necrosis, vascular injuries, and hematologic alterations and/or marked changes in neuromuscular transmission. Bites by pit vipers (e.g., rattlesnakes, cottonmouths, and copperheads) are marked usually, but not always, by instant severe pain. It is typical for swelling and edema to develop within 10 minutes, for ecchymosis to appear within 3–6 hours, and for blood-filled vesicles in the area of the bite to arise within 8 hours. Bites by some species causes tingling or numbness of the lips, fingers, and toes and a metallic taste in the mouth. Without immediate treatment, there may be localized thrombosis of vessels and muscle necrosis. Melana, hematuria, or frank bleeding from gums, along with severe hemolysis, can lead to cardiovascular collapse and renal failure. By contrast, the bite of the coral snake is associated with few immediate signs—mild or absent pain and little swelling. However, paresthesia and weakness of the bitten area develops within several hours, quickly followed by lethargy, generalized weakness, muscle incoordination, and increased salivation. Difficulty in swallowing and speaking, visual disturbances, and respiratory distress may ensue.

Whatever the species involved, patients should be administered ▶ ***first aid for snakebite*** and transported to a hospital immediately. Specific antivenoms should be administered at once. This presents a problem if the identification of the snake is uncertain. Fang marks can be helpful but are not conclusive, especially since, in many instances, the snake evenomates through only one fang puncture (fang puncture without any evenomation occurs in 20–40% of bites by crotalids and elapids). When there is doubt about the species or antivenom, two calls can be lifesaving: one to the local zoo and the other to the Oklahoma poison information center. If necrosis is present (it may not be with coral snake bites), extensive debridement is in order. Serious cases of snakebite may require antitetanus shots, broad-spectrum antibiotics, intensive care support, or amputation.

TABLE 11.4 POISONOUS SNAKES INDIGENOUS TO THE UNITED STATES

Common Name	Species	Western United States	Central United States	Eastern United States
Cottonmouths	*Agkistrodon pis-civorus*		TX, NE, IA, KS, OK, AK, MO, IL	TN, KY, NC, SC, GA, AL, MS, LA, FL, VA
Copperheads	*A. contortrix*		TX, NE, IA, KS, OK, AK, MO, IL	TN, KY, IN, OH, NC, SC, GA, AL, MS, LA, FL, PA, NJ, MD, DL, VA, WV, NY, CT, MA, RI, ME, NH, VT
Rattlesnakes				
Eastern dia-mondback	*Crotolus adaman-teus*			NC, SC, GA, AL, MS, LA, FL
Western dia-mondback	*C. atrox*	CA, NV, AZ, NM	OK, AK, TX	
Sidewinder	*C. cerastes*	CA, NV, AZ	UT	
Timber	*C. horridus*		TX, MN, WS, NE, IA, KS, OK, AK, MO, IL	TN, KY, IN, OH, NC, SC, GA, AL, MS, LA, FL, PA, NJ, MD, DL, VA, WV, NY, CT, MA, RI, ME, NH, VT
Ridge-nosed	*C. willardi*	AZ		
Rock	*C. lepidus*	AZ, NM	TX	
Speckled	*C. mitchelli*	CA, NV, AZ		
Black-tailed	*C. molossus*	AZ, NM	TX	
Twin-spotted	*C. pricei*	AZ		
Red diamond	*C. ruber*	CA		
Mojave	*C. scutulatus*	CA, NV, AZ, NM	TX	
Tiger	*C. tigris*	AZ		
Prairie	*Crotolus Viridus viridis*	OR, ID, AZ, NM, WY, UT, CO, MT	TX, SD, ND, NE, IA, KS, OK	
Grand Canyon	*C. V. abyssus*	AZ		
Southern Pacific	*C. V. helleri*	CA		
Great Basin	*C. V. lutosus*	OR, ID, CA, NV, AZ, UT		
Northern Pacific	*C. V. oreganus*	OR, ID, WA, CA, NV		
Massauga	*Sistrusus catenatus*	AZ, NM, CO	TX, WS, MN, NE, IA, KS, OK, AK, MO, IL	MI, IN, OH, NY, PA
Pigmy rattlesnake	*S. miliarius*		TX, OK, AK, MO	TN, NC, SC, GA, AL, MS, LA, FL
Coral snakes				
Western coral	*Elapidae Micru-roides euryxanthus*	AZ, NM		
Eastern coral	*E. Micrurus fulvius*		TX, AK	NC, SC, GA, AL, MA, LA, FL

TENDONS

Tendons are extensions of the epimysium that coalesce into a solid cord of connective tissue. They make the muscle attachments to skeletal parts for several reasons. Many muscles are too short to extend from one bone to another, and most are too bulky to pass over joints. Furthermore, muscle tissue is too delicate to withstand constant movement over bony prominences. Finally, tendon attachments allow muscles to cross the periphery of joints, enhancing rotational movement as well as stability.

Through tendon attachments to designated areas of periosteum (called "points of origin" and "points of insertion"), skeletal muscles use bones and joints as levers to create an impressive range of body movements (Table 11.5). All action is produced by pulling on the skeleton, since muscle cells can only shorten. For this reason, muscles usually work in pairs. To draw a handsaw through a woodcut, a group of

TABLE 11.5 ANATOMIC MOVEMENTS

Movement	Description	Example	Opposing Movement
Flexion	Bringing parts of limbs together.	Bending leg at knee.	Extension
Abduction	Moving an extremity away from the median plane.	Spreading fingers apart.	Adduction
Elevation	Raising a skeletal part.	Shrugging shoulders (raises scapula).	Depression
Protraction	Moving a skeletal part forward.	Sticking out tongue.	Retraction
Rotation	Partially revolving a body part around the long axis.	Turning head to one side.	Rotation (in opposite direction)
Supination	Rotating forearm.	Turning palms of hands up.	Pronation
Inversion	Rotating foot.	Turning soles of feet together.	Eversion
Circumduction	Complex movement involving elements of flexion, extension, abduction, and adduction.	Swinging arms in a circular motion.	Circumduction (in opposite direction)

Source: Silverstein A: *Human Anatomy and Physiology.* Wiley, New York, 1980.

forearm muscles (agonists) contract, while an opposite group of forearm muscles (antagonists) remain relaxed. To push the saw forward, antagonist muscles contract and agonist muscles relax.

Repeated or vigorous contractions of any one muscle group can cause tissues to tear along points of attachment, an injury known as a ***strain.*** Various types of strains are described in Table 11.6.

Complete separation of the muscle is described as ***severe strain.*** The most vulnerable muscles to this injury include the supraspinatus ***(torn rotator cuff),*** biceps ***(ruptured biceps),*** extensor pollicus longus ***(mallet finger deformity),*** and gastrocnemius ***(ruptured Achilles tendon).*** Usually an unmistakable picture develops at the area of injury, including sudden pain, dysfunction, a palpable defect, spasm, swelling, and ecchymosis. X-ray films may reveal ***avulsion fracture,*** whereby a small fragment of bone is torn away with the tendon attachment. Any severe strain warrants mangement by an orthopedist. Treatment involves surgical repair followed by immobilization until healing is underway.

In ***mild to moderate strains*** there is a stretching or partial tearing of musculotendinous fibers without complete separation. Symptoms include local pain aggravated by muscle contraction. Signs of spasm, swelling, ecchymosis, and some dysfunction may be noted. ▶ ***General measures for mild to moderate strains*** include rest, application of ice or heat, and muscle relaxants. Nonsteroidal anti-inflammatory (NSAI) agents may also be needed in either analgesic or anti-inflammatory doses. Some of the drugs available are listed in Table 11.7. They are divided into classes by increasing order of toxicity. Proper ▶ ***use of NSAI agents*** depends on careful selection (e.g., starting with a less toxic class), appropriate titration, and objective evaluation of therapeutic effects. If one drug does not work well, another drug from the next class should be tried. Patients should be followed for signs of adverse effects.

▶ ***Cervical strain*** is responsible for the common ailment known as "stiff neck."

TABLE 11.6 SOME TYPES OF STRAINS

Location	Etiology	Signs/Symptoms
Neck		
Upper trapezius and sternocleidomastoideus muscles	Sudden twist, forced hyperextension, or traumatic snap of the head.	Causes wryneck or acute torticollis, in which muscles on one side (tilted side) are in an acute state of spasm; marked pain in the area of contraction and continuing down one shoulder, with extreme limitation of movement in the cervical region.
Shoulder		
Glenohumeral joint (deltoid and rotator cuff tendons)	Usually the result of a violent pull to the arm, abnormal rotation, or a fall on an outstretched arm. Affects deltoid muscle superficially and tendons of rotator cuff internally (primarily supraspinatus muscle tendon).	Pain, loss of function (especially with the arm abducted or externally rotated), swelling, and point tenderness; passive movements seldom yield pain in strained condition.
Buttocks		
Gluteal muscles	Rare; gluteus maximus and gluteus medius muscles most often involved.	Pain and restriction of muscle function, hematoma and swelling of affected muscle, inability to bear weight on extremity due to pain in muscle. Voluntary contraction of muscle against resistance may be impossible or may produce severe pain.
Groin		
Inguinal region (iliopsoas, rectus femoris, and the adductor group: gracilis, pectineus, adductor brevis, adductor longus, adductor magnus)	Involving the musculature in the depression lying between the thigh and the abdominal region; overextension, especially in running, jumping, climbing, and twisting with external rotation, may result in "groin strain." Injury to adductor group more common than to iliopsoas.	Can appear as a sudden twinge or feeling of tearing during active movement or may not be noticed until after termination of activity; pain, weakness, internal hemorrhage present. Since patient is unable to pinpoint exact injury site, functional tests may be given to determine the extent of injury.
Thigh		
Hamstring muscle	Participation in active sports, especially running, may result in this strain. Deficiency in reciprocal or complementary action of opposing muscle groups (possibly due to fatigue, poor posture, uneven muscle strength, inflexibility, or poor form in athletic performance) is thought to contribute. Strain involves muscle at bony attachment or belly of tendon. This strain tends to become recurrent due to healing by inelastic, fibrous scar tissue.	Capillary hemorrhage, pain, and immediate loss of function, which vary with the degree of trauma; discoloration 1–2 days after injury has been incurred. Strain is preceded by a feeling of muscular fatigue or incipient spasm; sudden snap and/or sharp pain may occur at the time of severe strain, accompanied by loss of function; pain felt after an event has been completed usually indicates mild or moderate strain; stiffness and point tenderness occurring after the patient has cooled down from vigorous activity indicate mild strain; moderate strain is accompanied by severe pain persisting for several minutes after injury and loss of function on knee flexion.

TABLE 11.7 NSAI DRUGS

Class and Generic Name	Brand Name	Half-Life (hr)	Usual Maximum Daily Dose (mg)
Salicylates			
Aspirin	Bayer	3–16	2,600–5,200 (to 7,800 for acute rheumatic fever)
Choline magnesium trisalicylate	Trilisate	7–18	3,000
Diflunisal	Dolobid	8	3,000
Magnesium salicylate	Magsal	2–2.5	3,000
Salsalate	Disalcid	8	3,000
Oxicams			
Piroxicam	Feldene	44–50	20
Propionic acids			
Fenoprofen	Nalfon	3	3,200
Ibuprofen	Motrin, Rufen	2–3	2,400
Naproxen	Naprosyn, Anaprox	13	1,000
Indole analogues			
Indomethacin	Indocin	3–4.5	200
Sulindac	Clinoril	13	400
Tolmetin	Tolectin	1	2,000
Pyrazoles			
Oxyphenbutazone	Oxalid, Tanderil	72–96	400
Phenylbutazone	Butazolidin	84–96	400
Fenamic acids			
Meclofenmate	Meclomen	2–5	400
Mefenamic acid	Ponstel	2–5	1,250

Unlike other types of strain, it often develops without specific injury. To provide support and a wide range of movement for a (top-heavy) head, paravertebral neck muscles are exceedingly strong. They are also maximally burdened by everyday work. Prolonged or awkward positions, or exposure to air conditioning or fans, may be enough to cause spasm with overstretching of fibers. Neck strains are also related to falls, auto accidents (sudden deceleration), and athletic injuries (sudden thrusts or pulls on the arms). The predominant symptom is pain. It may localize along the neck as well as radiate to the occiput, between the shoulder blades, to the tops of the shoulders, or into the upper arms. Patients also complain of limited neck and shoulder motion. Crunching noises, "knots," spasm, and tenderness may all be observed. Patients with no signs of nerve root irritation (numbness, tingling, sensory loss, muscle weakness, atrophy, reflex changes in the extremity) should be treated with general measures for strains and given specific instructions for ▶***correct posture*** and neck exercises.

▶***Acute lumbar strain*** is unlikely to occur in athletes or young persons who are in good physical condition. However, in persons over age 30 who are overweight or seldom exercise, any sudden, excessive demand on the back such as lifting a heavy child, swinging a golf club, or raking leaves may precipitate spasm of the paravertebral muscles with overstretching of fibers. Symptoms of acute lumbar strain include intense pain, acute tightening, and almost paralyzing immobility of the low back. Patients tend to assume unnatural postures, particularly "scoliotic listing" (tilting to one side). Bending sideways or forward (but not backward) intensifies the pain. Muscles can be so taut that flexion of the spine becomes impossible and the patient can only bend from the hips or the lumbothoracic junction. The diagnosis is based on the history and x-ray films, which may show malalignment due to muscle spasm but no other abnormality. X-ray films are indicated in all new cases of sudden back pain to rule out compression fracture, metastatic bone cancer, spur formation, or disc narrowing. Unless spinal nerves are involved, reflexes, sensory testing, and straight leg raising should be normal. Patients with acute lumbar strain can be initially managed by bed rest, heat treatments, massage, muscle relaxants, and analgesics. In the absence of a firm mattress, patients should use a bed board or sleep on the floor. As soon as the pain slackens, gradual exercises should be initiated. Corsets or braces may be used for added support and comfort, but should be discontinued after short periods to avoid psychologic dependence. With these measures, acute symptoms usually subside in 3–10 days.

Recurrent lumbar strain is an initiating factor in ***low back syndrome.*** This problem is particularly prevalent in patients who are overweight and who have poor abdominal muscle tone. Due to added stress on the vertebral column, vertebral ligaments eventually become stretched or torn ***(lumbar sprain). Subluxation of a facet joint*** may follow, causing narrowing of the facet joints and nerve root entrapment. For this reason, patients with low back syndrome must be observed for neurologic symptoms and referred accordingly (see Chapter 12 and the later discussion). Otherwise, management of chronic lumbar strain centers on weight control, postural measures, faithful back exercises, and regular, sensible sports activity.

Unlike muscle tissue, tendon tissue is relatively avascular and has poor reparative ability. For this reason, ***tendinitis*** may follow a strain injury. This problem is also related to the aging process in that tendons lose collagen content and begin to fray along points of bony insertions, beginning in middle adulthood. Indeed, most cases occur after age 50. The most common types of tendinitis are described in Table 11.8. Initiating activities, signs, and symptoms, which are also described, form the basis for diagnosis. ▶ ***General measures for tendinitis*** include ice to ease pain and reduce swelling, followed by controlled range-of-motion exercises. Anti-inflammatory drugs, heat, massage, diathermy, local corticosteroid injections, and ultrasound are also used successfully. Of course, the activity that precipitated the problem should be discontinued until the patient regains normal joint motion and good strength without pain. An exercise program designed to strengthen involved muscles help prevent recurrent problems.

Sometimes inflammation of tendons is initiated by tissue deposition of calcium crystals, a condition called ***calcific tendinitis.*** The crystal formation causes sudden, severe pain that typically develops late at night and is unrelated to overactivity. Although the physical findings are consistent with the more common types of tendinitis, the unique history indicates the need for x-ray studies. If films show calcium deposits, needling of these deposits, local steroid injections, or even surgery may be necessary.

Although mentioned in Table 11.8, ▶ ***tennis elbow*** (lateral epicondylitis) warrants further discussion because of its common occurrence and chronic nature. The problem is initiated by a strain of the lateral forearm muscle caused by repetitive and/or strenuous supination of the wrist against resistance (e.g., hitting forehand ground strokes in tennis, using a screwdriver). Inflammation develops at muscle origins on the lateral epicondyle. It produces point tenderness, as well as pain radiating to the outer side of the arm and forearm that is sharply aggravated by dorsiflexion of the wrist. Wrist weakness may be pronounced. General measures for tendinitis should be initiated. Steroid injection into the lateral epicondyle may also be

TABLE 11.8 COMMON TYPES OF TENDINITIS AND TENOSYNOVITIS

Location	Etiology	Signs and Symptoms
Shoulder		
· Rotator cuff (supraspinatus) insertion into humeral head	Repetitive arm-raising activities contribute: hanging wallpaper, overhand tennis serves, freestyle swimming; also, faulty back posture.	Pain at tip of shoulder toward back, strongest between 70 and 100 degree of adduction; when asked to raise the arm, the patient manages only a shrug; rotation is also painful, and the patient will typically hold the arm braced across the chest wall.
· Insertion of biceps into bicipital groove	Overstress from bending elbow against resistance: curling weights, digging ditches, canoeing, doing construction work.	Symptoms may be similar to those of rotator cuff tendinitis; pain radiates along biceps, down forearm, and can be reproduced by flexing patient's arm against resistance; audible click sometimes noted as inflamed tendon slips out of bicipital groove with arm elevation.
Elbow		
· Insertions into medial and lateral epicondyle of humerus and head of radius; "tennis elbow"	Activities involving stressful or repeated twisting of wrist and forearm: racket sports, carpentry, mechanical work, use of screwdriver, hammer, masonry or garden tools.	Elbow pain increased by activity involving hand grip (patient may drop objects), tenderness over radial humeral head, lateral or medial epicondyles; no loss of elbow motion. Maudsley's test: pain produced by flexing middle finger against resistance while arm is held in extension. Mill's sign: pain produced by forced arm pronation against resistance while elbow is held in extension.
Wrist and hand		
· Insertion of long abductor, extensor, and flexor tendons into base of thumb; "washerwoman's sprain," "De Quervain's disease"	Wringing or kneading activities: pottery or bread making, guitar playing, garden pruning.	Swelling and tenderness of radial aspect of wrist; pain with grasping. Finkelstein's test: pain when hand in fist position is adducted. Tenosynovitis is associated with rheumatoid disease, gout, and disseminated gonorrhea.
· Insertion of extensor/flexor tendons to fingers into wrist	Stressful finger movements or grasping: playing musical instruments, typing, kneading bread, making pottery, weaving, or knitting.	Pain at ventral aspect of wrist when flexor tendons are affected and at dorsal aspect when extensors are involved; symptoms exacerbated by hyperextension/flexion of wrists and fingers; associated with radial nerve (carpal tunnel) or ulnar nerve syndromes; tenosynovitis is associated with pregnancy and menopause, rheumatoid disease, gout, and disseminated gonorrhea.
Hip		
Insertion of gluteal muscle tendons into trochanter	Walking, running (particularly on a banked surface); contributing factors include unbalanced abductor/adductor muscles, leg length discrepancies, gait problems.	Unilateral hip pain at lateral aspect of thigh radiating to lateral aspect of knee or, on occasion, to lower leg and ankle; pain exacerbated by extension of the leg; localized tenderness at region of greater trochanter; associated with bursitis in older patients.
Insertion of adductor tendons into pubic symphysis	Overstress from activities such as rock climbing, dance and stretching exercises, bicycling, rip kicking (as in swimming breast stroke).	Tenderness in groin area; abduction of hip and adduction against resistance produce pain.

TABLE 11.8 *(Continued)*

Location	Etiology	Signs and Symptoms
Knee		
Patellar tendon at insertion point into kneecap ("jumper's knee"), at body of tendon (patellar tendinitis), and at insertion point into tibial tuberosity	Active forceful knee extension from activities such as running and jumping, extended walking; contributing factors include inadequate warmup and stretching exercises.	Pain and point tenderness below kneecap, exacerbated by extension of leg; chondromalacia may be a complication; tendinitis at site of insertion into tibial tuberosity may lead to ossification (i.e., Osgood-Schlatter disease) in an adolescent.
Insertion of popliteal muscle tendon into lateral epicondyle of femur	Directly related to running on insides of feet (hyperpronation) and to running downhill or on banked surfaces.	Pain and tenderness localized to lateral aspect of knee at femoral epicondyle.
Insertion of sartorius, gracilis, and semitendinosus muscle tendons into medial border of tibial tuberosity; "anserine tendinitis"	Inadequate warmup and stretching prior to athletic activities; running on outsides of feet (hypersupination) contributes to the problem.	Pain localized to medial aspect of knee at tibial tuberosity.
Leg		
Insertion of tibialis posterior muscle tendon into interosseus membrane (between tibia and fibula) and tibial periosteum; "shin splints"	Running on hard or banked surfaces; contributing factors include poor conditioning, running on insides of feet or with toes pointed out, and wearing improper shoes.	Pain along lower two-thirds of inner tibial surface; as the problem first develops, soreness noted after running; later, pain develops during and after running; in severe cases, walking and stair climbing produce pain.
Ankle and foot		
· Insertion of toe extensor/flexor tendons into ankle; tibialis anterior tendinitis	Running or extended walking.	Pain and swelling on anterior portion of ankle; pain may be referred to top of foot and exacerbated by weight bearing and by flexion and extension of toes; no restriction of ankle movement.
· Insertion of tibialis posterior muscle tendon into navicular, cuboid, and cuneiform bones; tibialis posterior tendinitis	Skiing, running on banked surfaces; contributing factors include running on insides of feet, shoes with improper arch support, inadequate stretching prior to activity, flat feet.	Pain behind medial malleolus radiating into medial aspect of foot; tenderness and thickening at insertion point; localized edema and soft tissue swelling.
· Insertion of peroneii muscle tendons into toes	Skiing, running on banked surfaces; contributing factors include running on outsides of feet, poorly supportive shoes, inadequate warmup stretching.	Pain at lateral aspect of ankle referred to lateral dorsal surface of foot; tenderness and swelling behind lateral malleolus; pain exacerbated by inverting the foot and may restrict weight bearing.
· Insertion of gastrocnemius and soleus muscle tendons into heel; Achilles tendinitis	Uphill running; contributing factors include use of shoes with rigid soles or inadequate heel support, running on insides of feet (hyperpronation), high arches, tight hamstring and calf muscles.	Tenderness and swelling at back of leg above heel; chronic inflammation leads to mucoid nodule formation or painful bursa ("pump bump").

(·) = Possible site of tenosynovitis.

beneficial. Once pain has eased, patients should be started on exercises to strengthen forearm muscles. Use of a forearm strap during activities involving wrist supination is also helpful. The reason for this is not clear, though it is assumed that the strap redistributes stress points.

BURSA

Tendons that span freely movable joints are subject to much frictional stress. For lubrication, they are underpadded by tiny sacs called "bursae." There are approximately 156 bursae, each lined by a synovial membrane and filled with synovial fluid. Inflammation of an overlying tendon can extend to contiguous bursae, causing ▶ ***acute bursitis.*** In fact, tendinitis and bursitis often exist as concurrent or indistinguishable processes. The most common types are described in Table 11.9, along with the inciting activities, signs, and symptoms. As in tendinitis, treatment includes rest, anti-inflammatory medications, and heat.

Unlike tendinitis, all cases of bursitis warrant special diagnostic considerations. Because of the synovium, bursae are subject to the same problems as joints, including rheumatoid arthritis and gout. ***Septic bursitis*** may also occur, particularly in bursae lying close to skin surfaces. In fact, one study found 10 out of 30 cases of olecranon and prepatellar bursitis to be infectious, with fever, leukocytosis, and peribursal cellulitis being important distinguishing features. On the other hand, there may be no differentiating signs. Because misdiagnosis may end in fistula tracts or osteomyelitis, any swollen bursa, even if it is painless, should be aspirated. Patients with purulent aspirates and/or low bursal to serum glucose ratios and positive Gram stains must be treated with antibiotics for 10–14 days after cultures are obtained.

Recurrent inflammation of the bursa characterizes ***chronic bursitis.*** Flareups, each lasting for a few days to several weeks, lead to fibrotic changes of the bursa such as adhesions, villus tags, and calcium deposits. Known as ***calcific bursitis,*** the last condition is similar to calcific tendinitis, which was previously discussed. Whatever the pathologic change, pain is debilitating and muscle atrophy the rule. Furthermore, disuse because of pain may initiate a fibrotic process within the joint capsule referred to as ***adhesive capsulitis or frozen joint.*** Capable of forming in an alarmingly short time, these adhesions prevent normal joint movement after the pain and inflammation of the acute process have resolved. Without months (perhaps years) of rehabilitation and/or surgery, the dysfunction is permanent. For this reason, cases of chronic bursitis that fail to respond to medical treatment should be referred to an orthopedist. Surgical removal of a diseased bursa may be recommended, with the hope that a new bursa will form in its place.

One common complication of chronic bursitis is the ***bunion.*** The bursa located at the "ball" of the foot becomes inflamed, often from improperly fitting shoes (too small, too narrow) during the growth years. Highly arched feet, ankle pronation (rolling in), and long toes contribute to this condition. Unless walking, running, and all other forms of footwork are suspended, the injury is persistently irritated. The response in later years is an inflammatory reaction of surrounding tissues that causes the joint to enlarge and the toe to deviate inward ***(hallux valgus).*** One of the most important considerations in management is strict avoidance of ill-fitting shoes. Podiatry referral for orthotic devices and surgical correction may also be considered,

TABLE 11.9 COMMON TYPES OF BURSITIS

Location	Etiology	Signs/Symptoms
Shoulder		
Subacromial bursa beneath acromion overlying rotator cuff; lateral extension is termed the "subdeltoid bursa."	Secondary to rotator cuff tendinitis; poor posture and arm-raising activities such as painting, overhand tennis serves, and free style swimming may contribute.	Pain around head of shoulder, greatest when arm is elevated between 70 and 100 degrees and exacerbated by external rotation; tenderness, redness, and swelling over greater tubercle of humerus.
Elbow		
Olecranon bursa between epicondyles of humerus and adjacent to olecranon process of ulna.	Trauma, especially from prolonged leaning on elbows; common site for septic bursitis.	Pain on flexion or extension; passive movement shows range of motion to be unimpaired; enlarged bursa can be palpated between epicondyles with arm extended.
Hip		
Trochanter (multilocular) bursa covering lateral head of femur beneath gluteus maximus.	Secondary to or concurrent with trochanter tendinitis seen in runners with imbalance of adductor/abductor leg muscles or gait problems; leg length discrepancy is a contributing factor.	Hip pain radiating to lateral thigh and knee (with bilateral involvement in 10–15% of cases) aggravated by lying on side of hip and going downstairs; localized tenderness at lateral head of femur; discomfort greatest with extension of hip; no loss of range of motion.
Ischial bursa covering tip of ischium, overlying sciatic nerve and posterior femoral cutaneous nerve; underlies hamstring attachments	Due to activities involving violent hamstring contractions, such as cycling, rowing, uphill running, and possibly to prolonged sitting on hard surfaces or sitting on a wallet in a hip pocket. Called "weaver's bottom."	Pain in buttock radiating to posterior thigh; possible swelling over ischium.
Psoas (iliopectineal) bursa overlying lesser trochanter or femur beneath insertion of psoas muscle.	Dance exercises, cycling, and abnormal spine curvature contribute.	Pain and tenderness in groin radiating to front of thigh with weight bearing; pain reproduced by extension or flexion against resistance.
Knee		
Prepatellar bursa underlying kneecap	Due to direct trauma from fall or to prolonged kneeling on hard surfaces. Called "housemaid's knee" or "nun's knee."	Minimal pain except with extreme flexion or direct pressure; range of motion intact.
Deep infrapatellar	Due to stress from overuse of knee function, as in running, cycling.	Pain behind patella with forced flexion and extension.
Anserine bursa lying underneath tendon insertions to inner thigh muscles just below knee on medial side.	Due to stress from horseback riding or angular knee deformities secondary to obesity. Called "cavalryman's disease."	Medial knee pain, palpable swelling and tenderness over bursa.
Gastrocnemiosemimembranosis bursa at back of knee.	Trauma in young persons; rheumatoid processes in older age groups. Called "baker's cyst" or "popliteal cyst."	Palpable mass in popliteal space; inability to extend knee; when bursa is distended with fluid, it may interfere with walking.

TABLE 11.9 *(Continued)*

Location	Etiology	Signs/Symptoms
Ankle and foot		
Retroachilles bursa, retrocalcaneal bursa, and subcalcaneal bursa, which are closely situated around heel	Contributing factors are tight-fitting or high-heeled shoes, trauma from running or extended walking, and arthritic processes; associated with Achilles tendinitis. Calcification results in "pump bump." Called "policeman's heel" or "soldier's heel."	Considerable pain in back of heel radiating to ankle; swelling in area of Achilles tendon; calcified nodules may be palpable on bursa.
Metatarsal-phalangeal bursa and callus formation over ball of foot	Chronic irritation from poorly fitting shoes. Bunion.	Bony enlargement of joint; inward deviation of toe (valgus shift); chronic pain.

since bunions can lead to incapacitating osteoarthritis and spur formation ***(hallux rigidus).***

TENDON SHEATH

As a protective measure against constant friction, certain tendons in the shoulder, hand, hip, and foot are enclosed in a tendon sheath. A fibrous wall lined with synovial membranes, the sheath is actually a modified form of bursa. Sometimes, as a result of trauma, a portion of the synovial lining herniates to the outside of the tendon sheath. The membrane continues to produce synovial fluid, forming a fluid-filled sac that is logically called a ***synovial cyst.*** A ***ganglion*** develops if the pedicle connecting the cyst to its parent lining becomes walled off. With nourishment curtailed, the synovial lining then atrophies and the cyst becomes fibrotic. The ganglion not only feels rock hard but may reach sizable proportions and develop multilocular contours. Furthermore, while most ganglia are symptomatic, the location of others may cause joint dysfunction or symptoms of nerve pressure. Treatment should begin with conservative measures such as pressure bandages or tenotome rupture. Surgical removal is another possibility, though it is attended by a record of recurrence and complications. Years ago, people were known to treat ganglia by smashing down on them with the family bible (hence the folk name "bible bump"). However, this or any other treatment may be unnecessary. Ganglia often disappear spontaneously.

With its synovial lining, the sheath offers a potential space for arthritic complications known as ***tenosynovitis.*** Various types are described in Table 11.8. Along with all of the findings of tendinitis, tenosynovitis frequently presents with a friction rub due to an effusion within the sheath. The rub can be heard or felt on movement of the joint. Tenosynovitis usually develops secondary to trauma and can be treated as tendinitis. However, it also occurs with rheumatoid arthritis, SLE, gout, gonorrhea, and other bacterial infections. Special diagnostic and treatment measures are then needed.

▶ ***Tendinitis, bursitis, and tenosynovitis of the shoulder*** often coexist because of the joint's complex architecture. To begin with, the humeral head is much larger than the glenoid fossa of the scapula and is held in place by a single conjoined tendon of the rotator cuff muscles. This permits the widest range of motion of any joint in the body, but stability is sacrificed. Repeated overhead reaching or poor back posture can lead to ***rotator cuff tendinitis*** with secondary subdeltoid bursitis. As noted in Tables 11.8 and 11.9, the inciting activities, signs, and symptoms of the two problems are similar. Furthermore, encompassing the long head of the biceps muscle is a tendon sheath that is continuous with the joint capsule. When ***tendinitis or tenosynovitis of the biceps insertion*** develops from bending the elbow against resistance, the processes extend into the joint, mimicking or causing rotator cuff tendinitis/bursitis. Because of such interinvolvement, inflammatory conditions of the shoulder are particularly painful and prone to chronicity. Furthermore, reduced activity from pain quickly results in ***frozen shoulder*** (adhesive capsulitis). This syndrome, which is characterized by overall thickening of the joint capsule, inferior adhesion formation, and reduced synovial lubrication, leads to permanent restriction of shoulder movement. To prevent it, exercises are an important aspect of any shoulder treatment.

For unclear reasons, the tendon sheath sometimes thickens in areas where tendons of the palm pass through fibrous rings at the base of the thumb and fingers. This thickening is the cause of ***stenosing tenosynovitis,*** a condition characterized by pain with flexion of the finger or thumb. Furthermore, a callous-like nodule may eventually develop that slips back and forth through the fibrous ring, resisting movement as well as intensifying the pain. If the nodule catches on the distal side, the digit becomes locked into a flexed position and cannot be extended until the nodule is forced back through the ring. This produces a painful pop and provides the name ***trigger finger.*** Mild symptoms of stenosing tenosynovitis sometimes respond to a period of rest, heat, and anti-inflammatory agents. When it is incapacitating, the problem is best managed with local steroid injections or surgical decompression.

FASCIA

Fascia is a protective sheet of fibrous tissue that arises over the surface of muscles that are subject to a great deal of friction. In addition, closed layers of fascia pad the fingertips, which have no muscle tissue. An infection between these layers is called ***felon.*** The fingertip becomes red, tense, and exquisitely painful. Because a felon leads to rapid necrosis, it must be aggressively treated with surgical drainage and antibiotics. If drainage of a felon is persistent, x-ray films should be ordered to rule out osteomyelitis (see the later discussion).

Fasciitis may develop from excessive friction occurring with muscle overuse. The cardinal symptom is pain produced by a specific movement. The only sign is the development (in chronic cases) of ***bone spurs,*** which can be seen on x-ray films. Ice, anti-inflammatory agents, and rest are used in treatment. Orthopedic shoes or orthotic devices to correct pronated or varus foot formations may be useful in plantar fasciitis and/or heel spurs. In rare cases, steroid injections or surgical intervention may be needed.

Fibromyalgia (fibrositis, myofascitis, fibromyositis) is a rheumatic disorder affecting muscular connective tissues. Fibrocystic nodules (cord-like nodules of contracted muscle fibers or oval nodules of fibrofatty tissue) develop in areas of muscle insertion, producing "tender points" that set up a pain–spasm–pain cycle. The cause is unknown. Patients are typically women between 20 and 30 years old, men being affected only 15% of the time. They complain of diffuse muscle aches, as well as heightened pain and stiffness in certain areas (particularly the jaw, neck, back, elbows, and/or knees). They also complain of sleeping poorly and feeling tired on awakening. Symptoms are aggravated by cold or humid weather, overactivity, long periods of inactivity, and tension. On exam, muscle strength and neurologic and joint findings are normal. However, 4–40 tender points may be identified. Palpation in these areas produces pain and transient hyperemia. Laboratory tests are needed only when there is a suspicion of rheumatoid arthritis, lupus erythematosus, osteoarthritis, myositis, or another cause of musculoskeletal pain. Reassurance that the condition is benign and noncrippling is the most important aspect of management. Anti-inflammatory drugs, heat, massage, rest, and relaxation ameliorate the symptoms. Local steroid injections at obstinate trigger points are often curative.

FORMATION AND GROWTH OF BONE TISSUE

In the fetus, membranes and cartilage serve as a blueprint for skeletal development. They provide an environment for the formation of bone tissue by three cell types—osteoblasts, osteocytes, and osteoclasts. Osteoblasts secrete a gel-like substance (intracellular matrix) enriched with collagen fibers and laid out in long columns (trabeculae). The body supplies the matrix with calcium phosphate and calcium carbonate, which combine to form calcium salts. The collagen fibers somehow "seed" the calcium salts to form crystals (hydroxyapatites). The hydroxyapatites and collagen fibers are cemented together by a number of ingredients found in the matrix (iron, fluoride, sulfate, sodium, and magnesium), and the gel-like matrix "calcifies" (ossifies, mineralizes), forming a spicule.

Some osteoblasts become surrounded by the calcified material and trapped in small spaces called "lacunae." These cells become osteocytes. Through the development of long cytoplasmic processes, they communicate with osteocytes in neighboring lacunae. Meanwhile, untrapped osteoblasts swarm on spicule surfaces and begin to lay out new trabeculae in radiating patterns. Cancellous bone tissue forms as the spicules interlace. This lacy type of bone tissue remains in certain areas, providing space in the vertebrae, sternum, ribs, skull, hips, and epiphyses for red blood cell marrow. Lightweight and slightly flexible, it also modifies the ends of long bones for the purposes of weight bearing and articulation.

In other areas, osteoblasts fill in the porous spaces of cancellous bone to create compact (dense) bone tissue. They do so by laying down concentric "lamellae" of osteoid around blood vessels and nerves. Leaving a vertical shaft space for main vessels (Haversian canals) and a transverse shaft space for branching vessels (Volkmann's canals), they expand outward until one "Haversian system" becomes confluent with another, with osteocytes scattered throughout. The completed product is a dense tissue that makes up the thick outer portion (cortex) of skeletal bones.

As areas of the soft fetal skeleton are transformed into bone tissue, individual bones take shape. The process of bone formation from fetal membranes is known as "intramembranous ossification" and that from fetal cartilage is known as "endochondral ossification." Endochondral ossification also takes place along the cartilaginous plate between the head (epiphysis) and the shaft (diaphysis) of long bones. The growth of long bones continues until the cartilage plate is totally replaced by bone tissue (epiphyseal closure). Maturation is a long process, ending in men at around age 20 and in women at around age 18. Genetics and hormones (thyroid hormone, growth hormone, sex hormones, parathyroid hormone, and adrenosteroids) are important governing factors.

Calcium and phosphorus, the main minerals found in osteoid tissue, are crucial to bone formation. Obtained mainly from dairy foods, calcium must be absorbed from the gut for body use. Absorption, in turn, is stimulated by an active form of vitamin D. The two main sources of vitamin D are fortified foods and endogenous formation by skin that has been exposed to sunlight. Phosphorus is readily available in the diet and is directly absorbed. Needed for cellular metabolism as well as bone formation, calcium and phosphorus levels are carefully regulated by parathyroid hormone and excreted by the kidneys. When serum levels fall, parathyroid hormone stimulates the breakdown of bone tissue, releasing the minerals to keep serum levels within a normal range. Thus, low levels of calcium or phosphorus for any of the reasons listed in Table 11.10 lead to faulty mineralization, known as osteomalacia. Osteomalacia occurring during periods of active bone growth results in thin, softened bone tissue and the characteristic deformities of ***rickets.*** Unable to support an afflicted child's weight, the legs bow out and the thoracic spine curves abnormally. Fortunately, rickets is extremely rare in the United States. However, adult forms of the problem occur with some frequency. They are discussed in a later section.

Vitamin C is also crucial to the formation of bone tissue because, without it, the osteoblast cannot form sufficient quantities of matrix. ***Scurvy*** in childhood causes permanent malformations that include grossly enlarged heads of the long bones. Scurvy in adults may cause periosteal hemorrhage but is not otherwise responsible for bone changes. It is readily reversed by the provision of vitamin C.

MATURE BONE

The general features of mature bone are illustrated in Figure 11.6. The shaft of long bones (diaphysis) has a broad head (epiphysis) at either end. For the purpose of articulation, each epiphysis is uniquely shaped to fit the surface of communicating bones and constructed from lightweight, slightly flexible cancellous tissue. Here (and in the vertebrae, sternum, ribs, skull, and hips) cancellous tissue houses red

TABLE 11.10 CAUSES OF OSTEOMALACIA

- Inadequate calcium
  - Poor diet
  - Lactose intolerance
  - Pregnancy and lactation
- Vitamin D abnormalities
  - Deficiency
    - Dietary lack
    - Insufficient sunshine
  - Malabsorption
    - Sprue
    - Gastrectomy, small bowel bypass, small bowel resection
    - Bile salt deficiency
    - Pancreatic deficiency
- Impaired activation
  - Liver disease
  - Kidney disease
  - Parathyroid hormone deficiency
- Increased catabolism/excretion
  - Anticonvulsant, barbiturate use
  - Nephrotic syndrome
- Phosphate depletion
  - Malabsorption
  - Primary hypophosphatemia
  - Phosphate-binding antacids
  - Metabolic acidosis
  - Fanconi's syndrome

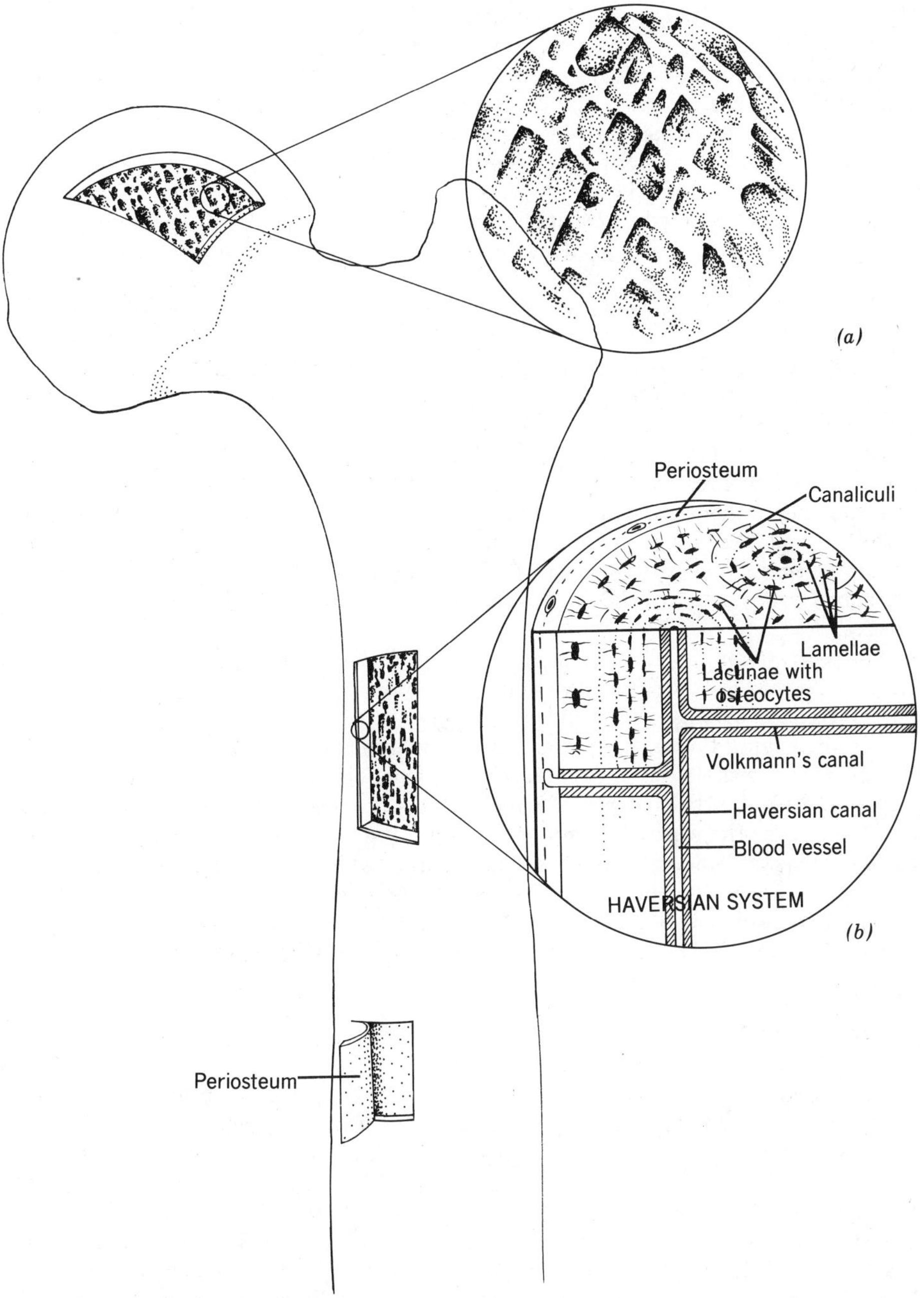

Figure 11.6 Mature bone: (*a*) cancellous bone; (*b*) compact bone.

blood cell marrow (hematopoietic tissue). Except for sharing space, the hematopoietic and skeletal systems function independently.

The center of the diaphysis is a space, the marrow cavity. A thick area of compact bone known as the "cortex" surrounds the marrow cavity, providing strength for weight bearing. Its outer surface is covered by the periosteum, a double-layered fibrous membrane. The cavity is packed with yellow marrow, a tissue whose sole purpose is support. Infection of the marrow cavity is called ***osteomyelitis.*** Most cases occur in children when organisms from a distant focus (e.g., lungs, kidneys, or intestines) are carried by the blood to seed the highly vascular areas of growing bones. Only 15% of acute osteomyelitis cases are encountered in adults, and these result from the contiguous spread of soft tissue infections. Once established in the marrow tissue, the infection travels laterally through Haversian and Volkmann's canals and eventually perforates the cortex. As pressure from inflammatory debris builds, the periosteum is lifted away and areas of sepsis extend longitudinally. This process is invariably accompanied by severe pain, fever, and tachycardia. Other signs include redness, swelling, or purulent drainage around the involved area of bone. Periosteal elevation with new formation is an early x-ray finding; actual bone lysis becomes radiographically evident 10–14 days later. Early hospital treatment with IV antibiotics is crucial. Pus that has collected beneath the periosteum must be evacuated through aspiration or surgical incision. Casting or splinting the involved extremity relieves pain and, according to some experts, enhances the healing process.

The periosteum has an inner layer, which is loose and elastic and pegs into the cortex with perforating (Sharpey's) fibers. Its outer layer is highly vascular and a key source of nourishment for underlying bone. In addition to protecting and nourishing underlying tissue, the periosteum augments the attachment of tendons and ligaments to the skeleton. In runners, chronic traction on the periosteum from unresolved tendinitis of the posterior tibeal attachments leads to ***shin splints.*** Persistent exercise despite the warning symptom of pain along the inner two-thirds of the shin causes abnormal bone formations in longitudinal patterns. This problem is particularly common among runners who have malalignment problems of the feet or who work out on hard or banked surfaces. It can be detected on bone scan or x-ray films. Treatment consists of rest, applications of heat, and use of anti-inflammatory agents.

BONE TURNOVER

The formation of bone tissue does not stop with growth. Weight-bearing activities incite osteoblasts to lay down trabeculae along shifting lines of mechanical stress throughout life (Fig. 11.7). Calcium and phosphorus are crucial to the mineralization of new trabeculae. As mentioned previously, calcium that is obtained mainly through dairy foods must be absorbed from the gut for body use; this absorption in turn, is stimulated by active forms of vitamin D. The two main sources of vitamin D are fortified foods and endogenous formation by skin that has been exposed to sunlight. Phosphorus is readily available in the diet and is directly absorbed. Needed for cellular metabolism as well as bone formation, both calcium and phosphorus are carefully regulated by parathyroid hormone and excreted by the kidneys. Thus, when serum levels fall, the hormone stimulates the breakdown of bone tissue, releasing the minerals to keep serum levels within a normal range.

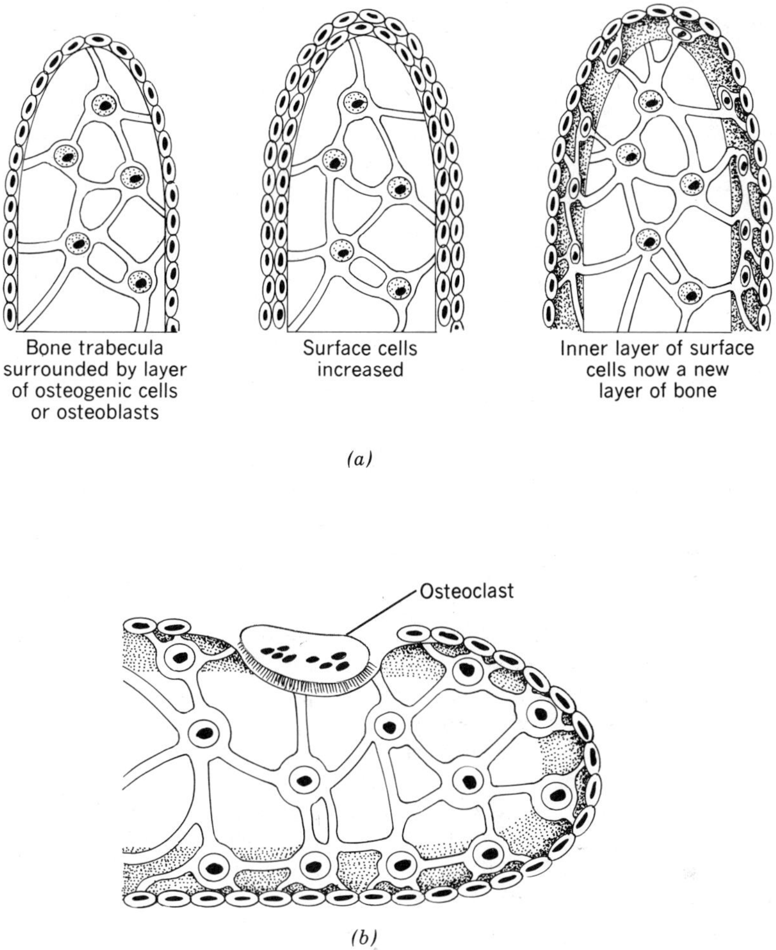

Figure 11.7 Bone deposition (*a*) and resorption (*b*).

If any of the conditions listed in Table 11.10 are present, ***osteomalacia*** develops. Old bone tissue is sacrificed and new trabeculae fail to harden properly. Mild forms of osteomalacia result in subclinical loss of bone mass. This often occurs, for example, during pregnancy and lactation. If the mother's increased needs for calcium are not met, her bone tissue undergoes accelerated breakdown to boost serum levels of this mineral. The slight sacrifice of bone mass remains unnoticed until further loss occurs around the time of menopause (see the discussion of postmenopausal osteoporosis).

More severe forms of osteomalacia result in softening of bone tissue and reduced bone mass ***(osteopenia);*** the latter can be demonstrated radiographically. Specific x-ray findings include loss of trabecular bone (washed-out, "ground-glass" appearance of the cortex) and/or abnormal deposition of bone around major blood vessels (pseudofractures). Some patients are asymptomatic, while others have varying degrees of bony achiness, muscular weakness, and general listlessness. Bony tenderness may be noted on exam. Serum calcium is low or normal, but never high. Serum phosphate is usually low except in the presence of significant renal failure. Alkaline phosphatase is elevated in more severe cases. Bone biopsy is sometimes required for confirmation. Newer noninvasive procedures are also available to measure bone mass [Norland-Cameron single-photon absorptiometry, quantitative computed tomography (CT) scans, and total body neutron activation analysis]. Definitive diagnosis is important if there is a question of an osteoporotic component. Osteomalacia, which must be addressed before osteoporosis will respond to therapy, is treated by correcting the underlying causes of calcium and phosphorus deficiency, including malabsorption syndromes. General measures are a diet high in calcium and vitamin D and supplements of both substances. Large amounts of vitamin D metabolites, once given automatically, are now known to cause serious toxicities and must be carefully managed.

If new bone tissue is formed continually thoughout life, what prevents the development of overly thick bones? The answer is an ongoing catabolic process (resorption) that destroys old bone in order to free space and minerals for new tissue. The destruction itself is conducted by a large multinucleated cell, the osteoclast (see Fig. 11.7). Actually, resorption and formation take place as coupled processes in microscopic areas of bone called "remodeling units." As long as these processes offset each other, bone mass remains constant. However, any of the conditions listed in Table 11.11 can cause excessive resorption and/or inhibited deposition, leading to a loss of bone mass referred to as ***secondary osteoporosis.*** Many cases are first discovered as an incidental finding on chest x-ray films that reveal a "codfish" appearance of the vertebrae (thinning of horizontal trabeculae accentuates the biconcavity of vertebral endplates) and/or translucency of the ribs. This codfish deformity also characterizes osteomalacia. Such radiographic changes indicate that 40–50% of bone has been lost in the thoracic vertebrae and ribs, and can therefore be expected along other areas of cancellous bone (lumbar vertebral bodies, humerus, distal radius, metacarpals, and proximal femur). Having a thin cortex, cancellous bone density can be readily reduced below the level required for mechanical support. Pathologic fractures may develop.

TABLE 11.11 CAUSES OF SECONDARY OSTEOPOROSIS

Cause	Example
Endocrine disease	Lack of androgens, hypopituitarism (with secondary gonadal failure), acromegaly, hypogonadism, thyrotoxicosis, excessive endogenous ACTH or corticosteroids (e.g., Cushing's disease), hyperparathyroidism, estrogen deficiency (not associated with normal menopausal processes), long-standing uncontrolled diabetes mellitus.
Metabolic disorder	Nutritional disturbances (chronic low intake of calcium, high intake of phosphate, protein starvation, ascorbic acid deficiency), malabsorption of calcium, acid-base imbalance, deficient production of 1,25-dihydroxyvitamin D.
Inactivity	Immobilization due to arthritis, prolonged bed rest, long-term use of casts or traction, paraplegia, degenerative muscle disease.
Developmental	Genetic disorders such as, osteogenesis imperfecta.
Drugs	Prolonged use of corticosteroids or heparin.
Cancer	Leukemia, myeloma, bone tumors.

Compression fractures, whereby vertebral bodies and corresponding portions of the vertebral column collapse, are inevitable and are often the presenting sign of osteoporosis. Patients experience an acute onset of back pain while resting, standing, or engaged in a routine daily activity. The pain usually corresponds to the area of injury except for high lumbar compressions, in which pain is usually referred to the lumbosacral region. It is typically aggravated by spinal movement, sitting, or standing and intensified to excruciating degrees by coughing, sneezing, or straining to move the bowels. Compression fractures in the lower thoracic/upper lumbar regions may also be marked by GI symptoms, since in rare cases they result in retroperitoneal hemorrhage with secondary ileus. By contrast, those in the midthoracic spine may produce little more than discomfort along the costal margins. Finally, multiple compression fractures are common and, in uncorrected osteoporosis, average six per every 10 years. With each fracture, patients lose 2–4 cm in height. Furthermore, fractures involving the thoracic spine cause the upper body to stoop forward progressively (***kyphosis*** or "dowager's hump"). Eventually, the lower ribs rest on the iliac crests and the abdomen protrudes due to downward pressure on the viscera. Severe kyphosis may interfere with cardiopulmonary function. Patients with any of these symptoms should be sent for spinal x-ray films. The crushing injury is confirmed by "anterior wedging" of vertebral spaces in the thoracic region or "ballooning" of vertebral spaces in the lumbar region. The acute phase is treated with analgesics, heat, and massage, with symptoms usually subsiding within a few weeks. Even more important, the underlying causes of the osteoporosis must be sought and corrected whenever possible.

In young adulthood, only a few remodeling units are active at any one time; bone turnover is low and skeletal mass remains constant. However, at around age 45, formation no longer compensates for resorption and skeletal mass begins to decline at a yearly rate of 1%. The cause of this age-associated decrease is only partially known. There is decreased calcium absorption from the GI tract. There is also an increased sensitivity to parathyroid hormone as levels of sex hormones fall. With estrogen withdrawal at the time of menopause, women undergo a 3-year period of accelerated bone resorption (2% per year). Women with submaximal bone masses may suffer a reduction to osteoporotic levels. Referred to as ***postmenopausal osteoporosis,*** the problem seems to be related to race, nutrition, activity level, and other factors listed in Table 11.12. It is responsible for 80% of the 1 million fractures sustained by women over age 50. Of these fractures, as many as 150,000 involve the hips, with a 15% mortality. Furthermore, 25% of all women over age 60 experience compression fractures. The signs, symptoms, and x-ray findings of postmenopausal osteoporosis are similar to those of the secondary forms of the disease (see the previous section). However, blood and urine tests should be normal.

The treatment for osteoporosis is divided into two phases. ▶***Preventive measures for postmenopausal osteoporosis*** center on developing and maintaining enough bone mass early in life to withstand the physiologic changes of aging. Instructions should also be given to increase the intake of calcium-rich foods in order to meet the Required Daily Allowance (RDA), particularly during pregnancy and lactation. In addition, daily supplementation of calcium is indicated for any woman with a calcium-poor diet and for all women over age 40. Furthermore, high-risk women may be given a course of estrogen during the climacteric and for a short period after menopause as a preventive measure. The treatment for ▶***established postmenopausal osteoporosis*** includes all preventive measures, as well as treat-

TABLE 11.12 RISK FACTORS FOR POSTMENOPAUSAL OSTEOPOROSIS

Caucasian race, particularly women of Northern European extraction
Family history
Small bone structure
Abnormal bone growth or skeletal abnormality of any type
Inadequate calcium intake: below 400–700 mg/day for children, 1,000–1,300 mg/day for adolescents, 400–800 mg/day for adults, 1,500 mg/day for pregnant women, 2,000 mg/day for lactating women, and 1,500 mg/day for postmenopausal women
Inadequate vitamin D [metabolite 1,25-(OH)2D3 needed for calcium absorption]: dietary intake below 400 IU for young adults, 800 IU for the elderly and meager exposure to sunlight
Residence in areas with unfluorinated water supplies
Multiple pregnancies and breast feeding without increased calcium intake
Heavy smoking
Bilateral oophorectomy without estrogen replacement
Sedentary lifestyle before menopause
Strenuous exercise after menopause

ment for acute compression fractures, carefully planned exercise, and safety precautions to guard against falls. Estrogen replacement is beneficial, especially up to 8 years following menopause, but must be weighed against the increased risks of endometrial cancer and cardiovascular complications. Fluoride therapy has been advocated but not yet aproved by the FDA. While it does seem to strengthen bones, tissue changes are somewhat abnormal. Overdoses may lead to ***fluorosis*** with paradoxic worsening of osteomalacia marked by vague pains in the small joints of the hands, feet, and ankles.

Excessive bone deposition occurs in ***Paget's disease.*** This seems to happen as a compensatory response to unexplained resorption. Increased rates of bone turnover (up to 20 times normal) result in thickened lamellae and neovascularization. Since osteoblasts secrete large amounts of alkaline phosphatase during matrix production, blood levels of this enzyme reflect disease activity. In the majority of patients, Paget's disease produces no symptoms and the diagnosis is made from incidental findings on x-ray films or blood screens. Yet, in some patients, involvement of the skull, spine, tibia, femur, and pelvis leads to serious consequences: compression syndromes of the spinal cord or posterior fossa, hearing loss, high-output cardiac failure, or fractures. Furthermore, pagetic bone has a malignant predisposition and 1% of patients develop sarcoma. Complicated cases require highly specialized care and intermittent hospitalization. Drugs that decrease osteoclastic activity (calcitonin, glucocorticoids, cytotoxic agents, and disodium etidronate) are sometimes used. Usually, however, Paget's disease can be managed by maintaining adequate hydration and prescribing analgesics for mild bone pain. Acetylsalicylic acid (ASA) relieves symptoms and, if given regularly, may even suppress disease activity.

Either osteoblastic or osteolytic activity may mark ***bone tumors.*** Both benign and malignant types are listed in Table 11.13. Osteolytic lesions cause bone destruction, hypercalcemia, and hydroxyprolinuria, while osteoblastic tumors cause radiodensities on x-ray films, increased alkaline phosphatase, and hypocalcemia. Primary malignancies are rare. The most noteworthy, ***osteogenic sarcoma,*** is in-

TABLE 11.13 BONE TUMORS: BENIGN (B) AND MALIGNANT (M)

Osteogenic	
B	Osteoid osteoma
B	Osteoblastoma (giant form of osteoid osteoma)
B	Osteoma (exostosis)
B	Osteochondroma (osteocartilaginous exostosis)
M	Osteosarcoma (osteogenic sarcoma)
M	Parosteal sarcoma (not common, "malignant analogue of osteochondroma")
Chondrogenic	
B	Enchondroma (enchondrosis; cartilage-forming hamartoma: excessive proliferation of cells that eventually reach maturity and cease reproduction; remains static from point when bone reaches maximal size, unless stimulated to begin neoplasmic growth)
B/M	Chondroblastoma (appears to be a hamartoma but occasionally have shown malignant changes)
B/M	Chondromyxofibroma (same as chondroblastoma)
M	Chondrosarcoma
Collagenic	
B	Nonosteogenic fibroma
B	Subperiosteal cortical defect
B	Angioma (often congenital; hemangioma or lymphangioma)
B	Aneurysmal bone cyst (nonneoplastic condition)
M	Fibrosarcoma
M	Angiosarcoma (rare form: hemangiosarcoma; originating from blood vessels)
Myelogenic	
M	Plasma cell myeloma (multiple myeloma, myelomatosis)
M	Ewing's tumor (Ewing's sarcoma)
M	Reticulum cell sarcoma (Hodgkin's sarcoma), mal. lymphoma
M	Lymphoma of bone
M	Hodgkin's disease
Others	
B	Benign chondroma
B	Giant cell tumor
M	Malignant fibrous histiocytoma
M	Mesenchymal chondrosarcoma (rare, distinct type of chondrosarcoma)
M	Chordoma (rare; develops from remnants of primitive notochord)
M	Malignant giant cell tumor (rare; existence is controversial)

frequent in persons over age 40 unless there is some predisposing factor (Paget's disease, radiation exposure, or bone infarction). Localized pain and swelling are often the only symptoms, but x-ray films can reveal profound changes. These include lytic lesions, bizarre densities, and complete destruction of the cortex with or without soft tissue penetration. If the tumor is found early, surgery can be curative. However, metastasis is extremely rapid and many patients already have lung involvement at the time of diagnosis. Advanced methods of chemotherapy now offer new hope.

Although primary malignancies are rare, ***bone metastases*** occur with considerable frequency, particularly from tumors of the breast, kidney, thyroid, prostate, and lung. Lymphomas, including Hodgkin's disease, and malignant carcinoid can also affect the skeleton. Whatever the primary site, the most common presenting symptom of bone involvement is pain from a pathologically induced fracture. Treatment of skeletal metastases is palliative: local radiation to reduce tumor size, mithramycin to control hypercalcemia, and L-dopa to relieve bone pain.

BONE REGENERATION

Bone tissue is unique in its ability to regenerate. When ***fractures*** occur, blood vessels in the periosteum, Haversian canals, and marrow space rupture. A blood clot (fracture hematoma) forms between areas of separated osteoid, pushing the periosteum and endosteum away from the cortex. Deprived of its blood supply, these areas of cortex become necrotic within 24–48 hours. Macrophages and osteoclasts enter to remove dead tissue and inflammatory debris. In response to osteoclastic activity, osteogenic cells from nearby bone permeate the fracture site. If the blood supply is good, they differentiate into osteoblasts that are capable of forming cancellous unions along the periosteum (external callus), marrow cavity (internal callus), and connecting fracture surfaces (intermediate callus) within 2 weeks. When the blood supply is inadequate, osteogenic cells differentiate into chondroblasts and hyaline cartilage is formed instead. The cartilage must be thoroughly vascularized by ingrowing capillaries before it can be replaced by cancellous bone. Although this process takes considerably longer, the final phases of healing are similar in uncomplicated, properly managed cases: cancellous bone converts to lamellar bone along lines of mechanical stress, and excess bone from callus formations is resorbed. The entire healing process takes place in 6–8 weeks in adolescents and in 10–14 weeks in adults. Exceptions occur in ***fibrous unions*** (the fractured ends unite with scar tissue), ***delayed unions*** (the fractured ends heal with normal osteoid tissue, but at a much slower rate than expected), or ***nonunions*** (the fractured ends fail to unite due to interposed soft tissue or infection).

There are more than 150 different types of bone fractures, and several classification schemes are used to describe them (Table 11.14). Presentations range from slight discomfort to life-threatening shock. The injured area may be deformed, swollen, and/or discolored. It may exhibit instability or protruding bone tissue, as well as producing a grating sound. If major nerves or vessels have been compromised (a medical emergency), the area may be marked by exquisite pain or absent sensation, paralysis, tingling, numbness, weak or absent pulse, cyanosis, and coldness. If obvious signs or symptoms occur, hospital transportation should be arranged for the patient and ▶ ***first aid for fractures*** should be administered. In less obvious cases, the diagnosis may depend on x-ray evaluation. Anteroposterior and lateral views are usually taken to include the joints above and below the point of injury. During any procedures, undue manipulation should be avoided. It can increase the injury by displacing fragments, damaging blood vessels and nerves, or forcing marrow into the venous circulation (see the discussion of fat embolism).

The principle behind fracture management is simple: maintain the fractured ends in proper alignment until healing occurs. However, applying this principle to patients with differences in fracture types and health status involves great skill. If the fractured ends are displaced, they must be restored to their normal position. This is sometimes accomplished through manipulation by hand (closed reduction) or by using a system of weights (traction reduction). However, compound and comminuted fractures or fractures with neurovascular complications must be surgically set (open reduction). They may also require internal fixation devices such as screws, plates, pins, wires, nails, or rods to help maintain the initial alignment.

Aligned fractures are immobilized with traction, splints, slings, and/or casts. ***Casts*** deserve a separate discussion because they may be the cause of serious complications that may be seen in a primary care setting. Several types of casting materi-

TABLE 11.14 TYPES OF BONE FRACTURES

Classification Method	Description
By severity	
Compound (open)	Break in skin present over fracture site with wound communicating from skin (externally) to fractured bone (internally), providing potential for infection from external environment. Wound may result from external trauma that penetrated skin and fractured underlying bone (e.g., bullet) or from ends of broken bone piercing the skin from within when fracture occurred. Broken ends of bone may or may not be visible through break in skin.
Simple (closed)	Uncomplicated fracture with skin intact over fracture site. Since no communicating wound exists, infection is not introduced into the fracture at the time of injury.
Complete	Fracture line extends entirely through bone substance; periosteum is disrupted on both sides of bone.
Incomplete (partial)	Fracture line extends partway through bone substance; continuity of bone is not completely disrupted.
Impacted (telescoped)	One bone fragment is forcibly driven into an adjacent bone fragment.
Comminuted	More than one fracture line exists, and bone fragments are crushed or broken into several pieces.
Displaced	Bone fragments are separated at the fracture line.
Complicated	Fracture is associated with injury to surrounding structure (e.g., adjacent organs, nerves, blood vessels, joints).
By direction of fracture line	
Linear	Fracture line runs parallel to long axis of bone.
Longitudinal	Fracture line extends in a longitudinal direction.
Oblique	Fracture line is at an oblique angle (about 45 degrees) to the bone shaft (axis).
Spiral (torsion)	Fracture line forms a spiral that circles the bone; results from a twisting force (e.g., while playing football or skiing).
Transverse	Fracture line is straight across the bone (at 90 degree angle to axis).
By force of production	
Shear	Fracture due to a glancing blow.
Angulation	Fracture that results from a force exerted when the bone is in an abnormal position.
Avulsion	Due to forcible tearing of tendon or ligament attachment.
Blowout	Results from blow that fractures floor of eye orbit.
Compression	Due to a crush injury.
Pathologic	Occurs in bones already weakened by disease.
March (fatigue)	Fracture of metatarsals due to long marches.
Missile	Fracture due to impact of a projectile (bullet, stone, metal fragment, arrow, etc.).
Stress	May occur in a bone subjected to prolonged muscular action to which it is unaccustomed.
After describing physician	
Colles'	Common type of fracture in which distal portion of radius is fractured within 1 in. of articular surface; typically characterized by a "silver fork" deformity caused by dorsal displacement of the distal fragment, with dorsal and radial deviation of the wrist and an abnormal radioulnar articulation.

TABLE 11.14 *(Continued)*

Classification Method	Description
Pott's	Occurs at distal end of the fibula and is often associated with rupture of the internal lateral ligament or chipping off of a portion of the medial malleolus or both; tibiofibular articulation is seriously disrupted; the foot is frequently displaced outward.
By general or specific anatomic location	
Articular (joint)	Involves the surface of a joint.
Extracapsular	Fracture near a joint that does not enter the joint capsule.
Intracapsular	Fracture within a joint capsule.
Shaft	Fracture limited to bone shaft.
Head	Fracture involves epiphysis of bone.
Condylar	Separation of a small fragment of bone (including the condyle) from the inner and outer aspects of the fractured bone.
Supracondylar	Fracture at the distal end of a bone.
Transcondylar	Fracture at the level of the condyles of a bone (or just above or below the condyles) and partially within the capsule.

als are available, but plaster of Paris is still the most commonly used. A stockinet is usually slipped over the area, and extra padding is placed on bony contours to prevent skin breakdown. The cast is then applied in layers. Neither too loose nor too tight, it extends to joints above and below the fracture site. Splints of wood, plaster, steel, or wire and/or walking heels can be added as the cast is being formed to lend additional strength. After the wet or so-called green cast has dried, the stockinet lining is doubled back or adhesive tape is added to "finish off" all rough edges and prevent crumbling plaster from falling under the surface, where it could damage the skin.

Cast-related complications include ischemia, nerve damage, infection, and cast syndrome (a potentially fatal vascular pooling sometimes seen in body casting). A neurovascular complication is characterized by exquisite pain or absent sensation, paralysis, tingling, numbness, weak or absent pulse, cyanosis, and coldness. Infection may be heralded by the onset of fever, redness, pain, and swelling of the casted area. In addition, areas of plaster may feel damp, or there may be frank drainage or an odor. Patients with cast syndrome develop nausea, vomiting, and altered mental status due to severe electrolyte imbalances and dehydration. To decompress nerves or blood vessels, the cast may have to be opened over bony prominences (windowed) or split into two sections (bivalved). It must be removed if infection or cast syndrome occurs. As an added precaution, women with casts of the lower extremities who are also using oral contraceptives should be advised to discontinue using the pills temporarily. Known to alter blood coagulability, estrogens may contribute to clot formation in an immobilized leg. If the pills are stopped, an alternative method of birth control should be provided.

A complication of fractures involving long bones is an acute respiratory distress syndrome called ***fat embolism.*** Fat cells from the marrow tissue enter the venous system and embolize to the lungs. For some reason, this is more likely to occur if the patient becomes hypovolemic. Plugged capillaries and damaged endothelium cause the arterial oxygen pressure (PaO_2) to fall, while released fatty acids produce capillary fragility and the classic finding of petechiae. In severe cases, fat globules travel to the brain (causing coma or hyperthermia), to the kidneys (causing lipuria or hematuria), or to the retina (causing blindness). Because the severity of the disease is directly related to the amount of marrow gaining access to the venous circulation, undue manipulation of fractured bones should always be avoided. As it is, fat embolism is a leading cause of all deaths related to skeletal injury.

JOINTS AND CONNECTING STRUCTURES

Joints formed between bones permit varying degrees of motion and are classified accordingly (Fig. 11.8). Synchondrosis is the temporary joint between the epiphysis and diaphysis of developing bones that closes once the bone reaches maturity. Like the pieces of a jigsaw puzzle, sutures are formed from the tight fittings of irregularly shaped bones. Synchondrosis and sutures have no axis of movement and are the strongest joints in the adult body.

Symphysis and syndesmosis joints are less rigid. In the symphysis, bones connect through a cartilage disc. During pregnancy, the disc in the symphysis pubis accumulates extra fluid and expands the pelvis in preparation for childbirth. In the syndesmosis, bones connect through ligaments; this, too, allows slight but critical degrees of movement.

Although defined as freely movable, diarthroses are subdivided into six groups according to their limitations of movement. The opposing bone surfaces are slightly curved in gliding joints, so there is rotation and sliding in all directions, but to restricted degrees. The saddle joint permits movement only in two planes at right angles; rotation is precluded because the bones fit snugly along convex and concave surfaces. The similar but much deeper configurations of hinge joints lock bones into a single plane of movement. In pivot joints, a ring-like fitting of one bone turns around the projecting part of another bone to enable axial movements. Ball-and-socket joints are just that—the rounded head of a long bone fits into the socket formation of a flat bone, allowing movement in a number of directions. A variation of this form (oval-shaped head, elliptically shaped socket) occurs in condyloid joints, restricting movement to right-angle planes.

Ligaments, which are made from dense connective tissue, lash bones together and, by spanning joints in key positions, help prevent undesirable movements. In the hip, for example, a somewhat circular placement of ligaments intertwines with the joint capsule, preserving rotation while keeping the femoral head pulled firmly into its socket.

To allow chest expansion with respiration, numerous "interchondral" ligaments attach the ribs to the sternum through small segments of "costal" cartilage. Inflammation of the sternum's connecting structures is called ***costochondritis.*** It affects women three times more often than men and usually occurs in persons over age 40. Pain in the chest wall is aggravated by deep breathing, coughing, and tenderness to pressure. The pain can develop acutely or insidiously and is often mistaken for angina, esophagitis, or pleurisy. Symptoms of costochondritis in younger persons, along with swellings of the upper costochondral junctions, characterize ***Tietze's syndrome.*** The cause is unknown, though it is suspected that violent coughing and direct trauma play a role. There may be spontaneous remission, or the lumps (show-

Class	Varieties	Some Examples
Synarthroses	Sutura Schindylesis Gomphosis Synchondrosis	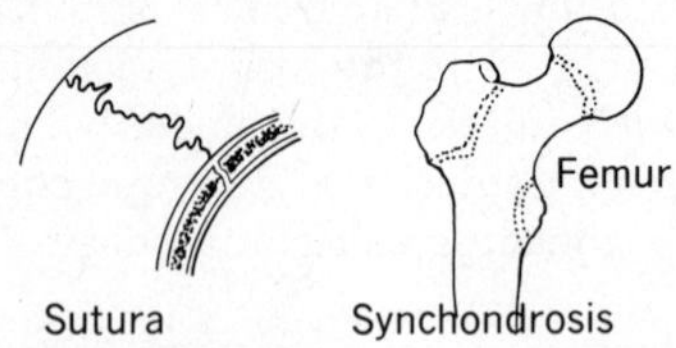
Amphiarthroses	Symphysis Syndesmosis	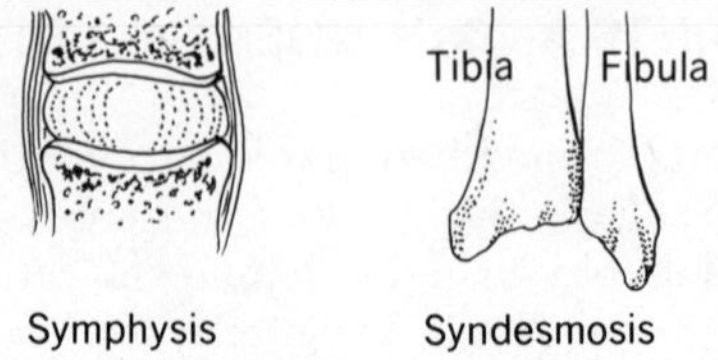
Diarthroses	Ginglymus (hinge) Trochoid (pivot) Condyloid Saddle Enarthrosis (ball and socket) Arthrodia (gliding)	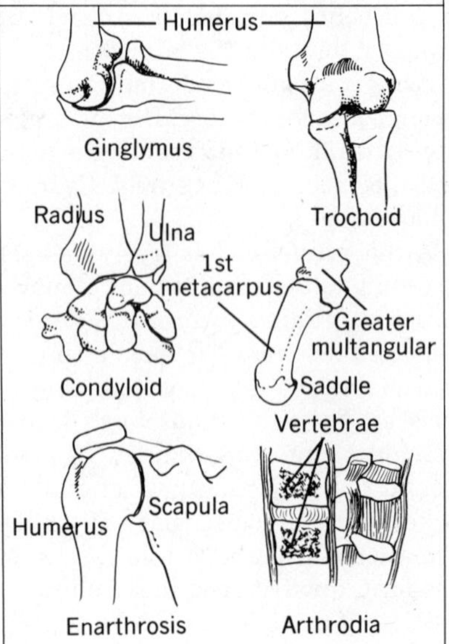

Figure 11.8 Types of joints.

ing minor inflammatory changes on biopsy) may persist for years. Both costochondritis and Tietze's syndrome are treated with heat, ASA, or NSAI drugs. Local injections of lidocaine or corticosteroids are occasionally helpful.

When ligament fibers are damaged from overstress, the injury is called a ***sprain.*** Some of the more common sprains are described in Table 11.15. They are classified as severe (third degree) if the ligament is completely severed, moderate (second degree) if it is partially torn, and mild (first degree) if it is badly stretched. ***Severe sprains*** can be recognized by loss of function and abnormal joint motion. Other signs include tenderness, extensive soft tissue swelling, and hemorrhage. Given these signs, an orthopedist should be consulted whether or not x-ray film show any abnormality. Surgery or a carefully designed program of immobilization followed by physiotherapy may be required. Without appropriate management, traumatic arthritis is likely to develop at some future time. Because the fibers have been only partially torn or stretched in ***mild/moderate sprains,*** there should be no signs of dysfunction or instability. Minimal tenderness and swelling are usually the only complaints. ▶ ***General measures for mild to moderate sprains*** include rest, ice, elevation, and compression for the first 24–48 hours. After that the patient should use warm soaks and start progressive activity until symptoms disappear.

Although described in Table 11.15 ***knee sprains*** warrant further discussion. In addition to external ligaments, the knee has medial and lateral "cruciate" ligaments inside the joint cavity for added protection against rotation. Forcible twisting motions or lateral blows to the knee may cause ***cruciate ligament damage*** as well as injury to the menisci ***(torn cartilage).*** Two C-shaped discs of cartilage, the menisci fill in the deep depressions along the medial and lateral surfaces of the knee joint. They absorb and redistribute about 60% of the forces imposed during weight bearing and are crucial to the normal kinetics of the knee. Complete tears with displaced fragments can cause locking, buckling, inability to bear weight, and the development of hemarthrosis within 6 hours of injury. Partial tears cause severe pain and the sensation that something is clicking in and out of place. The painful click can be reproduced on exam using either the McMurray or Apley tests. In long-standing cases, atrophy of the quadriceps muscle is noted. Tests to evaluate knee injuries and stability are described in Table 11.16. Suspected injuries to the meniscus or cruciate ligaments should be evaluated by an orthopedist. X-ray films using contrast fluid (arthrograms) or direct visualization with a specially designed endoscope (arthroscopy) is done to determine the degree of injury. Arthroscopy is preferred because tears can be excised or fragments removed at the time of diagnosis. Until recently, torn cartilage was surgically removed. However, by the mid 1970s, data had begun to reveal that a high proportion of persons with total menistectomy had developed significant osteoarthritis, some within 4 months of the procedure. Arthroscopic debridement preserving as much of the meniscus as possible is the present medical trend. Torn ligaments can be surgically reattached.

Ankle sprains account for one of the most common injuries seen in primary care settings and also deserve added attention. As a hinge joint created by mortar-like articulations of the distal tibia, fibula, and dome of the talus, the ankle can be dorsiflexed, plantarflexed, everted, inverted, and rotated. For stability, each motion is carefully limited by specific ligaments, some of which are reinforced by transverse muscle structures. When any ankle motion is forced beyond normal limitations, involved ligament structures stretch or tear. The most common injuries result from rolling in on the ankle (inversion sprain) and twisting the ankle (rotational injury).

TABLE 11.15 COMMON TYPES OF SPRAINS AND DISLOCATIONS

Location	Etiology	Signs/Symptoms
Jaw		
Temporomandibular joint ("TMJ syndrome")	Side blow to open mouth, forcing mandibular condyle forward and out of temporal fossa; sometimes yawning or opening the mouth too wide while eating; long-standing malocclusion, alteration of occlusion due to dental work (braces, new fillings, extractions), and night grinding contribute.	With sprain there is pain, spasm of surrounding muscles when mouth is opened too widely, radiating headaches and earaches. Signs of dislocation include locked-open position with jaw movement being almost impossible, and/or an overriding malocclusion of teeth.
Neck		
Cervical vertebrae ("whiplash injury")	Sudden twist, forced hyperextension, or traumatic snap of head (usually the result of a rear-end automobile accident). Injury to ligamentum nuchae and interspinous and supraspinous ligaments, and possible rupture of an intervertebral disc.	Cervical sprains appear as wryneck or acute torticollis: muscles on *tilted side* in acute state of spasm, marked pain in area of contraction and continuing down one shoulder, limitation of neck but not of shoulder movement. Cervical dislocation causes severe pain, spasm, deformity, and some paralysis; unilateral dislocation causes neck to be tilted toward dislocated side, with extreme muscle tightness on *elongated side* and relaxed muscle state on shortened side. (Note difference from wryneck and traumatic torticollis.)
Shoulder		
Sternoclavicular joint	Indirect force transmitted through humerus of shoulder joint or direct trauma (blow to clavicle) or by twisting or torsion of posteriorly extended arm. Depending on direction of force, medial end of clavicle can be displaced upward and forward, either posteriorly or anteriorly (most commonly upward and forward, slightly anteriorly).	Sprains are graded (in degrees) depending on extent of ligamentous involvement as follows: *First degree* (mild)—little pain and disability, some point tenderness, no joint laxity. *Second degree* (moderate)—inability to abduct shoulder full range or to bring arm across chest (indicates disruption of stabilizing ligaments), subluxation of sternoclavicular joint with visible deformity and swelling. *Third degree* (severe)—complete dislocation with gross displacement of clavicle at its sternal junction, swelling and disability (indicating complete rupture of sternoclavicular and costoclavicular ligaments); a posteriorly displaced clavicle may put pressure on blood vessels, esophagus, or trachea and may create a life-threatening situation.
Acromioclavicular joint	Direct blow to tip of shoulder that pushes acromion process downward or upward; force exerted against long axis of humerus. Arm position during indirect injury is one of adduction and partial flexion. With dislocation, the force is a similar direct blow that forces the acromion process downward, backward, and inward, while the clavicle is pushed down against the rib cage.	Sprains graded as above according to extent of injury: *First degree*—point tenderness and discomfort on movement at junction between acromion process and outer end of clavicle; no deformity (indicates only incomplete tear or stretching of acromioclavicular ligaments). *Second degree*—point tenderness on palpation, inability to fully abduct or bring arm across chest, definite displacement and prominence of lateral end of clavicle as compared to unaffected side (indicating rupture of supporting superior and inferior acromioclavicular ligaments). *Third degree*—rare dislocation involving rupture of acromioclavicular and coracoclavicular ligaments; gross deformity and prominence of outer clavicular head, severe pain, loss of movement, and instability of shoulder girdle.
Glenohumeral joint	Involves injury to articular capsule, usually resulting from violent force transmitted through long axis of humerus.	Pain, loss of function (especially with arm abducted or externally rotated), swelling, and point tenderness; pain results on passive movement.

TABLE 11.15 *(Continued)*

Location	Etiology	Signs/Symptoms
Anterior dislocation (subcoracoid dislocation)	Caused by abduction and external rotation of arm due to an abnormal force on the arm during execution of a throw, or to an arm tackle, or, less frequently, to a fall with inward rotation and abduction of the arm. First-time dislocations may be associated with a fracture; 95% of glenohumeral dislocations are anterior.	Humeral head is forced forward out of articular capsule, past glenoid labrum, and then up to rest under coracoid process, resulting in torn capsular and ligamentous tissue and possible tendinous avulsion of rotator cuff muscles and profuse hemorrhage. Humeral head may contact and injure brachial nerves and vessels (nerve damage in 5–14% of cases); bicipital tendon may be pulled from canal as a result of rupture of the transverse ligament. A flattened or indented deltoid contour is seen; palpation of the axilla reveals the prominence of the humeral head; patient is unable to place hand of affected side on opposite shoulder and carries arm in slight abduction.
Downward dislocation (subglenoid dislocation)	Rare; caused by hyperabduction of arm, which forces humeral head to position below glenoid cavity. Seizures are the most common mechanism of injury; 5% of glenohumeral dislocations are of this type.	Hyperabduction of arm forces humeral head to position below glenoid cavity, resulting in tear on inferior aspect of capsule and rupture of rotator cuff tendons, accompanied by profuse internal hemorrhage. Abduction and external rotation are limited; affected arm appears longer; neurovascular compromise is common.
Elbow	Injury may be caused by a fall on an outstretched hand with the elbow in extension, which forces elbow into sudden hyperextension and tears capsular and tendinous tissues anterior to joint, or by sudden or forceful abnormal pronation or supination or stretching while articulation is in position of full extension. Dislocation may also be caused by a severe twist while elbow is in flexed position. Bones of ulna may be displaced backward (most common), forward, or laterally.	Presence of pain when elbow is in position of 45 degree flexion with flexed wrist and extended fingers (if severe, fracture or epiphyseal separation should be suspected). Forward displacement of ulna or radius results in marked deformity, profuse hemorrhage, and edematous swelling; complications include injury to median and radial nerves and to major blood vessels, and, almost always, myositis ossificans.
Wrist		
Carpal bones	Caused by any abnormal forced movement of the wrist; falling on hyperextended wrist is most common, but violent flexion or torsion will also tear supporting tissue. Most common carpal bone dislocation is that of the lunate, resulting from a fall on an outstretched hand, forcing open the space between the distal and proximal carpal bones; with release of the stretching force, the lunate is dislocated anteriorly (palmar side).	Sprain exhibits generalized swelling, pain, tenderness, and inability to flex the wrist; there is also an absence of appreciable pain or irritation over the navicular bone (if sprain is severe, fracture should be suspected). Same symptoms are present with dislocation, and there is also difficulty flexing fingers and possibly numbness or even paralysis of flexor muscles due to lunar pressure on median nerve. This condition should be treated as acute.
Hand		
Phalanges	Sprain injury from blow to fingertip ("jamming" the finger) so that the joint is pushed together and often bent backward, or from violent twisting; force of injury is usually directed upward from the palmar side. Dislocations generally result from ball striking tip of finger from palmar side, displacing either the first or the second joint dorsally.	Pain and marked swelling centered on involved joint, possibly an inability to straighten or flex injured phalange, and deformity (an abnormal hard prominence or unusual angulation) may be present with dislocation. Possible rupture of flexor or extensor tendon and chip fractures in and around dislocated joint; hematoma.
Chest		
Costochondral separation or dislocation	Caused by direct blow, indirect trauma, violent muscular contractions, or general compression of rib cage such as might occur in football or wrestling.	Severe pain on inspiration, point tenderness and swelling on palpation (localization to area of rib cartilage distinguishes this injury from rib fracture), possible crepitus; separation resulting in dislocation of cartilage causes deformity and heals slowly, but without inhibiting normal functions.

TABLE 11.15 *(Continued)*

Location	Etiology	Signs/Symptoms
Back		
Thoracic vertebrae	Vertebral injury may be caused by violent hyperflexion or jackknifing of trunk, falling from a height and landing on feet or buttocks, sudden direct blow or twist.	Pain, acute muscle spasm, and local tenderness are symptoms of sprain; palpable or visible deformities and the prominence of spinous processes suggest dislocation or more serious vertebral injury. With all injuries to back, *suspect fracture and the possibility of spinal damage*, and, when necessary, transport the patient accordingly in such a way as to preclude twisting and to maintain the normal spinal curve.
Lumbosacral	Produced by abnormal strain exerted while trunk is twisted in one direction as hamstring muscles are pulling downward on pelvis on the opposite side. Predisposing anatomic vulnerability is generally present.	Injury occurs in the presence of anatomic vulnerability (an inelastic, structurally deformed, muscularly weak lower back or progressive bone degeneration). Symptoms include diffuse, dull ache in lower back (caused by irritation of the fifth lumbar nerve), spasm, point tenderness at lumbosacral junction, and restricted trunk movement; occurs most often in persons with lordosis.
Sacroiliac	Mechanism of injury is same as that of lumbosacral injury.	Same symptoms as above occur in the region of the junction formed by the ilium and sacrum; some authorities feel that this is actually a lumbosacral sprain.
Hip		
Junction of pelvis and femur	Tissue tears may result from any movement exceeding normal range of movement, such as a twist due to the impact of a moving object or to a forceful impact with an immobile object, or a situation in which the foot is firmly planted and the trunk is forced in an opposing direction. Dislocation may be the result of traumatic force directed along the long axis of the femur when the knee is bent, or a blow to an abducted, externally rotated thigh (anterior dislocation); or to one that is abducted and internally rotated (posterior dislocation).	Pain, muscle spasm, and restricted hip motion suggest sprain; dislocation is recognized by same symptoms, as well as by deformity: a flexed, abducted, and externally rotated extremity that appears longer than the uninjured limb is characteristic of an anterior hip dislocation, and a slightly flexed, abducted, and internally rotated extremity that appears shortened is indicative of a posterior dislocation. Palpation reveals that the head of the femur has been moved to an abnormal position. May be associated with a fracture or accompanied by possible damage to the sciatic nerve; requires immediate medical attention, or muscle contractures may complicate the reduction.
Separation of upper femoral epiphysis ("adolescent coxa vara")	Most characteristic of boys 10–16 years old who are also obese and display signs of Froehlich syndrome, or who are extremely tall for their age; rapid growth may predispose persons to the condition, and endocrine imbalance contributes to weakness in the area, so that mild trauma may initiate separation.	Head of femur is displaced backward and downward on neck of femur. Signs include complaint of pain in the hip or knee, slight limp (because of shortened femur), and external rotation of the extremity (may already be present or may occur in addition to abduction when the leg is brought into flexion).
Knee		
Medial collateral ligament	Direct blow from lateral side in an inward direction or severe inward twist. Severity depends upon knee position, previous injuries, strength of muscles crossing the joint, force and angle of trauma, fixation of foot, and conditions of ground surface. With repeated injury, deeper structures (anterior and posterior cruciate ligaments and medial or lateral menisci) may be affected.	Sprains of medial collateral ligament have as symptons severe pain and loss of function appearing immediately; discoloration and marked swelling due to profuse internal hemorrhage and effusion of synovial fluid into articular and tissue spaces (not usually present in first-time knee sprains) follow some time afterward; palpation reveals areas of point tenderness; patient unable to support weight flatfootedly (walks on toes).
Lateral collateral ligament	Blow from medial side or outward twist; less serious than medial collateral ligament sprain.	Symptoms are the same as for medial collateral ligaments.
Popliteal region	Blow delivered to anterior aspect of knee while foot is in stabilized position hyperextends knee.	Anteroposterior instability results; same symptoms as above.

TABLE 11.15 (*Continued*)

Location	Etiology	Signs/Symptoms
Patellar dislocation	Result of direct blow; poor quadriceps muscle tone, genu valgum (knock knees), or flattened lateral or medial condyle may predispose persons to this condition; displacement is lateral, as a rule, with patella resting on lateral condyle.	Pain, swelling, complete loss of function; patella residing in abnormal position.
Ankle		
Ankle joint	Sprain due to lateral or medial twist that results in external and internal joint derangement; dislocation results from blow from medial side or from sudden torsion.	Pain on weight bearing, swelling around ankle, especially laterally, limited range of movement, tenderness to palpation over involved ligaments, discoloration; patient may have heard a snap at the time of injury.
Foot		
Phalanges	Sprains to toes usually result from kicking an object or from a considerable force that extends the joint beyond normal range of movement or imparts a twisting motion to the toe.	Pain, swelling.

TABLE 11.16 TESTS TO DETERMINE THE EXTENT OF INJURY TO THE KNEE STRUCTURES

Purpose of Test	Description
To detect damage to collateral ligaments	Patient lies supine with both legs extended; examiner determines range of lateral mobility of affected leg as compared to normal leg.
To detect damage to medial ligaments	Examiner holds ankle firmly with one hand while placing other hand on lower lateral aspect of thigh; gently pushes medially on thigh while attempting to abduct leg. An intact ligament offers little movement.
To detect damage to lateral ligaments	Examiner changes hand positions and tests lateral ligaments in same manner as for medial ligaments.
To detect damage to cruciate ligaments (anteroposterior test)	Patient lies on back with injured leg flexed. Facing anterior aspect of patient's leg, examiner encircles upper portion of leg immediately below knee joint with both hands, fingers resting in popliteal space of affected knee and thumbs side by side directly over tibial tubercle. Examiner gently pulls tibia anteriorly and posteriorly; motion that exceeds $\frac{1}{4}$ in. may indicate looseness of (i.e., damage to) cruciate ligaments ("drawer sign").
To detect tear of meniscus (tibial rotation test)	Patient lies supine with injured leg fully flexed; examiner places one hand over patella, with fingers and thumb covering grasped knee, and with other hand holds patient's ankle. Ankle hand describes a small circle while knee hand feels for signs of abnormal clicking, grating vibrations, and pain sites.
To detect past damage to knee (atrophy measurement)	Knee injuries are almost always accompanied by marked decrease in girth of thigh musculature due to atrophy from favoring of a lower limb; most affected by disuse are quadriceps group ("antigravity muscles"), which assist in maintaining an erect, straight leg position. Measurement of circumference of both thighs (with tape measure around greatest circumference of thigh at measured distance from upper pole of patella) often detects existence of former leg injuries.

Rolling out on the ankle (eversion sprain) is less likely because this motion is quite limited in most persons. At the time of injury, patients experience sudden pain and often describe the sensation or actual sound of the ligament being torn. Swelling usually appears within minutes and is often accompanied by discoloration from extravasation of blood. If patients are seen immediately, palpation along the course of ligaments may reveal point tenderness or a gap indicating a tear. However, most patients wait a day or two before seeking medical attention. By that time, diffuse swelling and general ecchymosis prevent a precise clinical diagnosis. Signs of bone tenderness or deformity, joint instability, or crepitation are indications for orthopedist referral and x-ray studies (plain and stressed views). Specialists treat severe and moderate sprains with 1–2 days of elevation, ice packs, and ace bandaging. Adhesive strapping or a short leg walking cast and progressive ambulation follow over a 6-week period. After this time, if signs of instability persist, surgical reconstruction may be advised. Primary care providers can treat ▶***mild to moderate ankle sprains*** with elevation, compression, ice, and progressive activities. Muscle-strengthening exercises help prevent future injury.

Strains are often complicated by ***dislocations,*** in which case articulating bone surfaces slip out of place. Dislocations of the vertebrae, shoulders, clavicle, elbow, hip, patella, and fingers are not uncommon and are described in Table 11.15. Sometimes the disrupted surfaces snap back into alignment spontaneously. If not, the dislocation causes severe pain and could damage blood vessels or nerves. Patients should be sent for emergency x-ray films and reduction using specially prescribed maneuvers. Anesthesia and muscle relaxants may be needed to minimize further injury. Postreduction x-ray films are taken to rule out fracture resulting from manipulation, and the patient is treated for severe sprain.

In ***subluxations,*** the articulating surfaces are only partially separated but nonetheless are responsible for some significant clinical problems. Perhaps the most common is ***chondromalacia,*** a tracking abnormality of the knee cap (patella). The patella is a sesamoid (extra) bone that forms in areas of high friction. It is held in place between the femoral condyles by lateral and medial ligaments that minimize the possibility of lateral movements and hyperextension. Having also several tendon attachments to thigh and lower leg muscles, the patella glides up when the knee is extended and down when the knee is flexed. This action favorably alters compressive forces within the joint. In chondromalacia, the patella is displaced (usually laterally), and instead of gliding smoothly with knee movements, it scrapes against bone surfaces. The problem is common among runners. It causes crepitus and aching pain under or around the medial portion of knee. Symptoms are exacerbated by stair climbing or running. They may seem to ease during workouts on flat terrain, but any attempt to "work through" the injury only worsens the problem and could lead to an effusion or osteoarthritis. Patients with chondromalacia display a classic sign of apprehension when they contract the quadriceps to guard against lateral displacement of the knee cap during exam. Also, compressing the patella against the femoral condyle or extending the knee from 30 degrees of flexion to full extension against resistance reproduces the pain. Standard x-ray films of the joint tend to be normal, but tangential views (Merchant's or Sunrise) often reveal a deficiency of the lateral condyle and a "jockey cap" appearance of the patella. Treatment of chondromalacia consists of rest and the use of ice, followed by heat until all pain is gone. Progressive resistance exercises to strengthen the quadriceps muscle and orthotic devices for the knee or shoe to correct biomechanical problems are often helpful, but should be prescribed by an orthopedist or sports medicine specialist.

JOINT CAVITY AND SYNOVIUM

In all diarthrotic joints, a sleeve of connective tissue (joint capsule) encloses a potential space (joint cavity) between connecting bones. This is illustrated in Figure 11.9. Supplied with multiple nerve receptors, the capsule helps monitor joint position and relay pain messages. Whereas the outer layers of the joint capsule are composed only of fibrous bands, the inner layers become progressively more cellular, forming subsynovial tissue. The subsynovium consists of fibroblasts, fat cells, and a vast network of capillary endothelium. It is lined with the synovial membrane, which contains specialized fibroblasts (type B cells) and macrophages (type A cells). Type A cells secrete hyaluronic acid, which mixes with a dialysate (formed as plasma filters through the subsynovium) to make synovial fluid. Small quantities of synovial fluid lubricate and nourish the articular cartilage and defend the joint space against invading organisms. Volumes normally remain low in order to preserve negative pressure in the joint cavity. The negative pressure helps to stabilize articular sur-

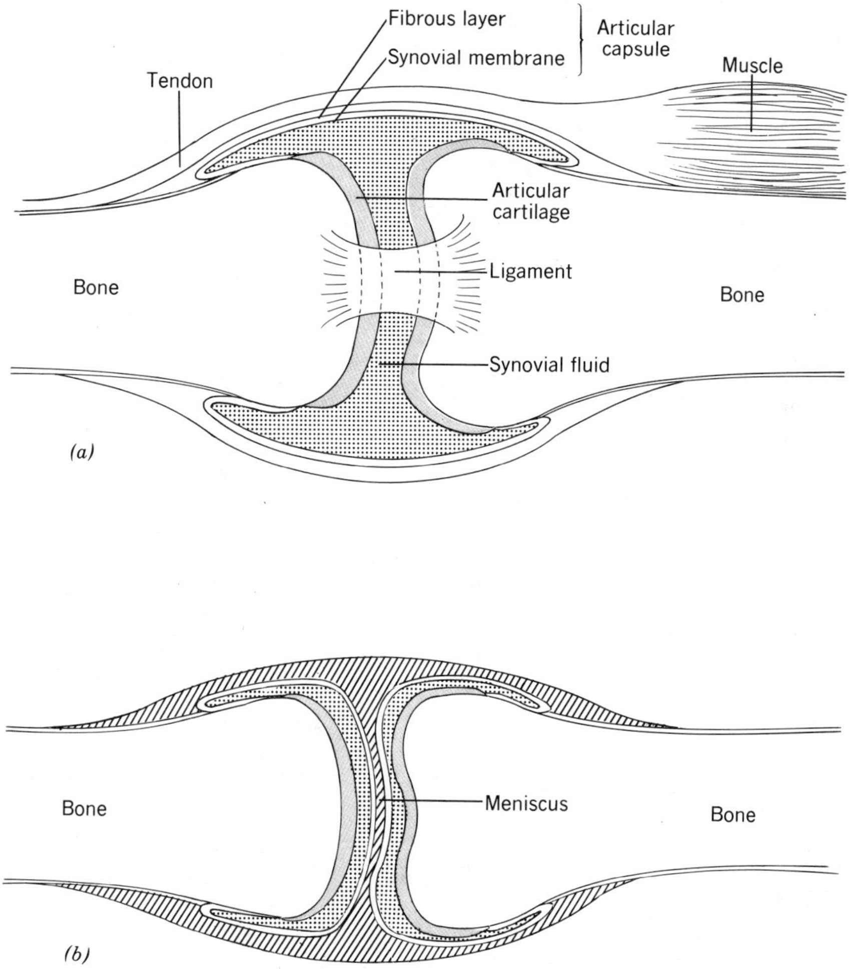

Figure 11.9 Joint cavity: (*a*) diarthrodial joint; (*b*) joint with meniscus.

faces against one another. It is also responsible for the noise produced when persons "crack their knuckles." When a relaxed joint is pulled suddenly, a bubble forms as a result of the widened pressure gradient and cavitates with the unmistakable sound. If repeated often enough, the process could presumably destroy the joint.

A ***synovial effusion*** occurs when increased amounts of fluid collect in the joint cavity. It changes joint pressures from negative to positive, producing significant discomfort. Patients tend to keep the joint slightly flexed, the position at which pressure remains minimal. In acute cases, full extension or flexion can actually increase pressures to levels high enough to rupture the joint capsule (an important thought to keep in mind during the exam). Other signs and symptoms vary according to the causative nature of the effusion. Associated with a number of pathologic disorders, effusions can be noninflammatory, hemarthrotic, or inflammatory (Table 11.17). A ***noninflammatory effusion*** is caused by edematous fluids from mechanical stress or metabolic disease, while a ***hemarthrosis*** develops from bleeding into

TABLE 11.17 TYPES AND CAUSES OF SYNOVIAL EFFUSIONS

Noninflammatory, group I—<5,000 WBC/cu mL		
Acromegaly	Hemochromatosis	Paget's disease
Amyloidosis	Hyperparathyroidism	Pancreatitis
Aseptic necrosis	Hypertrophic pulmonary osteoarthropathy	Sickle cell disease
Charcot's joints	Mechanical derangement	Traumatic arthritis
Ehlers-Danlos syndrome	Osteoarthritis	Villonodular synovitis and tumors
Epiphyseal dysplasias	Osteochondritis dissecans	Wilson's disease
Erythema nodosum		
Gaucher's disease		
Inflammatory, group II—3,000 to 50,000 WBC/cu mL; group III—75,000 WBC/cu mL (purulent)		
Ankylosing spondylitis	Fungal	Postsalmonella
Agammaglobulinemia	Mycoplasmal	Pseudogout
Behcet's syndrome	Bacterial (gonococcal, staphylococcal, tuberculosis, etc.)	Psoriatic arthritis
Carcinoid	treponemal	Regional enteritis
Gout	Juvenile rheumatoid arthritis	Reiter's syndrome
Erythema multiforme (Stevens-Johnson syndrome)	Leukemia	Rheumatic fever
Erythema nodosum	Multicentric reticulohistiocytosis	Rheumatoid arthritis
Familial Mediterranean fever	Palindromic rheumatism	Sarcoidosis
Giant cell arteritis	Polyarteritis	Scleroderma
Goodpasture's syndrome	Polychondritis	Serum sickness
Henoch-Schönlein purpura	Polymyalgia rheumatica	Shigella
Hydroxyapatite arthritis	Polymyositis	Sjögren's syndrome
Hyperlipoproteinemia	Postileal bypass arthritis	Subacute bacterial endocarditis
Hypersensitivity angiitis	Post-intra-articular steroid injection arthritis	Systemic lupus erythematosus
Infectious arthritis		Ulcerative colitis
Parasitic		Wegener's granulomatosis
Viral (hepatitis, mumps, rubella, etc.)		Whipple's disease
		Yersinia arthritis
Hemarthrosis, group IV—blood in synovial fluid		
Anticoagulant therapy	Idiopathic	Scurvy
Arteriovenous fistula	Myeloproliferative disease with thrombocytosis	Synovioma and other tumors
Charcot joint or other severe joint destruction	Pigmented villonodular synovitis	Thrombocytopenia
Hemangioma	Ruptured aneurysm	Trauma (with or without fractures)
Hemophilia or other bleeding disorders		Von Willebrand's disease

the joint as the result of a tumor, coagulopathy, trauma, or vascular disease. An ***inflammatory effusion*** evolves from defense reactions of the synovium against foreign stimuli such as bacteria, urate crystals, or antigens.

▶ ***Gout*** is caused by an inflammatory response to urate crystals in the joint space. It is not known whether the crystals form in the articular cartilage and break off or precipitate directly in the synovial fluid. Nor are the factors leading to crystal formation well understood, although it has been postulated that collagen turnover (from trauma or overuse), the temperature of the joint space (which tends to drop at night), and reduction of microvascular blood flow (as a consequence of aging) play significant roles. Even the well-known correlation with hyperuricemia has some mysterious anomalies. For instance, it is difficult to explain why most hyperuricemic patients never develop gout and why some patients have attacks at a time when their uric acid levels remained well below saturation. Nonetheless, hyperuricemia is a necessary precursor to gout and is actually considered the initial stage of disease. Serum levels of uric acid remain elevated (usually in ranges above 9 mg%) for an average of 20–30 years before the first attack occurs (see Chapter 8). Within minutes of crystal precipitation in the synovial fluid, neutrophils launch a phagocytic attack. Unfortunately, neutrophil lysosomes have a toxic interaction with the urate crystals and the cells break down, inducing a fulminant inflammatory response. This chain of events usually develops at night and seems to be set off by trauma, unaccustomed exercise, or ingestion of alcohol and rich foods. Characteristically, the first attack has an afebrile course and is monarticular. The big toe is involved 50% of the time, with the instep, ankles, heels, knees, wrists, fingers, and elbows being affected in decreasing order of frequency. After 1 day to several weeks, symptoms of a tumescent, exquisitely painful joint subside spontaneously. The patient then enters a problem-free stage of disease called the "intercritical period," which lasts for 6 months to 10 years. A small percentage of patients (7%) have no further episodes, but the majority suffer recurrent polyarticular attacks accompanied by fever. If the urate pool is extensive enough, the fine needle crystals begin to collect in cartilage, tendons, and soft tissues, causing ***tophi.*** These irregular deposits of chalky white material are most often found on the helix of the ear, fingers, knees, feet, forearm, elbow, and Achilles tendon.

The diagnosis of gout is strongly suggested by the history, the physical exam, and the presence of hyperuricemia, but to be confirmed, negative birefringent crystals must be demonstrated on analysis of synovial fluid. Synovial analysis also shows translucent yellow fluid of low viscosity, 2,000–50,000 leukocytes with more than 70% neutrophils, and negative cultures. Once gout has been established, patients should be advised to rest the joint as much as possible. Allopurinol (Zyloprim), probenecid (Benemid), or other antihyperuricemic drugs should neither be started, stopped, nor changed, since sudden fluctuations in serum urate levels can precipitate further attacks or worsen existing conditions. Colchicine administered in the first 12 hours produces such a dramatic response in cases of gout that the drug has been used diagnostically. Having few anti-inflammatory properties, it is ineffective in other forms of arthritis and probably works in gout by protecting leukocytes from toxic injury. However, some serious problems are associated with colchicine. The drug may have to be given IV because it is poorly tolerated in oral forms, and either route can cause bone marrow depression, alopecia, liver failure, seizures, paralysis, or respiratory distress. Consequently, NSAI agents are now preferred. Once the acute episode has resolved, prophylactic measures should be initiated. These include maintenance with colchicine or indomethacin, antihyperuricemic treatment, weight reduction or control, and avoidance of precipitating factors.

Calcium phosphate salts (CaPPi) can lead to crystal formation in tendons, ligaments, and articular cartilage. If these crystals break off into the synovial fluid, they invoke an inflammatory response similar in evolution but much less severe than that of gout known as ***pseudogout.*** Very little is known about the initiating factors, although some disease associations have been recognized. They are diabetes, rheumatoid arthritis, hyperparathyroidism, hypothyroidism, iron overload, and gout. Pseudogout typically affects the knees, hips, shoulders, elbows, ankles, wrists, and a number of bursae. It is not unusual to see a cluster pattern in which several joints flare up around the initial site of involvement. Acute symptoms of heat, swelling, stiffness, and pain last anywhere from 12 hours to 1 month or longer. They may be preceded by periods of transient stiffness or aching. Unlike gout, the diagnosis can be made by x-ray films, since CaPPi deposits produce a radiographic finding called ***chondrocalcinosis*** (coalescent or stippled calcifications that parallel articulating surfaces). The rhomboid, birefringent crystals can also be identified on synovial fluid analysis. Other analytic findings include a translucent yellow fluid of low viscosity, 2,000–50,000 leukocytes with more than 70% neutrophils, and negative cultures. Once the diagnosis has been established, associated disorders should be controlled and acute attacks managed by anti-inflammatory agents, aspiration of effusions, and local injections of corticosteroids.

Arthritis associated with autoimmune disease is common. Of the types noted in Table 11.17, ***rheumatoid arthritis (RA)*** has the most specific and destructive effect on joints. RA can appear at any time, but the peak onset occurs in the fourth decade. Women are stricken three times more often than men. Although the etiology of RA remains unknown, its pathogenesis has been fairly well established. Serum and joint fluid contain specific antibodies (rheumatoid factors) for IgM, IgG, and IgA. The antibodies form immune complexes that activate complement. A number of chemotactic and vasoactive factors are generated, drawing neutrophils into the joint. In phagocytosing the immune complexes, neutrophils not only create a great deal of cellular debris but also release enzymes (lysosomes). Both are damaging to synovial tissue. No doubt T-cell factors (lymphokines) also play a part in the genesis of inflammation. Eventually, the synovium develops large folds of villi called "pannus." Starting at the joint margins, pannus destroys articular cartilage and subchondral bone. The joint capsule and supporting ligaments, also weakened by inflammation, may fail to support the joint, resulting in subluxation. Alternatively, fibrous adhesions and new bone tissue may unite the opposing surfaces, causing ankylosis. The inflammatory process in RA is by no means confined to joints. Lymphocytes accumulate in muscle interstitium, leading to atrophy or myositis. Rheumatoid nodules (hard, nontender areas of fibrous tissue and cellular debris infiltrated by monocytes) develop under the skin or become attached to tendon or periosteum. They even appear in the pleura, lung parenchyma, heart valves or myocardium, and vocal cords. Vasculitis of small and medium-sized vessels occurs, which may be generally necrotizing or may lead to areas of local infarction (gangrenous changes of nails, fingers, toes, or skin around the lower extremities). Other complications of vasculitis include neuropathy, Sjögren's syndrome (occurs in 15% of patients), uveitis, or episcleritis. The latter problems are discussed in Chapters 3 and 1, respectively). ***Felty's syndrome,*** a combination of arthritis, splenomegaly, and neuropenia, may develop in persons with long-standing disease.

Thus, the presentation of RA can be quite varied. The majority of patients experience a prodrome of fatigue and weakness. Stiffness and vague arthralgias precede the appearance of joint swelling by several weeks. Occasionally, the disease declares itself suddenly with fever and acutely inflamed joints. A symmetric pattern involving several joints (particularly the hands and feet) or a single set of joints (commonly the knees) is classic, but asymmetric patterns do occur. If so, inflammation persists in the initially involved joints as other joints become affected, a characteristic that helps to distinugish RA from migratory polyarthritis. Temporomandibular, proximal interphalangeal, metacarpophalangeal, and metatarsophalangeal ligaments, wrist, knee, elbow, and ankle are the usual sites of involvement. Although cervical spine disease is common, the lower part of the spine is spared. Disease activity in any of these locations is marked by morning stiffness. During active inflammation, stiffness lasts for 1 hour or more; with improvement, it decreases significantly. On exam, the involved joints are warm, tender, and swollen. Overlying skin tends to be cyanotic, whereas marked erythema is unusual. A boggy synovium may be palpable around the joint margins, and adjacent muscles may be weak or atrophied. Range of motion, particularly extension, is often limited and contributes to the development of flexion contractures. Swan neck and boutonniere deformities of the hands and cock-up toes are a few. Contractures of the knees and hips hinder ambulation.

In diagnosing RA, a number of laboratory findings are important. Tests for rheumatoid factor are either positive at the onset of disease or tend to convert within the first year. Positive in other connective tissue disorders and several infectious diseases, rheumatoid factor supports but does not make the diagnosis. High initial titers indicate a serious clinical course, although subsequent titers correlate poorly with ongoing disease activity. On the other hand, the ESR is a fairly accurate parameter and is usually elevated with acute exacerbations. Antinuclear antibodies (ANA) are present in 25% of patients, and lupus erythematosus cells (LE prep) in 10–20%. Serum complement levels are rarely reduced. In early disease, joint x-ray films show only soft tissue swelling. Erosions of the joint margins are later findings, followed by narrowing of the joint space and destruction of subchondral bone. Synovianalysis reveals a turbid fluid of low viscosity with an elevated white blood cell count (ranging from 10,000 to 50,000). One-tenth of patients with RA have complete remissions or minimal symptoms, and another one-tenth suffer from unrelenting, crippling disease. The majority have a chronic course marked by periods of exacerbation and varying degrees of joint damage. Mild cases can be handled in primary care settings. ▶ ***General measures for RA*** include rest, anti-inflammatory drugs, and simple physical therapy measures. Inflammation and pain must be sufficiently controlled to preserve joint mobility and strength. If not, more aggressive therapy with gold salts, penicillamine, cytotoxic drugs, systemic or intra-articular corticosteroids, and professional physiotherapy may be needed. Surgery also has an important place in the management of severe cases. Synovectomy (removal of the synovial lining) not only diminishes pain but also retards the disease process. Instability problems and deformities can be corrected or destroyed joints replaced with a prosthesis. During the long and debilitating course of this disease, many patients may benefit from the work of ▶ ***arthritis organizations.***

Ankylosing spondylitis (Marie-Strümpell disease) is a chronic progressive form of arthritis distinguished by inflammation and ankylosis of joints, notably the spine. The cause is unknown, though persons with human leukocyte antigen (HLA)-B27 antigen are 300 times more likely than other persons to develop the disease. Ninety percent of these patients are men, most between the ages of 10 and 30. Symptoms begin with morning back stiffness and persistent episodes of low back aches, sometimes accompanied by pain in sciatic nerve distribution. Spreading to the upper back and sometimes the neck, they become progressively worse. In the later stages, hips, shoulders, knees, and sometimes more peripheral joints may also be affected. At first, findings may be limited to tenderness of the low back and flattened lumbar curvature from muscle spasm. Later, mobility becomes restricted, causing patients to bend forward as if they had a pole running down the spinal column. This is due to calcification and ossification of the intervertebral discs and surrounding connective tissues. Involvement of the costovertebral structures causes diminution of chest expansion with a decrease in vital capacity. The arthritic changes are often accompanied by fatigue, weight loss, and mild anemia. Heart complications (arrhythmias and aortic insufficiency) appear in less than 10% of cases and iritis in less than 25%. Diagnosis is based on lumbosacral spine films showing blurring of the sacroiliac joint margins, patchy sclerosis, fusion, or obliteration. Calcification of spinal ligaments may also be observed, along with demineralization and squaring of the vertebral bodies. In advanced disease, bony growths (syndesmophytes) weld the discs to vertebrae on each lateral aspect, the so-called bamboo spine. Except for the ESR, which may be elevated in 40% of cases, rheumatoid studies are diagnostically negative. In fact, the disease is often referred to as "seronegative arthritis." Treatment consists of anti-inflammatory drugs and exercises emphasizing good posture and complete range of back motion. Unfortunately, these measures do little to modify the progression of disease. The arthritis tends to smoulder for 10–20 years with varying degrees of damage and then remit. Patients with extensive involvement may need surgical procedures to straighten the spine.

Like ankylosing spondylitis, ***Reiter's syndrome*** is associated with HLA-B27. Occurring most commonly in young men, it may follow chlamydia infection or diarrhea due to *Shigella* or *Yersinia*. The exact cause, however, is not known. Initially, most patients experience a mild systemic illness marked by fever. A variable time later, they may develop urethritis, conjunctivitis (or, less commonly, uveitis), and/or arthritis. They may also experience an outbreak of skin lesions resembling pustular psoriasis, which are most apt to affect the glans penis, mucosa of the mouth, or nails. Carditis and aortic regurgitation have been reported as well. Although most of these conditions disappear within several days or weeks, the arthritis may persist for several months or even years. Typically asymmetric, it tends to involve the large weight-bearing joints (chiefly the knees and ankles). Ankylosing spondylitis is observed in 20% of patients. Recurrences of any or all manifestations are common, and progressive joint damage is seen in a number of patients. Diagnosis is based on the exclusion or rheumatoid, gonococcal, or other forms of arthritis. HLA-B27 testing is helpful. It is positive in 80% of white patients but only in 20–30% of blacks. Management centers on prompt treatment of any associated chlamydial infection (tetracycline or erythromycin) and anti-inflammatory drugs (specifically indomethacin or phenylbutazone).

Systemic lupus erythematosus (SLE) strikes 1 out of every 2,000 persons, 85% of whom are women. Most cases occur between ages 20 and 40, though SLE has been reported in all age groups. Familial and HLA-DR2/DR3 associations are high. The disease is characterized by the development of antibodies to nuclear material (ANA), "native" DNA (anti-DNA), and smooth muscle (anti-SM). A humoral attack is launched, causing disfiguration of targeted cells. This may be illustrated by the

LE cell phenomenon, in which leukocytes exposed to the serum of a lupus patient develop intranuclear inclusion bodies as a result of an antibody reaction to native DNA (LE prep). In addition to the humoral attack, antigen–antibody complexes become trapped in capillaries, producing vasculitis. This, in turn, is responsible for the major clinical manifestations. Patients usually present with articular pain, fever, anorexia, malaise, and weight loss. Common but varied skin lesions include the characteristic malar ("butterfly") rash, discoid lupus, fingertip changes (periungual erythema, nail fold infarcts, splinter hemorrhages), Raynaud's phenomenon, and alopecia (see Chapter 10). Vasculitis may complicate virtually every system, particularly the CNS, eyes, heart, lungs, kidneys, intestines, and blood. The role of various mediators of inflammation such as histamine or serotonin has been recently recognized. Damage to the glomerulus, for example, seems to develop following an intense inflammatory process provoked by the existence of local immune complexes. The diagnosis of SLE is based on criteria established by the American Rheumatism Association (Table 11.18). In most patients, the illness follows a mild chronic course in which periods of exacerbation become milder and less frequent. Such mild forms of SLE require little more than monitoring. A few patients suffer a virulent course marked by progressive renal disease and CNS involvement, requiring multispecialty care. All patients may benefit from the support and information provided by ► ***SLE organizations.***

Lupus-like syndrome can be induced by hydralazine, isoniazid, procainamide, and phenytoin, as well as many other drugs. It is distinguished from idiopathic SLE by the following features: (1) men and women are equally affected, (2) nephritis and CNS involvement rarely occur, (3) serum complement is unaffected, and (4) antibodies to native DNA are absent. Treatment consists of discontinuing the offending agent. Once this is done, the clinical features usually resolve at once. However, serologic abnormalities may persist for months.

The autoimmune etiology of ***scleroderma*** has not yet been proven but is strongly suspected. Appearing normally in the third to fifth decade, the disorder affects men two to three times more often than women. It is subclassified into three groups of patients. One group has slowly progressive disease with manifestations of calcinosis, Raynaud's phenomenon, esophageal dysfunction, scleroderma, and telangiectasia

TABLE 11.18 AMERICAN RHEUMATISM ASSOCIATION CRITERIA FOR THE DIAGNOSIS OF SLE[a]

Skin	Renal
Discoid lupus erythematosus	Proteinuria > 3.5 g/24 h
Malar rash	Cellular casts
Alopecia	CNS
Photosensitivity	Psychosis
Oral or nasal ulceration	Convulsions
Cardiovascular and pulmonary manifestations	Laboratory Findings
Raynaud's phenomenon	Positive LE prep
Pleuritis	Chronic false-positive test for syphilis
Pericarditis	Leukopenia < 4,000/cu mm
Musculoskeletal	Thrombocytopenia < 100,000 cu/mm
Nondeforming arthritis	Hemolytic anemia

[a]Minimum of four manifestations that develop concurrently or serially.

(CREST syndrome). Another group has manifestations limited to the skin ***(morphea scleroderma).*** As a probable variant, patients with ***esosinophilic fasciitis*** constitute a third category. Presenting with all the features of scleroderma, patients with this rare disease are found to have inflammation of fascia marked by eosinophil invasion. Fibrosis of connective tissue is the major histologic feature of other forms. In addition to polyarthralgia, patients with scleroderma present with Raynaud's phenomenon, subcutaneous edema, fever, and malaise. As the disease progresses, the skin becomes thickened and hidebound, with telangiectasia, pigmentation, and depigmentation. Thickening of skin on the fingers gives rise to the term ***sclerodactyly.*** GI involvement leads to dysphagia, hypermotility, and malabsorption diverticula. Cardiopulmonary disease is manifested as pulmonary fibrosis, pulmonary hypertension, pericarditis, and/or heart block. Often leading to hypertensive uremic syndrome, renal involvement indicates a grave prognosis. Laboratory studies in scleroderma patients reveal mild anemia, increased ESR, and hypergammaglobulinemia. Rheumatoid factor, LE prep, and ANA are frequently positive. The last shows a speckled or nucleolar pattern. If the kidneys are involved, proteinuria and cylindruria are found. Since there is no cure, treatment is largely symptomatic. Broad-spectrum antibiotics are given for malabsorption. Patients can obtain support and information from ▶ ***scleroderma organizations.***

Mixed connective tissue disease (MCTD) is a syndrome characterized by overlapping features of SLE, scleroderma, and myositis. The majority of patients are between 30 and 60 years of age. The diagnostic marker is extremely high titers of extractable nuclear antigen (ENA), which is associated with a speckled ANA pattern. Complement is normal and anti-DNA titers are unremarkable, though many patients have positive rheumatoid factor, high ESR, and hypergammaglobulinemia. If pulmonary and renal involvement remains minimal, the prognosis is good. The treatment is similar to that of SLE. Mild musculoskeletal manifestations can be controlled with NSAI drugs.

In normal states, synovial cells clear invading organisms through aggressive phagocytic activity and ***septic arthritis*** is rare. Infections develop only in joints that have been weakened locally (by trauma or joint disease) or systemically (by diabetes, alcoholism, malignancy, uremia, or immunodeficiency). Microbial agents enter the joint space by one of three routes: (1) direct inoculation by arthrocentesis, injections, or accidental puncture wounds, (2) local extension of soft tissue infections or osteomyelitis, and (3) blood-borne dissemination of a distant infection.

The third route is the one taken by the organism *Neisseria gonorrhoeae* to produce ***gonococcal septic arthritis.*** Accounting for 75% of all cases of joint infections, gonococcal septic arthritis typically strikes women less than 40 years old, the population most likely to have asymptomatic cervical gonorrhea. There is also a high occurrence during pregnancy and menstruation. This may be related to the altered pH of vaginal secretions, which enhances the opportunity for the infection to become established. Actually, *N. gonorrhoeae* commonly localizes in the pharynx, rectum, cervix, or urethra without spreading. Dissemination occurs for unclear reasons, although it has been shown that organisms responsible for systemic disease have unique nutritional requirements and seem resistant to the bactericidal action of normal serum. It produces migratory polyarthritis, which localizes in one or more joints and is complicated by tenosynovitis. Any joint can be affected, but the knees, wrists, and ankles are the most common. Characteristic vesiculopustular or hemorrhagic skin lesions may be sparsely distributed over the forearms and lower legs.

Systemic signs such as fever and chills can be extremely variable and, interestingly enough, leukocyte counts tend to be low or only moderately elevated. In fact, extremely high white blood cell counts are unusual.

Patients suspected of having gonococcal arthritis should be evaluated and treated with extreme urgency. Synovial cultures are mandatory, but given its fastidious nature, *N. gonorrhoeae* may be difficult to recover. Negative cultures have followed conclusive Gram stains of the fluid, and using a special high-sucrose medium, the organism has subsequently grown from reportedly sterile samples. Therefore, pharynx, cervix or urethra, rectum, blood, and skin lesions, as well as synovial fluid, should all be cultured. Positive yields from any one of these sources in the presence of acute arthritis is considered diagnostic. Patients should be hospitalized for immobilization and drainage of involved joints. Traditional treatment consists of parenteral penicillin until symptoms resolve, followed by a 10-day course of oral ampicillin. Good responses from oral, IM, and 3-day courses of antibiotics have also been reported. With appropriate care, the septic process resolves completely. Conversely, unattended infections can destroy joint cartilage and underlying bone within 48–72 hours.

Nongonococcal septic arthritis accounts for only 25% of acute joint infections. Of these, gram-positive cocci are recovered 80–90% of the time and gram-negative bacteria approximately 12% of the time. Clinical manifestations vary widely, depending on the patient's health status and on microbial factors such as virulence, bacterial debris, and toxin or enzyme production. Generally, there is an acute onset of heat, swelling, and pain confined to a single joint. Erythema may or may not be present, and systemic symptoms are often limited to a low-grade fever. These symptoms may easily be attributed to an exacerbation of RA or gout. Since persons with either disease are at high risk for developing joint sepsis, they must be evaluated with special attention. A clinical suspicion of septic arthritis should be followed up with arthrocentesis. Blood tests give little guidance, and x-ray films are diagnostic only after permanent damage has taken place. On the other hand, a septic process is immediately revealed by the evacuation of a purulent effusion containing more than 75,000 leukocytes (up to 75% neutrophils) and depressed glucose levels. Furthermore, Gram stains and cultures of the fluid are crucial for guiding antibiotic therapy. In rare cases, the cultures may yield tuberculosis (mycobacterium bacillus) or fungus (mycoses). In ***tubercular joints,*** the bacillus disseminates to the ends of long bones and destroys subchondral bone and articular cartilage before seeding the joint space. Infections from mycoses become established only in extremely compromised patients, most of whom are receiving steroids or chemotherapy. Whatever the organism, patients must be hospitalized to receive IV antimicrobials, joint drainage, and immobilization.

Viral arthritis is associated with several viral processes, the most common being hepatitis B, rubella, rubella vaccine, and mumps. Small numbers of reportable cases have also been attributed to adenovirus, echovirus, infectious mononucleosis, and varicella. Just how viruses induce joint inflammation is poorly understood, since only rubella has been consistently retrieved from joint fluid. This suggests mediation by immune complexes. Because diagnosis depends on recognition of the underlying viral entity, the patterns of involvement and prodromal symptoms listed in Table 11.19 may be helpful. Generally short-lasting, viral arthridities are best managed with ASA and rest.

A spirochete (*Borrelia burgdorferi*) transmitted by the tiny deer tick (*Ixodes dam-*

TABLE 11.19 VIRAL ARTHRITIS

Virus	Patients Who Develop Arthritis	Duration of Joint Symptoms	Joint Involvement
Hepatitis B	10–30%	7–180 days (14 average)	Symmetric or sometimes asymmetric, migratory, or additive; small, sometimes large joints; tendinitis; bursitis.
Rubella	15–35% of adult women; uncommon in men, children	5–30 days	Symmetric; knees, wrists, proximal interphalangeals; carpal tunnel syndrome; tendinitis.
Rubella vaccine	1–10% of children; even higher in women	7–21 days with common recurrences	Symmetric (proximal interphalangeals) or monarticular (knees); carpal tunnel syndrome.
Mumps	0.4%	2–90 days (14 average)	Migratory; large and small joints; tenosynovitis.
Smallpox	0.25–0.5%	Up to 60 days	Elbow, other large joints.
Adenovirus type 7	very rare	7–35 days; possible recurrences	Large and small joints.
Varicella	very rare	7 days	Knee and other large joints.
Infectious mononucleosis	very rare	6 days	Ankle.
Echovirus type 6	very rare	9 days	Large and small joints.

Source: Kelley WN, et al. *Textbook of Rheumatology*, Vol. II. Saunders, Philadelphia, 1981, p. 1587.

mini) has been identified as the cause of ▶***Lyme disease.*** Since 1976, when it was first described among several family members living near Lyme, Connecticut, thousands of cases have been reported, particularly along the northeast U.S. coast, Wisconsin, California, and Oregon. An immune mechanism is suspected, since most patients have the DRw2 alloantigen and evidence of circulating immune complexes. Ninety percent of the time, the first sign is the sudden appearance (in summer months) of a distinctive rash called ***erythema chronicum migrans (ECM).*** The rash begins as red macules that expand into large annular patches with raised borders and central clearings. From 3 to 20 days later, the neurologic, cardiac, or joint manifestations of Lyme disease develop in a limited number of cases. Neurologic signs include mild meningoencephalitis (fever, headache, stiff neck, nausea, and vomiting), cranial nerve palsies, and motor and sensory changes in the extremities. The cardiac abnormalities are atrioventricular conduction defects and electrocardiographic changes consistent with myocarditis or pericarditis. Both neurologic and cardiac complications tend to be self-limited. The arthritis, however, may be recurrent. Developing up to 2 years after the appearance of ECM, early attacks last only for several days and typically affect the knees, temporomandibular joint, wrists, and elbows. Involved joints are swollen and warm to the touch, but not erythematous. Attacks are painful, even crippling, but seem to have little residual effect. Joint damage is rare. Unlike RA, ANA and rheumatoid factor are negative. Furthermore, an asymmetric pattern is seen, and patients have no morning stiffness. Serologic tests measuring antibodies to the spirochete have been developed. To prevent or ameliorate the course of disease, treatment with tetracycline or penicillin should be initiated at the first signs of ECM.

ARTICULAR CARTILAGE

Articulating bone surfaces are coated with hyaline cartilage, which is chiefly composed of type II collagen and large molecular chains called "proteoglycans (PGs)." Extremely hydrophilic, PGs are largely responsible for cartilage compressibility; they release water during weight bearing and reabsorb it during deweighting. Shrinking of PG molecules with aging may be one of the earliest changes to occur in "***degenerative joint disease*** (DJD)." Once compressibility is lost, cartilage fibers begin to degenerate under the regular forces of joint movement. In this sense, the process is well described by the term "wear and tear arthritis." This expression is otherwise misleading, since joint activity creates the fluctuating pressures needed to pump nutrients from the synovial fluid to the chondrocytes of the articular cartilage. Having no vascular supply, articular cartilage probably depends on normal movement for nourishment, a theory supported by the deterioration that takes place whenever joints are immobilized by casts or bed rest.

While PGs lend resilience to articular cartilage, type II collagen fibers give it strength. These fibers are arranged in four distinct planes. This design helps to absorb and then to redistribute the forces of weight bearing. In an injured or unstable joint, forces impinge on the articular surfaces from unexpected directions and shear across the fibers, eventually destroying them. Deterioration of fibers also follows inflammatory arthritis, septic necrosis, diabetes, acromegaly, and skeletal deformities, a condition known as ***secondary osteoarthritis.*** It follows that secondary osteoarthritis is seen in all age groups, in both men and women, and would tend to develop in isolated joints. Conversely, ***primary osteoarthritis*** develops after age 50, afflicts women more frequently than men, and runs in families. It also has a distinct pattern of bilateral involvement characterized by bony swellings of the distal interphalangeal joints (Heberden's nodes) and of the proximal interphalangeal joints (Bouchard's nodes). The nodes develop gradually and without much pain. In primary osteoarthritis, wrists, elbows and shoulders are involved rarely and metacarpophalangeal joints not at all. It is estimated that 85% of persons over age 70 have some radiologic evidence of osteoarthritis. As cartilage surface is lost, the joint spaces appear to narrow on x-ray films. Unprotected, the subchondral bone becomes worn, glistening, and smooth (with an eburnated or ivory-like appearance on x-ray films). If the denuded bone is unable to withstand the intra-articular pressures of weight bearing, ***subchondral cysts*** or ***bone spurs*** may develop. Spur formations in the spinal column are known as "osteophytes." Surprisingly enough, patients with osteoarthritis remain relatively asymptomatic until the disease has reached an advanced stage. They then describe aching pain (most often of the spine, fingers, hips, and knees), which is greatest after exercise. Stiffness following inactivity usually disappears with minimal movement in 15–30 minutes. Tenderness, crepitus, limited range of motion, and joint enlargement are common findings, but systemic symptoms and extra-articular manifestations are notably absent.

X-ray changes confirm the diagnosis. In their absence, an inflammatory process should be ruled out with the appropriate tests (see the discussion of arthritis). ▶ ***General measures for osteoarthritis*** are designed to protect the joint from further destruction and to reduce pain. Weight reduction, physiotherapy, and exercise guidelines should be initiated. Heat can be given to relieve muscle spasm, but because muscle tone is important for joint stability, long-term use of muscle relaxants is ill-advised. Analgesics and anti-inflammatory drugs may help to relieve the symptoms of pain and stiffness. In severe cases, surgical removal of spur formations or even joint replacement may be required.

ANATOMIC SPACES FOR SPINAL CORD AND NERVE PASSAGE

A number of "anatomic spaces" are created by musculoskeletal structures for the protection of nerve passage. The most important of these exist in the spinal column. As illustrated in Figure 11.10, 33 vertebrae (5 of which make up the sacrum and 4 of which make up the coccyx) articulate one above the other in two distinct fashions. For flexibility, the vertebral facets unite through diarthrodial joints complete with joint capsules, synovial linings, and muscle and ligament attachments. For stability, the vertebral bodies are joined through symphysis unions, that is, via articulating plates (intervertebral discs). Together the bilateral facet joints and intervertebral joints comprise a three-joint complex at each spinal level.

The spinal cord passes down the middle of the three-joint complex through the central canal. It is protected by the vertebral bodies with their stable symphysis unions. Furthermore, each intervertebral disc consists of an outer layer of concentrically arranged ligament fibers (the annulus) and a center filled with a soft mucoid substance (the nucleus pulposus). Such modifications absorb the concussive shock created by jumping, running, and other movements that would otherwise be transmitted along the spinal cord to literally "rattle the brain."

Cord injury occurs from four types of mechanical trauma to the spinal column: (1) hyperflexion with fracture of the vertebral bodies and/or acute disc rupture, (2) hyperextension with fracture of the posterior bony elements and/or ligament disruption, (3) compression with explosion fracture of the vertebral body and/or ligament tearing, and (4) forceful rotation with disruption of entire ligamentous chains. Transection of the spinal cord causes immediate and total loss of neurologic function below the level of injury known as ***complete cord injury.*** With high lesions, intercostal muscles are paralyzed and patients may quickly die from cardiorespiratory instability. Those who survive remain quadriplegic. Lower lesions produce paraplegia. Other complications include ischemic changes of the skin, GI and GU dysfunction, spasticity, and muscle pain. Complete injuries are irreversible except for cases caused by ***concussive shock*** rather than actual transection. These rare patients begin to regain neurologic function immediately. Voluntary movement and preserved sensation below the level of the lesion at the time of injury are the hallmarks of ***incomplete spinal cord injuries.***

The spinal cord sends a major nerve root to either side of the body through the two lateral canals. Protected by these bony passages, exiting nerves provide sensory stimulation to a specific area of the body (dermatome), as well as motor innervation to particular sets of limb muscles (myotome). There is a lack of correspondence between dermatomes and myotomes that can be somewhat confusing.

Figure 11.10 Anterior, posterior, and lateral views of vertebral column. (From Crafts, *Anatomy*, 2nd ed. John Wiley & Sons, Inc., © 1985.)

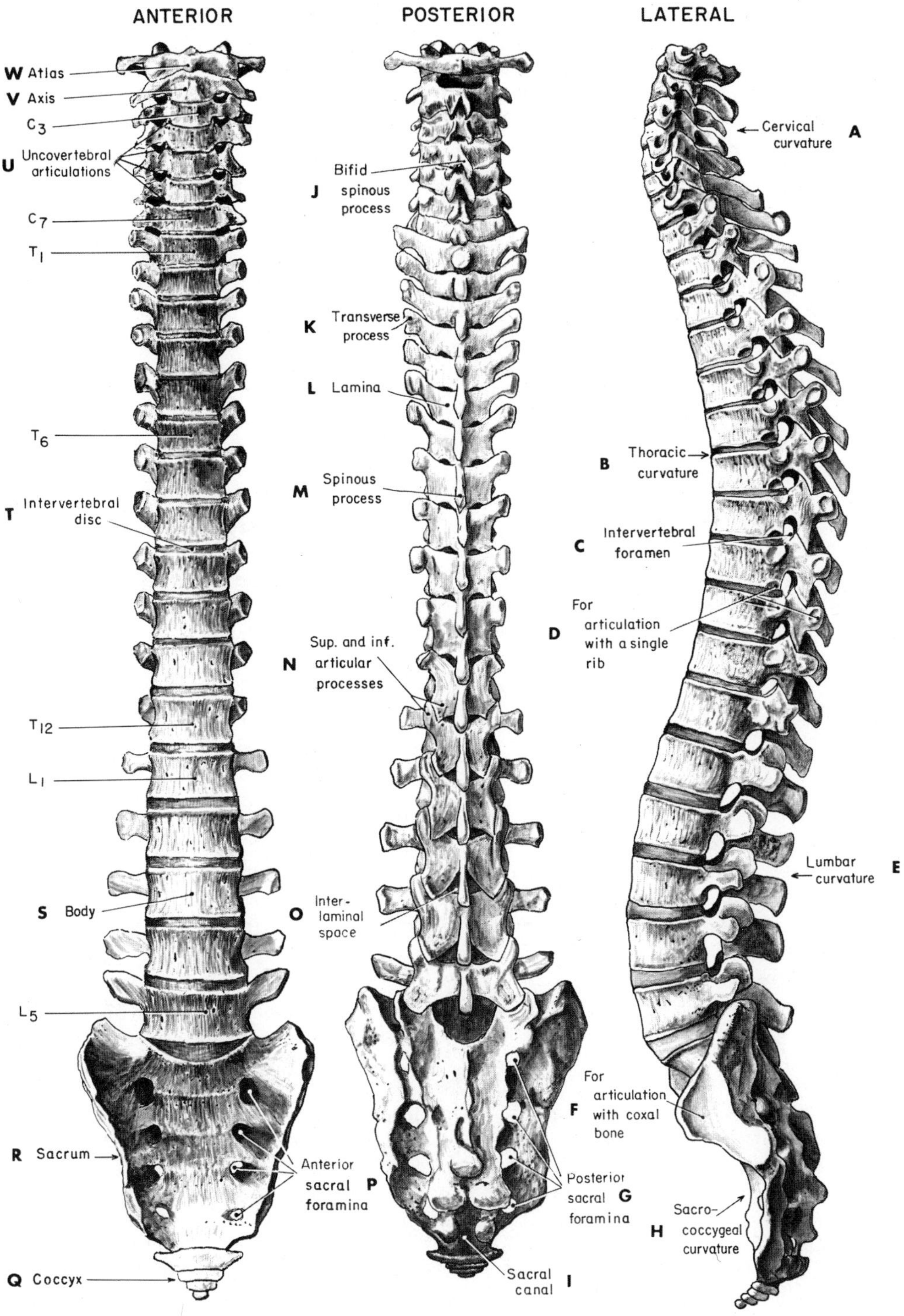
ANTERIOR
POSTERIOR
LATERAL
W Atlas
V Axis
C3
U Uncovertebral articulations
C7
T1
T6
T Intervertebral disc
T12
L1
S Body
L5
R Sacrum
Anterior sacral foramina
Q Coccyx
J Bifid spinous process
K Transverse process
L Lamina
M Spinous process
N Sup. and inf. articular processes
O Inter-laminal space
P
Sacral canal I
Cervical curvature A
B Thoracic curvature
C Intervertebral foramen
D For articulation with a single rib
Lumbar curvature E
F For articulation with coxal bone
Posterior sacral foramina G
H Sacro-coccygeal curvature

Spinal cord disorders (notably tumors) or bone disease (slipped or ruptured disc, osteophytes, inflammation, subluxation of the facet joint) may cause pressure to be exerted on the nerve roots exiting the spinal cord. If this happens, patients develop ***nerve root entrapment syndrome.*** The symptoms are variable, depending on which nerve root is involved and to what extent. For example, disturbance of the fifth lumbar nerve root causes weakness of extensor muscles of the great toe and altered sensation in the web space between the great and second toes. Irritation of the sciatic nerve ***(sciatica)*** produces a burning "pins and needles" sensation in the buttocks radiating into the groin or down the back of the leg toward the foot. Damage to the sciatic nerve causes numbness or a tourniquet sensation around the thigh or calf after walking a short distance, similar to intermittent claudication. In such cases, nerve origin can be differentiated from vascular origin by the presence of normal pulses, skin color, and texture. Furthermore, nerve root damage may lead to atrophy of thigh, calf, or gluteus muscles, along with loss of knee and ankle reflexes. Back pain is variable. It may be elicited by bending to the side, crossing the legs, sitting on soft surfaces, and straight leg raising. Symptoms of nerve root entrapment warrant evaluation by a neurologist. The first step is to identify the level of vertebral involvement by mapping the patterns of pain, sensation changes, and muscle dysfunction. Corresponding x-ray films of the spinal column follow and quickly reveal most skeletal changes. ***Slipped disc,*** which is relatively rare, may be suspected by the finding of a narrowed or altered configuration of the disc space. However, the more common disorder of ***ruptured disc*** (herniation of the nucleus pulposus) is not easily detected on routine x-ray films. The diagnosis may depend on CT scan, myelography, or isolated disk studies. This is also true for tumors of the spinal cord. Treatment of nerve root entrapment syndrome consists of correction of the underlying problem. It may involve bed rest, traction, or surgery. Some cases of ruptured disc are now being treated with injections of chymopapain, an enzyme specific for chondromucoprotein in cartilage. Called "chemonucleolysis," this procedure has a success rate comparable to that of surgery, but is less costly and is associated with fewer complications.

The major blood vessels and nerves supplying each arm pass beneath the clavicle through a space created by the scalene muscles and the first rib (the thoracic outlet). Compression of these neurovascular structures leads to ***thoracic outlet syndrome.*** Abnormal descent of the shoulder girdle (from aging, faulty posture, certain occupations, or chronic illness) is one cause. An extra "cervical" rib, highly positioned first rib, and "effort thrombosis" of the veins (from sudden or repetitive physical activity) are other causes. The condition is more common among women than among men, with a peak occurrence between ages 35 and 55. Patients present with pain in the area of compression, as well as referred pain to the base of the neck, axilla, and/or down the arm and into the hand. It may be accompanied by a pins and needle sensation, which is usually limited to the volar aspect of the fourth and fifth fingers. The paresthesia is usually aggravated by sleeping positions and prolonged use of the extremity. Patients also note increased sensitivity of hands and fingers to the cold. On exam, weakness and atrophy of muscles may be noted, but deep reflexes are rarely affected. Elevation of the arm may cause the fingers to become pale or blue. It may also cause a diminished pulse in the brachial artery or bruit development in the subclavian artery.

The clinical diagnosis of thoracic outlet syndrome is supported by x-ray findings and nerve studies that help pinpoint the area of compression to the shoulder girdle.

TABLE 11.20 PERIPHERAL NERVE ROOT ENTRAPMENT SYNDROMES

Entrapment Site/Syndrome	Clinical Manifestations
Axilla	
Radial nerve in axilla	Sensory loss in radial region; loss of elbow extension; wrist drop.
Midarm	
Radial nerve in spiral groove	Sensory loss in dorsum of hand on radial side; wrist drop.
Proximal forearm	
Anterior interosseous nerve	Index and middle fingers display weakness in flexion, extension, and pronation (abnormal "pinch sign").
Pronator (compression of median nerve)	Weakness in flexion and abduction of fingers; paresthesias in the thumb, first two radial fingers, and half of ring finger; pain and tenderness in proximal forearm.
Posterior interosseous nerve	Normal sensation; wrist drop.
Elbow	
Cubital tunnel (compression of ulnar nerve)	Wasting and weakness of hand muscles on ulnar side; sensory loss in small finger and half of ring finger; weakness in finger flexion.
Postcondylar groove (entrapment of ulnar nerve)	Wasting and weakness of hand muscles on ulnar side; weakness in wrist and finger flexion; sensory loss in small finger and half of ring finger; deformity of elbow joint.
Wrist	
Guyon's canal (compression of ulnar nerve)	Wasting and weakness of hand muscles on ulnar side; sensory loss in small finger and half of ring finger.
Carpal tunnel (compression of median nerve)	Wasting and weakness of hand muscles on radial side. Sensory changes in thumb, first two radial fingers and half of ring finger.
Pelvis and hips	
Obturator nerve	Weakness in adducting leg. Sensory loss over upper inner thigh.
Femoral nerve	Weakness and atrophy of quadriceps; sensory loss over anterior inner thigh.
Meralgia paresthetica (compression of lateral cutaneous nerve)	Numbness and sensory loss over anterior outer portion of thigh.
Common peroneal nerve	Altered gate; foot drop; sensory loss over dorsum of foot.
Ankle	
Tarsal tunnel (compression of posterior tibial nerve)	Weakness of foot muscles; numbness and tingling toes and sole of foot.

Venography or arteriography confirms any vascular obstruction. For treatment, patients are instructed to avoid any physical activity that precipitates or aggravates the symptoms. Exercises to improve posture and pillow arrangements (inverted V) that support the shoulder girdle at night are also helpful. Patients who do not respond to such conservative treatment may need surgery to widen the thoracic outlet.

Peripheral nerve entrapment syndromes are described in Table 11.20. ► ***Carpal tunnel syndrome*** is representative and common. A confined space formed by the bones of the wrist and the transverse carpal ligament is shared by flexor tendons and the median nerve. With inflammation of the tendon, pressure bears on the median nerve, resulting in numbness or burning pain on the palmar surface of the first three fingers. The numbness or burning tends to be most bothersome at night but can be elicited at any time by sustained flexion of the wrist or by tapping on the median nerve at its volar aspect (Tinel's sign). Thumb adduction is weakened and eventually thenar atrophy may develop. In evaluating carpal tunnel syndrome, a number of associated conditions should be considered, including pregnancy, RA, hypothyroidism, amyloidosis, gout, and acromegaly. The entrapment is diagnosed on the basis of a neurologic exam that has ruled out cervical radiculitis or thoracic outlet syndrome. It is also customary to measure the nerve conduction velocities of both motor and sensory nerves, as well as performing electromyography of the thenar and upper limb muscles. Patients with good motor function and only mild electrodiagnostic changes are treated with wrist splints, anti-inflammatory drugs, and local steroid injections. Those with weakness or significant test changes are advised to have hand surgery in order to decompress the nerve.

In the forearm and lower leg, sheets of fascia separate groups of muscles, major nerves, and blood vessels into the compartments described in Table 11.21. With no space for expansion inside these compartments, increased tension from any kind of muscle swelling causes ischemic changes known as ***compartment syndromes.*** These may be seen in runners who develop transient swelling from overusing a particular group of muscles. In such cases, treatment includes proper shoes, training surfaces, and stretching and strengthening exercises. However, compartment syndromes also develop from acute swelling following trauma or bone fractures. In these cases, symptoms of paresthesia, skin discoloration, sensory changes, or reduced pulses deserve immediate evaluation by an orthopedist. Surgical decompression of the fascia may be needed to prevent muscle infarction or nerve damage.

ACTIVITY

Normal function of the musculoskeletal system depends on activity. As noted in a previous discussion, the mechanical stress of movement and weight bearing is the key to mineralization of bone and nourishment of the articular cartilage. Stretching maintains the elastic properties of tendons, and regular use preserves muscle tone and strength. In contrast, ***prolonged confinement*** contributes to osteoporosis, osteoarthritis, contractures, muscle atrophy, and other complications. It is a problem of increasing concern to primary care providers as the trend toward home care of the sick and elderly increases. Scheduled visits or phone calls, written guidelines for patients and caregivers, and resource connections are important aids to management.

While normal musculoskeletal function can be maintained by general activity, enhanced function can be gained by specific exercises. ***Endurance training*** affects the aerobic threshold of muscle cell metabolism as follows. A muscle at rest extracts 25% of the O_2 in arterial blood supplied by the heart and lungs. Oxygen fuels the highly efficient Krebs cycle to generate cellular energy (because the Krebs cycle runs only on oxygen, it is referred to as an "aerobic pathway"). As muscle activity increases, higher percentages of O_2 are extracted from the blood. If the demand for O_2 exceeds the supply, anaerobic pathways of cellular metabolism take over. Besides generating two-thirds less energy, they produce the waste product lactic acid, which is blood borne to the liver for oxidation. An "oxygen debt" arises if the liver fails to

TABLE 11.21 COMMON SITES FOR COMPARTMENT SYNDROMES

Compartment	Location	Nerves	Muscles Contained	Function
Forearm				
Superficial volar	Beneath skin surface of forearm, palmar side.	Branches of median and ulnar nerves.	1. Flexor digitorum superficialis	Flexes middle fingers, hand, and forearm.
			2. Pronator teres	Pronates hand.
			3. Palmarus longus; flexor carpi ulnarus; flexor carpi radialus	Wrist flexors; aid in pronation and abduction of hand.
Deep volar	Behind superficial volar compartment just anterior to radius and ulna.	Branches of palmar interosseous nerve (from median nerve) and branch of ulnar nerve.	1. Flexor digitorum profundus	Flexes hand and distal phalanges.
			2. Flexor pollicis longus	Flexes thumb.
Leg				
Anterior	Runs parallel to tibia just beneath skin surface on lateral side.	Branch of deep peroneal nerve.	1. Tibialis anterior	Dorsiflexes, inverts foot.
			2. Extensor digitorum longus	Extends toes.
			3. Extensor hallucis longus	Extends large toe; dorsiflexes foot.
Lateral	Runs parallel to fibula just beneath skin surface lateral to anterior compartment.	Branch of superficial peroneal nerve.	1. Peroneus longus and brevis	Abducts, plantar-flexes foot; supports arches.
Superficial posterior	Just beneath skin surface of calf.	Branches of tibial nerve.	1. Soleus	Extends foot.
			2. Gastrocnemius	Extends foot; flexes leg.
Deep posterior		Branches of tibial nerve.	1. Tibialis posterior	Extends and inverts foot; maintains arches.
			2. Flexor digitorum longus	Flexes toes and extends foot.
			3. Flexor hallucis longus	Flexes large toe.

oxidize the lactic acid as fast as the muscle cells release it. Lactic acid then accumulates in the blood, causing neuromuscular irritability, fatigue, and weakness. It also produces metabolic acidosis. To buffer the falling pH, bicarbonate is reabsorbed from the kidney. This, in turn, raises body levels of CO_2, which must be eliminated by the lungs through hyperventilation.

Although endurance training has little effect on muscle size or strength, it improves cardiopulmonary performance. This, in turn, decreases myocardial oxygen requirements, lowering the heart rate and systolic blood pressure for submaximal workloads. Such changes reduce cardiovascular stress, protecting the heart against injury. Endurance training reduces cardiovascular risks in other ways as well. It raises high-density lipoproteins, lowers serum triglycerides, and is an important adjunct to weight control and possibly to smoking withdrawal. As an extra benefit, regular participants note enhanced self-esteem and higher energy levels.

In contrast to endurance training, ***isometrics*** (intense contractions repeated against resistance) cause muscles to increase in size and therefore in strength. They are used for ***body building*** as well as by athletes to enhance sports performance and endurance. In addition, isometrics are used in rehabilitation after injury, since the strengthening of muscles around joints adds to joint stability.

It is true that a relative lack of androgens prevents women and prepubescent youth from building muscles to the same extent as men. It is untrue that building muscles destroys tone and flexibility. Contrary to popular belief, weight lifters do not become "muscle bound." Nonetheless, weight training can result in muscle, tendon, or ligament damage, a fact confirmed by approximately 35,000 emergency room visits each year. Most injuries are confined to minor sprains and strains, but fractures and serious back, shoulder, and knee injuries also occur. Because isometric exercise increases peripheral resistance and causes a transient rise in blood pressure, it is also associated with significant cardiovascular risk. ***Weight lifter's blackout*** is a recognized syndrome attributed to a sudden decrease in cardiac output and/or arrhythmia. For someone with high blood pressure or a history of cardiac disease, its development could be fatal. Thus, ▶***exercise prescribing*** should be carefully tailored to each individual (Table 11.22).

TABLE 11.22 CONTRAINDICATIONS/LIMITING FACTORS TO STRENUOUS EXERCISE

- Contraindications
  - Cardiovascular
    - Poorly controlled dysrhythmias
    - Recent myocardial infarction (less than 8–10 weeks)
    - Symptomatic congestive heart failure (greater than class 11 per New York Heart Association classification)
    - New or unstable angina pectoris
    - Obstructive valvular or cyanotic heart disease
    - Second- and third-degree atrioventricular block
    - Active myocarditis
    - Pericarditis
    - Transient ischemic attacks
    - Thrombophlebitis
    - Exercise testing positive for (1) dysrhythmias including tachycardia and coupled or multifocal premature beats; (2) overt cardiac failure; (3) angina symptoms or dyspnea at low workloads (i.e., less than 4 METS); (4) ST depression greater than 4 mm; (5) ST elevation; (6) work capacity below 4 METS
  - Respiratory
    - Obstructive or restrictive pulmonary disease
    - Cor pulmonale
  - Metabolic
    - Poorly controlled diabetes
    - Active hyperthyroidism
    - Adrenal insufficiency
    - Hepatic insufficiency
    - Renal insufficiency
  - Musculoskeletal
    - Active arthritis
- Limiting factors
  - Cardiovascular
    - Poorly controlled hypertension at rest
    - Severe anemia
    - Medications altering hemodynamic response (notably beta blockers, ganglionic blockers, and vasodilators)
    - Exercise testing positive for (1) symptoms of angina and/or ischemic ST changes at intermediate workloads (i.e., 6–8 METS); (2) abnormally high blood pressure responses (i.e., above 225 mm Hg systolic or 120 mm Hg diastolic at intermediate workloads)
  - Respiratory
    - Poorly controlled exercise-induced asthma
  - Metabolic
    - Extreme obesity
  - Musculoskeletal
    - Osteoarthritis of weight-bearing joints
    - Osteoporosis
    - Postmenopause
    - Lumbosacral disk syndrome

The problems resulting from exercise programs are negligible compared to those occurring from ***accidental falls.*** Next to traffic accidents, falls kill more persons and are more costly than any other kind of accident. They take 10,000 lives and injure more than 13 million persons each year. The majority occur around the house rather than on the job or in public places and are the result of slips or trips at floor level, not falls from high places. Thus, ▶***preventing fall injuries*** centers on simple safety precautions at home. Such measures are particularly important for the elderly or for anyone with osteoporosis.

Motor vehicle accidents are responsible for 35,000 deaths and more than 50,000 injuries every year. Contrary to what might be expected, most fatalities occur within 25 miles of home, at speeds under 40 miles an hour, during the day, in dry sunny weather. Accident statistics reveal that ***seat belt use*** by all car passengers would reduce the number of deaths by 60–70% and the number of serious injuries by at least 50%. They are supported by collision studies. When a car traveling at 30 mph hits a wall or other stable object, it crushes in at the point of impact. Car seats, because they are padded, are anchored to the car frame, and are situated several feet from the front and back of the car, survive the crush better than any other part of an automobile's anatomy. Furthermore, the car slows down at the moment of impact, coming to a halt within 1/10th of a second. However, passengers who are not belted into seats (the most stable part of the car) continue to travel forward at 30 mph, colliding with anything in their path. This "second" or "human" collision is the source of injury. Within 1/50th of a second, passengers slam into the windshield with an impact equivalent to that of a fall from a three-story building. In side impact crashes, they slide across the seat, hitting car doors, the framework, or other persons. In rollover crashes, victims bounce off each other as well as off the car's roof, sides, and floor. Children held in the lap are in danger of being crushed by adult bodies. Even if adults are belted in place, the momentum of a sudden stop can increase the force of a 20-lb baby to 400 lb, far beyond the capability of human restraint. While any hard surface within the car may become an instrument of death, the chances of survival are even worse for the persons thrown out of the car. Being "thrown clear" is truly a misnomer, since persons are usually hurled into oncoming traffic, telephone poles, or trees, or across lacerating cement surfaces, and are 25 times more likely to die than those who remain in the car. Motorcyclists, who are thrown clear of their vehicles with almost every accident, have a fatality rate eight times that of automobile occupants. As the leading cause of death for Americans under age 35, motor vehicle accidents should be a major focus of primary care. Providers should actively promote ▶***seat belt use and motor vehicle safety.***

Details of Management

▸ *Muscular Dystrophy Organizations*

Laboratory Tests: None.

Therapeutic Measures: None.

Patient Education: Muscular Dystrophy Association, Inc.
810 7th Ave.
New York, New York 10019
Tel.: (212) 586-0808

This national headquarters can provide information about all local chapters of its organization.

Follow-up: As needed.

▸ *Primary Tetanus Immunization (Adults)*

Laboratory Tests: None.

Therapeutic Measures: Three doses of Td (tetanus and diphtheria toxoids combined and absorbed *for adult use*) as follows:

	Adult Dose	Schedule
Primary series 1 and 2	0.5 ml IM	6–8 weeks apart
First booster	0.5 ml IM	1 year
Subsequent boosters	0.5 ml IM	Every 10 years thereafter

Patients with serious clinical reactions to previous injections should receive a reduced dosage of plain (nonabsorbed) toxoid.

Patient Education: Immunizations are usually well tolerated. Nonetheless, inform patients that they may experience muscle achiness, localized redness and tenderness at the site of the injection, and low-grade fever. More serious reactions should be reported promptly. Inform patients that boosters may be necessary within 5 years with a deep or very dirty wound. Otherwise, boosters are required every 10 years.

Follow-up: None.

▸ *Tetanus Prevention in Wound Management*

Laboratory Tests: A test for serum hypersensitivity is needed if tetanus antitoxin is used.

Therapeutic Measures: Thoroughly clean and disinfect the wound; if necessary, surgically debride it and remove any foreign body as well. Give Td (tetanus and diphtheria toxoids combined and absorbed *for adult use*) and/or TIG as follows:

Immunization Status	Clean, Minor Wounds		All Other Wounds	
	Td	TIG	Td	TIG
Uncertain or known 0–1 dose in past	0.5 ml IM	None	0.5 ml IM	250 units IM
2 doses in past	0.5 ml IM	None	0.5 ml IM	None unless wound is more than 24 hours old
3 or more doses	None unless last dose given >10 years ago	None	None unless last dose given >5 years ago	None

When Td and TIG are given concurrently, separate syringes and separate sites should be used. If TIG is not available, give tetanus antitoxin, 3,000–5,000 units IM, only after serum antisensitivity testing.

Patient Education: Review dressing changes with patients. Explain Td immunization guidelines, stressing the importance of boosters.

Follow-up: As needed for wound care.

▸ *Myasthenia Gravis Organizations*

Laboratory Tests: None.

Therapeutic Measures: None.

Patient Education: Myasthenia Gravis Foundation
15 East 42nd St.
New York, New York 10010
Tel.: (212) 889-8157

Follow-up: None.

▸ *Muscle Cramps*

Laboratory Tests: None.

Therapeutic Measures: For nocturnal cramps, recommend the use of light bed covers (e.g., switching from several heavy blankets to a single electric blanket) loosely arranged (untucked or suspended from a foot board). Try quinine sulfate, 200 mg hs, or Benadryl, 50 mg hs (contraindicated in pregnancy). For cramps related to strenuous activity, advise adding extra salt to the diet before and after periods of exercise. Advise drinking to quench thirst. Premixed solutions containing water, salt, potassium, and glucose (e.g., Gatorade) readily replace lost fluids and electrolytes. Salt tablets are poorly absorbed from the stomach.

Patient Education: Explain the relationship of cramps to muscle irritability. Demonstrate maneuvers to relieve a cramped muscle (e.g., active, forceful dorsiflexion of the foot, repeated until the spasm breaks).

Follow-up: Advise patients to return in 2 weeks if cramps are unrelieved by these measures. Hypocalcemia, hypokalemia, or other metabolic imbalances should then be ruled out.

▸ *ALS Organizations*

Laboratory Tests: None.

Therapeutic Measures: None.

Patient Education: National ALS Association
185 Madison Ave.
New York, New York 10016
Tel.: (212) 679-4016

Follow-up: None.

▸ *Adult Polio Vaccination*

Laboratory Tests: None.

Therapeutic Measures: Because the incidence of poliomyelitis in the United States, is low, primary vaccination of adults is not recommended. However, patients who live in or travel to endemic/epidemic areas should receive either IPV ("killed" virus, Salk type) or TOPV ("live" virus, Sabin type) as follows:

Indication	Recommended Vaccine	Series
Continued exposure, never immunized	IPV (dose according to manufacturer's recommendations)	Three primary series: first and second doses 8 weeks apart; third dose 1 year after second dose; boosters every 5 years as long as exposure continues
Traveler, never immunized; >4 weeks before departure	IPV (dose according to manufacturer's recommendations)	2 doses at least 4 weeks apart
Traveler, never immunized; <4 weeks before departure	TOPV* 0.5 ml po	1 dose
Traveler, previously immunized	TOPV 0.5 ml po	1 dose

*Live vaccine should not be given to patients or household members of patients with immunodeficiency or immunosuppressive conditions such as AIDS, combined immunodeficiency, agammaglobulinemia, thymic abnormalities, leukemia, lymphoma, generalized malignancy, or immunosuppressive treatments (with corticosteroids, radiation, alkylating agents, antimetabolites).

Patient Education: Stress the importance of completing the immunization schedule.

Follow-up: As needed for boosters.

▸ *First Aid for Snakebite*

Laboratory Tests: None.

Therapeutic Measures: Immediately immobilize the victim, since activity will stimulate the spread of the poison. Place the bitten area below heart level (unless signs of shock are present) and keep the patient warm and as calm as possible. Remove watches, bracelets, rings, and other jewelry. If a medical facility can be reached within 30 minutes, transport the patient without further intervention. If not, apply a constriction band above the swelling caused by the bite. The band should be tight enough to impede lymph and superficial venous flow but loose enough to allow arterial and deep venous flow. Make an incision approximately $\frac{1}{8}$ in. deep and $\frac{1}{2}$ in. long through the fang marks. Press around the cut to make it bleed. Suction the wound using a device from a snakebite kit or your mouth (as long as the mouth and lips are free from open cuts or lesions). Unless performed within 30–60 minutes of envenomation, incision and suction is useless. Whenever possible, kill the snake and take it to the hospital for identification purposes. Do not give the patient any drugs or alcohol. During transport, reposition the band if swelling progresses above the point of constriction. A specific antivenin may be given by trained persons. Administration of antivenin must be preceded by hypersensitivity testing for horse serum (instructions and materials are included in each package of antivenin).

Patient Education: Emergency information about poisonous snakes and antivenins can be obtained from the following sources:

Bronx Zoo
Tel.: (212) 220-5063 or (212) 220-5100
Okalahoma City Poison Information Center
Tel.: (1-800) 522-4611 or (405) 271-5454

Follow-up: As needed.

▸ *General Measures for Mild to Moderate Strains*

Laboratory Tests: None.

Therapeutic Measures: The patient should rest the area of injury (specifically, discontinuing the precipitating activity) for 3–4 days. Prescribe ASA 325 mg, 2 tablets qid with meals and at bedtime, or ibuprofen (Motrin 400 mg) qid with meals and at bedtime for 2 weeks. If muscle spasm is present, prescribe a muscle relaxant such as Robaxin, 750 mg qid, or Flexeril, 10 mg tid, for the first few days (long-term use is not advised). The patient should apply heat or ice (whichever alleviates the symptoms) for 15 minutes tid and should return to full activity gradually.

Patient Education: Describe the strain and, if possible, use an anatomic illustration to point out the injured muscle or tendon.

Follow-up: None.

▸ *NSAI Agents*

Laboratory Tests: Periodic CBCs (every 2 weeks of therapy for the first month and every week thereafter) are recommended for patients taking pyrazolones.

Therapeutic Measures: Remember that gastric ulcers, renal failure, and hypertension can be exacerbated by NSAI agents. Keep a list of the commonly used NSAI drugs, grouped by classes in ascending order of toxicity similar to the one in Table 11.7. Individualize therapy as follows:

Drug selection: Rely on the patient's previous drug history (what anti-inflammatories have been used, how well they worked, associated problems) as an aid to present selection. Begin with less toxic drugs.

Initial dose: Start with the recommended dose for the specific condition. Prescribe pill use with meals to minimize gastric irritation.

Titration: Continue the starting dose for at least 1 or 2 weeks; then apply quantifiable measures to check the therapeutic effect (e.g., actual duration of morning stiffness, range-of-motion and muscle strength measurements). If improvement is unsatisfactory, increase the dose at weekly intervals but do not exceed the maximum daily allowance. At the first sign of side effects, return to the previous dose. With continued side effects, discontinue using the drug. Do not give phenylbutazone or oxyphenbutazone for more than 2 weeks at a time.

Changing drugs: If a poor therapeutic response occurs, choose a drug from the next class and begin the same titration procedure.

Patient Education: Take the medication with food to minimize gastric upset. Do not combine drugs. Report the symptoms of gastritis or other side effects and discontinue the drug at once.

Follow-up: Schedule visits every 1–2 weeks during the initial titration period and then every 3–4 months for medication review.

▶ *Cervical Strain*

Laboratory Tests: None.

Therapeutic Measures: General measures for mild strains as noted in the section on "General Measures for Mild Strains" (advise the use of moist heat rather than cold). Start the patient on an exercise program, providing a handout sheet with information such as the following:

EXERCISES FOR CERVICAL STRAIN*,†

Standing exercises (preferably done under a hot shower) as follows:

1. Stand straight and slowly turn the head as far as possible to the right. Return to the center position. Slowly turn the head as far as possible to the left. Return to the center position. Relax. Repeat.
2. Stand straight and slowly try to touch the chin to the chest. Slowly raise the head to the central position; then extend it backward until you are looking up at the ceiling. Relax. Repeat.
3. Stand straight and slowly try to touch the right ear to the right shoulder. Return to the central position. Slowly try to touch the left ear to the left shoulder. Relax. Repeat.
4. Stand straight and raise both shoulders as close to the ears as possible. Hold for 5 seconds. Relax. Stretch both shoulders backward as far as possible. Hold for 5 seconds. Relax. Repeat.
5. Stand erect and with one hand grasp the thumb of the other behind the back. Inhale, pull the thumb down, stand on the toes, and look at the ceiling. Hold for 2 seconds. Exhale and relax. Repeat.

*Refrain from any painful maneuvers. Gradually increase the number of repetitions as the condition improves. Always stop at the first signs of fatigue. Perform exercise 5 after every 2 hours of desk work.
†Information with illustrations available as tear-out sheets. Request "Helpful hints for a healthy neck" from Riker Laboratories, Northridge, California, 91324.

Floor exercises twice a day as follows:

1. With a small pillow placed under the neck, lie on the back and bend the knees. Inhale slowly until the chest is fully expanded. Exhale slowly. Repeat 10 times.
2. Turn onto the stomach. Clasp the hands behind the back. While inhaling, push the hands toward the feet, pinching the shoulder blades and lifting the chin off the floor. Hold for 2 seconds. Exhale and relax. Repeat.

Patient Education: Explain the vulnerability of neck muscles to strain. Have patients avoid cold air conditioning and fans that blow directly on them. Suggest the use of a specially contoured neck pillow (e.g., Jackson Cervipillow) for sleeping. Correct poor posture habits (see the next section).

Follow-up: As needed.

▶ *Correct Posture*

Laboratory Tests: None.

Therapeutic Measures: None.

Patient Education: Provide a handout sheet with following information:

MAINTAINING CORRECT POSTURE

Standing: Keep the neck drawn back and the chin tucked in. Try to thrust the shoulders and chin forward. Avoid carrying shoulder bags, brief cases, book bags, children, and so on on the same side all the time. Either switch sides frequently or use a backpack.

Sitting: Try to sit in straight-backed chairs with arm rests. Sit squarely in the chair with both feet touching the floor. Try to avoid slouching and crossing the legs.

Driving: Do not drive with the seat too far back or too low. If the seat cannot be adjusted to the right position, sit on a pillow or use a seat support. For extended drives, remove thick wallets or other objects from hip pockets.

Reaching: Stand on a stool to retrieve high objects. Avoid extended periods of overhead reaching or viewing.

Lifting: Lift by bending the knees rather than the back. Avoid lifting heavy objects.

Reclining: Do not lie on the sofa with the head propped up or forward with high pillows to read or watch television. Sit properly in a chair.

Sleeping: Never sleep in a chair. Use a bed board or firm orthopedic mattress. Use a proper pillow (3–4 in. thick, 6–7 in. wide, and 16 in. long). Place pillows under the neck, not the head, and position them to maintain neural alignment of the head and neck. Do not sleep on the stomach or with the arms extended overhead.

Follow-up: None.

▸ *Acute Lumbar Strain*

Laboratory Measures: Lumbosacral spine films.

Therapeutic Measures: Use general measures for strains. The patient should continue bed rest in a comfortable position until muscle spasm and acute pain have subsided. Start the patient on an exercise program, providing a handout sheet with information such as the following:

EXERCISES FOR LUMBAR STRAIN*,†

Floor exercises (can also be done in bed) twice a day as follows:

1. With the hands placed under the neck, lie on the back and bend the knees. Inhale slowly and press the small of the back against the floor, tightening stomach and buttock muscles. Hold for 5 seconds. Exhale and relax. Repeat.
2. With a small pillow placed under the neck, lie on the back and bend the knees. Grasp the right knee with both hands. Inhale slowly and pull the knee as close to the chest as possible. Exhale slowly, returning the leg to the starting position. Repeat with the left leg.
3. With a small pillow placed under the neck, lie on the back and bend the knees. Grasp the left knee with the left hand and the right knee with the right hand. Inhale slowly and pull the knees as close to the chest as possible. Exhale slowly, returning the legs to the starting position. Repeat.
4. Turn onto the stomach. Clasp the hands behind the back. While inhaling, push the hands toward the feet, pinching the shoulder blades and lifting the chin off the floor. Hold for 2 seconds. Exhale and relax. Repeat.

Standing exercises (can be done at work) as often as possible:

1. Stand straight with the back against a doorway, heels 4 in. from the frame. Inhale and press the small of the back against the door frame, tightening stomach and buttock muscles and allowing the knees to bend slightly. Hold for 5 seconds. Exhale and relax. Repeat.
2. Stand straight with the back against a doorway (heels 4 in. away), knees slightly bent, and hands extended to the opposite frame. Inhale and press the hands against one frame, flattening the neck and straightening the knees against the other frame. Hold for 5 seconds. Exhale and relax. Repeat.

*Refrain from any painful maneuvers. Gradually increase the number of repetitions as the condition improves. Always stop at the first signs of fatigue.
†Information with illustrations available as tear-out sheets. Request "Helpful hints for a healthy back," Pub. No. 91584 from Riker Laboratories, Northridge, California, 91324.

3. Stand straight and slowly try to touch the chin to the chest. Slowly raise the head to the central position; then extend it backward until you are looking up at the ceiling. Relax. Repeat.

Advanced exercises (only for pain-free, well-conditioned patients) as follows:

1. With a small pillow placed under the neck, lie on the back and bend the knees. Draw the right knee in to the chest. Inhale and slowly raise the leg as far as possible. Exhale slowly, bending the knee back to the chest and then to the starting position. Repeat with the left leg.
2. With a small pillow placed under the neck, lie on the back with the arms at the sides and the legs straight. Inhale and slowly raise the right leg as far as possible. Exhale, slowly reutrning the leg to the floor. Repeat with the left leg.
3. Stand in front of a chair. Assume a squatting position with the head flexed forward. Holding on to the chair for balance, bounce up and down three times. Stand and pause. Repeat.
4. With a small pillow placed under the neck, lie on the back and bend the knees. Inhale and pull up to a sitting position. Exhale and lie back. Repeat.

Patient Education: Explain the vulnerability of paravertebral muscles to strain. Correct poor posture habits (see the section on "Correct Posture"). Stress the importance of rest and sensible exercise.

Follow-up: As needed.

▸ General Measures for Tendinitis and Acute Bursitis

Laboratory Tests: None.

Therapeutic Measures: The patient should discontinue the activity that initiated the problem and rest the joint for 3–4 days. Prescribe NSAI drugs (indole analogues or pyrazolones seem to work best) for 7–14 days. Start Indocin 25 mg tid, Clinoril 200 mg bid, or Tolectin 400 mg tid (see Table 11.7). Heat or cold (whichever is more comfortable) should be applied for 20 minutes three times a day.

Patient Education: Explain the inflammatory nature of the problem. Use an anatomic drawing to point out the area of involvement.

Follow-up: As needed.

▸ Tennis Elbow

Laboratory Tests: None.

Therapeutic Measures: Use general measures for tendinitis/bursitis. After acute symptoms have resolved, start the patient on hand gripper exercises for 5–10 minutes four times a day. Exercises must be done with the elbow extended and the wrist flexed. Give racquet sports players the following advice:

1. Use a firm armband applied below the elbow for all racquet activities.
2. Use lightweight racquets with large enough grip sizes. Have tennis racquets strung at 55 lb tension or less (a heavy or high-strung racquet places added strain on the extensor muscles, as does a small grip size, which necessitates excessive hand squeezing).
3. Avoid exaggerated twisting of the wrist while serving and forceful pronation of the forearm on the backhand stroke. Consider taking professional lessons to help correct improper techniques.

Patient Education: Use an illustration of the elbow anatomy to explain the location and etiology of inflammation and strain.

Follow-up: If acute symptoms do not respond to general measures, refer patients for local injection of a steroid-lidocaine solution. Patients with no improvement after 6–12 months might consider surgery.

▸ *Tendinitis, Bursitis, and Tenosynovitis of the Shoulder*

Laboratory Measures: None.

Therapeutic Measures: Use the general measures for tendinitis and bursitis, along with concurrent exercises to prevent frozen shoulder. Give a handout with information such as the following:

SHOULDER EXERCISES*

1. Lean forward over a table and grasp its edge with one hand. Holding a 2-lb weight in one hand, swing the other arm forward and backward with the shoulder relaxed and the elbow straight. Swing the arm from right to left in front of the body. Finally, swing the arm in a circular motion, tracing small circle outlines at first, then larger ones. Repeat on the other side.
2. Stand sideways, at arm's length from the wall. Keeping the elbow straight, walk the fingers up the wall. Return to the starting position. Repeat, each time trying to climb a little higher. Perform the same procedure using the other arm and then while facing the wall.
3. Stand straight and raise both arms over the head, stretching them as far as possible.
4. Stand straight and stretch the arms out to the sides. Without bending the elbows, bring the arms together over the head and clap the palms. Repeat the procedure, clapping the back of the hands.
5. Stand straight and lock the hands behind the neck. Pull the elbows toward the back, thrusting the chest forward.

*Information with illustrations available as tear-out sheets. Request "Helpful hints for healthy shoulders," Pub. No. 91589 from Riker Laboratories, Northridge, California, 91324.

6. Stand straight and place the back of one hand on the small of the back. Gradually crawl the hand upward toward the opposite shoulder. Return the hand to the side. Repeat, using the other hand.
7. Stand straight with a towel thrown over the right shoulder. Hold the towel in front with the right hand. Reach around the back with the left hand and grasp the free end of the towel. Pull down on the towel in front as far as possible. Switch the towel to the left side and repeat the procedure.
8. Stand straight with the wrists crossed in front. Lift the arms above the head and stretch them backward as far as possible. Return to the starting position and repeat.

Patient Education: Use an anatomic drawing to point out the complicated structure of the shoulder and the various locations at which inflammation develops. Stress the importance of continuous exercise.

Follow-up: Shoulder ailments should be treated aggressively. Early referral is advisable for cases that do not show improvement within a few days. Steroid-lidocaine injections, professional physiotherapy, or surgery may be indicated.

▸ *Preventive Measures for Postmenopausal Osteoporosis*

Laboratory Tests: None.

Therapeutic Measures

Exercise: Start inactive patients on a sensible exercise program. Strenuous exercises such as long-distance running or competitive tennis promote bone maintenance during premenopausal years but may contribute to osteoporosis in postmenopausal women.

Dietary calcium: Maintain or increase the dietary intake of calcium to the RDA as follows:

Life Stage	Dose (mg)
Less than age 30	800
Age 30 through menopause	1,000
Pregnancy	1,500
Lactation	2,000
Postmenopause	1,500 + supplements

Supplemental calcium: Patients who dislike dairy products, who have lactose intolerance or are on a low-sodium diet, and all postmenopausal women are unlikely to meet their calcium needs through the diet and require supplements. Give the amount lacking in the diet (1,500 mg regardless of the diet to postmenopausal women) in the form of calcium carbonate, calcium lactate, or calcium gluconate divided into two, three, or four doses (generally before meals).

Calcium carbonate, which contains the highest amount of elemental calcium, necessitates the fewest number of pills (an important point for compliance and cost). However, it is also the most likey to cause gastric upset. Calcium can be obtained over the counter (crushed oyster shells), as a generic prescription (calcium carbonate 500 mg) or as a brand name (Os-Cal 500). It may also be given as a prenatal preparation, combined with multivitamins and minerals (e.g., Natalins, Prenate 90, or Mission Prenatal), or as a preparation combined with vitamin D (Calcet).

Vitamin D: This vitamin is essential for the absorption of calcium. About half of the amount needed for this purpose is obtained from fortified foods (cereals and milk) and the other half from sunshine conversion by skin. Maintain or increase the dietary intake of vitamin D according to the RDA as follows:

Age Group	Dose (IU)
Young adults	400
Elderly persons	800

Arrange periods of outdoor exposure (ideally, 30 minutes a day) for women confined or prone to indoor activity.

Estrogens: Unless contraindicated, maintain premenopausal women who have undergone hysterectomy/bilateral oophorectomy on estrogen therapy. Prescribe Premarin, 1.25 mg/day given cyclically (3 weeks on, 1 week off). For women who have not had hysterectomy, add Provera, 10 mg daily the third week (reduces the incidence of uterine cancer). Consider the same therapy for other patients at high risk (see Table 11.12) following natural menopause (beneficial for up to 8 years).

Patient Education: Explain the cause, prevalence, and complications of osteoporosis. Stress the importance of appropriate exercise, calcium intake, vitamin D and exposure to sunshine, and indications for estrogens to prevent bone loss. Provide a list of high-calcium foods such as the following:

CALCIUM CONTENT OF COMMON FOODS

Food	Calcium Content (mg)	Food	Calcium Content (mg)
Low-fat plain yogurt, 1 c	415	Dried almonds, $\frac{2}{3}$ c	254
Sardines (with bones), 3 oz	372	Cooked kale, 1 c	206
Low-fat fruit yogurt, 1 c	314	Cheddar cheese, 1 oz	204
Cooked collard greens, 1 c	304	Frozen yogurt, 1 c	200
Skim milk, 1 c	302	Ice cream, 1 c	176
Whole milk, 1 c	291	American cheese, 1 oz	174
Buttermilk, 1 c	285	Tofu, 4 oz	154
Canned salmon, 3 oz	285	Shrimp, 1 c	147
Swiss cheese, 1 oz	272	Low-fat cottage cheese, 1 c	138
Cooked turnip greens, 1 c	267	Cooked broccoli, 1 c	136

Follow-up: As needed for young women. For women on estrogen replacement therapy, review the medication every 3–4 months and do a complete gynecologic exam annually.

▸ *Established Postmenopausal Osteoporosis*

Laboratory Tests: X-ray films of the spine, wrist, or hands. More sophisticated tests include Norland-Cameron single-photon absorptiometry, quantitative CT scanning, and bone biopsy.

Therapeutic Measures

All preventive measures.

Additional calcium: Prescribe supplements: 1.5 g/day regardless of dietary intake.

Fluoride: Pending FDA approval. Prescribe in conjunction with calcium supplements (never alone): sodium fluoride, 1 mg per kilogram of body weight in three divided doses (solutions to be made up by the pharmacist). Calcium is best taken before meals and fluoride afterward. If patients develop fluorosis (wrist or ankle pain), discontinue the fluoride for several weeks and rechallenge at a lower dose.

Exercise: Prescribe 30 minutes of outdoor walking a day (additional benefit of sunshine exposure). Restrict athletic endeavors to nonstrenuous activities such as golf or swimming. Jogging, aerobics, and highly competitive racquet games should be avoided.

Compression fractures: Traction for compression or any other type of fracture is contraindicated. Prescribe bed rest in a horizontal position (with a small pillow under the head and intermittent use of a pillow under the knees) for 7–14 days until pain subsides. Give analgesics as needed (narcotics such as Tylenol with codeine, Percodan, or methadone seem to work best for elderly persons). Give Flexeril, 10 mg tid, or Robaxin, 750 mg tid, for muscle spasm. Advise the use of a sheepskin over mattress, deep-breathing exercises, stool softeners, and plenty of fluids to prevent some of the problems associated with prolonged bed rest. Begin mobilization as soon as the patient can turn in bed comfortably. Have the patient sit or stand for 10 minutes several times a day. Orthotic devices (rigid thoracicolumbar hyperextension or three-point, semirigid thoracicolumbar extension orthosis) may be helpful. Increase the duration of sitting/standing periods and begin progressive ambulation to patient tolerance. During early ambulation, suggest the use of low-heeled, soft-soled shoes with foam inserts (to cushion concussive movements) and a cane (to provide support). After acute symptoms have resolved, start the daily back exercises described in the section on “Lumbar Strain.”

Patient Education: See the section on “Preventive Measures for Postmenopausal Osteoporosis.” For patients suffering from compression fracture, use an anatomic drawing or x-ray film to point out the area of injury.

Follow-up: Same as noted under "Preventive Measures for Postmenopausal Osteoporosis." For patients who are taking calcium and fluoride supplements, schedule visits every 3–4 months for medication review. For patients suffering from compression fractures, schedule weekly phone calls until the patient is mobile.

▶ *First Aid for Fractures*

Laboratory Tests: None.

Therapeutic Measures: If a fracture is suspected, do not move the patient. Working with another person, splint the injured area as gently as possible. An air splint or a splint improvised from boards, rolled blankets, tools, newspapers, or magazines can be used. An improvised splint should be rigid enough to provide support and long enough to immobilize the joints above and below the injury. It should also be padded to ensure even contact and pressure on the limb and to protect bony prominences and/or wounds. Splint any dislocated joint as is—do not attempt reduction. Except for spinal injuries, splint malaligned bones after placing them in a position as close to normal as possible. To do this, grasp the affected limb gently but firmly, with one hand above and the other below the fracture location, and apply slight traction. As traction is being applied, have another person secure the splint. Arrange for immediate transportation to the nearest hospital.

Patient Education: Keep the patient as calm as possible. Describe any procedures as they are performed. Warn against undue manipulation of the fractured area to minimize the occurrence of fat embolism.

Follow-up: As needed.

▶ *General Measures for Mild to Moderate Sprains*

Laboratory Tests: None.

Therapeutic Measures: None.

Treatment Measures: Patients should refrain from the activity that initiated the sprain. They should apply ice to the injury for 15 minutes tid for the first 48 hours. Wherever feasible, apply an ace bandage, and elevate the injured area. If muscle spasm is present, prescribe Robaxin 750 mg or Flexeril 10 mg tid. Once swelling and pain have subsided, patients may find heat applied for 15 minutes tid more comfortable. Rehabilitation exercises should be used as necessary. The patient should return to full use of the injured area gradually.

Patient education: Use an anatomic drawing to explain sprains. Identify the location of the specific injury. Stress the importance of resting the area so that torn or stretched tissues can heal. Demonstrate prescribed rehabilitation exercises.

Follow-up: As needed. Refer patients with an unexpected course to an orthopedist.

▸ *Mild to Moderate Ankle Sprains*

Laboratory Tests: None.

Therapeutic Measures: Use general measures for sprains. Specific interventions are as follows:

First 48 hours: Immediately apply ice to the injured area for 20 minutes (ice whirlpool, crushed ice, or freeze pad). Reapply ice every 15 minutes tid. Following ice treatments, apply compression using an ace bandage or Unna boot (Medicopaste, Gelocast). Elevate the ankle above heart level as continuously as possible. Avoid weight bearing. If mobilization is necessary, use crutches.

Healing thereafter: After swelling and pain have subsided, apply heat for 15 minutes tid and begin gradual ambulation. Moderate sprains require ankle taping (with 1.5- or 2-in. adhesive tape) for continued compression and support.

Rehabilitation: Once the swelling and discoloration have resolved and the patient can bear weight without pain, begin the rehabilitation program. Give the patient a handout with instructions such as the following:

ANKLE REHABILITATION

1. Before starting strengthening exercises, do 5 minutes of stretching in all ranges of ankle motion tid for 1 or 2 days.
2. As long as pain or swelling does not recur, begin a daily routine of strengthening exercises. Sit on the edge of a high, stable bench or table with the knees bent and the feet swinging freely. Attach a 1-lb weight to the injured foot (ankle weights or a filled handbag may be used). For five repetitions each, evert, invert, and dorsiflex the foot. On the floor or stable bench, lie on the stomach and hang the weight over the ball of the foot. Flex the foot toward the ceiling five times. Gradually increase the number of repetitions for each exercise.
3. When you have worked up to 20 repetitions of each strengthening exercise, gradually resume sports activities. Tape the ankle or use an ankle support in the beginning.

Patient Education: Use an anatomical drawing to explain how prone ankle ligaments are to injury. Emphasize the importance of rehabilitation exercises in preventing chronic problems. Advocate use of properly fitted shoes that provide good foot and ankle support (high heels, clogs, and thongs should be avoided).

Follow-up: As needed. Refer patients in need for orthotics.

▸ *Gout*

Laboratory Tests: Uric acid levels. Definitive diagnosis depends on synovial fluid analysis.

Therapeutic Measures: Do not start, stop, or change therapy for hyperuricemia (can precipitate or worsen an attack). Prescribe Butazoladin 100 mg, 4 tablets to start followed by 1 tablet every 4 hours until the attack subsides (usually 4 days, never longer than 7 days) or indomethacin, 50 mg tid, until pain is tolerable (usually within 36 hours), then rapidly reduce and stop (usually in 3–5 days). An alternative therapy (although now rarely used) is colchicine 1 mg every 2 hours until pain subsides or signs of toxicity develop (nausea, diarrhea). The typical requirement is 4–8 mg. In addition to drugs, advise bed rest for 24–48 hours to minimize the chances of recurrence. Heat (or ice) and elevation of the affected joint may provide some relief.

Patient Education: Describe the disease process. Review medication use carefully, since toxicity is common.

Follow-up: Severe cases may require hospitalization for IV colchicine and IM pain medication. Reevaluate outpatients in 1–2 weeks. Start the treatment for hyperuricemia as necessary (see Chapter 8).

▸ *General Measures for RA*

Laboratory Tests: Joint x-ray films. CBC, ESR, rheumatoid factor, ANA. Synovial fluid analysis is helpful.

Therapeutic Measures

Rest: Complete bed rest during acute exacerbations and 2-hour rest periods daily for at least 2 weeks thereafter. Continue rest periods as needed.

Drugs: NSAI drugs as previously described. Consider adding indomethacin (Indocin) 50 mg at bedtime to relieve severe morning stiffness.

Physical therapy: In balance with rest requirements, start range-of-motion exercises designed to preserve joint motion and muscular strength. Radiant or moist heat (warm tub baths) preceding exercise periods usually produces a muscle-relaxing, analgesic effect. Some patients find that local application of cold packs relieves joint pain better than heat. As disease activity subsides and tolerance for exercise increases, introduce progressive resistance exercises. For a well-designed program containing specific instructions, request "Home Care Programs in Arthritis" from the Arthritis Foundation (see the following section for the address).

Splints: Splints are helpful for resting joints, reducing pain, and preventing contractures, but the type and use should be prescribed by a specialist. In general, the elbow and shoulder should not be splinted because frozen joints quickly develop in these regions. The hip and knee may be "splinted" by positioning alone (lying in a prone position for several hours a day on a firm bed). Prolonged sitting and the use of knee pillows have a negative effect.

Patient Education: Describe the pathophysiology of the disease. Emphasize that medications should be taken on a continuous basis during flareups, not only to relieve pain but to minimize inflammatory damage to joints. Stress the importance of proper rest and exercise. Teach patients the signs of drug side effects to be reported immediately.

Follow-up: Every 4 months and more often during exacerbations.

▸ *Arthritis Organizations*

Laboratory Tests: None.

Therapeutic Measures: None.

Patient Education: Arthritis Foundation
1314 Spring Street N.W.
Atlanta, Georgia 30326
Tel.: (404) 872-7100

Follow-up: As needed.

▸ *SLE Organizations*

Laboratory Tests: None.

Therapeutic Measures: None.

Patient Education: Lupus Foundation of America
11921A Olive Blvd.
St. Louis, Missouri
Tel.: (314) 872-9036

Follow-up: As needed.

▸ *Scleroderma Organizations*

Laboratory Tests: None.

Therapeutic Measures: None.

Patient Education: United Scleroderma Foundation
P.O. Box 724
Watsonville, California 95076

Follow-up: As needed.

▸ *Lyme Disease*

Laboratory Tests: Acute and convalescent (6 weeks after the onset of symptoms) titers for Lyme disease. Blood samples are being processed by the health departments of endemic states. Electrocardiogram if cardiac symptoms are present.

Therapeutic Measures: As soon as disease is suspected, start tetracycline, 500 mg qid, or penicillin V-K, 500 mg qid, for 10 days. Treat arthritis in the same manner as mild RA (see above).

Patient Education: Explain the disease process and transmission of the spirochete via deer tics. Inform patients that disease sequelae are self-limiting but may last for up to 5 years.

Follow-up: Hospitalization is required for patients with severe cases of encephalitis or cardiac complications. Other patients should be followed as needed.

▸ *General Measures for Osteoarthritis*

Laboratory Tests: Diagnosis based on joint x-ray films. ESR, rheumatoid factor analysis may be needed to rule out other cause of arthritis.

Therapeutic Measures

Exercise: Minimize occupational and recreational overuse of or trauma to affected joints. For example, patients with osteoarthritis of the knees should not jog and should limit stair climbing and prolonged standing. Active range-of-motion exercises and periodic stretching (e.g., getting up and moving around during commercials while watching TV) reduce the stiffness that follows periods of inactivity. Patients with osteoarthritis of the spine should be instructed on specific measures for posture, neck, and back care (see the sections on "Correct Posture," "Cervical Strain," and "Lumbar Strain").

Drugs: NSAI drugs given in analgesic or anti-inflammatory doses as described in a previous section.

Physical therapy: In addition to appropriate exercise, moist heat applied for 20 minutes four to six times daily usually produces a muscle-relaxing, analgesic effect. Some patients find that local application of cold packs relieves joint pain more effectively than heat.

Physical aids: Appliances to reduce the strain of weight bearing (braces, corsets, crutches, canes, walkers) can be helpful in certain cases, but the type and use should be prescribed by a specialist.

Diet: A well-balanced diet (no specific food contraindications). Weight control is important (due to decreased activity, most patients are overweight, which contributes to wear and tear on joints).

Patient Education: Explain the disease process, noting specifically the difference between osteoarthritis and a rheumatoid process. Stress the importance of therapeutic measures (particularly exercise guidelines), not only to prevent pain but also to minimize the progression of disease. Demonstrate exercises and the use of heat and cold. Review the side effects of prescribed drugs.

Follow-up: As needed. Patients with advanced joint degeneration should be referred to an orthopedist for surgical evaluation.

▸ *Carpal Tunnel Syndrome*

Laboratory Tests: Diagnosis can be made by the history and physical exam 95% of time. EMG may be needed to rule out (R/O) cervical root pressure.

Therapeutic Measures: The patient should splint the wrist at night. Unless the patient is pregnant, NSAI drugs (see the section "Use of NSAI Drugs") for 1–2 weeks and/or Lasix, 40 mg/day for 2–3 days can be given. If this does not work, give prednisone alone, 30 mg on day 1, 20 mg on day 2, and 10 mg on day 3.

Patient Education: Use an anatomic drawing to explain the problem. Review the associated causes. Give medication instructions.

Follow-up: Every 1–2 weeks for reevaluation and therapy change. If the above measures do not work, refer patients to an orthopedist for corticosteroid injections and/or surgical release.

▸ *Exercise Prescribing*

Laboratory Tests: Recommendations for asymptomatic patients are age related as follows:

Age	Recommended Tests
Under 30	None
30–39	Urine analysis, blood work,* resting EKG—repeat q2y
40–59	Urine analysis, blood work, resting and exercise EKG—repeat q2y
Over 59	Urine analysis, blood work, resting and exercise EKG—repeat yearly

Therapeutic Measures: History and physical exams as follows:

Age	Interval
Under 30	Once before starting (within the year)
30–59	Before starting (within 3 months) and q2y
Over 59	Before starting (within 3 months) and qy

The patient's history should concentrate on medication use and effort-related symptoms and the physical exam on cardiovascular, pulmonary, metabolic, and musculoskeletal function. Exclude patients with contraindications (Table 11.22) from exercise training. Refer patients with limiting factors to a professionally supervised program (e.g., YMCA, physical therapy department of a local hospital, cardiovascular fitness center). For all other patients, prescribe periods of an activity (one they enjoy) lasting for 30–40 minutes every day or every other day. Start patients at a level (intensity) of exercise that after 3 to 5 minutes results in a pulse rate of 60–85% of the maximum achieved on an exercise stress test. Five- to 10-minute rest periods may be needed in the beginning. Have patients continue at the beginning level for 4–8 weeks. If fitness improves, they may advance to a higher level. Provide a chart such as the following

*CBC, fasting SMAC (check glucose, cholesterol, triglycerides).

LEVELS OF FITNESS TRAINING*

Level	Activities
1	Walking (2–3 mph), outdoor bicycling (6 mph), stationary cycling (150–300 kpm), swimming using a kick board
2	Walking or jogging (4 mph), outdoor bicycling (8 mph), stationary cycling (450–600 kpm), swimming (treading water), light calisthenics
3	Walking or jogging (5 mph), outdoor bicycling (11–12 mph) stationary cycling (750–900 kpm), freestyle swimming (30 yd/min), tennis, badminton, hiking
4	Jogging or running (5.5–6 mph), outdoor bicycling (13 mph), stationary cycling (1,050 kpm), freestyle swimming (40 yd/min), vigorous calisthenics, rope jumping, cross-country skiing
5	Jogging or running (7 mph), stationary cycling (1,200 kpm), freestyle swimming (50 yd/min), basketball, soccer, handball, racquetball
6	Running, (8 mph), stationary cycling (1,500–1,650 kpm), freestyle swimming (50 yd/min), vigorous team sports (basketball, soccer, handball, racquetball) vigorous cross-country skiing or rope jumping
7	Running (10 mph), stationary cycling (1,800 kpm), trained athletic performance

*Patients with osteoarthritis of weight-bearing joints, osteoporosis, and postmenopausal women should limit vigorous exercise except for swimming.

Patient Education

Intensity of exercise: Teach patients to take their resting pulse (before exercise) by placing the fingertips of the right hand on the inside of the left wrist, counting the number of heartbeats for 15 seconds, and multiplying this number by 4. Instruct them to retake their pulse after 3 minutes of exercise and in the beginning to slow down if the pulse is more than 85% of the maximum achieved on the exercise stress test. With improved physical fitness, the pulse rate may approach but should not exceed 200 minus the age. Also inform patients to slow down whenever the intensity of exercise prevents easy talking or the ability to whistle (a sign of lactic acid accumulation) and to stop for any uncomfortable sensations, chest or stomach pain, cramps, or acute shortness of breath.

Warmup: Advise a brief warmup period to reduce musculoskeletal strain and prepare the cardiovascular system for the added workload. Give a handout with a sample 5-minute routine such as the following:

WARMUP EXERCISES

1. Stretch the arms, legs, and back (30 seconds each).
2. Do sit-ups with the knees bent (30 seconds).
3. Walk in a medium-sized circle at a fairly rapid pace (1 minute).
4. Alternate jogging/walking in a medium-sized circle (1 minute).
5. Jog at a very slow speed (1 minute).

Special considerations: Advise the use of good equipment (e.g., proper shoes and clothing, tuned bicycles). During warm weather, patients should exercise early in the morning or late in the afternoon. They should avoid prolonged exercise when temperatures exceed 80°F and humidity exceeds 75%. They should wear a face mask or mouth covering during extremely cold weather to warm the air entering the lungs. Road exercise at night or in inclement weather (rain, snow, ice) is ill-advised. Patients should refrain from smoking before exercise periods (for at least 1 hour). Replace the fluids, electrolytes, and calories expended during workouts.

Follow-up: As needed by the age groups for the history, physical exam, and laboratory tests.

▸ *Preventing Fall Injuries*

Laboratory Tests: None.

Therapeutic Measures: None.

Patient Education: Keep posted or provide handout information for patients such as the following:

Personal measures: Wear good, supportive shoes. Those with nonskid soles with low rubber heels and high ankle support are best. Keep laces properly tied. Shorten pants cuffs that are too long. Pace yourself. Be aware of your abilities and limitations. Ask for help whenever it is needed.

Floor space and walking surfaces: Take care when walking on floors that have been newly waxed but not buffed. Wipe up spills or wet spots on the floor immediately (use detergent or sawdust on oil and grease). Remove, skid-proof, or repair slippery, torn, or buckled rugs. Place nonskid treads in the tub and nonskid mats in the bathroom. Use caution when traversing areas with loose tiles, bricks, pavement, or floor boards or when descending steps. Avoid icy areas.

Obstacles: Keep unused articles properly stored, out of hallways and aisles and especially off stairs. Pick up toys, pencils, screws, and other small objects from the floor. Tape extension cords along baseboards. Avoid obstacle courses of furniture.

Repairs and projects: Keep your own flooring and steps well repaired and lighted. Sand or salt icy walkways. Always make proper use of a ladder to retrieve high objects or to engage in out-of-reach projects such as window washing.

Knowing the right way to fall: If you fall, the chances of injury can be reduced by (1) trying not to stiffen up and by (2) absorbing the impact with a spring-like action of the arms and legs or by rolling.

Follow-up: None.

▸ *Seat Belt Use and Motor Vehicle Safety*

Laboratory Tests: None.

Therapeutic Measures: Support actions and legislation regarding mandatory use of seat belts, car and road safety, emissions control, and drunk driving.

Patient Education: At the time of health maintenance visits, reinforce seat belt use. Review the definitions of illegal blood alcohol levels for drivers. Post charts that estimate the number of drinks and blood alcohol levels for each. Have on hand and demonstrate some of the over-the-counter devices that can be used to measure blood alcohol levels. Note the legal responsibility of hosts not to serve alcohol to underage persons and to prevent drunken guests from driving. Furthermore, urge drivers to do the following:

1. Keep windows, mirrors, and headlights clean. Wear sunglasses for high glare during the daytime but never at night. Views from windows and mirrors should be unobstructed.
2. Make sure that pets, children, and other passengers are properly restrained. Do not tolerate rowdy behavior in your car. Pack groceries, luggage, sports equipment, and so on securely.
3. Maintain your car in good running order, since breakdowns and/or faulty equipment are the source of many accidents. Do not run low on gas. Replace windshield wipers that streak. Keep the reservoir for windshield wiper fluid full. Repair any malfunction in the defrost system. Replace badly worn tires immediately, since they are prone to blowouts and provide inadequate traction. Have wheel alignment checked if the front tires are worn unevenly. Keep in the car at all times (a) a well-inflated spare tire and (b) an appropriate jack system in good working order. Check oil levels and replace oil according to the car owner's instructions. Replace fan belts every 4 years and frayed belts immediately. Also, replace dirty air filters. Keep the cooling system filled with appropriate antifreeze. Check the brake fluid level. Test brake function by keeping the accelerator depressed at 25 mph while applying steady pressure on the brakes. If the brakes are working properly, the car should come to and remain at a complete stop. Check for faulty shock absorbers (which are not only uncomfortable but dangerous) by pressing down on the bumper of the car. If the car bounces more than once, replace the shock absorbers. Keep safety flares and a working flashlight in the car at all times. Store the flares in the trunk or glove compartment, out of reach of children.

Follow-up: None.

BIBLIOGRAPHY

Aegerter E, Kirkpatrick JA Jr. *Orthopedic Diseases: Physiology, Pathology, Radiology*, 4th ed. Saunders, Philadelphia, 1975.

Agarwal A, Eisenbeis CH Jr. Office management of rheumatoid arthritis. *Family Practice Recertification*, (Oct.) 1979, 1(6):32–40.

Alcoff J, et al. Controlled trial of imipramine for chronic low back pain. *The Journal of Family Practice*, 1982, 14(5):841–846.

Altman R, Kaye J, McGinty JB. Arthroscopy/arthrography: When the knee needs a full evaluation. *Patient Care*, (Nov.) 1979, 20–38.

Amento EP. Skeletal problems associated with chest pain. *Chest Pain*, 6(5):1–8.

American Academy of Pediatrics. *Weight Training and Weight Lifting: Information for the Pediatrician.* AAP policy statement. July 1982.

American College of Sports Medicine. *The Recommended Quantity and Quality of Exercise for Developing and Maintaining Fitness in Healthy Adults.* ACSM position statement. Fall 1978.

American Heart Association (Committee on Exercise). *Exercise Testing and Training of Apparently Healthy Individuals: A Handbook for Physicians.* Dallas, 1972.

American Medical Association (Committee on Exercise and Physical Fitness). *Guide to Prescribing Exercise Programs.*

Baff SE, Weiss GB. Initial management of the common ankle sprain. *Physician Assistant and Health Practitioner*, (Nov.) 1982, 44–54.

Baker B. Manipulation for low back pain. *Aches and Pains*, (Aug.) 1983, 40–43.

Bates B. *A Guide to Physical Examination,* 3rd ed., Lippincott, Philadelphia, 1983.

Bayer AS. Nongonococcal bacterial septic arthritis: An update on diagnosis and management. *Postgraduate Medicine*, (Feb.) 1980, 67(2):157–165.

Bayer AS. Arthritis related to rubella: A complication of natural rubella and rubella immunization. *Postgraduate Medicine*, (May) 1980, 67(5):131–134.

Bayer AS. Arthritis associated with common viral infections: Mumps, coxsackievirus, and adenovirus. *Postgraduate Medicine*, (July) 1980, 68(1):55–64.

Beckenbaugh RD. Colles' fractures: A closer look. *Continuing Education*, (Dec.) 1980, 19–22.

Bergfeld JA, et al. Assessing and treating tennis elbow injuries. *PA Practice*, 1982, 1(2):15–17.

Bergfeld JA, et al. Managing carpal tunnel syndrome. *PA Practice*, 1983, 3–4.

Berkow RB (ed.). *The Merck Manual of Diagnosis and Therapy*, 14th ed. Merck Sharp & Dohme Research Laboratories, Rahway, N.J., 1982.

Bicknell JN. Nerve compression syndromes: Every active person is at risk. *Consultant*, (Feb.) 1982, 279–299.

Bluestone R. Physical diagnosis of rheumatic disease. *Consultant*, (Sept.) 1977, 66–73.

Bluestone R. Seronegative spondylarthropathies. *Hospital Practice*, (Oct.) 1979, 87–97.

Bogdonoff MD. Exercise as therapy: A burgeoning science. *Drug Therapy*, (Mar.) 1982, 52–54.

Bone scanning for stress fracture. *Emergency Medicine*, (Dec.) 1979, 49–52.

Brant KD, Fife RS. The diagnosis of osteoarthritis. *PA Practice*, 1983, 2(4):7–9.

Brewer EJ Jr, Nickeson RW Jr (with MD Lockshin, consulting ed.). Juvenile rheumatoid arthritis. *Physician Assistant and Health Practitioner*, (Mar.) 1981, 40–53.

Brody DM (KJ Bean, ed.). Running injuries. *Clinical Symposia*, 1980, 32(4):2–36.

Brown AM, Stubbs DW (eds.). *Medical Physiology*. Wiley, New York, 1983.

Bunch TW. Early therapy may increase strength, lessen discomfort when muscle weakness points to polymyositis. *The Journal of Musculoskeletal Medicine*, (May) 1984, 10–16.

Burkill ME. Rotator-cuff injuries and the acromial impingement syndrome. *PA Outlook*, (Nov.–Dec.) 1984, 2(6):7–12.

Cailliet R. Differential diagnosis: Examination of the shoulder. *Hospital Medicine*, (May) 1980, 26–31.

Calin A. Diagnosis, course, and management of Reiter's syndrome. *Continuing Education,* (June) 1982, 40–48.

Callen JP. Cutaneous manifestations of collagen-vascular disorders. *Continuing Education,* (Apr.) 1981, 31–39.

Chan DPK, Leung KYK. Managing RA of the cervical spine. *Consultant* (Mar.) 1980, 173–175.

Channing L. Bete Co., Inc. *How to Avoid Slips, Trips and Falls.* South Deerfield, Mass., 1982.

Clement DB, Taunton JE, Smart GW, et al. A survey of overuse running injuries. *The Physician and Sports Medicine,* (May) 1981, 9(5):47–58.

Conn HF, Conn RB Jr (eds.). *Current Diagnosis.* Saunders, Philadelphia, 1980.

Crafts RC. *A Textbook of Human Anatomy,* 3rd ed. Wiley, New York, 1985.

Crelin ES (IA Estler, ed.). Development of the musculoskeletal system. *Clinical Symposia,* 1981, 33(1):2–36.

Crouch JE, McClintic JR. *Human Anatomy and Physiology,* 2nd ed. Wiley, New York, 1976.

Delisa JA, Little J. Managing spasticity. *American Family Physician,* (Sept.) 1982, 26(3):117–122.

Delisa JA. Practical use of therapeutic physical modalities. *American Family Physician,* (May) 1983, 27(5):129–138.

Dembert ML. Lyme disease. *American Family Physician,* (June) 1982, 25(6):121–124.

Dietary phosphorus implicated in osteoporosis. *Hospital Practice,* (Dec.) 1981, 50–52.

Doody JB, Begley B. Juvenile rheumatoid arthritis. *PA Outlook,* (Oct.) 1983, 10–15.

Ebersold MJ. Neck injuries. *Continuing Education,* (May) 1982, 21–32.

Elias H, Pauly JE, Burns ER. *Histology and Human Microanatomy,* 4th ed. Wiley, New York, 1978.

Ellman MH, Neviaser RJ, Willkens RF. Nailing the elusive Dx in shoulder pain. (J Kent, ed.). *Patient Care,* (Mar.) 1985, 19:136–154.

Evens RP. Pharmacologic management of rheumatoid arthritis. *Therapeutics* (1981), 3–13.

Fager CA. Beware the quick fix for back pain. *Acute Care Medicine,* (June) 1984, 11–19.

Feagin J, Hlavac H, Miller HS, et al. Helpful hints for medical personnel treating joggers. *PA Practice,* 1982, 1(3):3–5.

Fischell T. Running and the primary prevention of coronary heart disease. *Cardiovascular Reviews and Reports,* (Mar.) 1981, 2(3):238–243.

Fletcher DJ. Exercise guidelines for the older patient. *Geriatric Consultant,* (Mar.–Apr.) 1984, 26–29.

Frame B. Vitamin D deficiency is not the only cause: Managing osteomalacia before deformities develop. *The Journal of Musculoskeletal Medicine,* (May) 1984, 19–30.

Franklin B, Rubenfine M. Losing weight through exercise. *Journal of the American Medical Association,* (July) 1980, 244(4):377–399.

Frary TN, Wessel A, Reimer L. Rhabdomyolysis and myoglobinuria: A report of five related cases. *Physician Assistant,* (Nov.) 1983, 90–102.

Fried JA, Bergfeld JA. The painful ankle: When to x-ray. *Hospital Medicine,* (Mar.) 1982, 106–123.

Friedman AP. Muscle contraction headache. *American Family Physician,* (Nov.) 1979, 20(5):109–113.

Friedman BJ, Knight K. Running for life, health, and pleasure. *American Journal of Nursing,* (Apr.) 1979, 602–607.

Friedman LW, Cassvan A. Guide to evaluation of low back pain and sciatica. *Hospital Medicine,* (June) 1980, 9–20.

Fuller E (staff ed.). Osteoarthritis, part I: What foreshadows osteoarthritis? *Patient Care*, (Feb.) 1981, 14–88.

Furst W, et al. Tetanus: Not too rare to be wary of. *PA Practice*, 1982, 1(2):1–3.

Geiderman JM, Dawson WJ. Diagnostic arthrocentesis: Indications and method. *Postgraduate Medicine*, (Aug.) 1979, 66(2):141–147.

Glass KD. Hand surgery: Why and when. Consultant, (Feb.) 1980, 71–85.

Gordan GS, Vaughn C. Osteoporosis: Early detection, prevention, and treatment. *Consultant*, (Jan.) 1980, 64–70.

Goroll AH, May LA, Mulley AG. *Primary Care Medicine: Office Evaluation and Management of the Adult Patient*. Lippincott, Philadelphia, 1981.

Graboys T. The economics of screening joggers. *New England Journal of Medicine*, (Nov.) 1979, 301(19):1067.

Gray H. *Anatomy of the Human Body*, 29th American ed. (CM Goss, ed.). Lea & Febiger, Philadelphia, 1973.

Greenberg M. The role of physical training in patients with coronary artery disease. *American Heart Journal*, (Apr.) 1979, 97(4):527–533.

Guyton AC. *Textbook of Medical Physiology*, 6th ed. Saunders, Philadelphia, 1981.

Hamilton WG (KJ Bean, ed.). Surgical anatomy of the foot and ankle. *Clinical Symposia*, 1985, 37(3):2–32.

Hanson PG, et al. Clinical guidelines for exercise training. *Postgraduate Medicine*, (Jan.) 1980, 67(1):120–138.

Harrell RM, Drezner MK. Postmenopausal and senile osteoporosis: A therapeutic dilemma. *PA Drug Update*, (Nov.) 1983, 25–38.

Harris ED. Decision points in the diagnosis and therapy of the rheumatic diseases (part I). *Continuing Education*, (June) 1981, 70–77.

Harris ED. Decision points in the diagnosis and therapy of the rheumatic diseases (part II). *Continuing Education*, (July) 1981, 104–109.

Hejna WF, Sinkora G. Chemonucleolysis of herniated lumbar discs. *American Family Physician*, (May) 1983, 27(5):97–103.

Hendrix PC, Malone T. Ankle sprains. *Physician Assistant and Health Practitioner*, (May) 1980, 22–29.

Hendrix PC, Malone T. Immediate care of soft tissue injuries. *Physician Assistant and Health Practitioner*, (Oct.) 1980, 63–69.

Hendrix PC, et al. Tennis elbow. *Physician Assistant and Health Practitioner*, (Sept.) 1980, 28–34.

Ho G Jr, Tice AD. Comparison of nonseptic and septic bursitis: Further observations on the treatment of septic bursitis. *Archives of Internal Medicine*, (Nov.) 1979, 139:1269–1273.

Hoffman GS. Tendinitis and bursitis. *American Family Physician*, (June) 1981, 23(6):103–110.

Hollander JL. Osteoarthritis: Perspectives on treatment. *Postgraduate Medicine*, (Nov.) 1980, 68(5):161–168.

Hoole AJ, Greenberg RA, Pickard CG Jr. *Patient Care Guidelines for Nurse Practitioners*. Little, Brown, Boston, 1982.

Horwitz CA. Laboratory diagnosis of rheumatoid diseases. *Postgraduate Medicine*, (May) 1980, 67(5):193–200.

Idzikowski JR. Meniscal disorders of the knee. *Physician Assistant and Health Practitioner*, (Feb.) 1983, 126–140.

Immunization today. *Emergency Medicine*, (Nov.) 1980, 72–77.

Isselbacher KJ, et al. *Harrison's Principles of Internal Medicine*, 9th ed. McGraw-Hill, New York, 1980.

Iversen LD, Clawson DK. *Manual of Acute Orthopaedic Therapeutics.* Little, Brown, Boston, 1977.

Jacobs B. *Low Back Pain.* American Academy of Family Physicians. Kansas City, Mo., Oct. 1978.

Jacobs R. Reiter's syndrome. *Drug Therapy,* (Aug.) 1983, 135–142.

Jones HR Jr (AH Trench, ed.). Diseases of the peripheral motor-sensory unit. *Clinical Symposia,* 1985, 37(2):2–32.

Kantor TG. Selecting the appropriate NSAID. *PA Drug Update,* (June) 1984, 44–50.

Kaplan FS (AH Trench, ed.). Osteoporosis. *Clinical Symposia,* 1983, 35(5):2–32.

Keene JS. Low back pain in the athlete from spondylogenic injury during recreation or competition. *Postgraduate Medicine,* (Dec.) 1983, 75(6):209–217.

Keim HA. Idiopathic scoliosis. *Myology,* 1978, 3(3):3–10.

Kelley WN, et al. *Textbook of Rheumatology,* Vols. I and II. Saunders, Philadelphia, 1981.

Khachadurian AK. Hyperuricemia and gout: An update. *American Family Physician,* (Dec.) 1981, 24(6):143–148.

Kornfeld P. Does the weakness stem from myasthenia? *Diagnosis,* (Oct.) 1983, 57–72.

Kraus H, Nagler W. Evaluation of an exercise program for back pain. *American Family Physician,* (Sept.) 1983, 28(3):153–158.

Krupp MA, Chatton MJ, Werdegar D (eds.). *Current Medical Diagnosis and Treatment 1985.* Lange, Los Altos, Calif., 1985.

Kurland RL, Pritchard DJ. Sprains of the lateral ankle ligaments. *Continuing Education,* (Dec.) 1980, 56–68.

Leitch CJ, Tinker RV. *Primary Care.* Davis, Philadelphia, 1978.

Levine AM. Spinal orthoses. *American Family Physician,* Mar. 1984, 29(3):277–280.

Levine I. Office surgery: Repairing the injured fingertip. *Patient Care,* (Oct.) 1977, 164–184.

Liederbach M. Sports medicine in action: A primer on aerobic dance. *Muscle and Bone,* 1983, 3(4):3–11.

Lightfoot RW Jr. Therapy of rheumatoid disease. *American Family Physician,* (Mar.) 1979, 19(3):186–196.

Litt JZ. Lupus erythematosus. *Cross Section,* 1982, 10(2):4–9.

Luckmann J, Sorensen KC. *Medical Surgical Nursing: A Psychophysiologic Approach,* 2nd ed. Saunders, Philadelphia, 1980.

Lyme disease: Spirochetes up to old ticks? *Journal of American Medical Association,* (Aug.) 1982, 248(7):812–813.

Marks JS. Early recognition of rheumatoid cervical myelopathy. *Internal Medicine for the Specialist,* (Apr.) 1984, 5(4):91–95.

Matsen FA. Compartmental syndromes. *Hospital Practice,* (Feb.) 1980, 113–117.

McIntosh H. Jogging thou shalt not kill (thyself). *Journal of the American Medical Association,* (June) 1979, 241(23):2547–2548.

McMicken DB. After the emergency. *Emergency Medicine,* (Apr.) 1979, 11:63.

McNeil Laboratories, Inc. *How to Get Along with Your Back.* Fort Washington, Pa.

Milhorn HT. Cardiovascular fitness. *American Family Physician,* (Sept.) 1982, 26(3):163–169.

Milvy P, Siegel AJ. Physical activity levels and altered mortality from coronary heart disease with an emphasis on marathon running: A critical review. *Cardiovascular Reviews and Reports,* (Mar.) 1981, 2(3):233–236.

Moskowitz RW. Management of osteoarthritis. *Hospital Practice,* (July) 1979, 75–87.

Muir BL. *Pathophysiology: An Introduction to the Mechanisms of Disease.* Wiley, New York, 1980.

Munsey WF. Foot problems in the overweight. *Postgraduate Medicine*, (Jan.) 1981, 69(1):33.

New tactics in the war on tetanus. *Emergency Medicine*, (Mar.) 1981, 73–78.

New York State Department of Health. *Walking: A Step in the Right Direction*. New York, May 1982.

Paffenbarger R, Hyde RT. Exercise as protection against heart attack. *New England Journal of Medicine*, (May) 1980, 302(18):1026–1027.

Patten BM. Inflammatory myopathy: A disease often missed. *Consultant*, (Feb.) 1980, 46–55.

Paulson JC, Beckenbauch RD. Rotator cuff tears. *Continuing Education*, (Dec.) 1980, 27–30.

Payne FE. A practical approach to effective exercises. *American Family Physician*, (June) 1979, 19(6):76–81.

Perlow NK (ed.). *Emergency First Aid for the Home*. Globe Communications Corp., Woodbridge, N.J., 1984.

Physical exercise and your health. *Physician Assistant and Health Practitioner*, (May) 1981, 77–78.

Pickering TG. Exercise and the prevention of coronary heart disease. *Cardiovascular Reviews and Reports*, (Mar.) 1981, 2(3):227–229.

Piper F. Guidelines for exercise prescribing. *Physician Assistant and Health Practitioner*, (May) 1981, 68–74.

Pisetsky DS. Treating arthritis in elderly patients. *PA Drug Update*, (Aug.) 1983, 26–36.

Polley HF, Hunder GG. *Rheumatologic Interviewing and Physical Examination of the Joints*. Saunders, Philadelphia, 1978.

Raffel GE. Fat emboli syndrome. *Physician Assistant and Health Practitioner*, (Sept.) 1982, 59–64.

Ramirez LF, Javid MJ. Chymopapain: A new alternative for herniated discs. *Drug Therapy*, (Mar.) 1984, 169–181.

Reid EL, Morgan RW. Exercise prescription: A clinical trial. *American Journal of Public Health*, (June) 1979, 69(6):591–595.

Roy S. How I manage plantar fasciitis. *The Physician and Sports Medicine*, (Oct.) 1983, 11(10):127–131.

Sager K. Senior fitness: For the health of it. *The Physician and Sports Medicine*, (Oct.) 1983, 11(10):31–36.

Sandzen SC Jr. Carpal tunnel syndrome. *American Family Physician*, (Nov.) 1981, 24(5):190–204.

Saunders EA. Ligamentous injuries of the ankle. *American Family Physician*, (Aug.) 1980, 22(2):132–138.

Schaller JG. Juvenile rheumatoid arthritis. *Pediatric Annals*, (Apr.) 1982, 11(4):375–380.

Schering Corporation. *Your Back and How to Care for It*. Pub. No. CE-473-11.74. Kenilworth, N.J., Nov. 1974.

Schurmann L. "Washerwoman's sprain": Working woman's pain. *Aches and Pains*, (Feb.) 1984, 14–20.

Schwartz GR, et al. *Principles and Practice of Emergency Medicine*, Vols. I and II. Saunders, Philadelphia, 1978.

Scott WR. Advances in myelography. *Continuing Education*, (Mar.) 1980, 43–48.

Seybold ME. Myasthenia gravis: A clinical and basic science review. *Journal of the American Medical Association*, (Nov.) 1983, 250(18):2516–2520.

Sheehan NJ, Mathews JA. Options for treating low back pain. *Drug Therapy*, (Mar.) 1983, 153–160.

Shellock FG. Physiological benefits of warm-up. *The Physician and Sports Medicine*, (Oct.) 1983, 11(10):134–138.

Sheon RP. Regional soft tissue rheumatic pain syndromes: A common challenge in daily practice. *Postgraduate Medicine*, (Nov.) 1980, 68(5):143–156.

Shephard RJ. Testing for fitness in the routine physical. *Diagnosis*, (Jan.) 1984, 157–172.

Sherman C. Managing pain in arthritis. *Aches and Pains*, (Feb.) 1984, 8–13.

Siegel IM. Muscular dystrophy: Multidisciplinary approach to management. *Postgraduate Medicine*, (Feb.) 1981, 69(2):124–133.

Silverstein A. *Human Anatomy and Physiology*. Wiley, New York, 1980.

Singer K. Knee pain: Diagnosis and management. *Myology*, Spring 1977, 2(2):3–11.

Skosey JL. Polyarthritis: How to select the right tests. *Consultant*, (Nov.) 1979, 45–56.

Staheli LT. Spinal deformity. *The Journal of Family Practice*, 1980, 10(6):1071–1075.

Steere AC, et al. Antibiotic therapy in Lyme disease. *Annals of Internal Medicine*, (July) 1980, 93(1):1–8.

Stein MD. Differentiating hip pain. *Aches and Pains*, (Feb.) 1984, 23–26.

Swezey RL. Rheumatoid arthritis: Long-range tips for a long-term problem. *Modern Medicine*, (Mar.) 1981, 44–52.

The checkout before the workout. *Transition*, (June) 1983, 36–43.

Trentham DE. Brief guide to office counseling: Gonococcal arthritis. *Medical Aspects of Human Sexuality*, (Mar.) 1982, 6(3):119–123.

Upton J, Littler JW, Eaton RG. Primary care of the injured hand, part 1. *Postgraduate Medicine*, (Aug.) 1979, 66(2):115–122.

Upton J, Littler JW, Eaton RG. Primary care of the injured hand, part 2. *Postgraduate Medicine*, (Aug.) 1979, 66(2):127–131.

U.S. Department of Transportation. *The Automobile Safety Belt Fact Book*. Pub. No. DOT-HS-802-157. Washington, D.C., May 1982.

U.S. Department of Transportation. *Safety Belt Fact Sheet*. Washington, D.C.,

U.S. Department of Transportation. *Safety Belts: A History Lesson for Adults*. Pub. No. DOT-HS-806-175. Washington, D.C., May 1982.

Varied regimens in RA and pseudogout evaluated. *Hospital Practice*, (Aug.) 1980, 44d–44k.

Walsh WM. Common shoulder ailments. *Continuing Education*, (Oct.) 1981, 62–72.

Ward PCJ. Interpretation of synovial fluid data. *Postgraduate Medicine*, (Sept.) 1980, 68(3):175–184.

Waterson M. Hot and cold therapy. *Nursing 78*, (Oct.) 1978, 46–49.

Weinberger AB. Scleroderma (systemic sclerosis): Part II. *Clinical Rheumatology*, (May–June) 1984, 102–128.

Weissman BN, Fingerg HJ. Radiography of the cervical spine for RA patients. *Consultant*, (Mar.) 1980, 179–186.

Whitman HH III, Case DB. New developments in the treatment of scleroderma. *Drug Therapy*, (Dec.) 1981, 97–104.

Williams GO. Management of spinal cord injury. *The Journal of Family Practice*, 1981, 12(2):231–237.

Williams RH. *Textbook of Endocrinology*, 5th ed. Saunders, Philadelphia, 1974.

Wyngaarden JB, Smith LH Jr (eds.). *Cecil Textbook of Medicine*, 16th ed., Vols. 1 and 2. Saunders, Philadelphia, 1982.

Yager MC, Ellison AE. Diagnosis and management of stress fractures. *Physician Assistant and Health Practitioner*, (Mar.) 1983, 16–22.

Yunus M, et al. Primary fibromyalgia. *American Family Physician*, (May) 1982, 25(5):115–121.

12

Central Nervous System and Hormone Control

Judy Barrigar-Hornibrook and Ellen Rich

Outline

- Sleep paralysis
- Hypnogogic hallucinations
- Sleep apneas (upper airway, central, mixed)
- Night terrors (nightmares)
- Dream anxiety attacks
- ► Sleep disorders organizations

Basal Ganglia

- Parkinson's disease
- ► Supportive care for Parkinson's disease
- ► Parkinson's disease organizations
- Drug-induced Parkinson's disease
- Huntington's chorea
- Essential tremor
- Senile tremor

Thalamus, Hypothalamus, Pituitary Gland, and Sympathetic and Parasympathetic Control

Cerebrospinal Fluid and Ventricular System

- Intracranial hypertension
- Hydrocephalus
- Pseudotumor cerebri

Vascular System

- Vascular headaches
- ► Classic migraine headache
- Migraine variations (common, basilar artery, ophthalmoplegic, hemiplegic)
- ► Cluster headaches
- Acute muscle contraction headache
- ► Chronic muscle contraction headache
- Cerebrovascular disease
- Cerebrovascular accident (CVA) (thrombosis, embolism, septic embolism)
- Transient ischemic attack (TIA)
- Intracranial hemorrhage
- Aneurysm rupture
- Subarachnoid hemorrhage

Protective Features (Skull, Meninges, and Blood–Brain Barrier)

- CNS injuries and infections
- Head injury
- Skull fracture (linear, comminuted, basilar, compound)
- Concussion
- Postconcussion syndrome
- Epidural hematoma
- Subdural hematoma
- Intracerebral hematoma
- Bacterial meningitis
- Viral (aseptic) meningitis
- Viral encephalitis
- St. Louis encephalitis
- Herpes encephalitis
- Brain abscess
- Rabies
- ► Antirabies measures
- Metabolic encephalopathy

HORMONE CONTROL

Hypothalamus and Pituitary

- Pituitary deficiency
- Pituitary dwarfism
- Psychosocial dwarfism
- Hypopituitarism in the adult
- Diabetes insipidus (DI)
- Hyperpituitarism
- Acromegaly
- Pituitary tumors
- Empty sella syndrome

Thyroid

- Hypothyroidism
- Cretinism
- ► Hypothyroidism in the adult
- Myxedema
- Myxedema madness
- Hyperthyroidism
- Graves' disease
- Thyroid storm
- Thyroiditis
- Hashimoto's thyroiditis
- Thyroid nodules and masses
- Goiter (endemic, sporadic)
- Thyroid carcinoma

Adrenals

- Addison's disease
- Adrenal cortical insufficiency
- Cushing's syndrome
- Natural Cushing's syndrome
- Iatrogenic Cushing's syndrome
- Primary aldosteronism

Conn's syndrome
Pheochromocytoma
Paraganglioma

Parathyroid Glands

Hyperparathyroidism
Primary hyperparathyroidism
Hypercalcemia
Hypoparathyroidism (surgical, idiopathic, functional, pseudohypoparathyroidism)
Hypocalcemia

BRAIN

Brain Tissues

The neuron (nerve cell) is the fundamental unit of the brain. There are four types. Motor (afferent) neurons send impulses to various parts of the body to initiate glandular activity and muscle contraction. Because of their distinctive shape, they are also referred to as "pyramidal cells." Sensory (efferent) neurons receive temperature, pressure, and pain sensations from the body and send them to the brain for interpretation. Cortical neurons interpret and store information for intellectual and emotional function, while internuncial neurons relay impulses. As illustrated in Figure 12.1, each neuron consists of a cell body and one or more processes known as "nerve fibers" (axons or dendrites). Dendrites receive impulses and conduct them toward the cell body; axons carry impulses away from the cell body. The main components of the cell body are the cytoplasm, made up of fats, carbohydrates, proteins, electrolytes, enzymes, organic salts, and water; the mitochondria, which secure energy from nutrients and oxygen and store it; and the nucleus, which controls the metabolic processes of the cell. Cell bodies are arranged in either cortical layers or relay centers called "nuclei." They form areas of the brain and spinal cord known as "gray matter." Some cell bodies have long axons covered with a layer of white fatty material called the "myelin sheath." Concentrations of these myelin-covered fibers form areas of white matter. Characteristic structures of gray and white matter constitute the various parts of the brain such as the cerebrum, basal ganglia, and medulla, illustrated in Figure 12.2 and discussed in later sections.

Neurons interpret and classify incoming stimuli from the body (chemical, electrical, mechanical, or thermal) and then either store the information for future reference or act upon it immediately. This is done through impulse transmission as follows. Because the cell membrane of the neuron is permeable only to certain substances, changes in intracellular-extracellular fluid electrical charges are possible. The main components of the intracellular fluid are chloride, potassium, and sodium ions and protein. The major extracellular ions are sodium, potassium, and chloride. Two ions, potassium and sodium, move across the cellular membrane. Potassium ions (K^+), found in large numbers intracellularly, readily traverse the cell membrane. Sodium ions (Na^+), the largest constituent of the extracellular fluid, can also cross the cell membrane, but an active transport system is needed for their movement.

When a cell is at rest (resting potential), the extracellular fluid contains more positively charged ions than does the intracellular fluid. When a stimulus of sufficient intensity stimulates the cell, depolarization occurs at the site of the stimulus. Figure 12.3 shows the sequence of changes along the axon as the impulse is transmitted. Sodium ions enter the axon of the cell at that segment. When this occurs, potassium ions leave in order for a positive-negative intracellular-extracellular ratio

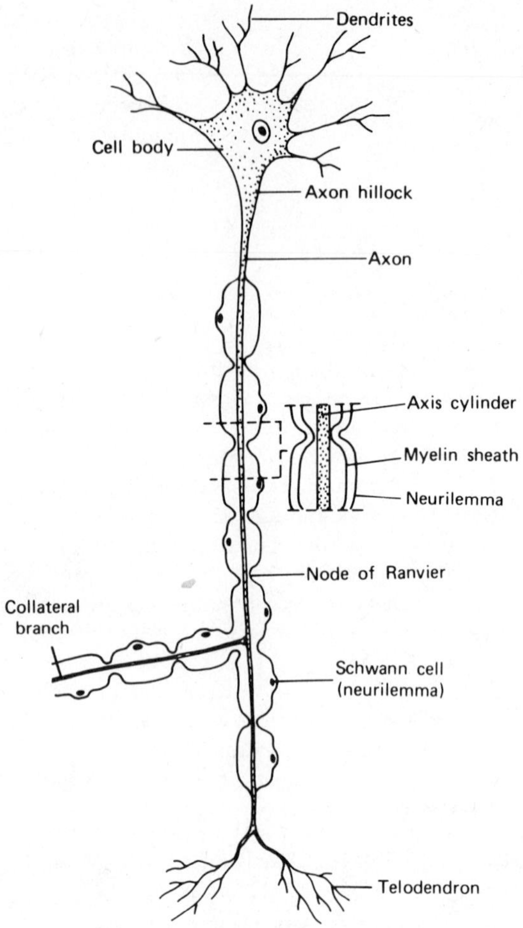

Figure 12.1 Typical motor neuron. (From Snyder, M, *A Guide to Neurological and Neurosurgical Nursing,* © 1983, John Wiley and Sons, Inc., New York.)

to be maintained. To return the segment of the cell to its prestimulus state, the sodium ions leave the cell assisted by a mechanism called the "sodium pump." Potassium ions then freely reenter the cell. Repetition of this process propagates the impulse along the axon. Synapses are essential in the transmission of impulses. Figure 12.4 shows a synapse. Note the relationships of its structures. Impulses may be transmitted across the synapse by either electrical or chemical processes, the latter being more common. A transmitter substance is released, diffuses across the synaptic gap, and changes the permeability of the cell membrane of the adjoining cell. Acetylcholine is the chief neurotransmitter. Other transmitter substances currently known are epinephrine, gamma-aminobutyric acid, glutamic acid, dopamine, and serotonin. The type of transmitter substance varies according to the area of the nervous system.

After one impulse has been transmitted, a time interval must elapse before the

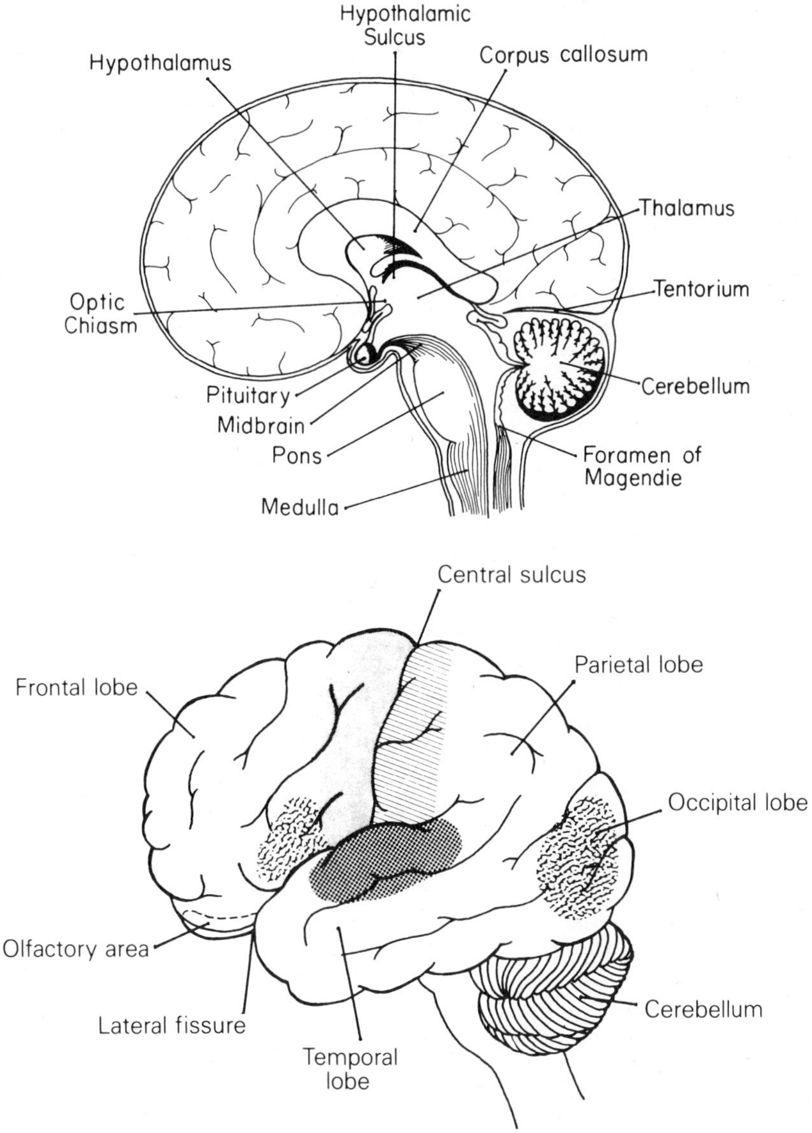

Figure 12.2 Parts of the brain. (From Snyder, M, *A Guide to Neurological and Neurosurgical Nursing,* © 1983, John Wiley and Sons, Inc., New York.)

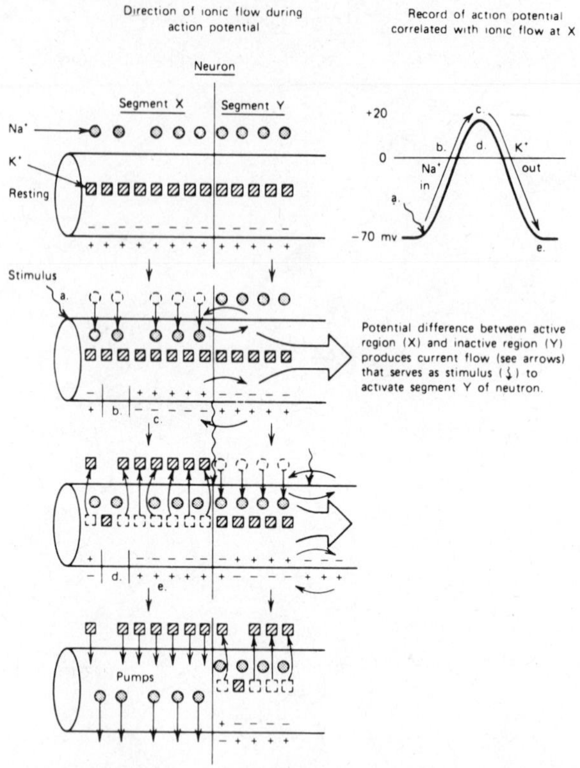

Figure 12.3 Action potential of a nerve cell. (From Snyder, M, *A Guide to Neurological and Neurosurgical Nursing,* © 1983, John Wiley and Sons, Inc., New York.)

neuron is capable of transmitting a second impulse; this interval is called the "refractory period." During the absolute refractory period, no impulse is capable of stimulating the cell. In the relative refractory period, an impulse of greater intensity than usual is required. The speed of transmission and length of refractory periods vary, depending on the diameter of the axon and the presence or absence of a myelin sheath. Large myelinated neurons conduct impulses the fastest.

Damage to or destruction of the myelin sheath can result from genetic or developmental failure ***(dymyelinating disease).*** More often, however, myelin forms normally but breaks down later in life. ***Multiple sclerosis (MS),*** the most common demyelinating disease, is 3 to almost 30 times more prevalent in northern (the United States and Europe) than in southern latitudes. Women are affected more often than men. Approximately 67% of cases begin between the ages of 20 and 40 years and 95% between 10 and 50 years. The average life expectancy for all patients is about 35 years after onset. Most patients are able to continue working, although occasional absences due to exacerbation of the disease can be expected. The etiology of MS has not been identified with certainty, since intensive research activity over the past several years has produced contradictory and controversial results. Several factors, however, have been indicated including allergy, immunologic abnormalities, genetic susceptibility and viruses. An infection of some type (i.e., upper respiratory

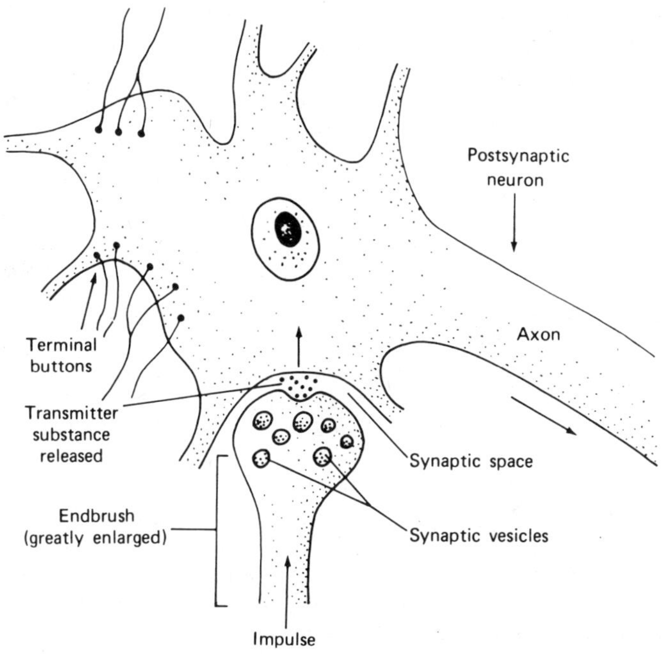

Figure 12.4 Structure of a synapse. (From Snyder, M, *A Guide to Neurological and Neurosurgical Nursing,* © 1983, John Wiley and Sons, Inc., New York.)

infection, influenza, urinary tract infection, gastroenteritis) precedes an initial attack or relapse in 10–40% of patients with MS. The onset of MS may be acute, with the appearance of symptoms within minutes or hours, or subtle, with symptoms gradually progressing over months. Most of these symptoms reflect involvement of the myelin in the central nervous system (CNS), but occasionally when nerve cell bodies are damaged, more serious signs (seizures, aphasia, neurogenic atrophy) are manifested. The clinical course of MS is characterized by exacerbations and remissions over a period of years. Neurologic deficits increase as lesions disseminate. Spinal nerve involvement is characterized by weakness of the lower extremities, spasticity, hyperreflexia, and pathologic reflexes. Total paralysis of a limb may be present. Urinary complaints such as frequency and urgency are common. Visual complaints (blurring, decreased acuity), cranial nerve signs, nystagmus, vertigo, and incoordination are prominent symptoms when the brain stem and cerebellum are affected.

Exclusion of other neurologic disorders such as vascular disease, degenerative disorders, and spinal cord, brain stem, or cerebellar tumors is essential in the diagnosis of MS (see discussions of associated disorders). Patients suspected of having MS should be referred to a specialist for a complete neurologic work-up and spinal tap. Abnormalities of the cerebrospinal fluid are reliable confirmations of pathology. They include increased IgG levels, the presence of discrete bands of IgG (oligoclonal bands) on protein electrophoresis, and mild lymphocytosis. Other diagnostic studies of value are computed tomography (CT) scans and evoked response potentials. Therapy to alter the course of MS is currently unsatisfactory. There is some evidence that adrenocorticosteroids or adrenocorticotropic hormone (ACTH) injections shorten the duration of acute exacerbations, but the treatments have no effect on the long-term outcome of the disease. The more important treatment task, however, is the management of MS-related disabilities. Pharmacologic agents may be administered to control spasticity and tremors. Medication, surgery, or intermittent daily catheterization avoids the collection of large amounts of residual urine and helps to prevent infection. Counseling about sexual problems, financial concerns, and physical disability will increase the patient's emotional security. ▶ ***MS organizations*** are valuable resources.

Vitamin B_{12} deficiency can lead to demyelinization of both sensory and motor neurons. Symptoms include symmetric numbness and tingling of the lower extremities, ataxia, mental disturbances, and loss of the vibration sense and deep reflexes. Unless it is corrected at an early stage, this vitamin deficiency can lead to permanent neurologic deficits. The problem is discussed at length in Chapter 7.

Neurons are supported by a special kind of connective tissue called "glia" ("neuroglia"). Outnumbering neurons by 10 to 1, glial cells include astrocytes, oligodendrocytes, ependymal cells, and microglial cells. Each has a special function described in Table 12.1.

Unlike neurons, glial cells and other types of brain tissue are capable of mitosis and thus are prone to neoplastic changes. Various types of ***intracranial tumors*** are detailed in Table 12.2. Most of them are characterized by insidious onset and progression of focal or general neurologic signs or both. Symptoms vary according to the type of tumor, its location, and its rate of growth. Common manifestations are headache, mental changes, speech, vision, and sensory disturbances, motor deficits, nausea and vomiting, seizures, stiff neck, and vasomotor and autonomic changes. Patients suspected of having intracranial tumor should be referred to a neurologist. Systemic and other cerebral disease must be ruled out. Skull x-ray films, electroencephalogram (EEG), cerebrospinal fluid (CSF) examination, CT scanning, and contrast and isotope studies will confirm the presence of a tumor and define its location and size. Most tumors can be surgically removed. Radiotherapy and chemotherapy are employed in conjunction with or as an alternative to surgery. Meningiomas, osteomas, neurofibromas, and pituitary tumors are nonmalignant and involve the least sacrifice of normal cerebral tissue. However, some of the gliomas are highly malignant and infiltrate brain tissue extensively. Often bilateral and sometimes extending into the ventricles and meninges, glioblastomas can reach enormous size

TABLE 12.1 FUNCTIONS OF NEUROLOGICAL CELLS

Type	Function
Astrocyte cells	Provide structural support Regulate the chemical environment of neurons Help nourish neurons
Oligodendrocyte cells	Myelin sheath for covering axons of cells in CNS
Ependymal cells	Line ventricles of the brain and central canal of the spinal cord; secretory and absorptive functions
Microglial cells	Phagocytosis

Source: M. Snyder (ed.), *A Guide to Neurological and Neurosurgical Nursing.* Copyright, 1983, John Wiley & Sons, New York. Used with permission.

TABLE 12.2 TYPES OF INTRACRANIAL TUMORS

Type	Description
Gliomas	
Astrocytoma	Composed of astrocytes; generally slow-growing; invasiveness may prevent complete removal by surgical excision; if enough is removed, prognosis is good; rarely, develops into highly malignant glioblastoma; most common in adults over 30 years of age
Ependymoma	Composed of ependymal cells; arises in the walls of the ventricles, filling and obstructing them, and eventually invades adjacent tissue; prognosis is poor; death usually occurs within 3 years of onset
Glioblastoma	Composed of very undifferentiated cells; most malignant glioma; very rapid growth; leads to tissue necrosis and is accompanied by brain edema; is usually located in cerebral hemispheres, is widely infiltrative, and may involve multiple lobes; complete surgical excision is impossible; prognosis is poor; death usually occurs within 6 months of onset
Medulloblastoma	Develops from primitive cells in the cerebellum; is highly malignant and frequently metastasizes to involve the cerebellum and spinal cord through the subarachnoid space; chiefly a tumor of childhood, but may occur in older patients
Oligodendroglioma	Composed of oligodendroglial cells; is similar to astrocytoma
Meningioma	Grows entirely outside the brain; is attached to the meninges; well encapsulated and highly vascularized, and may be calcified; most benign brain tumor, since it does not invade the brain; is often multiple; produces symptoms by compressing and distorting the brain; seizures frequently occur; not uncommon for tumor to erode overlying bone; complete surgical removal prevents recurrence
Pituitary adenoma	Arises from chromophobe, eosinophil, or basal cells
Chromophobe	Most common; produces symptoms by compressing the normal pituitary gland, optic chiasm, hypothalamus, and adjacent brain tissue
Eosinophilic	Symptoms are hyperpituitarism, acromegaly in adults, and giantism in children; does not generally compress
Basophilic	Is small; associated with Cushing's syndrome; does not compress
Acoustic neuroma	Benign neurofibroma of the eighth cranial nerve; arises within the internal auditory meatus; produces erosion and canal widening; progressive unilateral hearing loss, tinnitus, gait instability, hand clumsiness; is occasionally bilateral; treatment consists of surgical excision
Adnexal tumors	Include those originating in the pineal body and choroid plexus; rare; compression of ventricles leads to obstructive hydrocephalus; involvement of the pretectum of the midbrian leads to paralysis of vertical gaze; compression of the hypothalamus leads to precocious puberty or DI
Metastatic disease	Usually the result of primary tumors of the lung and breast, malignant melanomas, hypernephromas, and intestinal carcinomas; lesions are usually multiple

before being discovered. In such cases the prognosis is poor, with an average survival time of less than 6 months after diagnosis. On the other hand, tumors that can be totally excised usually do not recur.

Cerebrum

The cerebrum is divided into hemispheres, each containing five lobes: frontal, parietal, temporal, occipital, and limbic (see Fig. 12.2). Landmarks for delineating the boundaries of the lobes are shown. The cental sulcus (fissure of Rolando) separates

TABLE 12.3 DIVISIONS OF THE CEREBRUM

Division	Function
Frontal lobe—prefrontal area	Foresight Abstract thinking Judgment
Frontal lobe—prerolandic	Voluntary motor movement
Temporal lobe	Memory Visual association area Auditory association area
Parietal lobe	Recognition of pain, temperature, pressure, positions of body and limbs Body image
Occipital lobe	Vision
Limbic lobe (including cingulate gyrus, isthmus, parahippocampal gyrus, and uncus)	Emotions Drives Basic survival functions

Source: M. Snyder (ed.), *A Guide to Neurological and Neurosurgical Nursing.* Copyright, 1983, John Wiley & Sons, New York. Used with permission.

the frontal lobe from the parietal lobe. The temporal lobe is demarcated from the frontal lobe by the lateral fissure, or fissure of Sylvius. The parieto-occipital fissure separates the parietal lobe from the occipital lobe. Table 12.3 lists the specific functions of each cerebral lobe.

Functions of the right side of the body are mediated by the left cerebral hemisphere, and functions of the left side of the body are controlled by the right cerebral hemisphere. The term for this phenomenon is "contralateral control." Fibers to and from each hemisphere cross to the opposite side at various levels within the CNS.

Because their neurons are especially sensitive to biochemical changes, certain areas of the cerebrum are highly prone to seizure activity. They include the motor cortex, structures within the limbic system, amygdala, and hippocampus (nuclear aggregates within the parietal lobes). In the case of ***epilepsy,*** cell membranes remain in a chronic state of partial depolarization and increased permeability. This failure to recover after excitation is probably the result of sodium and potassium imbalances, although a disturbance of neurotransmitter function has been suggested in the pathogenesis of epilepsy. Sudden, excessive, and disorderly discharges from aggregates of these abnormally excitable neurons travel along neural pathways to normal cortical or spinal areas. Instantaneous disturbances of sensation, loss of consciousness, and convulsive movements, singly or in combination, result. Epileptic seizures are classified according to their focus of onset, clinical manifestations, and electroencephalographic changes. Table 12.4 presents the international classification of the epilepsies and their descriptions. Affecting approximately 2 million people in the United States, epileptic seizures can begin at any age, though 70–80% of patients experience their first episode before age 20. Seizures may occur many times daily or very infrequently. Episodes may be more frequent several days prior to a woman's menses. Pregnancy may increase or decrease their frequency. Nocturnal seizures are found in 20% of persons with epilepsy.

Symptomatic or ***acquired epilepsy*** can be linked to identifiable causes. Congenital malformation, prematurity, maternal infection (particularly rubella) or drug

TABLE 12.4 TYPES OF SEIZURES

Type	Age of Onset	Description	EEG Manifestations
Partial seizures	Ages 5–20 and older		
Simple partial seizures with motor signs		Focal motor symptoms with or without a march, turning of head or body, loss of posture, loss of speech	Unilateral spike or slow-wave discharge or both during seizures; local contralateral discharge between seizures
With somatosensory or special sensory symptoms		Hallucinations such as tingling, buzzing, lights flashing; visual, auditory, olfactory, gustatory, vertiginous	Same as above
With autonomic symptoms		Pallor, sweating, epigastric sensation, flushing, piloerection, pupillary dilatation	Same as above
With psychic symptoms		Dysphasia, dysmenesic, distorted cognition and affect, hallucinations	Same as above
Complex partial seizures		With or without impairment of consciousness, automatism	Unilateral or bilateral discharge, diffuse or focal, temporal or frontotemporal regions during seizures; unilateral or bilateral discharge, generally with the two sides discharging at different times, temporal or frontal regions between seizures
Partial seizures evolving to generalized seizures		Simple or complex; may evolve into generalized seizures	Discharge unilateral or bilateral, diffuse or focal, in temporal or frontotemporal regions; becomes secondarily and rapidly generalized during seizures; local contralateral, unilateral, or bilateral; generally two sides discharge at different times; temporal or frontal
Generalized seizures			
Absence seizures (petit mal)	Ages 5–20	Impairment of consciousness	Regular and symmetric 3-Hz spikes and waves may have 2- to 4-Hz spike and slow wave complexes, and may have multiple spike and slow-wave complexes, usually bilateral, during seizures; usually normal, although may have paroxysmal activity between seizures
Myoclonic seizures	Ages 5–20	Persistent, continuous spasms in unrelated muscles	Polyspike-and-wave, spike-and-wave, or sharp and slow waves during and between seizures

TABLE 12.4 *(Continued)*

Type	Age of Onset	Description	EEG Manifestations
Clonic seizures	Ages 2–20	Alternating contraction and relaxation of muscles; flailing and trembling	Fast activity and slow waves; occasional spike-and-wave during seizures; spike-and-wave or polyspike-and-wave discharges between seizures
Tonic seizures	Ages 2–20	Protracted muscle contraction and rigidity	Low-voltage, fast activity or a fast rhythm of 9–11 Hz or more, decreasing in frequency and amplitude during seizures; rhythmic discharges of sharp and slow waves, sometimes asymmetric; background abnormalities between seizures
Tonic-clonic seizures	Ages 2–20	Alternating stages of muscle rigidity and rhythmic flailing and trembling	Rhythm of 10 Hz decreases in frequency and increases in wave amplitude during the tonic stage and is replaced by slow waves during the clonic stage; polyspike-and-wave and spike-and-wave or sharp and slow wave discharges between seizures
Atonic seizures	Ages 2–20	Muscles lose normal tension; flaccid paralysis develops	Slow spike-and-wave discharges during seizures; polyspike and slow wave discharges during seizures

or alcohol abuse, and perinatal difficulties leading to birth trauma and asphyxia cause brain damage and later epilepsy. Febrile convulsions result in epileptic lesions in 2% of previously neurologically normal children. Head trauma and brain tumors are major causes of acquired epilepsies in adolescents and adults. Meningitic and encephalitic infections and brain abscesses frequently lead to epileptic seizures, as do cerebral degenerative and demyelinating diseases, cerebrovascular disease, and toxic or metabolic disorders (e.g., chronic drug intoxication, alcoholism, lead poisoning). Recently, the metabolic disorder nonketotic hyperglycemia has been causally implicated.

Specific structural or biochemical abnormalities cannot be determined in approximately 50% of patients with epilepsy. In such cases, the disorder is referred to as ***idiopathic.*** This failure to identify the etiology is due to the absence of a specific brain abnormality as described above. Many patients with idiopathic epilepsy may have a genetic predisposition, since the relatives of patients with epilepsy have a higher incidence of the disorder than individuals in the general population.

Generalized seizures are bilaterally symmetric and without local onset. About 90% of patients with such seizures experience their first attack before age 20, after which recurrence varies from minutes to years later. A ***tonic-clonic seizure,*** the most common and dramatic type of generalized seizure, may be preceded by a vague, indescribable feeling. In the majority of patients, however, sudden and intense electrical discharges overwhelm the brain's subcortical center and cause immediate unconsciousness. The standing or sitting patient may become injured from the fall following this loss of consciousness. A sudden shriek ("epileptic cry") produced by air being forced through the vocal cords as abdominal and chest muscles contract sometimes marks the beginning of the tonic stage of the seizure. This is followed by body muscle rigidity and cessation of breathing. Incontinence of feces and urine can occur. Patients often bite their tongues during this phase. Rhythmic trembling and flailing of the trunk and extremities, which characterize the clonic stage, follow within a few seconds to a minute. Saliva often froths from the mouth, and occasionally grunts are heard between convulsions. As the seizure ends, the patient begins to breathe deeply and all of the muscles relax. The entire attack lasts for approximately 2–5 minutes; in contrast, postictal confusion, drowsiness, sleep, and headache may persist for minutes to days. Between convulsions, about 25% of patients have EEG's within normal ranges.

Patients in ***status epilepticus*** remain unresponsive and in generalized seizure for long periods of time with only brief interruptions. Alternating tonicity and clonic movements, incontinence, severely disturbed breathing, high fever, excessive sweating, and blood pressure elevation are present. Cerebral damage and cardiac and renal failure result if emergency medical care is not given. Status epilepticus may begin spontaneously but most often follows a sudden withdrawal or a change in anticonvulsive medication.

Absence seizures (petit mal), beginning in childhood, rarely persist beyond age 30. Seizure onset is abrupt, with attacks lasting for no longer than 30 seconds (usually 10–20 seconds). Patients experience sudden lapses of consciousness, cease their activity, and stare blankly. Minor movements of the lips or hands and eye blinking and rolling are the only motor expressions. Attacks end as abruptly as they began, with no residual effects. Characteristically, their EEG's are grossly abnormal during the seizure. The frequency of petit mal seizures varies from a flurry every several days to 100 or more per day. A state of continuous attack, designated ***petit mal status,*** results in confusion, a dazed expression, and movements of the lips, arms, legs.

Although ***partial (focal) seizures*** occasionally spread rapidly to become generalized, they usually remain limited to one area of the brain and can be traced to specific lesions. Four types are recognized according to the main symptomatic manifestation (see Table 12.4). If the motor cortex is affected, physical manifestations in the form of trembling and repetitive or gross uncontrolled movements of the arms, legs, and trunk are noted. A ***simple partial motor seizure*** with a march (formerly called "Jacksonian motor seizure") begins with repetitive movements in one of three sites: the corner of the mouth, the thumb and index finger, or the great toe. The seizure progresses to the rest of the ipsilateral side. Occasionally, when seizure activity spreads to the opposite side, the patient loses consciousness and has a generalized tonic-clonic seizure. ***Simple partial sensory seizures*** may begin with numbness and tingling in the toes and fingers and progress in a march. Lesions of other sensory areas may produce disturbances of vision (flashing lights), hearing (buzzing), smell, taste, and balance. Common manifestations of ***simple partial autonomic seizures*** are epigastric sensations, pallor, sweating, flushing, piloerection, and pupillary dilatation. In instances of ***simple partial psychic seizure,*** disturbances of concentration and attention, memory lapse, dysphasia, perceptual difficulties, distortions of affect, and illusions or hallucinations are displayed. EEG changes during a simple partial seizure are often localized over the affected cerebral region. Also, diffusion of abnormal discharges from one hemisphere to the mirror point on the other is frequently demonstrated. Deeply situated lesions may produce no EEG changes.

The onset of a ***complex partial seizure*** is likely to be preceded by an aura, the most common of which is unpleasant epigastric sensations. Other signals of an impending attack are sensory hallucinations, unusual noises such as buzzing or ringing, or unpleasant odors. Immediate impairment of consciousness or simple partial seizure experiences (as described above) follow. Patients may appear to be in a dream state or report feelings of unreality or deja vu. Speech is often affected and visual distortions may occur. Involuntary semipurposeful motor behavior such as buttoning and unbuttoning a shirt or blouse is common. The seizure is followed by confusion, drowsiness, and an inability to remember what happened. Although complex partial seizures strongly resemble generalized seizures, they can be differentiated on the basis of EEG recordings. In addition, the immediate involvement of both cerebral cortices that is characteristic of generalized seizures is absent in complex partial seizures. As with generalized seizures, the frequency of focal attacks varies. ***Epilepsia partialis continua*** is a state of continuous focal seizure interrupted only briefly by nonseizure periods.

Any patient with a new onset of seizures should be immediately referred for neurologic work-up. This evaluation, consisting of thorough family, developmental, past and present medical histories, physical, neurologic, and psychologic examinations, blood chemistry and cerebrospinal fluid analysis, EEG, and roentgenogram studies (chest and skull x-ray films, CT scan) will determine whether the patient has a true epileptic disorder, a nonepileptic seizure disorder, or a condition that produces attacks resembling epileptic seizures. Many apparent epileptic seizures are manifestations of psychiatric disorders, syncope, or narcolepsy. The apparent seizure behaviors characteristic of these three and true epilepsy are compared in Table 12.5. Anticonvulsive drugs (Table 12.6) are prescribed, alone or in combination, to control epileptic seizures. The drugs of choice, which depend on the type of seizure, should be started slowly and their doses changed gradually. Rapid, frequent medication changes may precipitate seizure. Although drug therapy is often initiated by a neurologist, the primary caregiver may be called upon to provide ▶ ***supportive care for epilepsy,*** which includes monitoring drug levels and blood chemistry, instructing patients on emergency measures to take for a patient having a seizure, good health practices that help reduce the occurrence of seizures, and finally, counseling to facilitate adjustment to the disorder. In the last area, ▶ ***epilepsy organizations*** are important resources.

Any pathologic process affecting cerebral neurons can lead to a deterioration in mental process referred to as ***organic brain syndrome.*** Some of these processes are noted in Table 12.7. One of the most prominent clinical features is ***dementia.*** Early signs of dementia can be subtle, often going unrecognized. Relatives or close friends may be the first to detect the patient's lessening initiative, increased irritability, loss of interest, or inability to perform tasks at his or her usual level. Though such changes are also the hallmark of depression, certain distinctions can be noted (Table 12.8). As dementia progresses, memory failure, especially for recent events, becomes prominent. Other symptoms such as bewilderment in the face of a complex or new experience, marked mood fluctuations, and language difficulties emerge. In extreme cases, there is a loss of almost all intellectual abilities. The patient becomes bedridden, losing bowel and bladder control and eventually succumbing to pneumonia or

TABLE 12.5 COMPARISON OF EPILEPSY, SYNCOPE, PSYCHOGENIC DISORDERS, AND NARCOLEPSY

	Epilepsy	Syncope	Psychogenic	Narcolepsy
Onset	No warning; abrupt onset in most cases	Characteristic awareness of impending attack; fear or psychologic upset; face is pale or ashen white before the attack	Follows stressful circumstances	Triggered by joy, anger, amusement, or sadness
Attack	Involuntary	Involuntary	Voluntary, atypical behavior	Involuntary
	Loss of consciousness Injury occurs when the patient falls	Loss of consciousness	Falls to floor but does not sustain injury	Falls to knees and sometimes loses consciousness Cataplexy
	Body rigidness/convulsions, cataplexy No signs of vasomotor disturbance	Body limpness Signs of vasomotor disturbance include excessive sweating, bradycardia or tachycardia, and pallor	Rarely loses bladder and sphincter control	Loses bladder and sphincter control
EEG	Paroxysmal or focal discharges noted	Diffuse slow waves, asynchronous	Normal	Normal
Recovery	Postseizure confusion, headache, and drowsiness	Recovery of full consciousness and orientation is more rapid	No residual effects	No residual effects

another infection. The treatment and prognosis depend on the underlying processes, which are discussed throughout this chapter.

One of the most relentlessly progressive forms of cortical deterioration occurs in ***Alzheimer's disease.*** Accounting for over 50% of all cases of dementia, it affects 1.5 million people in the United States and 4 million throughout the world. It has been estimated to be the fourth most common cause of death in the elderly, with 100,000 succumbing annually. Alzheimer's disease generally begins after age 45; however, the onset may be later than age 60. Both sexes are affected equally. Although there is strong evidence of genetic transmission, the specific cause of Alzheimer's disease remains elusive. Slow viruses and autoimmune processes remain under investigation; aluminum toxicity, once suspected, has been ruled out. The existence of neurofibrillary tangles and senile plaques, characteristic of Alzheimer's disease, may provide etiologic clues in other disease states. In addition, recent advances in the detection of neurotransmitter and enzyme involvement may ultimately prove important. Pathologic changes in Alzheimer's disease are caused by substantial subcortical cell loss (specifically in the cholinergic system). Patients present with progressive dementia (see the previous discussion). They frequently fabricate elaborate stories to conceal their difficulties. Marked muscular rigidity and movement disturbances are present in the later stages. Patients with signs of Alzheimer's disease should have a psychiatric and/or neurologic evaluation to ascertain their mental status and rule out other neurologic or psychiatric processes. Brain biopsy is definitive, but most cases are diagnosed without it on the basis of exclusion. In the future, radionuclide imaging may become an invaluable diagnostic tool, as researchers using single-photon emission-computed tomography (SPEC) have identified characteristic scan patterns for Alzheimer's disease. In addition, a test that measures levels of acetylcholinesterase in spinal fluid may be available for diagnostic purposes (large-scale

TABLE 12.6 ANTICONVULSIVE DRUGS

Generic Name	Trade Name	Average daily dosage	Indications
Phenytoin	Dilantin	300–600 mg	Generalized tonic-clonic seizure Complex partial seizure Most effective when used in combination with phenobarbital or primidone
Phenobarbital	Luminal	100–300 mg	All seizure states Most effective in combination with other antieleptic drugs
Primidone	Mysolin	750–2,000 mg	Generalized tonic-clonic seizure Complex partial seizure Simple partial seizure Occasionally absence seizure
Carbamazepine	Tegretol	200–800 mg	Generalized tonic-clonic seizure Complex partial seizure Simple partial seizure
Clonazepam	Clonopin	3–12 mg	Myoclonic seizure Atonic seizure Absence seizure Some complex partial seizures
Ethosuximide	Zarontin	1,500 mg	Absense seizure Used in combination with Dilantin in mixed seizure states
Trimethadone	Tridione	1,200–2,400 mg	Absence seizure Myoclonic seizure Used in combination with Dilantin and phenobarbital
Valproic acid	Depakene	100–2,000 mg	Absence seizure Cautiously used in combination with phenobarbital and/or other antieleptic drugs for multiple seizures

clinical trials are now being conducted). There is no cure for Alzheimer's disease. However, ▶ ***supportive care for progressive dementia*** is essential. It includes (1) educating the patient and family about the illness and its course and encouraging them to express fears and concerns openly and (2) prescribing medications and environmental surroundings that maximize the patient's safety and well-being. In all of these areas, ▶ ***Alzheimer's disease organizations*** can be invaluable resources.

Pick's disease is much less common than and almost clinically identical to Alzheimer's disease. In contrast to the diffused degeneration that characterizes the latter, Pick's disease is marked by atrophy confined to the frontal and temporal lobes. No definite cause has been identified. Again, the symptoms, diagnosis and treatment are the same as for Alzheimer's disease.

The Cerebellum

The cerebellum is an infratentorial structure located below the occipital lobe. The vermis connects the two cerebellar hemispheres; the cerebellar peduncles connect the cerebellum with the remainder of the CNS. Unlike the cerebral hemispheres, each cerebellar hemisphere controls the body functions on the side where it is located

TABLE 12.7 MAJOR CAUSES OF DEMENTIA

Neurologic causes	Infectious causes
Alzheimer's disease	Syphilis
Parkinson's disease	Tuberculosis
Huntington's chorea	Cryptococcosis
Pick's disease	Viral diseases
Multiple sclerosis	Metabolic causes
Hydrocephalus	Hypothyroidism
Brain abscess	Cardiac, pulmonary, renal, and hepatic failure
Intracranial tumors	Electrolyte imbalance
Cerebrovascular disease	Toxins (medications, alcohol)
Chronic subdural hematoma	Nutritional deficiencies (vitamin B_{12}, thiamine)

(ipsilateral control). The main functions of the cerebellum are coordination of muscle movement, maintenance of equilibrium, and maintenance of muscle tone.

Cerebellar function is severely disturbed in ***Wernicke's encephalopathy*** and ***Korsakoff's psychosis*** (the ***Wernicke-Korsakoff syndrome***). Due to the lack of thiamine (vitamin B_1), these disorders are most often found in chronic alcoholics who have inadequate diets. Rarely is the Wernicke-Korsakoff syndrome associated with other forms of protracted malnutrition. The absence of thiamine results in major pathologic changes (i.e., proliferation of glial cells and blood vessels, with subsequent destruction of neurons). Drowsiness, apathy, and marked inattention make up the characteristic global confusional state of Wernicke's disease. Eye signs include ophthalmoplegia and nystagmus. Ataxia, usually confined to the legs, is always demonstrated as a gait disorder. Approximately 80% of patients with Wernicke's disease develop Korsakoff's psychosis, which is defined by memory loss (primarily for events just prior to disease onset), learning deficits, and confabulation. Other symptoms such as tachycardia, papillary atrophy of the tongue, angular stomatitis, a reddened and congested nose, and red blotches on the face caused by capillary dilatation accompany the acute phase. Wernicke-Korsakoff's syndrome is a medical emergency, and immediate administration of parenteral thiamine is required. Re-

TABLE 12.8 FEATURES DIFFERENTIATING DEMENTIA FROM DEPRESSION

Feature	Dementia	Depression
Onset	Unclear	Clear, recent, often a major psychologic event
Progression	Relatively steady decline	Uneven; often no progression
Patient insight	Often unaware of deficits, not distressed	Nearly always aware of deficits and quite distressed
Affect	Bland, some lability	Marked disturbance
Test performance	Good cooperation, stable achievement, little test anxiety, near-miss responses	Poor cooperation and variable achievement; considerable anxiety, "don't know" responses
Short-term memory	Often impaired	Sometimes impaired
Long-term memory	Unimpaired early in disease	Often inexplicably impaired

Source: D. S. Dahl, M.D., Diagnosis of Alzheimer's disease, part 2 of Alzheimer's disease: A five-article symposium, in *Postgraduate Medicine,* 73(4): April, 1983, a McGraw-Hill Publication, Minnesota. Used with permission.

covery, although slow (requiring weeks or months), is usually complete if treatment begins early enough. Global confusion states resolve in 1–6 weeks, eye signs in 2–3 hours, ataxia in 1–6 days, and mental symptoms in 3 weeks to 5 months. Without early treatment, residual gait and ocular disturbances and continued confusion and forgetfulness may be permanent. Patients with Wernicke-Korsakoff's disease pose a special management problem. Some of them require institutionalization. Others, having completely recovered from the acute stage, return to their previous drinking and eating habits. Placement in an alcoholism program or detoxification center or psychiatric consultation may be of minimal benefit. Close supervision by the primary caregiver or an enlisted family member or friend is often necessary, since chronic mental confusion and forgetfulness may interfere with health care. Approximately 15% of patients eventually die from the disease.

Cerebellar functions can also be compromised by MS, degenerative diseases, tumors, cerebrovascular disease, head injury, and other disorders described in other sections of this chapter.

Brain Stem and Cranial Nerves

The brain stem is located medially (toward the center of the body) to the cerebellum. Its divisions are the midbrain, pons, and medulla oblongata. No definite demarcations, such as those found in the cerebrum, separate these three divisions. Many vital body functions are controlled by the brain stem. Located in the medulla and pons are the cardiorespiratory centers.

The nuclei for 10 of the 12 cranial nerves, which have both motor and sensory functions, originate in the brain stem. Only the olfactory nerves (cranial nerve I) and the optic nerve (cranial nerve II) do not have their nuclei in this area of the brain. The specific locations for the origins of the cranial nerves are shown in Figure 12.5. Table 12.9 describes the cranial nerves in terms of their major functions, methods of examination, and typical symptoms of dysfunction.

Trigeminal neuralgia (tic douloureux), the most frequently encountered cranial nerve disorder, involves the sensory division (second and third divisions) of the fifth cranial nerve. Its onset is usually in middle to late life; however, it may occur at any age. The incidence in women is slightly higher than in men. The etiology of tic douloureux is not known. In rare cases, the trigeminal nerve is compressed by tumors or abnormal blood vessels or affected by lesions in the brain stem caused by MS or vascular accidents. Trauma and infections in the teeth, jaw, or adjacent paranasal sinuses may contribute to the condition. Some studies have suggested that tic douloureux is due to an excessive or paroxysmal discharge of impulses from the trigeminal nucleus. Patients report recurrent episodes of sharp, searing, burning, and stabbing pain that last for 1 to 15 or 20 minutes. During the trigeminal nerve attack, patients cease to talk, may rub or pinch the affected area, or may make violent convulsive facial movements (tic convulsif). The eye on the affected side often waters. Attack frequency varies from many times daily to several times a month. Although the interval between attacks is symptom free, a growing apprehension of impending pain prevails. Facial movement or chewing can trigger the neuralgia. Often patients refuse to eat in order to prevent exacerbation.

The diagnosis of tic douloureux can usually be made without difficulty from the description of the symptoms. Occasionally, other types of facial pain, particularly those caused by malocclusion, dental or sinus infection, herpes zoster, or other neu-

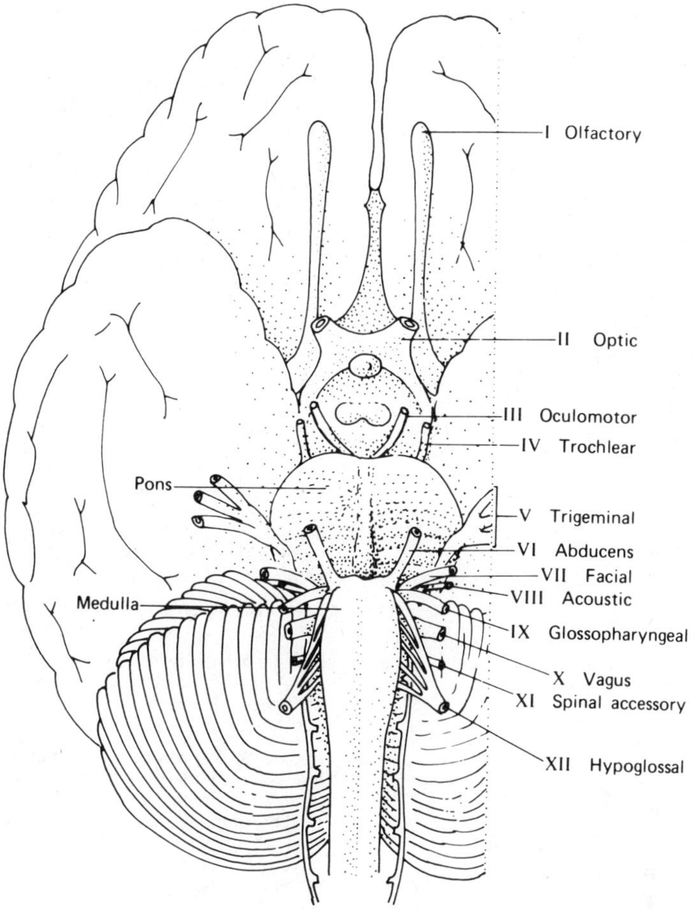

Figure 12.5 Cranial nerves. (From Snyder, M, *A Guide to Neurological and Neurosurgical Nursing,* © 1983, John Wiley and Sons, Inc., New York.)

ralgias must be ruled out. Nerve conduction and electromyographic studies are valuable diagnostic tools. Without adequate treatment, trigeminal neuralgia is characterized by periods of remission and exacerbation. Remission periods may be short or may last for months or years. Relapse is more frequent with aging, and permanent disappearance of symptoms is rare. Carbamazepine (Tegretol) is the treatment of choice. Starting with 100 mg bid, daily doses are gradually increased to 400–800 mg divided bid. A complete blood count (CBC) should be obtained before initiating the drug and after every 3 months of therapy due to an association (rare) of Tegretol with aplastic anemia. High doses of dilantin (approximately 800 mg daily) are a second choice. If medical therapy is ineffective, extracranial percutaneous thermal destruction of the affected nerve branch may be undertaken. Alcohol injections, partial section, decompression (freeing anomalous vessels, rhizotomy, or tractotomy) have also been employed.

TABLE 12.9 THE CRANIAL NERVES

Name		Functions	Method of Examination	Typical Symptoms of Dysfunction
I Olfactory	(s)[a]	Smell	Various odors applied to each nostril	Loss of sense of smell (anosmia)
II Optic	(s)	Vision	Visual acuity, map field of vision	Loss of vision (anopia)
III Oculomotor	(m)[b]	Eye movement	Reaction of light, lateral movements of eyes, eyelid movements	Double vision (diplopia), enlarged pupils, uneven dilation of pupils, drooping eyelid (ptosis), deviation of eye outward
IV Trochlear	(m)	Eye movement	Upward and downward eye movements	Double divsion, defect of downward gaze
V Trigeminal	(s, m)	Masticatory movements	Light touch by cotton baton; pain by pinprick; thermal reflex by hot and cold tubes; corneal reflex by touching cornea; jaw reflex by tapping chin, jaw movements	Decreased sensitivity or numbness of face; brief attacks of severe pain (trigeminal neuralgia); weakness and wasting of facial muscles; asymmetric chewing
VI Abducens	(m)	Eye movement	Lateral movements	Double vision, inward deviation of the eye
VII Facial	(m)	Facial movement	Facial movements, facial expression; test with sweet, salty, bitter substances on tongue	Facial paralysis
VIII Auditory vestibular	(s)	Hearing	Audiogram test hearing; test vestibular function by rotating patient or irrigating ears with hot or cold water (caloric test), looking for nystagmus	Deafness, sensation of noise in ear (tinnitus); disequilibrium, feeling of disorientation in space
IX Glossopharyngeal	(s, m)	Tongue and pharynx	Test pharyngeal or gag reflex by touching walls of pharynx (tested together with vagus)	Partial dry mouth, loss of taste (ageusia) over posterior third of tongue, anesthesia and paralysis of upper pharynx
X Vagus	(s, m)	Heart, blood vessels, viscera, movement of larynx and pharynx	Observe palate in phonation, palatal reflex by touching palate, shoulder muscles	Hoarseness, lower pharyngeal anesthesia and paralysis, indefinite visceral disturbance
XI Spinal accessory	(m)	Neck muscles, viscera, and soft palate	Movement, strength, bulk of neck, muscles, voice production	Wasting of neck with weakened rotation, inability to shrug, voice changes, soft palate, larynx, pharynx
XII Hypoglossal	(m)	Tongue muscles	Tongue movements; tremor, wasting, or wrinkling of tongue	Wasting of tongue with deviation to side of lesion on protrusion

[a] s = sensory
[b] m = motor

Seventh (facial) nerve injury produces paralysis of the facial muscles, with or without loss of taste on the anterior two-thirds of the tongue, and disturbance of lacrimal and salivary gland secretion. The superficial peripheral branches are subject to injury by stab or gunshot wounds, cuts, pressure of forceps at birth, and some operative procedures. Within the skull, the nerve may be damaged by tumors, aneurysms, meningitis, encephalitis, leukemia, osteomyelitis, herpes zoster, Paget's disease, sarcomas, or other bone tumors.

Paralysis of the facial nerve occurring without any known cause is called ***Bell's palsy.*** Since it often follows exposure to the cold (e.g., riding in an open car), it is thought to be due to swelling of the nerve within the stylomastoid foramen or bony facial canal. Bell's palsy occurs at all ages but is most common between 30 and 50. Both sides of the face are about equally affected. The onset of Bell's palsy is often signaled by facial stiffness or, rarely, pain. When the damage is severe, the muscles of the lower half of the face and occasionally of the lower lip sag; the normal folds and lines around the lips, nose, and forehead are absent; and voluntary movement of the facial and platysmal muscles is impossible. When patients try to smile, their lower facial muscles are pulled to the opposite side, so that they appear to have a protruding tongue or open jaw. Patients are also unable to close the affected eye. Attempts to do so cause the eyeball to be diverted upward and slightly inward (Bell's phenomenon). Excessive collection of tears, absence of corneal reflex due to paralysis of the upper lid, decreased saliva production, collection of saliva and food on the paralyzed side, and loss of taste are other symptoms. Partial injury may only produce weakness of the upper and lower halves of the face (the lower most frequently).

As with tic douloureux, the diagnosis of Bell's palsy is usually made without difficulty. Exceptions occur when only a minor degree of weakness is present or when there are other signs of cortical involvement. Patients should be referred to a neurologist for facial nerve excitability and electromyographic testing and institution of treatment. Essential local treatment of the facial muscles includes splinting the paralyzed muscles, daily massages (5 minutes twice daily, starting from the chin and lower lip up), and weak electrical stimulation. Eye patches are advisable for cornea protection. As the palsy begins to resolve, patients should practice various facial movements in front of a mirror. If Bell's palsy is diagnosed within the first 5 or 6 days, corticosteroids are often administered. Prednisone, begun at a dosage of 40–80 mg daily, is tapered over 10–14 days in an effort to reduce nerve swelling. Recovery from Bell's palsy is doubtful if the facial nerve has been severely damaged. In the majority of cases, however, partial or complete recovery is probable. Possible sequelae are abnormal movements (twitches) of the facial and labial muscles and disturbances of lacrimal and salivary gland secretion. In rare cases, synchronous blinking, labial twitching, and paroxysmal clonic contractions of all facial muscles stimulate focal Jacksonian seizures.

The reticular activating system (RAS), also located in the brain stem, consists of nuclei and fiber tracts. Impulses from all sensory organs and the spinal cord are received and integrated in the RAS and then transmitted to the cerebral cortex via the thalamus. In addition, signals from the cerebral cortex return to the RAS to be passed on to the lower nerve centers. This exchange is responsible for regulating the sleeping/waking process. If the influx of information into the RAS is continuous, the cerebral cortex remains alert; however, when it is at a minimum, the conscious mind is shut down and sleep occurs.

The average period of sleep for adults is 7.5 hours per night, with variations ranging from 3 or 4 to 12 hours. A single night of sleep consists of four to six cycles, each of which lasts for approximately 90 minutes. The first cycle begins at a sudden and precise moment (pinpointed on the EEG) when the person becomes disengaged from the external environment. The four stages of NREM sleep follow. These stages range from light sleep (stage I) to deep sleep (stage IV) and have characteristic EEG patterns. Arousal by external stimuli is difficult during stage IV. Sleep occurring during this time is therefore considered to be the most necessary. The cycle progresses back through the NREM stages to the first occurrence of REM sleep. Rapid eyeball movements, muscle twitches, penile and clitorial erections, and changes in heart and respiratory rates characterize REM sleep. CNS arousal and rapid neuron firing are reflected on the EEG, but voluntary movement is impossible and normal reflexes are blocked. Dreams are recalled in detail by persons awoken during this phase. The content of alternating NREM and REM sleep cycles changes as the night goes on. Stages III and IV are the longest in the early part of sleep and disappear toward morning. REM periods become longer as cycles progress and comprise approximately 25% of total sleep.

There has been much speculation regarding the significance of the two separate states of sleep. NREM sleep may facilitate biochemical restoration of the brain, while REM sleep is implicated in information storage and retrieval. Sleep deprivation studies have also suggested that dreaming, which occurs during the REM phase, is essential to psychologic health.

The quality and total length of sleep per night vary with age. Infants spend a disproportionate amount of their sleep in deeper stages or REM-like stages. By early adulthood, regular NREM/REM cycles emerge. During middle age, however, the time required to fall asleep increases, deep sleep is diminished (stage IV disappears by age 70), and sleep disturbances are more frequent and last for longer periods of time. Although daytime naps may compensate for these changes, they may also reduce the depth of sleep at night. These changes in sleep may contribute to the aging changes and the development of CNS defects. The quality of sleep is also affected by the presence of one of the ***sleep disorders*** described in Table 12.10.

▶ ***Insomnia*** is the most commonly reported sleep disturbance and is manifested as either difficulty in falling asleep or as frequent or early awakening. It may

TABLE 12.10 CHARACTERISTICS OF COMMON SLEEP DISORDERS

Disorder	Description
Insomnia	Characterized by difficulty in falling asleep, staying asleep, and/or awakening too early; underlying medical illnesses and drug or alcohol use should be explored; irregular schedules and poor sleep habits are common causes.
Narcolepsy	Characterized by excessive daytime sleepiness and sleep attacks, cataplexy, sleep paralysis and hypnagogic hallucinations, and identifiable sleep pattern abnormalities.
Sleep apnea	Characterized by daytime sleepiness and insomnia; patients may spend as much as 50–60% of sleep time with obstructed air flow; cycles of gasping, choking, and/or periodic loud snorting sounds occur.
Night terrors/nightmares	Sudden frightening awakenings; no dream recall; feelings of fear and physical discomfort.
Dream anxiety attacks	Less intense than night terrors; are normal efforts to control anxiety.

develop with underlying medical or psychiatric illness, or, more commonly, from irregular work and sleep habits. Although drug therapy has been a preferred treatment for insomnia, recent sleep research suggests several disadvantages: dependence is common; tolerance develops rapidly, reducing the drug's long-term effectiveness; effects of the drug last long after withdrawal; and the induced sleep does not follow normal sleep patterns. Behavioral therapy is a safe alternative. Supportive counseling is helpful, since insomniacs often become overly concerned about the effects of sleeplessness on their health.

Narcolepsy is a rare, progressive, and often disabling sleep disorder. It has four components, which occur together or in isolation: excessive daytime sleepiness and sleep attacks, cataplexy, sleep paralysis, and hypnagogic hallucinations. Daytime sleep attacks may be induced by either boring or monotonous situations or intense or exciting ones. Episodes occur in embarrassing, inappropriate, and even dangerous (driving a car) circumstances. Patients awaken after about 10–15 minutes fully alert and refreshed. ***Cataplexy*** is an important secondary symptom of narcolepsy. Loss of muscle tone or flaccid paralysis is triggered by strong emotions such as laughter, anger, fear, surprise, and exultation. Minor jaw sagging, head drooping, or total collapse may be exhibited. Typically, the patient remains fully alert but is unable to move. ***Sleep paralysis,*** a state of flaccid quadriplegia, occurs during transitions from wakefulness to sleep or sleep to wakefulness. The attacks are brief but frightening enough to cause patients to believe they are dying. Vivid and terrifying auditory or visual hallucinations ***(hypnagogic hallucinations)*** often accompany sleep paralysis. A number of patients with narcolepsy have episodes of amnesia or automatic behavior that may last for minutes or hours. The diagnosis is made from the presentation and from the documentation of abnormal sleep cycles (patients start with or go very quickly into REM sleep rather than beginning their first sleep cycle with an NREM period). The occurrence of cataplexy, sleep paralysis, and hypnagogic hallucinations is related to the fact that dreams occur and muscle activity is inhibited during REM phases. Long-term management of narcolepsy requires changes in lifestyle, as well as counseling and education of the patient and family. Amphetamines may be given for sleep attacks and tricyclic antidepressants for cataplexy.

Both excessive daytime sleepiness and insomnia may be symptoms of the ***sleep apneas.*** These sleep-induced respiratory disorders are characterized by a cessation of breathing during sleep for more than 10 seconds. These episodes occur more commonly in men and in older and/or obese persons. Patients may experience hundreds of episodes nightly and spend as much as 50–60% of their sleep time with obstructed air flow. Severe cardiac problems, hypertension, and sudden death can result. Collapse of the musculature of the nasopharynx due to profound loss of muscle tone is seen in ***upper airway sleep apnea.*** Complete obstruction, lasting for as much as 1 minute, precedes partial awakening, return of muscle tone, and a series of deep, loud, choking respirations. The patient usually falls asleep again and repeats the cycle. The reason for this disorder is not fully understood; however, it may be a result of the paralysis of skeletal muscles during REM phases of sleep. ***Central (diaphragmatic) sleep apnea*** occurs when the diaphragm stops moving during sleep. After about 15–30 seconds, respiration is restimulated by increased carbon dioxide in the blood. Diaphragmatic malfunction is believed to result from a temporary lapse in the transmission of neural impulses from the brain stem. ***Mixed sleep apnea*** is characterized by both the collapse of the nasopharynx musculature and the cessation of diaphragmatic movement. Profound excessive daytime sleepiness is the chief symptom of all of the sleep apneas. Loud snoring characterizes upper airway apnea and mixed sleep apnea. Although modified tracheostomy is the treatment of choice for upper airway and mixed sleep apneas, it is not helpful for central sleep apnea. Drug therapy (imipramine, protriptyline, or medroxyprogesterone) may be of some help. Care should be taken not to prescribe respiratory depressants for the symptomatic treatment of snoring or insomnia. Diaphragmatic pacemakers are being explored as a possible treatment mode.

Night terrors or ***nightmares*** are characterized by sudden, frightening awakenings and sensations of fear, physical discomfort, and chest pressure. There is usually no dream recall. These episodes take place during the deep stages of NREM sleep and probably indicate immature arousal mechanisms. ***Dream anxiety attacks*** are less intense and frightening, and represent normal efforts to control anxiety. Since they occur during REM sleep, they are easily remembered. Patients are unlikely to seek medical care for these disturbances. Supportive psychotherapy is offered to those who are sufficiently disturbed to seek help.

During the past 10 years, sleep research has given rise to sleep disorder centers. They are particularly helpful to clinicians who are faced with difficult or puzzling sleep disturbances. The Association of Sleep Disorder Centers will gladly provide information about available facilities. Other ▶ ***sleep disorders organizations*** are also helpful.

Basal Ganglia

The basal ganglia is a collection of nuclei (gray matter) lying deep within the white matter in each cerebral hemisphere. The basal ganglia structures are the caudate nucleus, putamen (these two structures make up the corpus striatum), and globus pallidus.

The basal ganglia is only one of the nuclear centers that comprise the extrapyramidal system. Other centers include the subthalamus, substantia nigra, brain stem nuclei, and reticular formations and other associated nuclei. Along with the cerebellum, the extrapyramidal system controls posture and motion and makes voluntary movements initiated by the pyramidal system (compromising motor and sensory neurons from the cortex and spinal cord) possible. Specifically, the basal ganglia facilitates smooth muscle movements and influences muscle tone and the processing of proprioceptive data needed for motor reflexes. Disturbance of extrapyramidal functioning, including that of the basal ganglia, makes voluntary movements difficult or impossible.

Parkinson's disease, the most common disease of the basal ganglia, is related to the loss of the neurotransmitter substance dopamine. Dopamine is required in the basal ganglia to carry out its motor functions and to maintain the connection between the proprioceptive sensory system and the motor system. It also balances the activity of another neurotransmitter, acetylcholine. Dopamine is manufactured and stored in an area of the midbrain around the cerebral penduncles called the "substantia nigra." Neuronal fibers project from this structure to the corpus striatum (nigrostriatal pathway), where they release the dopamine. Degeneration of the substantia nigra may occur as a sequela to encephalitis, syphilis, or viral infection or as a result of tumors, arteriosclerosis, or aging. Carbon monoxide, lead, and magnesium poisoning are also known causes. Enzymes that destroy waste products of nigral cell metabolism are decreased as a result of deterioration. Toxic substance buildup leads to cell destruction and halted production of another enzyme essential to dopamine production. Dopamine is reduced by over 90% or often to undetectable amounts and thus cannot be supplied to the basal ganglia.

Parkinson's disease typically begins between ages 50 and 65, and affects both sexes (men slightly more often than women) and all races. It is characterized by very gradual progression and a prolonged course. Usually 10–20 years elapse before symptoms are disabling. The principal features are tremor, muscular rigidity, akinesia, facial immobility, and postural abnormalities. The "pill-rolling tremor," a rhythmic, alternating flexion and extension of the fingers, is an early symptom. This tremor stops during voluntary movement or sleep but reappears when the limb is unsupported at rest. Patients can alleviate minimal tremors by resting their hands and arms on tables or chairs or by keeping them in their pockets. Eventually, however, the tremors become gross and disabling. The head, lips, tongue, and feet may also be affected. Muscular rigidity results when muscle tone increases in both the extensor and flexor muscles simultaneously. It first appears in the proximal limbs and neck muscles, and is most evident on passive movement of the joint. Rather than a smooth, flowing motion, movement is characterized by a series of interrupted jerks (cog-wheel phenomenon). Akinesia or lack of spontaneous movement is also characteristic of Parkinson's disease. Initiation of movement is slow, and once motion does begin, patients find themselves suddenly and unexpectedly "frozen" or unable to move. Periods of motionlessness, perhaps for hours, may develop. Speech becomes slow and monotonous. Facial immobility is characterized by infrequent blinking, lack of expression, and dulling of facial features. Patients become stone-faced. Postural abnormality is demonstrated in a variety of ways, one of which is a head loll. Also, when standing, patients may gradually bend forward until they find themselves on their knees. Difficulties in maintaining equilibrium are evident from the inability to sit or stand unsupported and the failure to catch themselves when pushed forward or backward. Distinctive walking patterns develop as a result of balance problems. Footsteps usually become short and shuffling. Some patients, once they begin walking, may take faster and faster steps and end up running forward. Symptoms that occur with some variability are dementia, depression, pupillary abnormalities, tics, diaphragmatic spasms, and repetitive speech. A characteristic handwriting change, micrographia (letters become progressively smaller), may also be evident.

There is no known cure for Parkinson's disease, probably because the etiologic factors and progression are still not fully understood. Treatment is therefore symptomatic. Amantadine seems to improve mild symptoms (its mode of action is unknown). Anticholinergic drugs (e.g., Cogentin, Artane) reduce the heightened cholinergic activity occurring in the presence of decreased dopamine. A number of drugs that affect dopamine (levodopa, carbidopa, bromocriptine) may also be used. In patients with severe Parkinson's disease, combining and titrating these agents can be a complicated task. It is best managed by a neurologist. ▶ ***Supportive care for Parkinson's disease*** is an important aspect of primary care. ▶ ***Parkinson's disease organizations*** can also prove helpful.

Ingestion of various drugs, particularly major tranquilizers that include reserpine and several phenothiazine and butyrophenone derivatives, is associated with ***drug-induced Parkinson's disease.*** Rather than causing damage to the substantia nigra and halting dopamine production, these drugs block dopamine activity. The symptoms are difficult to distinguish from those of Parkinson's disease but are reversible once the drug is withdrawn. Occasionally, however, they may persist for months or become permanent. In view of these side effects, care should be taken in administration, and long-term treatment should include drug-free periods.

Huntington's chorea (hereditary chorea), a progressive degenerative disease of the basal ganglia (particularly those in the caudate and putamen), is caused by inheritance of a single dominant autosomal gene from either parent. Since onset is usually between the ages of 35 and 39, patients may unknowningly pass it on to their children. Mental deterioration and rapid, involuntary jerks of the limbs during voluntary movement called "choreiform movements" progress together. Occasionally, one precedes the other by several years. There is no effective treatment for Huntington's chorea. Several drugs, however, may prove helpful in decreasing the symptoms. It is interesting to note that some of them, including reserpine, phenothiazines, and butyrophenones, are known to cause secondary parkinsonism. Also noteworthy is the fact that some patients with Parkinson's disease receiving dopamine-replacing drugs develop choreiform disorders. Taken together, these findings may provide clues to a more effective treatment of both disorders. In the meantime, genetic counseling for patient's with Huntington's chorea remains the most important weapon for its control.

Although no specific pathologic lesions have been found in the brains of patients with ***essential tremor,*** it has been suggested that this condition is related to Parkinson's disease. Essential tremor is one of the most common disorders of movement and has a strong familial incidence. Tremor, predominantly involving the hands, usually begins before age 25 (the trunk and legs are not usually involved). It is most obvious when there is voluntary movement, when the arms are unsupported, or during fine manipulation. A nodding head tremor and shakiness of speech often occur. As more body parts become affected and the intensity of the tremor progresses, patients become physically and socially disabled. It is important to differentiate essential tremor from parkinsonism. The distinguishing characteristics are earlier age of onset, lack of severe progression, akinesia, rigidity or postural abnormalities, and the presence of a strong familial tendency. There is no curative therapy for controlling the tremor, although some pharmaceutic agents (notably beta blockers such as propranolol) are helpful.

Involving both cerebral and basal ganglia structures, ***senile tremor*** is frequently found in elderly patients. Rapid tremor of the head and arms occurs only with voluntary movement at first, but as the disease progresses, it becomes more constant and is present even when the limb is at rest. There is no effective treatment. Some relief may be achieved with propranolol or other beta blockers. Assuring patients that they do not have Parkinson's disease is important.

Thalamus, Hypothalamus, Pituitary Gland, and Sympathetic and Parasympathetic Control

Located deep within the cranium are the thalamus, hypothalamus, and pituitary gland (Figure 12.2). The thalamus serves as the chief relay station for sensory fibers. The hypothalamus is involved in regulation of temperature and fluid balance. Along with the pituitary gland, it regulates hormonal activities throughout the body. Hormone control is discussed in a later section. The hypothalamus also regulates activity of the sympathetic and parasympathetic nervous systems.

Figure 12.6 shows the fibers of the parasympathetic and sympathetic nervous systems and the structures they innervate. Note that the preganglionic fibers of the parasympathetic nervous system are long, whereas the postganglionic fibers are short. The reverse is true in the sympathetic nervous system. Parasympathetic fibers originate primarily in cranial nerves VII, IX, and X and in the sacral area of the spinal cord. The chief function of the parasympathetic nervous system is the regeneration of body energy stores.

Sympathetic fibers exit mainly from the cervical and thoracic areas of the spinal cord. Many functions of the sympathetic nervous system prepare the body to handle stressful situations. Stimulation from the adrenal glands releases adrenaline which causes blood and body energy stores to be allocated to essential organs such as the brain, heart, lungs, and skeletal muscles. Increased vascular tone and cardiac output, gluconeogenesis, and increased oxygen intake due to increased ventilatory rate and volume also occur in response to secretion of adrenaline. The parasympathetic and sympathetic nervous systems exert the body effects, often antagonistic, noted in Table 12.11.

Cerebrospinal Fluid and Ventricular System

The brain is cushioned by cerebrospinal fluid (CSF), a clear liquid made up of small amounts of protein, sugar, and ions of salts. CSF is manufactured within and circulates through small spaces called "ventricles." Formed in the choroid plexuses, located principally in the lateral ventricles, it flows through the foramen of Monroe to the third ventricle and then through the aqueduct of Sylvius to the fourth ventricle. Passing through two or more foramina (Magendie and Luschka), it enters the subarachnoid space and circulates down the spinal column and back to the lateral ventricles. Although 500–700 mL of CSF is manufactured each day, only 140–150 mL circulates at any one time. The remainder is absorbed through arachnoid villi into the venous circulation.

Increased CSF pressure is referred to as ***intracranial hypertension.*** The problem may result from increased production, defective absorption, or obstructed circulation of CSF. Major causes of obstruction are neoplasms, congenital malformations, and posttraumatic or postinflammatory lesions. Infants and young children with intracranial hypertension may develop ***hydrocephalus*** marked by increased head growth rate and size and distended scalp veins. Older children and adults develop headache, double vision, blurred vision, nausea, and vomiting. Eye exam reveals papilledema and an extended blind spot. A detailed neurologic study is necessary to determine the underlying cause. Skull x-ray films, CT scans, carotid angiography, and air contrast studies are useful in determining the presence of obstruction, the amount of ventricular enlargement, and the degree of subarachnoid space compromise. Treatment is aimed at the underlying cause. Surgical shunting procedures may be indicated to reduce the volume and pressure of CSF.

Pseudotumor cerebri is characterized by increased intracranial pressure in the absence of lesions or ventricular enlargement. Idiopathic disease is fairly common, particularly among young, overweight women. Secondary disease is associated with thrombosis of the transverse venous or sagittal sinus, chronic pulmonary disease, hypoparathyroidism, Addison's disease, and drug use (nalidixic acid, tetracycline, oral contraceptives, withdrawal of long-term steroids). The signs and symptoms are usually confined to headache, diplopia, and papilledema. Patients should have a CT

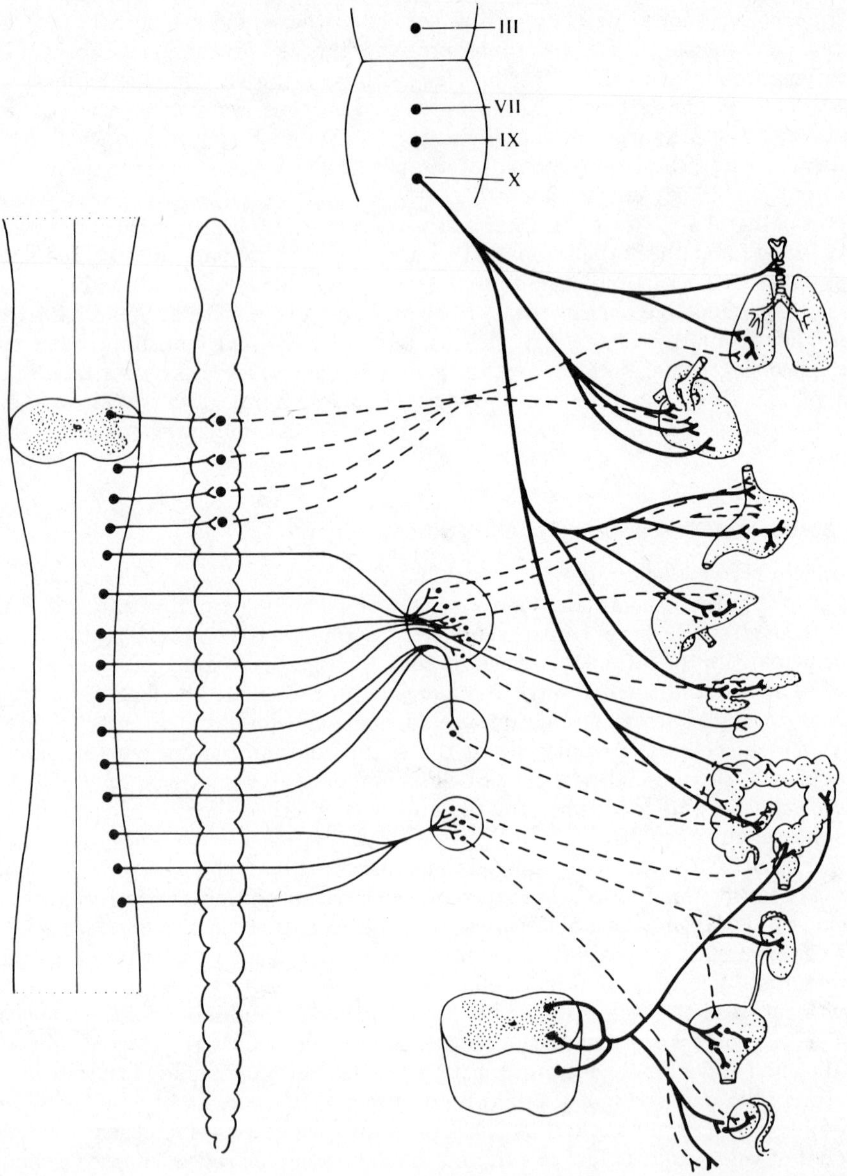

Figure 12.6 Sympathetic and parasympathetic nervous systems. (From Snyder, M, *A Guide to Neurological and Neurosurgical Nursing,* © 1983, John Wiley and Sons, Inc., New York.)

TABLE 12.11 EFFECTS OF AUTONOMIC STIMULATION ON SELECTED BODY ORGANS

Organ	Sympathetic Effect	Parasympathetic Effect
Pupil	Dilatation	Contraction
Ciliary process of eye	None	Excitation
GI glands	Inhibition or no effect	Copious secretions of serous fluids and enzymes
Salivary glands	Thick, viscous secretion	Serous or watery secretion
Sweat glands	Copious secretion	None
Heart	Increased rate and force of contraction	Decreased rate and force of contraction
Lungs	Constriction of blood vessels, dilatation of bronchi	Constriction of bronchi
GI muscle	Inhibition of peristalsis, stimulation of sphincters	Stimulation of peristalsis, inhibition of sphincters
Liver	Release of glucose	None
Penis	Ejaculation	Erection
Muscles	Constriction of abdominal muscles, constriction or dilatation of smooth muscles, depending on receptors in tissues	None
Bladder	Uncertain	Stimulation of smooth muscle for emptying and contraction of detrusor muscle, relaxation of internal sphincter

Source: M. Snyder (ed.), *A Guide to Neurological and Neurosurgical Nursing.* Copyright, 1983, John Wiley & Sons, New York. Used with permission.

scan and lumbar puncture to rule out lesions or infection. Treatment begins by discontinuing any causative drug and/or correcting any endocrine disturbance. Medical measures include acetazolamide or furosemide (lowers the production of CSF), repeated lumbar punctures (lowers intracranial pressure), and oral corticosteroids (reduces papilledema). Weight reduction is important for obese patients. If medical approaches fail, shunt placement may be necessary to preserve vision.

Vascular System

Blood reaches the brain through two major channels: the vertebral system and the carotid system. The vertebral arteries originate from the subclavian arteries, as shown in Figure 12.7. Before entering the brain, the two vertebral arteries join to form the basilar artery. The internal carotid arteries are branches of the common carotid arteries; the common carotid arteries arise from the arch of the aorta. At the base of the brain, the posterior communicating arteries connect the basilar artery with the right and left internal carotid arteries, and the anterior communicating artery connects the right and left anterior cerebral arteries. Called the "circle of Willis," this arrangement provides several routes of circulation to brain structures. Blood leaves the brain through the thin-walled vessels located in the subarachnoid space. These vessels eventually cross the subdural space and empty into venous sinuses that connect with the internal jugular vein. A small amount of venous blood leaves the brain via the emissary veins.

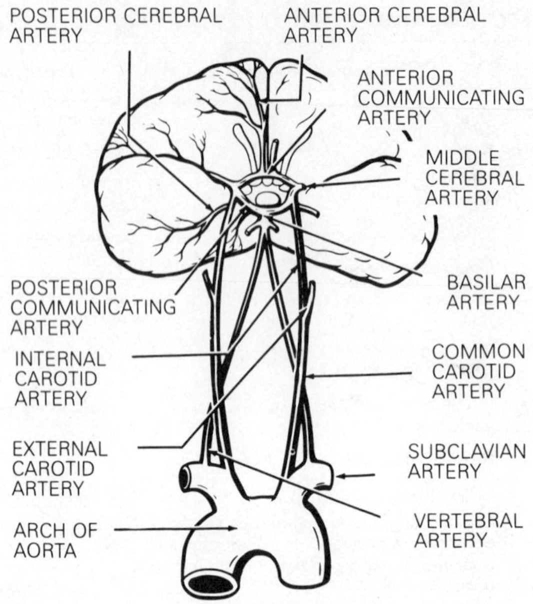

Figure 12.7 Vascular supply of the brain. (From Snyder, M, *A Guide to Neurological and Neurosurgical Nursing,* © 1983, John Wiley and Sons, Inc., New York.)

Cerebral tissue is unable to store adequate amounts of oxygen, glucose, and other nutrients to maintain its high metabolic rate. Approximately 20% of the oxygen and 25% of the glucose consumed by the body are used by the brain. The brain, therefore, receives about 20% of the total cardiac output. Blood flow to the brain is controlled to some extent by the rise and fall of cerebral carbon dioxide levels, increasing when these levels rise.

Vascular headaches result from constriction of arteries within the brain. The most common type is the ▶ ***classic migraine headache.*** It affects about 15% of the population 40 years of age and under, with the highest incidence between 20 and 35. Although usually beginning in puberty, the initial attack can occur any time between the ages of 5 and 30. Women are affected more often than men. Migraine may subside in women following menopause. More than half of the patients with migraine have a family history of the disorder. The incidence of hypertension, myocardial infarction, and death is increased in individuals who have migraines. Vascular changes in the extracranial, pial, basal, scalp, and parenchymal arteries correspond to the three phases of the migraine attack. In the initial phase, trigger factors begin a series of local and systemic changes. Although stress is the major initiating factor, a migraine attack characteristically begins after stress resolves. Rapid changes in hormonal levels may account for migraines accompanying ovulation and premenstruation. Increased blood glucose levels in patients fasting for long periods also lead to migraine attacks. Foods high in vasoactive substances are listed in Table 12.12, along with medical conditions and medications that may trigger migraines. Systemically, aggregated platelets release serotonin, a cerebral vasoconstrictor. Along with other neurogenic stimuli, serotonin initiates vasoconstriction of inner-

TABLE 12.12 FACTORS THAT TRIGGER MIGRAINE HEADACHE

Stress; migraine begins when stress is resolved	Medical conditions Depression Moderate to severe hypertension Collagen disorders Febrile conditions
Rapid changes in hormonal levels (ovulation, menstruation)	
Rapid changes in blood sugar level (after oversleeping or fasting)	Medications Reserpine (serotonin releaser) Nitroglycerine (vasodilator) Antihypertensive drugs causing vasodilatation Ergotamine (excessive amounts lead to rebound headaches) Oral contraceptives (particularly estrogen)
Foods with high tyramine content Alcohol Chocolate Nuts Cirtrus juices (large quantities) Aged cheese	
Physical stimuli Bright sunlight Stuffy rooms	

vated cerebral arteries, causing reduced cerebral blood flow and localized ischemia. This aura stage is characterized by focal neurologic signs and symptoms such as lateralized numbness or weakness, transient aphasia, thickness of speech, or vertigo. Blurred or cloudy vision with superimposed zigzag lines, sometimes of various colors and usually only in one visual field, often occurs. Episodes usually last for 15 to 30 minutes and signal the impending headache. In response to the effects of decreased blood flow (anoxia and acidosis), noninnervated parenchymal arteries dilate. Dilatation is initiated by serotonin-induced prostaglandin release and a drop in blood serotonin levels. Vasodilatation, sensitization of pain receptors in the blood vessels, and sterile inflammation around the vessels (induced by serotonin and other vasoactive substances) lead to throbbing and sometimes excruciating pain. The migraine headache may be limited to one side at first, but spread to the other side often follows. Nausea, photophobia, vomiting, diarrhea, vertigo, tremors, excessive perspiration, and chills frequently accompany the headache. The headaches are generally brief, most subsiding within 6 hours. During the postheadache phase of migraine, blood serotonin levels and vessel size return to normal. There is residual inflammation and edema, and the scalp may remain tender to the touch. Patients are usually exhausted, and some experience euphoria. Physical efforts such as bending over, lifting, or running may precipitate another attack.

Migraine headaches usually require pharmacologic intervention: beta blockers, amitriptyline for prophylaxis, vasoconstrictors (e.g., ergotamin tartrate) to abort impending attacks, and analgesics to relieve pain during attacks. Careful drug supervision is needed for patients who have frequent migraines.

Variations of the classic migraine syndrome are ***common migraine, basilar artery migraine, ophthalmoplegic migraine,*** and ***hemiplegic migraine.*** They are described in Table 12.13.

Closely related to but distinguishable from migraine headaches are ▶***cluster headaches.*** The onset is usually within 2–3 hours after falling asleep (during REM sleep), and is occasionally precipitated by consumption of alchohol, tyramine-containing foods, nitroglycerine, or histamines. Attacks during waking hours are uncommon. Headaches recur nightly for several weeks or months and then disappear for a period ranging from 6 months to years. In rare cases, attacks continue for years (chronic cluster headache). Most patients who experience cluster headaches are be-

TABLE 12.13 FOUR VARIATIONS OF MIGRAINE HEADACHE

Type	Description
Common migraine	More frequent than classic migraine; some behavior changes precede it (depression to exhilaration); prodrome of somatic neurologic symptoms is absent; present on awakening and intensifies, necessitating retreat to a darkened room and use of ice packs; attacks last for periods ranging from hours to days or weeks; anorexia and nausea or vomiting often accompany headache; attacks are infrequent during adolescence, become bimonthly during young adulthood, and are nearly continuous ("migraine storms") from ages 30 to 40; there is partial or total relief during pregnancy, but attacks return with a vengeance postpartum.
Basilar artery migraine	The prodrome consists of vertigo and tinnitus, bilateral visual blurring and diplopia, dysarthria, unsteadiness, bilateral paresthesia, and occasional unconsciousness; there is transient global amnesia in rare cases during the prodrome; prodrome gives way to a throbbing occipital headache of varying length; there is no residual defect; generally occurs in girls under age 21.
Ophthalmoplegic migraine	Symptoms resemble those of a carotid aneurysm, since headache, extraocular paralysis, ptosis, ocular muscle weakness, and pupillary changes occur on the same side; begins with focal head pain around the eye accompanied by nausea, vomiting, and photophobia; extraocular paralysis begins 1–2 days later as headache is subsiding; symptoms may last for periods ranging from hours to days or weeks; onset occurs in childhood.
Hemiplegic migraine	Begins as a sudden attack of hemiparesis or hemiplegia, often accompanied by aphasia and confusion; these symptoms give way to a contralateral throbbing headache; symptoms may persist for several days; on rare occasions, hemiparesis does not resolve.

tween the ages of 20 and 30, and 90% are men. Increased blood levels of histamine and serotonin have been found in patients with cluster headaches. As in migraine attacks, they cause vasoconstriction and inflammation of cerebral vessels. Their levels remain high throughout the cluster headache period and drop when the headaches disappear. Cluster headaches are characterized by excruciating, boring pain that begins behind or around one eye and then spreads over the affected side. The painful area may include the forehead but is rarely bilateral. Associated symptoms include temporal artery bulging and pulsating, drooping, swelling, and redness of the eyelid, pupillary constriction, conjunctival injection, tearing, flushing of the side of face, sweating, nasal congestion, and rhinorrhea. Due to the severity of the pain, immediate treatment is necessary. Analgesics or ergotamine tartrate can terminate headaches, though the amounts needed could prove dangerous. Prophylaxis may therefore be a more desirable approach. The agents used include prednisone, lithium, methysergide, and indomethacin.

Some vasoconstriction also accompanies ***acute muscle contraction headache.*** However, muscle tension is its most prominent feature. Stress and depression, the most significant causative factors, trigger a generalized, steady, nonpulsating headache. Bitemporal or occipital tightness is also reported. Pain may spread to the neck and upper back. Palpation of the affected area may reveal one or more nodules (areas of sharp, localized tenderness). Pressure on these areas may cause the pain to spread. Patients complaining of continuous pain that does not respond to the usual analgesia may have ▶ ***chronic muscle contraction headache.*** Sleep disturbances often accompany this type. However, these headaches may be more closely related to underlying stress or depression. Simple muscle contraction headaches respond to over-the-counter analgesics. Patients suffering from chronic headache are more likely to seek medical advice. Analgesia, relaxation training, biofeedback, and counseling are the suggested treatment measures.

Collectively referred to as ***cerebrovascular disease,*** any defect, obstruction, or rupture of blood vessels within the brain can reduce blood to tissues, depriving them of necessary oxygen and nutrients. Deprivation, if severe and prolonged enough (10–15 minutes), leads to cerebral dysfunction and tissue death (infarction) known as ***cerebrovascular accident (CVA)*** or ***stroke.*** Cerebrovascular disease is the most common neurologic disorder in adults, accounting for about 50% of all patients hospitalized for neurologic disorder. Prominent risk factors are hypertension, diabetes, and combined smoking/oral contraceptive use. The problem accounts for approximately 250,000 deaths per year in the United States. Many survivors are totally disabled and dependent on others for activities of daily living.

A stroke resulting from clot formation is called ***cerebral thrombosis.*** It is usually caused by atherosclerotic disease whereby plaques form in arterial walls, instigating platelet aggregation and thrombus formation. However, thrombosis can also develop in the wake of inflammatory vessel disorders (syphilis, tuberculosis, or arteritis), as well as with cranial trauma. In general, the symptoms of cerebral thrombosis are headache, drowsiness, double vision, and convulsions. More specific deficits are dependent on the location of the thrombus and the size of the resultant infarction. Such symptoms usually develop rapidly. However, they may also develop over a period of time with step-like changes, particularly in the case of atherosclerotic disease. In the latter case, thrombus formation only partially occludes the artery, causing mild neurologic signs and weakness and prompting the development of collateral circulation. Then, even though the thrombus evolves and stroke ensues, patients may regain some function.

Embolic stroke develops abruptly, progresses rapidly, and reaches a maximum within a short period of time. Neurologic disturbances due to embolic stroke closely resemble those associated with thrombosis. In most cases, emboli are fragments that have broken away from a thrombus within the heart. Approximately 50% of all cases are associated with chronic atrial fibrillation due to atherosclerotic or rheumatic heart disease. Other types of coronary pathology (e.g., hypertensive, congenital, or syphilitic) causing atrial fibrillation can also lead to embolism. Thrombi formed on the damaged endocardium following myocardial infarction and those associated with severe mitral stenosis (with or without atrial fibrillation) are occasional sources of emboli. Emboli consisting of other material (fat, air, vegetations from infectious processes, and tumor cells) or originating in pulmonary, carotid, or thoracic arteries are less frequent. The amount of tissue damage depends on the size of the embolus and the vessel affected. Small emboli occlude vessels of lesser diameter, and the resultant strokes clear quickly or may not be detected at all. In contrast, large emboli block major vessels, resulting in widespread, permanent damage. In addition, if a small vessel to a major area is occluded, such as the frequently affected internal capsule, major deficits will result. Sparing of tissues distal to the obstruction is not as likely as in thrombosis, since the rapidity with which occlusion occurs does not allow the development of compensatory collateral blood flow. Emboli dissipate or become lodged in blood vessels, and, along with fibrous material supplied by the vessel wall and clotting factors, form plugs that lead to further infarction.

In the case of ***septic embolism,*** fragments dislodge from infectious processes (usually of the endocardium). Single or multiple, small septic infarcts develop. Further complications such as embolic meningitis and encephalitis or cerebral hemorrhage are common. Aggressive antibiotic treatment is needed in conjunction with stroke management procedures.

Approximately 25% of patients succumb to their first thrombotic or embolic stroke. Mortality rises sharply with age (near 50% in patients over 70) and in the presence of preexisting cerebrovascular disease, coma, or marked neurologic deficit. Of those who do survive a first attack, one-fifth suffer another CVA within the next 12–24 months. Treatment of cerebral infarction due to thrombi or emboli is aimed at preserving life, limiting the amount of damage, and lessening the disability. Arterial occlusion is confirmed by arteriography. There is a risk, however, of dislodging a plaque, resulting in further neurologic damage. CT scanning is useful for defining the area and extent of infarction. Cerebral edema, which accompanies all strokes to some degree, adds to the deficits. In cases of extensive edema, herniation with brain compression occurs. Measures to reduce increased intracranial pressure are necessary. Physical therapy should begin within a few days after there is no longer evidence of increasing stroke. Anticoagulation drug therapy may be effective in reducing the likelihood of recurrence. In some instances, surgical revascularization procedures may be used to improve circulation.

Transient ischemic attack (TIA) reflects evolving thrombi or rapidly dissolving microemboli. It develops suddenly, lasts for periods ranging from 5 minutes to several hours (never more than 24), and resolves completely. The symptoms depend on the arterial system affected. Carotid artery involvement causes ipsilateral blindness and contralateral hemiparesis, often with paresthesias. When the vertebrobasilar system is involved, patients display symptoms of brain stem dysfunction: confusion, vertigo, binocular blindness, or diplopia, as well as weakness and paresthesias (usually bilateral). Approximately 80% of patients suffering from TIAs have CVAs. Thus a neurologic consultation for diagnosis and initiation of treatment is in order. Surgery (endarterectomy) and anticoagulant drug therapy are frequently prescribed treatment modes.

Intracerebral hemorrhage accounts for about 10–20% of all CVAs. Bleeding into cerebral tissue most often results from hypertensive vascular disease (see Chapter 6). Moderate to severe hypertension causes thickening, degeneration, and eventual rupture of small cerebral arteries. Signs evolve over an hour or two and include headache, nausea and vomiting, and decreased responsiveness. Specific neurologic deficits emerge, indicating the area of the brain affected. Cerebral edema is a complication. Extension of bleeding into the ventricles may occur and indicates a poor prognosis. The overall mortality of patients with intracerebral hemorrhage due to hypertensive vascular disease is 50%. Older age groups have corresponding higher mortalities.

Aneurysm rupture is the most frequent cause of ***subarachnoid hemorrhage.*** Intracranial pressure increases, causing sudden loss of consciousness. Rapid elevation with subsequent herniation may cause death. Irritation of tissue (meninges and blood vessels) leads to severe headaches and nuchal rigidity. The initial symptom is a sudden, violent headache. Its location suggests the rupture site. Extension of bleeding into the cerebral tissue may result in lateralization of the neurologic signs. Although aneurysm may occur at any age, middle age is the most common time for rupture. Subarachnoid hemorrhage can take place during sleep but usually occurs while the patient is engaged in daily activity. The onset may be during straining at stool, heavy lifting, or coitus. There is a 45% mortality for each episode of subarachnoid bleeding due to ruptured aneurysm. Recurrence of bleeds is common in one-third of patients within 2 weeks of the first attack; 20% have second bleeds within 3–4 weeks. Unfortunately, there is no way to predict which patients are susceptible to further hemorrhage or when it will occur. Hospitalization and care by a neurologist and neurosurgeon are essential. CT scans are utilized for diagnostic confirmation. Continued judicious management of the underlying medical disorders is an important consideration for primary caregivers. Because recurrent hemorrhage is a danger in cases of subarachnoid aneurysm rupture, careful posthemorrhage management is recommended. Patients should have total bed rest for several weeks following the initial episode and should avoid potentially dangerous activities.

Protective Features (Skull, Meninges, and Blood–Brain Barrier)

For protection, the brain is encased in a thick bony helmet, the skull. Beneath the skull are three meningeal layers that cover the brain and spinal cord and protect the underlying structures. The meningeal layers also protect the underlying blood vessels. The thick outer covering is called the "dura mater." The middle layer is called the "subarachnoid meninges." Though only a potential space exists between the dura and the arachnoid, a space beneath the arachnoid ("subarachnoid space") provides a channel for the flow of CSF. Closely adherent to the brain and cord is the "pia meningeal layer," which is a thin, delicate structure. Because the meninges contain many nerve endings, they are extremely sensitive to stimuli. Two large infoldings of the meningeal layers are found in the cranial vault. The falx separates the right and left hemispheres of the cerebrum. The infolding that separates the occipital lobe from the cerebellum is called the "tentorium."

A mechanism that protects the brain from direct damage caused by organisms and toxic substances present in the bloodstream is the blood–brain barrier. This barrier also protects against indirect damage resulting from inadequate supplies of oxygen, glucose, amino acids, and other essential nutrients (regulatory interface). The mechanisms involved are anatomic specializations of the cerebral capillaries and adjacent endothelial cells such as nonfenestration, tight junctions at the interface, and a dense basement membrane with astrocytic processes on the outer surface that restrict intercellular diffusion. These same features are found in the epithelial cells of the choroid plexus, providing a barrier between the blood and the CSF. Lipophilic (liposoluble) compounds, such as oxygen and carbon dioxide, traverse the barrier easily, while many hydrophilic (water-soluble) substances, such as acids, hydrogen, and microorganisms, enter slowly or not at all. Adequate supplies of essential hydrophilic metabolites such as glucose and amino acids are brought into the brain via a carrier-mediated transport system in cerebral capillaries much like that found in renal tubules. The blood–brain barrier is not fully developed in children. Thus, they are more vulnerable than adults to toxic substances and organisms in the bloodstream. Despite these specially designed protective features, a number of ***CNS injuries and infections*** occur. In fact, ***head injury*** is the leading cause of death in persons aged 1 to 44. About 7 to 10 million people in the United States receive medical care for head injuries sustained in motor vehicle and industrial accidents, assaults, falls, and sports injuries annually. When the head is forcefully struck, it either bends to absorb the shock or cracks (skull fracture). ***Linear fractures*** appear as distinct straight lines with parallel margins on x-ray films, while multiple bone fragments characterize ***comminuted fractures.*** Bone fragments are sometimes driven in, compressing or tearing the underlying tissue, a condition referred to as a ***depressed fracture. Basilar fractures,*** occurring at the base of the skull, are not readily detected on routine x-ray films but can sometimes be reliably diagnosed clinically (signs include rhinorrhea, otorrhea, or ear hemorrhage, postauricular hematoma, leakage of blood from the anterior fossa into periorbital tissues). Finally, a ***compound fracture*** is accompanied by a scalp laceration and involves the paranasal sinuses and ear cavity as well as the skull. Direct damage to brain cells is certain in cases of compound fractures. Other complications may include scalp infection, osteomyelitis, and meningitis (most often staphylococcal). Closed head injuries can also result in contusion, laceration, hemorrhage, edema, and herniation of cerebral tissues as the brain is sent into motion against the sharp, irregular surfaces inside the cranial cavity (orbits, sphenoid ridge, falx, and tentorium).

Concussion, an immediate and transient impairment of neural function (e.g., alteration of consciousness, disturbance of vision and/or equilibrium), is common following a moderate to severe blow to the head. Even though skull fracture or gross brain injury is absent, microscopic changes that may cause permanent damage can be sustained. Unresponsiveness may last for periods ranging from seconds to hours. Amnesia for events that occurred just before (retrograde) or after (posttraumatic) the accident is common. Concussions are classified according to the severity of the injury and the resultant neurologic dysfunction, as described in Table 12.14. ***Postconcussion syndrome*** is not uncommon. Characterized by irritability, fatigue, inability to concentrate, and giddiness, it may receive less attention than warranted because the patient "looks fine."

Epidural hematoma, hemorrhage between the dura meningeal layer and the skull, most frequently occurs in the temporal area, since fracture of the temporal bone severs the middle meningeal artery. After a brief period of unconsciousness, the patient may experience a period of alertness. As the clot increases, however, decreased arousal and other signs of increasing intracranial pressure are noted. Prompt surgical intervention is required, since epidural hematomas rapidly jeopardize the patient's life. Recovery depends on the promptness of surgical intervention to lessen the amount of damage to brain tissue.

A blood clot between the dura and the subarachnoid space, or ***subdural hematoma,*** may be acute, subacute or chronic. Acute subdural hematomas occur within the first 24 hours following the trauma and subacute hematomas within 10 days. Chronic subdural hematomas, however, may be found weeks or months following an accident or fall. Subdural hematomas are usually the result of venous bleeding;

TABLE 12.14 TYPES OF CONCUSSIONS

Grade	Description
I	Transient confusion; rapid return to normal consciousness; no amnesia
II	Increased confusion; some residual amnesia (posttraumatic only)
III	More pronounced initial confusion; greater degree of amnesia (posttraumatic and retrograde)
IV	Classic concussion; brief loss of consciousness; variable period of subsequent confusion; some degree of amnesia (both posttraumatic and retrograde)

hence, the symptoms and signs are not manifested as rapidly as in epidural hematomas. A high level of suspicion should be maintained in regard to alcoholics who frequently do not report any antecedent trauma. Symptoms depend on the location of the hematoma as it expands and presses on underlying brain tissue. Again, surgical intervention, usually burr holes, is required to remove the accumulated blood. If done before there is permanent damage to brain tissue, the outcome is good.

Intracerebral hematoma is most common in missile injuries (gunshot wounds, depressed skull fractures, etc.). The signs and symptoms depend on the area of the brain involved. Patients with intracerebral hematomas usually have a poorer prognosis than those with epidural or subdural hematomas. Substantial neurologic deficits often remain in the few surviving patients.

Meticulous evaluation of every patient with a head injury helps to improve the ultimate prognosis. This is best accomplished in an emergency room and subsequent hospital observation. Diagnosis is made by neurologic examination, careful and frequent neurologic assessments, and diagnostic tests. The CT scan is frequently used, and angiography is used if definitive diagnoses cannot be made via the CT scan. Treatment aims at reducing or preventing large increases in intracranial pressure, since such increases interfere with cerebral perfusion and put the entire brain at risk for permanent damage. In addition to surgical intervention, treatment methods include the use of hyperosmolar solutions (such as mannitol), diuretics, corticosteroids, fluid restriction, ventilatory assistance, elevation of the head of the bed, use of a hyperthermia blanket, and administration of muscle relaxants.

Following head injury, ***bacterial meningitis*** may develop. This acute infection of the arachnoid, pia mater, and CSF in adults is usually traced to pneumococci, *Hemophilus influenzae,* or meningococci. Besides trauma, the organisms may reach the CNS through (1) bloodstream invasion by the bacteria; (2) contiguous spread of infection from middle ear, paranasal sinuses or brain abscess; or (3) congenital neuroectodermal defects and craniotomy sites. A majority of patients with meningitis caused by the three common forms of bacteria have an antecedent or concurrent upper respiratory tract infection, acute otitis (or mastoiditis), or pneumonia. Fever, nausea and vomiting, irritability, restlessness, and generalized headache and weakness are common symptoms irrespective of the etiology. Neck and spinal column stiffness are usually present as well. These manifestations may be obscured, however, in the very young or debilitated patient. Confusion and loss of consciousness develop as the illness progresses. Seizures may occur in the acute phases. Extremely rapid onset, the presence of petechial, purpuric, or ecchymotic skin rashes, and circulatory collapse almost always indicate meningococcal infection. Prompt treatment is of the utmost importance because of its rapid progression. Cranial nerve abnormalities occur in 10–20% of patients with bacterial meningitis but disappear after recovery. Partial or total sensorineural hearing loss, which may be irreversible, affects approximately 20% of patients over the age of 3. These losses are not associated with concurrent otitis media. Hemiparesis, dysphasia, and visual field defects develop in about 15% of patients.

Bacterial meningitis is a life-threatening emergency. Patients should be hospitalized for a spinal tap and the initiation of antimicrobial therapy. CSF exam is necessary for diagnosis. Characteristic changes are described in Table 12.15. Gram-stained smears of CSF sediments and cultures of CSF reveal the etiologic agent in 70–80% of cases. Additional laboratory testing is useful for diagnosis and treatment. Blood cultures are positive in 40–60% of patients with *H. influenzae* and may be the

TABLE 12.15 CSF FINDINGS IN BACTERIAL AND VIRAL MENINGITIS

	Bacterial	Viral
Intracranial pressure (mm H_2O)	200–300	90–200
White blood cell count (cells/ mm^3)	100–5,000; usually more than 80% neutrophils	10–1,000; mostly mononuclear
Glucose (mg/dL)	Reduced; less than 40	Normal; occasionally low in mumps and lymphocytic choriomeningitis (LCM) virus
Protein (mg/dL)	100–1,000	50–100
Organisms	Found on Gram stain in 80% of cases; found on culture in 80–90% of cases	LCM and herpes virus isolated from CSF (enteroviruses isolated in stool)

only conclusive test in cases of meningococcal or pneumococcal meningitis (if CSF culture are negative). White blood cell counts are generally elevated. Elevation of lactic dehydrogenase (LDH) may be observed. X-ray films of the chest, skull, and sinuses may provide clues to the location of the primary infection. Antibiotics are administered intravenously for 10 days or more. Penicillin G, ampicillin, and/or chloramphenicol are the drugs of choice, although some bacterial infections may require others (Table 12.16). Prompt treatment is essential to combat complications such as shock, coagulation disorders, endocarditis, and pyogenic arthritis. Mortality is also greatly reduced (that from *H. influenzae* is below 5%, from meningococcal meningitis about 10%, and from pneumococcal meningitis about 20%). In addition to delay of treatment, poor prognostic factors include advanced age, the presence of other areas of infection, underlying diseases (leukemia or alcoholism), and coma.

A number of viruses have been associated with ***viral (aseptic) meningitis*** (Table 12.16). Mumps and poliomyelitis (or other enteroviruses) remain common causes. In addition, infection due to herpes simplex virus has sharply increased in recent years. In general, viral meningitis occurs more frequently during the late summer and early fall in patients under 40. This pattern is mediated to some extent by the type of viral agent and its method of contagion. Once viruses gain access to the body, they replicate in the cells at the site of entry (respiratory tract, GI tract, skin, muscle), disseminate via the bloodstream, and invade the CNS. Symptoms have an abrupt onset and may persist for periods ranging from 3 days to 2 weeks. As with bacterial meningitis headache, fever and neck stiffness are major complaints. In contrast, however, temperature elevations above 40°C are rarely seen and neck stiffness may be present only on extreme flexion. Kernig's sign may or may not be elicited. Other symptoms include general malaise, sore throat, nausea and vomiting, drowsiness, and abdominal pain. Viral meningitis caused by several of the enteroviruses has associated skin rashes that usually appear with fever and resolve in 4–10 days. The diagnosis is confirmed by CSF exam. Changes in CSF fluid in cases of viral infection must be distinguished from those in bacterial meningitis (Table 12.15). Specific antiviral therapy is not available for viral meningitis. Treatment is therefore supportive. Bed rest is important. Analgesics for headache and fever are helpful but should be limited. A slightly elevated temperature may actually be therapeutic because viruses are destroyed easily by heat. Hospitalization may be necessary only if symptoms are severe or if focal neurologic signs are manifested. Full recovery

TABLE 12.16 TYPES AND TREATMENTS OF MENINGITIS AND ENCEPHALITIS

Pathogen	Method of Contagion	Drug of Choice
	Bacterial	
Streptococcus pneumoniae	Direct contact or contiguous infection from otitis media, mastoiditis, sinusitis, pneumonia; head trauma	Penicillin G
Streptococci		
Groups A and B	Direct contact: otitis media, mastoiditis, sinusitis; peritonsillar abscess	Penicillin G
Nongroup A and B	Direct contact: upper and lower respiratory tracts; endocarditis	Penicillin G, gentamycin
Staphylococcus aureus	Complication of neurologic procedure; penetrating head wound; direct contact or contiguous infection from upper respiratory tract	Nafcillin
Neisseria meningitidis	Direct contact: upper respiratory tract	Penicillin G
Hemophilus influenzae	Direct contact: upper respiratory tract	Ampicillin, chloramphenicol
	Spirochete	
Lyme disease	Tick bite	Tetracycline, penicillin
	Viral	
Enteroviruses Polioviruses Coxsackieviruses Echoviruses	Direct contact: respiratory tract, fecal material; replication in intestinal tract Contiguous infection spread from myocarditis, pericarditis	None
Togaviruses (arboviruses)		None
Eastern equine	Mosquitoes	
Western equine	Mosquitoes	
Venezuelan equine	Mosquitoes	
St. Louis	Mosquitoes	
Powassan	Tics	
California	Mosquitoes	
Herpes virus		Adenine arabinoside
Herpes simplex		
Type 1	Direct contact: respiratory	
Type 2	Sexual contact	
Varicella zoster	Direct or direct droplet contact; rarely, droplets are airborne	
Cytomegalovirus	Congenital, vaginal canal; breast feeding; blood transfusions	
Myxoviruses and paramyxoviruses		None
Influenza	Direct contact via respiratory tract or with nasopharyngeal or bronchial secretions	
Parainfluenza	Same as influenza	
Mumps	Same as influenza	
Measles (rubeola)	Same as influenza	
Adenovirus	Direct contact via respiratory tract	None
Lymphocytic choriomeningitis virus	Fecal contamination by infected rodents, dust, and food	None

follows in 5–14 days, although fatigue, lightheadedness, and weakness may persist for months.

Although it was once believed that viruses could not penetrate the blood–brain barrier, it is now evident that in some cases they invade the parenchyma of the brain by infecting and passing through capillary endothelial cells. Subsequent infection develops in the surrounding glial cells and neurons, resulting in ***viral encephalitis.*** The causes are noted in Table 12.16. The most common epidemic form in the United States is ***St. Louis encephalitis.*** Transmitted through mosquito bites, it appears almost exclusively in the summer months. ***Herpes encephalitis*** (caused by herpes simplex virus) also occurs with some frequency and may be seen at any time of the year. Patients present with headache, fever, and neck stiffness. In cases of herpes encephalitis, they may exhibit bizarre behavior, hallucinate, or become aphasic. As the disease progresses, patients develop lethargy, eventually becoming confused and stuporous and eventually comatose. Herpes encephalitis can be treated with adenine arabinoside; however, antiviral therapy is unavailable for the other viruses. Vigorous inhospital supportive care and avoidance of complications is all that can be done. Recovery is possible even after prolonged periods of coma, although neurologic or psychiatric disorders and parkinsonism are frequent sequelae. The overall prognosis depends on the etiologic agent. Herpes infection is associated with a 50% mortality, with a high rate of recurrence in survivors. On the other hand, death from mumps-caused encephalitis is rare and recurrence is infrequent. Mortality for other viruses ranges from 0.5 to 50%.

Brain abscess, the most common parameningeal infection, develops in much the same ways as meningitis or encephalitis. Approximately one-third of these cases are due to pathogens from the lungs or heart or to distant infectious processess (burns, pelvic infection) that gain access to the brain by breaking through the blood–brain barrier. Contiguous infection spread from the middle ear, mastoid cells, sinuses, mouth, face and scalp, craniotomy wounds, metastatic processes, and penetrating head wounds accounts for 30–50% of abscesses. Although brain abscesses can occur at any age, they are most common between ages of 20 and 50. Formation of a brain abscess extends over several weeks to months. A poorly defined area of bacterial encephalitis gradually becomes liquefied, causing tissue death. As time passes, some of these areas develop thick outer shells, while others spread into central white matter and penetrate the ventricular wall. Acute meningitis results in the latter cases. Headache, the most common initial symptom, may not be recognized as serious because attention is directed to the primary infection. The headache is usually localized on the side of the abscess. As infection progresses, however, it often generalizes and increases in severity. Along with headache, other early symptoms suggest meningitis or stroke and subside or respond to antimicrobial treatment. Within a few weeks, however, growing intracranial pressure causes nausea, vomiting, drowsiness, bradycardia, confusion, and stupor. Specific neurologic signs develop and indicate the location of the abscess. Patients exhibiting these symptoms should be hospitalized.

The diagnosis of brain abscess is based on clinical findings and diagnostic tests. CT scanning provides the most extensive information about the size and location of the abscess. Lumbar puncture may not be advisable due to elevated intracranial pressure. Surgical drainage is the most widely used intervention in cases of brain abscess. Gram-stained smears and cultures of the aspirated fluid isolate the pathogen. Streptococci, often non-group A or anaerobic strains, are implicated in most cases. Based on these findings, antibiotic therapy is initiated. When left untreated, brain abscess leads to death. With the introduction of CT scanning and the use of antibiotics, mortality has decreased. Seizures are a common sequela; therefore, anticonvulsive therapy may be indicated.

There is little protection against the bullet-shaped rhabdovirus that causes ***rabies,*** since this virus is transmitted along the peripheral nerves to the gray matter of the brain. The most common mode of entrance into the body by far is the bite of a rabid animal, particularly wild skunks, raccoons, foxes, bats, coyotes, and wolves. Less often, animal rabies is found in dogs, farm animals, rodents, and rabbits. In rare cases, airborne viruses are inhaled or come in contact with open wounds and mucous membranes. The incubation period in humans, which varies from 10 days to over 12 months, is related to the amount of virus introduced and the severity of the wound. During this time, the virus replicates in the skin and muscle at the site of invasion, travels to the gray matter where replication continues, and returns to the body (again along peripheral fibers). In 90% of cases, the prodromal phase of rabies begins 14–90 days afer exposure. Malaise, fever, fatigue, nausea and vomiting, sore throat, nonproductive cough, and paresthesia characterize this period. Intermittent pain, tingling, or burning around the bite is diagnostically significant. Rabies progresses to the excitation or encephalitic phase, which is marked by convulsions, hypersensitivity to light and noise, active deep tendon reflexes, Babinski sign, neck stiffness, and focal paralysis. Spasm of respiratory muscles leads to shallow, and irregular breathing and paralysis of the speech muscles result in hoarseness and voice loss. In a majority of cases, contractions of the mouth, pharynx, and larynx on drinking and later at the sight of liquid are noted. Symptoms of excitation usually give way to generalized flaccid paralysis shortly before death. The usual course of rabies (if untreated) from prodrome to death is 4 to 20 days.

The diagnosis of rabies is based on the source of the bite (animal species, unprovoked attack), the prevalence of rabies in the area, and laboratory findings. Following an attack, domestic animals should be observed by a veterinarian for 10 days. If signs of rabies develop during that time, the animal is killed and the head sent for autopsy. Observation of wild animals is not recommended. They should be killed immediately upon capture, decapitated, and sent for laboratory exam. If antirabies treatment is instituted early, recovery is probable. Once signs of the disease are evident, this is less likely. ▶***Antirabies measures*** begin with immediate local treatment of the wound (refer to the discussion of the skin for laceration care). In addition, all patients licked, scratched, or bitten by suspicious animals should receive an antirabies vaccine. Human diploid cell vaccine (HDCV) and human rabies immune globulin (RIG) are the preferred vaccines because they produce the fewest side effects. Preexposure prophylaxis for high-risk persons (veterinarians, animal handlers, laboratory workers, trappers, taxidermists, and cave explorers) is recommended. Finally, all domestic animals should receive antirabies vaccine according to a veterinarian's recommendations.

Decreased cardiac output, pulmonary failure, severe anemia, insulin overdose, pancreatic adenoma, and liver failure reduce or eliminate oxygen and glucose supplies to be transported by the blood–brain barrier into the brain. High levels of acidity and alkalinity that accompany the accumulation of certain pancreatic, liver, and kidney diseases and toxic metabolic products (urea, creatine, and ammonia) during renal and hepatic failure may overwhelm and break through the blood–brain barrier. In such cases, ***metabolic encephalopathy*** results. Although focal or lateralized signs of cerebral disease and cellular changes in spinal fluid are absent, consciousness is invariably impaired. Alterations in consciousness range from restlessness, agitation, delirium, and apathy to confusion or coma. Generalized or multifocal convulsions are common. Disturbance of muscle tone is often demonstrated as paratonia, primitive sucking, snouting and grasping reflexes, involuntary movements, and, most commonly, "metabolic flap" (flapping tremor). In many cases of metabolic encephalopathy damage is irreversible. Careful management of underlying disease (see the relevant chapters) and appropriate treatment of hypoxia, hypoglycemia, hypercapnia, or toxin invasion at the earliest possible moment will prevent and limit injury.

HORMONE CONTROL

Hypothalamus and Pituitary

The hypothalamus, a small portion of the diencephalon, rests on the floor of the brain's third ventricle (Fig. 12.8). It contains neurons that function both as electrically excitable nerves and as glands that synthesize and secrete hormonal substances. Thus, the hypothalamus serves as an intermediary between the nervous and endocrine systems. Most of the hormones produced are termed "regulating hormones," since they influence a chain of hormonal events in other organs. They include corticotropin-releasing factor (CRF), prolactin inhibitory factor (PIF), human growth hormone-releasing factor (HGHRF), melanocyte stimulation hormone-releasing factor (MSHRF), melanocyte-stimulating hormone inhibitory factors (MSHIF), luteotropin-releasing factor (LRF), follicle-stimulating hormone-releasing factor (FSHRF), and thyrotropin-releasing factor (TRF).

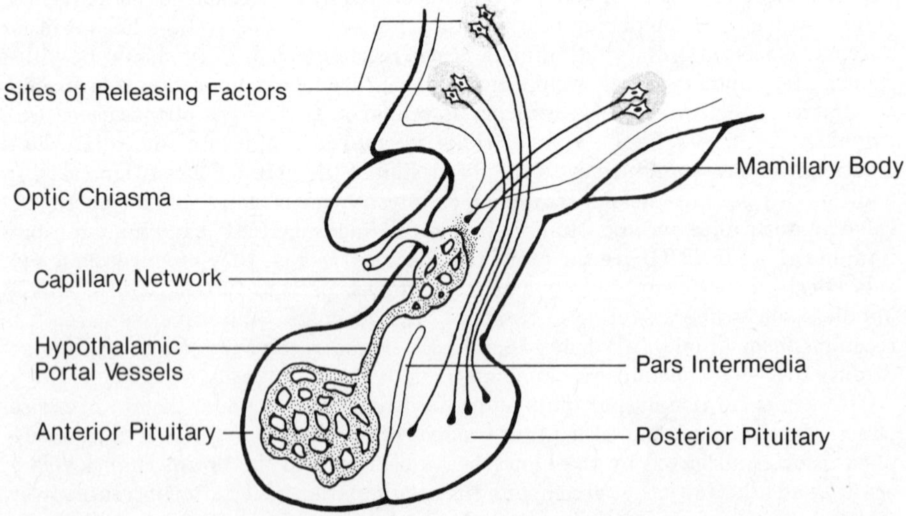

Figure 12.8 Hypothalamus and pituitary. (From Butnarescu, GF, and Tillotson, DM, *Maternity Nursing: Theory to Practice,* © 1983, John Wiley and Sons, Inc., New York.)

The infundibular stalk connects the hypothalamus to the pituitary gland. About 1.3 cm in diameter, the pituitary is located in the bony sella turcica. Secretions from the hypothalamus are carried via the hypophyseal-portal circulation to the anterior lobe of the pituitary (adenohypophysis). Cell bodies of the hypothalamic neurons terminate directly in the posterior lobe of the pituitary gland (neurohypophysis).

Neurons of the anterior pituitary are electrically excitable and are influenced by impulses from other brain areas and by hormonal feedback. Glandular cells of the adenohypophysis produce tropic hormones that stimulate other endocrine glands. Named by laboratory stains, glandular cells include (1) acidophils that produce human growth hormone (HGH) and prolactin; (2) basophils that secrete thyroid-stimulating hormone (TSH), adrenocorticotropic hormone (ACTH), melanocyte-stimulating hormone (MSH), luteinizing hormone (LH), and follicle-stimulating hormone (FSH); and (3) chromophobes that are probably involved with ACTH production. Cell bodies of the hypothalamic neurons, located in the posterior lobe of the pituitary, release antidiuretic hormone (ADH) and oxytocin when stimulated.

Hormones are released in response to signals received via the bloodstream, nervous system, or hypothalamus. The endocrine glands usually respond via a negative feedback mechanism whereby secretion is halted when hormone levels are adequate but stimulated as these levels drop. Sex hormones, secreted by the ovaries and testes, and insulin, secreted by the pancreas, are discussed in Chapters 5 and 9, respectively.

Pituitary deficiency (hypopituitarism) may be manifested as a shortage of one or many hormones. In childhood, it results in ***pituitary dwarfism.*** GH, described in Table 12.17, is the most sensitive of the pituitary hormones to pituitary compromise, and levels may plunge while normal amounts of other hormones are secreted. Causes of pituitary dwarfism include idiopathic hypopituitarism, intracranial lesions, or a reversible condition known as ***psychosocial dwarfism,*** where a child continuously exposed to an abusive and neglectful environment will fail to produce

TABLE 12.17 GROWTH HORMONE

			Clinical Manifestations of:	
Effects	**Mechanisms**	**Regulation**	**Hypo-secretion**	**Hyper-secretion**
Increases growth rate of soft and hard tissues. Maintains tissue size after maturity.	Increases entrance rate of amino acids into cells. Increases rate of protein synthesis. Stimulates adipose tissue to release fats (lypolysis), thereby supplying free fatty acids to bloodstream. Stimulates the breakdown of glycogen to glucose (hyperglycemic effect). Decreases rate of carbohydrate utilization throughout the body. Stimulates cellular hypertrophy and hyperplasia. Increases rate of mitosis. Increases tissue and organ weight. Increases tissue protein. Increases amount of water retained by tissues.	Secretion increased by human growth-releasing factor (HGHRF) when blood sugar falls or amino acid consumption rises (with stress, exercise). Secretion decreased by human growth-inhibiting factor (HGHIF) when blood sugar is abnormally high.	Dwarfism	Giantism (in children), acromegaly (in adults)

adequate levels of HGH. The child with pituitary dwarfism is normally proportioned, but the stature is short and a plateau effect may be noted on the growth chart. Premature wrinkling of the skin may be present. If the condition continues through the pubertal years, sexual development is likely to fail. It is important to rule out other conditions that interfere with growth such as primary hypothyroidism, nutritional deficiency, cardiac or renal disease, or familial short stature. If the last is the case, the child may fall below the lower line on the growth chart, but in a parallel fashion as opposed to a noticeable leveling off. The diagnosis is confirmed by measuring HGH by radioimmunoassay before and after a stress challenge. Normally, HGH levels will rise by at least 7 ng after induced stresses such as insulin hypoglycemia or administration of levodopa or arginine. Failure to increase sufficiently is diagnostic of HGH deficiency. Since the development of synthetic HGH, treatment is available for all children in need. Monthly injections will maintain a near-normal level of growth, with the best results derived when treatment is implemented earlier in the life cycle. Replacement of other hormones is necessary if they are also affected by the hypopituitarism. Changes in environment have been shown to reverse the HGH deficiency peculiar to psychosocial dwarfism.

Hypopituitarism in the adult may be caused by hypothalamic failure, tumors (particularly chromophobe adenomas), ischemic necrosis of the gland due to infection, carotid aneurysm, or carcinomatous metastases. A fourth cause, more prevalent in Third World countries than in the industrialized world, is postpartum necrosis to the pituitary. The pituitary swells during pregnancy and is believed to be more susceptible to necrosis during the postpartum period. If damage is limited to the anterior pituitary, noticeable symptoms are a gradual loss of pubic and axillary hair, loss of libido, and weakness. Men with hypopituitarism may notice that they need to shave less frequently than formerly, and women experience oligo- or amenorrhea. Symptoms of hypothyroidism and hypoadrenalism are likely to appear (see the later section). Treatment consists of hormonal replacement (androgens, estrogens, cortisone, thyroid hormone) and tumor removal, if possible.

If the posterior pituitary is compromised, insufficient amounts of antidiuretic hormone (ADH) are released, resulting in ***diabetes insipidus (DI).*** As described in Table 12.18, ADH regulates water conservation by the kidney. In addition to the contributing conditions discussed above, DI may be idiopathic, familial (rare), or caused by trauma to the neurohypophysis. Trauma-induced DI may be reversible. All types are typified by thirst, especially for water, and by excretion of voluminous amounts of urine (3–18 L/day). The onset of symptoms may be abrupt. The presence of nocturia is common, and this helps to distinguish it from psychogenic polydipsia. The major danger with DI is the consequence of inaccessibility of water. In severe cases, fluid loss without replacement can result in circulatory collapse or hypertonic encephalopathy within hours. Laboratory testing reveals urine specific gravity of less than 1.005 and urine osmolality of less than 200 mOsm per kilogram of water. Serum sodium is generally elevated. Provocative testing can be done by closely monitoring the patient during water deprivation and evaluating the specific gravity, which would rise in the normal individual. Changes in specific gravity can also be quantitated in response to injected ADH. A normal response only after injection indicates DI. In mild cases where some ADH production remains, the drug chlorpropamide acts both to stimulate ADH secretion and to enhance the effect of existing ADH on the collecting ducts. In the absence of endogenous ADH, supplemental ADH can be administered in the form of a nasal spray or intramuscular injection.

TABLE 12.18 ANTIDIURETIC HORMONE (ADH)

Effects	Mechanism	Regulation	Clinical Manifestations of: Hypo-secretion	Clinical Manifestations of: Hyper-secretion
Maintains appropriate tonicity of urine. Conserves body water. Maintains blood pressure in case of severe volume depletion.	Increases water permeability of renal collecting ducts. Enhances active transport of NaCl from ascending limb of Henle to interstitial spaces of kidney. Directly constricts vascular smooth muscle.	Hypothalamic receptors directly stimulated by plasma osmolarity and baroreceptors to release ADH in posterior pituitary. Secretion increases when blood osmolarity is high (dehydration) or when blood pressure suddenly decreases. Secretion halted when blood osmolarity is low (dilution).	Pituitary DI	Inappropriate ADH syndrome

Hyperpituitarism in the adult may result in prolonged, excessive secretion of HGH, with bony overgrowth of skin, cartilage, subcutaneous tissue, and internal organs that characterizes ***acromegaly.*** Acidophil cell adenoma or hyperplasia are the usual causes. Although nonmalignant, such tumors may impinge on the nearby optic chiasma and cause neurologic symptoms. The onset of acromegaly is insidious and the progression is slow. Men are affected more frequently than women, with onset usually occurring during the third and fourth decades. An acromegalic may note change in features only when comparing his or her present appearance to that of old photographs. Bony enlargement is most noticeable distally on the hands, feet, and face. The skin thickens, skin folds are accentuated, and large, meaty hands and features are observed. The patient may notice the need for larger glove or shoe sizes and the tightening of rings. Other early symptoms include excessive sweating, paresthesia of the hands and feet, and hypogonadism manifested by loss of libido and amenorrhea. If the tumor is impinging on nervous tissue, headaches, loss of visual fields, and decreasing visual acuity are warning signals. As deep layers of joint cartilage proliferate, articular cartilage becomes thin and acromegalic arthritis may occur as joint pain and stiffness. Organs such as the lungs, liver, heart, spleen, and intestine can enlarge from two to five times the normal size. A late complication is osteoporosis. Huskiness of the voice, recent onset of snoring, spreading of the teeth and bite, and an unpleasant body odor are additional manifestations of acromegaly.

The course of acromegaly is variable, ranging from chronic, lasting for more than 50 years, to fulminant, where a rapidly growing tumor can lead to death caused by tumor hemorrhage, hypertension, or heart failure (acromegalic heart disease) within 3 years of onset. Again, the onset is often difficult to determine due to the subtlety of symptom development, and clinicians should be alert in order to recognize acromegaly as early as possible. Radioimmunoassay of serum HGH will reveal elevation in the acromegalic. An abnormal visual field exam and positive skull x-ray films indicate an enlarging tumor. Transsphenoidal resection or cryosurgery is undertaken for small tumors and transfrontal surgery for large tumors. If the patient is a poor surgical candidate, irradiation of the pituitary can control abnormal HGH secretion in most cases.

Basophilic, acidophilic, and chromophobe adenomas are the different types of

pituitary tumors. Malignancy of the pituitary is rare. Men are more commonly affected than women, with the usual age at onset being between 30 and 60. The signs and symptoms of endocrine insufficiency develop early but are often so subtle that the patient may not even seek medical care. Gonadal, thyroid, and, less often, adrenal insufficiency will develop. Prolactin-secreting microadenomas cause galactorrhea. It is the neurologic symptoms that often bring the patient to the health care provider and lead to diagnosis. These include loss of visual fields, usually bitemporal hemianopia (which may be unnoticed by the patient), failing visual acuity, headache, and, in severe cases, paralysis of cranial nerves III, IV, and VI (oculomotor, trochlear, and abducens). The headache has no typical form. Some patients with pituitary tumors are asymptomatic. The risks of untreated pituitary tumors are continued growth, causing irreversible neurologic damage, and pituitary apoplexy. Pituitary apoplexy is caused by tumor infarction, hemorrhage, or necrosis; blindness, coma, and death may follow. Frontal and sagittal skull x-ray films, CT scanning, and carotid artery angiography are used to demonstrate changes in tissues surrounding the tumor, such as an enlarged sella turcica or tumor extension into a nearby sinus. The ***"empty sella syndrome"*** is found in one-fourth to one-third of patients with enlarged sella turcica. These patients may have normal or diminished pituitary function. Since there is no tumor in these cases, surgery is not indicated; if it is performed, complications such as CSF fistula formations can occur. Thus, a CT scan is performed to rule out the empty sella syndrome. If this syndrome is found, hormonal replacement is rarely indicated for those with hypopituitary function. Transsphenoidal adenomectomy, preferably with microsurgical techniques, is curative in most instances. Irradiation of the pituitary can arrest tumor growth. Patients should be monitored after treatment for secondary hypopituitarism.

Thyroid

TSH is promptly released from the adenohypophysis in response to secretion of TRH by the hypothalamus. The thyroid gland reacts by augmenting the circulating levels of free thyroid hormones, which then feed back to the hypothalamus and anterior pituitary to discourage further secretion of TRH or TSH.

The two lateral lobes of the butterfly-shaped thyroid gland lie on either side of the trachea, with a connecting isthmus below the cricoid cartilage in the neck (Fig. 12.9). A pyramidal lobe may be present; if so, it extends upward from the isthmus. Within the follicles, spheroid sacs that compose thyroid tissue manufacture three thyroid hormones; tetraiodothyroxine (thyroxine, T_4), triiodothyronine (T_3), and thyrocalcitonin (calcitonin). These hormones are described in Table 12.19. Iodine and the amino acid tyrosine, obtained from the diet, are crucial to the synthesis of the thyroid hormones, which are stored as the protein thyroglobulin within the colloidal portion of the follicle. The thyroid picks up and efficiently concentrates one-third of the ingested iodine, the rest being lost in the urine. When stimulated by TSH, the thyroid initiates hormone synthesis and secretion into the bloodstream. Although it composes less than 5% of the total circulating thyroid hormones, T_3 is three to five times more active biologically than T_4. More profuse but far less potent, T_4 can be converted by the liver and kidneys by deiodination to form T_3. Once in the bloodstream, all but a fraction of 1% of the thyroid hormones are bound to a serum protein, thyroxine-binding globulin (TBG). Only the tiny amounts of "free" hormone are registered by the hypothalamus; high amounts of TBG alone will not cause suppression or curtailment of TRF release.

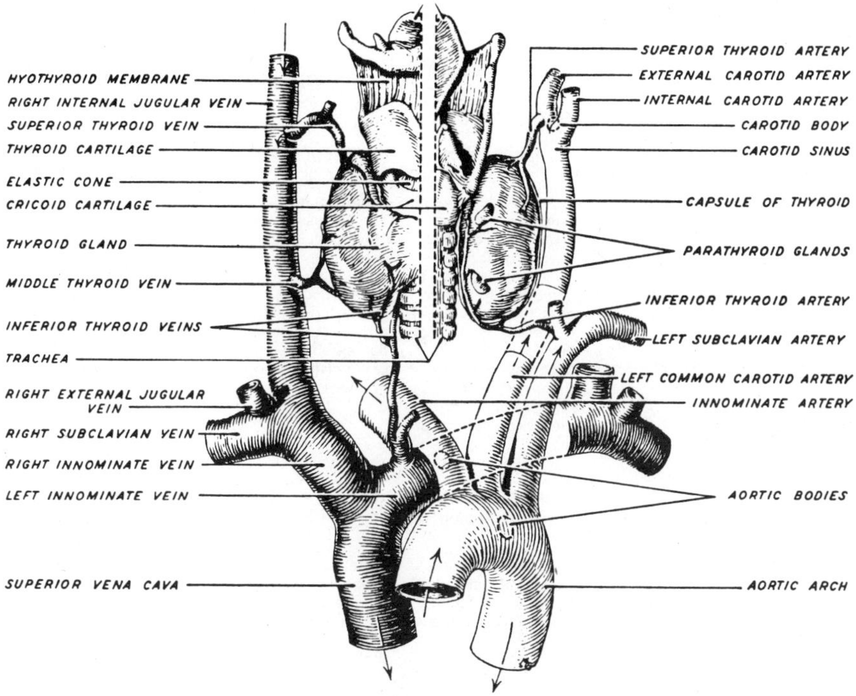

Figure 12.9 Thyroid and parathyroid glands. (From Brown, AM, and Stubbs, DW, *Medical Physiology,* © 1983, John Wiley and Sons, Inc., New York.)

A deficiency of thyroid hormones results in the clinical entity ***hypothyroidism.*** Infants are carefully screened for this condition, since deprivation of T_3 and T_4 in the first few years of life can have devastating effects. The incidence of congenital hypothyroidism is approximately 1 per 5,000 live births annually. Normal development of the CNS and skeleton does not occur, resulting in irreversible mental retardation and stunted growth known as ***cretinism.*** Widespread screening programs and prompt hormonal replacement therapy ensure normal development of the hypothyroid child. Delay of treatment past the sixth week of life is strongly associated with an increased rate of mental retardation.

The effects of ▶***hypothyroidism in the adult*** are often much more subtle. The onset of symptoms may be insidious and gradual. The various etiologies of hypothyroidism, enumerated in Table 12.20, share the net effect of insufficient circulating thyroid hormone to meet cellular metabolic needs, with diminished energy production, lethargy, weakness, fatigue, vague aches and pains, and cold intolerance often attributed by the patient to other causes. In more severe cases, a mucinous fluid accumulates in the interstitial spaces, causing a nonpitting swelling of the skin and other subcutaneous tissues. This condition, known as ***"myxedema,"*** gives a puffy appearance to the face (especially the periorbital area) and extremities. When deposited in the larynx or oropharynx, the fluid contributes to the hoarse, husky vocal changes associated with hypothyroidism. It also produces a modest weight gain, usually of 5–10 lb. Loss of appetite is common. Heart rate and output are decreased, the extreme consequence being congestive heart failure. The low metabolic rate

TABLE 12.19 THYROID HORMONES

Hormone	Effect	Mechanism	Regulation	Clinical Manifestations of: Hyposecretion	Clinical Manifestations of: Hypersecretion
T_3 and T_4 (via TSH)	Controls rate of body metabolism/energy production. Helps regulate tissue growth. Increases CNS reactivity. Ensures adequate heat production.	Increases cellular enzymatic activities. Increases rate of glucose absorption from GI tract. Increases rate of glucose utilization by cells. Increases rate of carbohydrate metabolism. Encourages lypolysis. Encourages protein breakdown for energy production. Increases pulse and cardiac output. Increases GI motility and secretions. Increases synaptic activity influencing reaction times.	Secretion increased by TRF (causes release of TSH) when level of circulating thyroid hormone is low or when there is cooling of preoptic area of hypothalamus. Secretion decreased when level of circulating thyroid hormone is high.	Hypothyroidism, cretinism	Hyperthyroidism
Thyrocalcitonin	Maintains homeostasis of blood calcium and phosphate levels.	Accelerates absorption of calcium by bone. Inhibits bone breakdown. Inhibits parathormone.	Negative feedback based on serum calcium levels. Secretion increases when blood calcium is high. Secretion halts when blood calcium is low.	Not established	Not established

causes decreased oxygen and energy availability and may result in angina pectoris or myocardial infarction in the high-risk individual. Low levels of T_3 and T_4 are associated with high blood lipid levels, especially cholesterol, thus accelerating the development of atherosclerosis and coronary artery disease. Other cardiovascular changes include increased capillary fragility, decreased systolic blood pressure, possibly mild elevation in diastolic blood pressure, anemia, pericardial effusion, and cardiomegaly. The skin becomes dry and inelastic, the hair brittle and sparse. An orange discoloration of the skin, caused by carotene deposition, may be observed. Thyroid hormone is necessary for the conversion in the liver of beta carotene to vitamin A, hence the hypercarotenemic state with a possible associated deficiency of vitamin A. The thyroid gland may be enlarged or normal in size. GI motility is slowed and constipation is the rule. The patient is usually apathetic; however, an extreme form of psychotic withdrawal, known as ***myxedema madness,*** may occur. Hypothyroidism in the elderly may be manifested subtly as hearing impairment, decreased calculation skills, failing memory, or somnolence, leading to a misdiagnosis of senility. In very severe cases, hypoxic "myxedema coma" carries a high mortality. Other symptoms include ataxia, menorrhagia, loss of fertility and/or libido, greater susceptibility to infection, and increased sensitivity to CNS depressants. A diagnostic sign of hypothyroidism is a prolonged deep tendon reflex relaxation phase.

Once the clinician suspects hypothyroidism, the diagnosis can be confirmed by laboratory analysis. Initial testing is done to determine the free fraction of T_4 (free T_4 index). This is commonly achieved by measuring total T_4 (including protein-

TABLE 12.20 CAUSES OF HYPOTHYROIDISM

Primary congenital	Exposure to goitrogens (thiocyanate, perchlorate, cobalt, aminoglutethimide)
Thyroid dysgenesis or agenesis	Drug induced (lithium carbonate, sulfonamides, phenylbutazone, antithyroid drugs and others)
Maternal use of antithyroid drugs	Cancer of the thyroid
Enzyme defects causing impaired synthesis of thyroid hormones	Infiltrative disorders of the thyroid
Primary acquired	Secondary
Idiopathic	Hypothalamic dysfunction
Radioactive iodine treatment of hyperthyroidism	Pituitary dysfunction
Thyroiditis (autoimmune or subacute)	
Iodine deficiency	

bound T_4) and resin T_3 uptake (a percentage value reflecting occupied thyroxine-binding sites in the patient's serum). Serum poorly saturated with T_4 will attract radioactive T_3; thus, less is left for the resin to pick up. The lower the percentage (less T_3 picked up by the resin), the more binding sites are available (serum thyroid-binding proteins hungry for the short supply of thyroid hormone). Since numerous factors can affect the amount of plasma proteins, the resin T_3 uptake and total T_4 values are combined to form an indirect measure of free T_4. Free T_4 can also be directly measured. In a hypothyroid patient, one expects to find a low total T_4, a low T_3 resin uptake percentage, and a low calculated free T_4. Further evaluation includes measurement of TSH; this is increased in primary hypothyroidism as a well-functioning anterior pituitary attempts to stimulate a failing thyroid gland. An increased TSH level and borderline or low normal free T_4 are still strongly indicative of hypothyroidism. If the problem is at the level of the pituitary gland (secondary hypothyroidism), an assay of TRH may be increased with low TSH and free T_4. In hypothalamic failure, all values are diminished. Measurement of the TSH response to injected TRH has been found to diagnose hypothyroidism in cases where other laboratory results have been within normal limits.

Treatment of hypothyroidism consists of thyroid hormone replacement and amelioration of the underlying cause, if possible. Both synthetic and natural (made from desiccated thyroid gland) thyroid hormones are inexpensive and readily available. The synthetic form (usually levothyroxine) appears to have an even more physiologic effect. Desiccated thyroid contains some free T_3, which may cause symptoms of hyperthyroidism (see the next section) 2–4 hours following administration. The patient's clinical picture and blood tests can be used to monitor therapeutic levels of replacement hormones.

At the opposite end of the spectrum lies ***hyperthyroidism,*** a hypermetabolic state produced by excessive quantities of circulating thyroid hormones. Table 12.21 lists some of the diseases associated with hyperthyroidism in order of incidence.

Graves' disease is the cause of approximately 85% of cases of hyperthyroidism. Although the precise etiology has not been established, Graves' disease is generally

TABLE 12.21 CAUSES OF HYPERTHYROIDISM

Graves' disease	Subacute thyroiditis
Toxic goiter	TSH-secreting tumor of the pituitary
Toxic adenoma	Thyroid carcinoma
Iodide-induced hyperthyroidism	

assumed to have an autoimmune basis, since non-TSH long-acting thyroid-stimulating immunoglobulins are found in the serum of most patients. Women are affected 10 times as frequently as men, with disease onset peaking between the ages of 30 and 40. A genetic predisposition has been established. Mild weight loss and anxiety may be the only indicators of early hyperthyroidism; later in the disease, the clinical picture can become quite dramatic. Symptoms of this hypermetabolic state include nervousness, tremor, emotional lability, increased appetite with weight loss, rapid speech, heat intolerance, and increased perspiration. The cardiovascular system is in high gear, and the patient may experience tachycardia, palpitations, and arrhythmias (usually of atrial origin). Objective investigation may reveal cardiomegaly, accentuated first heart sound (S1), increased systolic and decreased diastolic blood pressures, and, in some cases, congestive heart failure. Hypermotility of the GI system frequently causes diarrhea and perhaps nausea and vomiting. In contrast to the dry, brittle skin and hair changes of hypothyroidism, one observes smooth, warm, moist, flushed skin and fine, soft hair. A painless separation of the distal portion of the nail plate from its underlying bed, called "onycholysis," characteristically initially affects the fourth digit most frequently. Later, the separated portion may become smooth and concave. Menses may be scant or cease. Muscle weakness and even atrophy may be present. However, a strongly accelerated Achilles reflex may be observed. Eye changes are characteristic of Graves' disease. These include unilateral or bilateral lid lag, protrusion of the globe (exophthalmos), dry or gritty-feeling eyes, photophobia, and diplopia. The patient may need to tape the eyelids closed at night to avoid drying and desiccation of the cornea. The thyroid is usually enlarged from one and a half to five times the normal size, with an audible bruit in some cases. Not every hyperthyroid individual manifests all of these symptoms. In the elderly, hyperthyroidism may be masked and may present only with depression, weight loss, congestive heart failure, and/or atrial fibrillation. The recent onset of atrial fibrillation in an elderly patient mandates laboratory testing for hyperthyroidism, which is a reversible cause of this arrhythmia.

Thyroid storm or thyrotoxic crisis is an extreme hypermetabolic state triggered in the uncontrolled or poorly controlled patient by surgery or intercurrent medical illness (usually sepsis). Elevated temperature, perhaps as high as 106°F, delirium, and/or coma typify this life-threatening condition. Other symptoms include irritability, restlessness, tachycardia, hypotension, vomiting, and diarrhea. In these patients, emergency measures may be taken to correct hypotension and possible shock and to reduce body temperature. Large doses of thyroid-suppressing medication must be administered immediately to slow the metabolic rate. Administration of iodide in the thyrotoxic patient can have a rapid inhibitory effect on thyroid hormone output. Since this effect is transitory, iodide may be given initially in addition to other antithyroid agents. Careful presurgical thyroid suppression can prevent the onset of thyroid storm. Calculation or direct measurement of free T_4 often yields an elevated value in the hyperthyroid patient. However, in some cases, only free T_3 may be increased; thus, if hyperthyroidism is clinically suspected and the free T_4 level is normal, free T_3 should be assessed. If doubt still remains, the change in TSH in response to TRH administration can clarify the diagnosis. Since TSH is undetectable or low in normal and hyperthyroid individuals, measurement of TSH alone is not worthwhile. However, if the TSH response to stimulation by intravenous TRH is absent or diminished, hyperthyroidism is likely. An autoimmune basis for thyroid dysfunction can be documented by identifying serum antithyroid antibodies (such as antithyroglobulin, anticytoplasmic, or antimicrosomal antibodies) having significant titers.

Treatment of Graves' disease is aimed at reducing thyroid hormone output by either chemotherapeutic suppression of hormone synthesis or by destruction or removal of thyroid tissue by radioactive iodine or surgery. Propylthiouracil (PTU) and methimazole are two agents that can be used individually for long-term antithyroid therapy, PTU being considered safer. When a euthyroid state is reached, a low maintenance dose is continued, sometimes combined with exogenous thyroid hormone; this addition may help avoid "burnout" hypothyroidism. The latter complication is common in hyperthyroidism, either as a consequence of thyroid suppression or as the natural endpoint of disease. The antithyroid medications can help produce the euthyroid state but may not help prevent future exacerbations. Leukopenia (mild to marked) with rare agranulocytosis, hypersensitivity reactions, and hepatitis are adverse drug effects that may warrent discontinuation or close observation. Treatment during pregnancy is controversial, since the drugs may cause hypothyroidism in the fetus. Radioactive iodine (^{131}I), administered orally, is a very effective ablative treatment of hyperthyroidism and is especially convenient for patients who are a poor surgical risk. A recognized drawback is the high incidence of subsequent hypothyroidism: 15–20% in the first year and 70–80% after 20 years. Radiation thyroiditis is a complication that may occur, causing excessive release of thyroid hormone in the blood 7–10 days after treatment—a potentially dangerous problem for the patient with cardiac disease. Carcinogenic or leukemic effects of therapeutic dosages of ^{131}I have not been established. However, this treatment is now considered the primary therapy for everyone, including children and young adults, with the exception of pregnant women. Subtotal thyroidectomy, the classic ablative therapy, is now employed mainly during pregnancy or for large goiters not responding to thyroid medications. Late hypothyroidism is less common than with radioactive iodine administration. Since surgery may trigger thyroid storm, patients must be brought to the euthyroid state preoperatively by antithyroid medications. Then iodide is administered concurrently to cause involution of the gland. Propranolol has been used prior to surgery to control symptoms; however, it does not induce a euthyroid state. Hemorrhage, laryngeal nerve damage, and hypoparathyroidism are the principal complications of thyroidectomy.

Inflammation of the thyroid gland, or ***thyroiditis,*** may be caused by a variety of processes including bacterial or viral infection, autoimmune response, and invasive fibrosis, as described in Table 12.22. Women are more commonly affected than men. The thyroid gland is usually enlarged or otherwise abnormal to palpation. Symptoms may range from hypo- to hyperthyroidism, depending on the etiology. Thyroid autoantibodies are found in the sera of patients with autoimmune thyroiditis, most commonly ***Hashimoto's thyroiditis.*** Systemic complaints such as fever, aches, and malaise are often present in subacute thyroiditis. The prognosis is generally quite good once the appropriate diagnosis is made and treatment is instituted as outlined in Table 12.22.

There are various etiologies for ***thyroid nodules*** or ***thyroid masses. Endemic goiter*** is an enlargement of the thyroid caused by a dietary iodine deficiency. Failure to consume 100 μg/day of iodine results in decreased production of T_4. Iodine is still scarce in some regions, including the Andes and the Himalayas. Low levels of T_4 feed back to the anterior pituitary, and TSH is released in greater amounts. T_3 levels can be normal; thus, patients may be euthyroid. Continual overstimulation by TSH

TABLE 12.22 TYPES OF THYROIDITIS

Type	Etiology	Histopathology	Incidence
Subacute nonsuppurative	Unknown, but associated with recent viral infection.	Leukocyte and multinucleated giant cell infiltrate.	Not rare. Occurs in third to fifth decades. F:M[a] = 4:1.
Subacute lymphocytic	Possibly autoimmune.	Lymphocytic infiltration.	Incidence increasing. F:M = 2:1.
Acute	Bacterial infection.	Bacteria isolated. White blood cells increased.	Rare.
Chronic (Hashimoto's)	Autoimmune.	Lymphocyte, plasma cell infiltrates. Fibrosis of germinal centers.	Not rare. Increases with age. F:M = 5:1.
Chronic (Riedel's)	Unknown.	Fibrosis of thyroid tissue and possibly trachea.	Rare.

[a] Female : Male.

causes hypertrophy and hyperplasia of the thyroid gland. Low levels of thyroid hormones also result from impaired hormone synthesis; in this case, TSH is released in large quantities, causing ***sporadic goiter.*** Both sporadic and endemic goiters may begin with a diffusely enlarged thyroid. Later, large follicles can form, while other areas of the gland may atrophy or fibrose. The goiter is then termed "multinodular." Long-term high TSH levels may cause increased production of T_4 by an active follicle, leading to symptoms of hyperthyroidism. The thyroid gland may become so large that dysphagia and/or respiratory obstruction present in extreme cases. Most commonly, a goiter is discovered in an asymptomatic patient during routine exam. Treatment of endemic goiter consists of iodine supplementation either in foods or by injection of iodinated oil. Sporadic goiter is treated on the basis of glandular function. If the patient is euthyroid and less than age 40, suppression of TSH by thyroid hormone administration may cause regression of the goiter. Care must be taken with the elderly or those with cardiac disease, since hormone supplementation may result in hyperthyroidism. If the thyroid is hyperfunctioning, radioactive iodine and antithyroid drugs are used; if it is hypofunctioning, thyroid hormone supplementation is required. Surgery is indicated if tracheal or esophageal obstruction is present.

Of prime importance is the differentiation between ***thyroid carcinoma*** and benign thyroid growths. Solitary nodules are more suggestive of malignancy, although thyroid cancer is low in incidence (0.5% of all malignancies). Palpable thyroid nodules may be found in 4% of the general population, especially in women. Follicular and papillary carcinomas constitute approximately 80% of thyroid cancers; if appropriately diagnosed, these tumors respond well to therapy. Benign thyroid tumors are commonly follicular adenomas, most of which do not overproduce thyroid hormones; however, those that do may precipitate symptoms of hyperthyroidism. Usually the patient is unaware of the existence of a thyroid nodule, which is typically discovered during routine physical exam. Since only 20–30% of surgically removed tumors are malignant, the trend has shifted to diagnosis based upon less invasive techniques.

Presentation	Thyroid Function	Treatment	Course
Tender, large thyroid. Systemic symptoms (fever, chills).	Mild increase; decrease may follow illness.	Analgesics, steroids.	Self-limiting.
Symptoms of hyperthyroidism.	Increased; late decrease possible.	Inderal, steroids to shorten course of disease.	Symptoms resolve within a few months to 1 year.
Fever; tender, large thyroid.	Normal.	Antimicrobials.	Rapid response to appropriate treatment.
Firm, symmetrically enlarged thyroid. Symptoms of hypothyroidism.	Decreased.	Thyroid hormone replacement.	Good prognosis with treatment.
Very firm thyroid. Onset may be sudden. Symptoms of hypothyroidism.	Decreased.	Surgery if fibrosis causes tracheal obstruction. Steroids may be beneficial.	Variable.

Historical factors more suggestive of malignancy include an age less than 14, male gender, a family history of thyroid carcinoma, and a personal history of therapeutic doses of ionizing radiation to the head or neck area. Women with solitary thyroid nodules more frequently have benign lesions. Occasionally, what is believed to be a solitary nodule may be one palpable nodule of a multinodular goiter, a benign condition. A family history of goiter or an environmental iodine deficiency points to a nonmalignant nodule. Thyroid carcinomas tend to feel hard and fixed. Accompanying cervical lymphadenopathy is strongly indicative of malignancy, as are hoarseness and laryngeal nerve paralysis. Radioisotope scanning of the thyroid that reveals a cold (hypofunctioning) nodule suggests a greater chance of carcinoma. Ultrasonography can help distinguish mixed or solid growths from cystic growths. If they are less than 4 cm in diameter, cystic growths are considered benign.

Fine needle aspiration with cytologic exam by an experienced pathologist can definitively diagnose most thyroid nodules without the risks of surgery. In the younger patient without cardiac disease, suppression of TSH by thyroid hormone supplementation may distinguish TSH-responsive follicular adenomas that may shrink with hormone suppression from carcinomas that continue growing or remain the same size. On the basis of a careful consideration of historical data, physical exam, and laboratory testing, those at high risk of thyroid carcinoma should have surgical removal of the nodule, frozen section specimen exam, and further excision of thyroid or surrounding tissue. Radioactive iodine therapy may help control metastatic growth. Treatment of adenomas is based on thyroid function and the size of the nodule. Large nodules that are cosmetically unattractive or cause tracheal or esophageal obstruction should be surgically removed.

Adrenals

The anterior pituitary hormone, adrenocorticotropic hormone, is aimed at a target organ, the adrenal gland, and specifically the adrenal cortex. The adrenals are two 5

TABLE 12.23 ADRENAL HORMONES

Hormone	Effect	Mechanism	Regulation	Clinical Manifestations of: Hypo-secretion	Hyper-secretion
Glucocorticoid (principally cortisol) via ACTH	Promotes normal metabolism. Provides energy in form of glucose. Aids body resistance to stress. Anti-inflammatory.	Retards uptake and use of glucose by muscle cells. Stimulates gluconeogenesis in liver. Mobilizes fatty acids from adipose tissue. Sensitizes blood vessels to vasoconstrictors. Helps maintain blood pressure. Decreases inflammatory blood vessel dilatation and edema. Increases appetite.	Negative feedback based on low levels of circulating glucocorticoids. Stress (often perceived by hypothalamus). Secretion increases in early morning and in response to stress or low levels of circulating cortisol. Secretion decreases in evening and in response to high levels of circulating cortisol.	Adrenal insufficiency (Addison's disease)	Cushing's syndrome
Mineralocorticoid (principally aldosterone)	Conservation of sodium and water. Elimination of potassium.	Acts on kidney tubules to increase reabsorption of sodium/water and decrease reabsorption of potassium. Conserves sodium in sweat glands, epithelial cells, and GI tract.	Renin-angiotensin pathway. Secretion increases when blood volume/pressure fall or when extracellular potassium level rises. Secretion decreases when blood volume/pressure remain normal or when extracellular potassium level falls.	Hypotension, hyponatremia, hyperkalemia.	Conn's syndrome, hyperaldosteronism, hypertension.

× 3 × 1 cm vascular organs located superiorly to each kidney. Each adrenal is divided into two sections that differ in both structure and function: the inner core, called the "adrenal medulla," and surrounding this, the "adrenal cortex." The adrenal cortex itself is divided into three discrete zones. The outermost zone, the zona glomerulosa, has cells that secrete mineralocorticoids. The inner zone, or zona reticularis, synthesizes and secretes sex hormones (see Chapter 9). Between these lies the wide zona fasciculata; this is the area that secretes glucocorticoids in response to stimulation by the pituitary hormone, ACTH. Table 12.23 discusses the function and regulation of the adrenal hormones.

Damage to the adrenal cortex results in insufficient secretion of adrenal cortical hormones regardless of pituitary stimulation. Causes of ***Addison's disease*** (primary adrenocortical insufficiency) include granulomatous destruction of the adrenal cortex (tuberculosis, disseminated fungal infection), idiopathic destruction (believed to be autoimmune in nature), and, rarely, amyloidosis, adrenal apoplexy or metabolic tumors. ***Adrenal cortical insufficiency*** can also be induced by secondary means: suppression of hormone secretion by the intake of exogenous glucocorticoids or pituitary failure. If the pituitary is hypofunctioning, one would also expect to find concurrent abnormalities in other glands, notably the thyroid. Clinical manifestations of adrenal cortical insufficiency usually do not surface until over 90% of cortical tissue has been damaged. Symptoms may develop insidiously. Lack of glucocorticoids results in loss of appetite, weakness and fatigue, inability to maintain adequate blood sugar levels during fasting, and inability to withstand stress. Stresses such as infection, surgery, injury, or vomiting, which are tolerable by the healthy individual, can result in shock or even death for the patient with adrenal insufficiency. The pituitary tries to stimulate the failing adrenals by secreting more ACTH; at the same time, melanocyte-stimulating hormones are released from the adrenohypophysis. This causes the skin changes associated with hypoadrenalism—bronzing of exposed areas, increased pigmentation of skin creases and friction areas, and possibly blue, gray, or brown spots on the lips or in the mouth. In cases of glucocorticoid deficiency due to pituitary failure, these skin changes are not present. Since the testes produce most of their androgens, men are clinically unaffected by decreased output. Women, however, may exhibit loss of pubic or axillary hair, since the adrenals produce the majority of their androgens. Lack of adequate aldosterone secretion results in sodium wastage, with concurrent loss of water from extracellular fluid and retention of potassium. Depletion of blood volume causes hypotension and finally decreased cardiac output, sometimes associated with diminution of heart size. Cardiac manifestations of hyperkalemia can further complicate the clinical picture.

Proper diagnosis of adrenal cortical insufficiency is important, since presenting symptoms represent vague and often common complaints, and failure to initiate appropriate therapy in time puts the patient in a clearly life-threatening situation. The diagnosis is made by the symptoms and by a laboratory observation of plasma cortisol levels after 8 hours of continuous IV infusion of 50 units of ACTH. Persons with Addison's disease will show little or no rise in cortisol level, while those with a normal adrenal response will increase their cortisol levels by approximately 30 μg/dL. Those with adrenal suppression due to hypopituitarism or prolonged corticosteroid therapy will show an intermediate but normal rise, although with daily ACTH administration these values will gradually increase to normal. Treatment is straightforward, and consists of hormonal replacement and a diet containing adequate amounts of sodium chloride and fluids. Mineralocorticoid replacement, such as 0.1 mg fludrocortisone, is administered daily, along with 20 mg supplemental cortisol in the morning and 10 mg in the late afternoon. The dosage of cortisol must be increased during times of stress, notably with infection and surgery. For emergency aid in situations of unanticipated stress, a card or bracelet identifying the patient's problem, along with a syringe of dexamethasone and instructions for its use, can be lifesaving.

As one often observes in endocrinology, glandular hyperfunction will produce a clinical entity somewhat opposite to that seen in hypofunction. ***Cushing's syndrome*** represents a condition of glucocorticoid excess. ***Natural Cushing's syndrome*** is caused by cortisol-producing adrenal cortical tumors, pituitary overproduction of ACTH (frequently pituitary microadenomas), or nonpituitary (ectopic) ACTH production, usually by tumors located elsewhere in the body. The pituitary form of Cushing's syndrome, which is the most common, is seen frequently in women of childbearing age. Adrenal tumors are more often observed in childhood, while ectopic ACTH production is more likely to be found in the adult man. ***Iatrogenic Cushing's syndrome*** is caused by prolonged administration of pharmacologic glucocorticoids. Cortisol excess causes catabolism of proteins and thus a wasting of various body tissues. When it is present in the bone, osteoporosis is found; when skin thins and capillaries weaken, ecchymoses may occur. Purple striae appear in areas of recent weight gain. The appetite is increased and the blood sugar remains elevated, with onset of mild diabetic symptoms. Weight gain is noted in central areas of the body; one observes the characteristic "moon facies," "buffalo hump," and adipose deposition in the supraclavicular and abdominal areas. The extremities tend to remain slim. Hypertension is common, and personality changes ranging from mild to major depression or psychosis, may be present in more than 50% of patients with Cushing's syndrome. Cushingoid children are likely to experience linear growth retardation, often following the onset of obesity. Cortisol suppresses the body's inflammatory response, and when cortisol levels are elevated over time, antibody production and lymphocyte proliferation are impaired. The patient with Cushing's syndrome is thus immunosuppressed and poorly prepared to control infection. If androgen levels are elevated, the woman is likely to experience oligomenorrhea or amenorrhea. A mild virilism also occurs, manifested as acne, facial hirsutism, and thinning of scalp hair.

The presence of the multiple signs and/or symptoms listed above suggests a diagnosis of Cushing's syndrome. Confirmation by laboratory testing is based upon elevated serum cortisol levels, especially toward evening when these levels naturally fall, and urinary steroid metabolites. It is important that these specimens be collected when the patient is in a nonstressed state, since stress will increase these values in the normal individual. The dexamethasone suppression test determines whether Cushing's is caused by pituitary ACTH excess. Dexamethasone, a potent glucocorticoid, is administered and levels of ACTH and cortisol are measured. In the normal individual, ACTH secretion will decrease due to the rising blood glucocorticoid levels. Cortisol production should fall off due to reduced ACTH stimulation. Abnormal responses to the dexamethasone suppression test are presented in Table 12.24. Pregnancy or the intake of synthetic estrogens can alter the results of glucocorticoid assays.

The treatment of Cushing's syndrome is dependent on the cause. Excessive pituitary ACTH production or Cushing's disease in children is treated by radiotherapy, and in adults by transsphenoidal microdissection of the pituitary with removal of the adenoma. If a tumor cannot be found, the pituitary may be removed, but the patient will lose reproductive capability and be dependent on lifelong hormonal supplementation. Large doses of radiation have been used in adults; however, hypopituitarism is often a consequence. Removal or ablation of adrenal cortical tissue halts cortisol production, but adenomas remain and hypersecrete ACTH. Adrenocortical tumors should be surgically removed. Benign adrenal adenomas may be bilaterial; thus, appropriate surgical plans must be made. For the poor surgical candidate, various adrenal inhibitory drugs, such as metyrapone, may be successful. The neoplasm

TABLE 12.24 EFFECTS OF THE DEXAMETHASONE SUPPRESSION TEST

Condition	ACTH Response	Cortisol Response
Adrenal neoplasm	Suppression; pituitary responds.	No suppression; abnormal adrenal response.
Ectopic ACTH	No suppression; areas of ectopic production do not respond to feedback.	No suppression; ACTH levels still high and stimulate cortisol production.
Pituitary hypersecretion of ACTH (Cushing's syndrome)	Some suppression; modified but abnormal pituitary response.	Suppression; adrenals respond normally.
Normal	Suppression.	Suppression.

causing ectopic ACTH secretion needs to be surgically removed. If metastasis prevents this, adrenalectomy or adrenal suppressive medications will treat elevated cortisol levels.

Some disorders of the adrenal gland cause hypersecretion of aldosterone, or ***primary aldosteronism.*** The most common etiology is an aldosterone-secreting adrenal adenoma known as ***Conn's syndrome,*** which affects women twice as often as men. Other causes include adrenal hyperplasia and idiopathic hyperaldosteronism. Secondary aldosteronism involves hypersecretion of aldosterone stimulated by an extra-adrenal source. It is discussed in Chapter 8. Signs and symptoms of primary hyperaldosteronism are predictable if one understands the physiologic effects of aldosterone. Sodium is retained by the renal distal tubules in exchange for hydrogen and potassium ions. The sodium-potassium ratio is also altered in saliva and GI secretions. Potassium depletion in muscle tissue causes general muscle weakness and fatigue; in cardiac muscle, premature contractions and arrhythmias may occur. Extracellular fluid volume expands with sodium reabsorption, although, due to the "escape phenomenon," a balance is eventually struck and edema rarely results. Mild to moderate diastolic hypertension is the rule, but the exact mechanism is unknown. It is usually not severe, but patients frequently suffer headaches. Primary aldosteronism is responsible for disease in only 1% of hypertensives. Complications of uncontrolled hypertension—namely, cardiomegaly, impaired renal function, stroke, and congestive heart failure—represent the major health threats of hyperaldosteronism. Hypertensive individuals should be screened upon diagnosis for serum postassium levels while taking in normal amounts of sodium and in the absence of potassium-wasting diuretics. If these persons are using diuretics, they should be discontinued for 10 days and potassium supplements given for the same period of time. Persistent hypokalemia indicates the need for further work-up to rule out primary hyperaldosteronism. Chronic overingestion of licorice can mimic this disease, so a diet history must be included. Initially, plasma renin levels are monitored in response to volume depletion. High plasma renin activity is associated with secondary hyperaldosteronism and some cases of essential hypertension. Abnormally low renin activity suggests primary hyperaldosteronism; if this is found, the patient's plasma aldosterone level is assessed following intravenous saline loading. Normally, aldosterone secretion would be suppressed and levels would dip.

High levels of aldosterone in response to saline loading confirm the diagnosis of primary hyperaldosteronism. Adrenal venous catheterization is then used to locate tumors. Treatment consists of surgical removal of the adrenal gland containing the adenoma, if present. If adenomas are bilateral, surgery is deferred, since medical control of symptoms offers a better alternative than bilateral adrenalectomy with resulting total adrenal insufficiency. Drug therapy is also employed when no tumor has been isolated, as in the case of bilateral adrenal hyperplasia. Spironolactone, 25–100 mg every 8 hours, antagonizes aldosterone activity, reducing blood pressure and normalizing the electrolyte imbalance. A sodium-restricted diet is recommended. Major drawbacks to chronic spironolactone therapy are gynecomastia, decreased libido, and impotence in the man.

In the core of the adrenal gland lies the adrenal medulla, an active portion of the sympathetic nervous system. Preganglionic nerve fibers, functionally and structurally similar to sympathetic nervous system fibers originating from the spinal cord, innervate the adrenal medulla's chromaffin cells. These cells possess the ability to synthesize epinephrine from norepinephrine, unlike CNS tissue, in which the formation of norepinephrine is the final step. Both of these hormones are called "catecholamines" and, once formed, are stored in intracellular granules. When CNS catecholamines are released, rapid reuptake into the nerves occurs and only trace amounts ever reach the bloodstream. The adrenals secrete catecholamines directly into the circulation. Thus, their action is more prolonged and they can influence all body cells. After exerting their peripheral effects, epinephrine and norepinephrine are metabolized mainly in the liver to inactive compounds, which are excreted in the urine. Both epinephrine and norepinephrine have alpha-adrenergic effects—namely, vasoconstriction of all blood vessels, increased cardiac activity, GI tract inhibition, pupillary dilatation, and decreased urinary output, among others. Epinephrine has both alpha and beta influences. The additional responses are vasodilatation in skeletal and muscle tissue, greater cardiac muscle strength, and bronchial and myometrial relaxation. Epinephrine is also a more potent sympathetic stimulant, although its vasoconstrictive effect is weaker than that of norepinephrine.

Catecholamine-producing tumors made up of sympathetic nervous system cells are called ***pheochromocytomas.*** The most common site for pheochromocytoma is the adrenal medulla. ***Paragangliomas*** are extra-adrenal catecholamine-producing tumors (also classified as pheochromocytomas) arising from neural crest cells surrounding the sympathetic ganglia along the aorta or inside blood vessel walls and, rarely, in the bladder. The incidence of pheochromocytoma is low, and children and young adults are most commonly affected. Often the diagnosis is made during pregnancy, since blood pressure is monitored more regularly and the pressure of the enlarging uterus may stimulate more frequent hormonal release from the tumor. There is a hereditary component to pheochromocytoma related (in descending order of frequency) to simple familial pheochromocytoma, multiple endocrine neoplasia, neurofibromatosis, and von Hippel-Lindau disease, a hereditary preneoplastic syndrome. Knowlege of the family history is helpful in diagnosis and treatment, since the tumor location and behavior tend to be consistent. The classic symptoms of pheochromocytoma are headache, tachycardia, and sweating. Hypertension is universal, although between attacks the blood pressure may be normal. Less than 1% of hypertensives are found to have pheochromocytoma. If the tumor secretes predominantly norepinephrine, symptoms may be minimal and may mimic essential hypertension. When epinephrine is the main hormone secreted, a paroxysm may produce flushing, nervousness, angina pectoris, and heat intolerance in addition to the three cardinal symptoms. Over time, weight loss may occur and postural hypotension is common. Attacks may be very rare, with years between occurrences, or take place as often as 25 times per day. Symptoms occur suddenly and last for periods ranging from less than 1 minute to over a week, but usually resolve within hours.

Recognition of pheochromocytoma is important, since treatment is successful in more than 90% of patients and failure to treat can lead to malignant hypertension and death. During a severe attack, the systolic blood pressure may exceed 300 mg Hg, with myocardial infarction and shock being possible sequelae. A single well-collected 24-hour urine specimen to test for elevated levels of catecholamines and their metabolites (norepinephrine, epinephrine, metanephrine, vanillylmandelic acid) confirms the diagnosis. In rare cases, a 6-hour urine collection immediately following an attack will be needed to document the existence of pheochromocytoma. Some pharmacologic agents, such as methyldopa, levodopa, monoamine oxidase inhibitors, clofibrate, and nalidixic acid can falsely elevate or diminish urinary catecholamine levels. A work-up for pheochromocytoma is indicated in hypertensive patients with suspicious symptoms, labile, moderate or severe hypertension, or those unresponsive to antihypertensive drugs. Less than 10% of pheochromocytomas are found to be malignant. Since the cellular appearance of benign pheochromocytomas is bizarre, malignancy is established only when metastases are identified. Surgical removal of the tumors is the treatment of choice; it is effective in symptom resolution and blood pressure regulation. For 1–2 weeks prior to surgery or invasive diagnostic testing, the alpha-blocking agent phenoxybenzamine is administered to lower the blood pressure and to allow the intravascular fluid volume to normalize. Even with appropriate preoperative measures, there is still a threat of marked rebound hypotension, which is treated with volume expansion and pressor agents. Hypertensive crisis prior to medical or surgical intervention is treated on an emergency basis with IV vasodilatory agents.

Parathyroid Glands

The small, round parathyroid glands are embedded, two to a lobe, in the posterior surfaces of each lateral thyroid lobe. "Principal" or "chief" cells in the parathyroids secrete parathyroid hormone (PTH) directly into the bloodstream in response to lowered serum ionized calcium levels. PTH function and regulation are described in Table 12.25. Oxyphil cells and "clear" cells are also present in the parathyroids; however, their functions are still unknown.

There are several clinical types of ***hyperparathyroidism*** (Table 12.26). ***Primary hyperparathyroidism*** arises when an abnormally high amount of PTH is released with no decrease in serum calcium levels. A solitary adenoma is the etiology in 85–90% of cases. Chief cell hyperplasia is the next most common cause, and carcinoma of the parathyroid is the rarest. Risk factors may include a family history of primary hyperparathyroidism or previous irradiation of the neck area. Most pa-

TABLE 12.25 PARATHYROID HORMONE

			Clinical Manifestations of:	
Effects	**Mechanism**	**Regulation**	**Hypo-secretion**	**Hyper-secretion**
Controls homeostasis of calcium and phosphate in blood.	In presence of vitamin D, enhances calcium, magnesium, and phosphate absorption from intestines into the bloodstream. Increases number and rate of activity of osteoclasts to cause release of calcium and phosphate into the bloodstream. Promotes reabsorption of calcium and magnesium from the kidney tubule. Inhibits phosphate and bicarbonate reabsorption by the proximal tubule, thus increasing renal excretion. Stimulates synthesis of 1,25-dehydroxycalciferol.	Negative feedback based on serum calcium level. Secretion increases when blood calcium ion level falls. Secretion decreases when blood calcium ion level is adequate.	Hypoparathyroidism	Hyperparathyroidism

TABLE 12.26 FORMS OF HYPERPARATHYROIDISM

Type	Mechanism	Etiology	Effect on Serum Calcium
Primary hyperparathyroidism	Excess PTH production by lesion in the parathyroid gland	Parathyroid adenoma, carcinoma, or hyperplasia.	Usually elevated
Secondary hyperparathyroidism	Excess PTH production in response to feedback signals; normal functioning of parathyroid.	Hypocalcemia, hyperphosphatemia, hypomagnesemia secondary to renal failure, osteomalacia.	Normal or low
Hypercalcemia of malignancy (previously ectopic or pseudohyperparathyroidism)	Malignant tissue secretes PTH-like substances.	Malignancy produces osteoclast-activating factor (OAF) and other unknown substances.	High
Tertiary or autoimmune hyperparathyroidism	Parathyroid gland becomes hyperplastic in response to high PTH levels and begins to function autonomously.	Renal failure	High

tients with primary hyperparathyroidism have few or no symptoms; in fact, most cases are now discovered on routine assay of serum calcium. Symptoms may be vague and physical signs are usually absent. When present, signs and symptoms are related to ***hypercalcemia*** (see Table 12.27) and/or osteitis fibrosa cystica, typical bony changes associated with primary hyperparathyroidism. These abnormalities include bony cysts, subperiosteal bone resorption, and erosion of portions of the distal phalanges and clavicles. The severity of symptoms increases with the serum calcium level, although there is a great deal of individual variation. When an elevated serum calcium level is detected, this test must be repeated at least twice to confirm hypercalcemia. Once this condition is established, the history and physical exam should be reviewed, with closer attention paid to the family history and to signs and symptoms suggestive of hyperparathyroidism or malignancy. Use of thiazide diuretics, doses of vitamin D exceeding 10,000–50,000 units/day, and intake of more than 5 g/day of calcium carbonate can also cause hypercalcemia. Radioimmunoassay of serum parathyroid hormone (iPTH) revealing an elevated level in combination with hypercalcemia is quite accurate in diagnosing primary hyperparathyroidism; if serum iPTH is not inappropriately elevated for the coexistent level of calcium, another cause of hypercalcemia must be sought.

Surgical removal of diseased parathyroid tissue (parathyroidectomy) is the treatment of choice. It is important that the surgeon have a great deal of experience with recognition and removal of abnormal parathyroid tissue. If tumors are found in multiple glands, there is a chance of disease recurrence. Postoperative hypocalcemia may occur as "hungry bones" draw calcium from the bloodstream. Bone changes associated with osteitis fibrosa cystica, unless dramatic, tend to improve during the months after surgery. In general, symptoms of hypercalcemia, if any, do resolve, except for severe nephropathy due to calcification.

Hypoparathyroidism is deficient secretion of PTH. The most common etiology, ***surgical hypoparathyroidism,*** is caused by previous parathyroidectomy or other anterior neck surgery that may have compromised the blood supply to the parathy-

TABLE 12.27 SYMPTOMS OF HYPERCALCEMIA

Central nervous system	Renal
Loss of sense of smell	Polyuria
Impairment of recent memory	Polydipsia
Poor mentation	Stone formation
Fatigue	Nephrocalcinosis
Apathy, depression	Reduced glomerular filtration rate
Personality changes	Cardiovascular
Somnolence	Hypertension association
Coma	Gastrointestinal
Neuromuscular	Anorexia
Muscle fatigue	Nausea, vomiting
Arthralgias	Dyspepsia
Weakness	Increased incidence of pancreatitis
Hypotonia	Skin
Gout	Severe pruritus
Pseudogout	
Periarticular calcifications	

roids. Congenital absence of the parathyroid gland is the cause of ***idiopathic hypoparathyroidism. Functional hypoparathyroidism*** occurs when there is severe, prolonged hypomagnesemia, since magnesium must be present in order for the parathyroids to release PTH. This does not represent a glandular failure, since it is easily correctable with magnesium infusion. ***Pseudohypoparathyroidism*** is a rare hereditary disorder in which symptoms of hypoparathyroidism are secondary to a deficient end organ response to PTH. The severity of the clinical symptoms of hypoparathyroidism is dependent on the degree and chronicity of ***hypocalcemia.*** Insufficient PTH secretion results in hypocalcemia by allowing calcium to be lost via the kidneys while phosphate is retained, reduced calcium uptake from the GI tract, and calcium storage in the bones. Hypocalcemia lowers the excitation threshold and causes a repetitive reaction to a single stimulus in sensory and motor fibers. Neuromuscular signs are more pronounced when serum calcium falls rapidly, for example, following anterior neck surgery. In extreme cases, incessant activity of nervous tissue is provoked. This excitability is manifested as numbness or tingling around the mouth, fingertips, or feet and as tetany. An attack of tetany may progress from muscle spasm of the face and extremities to contorted posturing of the hands and arms, whereby all involved joints are flexed except for the interphalangeal joints and the thumb, which is adducted. The seizure threshold is also lowered; epileptiform seizures are not uncommon. Latent tetany may be detected by a positive Chvostek's sign and, most accurately, by a positive Trousseau's sign. Trousseau's sign is elicited by inflating a sphygmomanometer cuff around the arm to above the patient's systolic blood pressure for more than 2 minutes. Sustained spasm of the opposite wrist, which ceases only after cuff deflation, constitutes a positive response. Other manifestations of hypocalcemia are basal ganglia calcification associated with parkinsonian symptoms, increased susceptibility to *Candida* infections, lenticular cataract, intestinal malabsorption, and occasionally psychiatric disorders.

When present during formative years, hypocalcemia may cause improper development of the teeth and skeleton. Short, stocky stature with characteristically shortened fourth and fifth metatarsals or metacarpals are classic findings. Low serum calcium levels, usually combined with high serum phosphate levels, are suggestive of hypoparathyroidism. Further investigation should include iPTH; low or undetectable levels help confirm the diagnosis. Normal serum magnesium levels will rule out hypoparathyroidism secondary to hypomagnesemia. If iPTH is elevated, one must suspect pseudohypoparathyroidism. Treatment is aimed at maintaining low normal values of serum calcium via the administration of vitamin D and calcium supplements. Therapy with PTH is impractical, so patients remain in a calcium-wasting state and are at risk for renal lithiasis. Lenticular cataracts may not improve with treatment. Vitamin D_2 (ergocalciferol) is given in large doses ranging from 50,000 to 100,000 units/day. An undesirable effect is vitamin D intoxication, which may produce a prolonged state of hypercalcemia, since excess vitamin D can be stored for months. Monthly monitoring of serum calcium levels is important to avoid this situation. Some patients can be maintained on a regimen consisting only of calcium supplementation (1–2 g elemental calcium per day), aluminum hydroxide gel to bind intestinal phosphates, and a diet limited in phosphates (less meat, dairy products, and sodas). Complications of vitamin D administration would thus be eliminated.

Details of Management

▸ *MS Organizations*

Laboratory Tests: None.

Therapeutic Measures: None.

Patient Education: National Multiple Sclerosis Society
205 East 42nd Street
New York, New York 10017
Tel.: (212) 986-3240

Follow-up: Help patients make contact as needed.

▸ *Supportive Care for Epilepsy*

Laboratory Tests: Serum drug toxicity levels. A CBC and liver evaluation are recommended periodically at the discretion of the supervising physician. Patients on Tegretol should have a CBC every 2 weeks for 2 months and then quarterly thereafter.

Treatment: Under direct supervision of a physician, adjust anticonvulsive drug dosages in accordance with serum drug levels. Therapeutic serum values vary among clinics and laboratories.

Patient Education: Stress the importance of taking anticonvulsive medications as directed to prevent seizures, since the largest number of treatment failures are due to noncompliance. Explain the signs and symptoms of drug toxicity listed below to the patient and his or her family or friends.

Anorexia	Fever
Visual symptoms (specifically, double vision)	Drowsiness
	Rash
Numbness of extremities	Ataxia
Dizziness	Irritability
Behavioral problems	Gastric distress

The following emergency procedures for the seizing patient should be well understood:

1. Place the seizing patient on the floor or on a bed.
2. Remove glasses and loosen the clothing around the head and chest.
3. Avoid any attempt to place spoons, tongue blades, or other objects in the patient's mouth, since this previously recommended measure can injure the patient (e.g., broken teeth) and the helper (serious bites).
4. Be sure that the patient's head is protected at all times, and guide or control the patient's body movements to prevent injury.
5. Do not forcibly restrain the patient, since such action will worsen the convulsion.
6. Although the patient may show signs of airway obstruction or other respiratory abnormalities, normal breathing will resume when the attack is over.
7. After the seizure, turn the patient on the side to allow any saliva, mucus, food, or vomitus that has collected to drain.
8. The patient should rest undisturbed; immediate rising and walking may precipitate another seizure.
9. If the person with epilepsy can foresee that an attack is imminent, he or she should find a quiet place and lie down.
10. Call for help if the person having the seizure injures himself, does not start breathing after the seizure, or passes from one seizure to another without regaining consciousness.

Stress the importance of adequate and regular meals and getting enough sleep. Long periods without nourishment or rest increase the chances of having an attack. Most persons with epilepsy report that they feel better and more energetic if they are active. Therefore, assist the patient in working out a moderate, regular exercise program, keeping in mind the severity of the individual's disorder. Activities such as swimming, bike riding, and jogging are acceptable, provided that the patient is accompanied by someone who is aware of the condition and is able to provide emergency care if needed. Also, advise the patient to avoid crowded, noisy recreational areas or dangerous activities (scuba diving, mountain climbing, hang gliding, water or snow skiing) in which momentary loss of consciousness could result in injury or death.

Driving should be avoided unless the patient has been seizure free for at least 6 months (individual states set their own requirements). Jobs such as the operation of heavy machinery, those performed underground or underwater, or any others in which there is potential danger should be avoided.

Couples in whom one or both partners has epilepsy and who wish to have children should be advised that 6% of children with one epileptic parent and 10–12% of children with two epileptic parents will develop the disorder. In addition, women with epilepsy have a slightly higher than normal risk of maternal complications during pregnancy and delivery. Finally, anticonvulsive medications contribute to the risk of fetal abnormalities. Other educational or supportive information can be obtained from the organizations listed below.

Follow-up: As needed based on the stability of the serum drug level and the frequency of seizures. More frequent visits are necessary if the drug levels and symptoms are poorly regulated.

▸ *Epilepsy Organizations*

Laboratory Tests: None.

Therapeutic Measures: None.

Patient Education: American Epilepsy Society
Department of Neurology
Reed Neurological Research Center
710 Westwood Plaza
Los Angeles, California 90024
Tel.: (213) 825-5745

Epilepsy Foundation of America
4351 Garden City Drive
Landover, Maryland 20781
Tel.: (301) 459-3700

Follow-up: Help patients make contact as needed.

▸ *Supportive Care for Progressive Dementia*

Laboratory Tests: None.

Therapeutic Measures: Focus on relieving symptoms and improving some aspects of behavior. Prescribe a mild tranquilizer such as Haldol, 1 to 2 mg daily, or Navane, 1 tablet once or twice a day, to reduce agitation, anxiety, and unpredictable behavior (watch carefully for evidence of side effects). For depression, prescribe a tricyclic or other antidepressant in individualized dosages so as not to cause undue sedation (see Chapter 13). Familiar surroundings minimize the patient's fear, confusion, and discomfort. Therefore, home care is preferable to institutionalization when family members and/or friends are willing and able to help.

Patient Education: Family members and friends should fully understand the nature of the disease. They may also benefit from the following guidelines:

1. Encourage the patient to use his or her preserved abilities as much as possible while reducing the patient's need for lost functions.
2. Avoid stressful situations such as unfamiliar places, persons, or circumstances.
3. Continually orient patients by providing social stimulation, a calendar, a clock, and a daily newspaper.

4. Treat medical problems promptly, since any illness may exacerbate dementia. Carefully monitor all medications, and do not let the patient take any that have not been prescribed by a doctor or primary caregiver.
5. Provide regular, nourishing meals; avoid alcohol.
6. Regulate sleeping patterns by keeping the patient active during the day and putting him or her to bed at an appropriate time.

Families and friends of patients with Alzheimer's disease or other such disorders can contact the organizations below, which will provide valuable information and put them in contact with support groups in their own communities.

Follow-up: As needed.

▸ *Alzheimer's/Dementia Organizations*

Laboratory Tests: None.

Therapeutic Measures: None.

Patient Education: Alzheimer's Disease and Related Disorders Association, Inc.
360 North Michigan Ave.
Chicago, Illinois 60601
Tel.: (800) 621-0379

National Geriatrics Society
212 West Wisconsin Ave., 3rd Floor
Milwaukee, Wisconsin 53203
Tel.: (414) 272-4130

Follow-up: As needed.

▸ *Insomnia*

Laboratory Tests: None.

Therapeutic Measures: Take a careful history to evaluate the patient's patterns of wakefulness and sleep. Care should be taken in prescribing pharmacologic agents for the treatment of insomnia due to their addictive properties. However, if a situational crisis or change is unlikely to resolve quickly or the drug will be well tolerated and taken responsibly by the patient, prescribe temazepam (Restoril) or a similar mild sedative-hypnotic. Mild tranquilizers such as Ativan or Librium are to be taken hs as an alternative. Teach patients the fundamentals of relaxation therapy (see Chapter 13).

Patient Education: Give patients suffering from insomnia the following instructions:

1. Establish a regular sleep routine by going to bed and rising at about the same time every day.
2. Make your sleeping conditions as comfortable as possible. Separate sleeping arrangements may have to be made if you share a bed or room with a snoring or restless partner. Wear loose-fitting night clothes.
3. Keep your bedroom darkened, shades or blinds will prevent street lights or the sun (if you sleep during the day) from keeping you awake.
4. Keep your bedroom as quiet as possible. If outside noises cannot be blocked, cover them with a steady noise such as that of a fan.
5. Avoid drinking alcohol before going to bed.
6. Avoid mental stimulation during the hour just prior to going to bed.
7. Do not use your bedroom for working or watching TV.
8. If you cannot sleep, get up and engage in a relaxing activity such as reading until you are sleepy.
9. Avoid daytime naps.
10. Avoid caffeine-containing beverages after lunch.
11. Get regular exercise each day.

Follow-up: As needed.

▸ Sleep Disorders Organizations

Laboratory Tests: None.

Therapeutic Measures: None.

Patient Education: Association of Sleep Disorders Centers
TD 114 University Medical Center
Stanford, California 94305
Tel.: (415) 723-7458

American Narcolepsy Association
P.O. Box 5846
Stanford, California 94305
Tel.: (415) 723-4000

Narcolepsy and Cataplexy Association of America
1410 York Avenue, Suite 2D
New York, New York 10021
Tel.: (212) 628-6315

Follow-up: As needed.

▸ Supportive Care for Parkinson's Disease

Laboratory Tests: Per neurologist.

Therapeutic Measures: Per neurologist.

Patient Education: Encourage patients to develop exercise routines to minimize symptoms as follows:

1. For stooping: press your spine against a wall or door jam several times daily.
2. For shuffling: line up books at regular intervals on the floor and raise your feet over them as you walk.
3. For difficulty in speaking, read aloud.
4. For difficulty in rising from chairs, stand up by leaning forward 45 degrees and pushing up with your hands.
5. For improved facial control and expression, hold a sound (vowel sounds are best) for 5 seconds.
6. For improved lung capacity, do deep diaphragmatic breathing.
7. For tongue control, extend the tongue to the nose and chin and laterally.
8. For voice tone, sing the scales.
9. For muscle rigidity and improved control, do range-of-motion exercises for the entire body, including systematic rotation, flexion, and extension.

Other exercises may be recommended by a physical therapist. Instruct the patient to drink adequate fluids to combat constipation. Home modifications that are of great help include handbars and rails, especially in the bathroom, a raised toilet seat, and furniture that is not difficult to rise from (e.g., chairs whose back legs are 2 in. higher than their front legs). Emphasize to the family and friends the importance of sensitivity and support.

Follow-up: Schedule visits every 4–6 months for stable patients.

▸ *Parkinson's Disease Organizations*

Laboratory Tests: None.

Therapeutic Measures: None.

Patient Education: The American Parkinson's Disease Association
116 John Street
New York, New York 10038
Tel.: (212) 732-9550

The Parkinson's Disease Foundation
Columbia-Presbyterian Medical Center
640 West 168th Street
New York, New York 10032
Tel.: (212) 923-4700

The National Parkinson's Foundation
111 Park Place
New York, New York 10007
Tel.: (212) 374-1741

The United Parkinson's Foundation
220 South State Street
Chicago, Illinois 60604
Tel.: (312) 922-9734

Follow-up: Help patients and family members make contact as needed.

▸ *Classic Migraine Headache*

Laboratory Tests: None.

Therapeutic Measures

Prophylaxis: Prescribe propranolol (Inderal), 20 mg three times a day, increasing in 2 weeks to 80–200 mg/day in divided doses as needed, or Elavil, 25–100 mg given hs, or methysergide, 4–8 mg/day given for 5–6 months, followed by a drug holiday for at least a month. Avoid triggering factors (see Table 12.12).

Abortive therapy: If the migraine is very mild, prescribe aspirin, 600 mg every 4 hours, or acetaminophen, 600 mg every 4 hours. For moderate to severe attacks, prescribe ergotamine tartrate (cafergot, Wigraine), 2 mg sublingually at onset and 1 mg every ½ hour (maximum, 6 mg/day or 12 mg/week) or 1–2 mg rectal suppository initially, repeated 1 hour later as needed (maximum, 4 mg/day or 10 mg/week). Ergotamine given for 2 consecutive days causes rebound headaches and therefore may not benefit a patient who experiences more than two migraines a week. In such cases, prescribe dihydroergotamine mesylate, 1 mg IM at onset and 1 mg every hour (maximum, 3 mg/day or 6 mg/week). Chlorpromazine 25 mg may be given to relieve associated nausea (most effective IM).

In addition to the above-mentioned drugs, various combinations of ergot, barbiturates, and atropine-like medications (Bellergal and Bellergal-S) have been found to be effective. Biofeedback and other relaxation techniques are useful as both preventive and abortive measures.

Patient Education: Avoid those factors that trigger migraines (see Table 12.12). Be able to recognize the signs of an impending attack in order to begin therapy as soon as possible. These include numbness or weakness on one side of the body, transient aphasia, thickness or speech or vertigo, or visual distortions (blurred or cloudy vision, bright flashing lights, bright colors, or zigzag lines). Increased hunger, nervousness, or alterations of moods may start a day before the migraine. Use drugs only as directed. Rebound headaches will occur if ergotamine tartrate is used 2 days in a row. Overuse may also cause dangerous vasconstriction of extremities. Side effects include abdominal cramps, epigastric discomfort, diarrhea, nausea, vomiting, drowsiness, or painful uterine contractions.

Follow-up: As needed.

▸ *Cluster Headaches*

Laboratory Tests: None.

Therapeutic Measures

Prophylaxis: Prescribe lithium carbonate, 300 mg two to eight times daily, until therapeutic blood levels have been reached (under 1 mEq/L). Observe special considerations for lithium therapy such as avoiding salt depletion and ongoing blood monitoring (see Chapter 13). As an alternative for short-term headaches, prescribe prednisone or methysergide (Sansert), 4–8 mg/day, or ergotamine tartrate, 1 mg three times a day for 1 week and 1 mg twice daily for the duration of the cluster period.

Abortive therapy: Prescribe ergotamine tartrate as described for migraine for mild to severe cluster attacks. Due to the rapid speed with which severe headache develops, administration by suppository allows the medication to enter the bloodstream quickly. Less nausea and vomiting will occur if dihydroergotamine as described for migraine is given parenterally. Oxygen by mask, 8–10 L/min for 5 minutes, is useful when drugs are not.

Patient Education: Avoid those factors that trigger cluster headaches (notably consumption of alcohol). Nitroglycerine use may be associated with the problem. Since there are no prodromal symptoms and since the onset of severe pain is rapid, seek help at the first sign of headache. Be prepared for possible side effects of the medications such as abdominal cramps, epigastric discomfort, diarrhea, nausea, vomiting, drowsiness, and painful uterine contractions.

Follow-up: As needed.

▸ *Chronic Muscle Contraction Headaches*

Laboratory Tests: None.

Therapeutic Measures: Headache occurrence can often be resolved by discussion and counseling. After gaining the patient's confidence, explore his or her marital, occupational, and social relationships, life stresses, personality traits, methods of coping, and sexual problems. Aid the patient in identifying the cause of headaches and solving the problem. If severe emotional problems surface, a psychiatric referral may be in order.

As an adjunct to counseling, Elevil 25–100 mg/day hs may prove helpful. For pain, start with mild analgesics (acetylsalicylic acid or Tylenol). If these fail to provide relief, prescribe Fiorinol (also contains caffeine), 1 or 2 tablets every 4 hours, not to exceed 6 tablets a day, or Axotal, 1 tablet every 4 hours, not to exceed 6 tablets a day (habit-forming).

Referral for relaxation training through biofeedback is beneficial for some patients.

Patient Education: Identification of the underlying causes of headache is essential. Try to identify problems at home or work that are causing emotional stress. Seek professional help if these problems are overwhelming or cannot be solved. Be prepared for possible side effects of the medication.

Follow-up: Frequent visits may be necessary until the underlying psychogenic problems are resolved. The patient should return or be called 1 month after problem resolution to check on the patient's continued health.

▸ *Antirabies Measures*

Laboratory Tests: In cases of attack by stray or wild animals, the animal's head should be sent to a laboratory for confirmation of rabies. A serum antibody sample should be drawn on a previously vaccinated patient to ascertain and document the patient's immune status.

Therapeutic Measures

Preexposure prophylaxis: Recommend immunization for veterinarians, laboratory workers exposed to rabies virus, or other high-risk persons as detailed below.

1. Give human diploid cell vaccine (HDCV), three 1-mL injections on days 1, 7, and 21 or 28.
2. Do serum antibody tests 2–3 weeks after the last shot. If antibodies are inadequate, give one booster.

Rabies exposure: If the attack is made by a healthy domestic animal, (1) thoroughly clean the wound with soap and water, (2) give diphtheria and tetanus toxoid for adult use (see Chapter 11) if it has been 5 years since the last immunization, and (3) have the animal observed for 10 days by a veterinarian and await the report. If the attack is made by a stray or wild animal, follow the above procedures but, instead of observation, have the animal decapitated immediately and send the head for detection of rabies. Start antirabies immunization with rabies immune globulin (RIG) and human diploid cell vaccine (HDCV) at once. If no rabies is seen, the rabies regimen can be discontinued. If the animal is a skunk, bat, fox, coyote, raccoon, bobcat, or other carnivore that cannot be captured, proceed with the entire rabies series (rabies is almost never seen in squirrels, hamsters, guinea pigs, gerbils, chipmunks, rats, mice, or rabbits). To patients who have never been immunized:

1. Give RIG, 20 IU/kg, immediately after exposure, half of the dose infiltrated into the wound and the other half given IM.
2. Give HDCV, five 1-mL IM injections on days 1, 3, 7, 14, and 28. Do antibody tests on day 28. If the antibody response is inadequate, give additional boosters and repeat levels in 2–3 weeks. Cases of inadequate antibody response must be reported to the Center for Disease Control at (404) 329-3737.

To previously immunized patients with adequate antibody titers:

1. Give HDCV, 1 mL IM immediately, followed by a second dose in 3 days.
2. Do serum antibody tests 2–3 weeks after the second dose. If antibodies are inadequate, give a booster of 1 mL.

Patient Education: Be sure that domestic animals are properly immunized against rabies according to a veterinarian's advice. Seek medical attention immediately after an attack by a strange animal. Be sure to complete all immunization schedules.

Follow-up: None is necessary after completion of immunization schedules.

▸ *Hypothyroidism in the Adult*

Laboratory Tests: T_3 resin uptake, total T_4, free T_4 by calculation. TSH and TRH. TSH response such as a change in TSH to injected TRH. Do tests one at a time, moving down the list if hypothyroidism is suspected and the initial studies are inconclusive.

Therapeutic Measures: L-Thyroxine, 0.05 mg/day for 1 month, then build up to 0.10–0.15 mg/day over the next 2–3 months. Serum TSH values will fall to normal as adequate therapeutic levels are reached. In the elderly or individuals with significant cardiac disease, start with a lower dosage and titrate with gradual increments.

Patient Education: Explain the importance of compliance with the hormone replacement schedule and the consequences of failure to comply. Teach patients the signs of hyperthyroidism and tell them to report these promptly. Patients should tell all medical personnel about their medical condition and the type and dosage of medication taken. A Medic-Alert identity tag describing the illness and medication should be worn.

Follow-up: In the beginning, close follow-up for medication titration is needed. Watch closely for patients who stop taking the medication periodically, since this may lead to a state of hypothyroid apathy and further neglect of the therapeutic regimen. Once the proper dosage has been established, serum T_4 and T_3 should be monitored every 12 months or less if the patient's clinical status changes. Closer follow-up of the clinically unstable or poorly compliant patient is necessary.

BIBLIOGRAPHY

Adams HP. Transient ischemic attacks: Differentiation and treatment. *Postgraduate Medicine,* (Feb.) 1971, 69(2):157–166.

Ariel IM. Tumors of the peripheral nervous system. *Ca—A Cancer Journal for Clinicians,* (Sept.–Oct.) 1983, 33(5):282–299.

Baker CC. Headache: Differentiating the causes. *PA Practice,* 1985, 3–6.

Bates B. *A Guide to Physical Examination,* 3rd ed. Lippincott, Philadelphia, 1983.

Baylis RIS, et al. Solving thyroid dysfunction puzzlers. *Patient Care,* (Feb.) 1980, 44–71.

Berger JA, et al. Letter to the editor. *Journal of the American Medical Association,* (Feb.) 1982, 247(7):979.

Berkow RB (ed.). *The Merck Manual of Diagnosis and Therapy,* 14th ed. Merck Sharp & Dohme Research Laboratories, Rahway, N.J., 1982.

Blonde L, Riddick FA Jr. Hypothyroidism: Clinical features, diagnosis, and therapy. *Hospital Medicine,* 52–63.

Brodoff AS. Using the history to classify epilepsy. *Patient Care,* (July) 1983, 21–68.

Brodoff AS. Helping your patient live with epilepsy. *Patient Care,* (Sept.) 1983, 171–181.

Brown AM, Stubbs DW (eds.). *Medical Physiology.* Wiley, New York, 1983.

Burke MD. Calcium and phosphorus studies: Interpretation of results for further testing. *Postgraduate Medicine,* (July) 1980, 68(1):69–78.

Burke MD. Adrenal dysfunction: Test strategies for diagnosis. *Potgraduate Medicine,* (Jan.) 1981, 69(1):155–170.

Compendium of Patient Information. Biomedical Information Corporation, New York, 1983.

Conn HF, Conn RB Jr (eds.). *Current Diagnosis.* Saunders, Philadelphia, 1980.

Cook DM. Pituitary tumors: Diagnosis and therapy. *Ca—A Cancer Journal for Clinicians,* (July–Aug.) 1983, 33(4):215–231.

Crafts RC. *A Textbook of Human Anatomy,* 3rd ed. Wiley, New York, 1985.

Crouch JE, McClintic JR. *Human Anatomy and Physiology,* 2nd ed. Wiley, New York, 1976.

Diamond S, Medina JL. Headache. *Clinical Symposia,* 1981, 33(2).

Dluhy RG, Williams GH. Adrenal causes of hypertension. *Medical Times,* (Nov.) 1980, 108(11):61–70.

Donovan WH, Bedbrook G, (B. Bekiesz, ed.). Comprehensive management of spinal cord injury. *Clinical Symposia,* 1982, 34(2):2–36.

Dowie E. Rabies. *Physician Assistant and Health Practitioner,* (July) 1982, 28–34.

Drayer JIM, Weber MA. Antihypertensive therapy in patients with mineralocorticoid excess. *PA Drug Update,* (Jan.) 1983, 51–62.

Elias H, Pauly JE, Burns ER. *Histology and Human Microanatomy,* 4th ed. Wiley, New York, 1978.

Erkert JD. Alzheimer's disease. *Physician Assistant,* (Apr.) 1983, 13–24.

Facer GW. Facial nerve paralysis: Is it always Bell's palsy? *Postgraduate Medicine,* (Feb.) 1981, 69(2):206–216.

Feinberg JF. The Wernicke-Korsakoff syndrome. *American Family Physician,* (Nov). 1980, 22(5):129–133.

Fekety R. Rabies prevention guidelines. *PA Drug Update,* (Oct.) 1982, 34–42.

Ferriss GS. Narcolepsy. *Continuing Education,* (May) 1982, 41–52.

Fisher MA, Gorelick PB. Entrapment neuropathies: Differential diagnosis and management. *Postgraduate Medicine,* (Jan.) 1985, 77(1):160–174.

Fisk AA, et al. Alzheimer's disease: A symposium. *Postgraduate Medicine,* (Apr). 1983, 73(4):204–255.

Friedman WA. Head injuries. *Clinical Symposia,* (Sept.) 1983, 35(4).

Gill GN. Diagnosing and treating Cushing's syndrome. *Consultant,* (Mar.) 1980, 50–61.

Goldberg S. Principles of neurologic localization. *American Family Physician,* (Apr.) 1981, 23(4):131–141.

Gorroll AH, May LA, Mulley AG. *Primary Care Medicine: Office Evaluation and Management of the Adult Patient.* Lippincott, Philadelphia, 1981.

Gray H. *Anatomy of the Human Body,* 29th American ed. (CM Goss, ed.). Lea & Febiger, Philadelphia, 1973.

Griffiss JM, Craig CP, Johnson JE III. Tailoring drug therapy in meningitis. *Patient Care,* (May) 1983, 17(10):63–92.

Guyton AC. *Textbook of Medical Physiology,* 6th ed. Saunders, Philadelphia, 1981.

Hall M. New heights for growth hormone deficient children. *Nurse Practitioner,* (Nov.–Dec.) 1982, 26.

Hallal JC. Thyroid disorders. *American Journal of Nursing,* (Mar.) 1977, 77(3):418–432.

Hart RG, Sherman DG. The diagnosis of multiple sclerosis. *Journal of the American Medical Association,* (Jan.) 1982, 247(4):498–503.

Hilyard N. Diagnostic protocol: Solitary thyroid nodules in adults. *Nurse Practitioner,* (Feb.) 1983, 14–15.

Hoole AJ, Greenberg RA, Pickard CG Jr. *Patient Care Guidelines for Nurse Practitioners.* Little, Brown, Boston, 1982.

Isselbacher KJ, et al. *Harrison's Principles of Internal Medicine,* 9th ed. McGraw-Hill, New York, 1980.

Jones HR Jr (Trench AH, ed.). Diseases of the peripheral motor-sensory unit. *Clinical Symposia,* 1985, 37(2):2–32.

Jones JM. Current strategies in the pharmacologic management of vascular headaches. *Physician Assistant,* (Feb.) 1985, 43–75.

Kabadi UM. Laboratory tests for evaluating thyroid therapy. *American Family Physician,* (Sept.) 1982, 26(3):183–188.

Kolb B, Whishaw IQ. *Fundamentals of Human Neurophysiology.* Freeman, San Francisco, 1980.

Kramer M, Kupfer DJ, Pallak CP. When the patterns of sleep go askew. *Patient Care,* (Aug.) 1980, 122–178.

Krupp MA, Chatton MJ, Werdegar D (eds.). *Current Medical Diagnosis and Treatment 1985.* Lange, Los Altos, Calif., 1985.

Kunkel RS. Eleven clues to cluster headache: And tips on drug Rx. *Modern Medicine,* (Nov.–Dec.) 1980, 26–32.

Larson PR. A common endocrine disease in all age groups: Hypothyroidism. *Medical Times,* (Nov.) 1980, 108(11):47–60.

Locke W. Management of hyper- and hypothyroid conditions. *Postgraduate Medicine,* (Mar.) 1982, 71(3):118–129.

Luckmann J, Sorensen KC. *Medical Surgical Nursing: A Psychophysiologic Approach,* 2nd ed. Saunders, Philadelphia, 1980.

Lum G. The differential diagnosis of hypercalcemic disease. *Laboratory Management,* (Mar.) 1983, 29–40.

Malhotra AS, Goren H. The hot bath test in the diagnosis of MS. *Journal of the American Medical Association,* (Sept.) 1981, 246(10):1113–1114.

Merrit HH. *A Textbook of Neurology.* Henry Kimptor, London, 1979.

Miller JM. Thyroid nodules: Needle biopsy to separate candidates for surgery. *Diagnosis,* (Nov.) 1980, 16–21.

National Association of State Public Health Veterinarians, Inc. Compendium of animal rabies vaccines, 1983. *Morbidity and Mortality Weekly Report,* (Dec. 31) 1982, 31(51):685–695.

Neelon FA. Nail changes in thyroid disease. *Drug Therapy,* (Nov.) 1980, 153–155.

Nora LM, Weiner WJ. Parkinson's disease, parkinsonism, and the evaluation of tremor. *Continuing Medical Education,* (June) 1983, 575–581.

Palmer GC. Clinical pharmacology of anticonvulsants. *Continuing Education,* (Feb.) 1980, 71–83.

Penry JK, Porter RJ. Epilepsy: Mechanisms and therapy. *Medical Clinics of North America,* (July) 1979, 63(4):801–811.

Plotkin SA. Rabies vaccintion in the 1980's. *Hospital Practice,* (Nov.) 1980, 65–72.

Reed JW, McCowen KD. Hyperthyroidism and thyroid cancer: A report of three cases. *Postgraduate Medicine,* (Feb.) 1980, 67(2):169–172.

Rizzolo PJ, Fischer PM. Re-evaluation of thyroid hormone status after long-term hormone therapy. *The Journal of Family Practice,* 1982, 14(6):1017–1021.

Roof BS, Lichtenstein LS. Primary hyperparathyroidism: Clinical diagnosis and management. *Continuing Education,* (May) 1982, 53–64.

Rubenstein E, Federman D. *Scientific American Medicine.* Scientific American, New York, 1985.

Safrit HF. Diagnosis and management of Graves' disease. *Hospital Medicine,* (Oct.) 1979, 74–87.

Sagel J. Hypothalamic regulatory hormones: Their clinical application in hypothalamic, pituitary, and end organ diseases. *Continuing Education,* (June) 1982, 74–78.

Schwabel ST. The solitary thyroid nodule: Malignant or benign? *Physician Assistant,* (July) 1983, 28–42.

Sherman C. Trigeminal neuralgia. *Aches and Pains,* (Feb.) 1984, 35–38.

Silverstein A. *Human Anatomy and Physiology.* Wiley, New York, 1980.

Snyder M (ed.). *A Guide to Neurological and Neurosurgical Nursing.* Wiley, New York, 1983.

Speed WG III. Ergotamine and beta blockers for migraine. *Modern Medicine,* (Feb.) 1985, 59–66.

Stabile N. Adrenal disease and suppression: Natural and iatrogenic. *PA Outlook,* (Nov.) 1983, 3–7.

Stuart PM. Update on managing parkinsonism and tardive dyskinesia. *Consultant,* (June) 1983, 51–80.

Thorn GW, et al. Diagnostic approach to endocrine disorders. *Medical Times,* (Nov.) 1980, 108(11):28–32.

Tortora G, Anagnostakos N. *Principles of Anatomy and Physiology.* Harper & Row, New York, 1981.

Usdin E, Hawkins D (eds.). *The Office Guide to Sleep Disorders.* KPR Infor/Media Corp., New York, 1980.

Varma SK. Endocrine diseases and autoimmunity. *Cutis,* (Feb.) 1981, 27:127–134.

Vinicor F, Cooper J. Early recognition of endocrine disorders. *Hospital Medicine,* (Dec.) 1979, 38–47.

Vogel R. Peripheral nerve entrapment syndrome. *American Family Physician,* (Nov.) 1983, 28:130–135.

Williams RH. *Textbook of Endocrinology,* 5th ed. Saunders, Philadelphia, 1974.

Wyngaarden JB, Smith LH Jr (eds.). *Cecil Textbook of Medicine,* 16th ed., Vols. 1 and 2. Saunders, Philadelphia, 1982.

13

Psychology

Carla Greene and Connie Main
Wes McGovern, Special Consultant

Outline

THOUGHT

Mental retardation (severe, profound, moderate)
Down's syndrome
Borderline intelligence
Schizophrenia
Neologisms
Thought broadcasting, insertion, withdrawal
Hallucinations
Paranoid schizophrenia
Antipsychotic medications
Dystonia, akathesia, tardive dyskinesia
▶ Organizations for mental illness
Coordinated care of the schizophrenic patient

EGO AND PERSONALITY

Ego defense mechanisms
Personality disorders
Antisocial/psychopathic personality disorder
Alcoholism
▶ Office management of alcohol abuse
▶ Alcohol treatment programs and support groups
Drug abuse
▶ Drug abuse organizations
Drug overdose
Drug withdrawal
Sedative-hypnotic withdrawal
Benzodiazepine withdrawal
Narcotic withdrawal
Methadone clinics

SEXUALITY

Satisfaction with sexual relationships
Psychosexual disorders (gender identity, paraphilia, ego dystonic homosexuality, psychosexual dysfunction)

Rape
Rape trauma syndrome
► Proper care of the rape victim

FEELINGS

Anger
Grief reactions
Affective disorders
Depression (reactive, secondary, postpartum, primary)
Depression in the elderly
► Office management of depression
Antidepressant drugs
ECT or "shock therapy"
Atypical depression
Bipolar (manic) depression
Lithium
► The patient taking lithium
Lithium toxicity
Suicide
► Suicide prevention

STRESS

Psychophysiologic disorders
Anorexia nervosa
Bulimia
► Anxiety reaction
► Panic attack
Anxiety disorders (phobic, counterphobic behavior, obsessive-compulsive disorder)
Dissociative disorders (somnambulism, amnesia, anterograde amnesia, multiple personality)
Somatiform disorders (somatization, psychogenic pain, hypochondriasis, conversion)
Malingerer
Munchausen's syndrome
► Stress reduction

FAMILY SYSTEMS

Domestic violence
► Organizations for abused adults
Incest or sexual abuse
► Organizations for victims of childhood sexual abuse

DEVELOPMENTAL MILESTONES

Developmental crisis
Midlife crisis
Death
► Considerations for the dying patient

Each person has a distinct psychologic makeup, that is, the way he or she thinks, feels about, and relates to the world. These processes vary from time to time and from person to person. Nonetheless, there are certain signs of psychologic health. For the most part, mentally healthy persons are eager to learn and grow. By using information and imagination, they can formulate questions, come up with ideas, and judge situations. This helps them to deal with life realistically rather than in terms of how they wish it were or expect it to be. Mentally healthy persons are interested in the world. They work, make friends, and enjoy good times. Recognizing the uniqueness of themselves and others, they can give and accept warmth. They take responsibility for their thoughts, feelings, and behavior, understanding that this is often difficult or painful.

Mental health is an area of prime concern to the primary care provider. Intelligence, personality and ego strengths, and support systems must be taken into account when planning medical intervention. This is important for all patients, but particularly for the patient already under treatment for a psychiatric illness. As the trend to release people from institutions into the community continues, primary care providers will be seeing more patients with chronic psychiatric disorders. Most of these patients will be maintained on medications and special treatment programs. It is thus imperative that their medical care be coordinated with their psychiatric care.

A number of medical illnesses may precipitate psychologic symptoms (Table 13.1). By the same token, medical complaints may be presenting symptoms of depression, anxiety, hypochondriasis, and many other psychiatric problems. The criteria for mental illness focus on relatively enduring psychologic syndromes or behavior patterns that provoke subjective distress, impair social relations, and/or disrupt day-to-day functioning. Attempts to classify such syndromes and patterns run the risk of labeling patients and detracting from the uniqueness of individuals and their problems. Nonetheless, classification systems enable clinicians to diagnose, communicate about, study, and treat various mental disorders.

One of the most widely used systems is the American Psychiatric Association's third edition of the *Diagnostic and Statistical Manual of Mental Disorders* (DSM-III). Its classifications are descriptive and allow for various theoretical explanations, noting that in many instances the etiology or the exact pathophysiologic process is unknown.

DSM-III uses the term "psychotic" to describe either an isolated behavior or a general disorder that is characterized by gross impairment of reality testing. Evidence of such impairment includes delusions (false, fixed beliefs based on incorrect inferences and not ordinarily accepted by other members of the person's culture or subculture) and hallucinations (sensory perception without external stimulation of the relevant sensory organ).

The term "neurosis" has been dropped in DSM-III. In its place are the terms "neurotic disorder" and "neurotic process." Neurotic disorder is marked by distressful and alienating behavior. The behavior does not actively violate social norms, although it may be disabling to the individual. Reality testing remains basically intact. The neurotic process is the etiology—unconscious conflicts, anxiety, the use of defense mechanisms, or a personality disturbance. Such a process is one of many factors involved in the development of neurotic disorders.

As noted throughout this chapter, many psychiatric problems can be handled in primary care settings. Primary care providers must also be able to refer those problems that require special care to the appropriate source. The modes of treatment described in Table 13.2 are practiced by various professionals. As a physician with at least 3 years of psychiatric residency, the psychiatrist treats patients requiring medications, electroconvulsion, or involved psychotherapy. Psychologists (with a master's degree or Ph.D.) administer and interpret psychologic tests and practice psychotherapy. Psychotherapy can also be undertaken by social workers, clinical nurse specialists, and by marriage, family, and mental health counselors. Having undergone several years of training in a psychoanalytic institute and personal analysis, the psychoanalyst (psychiatrist, psychologist, psychiatric nurse, or social worker) engages in long-term, in-depth therapy.

THOUGHT

There are three aspects of thought (cognition). These include the degree to which one is able to comprehend, remember, synthesize, and apply information (intelligence), how one thinks (thought process), and what one thinks about (thought content).

Intellectual performance is measured in terms of an intelligence quotient (IQ),

TABLE 13.1 MEDICAL CONDITIONS THAT CAUSE PSYCHIATRIC SYMPTOMS

Condition	Psychiatric Symptoms
Metal Reactions	
Lead	Irritability, restlessness, symptoms of acute psychosis
Manganese	Emotional instability, hallucinations, impulsiveness, aggressiveness, irritability
Mercury	Lethargy, irritability, auditory hallucinations, paranoid delusions
Thallium	Paranoid ideation, depression
Environmental hazards	
Carbon disulfide	Irritability, mood swings, confusion, personality changes
Organophosphates	Decreased memory and concentration, auditory hallucinations
Drug reactions	
Corticosteroids	Euphoria, symptoms of acute schizophrenia
Digitalis	Apathy, memory loss, confusion, lability, symptoms of psychotic depression or schizophrenia
Antabuse	Delirium, agitation, and mood swings mimicking schizophrenia or manic-depression
Isoniazid	Disorientation, delirium, paranoid ideation, euphoria that resembles schizophrenia or manic psychosis
Levodopa	Depression, delirium, restlessness, euphoria, auditory hallucinations
Aldomet	Decreased mental acuity, nightmares, reversible depression or psychosis
Inderal	Depression, withdrawal, lassitude, auditory hallucinations
Reserpine	Severe depression, psychomotor retardation, suicide ideation, nihilistic delusions
Nutritional deficiencies	
Niacin	Insomnia, confusion, delusions resembling those of acute psychosis
Pyridoxine	Visual hallucinations and confusional states similar to those of acute psychosis
Thiamine	Decreased memory, confabulation, auditory and visual hallucinations
Vitamin B_{12}	Apathy, mood swings, delusions and hallucinations similar to those of acute psychosis
Endocrine disorders	
Cushing's syndrome	Bizarre somatic delusions, anxiety, thought dysfunctions similar to those of schizophrenia
Addison's disease	Depression, negativism, apathy, paranoia, confusion, and agitation
Hyperthyroidism	Anorexia, fatigue, and withdrawal resembling psychotic depression; clouded sensorium, paranoia, somatic delusions and thought disorders similar to those of psychosis
Hypothyroidism	Paranoid and belligerent behavior; anxiety, irritability, somatic delusions and hallucinations
Systemic disorders	
Huntington's chorea	Mood swings, delusions, and auditory hallucinations
Wilson's disease	Explosive mood swings, decreased memory and intellectual function, antisocial behavior
Alzheimer's disease	Dementia, depression, cognitive deterioration, paranoid delusions
Encephalitis	Symptoms resembling those of psychotic depression, stupor, coma
Epilepsy	Impulsive outbursts of anger that may be confused with personality disorder; amnesia for the event

TABLE 13.1 *(Continued)*

Condition	Psychiatric Symptoms
Normal pressure hydrocephalus	Agitation, insidious dementia, psychotic symptoms
Systemic lupus erythematosus	Thought disorders, depression, confusion
Meningitis	Acute psychotic symptoms including disorientation, hallucinations, and agitation
Neurosyphilis	Memory defects, bizarre dress, personality changes much like those of chronic schizophrenia
Porphyria	Mood swings, outbursts, withdrawal that may resemble conversion reaction, anxiety attack, or a manic or depressive episode
Multiple sclerosis	Personality changes, mild euphoria, depression, inappropriate behavior
Tumors	
Intracranial	Depression, anxiety, decreased memory and consciousness
Adrenal	Severe agitation, anxiety, or panic during attack
Pancreatic	Depression, decreased drive, sense of doom

Source: Based on Psychiatric emergency, *Patient Care,* (November) 1980,

determined through such tests as the Wechsler Intelligence Scale for Children (WISC), the Wechsler Adult Intelligence Scale (WAIS), and the Stanford-Binet Intelligence Scale. The WAIS includes verbal, performance, and written subtests that concentrate on a specific area of cognitive ability. For example, general knowledge may be assessed by questions such as "Who wrote Hamlet?", "Name five large cities," and "What are the colors of the American flag?" Recent and remote memory might be tested by asking subjects to repeat material given during the interview and to recall the birth dates of their children. Attention and concentration may be evaluated through serial repetition.

Thought process and content are noted by asking the person to respond to hypothetical situations ("What would you do if you noticed a fire in a theater?"); by checking the ability to discriminate between essential and nonessential elements in a series of incomplete picture cards (picture completion test); and by a number of projective and nonprojective tests (Rorschach, Thematic Apperception, and Sentence Completion). The latter are discussed more thoroughly in the section on personality.

Cognition is influenced by physical status, environmental exposure, and social interactions, and is inborn in that the nervous system is genetically determined. Beginning in infancy and continuing throughout life, it develops in stages. When one cognitive stage has been successfully completed, the individual moves on to a more complex one and, it is hoped, has the ability to balance and integrate new experiences with those of the past.

During the first 2 years of life, children are preoccupied with their senses and motor activities. They achieve a rudimentary understanding of time, space, and causality. For example, they come to realize that an object exists even though it may be out of sight. Children of this age reason through mental images and begin to acquire concepts of form, color, size, and early language skills.

From 2 to 7 years, they refine language skills and are able to reason through words as well as mental images. During this stage, thinking is directly related to the

TABLE 13.2 TREATMENT APPROACHES USED IN PSYCHIATRIC DISORDERS

Type of Therapy	Description	Target Population	Rationale
Insight/cognitive		Most appropriate for mildly disturbed persons; not always helpful with more severe disturbances (psychoses), or with retarded or autistic individuals, because it requires some ability to understand personal behavior and motivational factors. It is, however, an appropriate therapy for victims of violent crimes (e.g., assault, rape) and for persons experiencing difficult life changes or crises, such as the death or impending death of a close friend or relative, an illness that causes a radical change in lifestyle or is terminal, unemployment, relationship problems, or depression (in severe depression, one of the cognitive therapies may supplement chemotherapy).	Basic assumption in cognitive approaches is that many emotional and psychologic problems can usually be resolved by exploration and understanding of the meanings of personal behavior and feelings; the ability to communicate feelings and participate in resolution of problems is a prerequisite for this type of therapy.
Psychoanalysis (Freudian)	The individual relaxes and speaks about whatever comes to mind and the therapist interprets, pointing out meanings and associations. Past life events, childhood memories, and dreams are considered to be sources of relevant information about present difficulties.		
Client-centered (Rogerian)	Therapist's role is nondirective, involving rephrasing and clarifying the information that the client provides about his or her life, without explaining or evaluating the person or his or her thoughts, feelings, or statements. Usually the individual, rather than the therapist, decides which experiences are discussed, and the emphasis is on clarification of the client's interpretations of these experiences, rather than on those of the therapist. Therapy most often focuses the discussion on *present* experiences and feelings, rather than childhood experiences.		
Behavioral			The maladjusted person is seen as different from normal only in having failed to learn behaviors useful for coping with everyday life situations or in having learned faulty or inefficient coping styles that are maintained through habit or some form of reinforcement; rather than attempting to bring about cognitive change, the therapist tries to modify behavior directly by manipulation of environmental reward and punishment contingencies.
Systematic desensitization (SD)	Individuals are taught (through relaxation exercises, hypnosis, biofeedback, etc.) to associate relaxation with situations that previously induced fear or anxiety, with the end result of completely eliminating the anxious response.	SD is useful for isolated problems that are conditioned avoidance responses, such as phobias, and is not limited to any one target population. However, it is not designed to resolve complex psychologic disturbances.	
Aversion therapy (AT)	Punishment (removal of positive reinforcement or use of aversive stimuli) is used to lessen the "desirability" of stimuli that elicit undesirable behavior. Possible aversive stimuli are mild electric shock or drugs or odors that induce nausea; these methods raise the issues of ethics and informed consent, and generally an alternative approach is preferable.	AT is generally used when other therapies are ineffective. It has produced results in very difficult cases, such as autistic, severely retarded, or psychotic individuals who are unresponsive to other therapeutic interventions. Currently being used for treatment of child sexual abuses.	
Differential reinforcement of other responses (DOR)	An alternative to AT in which behaviors alternative to and incompatible with undesirable behaviors are reinforced. For example, if the problem is antisocial behavior, the individual will be rewarded for all constructive behaviors exhibited, and at the same time, any reinforcement (usually attention) for the undesirable behavior will be eliminated.	May be used with autistic, psychotic, or retarded individuals or with young children. Effective for behavioral problems.	

TABLE 13.2 *(Continued)*

Type of Therapy	Description	Target Population	Rationale
Implosive therapy (flooding)	The therapist deliberately attempts to elicit anxiety by asking the client to imagine in detail (or relive, in the case of actual past experiences) anxiety-producing situations that he or she would ordinarily avoid thinking about. The assumption is that repeated exposure to the imagined scenes in a safe setting will cause the stimulus to lose some of its power to elicit anxiety, and avoidance responses (defenses) will become unnecessary and disappear.	Most appropriate for mildly disturbed (not psychotic) persons. Used with isolated problems such as phobias or disturbing memories (e.g., of a rape or similar experience).	
Biologically based therapies			
Chemotherapy	The following medications are used to treat psychological disorders:		Pharmacologic therapy often reduces the severity and chronicity of many types of illnesses (particularly the psychoses), making outpatient management of many individuals possible. However, drugs tend only to alleviate the symptoms of the difficulty; they do not help the individual understand personal or environmental factors that may have contributed to the problem or that may have developed secondary to the disturbance. For this reason, adjunct therapies (such as cognitive and behavioral therapies) are indicated, whenever possible, to render the benefits of drug therapy more permanent and sometimes to eventually eliminate the need for the drug.
	1. *Antipsychotic compounds* (neuroleptics or major tranquilizers) are used to calm the patient, as well as to alleviate the intensity of schizophrenic symptoms (extreme agitation, delusions, hallucinations, bizarre behavior). These include drugs from the phenothiazine family and others such as haloperidol (Haldol). Major disadvantages are side effects such as dry mouth and throat, muscle stiffness, jaundice, and extrapyramidal symptoms (parkinsonism, tardive dyskinesia). Not a cure for schizophrenia; symptoms are only suppressed.	1. For use with major psychologic disorders (the schizophrenias).	
	2. *Antianxiety compounds* (anxiolytics or minor tranquilizers, sedatives) reduce tension without affecting psychotic symptoms. These include barbiturates, meprobamates, and benzodiazepine derivatives. Major disadvantages are limiting side effects such as drowsiness, lethargy, restlessness, dizziness, and the risks of toxicity and drug dependence	2. Used in nonpsychotic conditions in which tension and anxiety are significant components, such as neurotic and psychosomatic disorders, and also as supplementary treatment in some neurologic disorders for control of convulsive seizures, and as sleep inducers. Not appropriate for psychoses.	
	3. *Antidepressant compounds* are mainly used with unipolar psychotic depressions and include tricyclics and MAO inhibitors. Among the multiple side effects of tricyclics are those due to anticholinergic activity (dry mouth, blurred vision, urinary hesitation, constipation), cardiac disturbances, orthostatic hypotension, hy-	3. Used in treatment of psychotic depression, particularly unipolar types; may be used initially to relieve the symptoms and stabilize the patient, and may then be supplemented by another approach, such as a cognitive therapy.	

TABLE 13.2 *(Continued)*

Type of Therapy	Description	Target Population	Rationale
Chemotherapy (*cont.*)	pertension, and precipitation or aggravation of glaucoma. MAO inhibitors are generally used only after tricyclics have proven ineffective because of serious side effects involved with their use, including the possibility of severe hypertensive reactions (accompanied by hypertensive encephalopathy and cerebrovascular accidents). The use of MAO inhibitors requires certain dietary restrictions as well. Both classes of drugs have the disadvantage of being slow-acting.		
	4. Regular maintenance doses of *Lithium* modulate or prevent cycles of mania and/or depression when these are symptoms of a bipolar affective disorder. Alleviation of these symptoms makes it possible to employ other therapies more effectively (e.g., individual psychotherapy). There are multiple side effects and potential toxicity unless use is carefully monitored.	4. Used with bipolar affective psychoses (i.e., those that include periods of mania as well as depression).	
ECT	Following premedication with a muscle relaxant, an electric current is passed from one side of the patient's head to the other (approximately 160 V lasting for up to about 1.5 seconds); immediately losing consciousness, the patient undergoes a marked tonic (extensor) seizure of the muscles, followed by a lengthy series of less severe clonic (contractile) seizures. The patient has amnesia upon awakening several minutes later, and confusion usually persists for about an hour. A modification of the technique is unilateral ECT, in which the current is passed through the nondominant side of the brain; this method seems to be just as therapeutically effective as bilateral ECT, but memory impairment is less severe.	Sometimes dramatically effective in resolving psychotic states, especially the affective ones (involving depression and/or mania), and, less, often the schizophrenias; benefits may be only temporary, however, Not a frequent choice of therapy, but it may be used in cases where drugs are too slow in relieving the symptoms, especially those of a depression that is potentially suicidal.	Developed as a result of an early (erroneous) observation that schizophrenia rarely occurred in individuals with epilepsy. It was thought that if schizophrenia and epilepsy were incompatible, then induced convulsions might cure the psychosis. The therapeutic effect is unclear, but may be due to induced biochemical changes in the brain at the synaptic junctions.
Megavitamin therapy	Dietary changes and administration of large doses of vitamins and minerals	Chronic schizophrenia, senility, alcoholism	Niacin is thought to relieve schizphrenic symptoms, zinc and manganese to control senility, and a high-protein, vitamin-enriched diet to remove the craving for alcohol. Generally discredited.

TABLE 13.2 *(Continued)*

Type of Therapy	Description	Target Population	Rationale
Group therapy		More appropriate for mildly disturbed individuals, but some have been used successfully with psychotic patients.	
Psychoanalytic client-centered, and behavioral	All of these therapeutic approaches have been adapted for use with groups; the same emphases and therapeutic methods are incorporated, but the group members are all clients; most typical group size is 8–12 members, in addition to the therapist or "leader."		Advantages include efficiency (one therapist can deal simultaneously with several patients), an opportunity for patients to share and benefit from the experiences of others, multiple support and feedback sources, and practice in relating to others.
Psychodrama	Developed by J. L. Moreno as a way for clients to move beyond talking about their feelings and reactions to experiencing them actively in the process of therapy. The client, with the assistance of other group members who play the roles of significant persons ("actors"), is encouraged to act out problem situations from his or her own life; the therapist makes comments and suggestions as they proceed.		The intent is that genuine feelings and thoughts will emerge as the actors become involved in their parts; these are discussed and alternative responses are tried out. In the course of a few group sessions, a member may gain a great deal of insight into his and others' behaviors and feelings, and has the opportunity to act out even unacceptable responses in a setting that simulates real life but is more sheltered.
Encounter groups	The leader is basically nondirective and is usually responsible for screening group members; scheduling meetings; and establishing a psychologically safe climate in which participants feel safe enough to drop facades, express their true feelings, and experiment with new ways of interacting; the leader models this openness in his or her own communications and encourages members to give descriptive feedback ("It made me feel angry when you said that") instead of evaluative feedback ("You are inconsiderate"); nonverbal "exercises" may be used to facilitate trust, awareness, and communication.		Emphasis is on providing an intensive group experience that helps members work through emotional problems and achieve more adequate coping techniques; it is superior to individual therapy in providing an environment that is similar to social reality, but its healing capacity generally surpasses that of conventional reality because of its demands for openness and honesty.
Sociotherapies			
Couple or marital therapy	Typically both marriage partners are seen together; focus of therapy is on clarification and improvement of communications and the relationship between them. Various approaches have been used, including insight and behavioral therapies and videotape recordings of the sessions, which can be played back later for the purpose of getting insight and feedback about interactions that take place in the therapy session.	Not advisable as the initial therapy for cases involving spouse abuse, since the involvement of both members in the treatment suggests that the abuse is somehow the fault of both; individual therapy is indicated for the wife initially in order to help her recognize that the problem is her spouse's and that she does not somehow deserve the abuse; joint therapy may be used later. Marital therapy is helpful for most other difficulties centering on a couple's relationship.	Often the emotional involvement of marriage partners in their relationship makes it difficult for them to perceive their interactions objectively; they may see faults in their partner but do not recognize what they do to contribute to their spouse's behavior. Therapy provides a setting in which feelings can be expressed, encouraging careful listening to the needs and feelings of each member and honest feedback.

TABLE 13.2 (*Continued*)

Type of Therapy	Description	Target Population	Rationale
Family therapy	Most widely used approach is "conjoint family therapy," developed by V. Satir, with emphasis on improving faulty communications, interactions, and relationships between family members and promoting a family system that is more beneficial for all of its members. The client is the entire family as a unit, rather than individual members.	Therapy is typically begun when one child (the "identified patient") displays signs of disturbance.	It has been discovered that many persons who make considerable progress in individual therapy will have a relapse upon returning home. This is attributed by many to the fact that whatever symptoms the child has developed have either been caused by or incorporated into the function of his or her particular family system; if changes are to occur in the individual, the family system must also change to accommodate them. Therefore, most family therapists feel that the entire family should be directly involved in the therapy if there is to be lasting improvement.
Hospital approaches		May be used with any hospital (psychiatric) population.	
Milieu therapy[a]	Focus is on structuring the patient's environment (milieu) to provide clear communication of expectations and to involve the patient in the treatment and in participation in the therapeutic community via the group process. All members of the community (staff and patients) are perceived as participants in the healing process, as opposed to a few trained therapists.		The entire facility is regarded as a therapeutic community; emphasis on developing a meaningful and constructive environment in which patients participate in regulating their own activities. Self-reliance and the formation of socially acceptable interpersonal relationships are encouraged.
Social learning[a] (e.g., "token economy")	Uses learning principles and techniques (e.g., positive reinforcement of acceptable behaviors and nonreinforcement of nonacceptable behaviors) to shape more socially acceptable behavior.		Some individuals who stay in mental hospitals for long periods become passive, having lost the motivation or self-confidence to attempt reentry into society. Behavioral approaches help individuals learn or maintain appropriate and efficient interactional skills so that they can function outside of the hospital environment.
Traditional[a] mental hospital treatments	Include chemotherapy, occupational, recreational, and activity therapies (for exercise, learning skills, and use of creativity), and individual or group therapy.		Intent of intensive inpatient treatment is to prevent a serious disorder from becoming chronic and to enable the individual to return home as soon as possible. Activities such as recreational therapies are intended to keep the patient active and to provide experiences that are similar to those the patient might choose outside of the institution.
Adjunct techniques			
Biofeedback	Involves amplifying minute changes occurring in the body or brain and displaying them to the individual who experiences them by some signal,	Useful in treatment of hypotension, hypertension, circulatory problems, and heartbeat irregularities, and in training individuals to slow their heart	Voluntary control of some physiologic processes can eliminate the need for chemical therapies for some disorders; also, training in relax-

TABLE 13.2 *(Continued)*

Type of Therapy	Description	Target Population	Rationale
Biofeedback (*cont.*)	such as a tone or light. Many persons can learn to exert voluntary control over internal bodily processes by means of such feedback.	rates. May be used with systemic desensitization to elicit a relaxation response.	ation can be accomplished with this technique.
Hypnosis	Hypnotherapy involves induction of an altered state of consciousness in which there is extreme suggestibility. The therapist helps bring about this state by enlisting the subject's cooperation and eliminating any fears of the technique. Completely relaxed in a comfortable position, the subject's attention is focused so that irrelevant stimuli are tuned out, and activities are directed by the therapist by means of suggestions. *Narcosynthesis,* the administration of a hypnotic drug prior to hypnosis, may be used with subjects who are particularly resistant to suggestion. Sodium amytal, paraldehyde, and sodium pentothal have been used for this purpose.	Of all psychologic problems, conversion disorders are the most responsive to hypnosis, but prolonged analysis is required to discover the personality problem causing the condition. Hypnosis may be used successfully with anxiety neuroses, is dramatically effective with traumatic neuroses, and is almost as effective with psychosomatic disorders. Character disorders, obsessional neurosis, and anxiety hysteria characterized by phobia respond poorly to this therapy. The use of posthypnotic suggestion with alcoholics has been successful for strengthening the individual's ability to abandon drinking, but the use of hypnosis as an isolated therapy with most habit disturbances and symptoms, such as excessive smoking, overeating, drug addictions, insomnia, nail biting, enuresis, stage fright, and stuttering, is not advisable, since it will not extend beyond mere symptom removal. Since such symptoms are indications of deeper psychologic disturbances, the individual should be encouraged to explore the sources of the symptoms through more in-depth analysis. The effectiveness of hypnosis in treatment of the psychoses is limited, but it has been employed as an adjunct therapy with other treatments.	This technique has been employed to bring about recall of repressed memories; by reliving a traumatic experience during the hypnotic state, a subject is able to discharge the emotional tensions associated with it and is freed to assimilate the experience into his or her self-concept. Hypnosis is also used to bring about "hypnotic age regression," in which individuals are told that they are once again a certain age and will subsequently behave, think, and talk in much the same way as they did at that age. Regression to an age just prior to the time of the onset of a phobia may reveal the traumatic experience that precipitated it. Subjects may then be desensitized to the traumatic experience by reliving it through hypnosis. Also, suggestions can be made by the therapist while subjects are in the hypnotic state about behaviors that they are to carry out later in the waking state; this technique (posthypnotic suggestion) is useful in eliminating certain isolated habits or symptoms but must always be supplemented by a therapy that enables exploration of the underlying sources of the problem, since amelioration or removal of symptoms will probably be ineffective or temporary unless a fundamental change in the person's coping patterns is effected.

[a] One study comparing these three hospital approaches showed that 70% of released patients of *milieu therapy* remained continuously in the community and over 90% of those from the *social learning* program had the same results, as opposed to less than 50% for those in the *traditional* treatment program.

senses (prelogical). The child believes that anything that moves has life. After age 7, children develop the capacity to relate experience to an organized whole without direct involvement of the senses. By 11 years of age, they can deal with immediate concepts in solving problems, but reasoning is inductive rather than deductive. From 12 to 15 years, the child develops the capacity for deductive or abstract hypothetical reasoning.

In cases of ***mental retardation,*** IQ levels are below 70. Affecting 3% of the U.S. population, the problem is caused by genetic defects, infections, toxic exposure, birth

TABLE 13.3 CAUSES OF MENTAL RETARDATION

Genetic factors	Metabolic imbalances
Down's syndrome	Phenylketonuria (PKU)
No. 18 trisomy syndrome	Hypothyroidism (cretinism)
Tay-Sachs disease	Hyperbilirubinemia
Klinefelter's syndrome	Anemia
Niemann-Pick disease	Hypoxia
	Birth trauma
Infectious agents	Malnutrition
Maternal rubella	
Maternal syphilis	Toxic substances
Encephalitis	Carbon monoxide, lead, other poisons
Meningitis	Vaccines
	Teratogenic drugs

trauma, physical injury, radiation during pregnancy, and malnutrition (Table 13.3). Patients with ***severe retardation*** (IQ 20–35) or ***profound retardation*** (IQ under 20) are usually institutionalized. Limited self-help skills, rudimentary speech, and occasionally supervised occupational tasks are the best that can be hoped for. Sensory defects, motor handicaps, central nervous system (CNS) pathology, seizures, deafness, cataracts, and other physical problems are common. The life expectancy is short. Though learning is slow, individuals with ***moderate mental retardation*** (IQ 36–51) achieve a fair command of the spoken language, and many acquire simple literacy skills. Other goals include partial independence in daily routines, acceptable behavior, and limited work skills. These individuals tend to be ungainly and have poor motor coordination. Personality types range from affable or vacuous to aggressive or hostile. Relatively few cases fall into the moderate and more severe categories, and these are usually diagnosed in infancy. Genetic defects account for most of them. In the most common, ***Down's syndrome,*** patients have 47 chromosomes instead of the normal complement of 46 due to a trisomy of chromosome 21. The risk of this mutation increases with the age of the mother and reaches 1 in 50 when pregnancy occurs past age 40. The syndrome results in a number of physical changes as well as mental retardation. Slanting "mongoloid" eyes, thickened eyelids, broad, flattened head and facial features, enlarged tongue, short neck, and stubby fingers typify the appearance of persons with Down's syndrome. Congenital heart defects, circulatory and respiratory problems, and gastrointestinal complications are also common.

The majority of cases (almost 80%) fall into the category of ***mild retardation*** (IQ 52–68). The former subdivision of "borderline retardation" has been relabeled ***borderline intelligence*** (IQ 68–83). It is unusual for these disabilities to become evident during the early years; it is not until the child enters school and demonstrates learning difficulties that most cases are diagnosed. Mildly retarded adults function at the intellectual level of an 8- to 11-year-old and at the social level of an adolescent. With early diagnosis, parental support, and special educational programs, many of them achieve simple academic and occupational skills and become self-sufficient. In dealing with patients of borderline or low intelligence, primary care providers should make certain adjustments in the administration of their care. Instructions should be consistent with the individual's verbal and conceptual skills. Helping the patient focus his or her attention and subdividing care into manageable components is also important.

Schizophrenia is a chronic mental disorder characterized by distorted thought,

TABLE 13.4 SUBTYPES OF SCHIZOPHRENIA

Subtype	Essential Feature
Disorganized	Absence of systematized delusions. Frequent incoherence. Blunted, silly, or inappropriate affect.
Catatonic	Nonreactive. Rigid posture or excited, purposeless motor activity with a bizarre and inappropriate posture. Mutism or negativism.
Paranoid	Delusions and/or hallucinations of a grandiose, persecutory, and jealous nature.
Undifferentiated	Mixture of disorganized, catatonic, and paranoid tendencies.
Residual	Eccentric behavior, blunted affect, loose associations, and social withdrawal without true psychotic change.

emotion, and behavior, all of which lead to impaired social functioning. Since the symptoms are varied, various subtypes have been described (Table 13.4). Several factors probably interact in the development of schizophrenia. A genetic role is suggested by twin studies and by the fact that many children of schizophrenic parents develop the disorder even if they are removed from parental influence. Complications during pregnancy or birth are also associated with the disorder. Schizophrenic patients apparently have abnormal amounts or types of neurotransmitters in the brain (dopamine has received particular attention). This is thought to diminish their ability to handle changing or stressful situations. Unhealthy family environments and developmental crises are leading precipitating factors. A number of patients have a history of being shy, oversensitive, or loners. The majority of schizophrenic patients are found in the lower socioeconomic classes. Since many of them were born into more affluent families, this situation is probably the result, not the cause, of their illness. Autism and childhood schizophrenia occur but are relatively uncommon. Adolescence, a time of rapid physical, cognitive, and emotional growth, is a fairly vulnerable period. However, early adulthood accounts for most cases. Men are at highest risk during their twenties and thirties, and women during pregnancy, the postpartum period, and menopause.

Except for an association with menopause, schizophrenia rarely strikes for the first time over age 45. A disturbance of thought is an important symptom. Associations are often incorrect, incoherent, or even bizarre. Speech patterns do not follow conventional semantic rules, and in extreme cases, patients invent new words ***(neologisms).*** "Thought blocking," an abrupt stoppage of speech flow, is often displayed. Delusions, with or without hallucinations, signal serious degeneration of thought content. Often schizophrenics believe that their thoughts are being broadcast to the world ***(thought broadcasting),*** that mental images that are not their own are being inserted into their minds ***(thought insertion),*** or that images are being removed from their minds ***(thought withdrawal).*** Delusions are common, the usual themes being jealousy, persecution, control, grandeur, or nihilism. Auditory ***hallucinations*** (typically voices) constitute the most common perceptual disturbances. Some patients have difficulty localizing the source of "voices," while others perceive them to be coming from light fixtures, shut-off televisions, or imaginary telephone receivers. Often described as belonging to friends, relatives, enemies, or God, the voices direct comments, usually derogatory, at the patient. Visual, olfactory, and tactile hallucinations are also experienced. In other words, schizophrenics may see and hear persons or things that are not there, smell noxious gas, or taste poison in their food. The emotional expressions (affect) of schizophrenics are commonly blunted or inappropriate. For example, if confronted with news of a friend's death, a schizophrenic may respond with a blank stare or laughter. Physical and emotional withdrawal increases as patients become engrossed in their own delusions, hallucination, thoughts and feelings. Such "autism" is a cardinal sign, warranting psychiatric evaluation.

For the most part, schizophrenics pose no threat of danger to others. An exception is ***paranoid schizophrenia.*** These patients show a history of growing suspicion and interpersonal difficulty. Eventually they are dominated by absurd, illogical, and changeable persecutory delusions. Paranoid schizophrenics complain of being watched, followed, talked about, poisoned, or influenced by some supernatural force. Often they believe this is because they possess remarkable qualities or are great persons. As all attention becomes centered on these delusions, critical judgment is lost and behavior becomes erratic, unpredictable, and sometimes dangerous.

Antipsychotic medications have brought new hope to patients suffering from schizophrenia. Prior to the introduction of reserpine in the 1930s, patients with schizophrenia spent their lives deteriorating in mental institutions. Reserpine actually had few antipsychotic properties but was important in setting a historical precedent. It led to a search for more effective medications, which finally led to the discovery of the phenothiazines in the 1950s. Today, at least nine classes of antipsychotic medications (neuroleptics) exist, five of which are used in the United States (Table 13.5). The term "major tranquilizer" is misleading in that a withdrawn patient who takes it may become more active. The various drugs work by blocking specific neurotransmitters in postsynaptic junctions of the CNS. For example, Thorazine blocks mainly noradrenaline, while Haldol specifically blocks dopamine. The drugs may also interfere with alpha-adrenergic mechanisms, as suggested by their hypotensive effects. Finally, they increase the turnover of catecholamines and the intraneuronal levels of adenosine triphosphate (ATP). By decreasing the symptoms of hallucinations and delusions, antipsychotic medications make the patient more amenable to occupational and recreational programs. This, in turn, permits hospital discharge once the active phase of the illness is over. Although patients continue to have some aberrant thought patterns and contents, maintenance drug therapy ensures minimal disturbance and some independence. If it is discontinued, however, relapse rates are high. The symptoms of relapse usually are similar to those that lead to the initial diagnosis. Many studies have raised a question about the value of psychotherapy for schizophrenia in relieving psychotic symptoms. Patients receiving drugs alone were shown to improve markedly, but no less so than those receiving drugs plus psychotherapy. On the other hand, there was rapid deterioration in schizophrenics receiving psychotherapy alone. These studies did, however, find that group and/or family therapy helped schizophrenics in remission to remain in the community.

Although there is no doubt about the efficacy of neuroleptic drugs, numerous side effects may limit their use. Some patients develop spastic muscle jerking ***(dystonia)*** or restless sensations and jitters ***(akathesia)*** when they first start taking the drugs. Others show parkinsonian symptoms such as tremors, rigid posture, and shuffling walk. Hypotension, palpitations, sweating, dry mouth, and other cholinergic effects are common. Sun sensitivity and rashes are experienced by a limited number of patients. These acute side effects usually disappear on their own, by lowering the dose, or by switching drugs. They can sometimes be reversed by concurrent treat-

TABLE 13.5 ANTIPSYCHOTIC DRUGS USED IN THE UNITED STATES

Generic Drug (Sample Brand Name)	Common Dose Range (mg daily)
Aliphatic phenothiazines	
Chlorpromazine (Thorazine)	50–1,200
Promazine (Sparine)	25–1,000
Triflupromazine (Vesprin)	50–150
Piperidine phenothiazines	
Thioridazine (Mellaril)	50–800
Mesoridazine (Serentil)	50–400
Piperacetazine (Quide)	10–160
Piperazine phenothiazines	
Trifluoperazine (Stelazine)	5–80
Perphenazine (Trilafon)	12–64
Fluphenazine (Prolixin)	1–20 every 1–3 weeks
Acetophenazine (Tindal)	40–80
Butaperazine (Repoise)	15–100
Carphenazine (Proketazine)	25–400
Prochlorperazine (Compazine)	10–150
Aliphatic thioxanthenes	
Chlorprothixene (Taractan)	25–600
Piperazine thioxanthene	
Thiothixene (Navane)	5–30
Butyrophenones	
Haloperidol (Haldol)	5–80
Dihydroindolones	
Molindone (Moban)	15–225
Dibenzoxazepines	
Loxapine (Loxitane)	20–250

ment with anticholinergic drugs such as Cogentin or Artane. However, ***tardive dyskinesia,*** which afflicts about 5% of all persons taking antipsychotic medications, may be a permanent side effect. These rhythmic movements can develop anytime during therapy, and, strangely enough, often appear when the drug is withdrawn or the dose lowered. They characteristically involve the mouth, with some order of lip smacking, sucking, chewing, or tongue protrusion. Grimacing, blinking, frowning, and writhing body motions also occur. In extreme cases, dyskinesia interferes with talking and swallowing. At the present time, there is no way to predict who will develop the problem and no effective treatment. For this reason, the American Psychiatric Association (APA) advises that patients sign an informed consent regarding the possible development of tardive dyskinesia before initiating neuroleptic drugs.

► ***Organizations for mental illness*** offer many resources for patients and families. In addition, primary care providers are important participants in ***coordinated care of the schizophrenic patient.*** Health maintenance and acute care intervention are crucial, since physical illness can compound mental health problems. Furthermore, therapy with psychotropic drugs requires special screening exams and routine follow-up to monitor the blood for therapeutic levels and adverse effects such as liver dysfunction or blood dyscrasias. The psychiatric specialist often delegates these tasks to primary care providers. Patient visits can be used to encourage compliance and to observe for signs of relapse.

EGO AND PERSONALITY

Referred to as "personality traits," abilities, interests, values, temperament, and self-concept are some of the factors that constitute behavioral character—that is, personality. In rare cases, a single "cardinal" trait dominates nearly all of an individual's actions. Examples of this phenomenon enrich our language: Machiavellian, sadistic, quixotic. However, most persons are guided by several "central traits" and a number of less consistent "secondary traits." Some of these are outgoing/reserved, submissive/aggressive, serious/happy-go-lucky, tough-minded/sensitive, conservative/experimental, group oriented/self-sufficient, trusting/suspicious, spontaneous/self-controlled, and relaxed/tense.

A number of theories have emerged concerning the formation of personality. Some stress the importance of genetically determined factors such as intellectual capacity, facial features, and body build. One study concluded that plump "endomorphic" persons are sociable and pleasure-seeking, muscular "mesomorphic" persons are aggressive and achievement-oriented, and slender "ectomorphic" persons are sensitive and withdrawn (Sheldon, 1954). Later studies concurred that physical and personality characteristics are correlated but disagreed that one determines the other in such a simplified fashion. It has also been suggested that the society may be a key determinant of personality. Individuals coming from closed groups that assume the major responsibility for educating their young share many common personality traits. In a society such as ours, where children have diverse social contacts, individual differences are more likely. Furthermore, personality may be influenced by societal roles, such as child, student, worker, spouse, parent, or senior citizen.

In contrast to the idea of personality development, Barry Brazelton, Penelope Leach, and other contemporary psychology workers suggest that basic personality is born, not made. This belief is supported by the Chess-Thomas study, which followed subjects from infancy to early adulthood. The study concluded that distinct behavioral characteristics can be noted soon after birth and that these characteristics persist through several stages of growth and development. Many of the observed infants displayed characteristics that clustered into noticeable patterns. Forty percent could be described as "easy" children with regular schedules, a positive approach to change, and mild mood swings. Ten percent were "slow to warm up" children who manifested mildly negative responses to new stimuli. Fifteen percent were "difficult" children characterized by irregular patterns of eating and sleeping, slow adaptability, and intensely negative moods. Having little relationship to sex (e.g., girls are not easier than boys) or birth order (the first born are not more difficult than later children), these patterns remained fairly constant throughout childhood and adolescence and into early adulthood. However, these characteristics alone did not predict the child's adjustment. It was found that even easy children developed problems when the parents' demands and expectations failed to fit the child's style of behavior. On the other hand, difficult children remained problem free as long as their parents accepted and appreciated their special natures. This "goodness of fit" between parent and child proved to be a stronger determinant of the child's eventual well-being than a parent's divorce or death. It is no doubt important with peers and teachers as well. The child who is accepted and encouraged responds differently from the child who is rejected, mistreated, or overprotected.

A number of tests measure personality traits. Projection tests employ ambiguous stimuli such as ink blots (Rorschach), pictures (Thematic Apperception), and phrases (Sentence Completion) to elicit information about an individual's conflicts, motives, intellectual level, and coping techniques. Nonprojection tests use a more structured approach, employing questionnaires, self-inventories, and rating scales. Examples include the Minnesota Multiphasic Personality Inventory, the Comrey Personality Scale, and the Q-sort.

Facets of personality are also assessed through direct observation of patient behavior. Formal descriptions cover personal hygiene, aggressiveness, emotional responses, reality testing, physical and motor activity, and sexual tendencies. Observations made at work, at home, or in other natural settings provide the most information. Finally, information about a patient's personality can be derived from talks with family members, friends, or fellow workers.

Many of the major theories about personality development center on ego, a person's sense of security and self-esteem. In Freudian terms, the ego emerges in stages of early life to help a child balance his instincts (id) with the demands of his expanding world (superego). If expected conflicts between the id, ego, and superego are not worked out in childhood, deep-seated problems may emerge in later life. Psychoanalysis is the therapeutic approach based on uncovering such conflicts. Later, Erik Erikson, Sullivan, and many other theorists also stressed the importance of ego development but described it in terms of psychosocial functions. In other words, a person with a healthy ego is able to:

1. Recognize the self as a distinct and unique person.
2. Appraise his or her own strengths and weaknesses.
3. Deal with the frustration and anxiety of day-to-day living.
4. Direct urges, behavior, and feelings appropriately.
5. Form friendships.
6. Continue to learn.
7. Communicate effectively.
8. Work productively and creatively.
9. Function within societal or cultural norms.
10. Increase competency and control over one's life.

The ego acquires a number of ***defense mechanisms*** (Table 13.6). These usually operate at an unconscious level, and several may be used simultaneously or in close succession. They normally become manifest whenever an individual is threatened with overwhelming stress. Although defense mechanisms always distort reality, they may provide the only means an individual has for coping and should never be exposed. It is far more important to help the patient identify and work through the underlying problem. Every ego calls a defense mechanism into play at some time. However, overuse of such mechanisms, particularly of projection and fantasy, is likely to lead to delusions and hallucinations. In addition, complete psychologic disintegration can occur. Such patterns require more extensive psychiatric evaluation and treatment.

Immature and distorted personality development leads to ***personality disorders.*** The symptoms of the various subtypes are described in Table 13.7. They rarely exist in pure form, as exemplified by a paranoid person who exhibits compulsive

TABLE 13.6 DEFENSE MECHANISMS

Mechanism	Illustration
Repression The involuntary exclusion of painful or conflicting thoughts and memories.	A woman cannot recall the night her house was burglarized and she was raped.
Suppression Conscious exclusion of anything undesirable.	A student "forgot" to bring his report card home.
Identification Unconscious attempt to become like someone admired.	A young tennis player assumes some of the court mannerisms of Jimmy Conners.
Introjection Person incorporates not only the mannerisms, but also the values of someone else in an intense type of identification.	Like his father, Joe smokes a pipe, belongs to a country club, and feels that blue-collar workers are inferior.
Displacement Transferring an emotional response from its source to another, usually more neutral, object.	Gretchen snaps at her secretary after being criticized by her own boss.
Projection Attributing one's own thoughts or impulses to another person.	Paula is jealous of Jane's attractiveness and tells her friends that Paula is jealous of her.
Reaction Formation The development of conscious attitudes and behavior that are the opposite of one's real feelings.	Karen fantasizes about being seductive but dresses in a prudish manner.
Undoing An act or communication that partially negates a previous one.	Barbara is sarcastic to her mother and later that day cleans her room and washes the family dishes.
Regression A retreat in the face of stress to behavior that marked an earlier stage of development.	David, who is in the hospital with pneumonia, tips over his food tray when his roommate changes the TV channel.
Sublimation Finding expression for a drive that is usually blocked by society.	John, who enjoys physical violence, becomes a professional football player.
Compensation Placing emphasis on certain aspects in an attempt to cover up perceived deficiencies.	Peter, who is quite shy, memorizes jokes to use in conversations.
Rationalization Finding acceptable reasons to justify unacceptable feelings, behavior, or motives.	Betty justifies the purchase of a dress she cannot afford by reasoning that the sale price is a bargain.
Isolation Isolating emotions from a painful, unacceptable thought or event.	Karl stares with detachment at his mother's casket.
Denial Avoiding recognition of unacceptable realities.	A mother continues to plan for the hospital discharge of her dying child.

TABLE 13.7 PERSONALITY DISORDERS

Subtype	Essential Features
Paranoid	Pervasive, unwarranted suspiciousness and mistrust of people. Hypersensitivity.
Schizoid	Incapable of forming social relationships. Absence of warmth or tenderness. Indifference to praise, criticism, or feelings of others.
Schizotypal	Odd thinking, perceptions, speech, and behavior. Symptoms not severe enough to meet the criteria for schizophrenia.
Histrionic	Overly dramatic and reactive. Demanding, egocentric, inconsiderate, manipulative, self-indulgent, and/or dependent behavior. Disturbance in interpersonal relationships.
Narcissistic	Grandiose sense of self-importance or uniqueness. Preoccupation with fantasies of unlimited success. Exhibitionistic need for attention and admiration. May alternate between overidealization and devaluation. Interpersonal relationships disturbed by exploitiveness and demands of entitlement.
Antisocial	Persistently engages in behavior that violates the rights of others. Unable to maintain jobs or develop interpersonal relationships.
Borderline	Unstable moods and self-image marked by feelings of emptiness or boredom. May be unable to tolerate being alone.
Avoidant	Low self-esteem. Hypersensitivity to possibility of rejection, humiliation, or shame, leading to social withdrawal despite the desire for affection and acceptance.
Dependent	Lacks self-confidence and self-reliance. Passively allows others to assume responsibility for major areas of his or her life.
Compulsive	Perfectionist. Devotion to work and productivity to the exclusion of pleasure. Insists that others submit to his or her own preoccupation with trivial details, schedules, order, rules. Restricted ability to express warm and tender feelings. Indecisive.
Passive-aggressive	Resistant to demands for adequate social or occupational performance. Expresses resistance indirectly through procrastination, dawdling, stubbornness, forgetfulness, or intentional inefficiency.

behavior. In general, however, patients display irresponsible, impulsive, selfish, and manipulative patterns of behavior that develop by adolescence. This distinguishes personality disorders from many other psychologic disorders in which an established personality decompensates in the face of overwhelming anxiety. On the other hand, persons with personality disorders are at risk for the development of further problems such as somatic complaints, anxiety, or depression. The most common type of personality disorder is the ***antisocial*** or ***psychopathic personality.*** This category includes con artists, self-gaining religious figures, imposters, drug dealers, and unethical professionals, as well as the stereotyped criminal. In the United States, the number of psychopaths is estimated to be over 5 million. Most of them are young men. Their outstanding characteristics are marked lack of ethical or moral development, lack of conscience, irresponsible, impulsive, and socially disapproved behavior patterns, and an inability to maintain interpersonal relationships.

Since many individuals with personality disorders function fairly well, they rarely come to the attention of mental health centers. Those who come into conflict with the law may participate in rehabilitation programs. Very few of these programs have proven successful. Traditional psychotherapy, electroshock treatment, and drug therapy have fared no better. More recently, behavioral techniques have shown promise. These therapies, however, deal with specific maladaptive behaviors and fail to change the total lifestyle. Many psychopathic personalities improve on their own after the age of 40. However, an increased effort to develop more effective treatment programs is needed.

Personality disorders are often associated with ***alcoholism,*** which has been defined as a chronic behavioral disorder. Although our society generally accepts the use of alcoholic beverages under certain circumstances as normal and appropriate, using alcohol self-destructively or to the detriment of one's relations with others is regarded as a serious problem. It is estimated that as much as 7% of our adult population suffers from alcoholism, and this condition is a leading cause of death. In addition, its toll on the families of alcoholics and on the economy is staggering. The skid row bum accounts for only a small proportion of the alcoholic population. The more typical alcoholic is an involved community member who is married and employed. Vast numbers, perhaps as many as 4 million, are undiagnosed "closet drinkers," many of whom are women. Recent widows or women with a personal or family history of depression are particularly vulnerable to alcohol problems. Children and spouses of alcoholics or rigid abstainers have a greater than normal chance of becoming alcoholic.

Alcoholism presents in different ways. The most subtle pattern consists of heavy, frequent, but controlled drinking. Actual intoxication is unusual, as are withdrawal symptoms. Drinking frequently in response to a recognized stress causes little change in social or psychologic function. A second pattern occurs when persons have lost control of their drinking. These individuals may sneak drinks, gulp them, drink alone, or drink without eating. They may experience mild withdrawal symptoms and diminished functioning, miss work frequently, and have feelings of remorse, resentment, and anxiety. In this pattern, persons organize their lives around getting and drinking alcohol. Even though they drink without enjoyment, they feel compelled to drink constantly and are intoxicated for long periods. They experience major withdrawal symptoms, personality disintegration, and physical deterioration. Problem drinking in the earlier stages can be identified by the answer "yes" to more than two of the following questions:

1. Have you ever thought you should cut down on your drinking?
2. Have you ever been annoyed at the complaints of others about your drinking?
3. Have you ever felt guilty about your drinking?
4. Do you ever take morning "eye openers"?

In the later stages of alcoholism, organ damage such as liver disease, as well as nutritional deficiencies, pancreatitis, gastritis, or gastric ulceration, will be seen.

▶ ***Office management of alcohol abuse*** begins by approaching the problem in a manner that neither supports the patient's denial nor forces premature acceptance. This can be accomplished by centering the discussion on the destructive consequences of drinking without rejecting or judging the person and by exploring other ways of dealing with stress or psychologic problems. Librium may be needed to decrease anxiety and withdrawal symptoms. Since there is potential for drug abuse, it should be given only for acute withdrawal problems. Antabuse has a place in helping patients maintain hard-earned sobriety. In conjunction with alcohol ingestion, the drug causes acetaldehyde to accumulate, bringing on nausea, vomiting, sweating, a throbbing headache, and other deterring symptoms. It is contraindicated in patients who are intoxicated or who have heart disease, diabetes, cirrhosis, organic brain syndrome, or psychosis. Although office measures represent a positive step, more specialized and intensive approaches are needed by most addicted drinkers. Wherever possible, referrals should be made to one or more ▶ ***alcohol treatment programs and support groups.*** Alcoholics Anonymous, the most widely known, uses a self-help group format. Groups help the patient improve social skills, provide personal support and acceptance, and foster a sense of self-worth. Al-Anon and Al-Ateen groups are available for the families and children of alcoholics. For patients who do not function well in group settings, individual or family therapy can be arranged privately or through community mental health centers. Behavior modification programs are another possibility. Therapists identify the factors that precipitate or discourage drinking for each individual. Then they devise a "drinking schedule" that emphasizes rewards for controlled drinking. No matter which treatment is undertaken, relapses are common. Professionals need to be aware of this fact and not to view it as failure.

Like alcoholism, ***drug abuse*** is a socially deviant behavior frequently associated with personality disorders. It is defined as any pattern of substance use that continuously or intermittently interferes with an individual's ability to function. According to the psychiatric classification, the pattern of drug use may be variable but must last for 1 month or longer. Addiction problems are poorly understood but seem to arise from a subtle interplay of social and psychological factors. Among these are:

1. Impulsive behavior, difficulty in delaying gratification, antisocial personality, and a tendency to seek sensation.
2. A high value on noncomformity, with little commitment to socially desirable goals.
3. A sense of heightened stress, lack of self-esteem, and marked depression or anxiety.
4. Physical or sexual abuse in childhood and sharply conflicting parental expectations.
5. Feelings of social alienation.

As described in Table 13.8, the signs of drug abuse may vary according to the administration and drugging effect of specific substances. By contrast, behavior characteristics are fairly general. Drug abusers usually have an overall change in temperament, becoming withdrawn or volatile. To take drugs, the user may disappear at odd times into locked rooms, basements, or parked cars and emerge with a notable change in mood. School or work performance declines, while money borrowing or petty stealing increases. Appearance and grooming deteriorate. Sunglasses (to hide pupillary changes) or long-sleeved shirts (to hide injection marks) may be worn constantly. There may be furtiveness regarding activities and possessions, or there may be an open association with known addicts and pushers. Such behavior changes lead to conflicts at home, on the job, or with the law. Physical problems include injury, malnutrition, and serious infections (abscesses, hepatitis, osteomyelitis, AIDS, etc.). Drug abusers are often considered criminals rather than persons in need of treatment. Patients indicating a willingness to be helped should be referred to one of the ▶ ***drug abuse organizations.*** Most communities offer residen-

TABLE 13.8 COMMON STREET DRUGS

Substance	Street Names	Methods of Administration
1. Opium (paregoric)	Blue velvet (paregoric and pyribenzamine, an antihistamine, mixed and injected)	Oral, smoked, injected
Morphine	"M"	Injected, smoked
Codeine	Turps (elixir of terpin hydrate with codeine, a cough syrup)	Oral, injected
Heroin	Scag, smack, horse, lemonade (poor quality), dynamite (high quality)	Injected, sniffed
Meperidine (Demorol)		Oral, injected
Methadone	Meth, dollies	Oral, injected
2. Barbiturates	Barbs, yellow jackets, red devils, blue angels, rainbows, goofballs	Oral, injected
Minor tranquilizers	Downers	Oral
3. Amphetamines	Pep pills, jolly beans, crystal (methedrine), speed, uppers, bennies, dexies, meth, purple hearts, bombita (amphetamine injection, sometimes taken with heroin)	Oral, injected, sniffed, absorbed through genital mucosa; paraphernalia, if drug is injected, includes eye droppers and needles
Cocaine/crack	Snow, crack	Injected, sniffed, absorbed through genital mucosa; smoked; paraphernalia includes syringes, bent spoons, bottle caps, eye droppers, needles, glass pipes
4. Lysergic acid diethylamide (LSD)	"25," acid	Oral, injected; commonly taken as a liquid on a sugar cube
Mescaline	Mesc	Oral, injected
Phencyclidine	PCP, angel dust	Oral, injected, smoked
5. Marijuana	Joint, "J," grass, pot, reefer, gage, stick, weed, hay, roach	Smoked, ingested; paraphernalia includes rolling papers, "roach" holders ("clips")
Hashish	Hash	Smoked, ingested

Key: 1. Narcotics
2. Depressants
3. Stimulants
4. Hallucinogens
5. Cannabis

Source: Adapted from Oral Vistaril chart by Pfizer Laboratories Division ("Controlled Substances: Uses and Effects"). Pfizer, New York, 1982.

Signs of Use	Signs of Overdose	Signs of Withdrawal
Pupils constricted and unresponsive, respiratory depression, hypothermia, hypotension, inflamed nasal mucosa from inhaling powder, "track marks" on arms or less apparent areas of body (backs of legs, ankles), euphoria, disorientation, drowsiness, lethargy, nausea.	Slow, shallow breathing, clammy skin, convulsions, coma, possibly death.	Watery eyes, runny nose, yawning, loss of appetite, irritability, tremors, panic, chills, sweating, cramps, nausea.
Symptoms mimicking drunkenness without odor of alcohol on breath, slurred speech, staggering or stumbling, tremulousness, drowsiness and inability to remain awake, lethargy, depression, disorientation, respiratory depression.	Shallow respiration, cold clammy skin, dilated pupils, weak rapid pulse, respiratory collapse, coma, possible death.	Anxiety, insomnia, tremors, delirium, convulsions, possible death.
Skin tracks, increased alertness, excitation, euphoria, dilated pupils, increased pulse rate and blood pressure, insomnia, loss of appetite, chain smoking, difficulty sitting still.	Dry mouth and nose (frequent licking of lips), bad breath, flushed face, fever, sweating, rapid pulse, headache, excessive activity, irritability, argumentativeness, nervousness, paranoid ideation, hallucinations.	Apathy, long periods of sleep, depression, emotional instability, disorientation, irritability.
Illusions and hallucinations, anxiety, distorted sensory perception and cognition; occasional "flashbacks" later on (while not using the drug).	Pupils dilated with LSD and constricted with PCP. Excessive sweating, increased pulse and blood pressure, agitation, flushing. Possible fever, nausea, and vomiting. Occasional paresthesias, more intense "trip" episodes, psychosis, possible death.	No known withdrawal syndrome.
Euphoria, relaxation of inhibitions, silliness, disoriented behavior, increased appetite, dilated pupils, conjunctival irritation, distorted perception, dry mouth, mild hypotension, burnt rope odor.	Fatigue, stupor, paranoia, possible psychosis.	Insomnia, hyperactivity, decreased appetite.

tial outpatient programs (e.g., methadone clinics) or halfway houses. Psychotherapy is useful if backed by programs supporting a change of lifestyle. Self-help groups such as Narcotics Anonymous, are also effective.

Drug overdose is a life-threatening condition. Presentations range from stupor and unconsciousness to panic states, hallucinations, and uncontrollable agitation. The signs of intoxication produced by a specific drug may be muddled by the simultaneous use of several drugs. Studies show that 90% of narcotic addicts abuse alcohol, and 75% of them abuse sedative-hypnotics. In the case of overdose, emesis, gastric lavage, specific antidotes such as Narcan, or even dialysis may be necessary. A history of past and present patterns of abuse, identification of drugs brought in with the patient, or toxicology screens can help determine the best measure. Exact information can also be used to determine the appropriate amount of antidote to be given. Too much, too fast can throw the patient into immediate withdrawal.

Drug withdrawal is another complication of abuse. ***Sedative-hypnotic withdrawal*** is among the most common and has the most potential to produce serious complications. Symptoms begin 24 hours after the last dose. Patients are diaphoretic, restless, and irritable. Temperature, pulse, and respiratory rates may be elevated and pupils dilated. Advanced states of withdrawal are marked by hallucinations, muscle fasciculations, seizures, and hypotension. Patients should be hospitalized. As soon as overdose, trauma, or an infectious process is ruled out, they can be given a test dose of oral pentobarbital. If a starting dose of 200 mg produces intoxication, dependence is an unlikely cause of symptoms. Patients who show no signs of intoxication after 1 hour are given 200-mg doses every hour until they become mildly intoxicated. The amount needed to arrive at this state (rarely more than 600 mg) determines the initial stabilizing dose. Stabilizing doses are repeated every 6 hours, provided that patients remain easily arousable. They allow psychologic and physiologic relaxation, thus minimizing complications such as trauma, rhabdomyolysis, hyperthermia, and aspiration. Once the patient is stable for 24 hours, controlled reduction of the pentobarbital may begin on an outpatient basis. Doses are reduced by approximately 10% or 100 mg/day over the course of 2–3 weeks. During this period, some specialists substitute 30 mg of phenobarbital for every 100 mg of pentobarbital because it fails to produce a pleasurable "nod" and has little street value.

It is now known that a life-threatening syndrome may accompany ***benzodiazepine withdrawal.*** This syndrome is seen with illicit drug use but also results from prescribed therapy. Given for psychiatric disorders or, ironically enough, for dependence on alcohol or other substances, benzodiazepines (Librium, Valium, Serax) are among the most widely prescribed drugs in the world. Symptoms begin within days of discontinuing short-acting agents, but up to weeks after discontinuing long-acting drugs. Seizures may occur along with hallucinations, hyperactivity, confusion, and disorientation. Advanced complications due to benzodiazepine withdrawal require admission to a hospital for supportive care. Milder symptoms can be managed by slowly tapering the drug. Although propranolol helps control tremor, tachycardia, and hypertension, its use is limited by its worsening effect on anxiety and dysphoria.

Narcotic withdrawal is less dangerous. Aside from agitation, the patient's mental status remains normal. Elevations of pulse rate, blood pressure, and respiration occur, but body temperature usually remains normal. Seizures develop only in neonates. Yawning, goose bumps, and watery eyes and nose are annoying problems.

Uncomfortable developments are nausea, vomiting, stomach cramps, and diarrhea. Narcotic withdrawal can be managed on an outpatient basis. It is one of the functions of ***methadone clinics.*** An initial dose of methadone (an oral narcotic) is determined according to the patient's habit. The doses are gradually tapered over the course of several weeks to months. Patients are given ongoing psychosocial support and are sometimes prescribed clonidine or benzodiazepines to minimize the physical discomfort. However, in many instances, drugs are never completely withdrawn, and the clinics assume the responsibility of maintaining addicts on methadone for indefinite periods. For this reason, methadone clinics are the subject of much controversy. Some experts argue the worth of substituting one habituating drug for another. Others maintain that close supervision and oral drug use help prevent problems such as stealing, prostitution, and health deterioration related to illicit intravenous (IV) use.

SEXUALITY

The groundwork for sexual intimacy is laid at birth. Infants develop trusting and intimate relationships by sensing that their biologic needs and tensions are acceptable and appropriate and will elicit a positive response. Toddlers gain an appreciation of the anatomic, behavioral, and biologic differences between males and females and become aware that they are either a girl or a boy before they classify themselves as Catholic or Jewish, white or black.

Although masculine or feminine traits and an interest in the opposite sex are expressed by preschoolers, children between the ages of 6 and 10 are more likely to disavow sexual interest and seek out playmates of the same sex. Still, they engage in romantic fantasies (princes coming to the rescue of princesses). With the development of secondary sex characteristics and specific sex drives, adolescents struggle to achieve a satisfying and socially acceptable sex role. Through close relationships with members of the opposite sex based on mutual regard rather than infatuation, they prepare for responsible sexual contact.

Sexuality has traditionally been correlated with "gender identity." Categories of masculinity and femininity emerge from the cultural framework in each society. In Western cultures, competitiveness, aggressiveness, and intelligence are ascribed to men, while gentleness, passivity, and warmth are considered female traits. Sex role stereotyping has been perpetuated by both men and women. Recently, changes in social norms have resulted in a blurring of traditional sex roles and in a wider acceptance of a variety of styles or sexual partnerships among adults. For example, homosexuality is no longer considered evidence of a psychiatric disorder. Theorists have suggested the concept of androgeny, the possession of human rather than masculine or feminine traits. There is some concern, however, that a strict application of this theory will compromise a child's developing sense of identity, since normal development arises from clear messages that the child is male or female.

Satisfaction with sexual relationships is determined by more than the experience of physical arousal and release. It includes feelings of happiness, and intimacy as well. The individuals involved merge and separate without intolerable anxiety and regard one another as companions, not parental substitutes. Sexual activity is based on mutual consent and is a physically and psychologically positive, not harmful, experience. It is important that the health care provider be adept at assessing sexual problems or conflicts that patients may have. The extent of the assessment is based on the patient's needs and may change over the course of long-term care. For example, experiences such as a mastectomy, coronary bypass surgery, divorce, or separation may alter the patient's sexual self-image. However, patients may not bring up the topic of sex because of their own embarrassment or lack of understanding about the psychology and physiology of sexual functioning. Patients describing the sexual problems of a "friend" may in fact be relating their own problems. Clinicians should be aware of verbal and nonverbal hidden messages that may indicate unmet sexual needs. Remarks such as "I'm not the woman I used to be" or lack of eye contact when undergoing a physical exam, blushing, or monosyllabic responses to questions about sexuality may indicate discomfort about sex.

Primary care providers may find the topic guidelines listed in Table 13.9 helpful for general assessment of the patient's sexuality. The more specific history may reveal characteristics of one of the ***psychosexual disorders*** described in Table 13.10. In ***gender identity disorders,*** patients feel that their psychologic makeup is incongruent with their anatomic sex. They assume the role of the opposite sex and may undergo sex change operations. This disorder is rare and should be distinguished from the inadequacy many persons experience concerning fulfillment of sex role expectations. Patients with ***paraphilia disorders*** employ bizarre imagery and/or acts (repeated involuntarily) in order to achieve sexual excitement. These individuals do not regard themselves as ill. If they seek help, it is usually because their behavior has created a social or legal conflict. Patients with ***ego dystonic homosexuality*** (an example of "other psychosexual dysfunctions") experience difficulty in accepting their homosexual impulses. They make persistent but unsuccessful attempts to achieve heterosexual arousal. For patients with any of these dysfunctions, referral to a qualified sex therapist may be extremely beneficial. The purpose of therapy is not necessarily to change existing behavior but to help patients work out conflicts and avoid compromising their social and occupational functioning.

Psychosexual dysfunction, the most common type of psychosexual disorder, may also be revealed by the patient's history. It is the inability to perform sexually due to lack of arousal, premature ejaculation, or failure to achieve orgasm. The problem may be lifelong or may develop after a period of normal functioning. It may occur always, occasionally, or only in certain situations or with certain partners. The first step in any case of sexual dysfunction is to rule out an organic cause, since medications, hormone changes, diabetes, and other conditions may be involved (see

TABLE 13.9 HELPFUL APPROACHES IN ASSESSMENT OF SEXUALITY

Knowledge, concerns, and attitudes

What do you know or not know about sex? What are your sexual concerns and goals? What are your present sexual beliefs, values, and attitudes? How were they influenced by those observed during your developmental years? Are you comfortable with them?

Relationships

With whom do you have sexual relationships? What is the type and quality of each relationship? Are there any recurrent problems?

Sensuality

Which experiences have been sexually satisfactory? Which have not? Do any techniques or environments improve or hinder sexual expression? Is there any effect due to illness, disability, surgery, drugs, or alcohol on your self-image or sexual relationships? If so, do you have someone (partner, physician, friend) to turn to for help or advice? Would you be able to accept their recommendations?

TABLE 13.10 PSYCHOSEXUAL DISORDERS

Type	Essential Features
Transsexualism (gender identity disorder)	Unhappiness with anatomic sex. Persistent wish to assume genitals and characteristics of opposite sex.
Fetishism (paraphilia)	Dependence on an unlikely object (fetish) to achieve sexual excitement.
Tranvestitism (paraphilia)	Dressing as a woman by a heterosexual man for the purpose of sexual excitement.
Zoophilia (paraphilia)	Use of animals as the preferred or exclusive method of achieving sexual excitement.
Pedophilia (paraphilia)	Fantasizing about or engaging in sexual activity with prepubertal children as the preferred or exclusive means of achieving sexual excitement.
Exhibitionism (paraphilia)	Exposing penis to various strangers for the purpose of achieving sexual excitement without further attempt at sexual activity.
Voyeurism (paraphilia)	Watching unsuspecting strangers disrobe or engage in sexual activity as the sole or preferred means of achieving sexual excitement.
Masochism (paraphilia)	Receiving humiliation or physical punishment for the achievement of sexual excitement.
Sadism (paraphilia)	Inflicting humiliation or physical punishment for the achievement of sexual excitement.
Frigidity/impotence (psychosocial dysfunction)	Failure to achieve or maintain physiologic responses to sexual stimulation (erection in the man, lubrication in the woman).
Inhibited female orgasm (psychosexual dysfunction)	Failure to achieve orgasm following normal excitement phase.
Inhibited male orgasm (psychosexual dysfunction)	Delayed or absent ejaculation following normal erection.
Premature ejaculation (psychosexual dysfunction)	Ejaculation occurring before it is desired due to persistent absence of control.
Functional dyspareunia (psychosocial dysfunction)	Pain, without a functional basis, consistently experienced with coitus by either the man or the woman.
Functional vaginismus (psychosexual dysfunction)	Persistent involuntary spasm of the vaginal musculature at the time of sexual activity that interferes with coitus.
Ego-dystonic homosexuality (other psychosexual dysfunction)	Attempts to engage in heterosexual arousal by a homosexual who has been unable to resolve conflicts about his homosexuality.

Chapter 9). Once this has been done, referral to a sex therapist can be extremely beneficial. Using a detailed and direct sexual history, specialists determine which aspect of the sex act—arousal, ejaculation, or orgasm—is dysfunctional. Through counseling sessions, they help patients understand the circumstances that may have contributed to the problem's evolution and then prescribe a specific course of therapy. For example, patients with arousal or orgasm failure may be encouraged to masturbate or fantasize. Those who experience performance anxiety or premature ejaculation learn how to give and receive pleasurable stimuli without engaging in intercourse.

Victims of rape may undergo an alteration in their image of sexuality. However, ***rape*** (defined as any form of sexual intercourse imposed without consent) is an act of violence, not of sex. Rapists may assault men and children, but their usual targets are adult women (50% of rapes involve acquaintances). It has been estimated that one out of every two women will be attacked during her lifetime. The medical effects of rape are many and far-reaching. Nearly all victims sustain genital injuries, one-fourth receiving other bodily injuries as well. Venereal disease is a consequence in 5% of cases. In addition, victims pass through a sequence of psychologic phases referred to as ***rape trauma syndrome.*** The acute phase involves the immediate response to the assault. Some women show signs of intense distress such as shock, disbelief, emotional breakdown, and disruptions of eating, sleeping, or other patterns of normal behavior. The distress may prevent them from seeking medical attention, reporting the crime to the authorities, or even telling friends or family members. Victims who do report the crime may have difficulty recalling details, since recounting the assault exposes them anew to a degrading and frightening experience. On the other hand, they may be surprised at the depth and uncontrolled nature of the anger that may surface. This anger may be directed at all men or, paradoxically, at those individuals who are trying to help. By contrast, some victims repress their immediate distress. Able to talk about the attack in a controlled manner, without revealing to themselves or others the full extent of their reaction, these victims are often among those who have feelings of guilt or self-blame. Although less than 5% of rapes may be classified as victim precipitated, many women harbor the notion that they may have provoked the attack, particularly when the assailant was known. Shame may also stem from responding to the attack in an unanticipated manner such as by panicking or submitting without a struggle.

Several days to 2 weeks later begins a period of adjustment, the second phase of rape trauma syndrome. The initial terror fades and the victim returns to her usual life pattern, attempting to behave as if all were well. Hopefully, in time, she regains a sense of security and self-esteem. Unlike the acute phase, when reluctance to recount the details of the assault is typical, victims may want to talk more fully about what has happened. Unfortunately, many women never fully resolve their feelings about the rape. They display a lingering mistrust or anger toward all men and develop persistent anxiety, depression, and/or phobias (particularly an inordinate fear of crowds or of staying at home alone). Sleep is often interrupted by vivid dreams and nightmares that reenact the event. Sexual fears, a decline in libido, and withdrawal from intimate sexual contact are common. In addition, their functioning at work and at home may be impaired; frequent moves or other changes in lifestyle may predominate. Whether coping responses are ultimately positive or negative depends on the woman's age and prior experiences, her psychologic stability (including the ability to adapt to stress), and the specific circumstances and details of the event. ▶ ***Proper care of the rape victim*** is another influential factor. Victims treated to correct protocols for obtaining a history and exam, collecting and recording evidence, preventing venereal disease or an unwanted pregnancy, and understanding, emotional support, and counseling may recover faster and more fully than those who are less well treated.

FEELINGS

Feelings have been divided into three groups. Those in the first group (anger, anxiety, shame, pride, and guilt) protect the survival of the individual and the community. Those in the second group (envy, boredom, fatigue, irritation, or unrest) warn the individual that goals are not being met. Finally, those in the third group (pleasure, elation, hurt, sadness) provide motivations that are used ultimately to measure the value of life.

Feelings are communicated through affect, that is, facial and body expressions. Affect makes it possible for individuals to sense in one another delight, love, appreciation, respect, anger, or danger. By helping persons know that they have made contact and are being understood or ignored, appreciated or rejected, affective response is the basis for learning reinforcement and conscience development. To this end, correct communication of a wide range of feelings is obviously important.

Anger is a normal human reaction that serves certain necessary purposes. It tends to vitalize a person, giving him or her a sense of power and control in the face of an acute concern. When directly expressed, it alerts others to the same concern and thus helps to elicit supportive interest. Such important adaptations are not available to persons who have difficulty expressing anger. Ineffective and overburdened by internalized concerns, such persons may benefit from assertiveness training. Role playing and practice in real-life situations can help them express their rights and considerations.

Moods of sadness are experienced by everyone at some time. Those that mark normal responses to death are called ***grief reactions.*** Actually, grief reactions develop in the face of any kind of loss or change, real or symbolic. They follow alterations in self-image (due to surgery, trauma, or illness) and accompany developmental milestones (lost youth, menopause, the "empty nest"). Paradoxically, they also herald successes such as job advancement or the evolution of intimate sexual relationships. The feelings of sadness and depression help persons cope with difficult situations by forcing them to withdraw from the difficulty until they are ready to deal with it constructively. Then, by working through feelings of depression, people accept and adapt to the new situation. An essentially healthy process, grief reactions are self-limiting and rarely last longer than 6 weeks. They are best managed by counseling, understanding, emotional support, and minimal drugs. While antidepressants are not indicated, anxious patients may benefit from short-term use of a benzodiazepine (Serax or Librium).

A mood of sadness that persists and becomes pervasive may mark an ***affective disorder*** Table 13.11). Heading the list of affective disorders, ***depression*** is considered unhealthy whether or not it is related to a specific situation (***reactive depression).*** Striking 15–30% of the population, it is the most common psychiatric illness and the fourth most common reason for primary care visits. Every year, 8 million persons seek treatment and another 12 million need attention that they never receive. A small number of them suffer from ***secondary depression.*** Medical and mental conditions that cause depression include endocrine disturbances (hypothyroidism, Cushing's syndrome), cancer of the lung or pancreas, viral illnesses (mononucleosis, influenza, and hepatitis), and drugs (most antihypertensives, birth control pills, corticosteroids, alcohol, sedative-hypnotics, and stimulants). Depression may also be a component of psychotic illnesses, notably schizophrenia, or may be misdiagnosed as dementia (see Chapter 12). Most cases, however, are primary, their exact etiology being unknown. Alterations in the metabolism of thyroid, cortisol, and sex hormones, as well as decreases in certain brain amines, have been hypothesized as the cause. It is known that there is a familial association and that the persons most prone to depression are conscientious, hard-working, and "obsessive-compulsive" personality types. Those who are only concerned with their immediate needs are less likely to develop a serious depression. The problem involves women twice as often as men and older persons more than young ones. It also seems to be modified by life stages.

Developing at any time within 6 months of childbirth, ***postpartum depression***

TABLE 13.11 AFFECTIVE DISORDERS

Type	Essential Features
Major depression	Patients have feelings or worthlessness or guilt that may be delusional. Mood is dejected. Speech is absent or slow and monotonous. Sleep disturbance (difficulty falling asleep, waking in the middle of the night, or rising early in the morning) is common. There may be psychomotor agitation (pacing, hand wringing, constant manipulation of hair, skin, or clothing) or psychomotor retardation (decreased energy and slowed body movements) Thinking is characterized by poor concentration and preoccupation with death. Suicide attempts are likely.
Bipolar disorder	Patients have mood swings between major depression (see above) and manic episodes. During manic episodes, they have an inflated self-esteem that is often delusional. Mood is marked by euphoria, expansiveness, cheerfulness, and enthusiasm. It is labile, with rapid shifts to anger or irritability. Patients are hyperactive, as demonstrated by their participation in multiple activities, excessive planning, and decreased need for sleep. Speech is loud, rapid, and difficult to interrupt. Thinking is easily distracted by external stimuli and characterized by abrupt, disconnected changes in topics (flight of ideas).
Cyclothymic disorder	Chronic mood disturbance of at least 2 years' duration involving numerous periods of depression that are not serious enough to meet the criteria for a major depression.
Dysthymic disorder	Chronic disturbance of mood characterized by loss of interest or pleasure in usual activities and pastimes. Symptoms are not serious enough to meet the criteria for a major depression.

is precipitated by the stress of fluctuating hormone levels, pregnancy, delivery, and motherhood superimposed on a vulnerable personality. It is most likely to occur after the birth of the first child or a child delivered late in life. Showing disinterest initially, the mother may later become preoccupied with the infant and with the responsibilities of parenthood. Bizarre behavior or complete withdrawal may follow. In advanced stages, the woman may experience delusions or hallucinations that often center on a fear of death and malformation from childbirth. Although violent actions against the baby rarely occur, thoughts of suicide/homicide are common. Unlike "maternity blues" (short-lived but overwhelming emotions experienced by most new mothers on the third day postpartum), postpartum depression is a serious condition requiring immediate psychiatric evaluation.

Most cases of ***primary depression*** present in middle age between the ages of 40 and 60. ***Depression in the elderly*** is a distinct problem affecting 10–20% of those over age 65. In fact, elderly persons account for one-fourth of all suicides. These high rates are definitely related to the many losses incurred by aging people in our society—family position, employability, financial stability, friends, health, and familiar home settings. Biochemical changes may also contribute to the problem. There is evidence that brain levels of serotonin, norepinephrine, and dopamine decrease with aging, while that of monoamine oxidase increases. Testosterone, progesterone, and estrogen changes are well established.

Whatever the age of the victim, the onset of depression is insidious, early symptoms stemming from increased anxiety. Sleep disturbance is particularly common. Many patients have no trouble falling asleep but awaken at around 2 A.M. and are unable to fall asleep again until 5 or 6 A.M. Others find themselves sleeping excessively. Poor concentration and indecisiveness are important clues. Patients can no longer sit through a television show or read a newspaper. Although they continue to make major decisions, they agonize over minor ones—what clothes to wear and what to order for dinner. In these early stages, patients may still be able to focus on things that are bothering them. However, as depression progresses, specific sources of anxiety become buried and somatic complaints may develop. Indigestion, nausea, and diarrhea are the most frequent, followed by dizziness, shaky spells, blurred vision, lightheadedness, fatigue, palpitations, and cough. Patients often have fears of serious disease, loss of appetite, and decreased libido. One or several of these symptoms may be experienced over time. Persistent, severe menopausal symptoms are another clue. Although the belief that menopause precipitates depression is no longer accepted, it has been shown that depression may heighten the woman's sensitivity to the physiologic changes of menopause, leading to pronounced complaints of menstrual irregularity, and hot flashes. A sense of overall helplessness and futility signals more advanced stages of depression. Patients express notions of unworthiness and guilt. They look and feel troubled, down, flat. In withdrawing, many turn to alcohol or drugs. Thoughts of death may become pervasive.

The first step in treating depression is recognition. This may be a problem, particularly with older patients. Though the elderly present with classic signs of anxiety—appetite changes, lost libido, sleep disturbance, lethargy, and somatic complaints—the mood component of their depression may be less distinct. The second step is to rule out a variety of medical and mental conditions responsible for secondary depression (see the previous discussion). Once this has been done, the diagnosis is basically clinical and can be aided by information provided by psychologic testing as well as interviews with family members and friends. The dexamethasone suppression test may add supportive evidence, but the findings can be extremely variable. Given a single dose of dexamethasone at midnight, most depressed patients demonstrate a marked suppression of plasma cortisol over the next 24 hours. However, those with pituitary-adrenal disinhibition may have increased levels 11–16 hours after administration. The test is also altered by certain drugs (e.g., Dilantin and barbiturates) and by a number of medical disorders (e.g., diabetes, fever, and Cushing's syndrome). Other tests measuring metabolites of norepinephrine (MHPG) or serotonin (5-HIAA) are also available. Depressed patients should be referred for psychiatric care. Many, however, are unable to afford or unwilling to accept it.

Unless patients are severely depressed or suicidal, ▶ ***office management of depression*** represents a viable alternative. Frequent, short visits should be arranged, and unless contraindicated (by known hypersensitivity, pregnancy, or conditions aggravated by atropine-like or quinidine-like actions or liver disease), one of the tricyclic or tetracyclic ***antidepressant drugs*** described in Table 13.12 should be started. All of these drugs work by blocking the "amine pump" for neurotransmitters, but some selectively increase norepinephrine, others serotonin. Although antidepressant effects cannot be expected for 2–3 weeks, patients should feel less anxious and note improved sleeping patterns almost immediately. If there is no response after 1 month, a different tricyclic drug should be tried. If there is still no response, referral to a psychiatrist is indicated. In 70% of uncomplicated cases, remission occurs within 2 months. Drug therapy should continue for another 3–6 months to reduce the chance of relapse. Daily doses can then be tapered, and if patients continue to do well, the drug can be gradually withdrawn. However, periodic reassessment should continue.

Signs of severe depression or suicidal intent require immediate psychiatric evalu-

TABLE 13.12 ANTIDEPRESSANT DRUGS

Class and Name	Trade Name	Daily Dose Range (mg)	Anticholinergic Activity	Distinguishing Characteristics
Tricyclics				
Amitriptyline	Elavil, Endep, Amitril	75–300	5+	More cardiotoxicity; very sedating.
Amoxapine	Asendin	75–300	2+	New; faster onset of action; less cardiotoxicity reported.
Desipramine	Norpramin, Pertofrane	75–200	1+	Low side effect profile; little sedation.
Doxepin	Adapin, Sinequan, Curetin	75–300	2+	Less quanethidine inhibition; commonly used in elderly and cardiac patients; sedating.
Imipramine	Imavate, Janimine, Presamine, Tofranil, SK-Pramine, Antipress	75–300	4+	The standard antidepressant; midrange in side effects.
Nortriptyline	Aventyl, Pamelor	75–100	3+	Lower dosages; therapeutic blood levels are more established.
Protriptyline	Vivactil	20–60	3+	Lowest-dose form; little sedation.
Trimipramine	Surmontil	75–300	4+	New; short half-life; sedating.
Tetracyclic				
Maprotiline	Ludiomil	75–300	2+	New; less cardiotoxicity reported; sedating.
Triazolopyridine				
Trazodone	Desyrel	150–600	1+	Newest; much lower cardiotoxic effect reported; sedating.
MAO inhibitors				Due to high toxicity, MAO inhibitors are used only when tricyclics have proven ineffective.
Isocarboxazid	Marplan	10–30	Significant	Antidepressant effect often slow to appear; 3- to 4-week trial is necessary in most cases.
Pargyline	Eutonyl	10–200	Significant	Used in treatment of hypertension; therapeutic effect slow to appear and residual effects persist for 3 weeks after discontinuation.
Phenelzine sulfate	Nardil	7.5–90	Significant	Therapeutic effect may not be seen until 60 mg has been given daily for 4 weeks or more.

TABLE 13.12 (*Continued*)

Class and Name	Trade Name	Daily Dose Range (mg)	Anticholinergic Activity	Distinguishing Characteristics
Tranylcypromine sulfate	Parnate sulfate	10–30	Significant	More rapid onset of action than with other MAO inhibitors; more likely to cause hypertensive crisis; for use with severely depressed hospitalized patients.
Lithium				
Lithium carbonate	Eskalith, Lithane, Lithobid, Lithonate, Lithotabs, Pfi-Lith	600–900 + increased over a 7- to 10-day period until adequate serum level is obtained	Not applicable	Appropriate only for bipolar disorders (those that include both manic and depressive phases). Lithium has a 4- to 10-day latency period, so administration of haloperidol (5–10 mg IM prn, up to 80 mg/day) or some other neuroleptic may initially be necessary until manic psychosis is under control. Because the therapeutic serum level is close to the toxic level, it is imperative that blood serum levels be carefully monitored (one to two times per week during initiation of therapy and 3–4 times a year once stabilized).
Lithium citrate	Cibalith-S		Not applicable	

Sources: Lippman S: Antidepressant pharmacotherapy, *American Family Physician,* (June) 1982, 145–153. Loebl S, Spratto G: *The Nurse's Drug Handbook,* 3rd ed. Wiley, New York, 1986. Berkow RB et al.: *The Merck Manual of Diagnoses and Therapy,* 14th ed. Merck Shark & Dohme Research Laboratories, Rahway, N.J., 1982.

ation. Patients are usually hospitalized for close observation and aggressive therapy. Electroconvulsive treatment ***(ECT or "shock therapy")*** may be used because it is consistently more effective than either tricyclics or monoamine oxidase inhibitors in relieving severe depression. An electric current is passed through the brain, causing a brief (5- to 20-second) CNS seizure. Although ECT has a success rate approaching 70%, it is generally reserved as an emergency measure for patients who are at risk of suicide and also for those with prolonged, severe depression who have not responded to adequate trials of antidepressant medication and who cannot tolerate chemotherapy (e.g., some elderly patients) or for whom drug therapy is not recommended (e.g., pregnant women). Among the factors that have been identified as being predictive of successful ECT therapy are a family history of depression, early morning awakening, delusions, and psychomotor retardation. Substituting the technique of unilateral nondominant hemisphere ECT for the earlier bilateral technique has significantly decreased the side effect of memory loss, although some amount still occurs. However, unilateral ECT is slightly less effective and may require more than the usual 9–12 treatment sessions (usually three per week). Brain tumor, cerebral aneurysm, and other CNS lesions (sometimes revealed on an electroencephalogram, which is part of the pretreatment laboratory workup) are positive contraindications for ECT. Other relative contraindications include recent myocardial infarction and decompensated heart failure.

Some patients develop hysteria-like features known as ***atypical depression.*** Phobias or personality traits such as compulsiveness become exaggerated. Instead of the more usual manifestation of appetite loss, these patients develop hyperphagia. Nighttime and binge eating is particularly common. Patients with these signs and symptoms should be referred to a specialist. They often require monoamine oxidase inhibitors, stronger antidepressants with more worrisome side effects.

Bipolar (manic) depression is marked by mood fluctuations between depression and mania. During manic episodes, patients feel elated, full of enthusiasm and high self-esteem. With unstoppable energy, they make grandiose plans, undertake multiple projects, and interact with everyone, including strangers. Although little time is spent resting, they do not feel tired. Hyperactivity is further evidenced by pressured speech (loud, rapid, and difficult to interrupt), easy distractibility, and a flight of ideas (abrupt changes in topics). With judgment impaired, the risks of substance abuse, gambling, and dangerous or disorderly conduct increase. Bipolar disorders also require referral. These patients are usually treated with ***lithium.*** It is the only drug that prevents swings between acute mania and depression; the effectiveness of Haldol and other neuroleptics is limited to manic symptoms. Since lithium has a 4- to 10-day lag period before producing a response, it may be started in combination with shorter-acting drugs (either tricyclic antidepressants or antimania agents, depending on the phase of the disease). Once the patient is stabilized, the other drug can be discontinued. Patients with frequent mood swings are maintained on lithium. In those with infrequent swings, the drug is withdrawn after several months and restarted as needed.

► ***The patient taking lithium*** must be closely followed for signs of toxicity or other problems. Contraindications to lithium use include cardiovascular disease, renal dysfunction, first trimester of pregnancy, and hyponatremia. The drug is normally well tolerated, although many patients note polyuria, polydipsia, hand tremor, and mild nausea at the beginning of treatment. These side effects are usually transient but sometimes continue throughout therapy. Weight gain may occur with long-term treatment. Complications include hypothyroidism (with or without goiter), dermatologic reactions, nephritis, and hypercalcemia. Narrow to begin with, the range of ***lithium toxicity*** is further reduced by salt depletion. For this reason, patients should not be given thiazide diuretics or placed on salt-restricted diets. They should also be carefully monitored in the event of dehydration. Early symptoms of toxicity (tinnitus; gastrointestinal disturbances; muscle irritability, stiffness, or weakness; dizziness; or ataxia) should be treated by briefly stopping the drug or reducing the dosage. Progressive intoxication causes serious cardiovascular and neuromuscular complications. Without emergency measures for overdose, the patient may die.

Fifteen percent of all serious depressions end in ***suicide.*** Each year, more than 25,000 Americans (mostly men) kill themselves and three times as many make an attempt (mostly women). The incidence of suicide increases with age, the highest rates occurring in persons over 85. Professional persons and minorities (the suicide rate for American Indians is five times the national average) are other groups at high risk. Most suicides stem from a sense of hopelessness in the face of an overwhelming situation. When the central fact of life is physical decline, financial insecurity, disease, loneliness, or loss of self-esteem, death may be chosen as the best alternative. This is particularly true if depression or alcoholism exists. Occasionally, persons commit suicide as a rash response to momentary frustration or anger.

Certain signs may indicate suicidal behavior. These include exacerbation of depressive symptoms such as disruption of sleep patterns, poor appetite or compulsive overeating, and neglected hygiene. Patients may also show heightened feelings of sadness, hopelessness, and persecution. They may display unexplained euphoria or excitement. The disposition of possessions and unfinished business and sudden calmness in a previously agitated person are especially telling. Suicide threats are followed by an attempt 70% of the time. They may be overt statements of intention or mysterious references to long trips or absences. It is interesting to note that the elderly rarely give any verbal forewarning. The suicide plan provides important information about how imminent or successful the act will be. For instance, the man stating that he has a gun hidden away and has raised it to his head a few times is probably at higher immediate risk than the girl who states that she plans to suffocate herself with a paper bag. Professional help should be sought in any case where suicide is a possibility. Suicide hotlines, emergency rooms, mental health clinics, or private physicians can be called at any time. All weapons (especially guns) and potentially dangerous medications should be removed. The patient's family and friends should be educated about ► ***suicide prevention.***

STRESS

Stress is a normal occurrence. It activates an internal alarm system that warns persons that their physical or emotional security is being threatened. The nervous system sends messages to the hypothalamus, which, in turn, stimulates the pituitary and adrenal glands to release several hormones into the bloodstream. Cortisol increases blood sugar and speeds up body metabolism. Epinephrine helps supply muscle and brain tissue with extra glucose, while norepinephrine speeds up the heart rate and raises the blood pressure. Morphine-like painkillers called "endorphins" are also released, which may explain why persons can be severely injured without feeling any pain. Last but not least, the excess amount of epinephrine has an anticholinergic effect at neuromuscular junctions. This causes pupils to dilate, mouth secretions to dry up, underarms to perspire, and digestive functions to cease. These changes prepared primitive man for fight or flight. However, these powerful hormones were dissipated in the subsequent skirmish or flight that followed. Having learned to repress their physical responses to disequilibrium, modern persons are less likely to expend the hormones generated in the course of stress. High levels disrupt normal functioning and after extended periods of time cause permanent tissue changes. Ulcers, hypertension, headaches, muscle spasm, regional enteritis, ulcerative colitis, asthma, obesity, cardiac arrhythmias, angina, dermatitis, palpitations, and a number of other physical ailments known as ***psychophysiologic disorders*** may result. Infections and cancer might well be added to the list, since it is now known that stress inhibits leukocyte migration and T-lymphocyte activity.

The physiologic changes of stress are also implicated in psychologic problems. The low levels of serotonin and norepinephrine seen in depression and the excess dopamine associated with schizophrenia have already been discussed. Recent studies suggest that stress-related hypothalamic dysfunction may be involved in the development of ***anorexia nervosa.*** Anorexia is a poorly understood disease of increasing prevalence. Women in their thirties and men are occasionally affected, but the typical patient is a girl between 12 and 20. While their personality profiles are basically normal, these girls tend to be perfectionists who are eager to please and well behaved. Family environments are often overprotective and rigid. One theory is that changes, including body changes with puberty, are particularly stressful for children with such backgrounds. In keeping with this theory, weight loss usually begins within a year of some traumatic event (death in the family, the mother's pregnancy, or a sibling's marriage) and is centered on an altered body image. It often follows family chiding about being overweight. Even after reaching their ideal weight, patients feel they are too heavy and continue to limit their food intake to 600 or 700 calories/day. Bulimia (see the next section) and laxative abuse are common. Other signs of compulsive behavior such as repetitive stair climbing or all-night studying may become evident. Depression or schizophrenic behavior and physical changes follow. The skin takes on a dirty, rough appearance and may desquamate. Lanugo-like hirsutism develops over the trunk, extremities, and face, while scalp hair falls out. Hypothermia, hypotension, and bradycardia develop with continued starvation. Interestingly enough, amenorrhea begins before significant weight loss in 50% of anorexics and continues after recovery. This fact, along with many cases of unexplained hypercarotenemia and edema, raises the possibility that a stress-induced hypothalamic dysfunction leads to cachexia.

Patients suspected of having anorexia should be referred to a psychiatrist for evaluation. Many are hospitalized for extended periods (the average stay is 3 months). A broad range of treatments may be combined, including IV or forced feeding, hormone therapy, antidepressants or ECT, hypnosis, family therapy, and behavior modification. About 60% of these patients recover completely. The rest (particularly men, the originally overweight, laxative abusers, or bulimic patients) have recurrent problems, and as many as 5–20% eventually die.

Bulimia may exist as a component of anorexia or as a separate illness. Patients consume large quantities of high-calorie foods and then induce vomiting by tickling their throats or by taking cathartics. Abuse of laxatives and diuretics is not uncommon. The psychopathology is similar to that of anorexia, except that bulimics have an exaggerated fear of becoming fat, whereas anorexics are obsessed with becoming thin. Patients often maintain near normal body weight, and diagnosis may be difficult due to the secretive nature of the binging and purging. Some, however, develop severe alkalosis, electrolyte disturbances, and bowel irregularities. They also present with tooth erosion (from vomiting and excessive tooth brushing following emesis), chronic sore throat, and painless parotid swelling. Many cases are first recognized by dentists and oral surgeons. Treatment consists of emotional support, psychotherapy (individual, group, family), nutritional counseling, and close follow-up.

A stressful stimulus can arouse conflict, the simultaneous existence of opposing goals, motives, or needs. This conflict, which can be either conscious or unconscious, causes ambivalence and indecision. It can lead to a state of physical and psychologic disequilibrium known as ▶ ***anxiety reaction.*** At mild levels, anxiety can be desirable because it creates tension that promotes learning and adaptation. However, higher levels of anxiety narrow perceptions and decrease the ability to concentrate. Patients feel uneasy or restless and have a vague sense of foreboding. In addition to accident proneness, they become irritable, easily startled, or quickly moved to tears. Fears of strangers or animals, of crowds, or of being left alone become exaggerated. "Tunnel vision" (focusing on details to the exclusion of all else) may develop. Unlike fear, these subjective experiences cannot be related to any specific object or event. Often they are sublimated or attributed to a number of physical symptoms, some of which can be quite alarming. Pressure or pain in the chest, a choking sensation, tachycardia, palpitations, dizziness, and flushing or pallor, are common acute symptoms. Sleep becomes broken, unsatisfying, filled with disturbing dreams, and shortened by difficulty falling asleep or by early morning awakening. Tightening of facial muscles, along with clenching and grinding of the teeth, may lead to neck pain and headaches. Weight loss, bowel changes, amenorrhea, sexual dysfunction, fatigue, and loss of interest in work or usual activities signal more chronic states of anxiety. Anxious patients may be noted to have a hand tremor, moist palms, an unsteady voice, and fidgety body movements. They often have irregular breathing, tachycardia (ST-T wave changes can occur), and elevated blood pressure. Several organic problems have similar clinical pictures and must be excluded in order to make the diagnosis of anxiety. Hyperthyroidism, myocardial infarction, congestive heart failure, anemia, adrenal insufficiency, hypoglycemia, cerebral arteriosclerosis, and labyrinthitis are the most notable. Drug reactions must also be taken into account.

Patients with anxiety reaction precipitated by episodic stress may respond to simple reassurance. Their symptoms usually lessen once the problem or conflict is revealed and the fear of a serious physical problem is removed. Unlike cases in which anxiety is part of a personality trait (obsessive-compulsive or somatiform disorders), these patients may benefit from short-term use of antianxiety medication. A number of drugs have antianxiety properties, including phenobarbital, phenothiazines, and tricyclic antidepressants. Those used specifically for anxiety (minor tranquilizers) are described in Table 13.13. Since sedation, disturbed sleep patterns, depression, and habituation may result, antianxiety drugs must be judiciously prescribed. While patients are taking them, their progress should be closely watched. Open-ended prescriptions are never justified.

Extremely high levels of anxiety may lead to a ▶ ***panic attack.*** Patients develop sudden terror or a sense of imminent catastrophe that arises for no evident reason. They break out in a sweat and experience tachycardia, palpitations, and chest pain described as sharp and sticking. Generalized motor weakness, nausea, and occasionally diarrhea occur. Air hunger leads to hyperventilation and can result in respiratory alkalosis. This problem compounds the discomfort by causing muscular stiffness in the extremities and numbness or tingling around the mouth, fingers, or toes. Patients undergoing this terrifying experience are convinced that they are about to die. They have a feeling of unreality and of losing contact with their surroundings. They become uncontrollable and violent or lose consciousness. Although panic attacks are self-limiting (lasting anywhere from a few minutes to a couple of hours), they represent a psychiatric emergency. Patients should be isolated in a safe room and sedated with diazepam (Valium) or chlordiazepoxide (Librium) as soon as possible. Calming reassurance from someone who remains several feet away is extremely important. A psychiatric consultation should be immediately arranged, since the attack may be a precipitating sign of psychosis. The consultation is further warranted by the fact that the problem tends to be recurrent. Thus, psychotherapy or administration of an antianxiety medication may be necessary.

TABLE 13.13 ANTIANXIETY AGENTS

Generic Name	Trade Name	Uses
Alprazolam	Xanax	Anxiety associated with depression
Chlordiazepoxide	Librium	Neurotic depression, anxiety, tension, acute alcohol withdrawal symptoms
Chlormezanone	Trancopal	Mild anxiety and tension
Clorazepate dipotassium	Tranxene	Anxiety disorders, acute alcohol withdrawal, adjunctive treatment for seizures
Clorazepate monopotassium	Azene	Anxiety, psychoneuroses including anxiety neurosis, acute alcohol withdrawal symptoms
Diazepam	Valium	Tension, anxiety, acute alcohol withdrawal, muscle relaxant, anticonvulsive, preoperative medication, adjunctive therapy for cardioversion
Flurazepam hydrochloride	Dalmane	Simple insomnia
Halazepam	Paxipam	Short-term relief of anxiety
Hydroxyzine	Atarax, Vistaril	Anxiety and tension associated with psychoneurosis, agitation, alcohol withdrawal, postpartum adjunctive medication, allergic pruritus, preoperative sedation
Lorazepam	Ativan	Tension, anxiety, agitation, irritability, insomnia
Meprobamate	Miltown, Equanil	Minor tension and anxiety, neurotic anxiety, simple insomnia, muscle relaxant, premedication for ECT
Oxazepam	Serax	Mild or moderate anxiety, tension, irritability, agitation, depressive anxiety, adjunct for acute alcohol withdrawal
Prazepam	Centrax	Situational, functional, or organic anxiety disorders
Temazepam	Restoril	Simple insomnia
Tybamate	Tybatran	Short-term relief of anxiety

Anxiety reaction (generalized anxiety) is characterized by persistent anxiety of at least 4 weeks' duration with somatic and psychic manifestations (motor tension, autonomic hyperactivity, apprehension, a feeling of dread). It is one of the ***anxiety disorders*** described in Table 13.14. ***Phobic disorders*** are characterized by an irrational fear of relatively harmless objects or situations. Affecting less than 1% of the population, these anxiety-producing fears occur more frequently in women than in men, and familial tendencies are high. The phobia itself is a learned defense mechanism. A forbidden or threatening drive is displaced to a specific symbol, which is usually determined by a chance exposure at a time when the anxious impulse first appeared. Thereafter, patients learn to protect themselves from the threatening drive by fearful avoidance of the symbol. This may lead to reduction of normal functioning or to ***counterphobic behavior.*** The latter describes a deliberate, often dangerous, exposure to phobic fears. A good example is an individual who is afraid of snakes but becomes the owner of poisonous reptiles. Usually beginning in early adulthood, most phobias have a chronic course marked by exacerbations and remissions. A sudden outbreak may herald the onset of schizophrenia, while persistent problems may lead to depression. Patients should therefore be referred for psychiatric treatment. Many will benefit from insight psychotherapy or behavior therapy in which they confront their fears while using relaxation techniques (including hypnotism). Flooding is an extreme form of behavioral therapy based on prolonged, intense

TABLE 13.14 ANXIETY DISORDERS

Type	Essential Features
Agoraphobia	Marked fear of being alone or in public places. Patients may insist that they be accompanied on public transportation, bridges, or tunnels and in crowds. Depression is usually associated.
Social phobia	Marked fear of social interactions or of being humiliated or embarrassed by others.
Simple phobia	Marked fear of certain objects or situations (e.g., snakes, carnivals).
Panic disorder	Unpredictable, recurrent attacks of panic-level anxiety unrelated to any specific cause.
Obsessive-compulsive disorder	Anxiety manifested by excessively troublesome thoughts (e.g., contamination) and actions (e.g., hand washing).
Generalized anxiety disorder	Pervasive anxiety lasting for more than 1 month unrelated to any specific cause.

exposure to the phobic stimulus. Minor tranquilizers and antidepressants are also used in treatment.

In ***obsessive-compulsive disorder*** an obsession (word, image, idea) or compulsion (repetitive impulse, action) represents an attempt to undo anxiety generated by some forbidden drive. As an example, a twin thinks of his brother's death every time he picks up the mail. To quell the thought, he checks the post box repeatedly. Although he recognizes that the idea is unreal and the subsequent action nonsensical, he cannot rid himself of this pattern. The problem is quite rare, affecting only about 0.05% of the population, men and women alike. It is most common among intelligent individuals from upper socioeconomic levels. Symptoms begin in early adolescence or later. Although they tend to run a chronic course, improvement is seen in 25% of the patients with early treatment. Supportive therapy with an emphasis on reassurance and encouragement seems to give the best results. Behavioral therapy and flooding have also been used. Treatment emphasizes the patient's strengths and encourages verbalization of feelings.

Overwhelming stress may lead to a ***dissociative disorder.*** Patients banish anxiety-provoking memories, feelings, ideas, or perceptions from their conscious minds in a number of ways, all centered on the defense mechanism of dissociation. One of the most dramatic forms is ***somnambulism*** (sleepwalking). After going to sleep normally, patients arise and engage in complex activities that, in many cases, dramatize a past, recent, or anticipated emotionally traumatic event. During this time, they remain unresponsive to external stimuli, and upon awakening remember nothing of the experience. The most common form is ***amnesia.*** Loss of memory for past events may cover a period of several hours to several weeks. With ***anterograde amnesia,*** patients experience an ongoing memory loss and are unable to recall thoughts, feelings, or actions from moment to moment. Less commonly, a ***fugue state*** may evolve in which the individual loses all recollection of past identity. Unaware of any change, he or she disappears from the job and family, beginning a completely new existence at a distant location. A similar change of identity occurs in ***multiple personality,*** an extremely rare phenomenon. Memory loss and personality changes occurring in dissociative disorders must be distinguished from those accompanying organic brain disease (see Chapter 12). The work-up may require

TABLE 13.15 SOMATIFORM DISORDERS

Type	Essential Features
Somatization	Patients develop multiple complaints such as double vision, fainting, memory loss, nausea, abdominal bloating, palpitations, and so on before age 30. Medical attention is repeatedly sought, but no physical disorders can be found.
Psychogenic pain disorder	Patients have persistent complaints of severe pain not explained by any physical disorder.
Hypochondriasis	An exaggerated interpretation of physical signs or sensations stemming from preoccupation with the possibility of a serious disease.
Conversion	Real functional disturbances (paralysis, blindness, vomiting) with no physical basis. Disorder arises from an extreme psychologic conflict (e.g., a mother who witnessed the murder of her young child goes blind).

electroencephalography and computed tomography scanning to rule out physiologic problems. In the absence of physical abnormalities, psychotherapeutic referral is indicated. Effective treatments include hypnosis, family therapy, and environmental manipulation to lower stress levels (job changes, homemaking assistance, etc.). The symptoms may be recurrent unless more effective coping mechanisms are learned.

Somatiform disorders include ***somatization, psychogenic pain disorder, hypochondriasis,*** and ***conversion disorder*** described in Table 13.15. The etiology is unknown, though it may be related to narcissistic personality types that are marked by excessive concern with the self and with the gratification of dependency needs. Patients have a number of physical complaints for which there are no organic patterns or findings. Covering a wide variety of body parts, the complaints usually involve the head, neck, chest, and abdomen, and are described in minute detail. The problem usually appears by adolescence or young adulthood, and the course tends to be chronic.

Patients with somatiform disturbances are extremely resistant to medical reassurance and are poor candidates for antianxiety medications. These medications not only tend to reinforce maladaptive behavioral patterns but may also lead to dependency. Confrontation causes little change and may prompt the individual to seek care from several sources. This is detrimental, since a long-term relationship with a supportive primary care provider is extremely important. Appropriate reinforcement is crucial. Attention and praise should be given to encourage adaptive behaviors like work, conversation, and exercise. They should be withheld when patients revert to somatization and self-pity. Psychiatric referral should always be encouraged. However, patients find a psychogenic diagnosis extremely threatening, since belief in their symptoms has developed as a way to avoid responsibility through illness and thus manage underlying anxieties. Hypnosis is often helpful in removing the symptoms and getting the person through an immediate crisis, but more extensive psychotherapy is necessary to discover and alleviate the conditions that seem to have influenced the development and maintenance of such a coping response pattern and to assist in developing a more adaptive response style. In recent years, behavior modification has been successful in the treatment of pain behavior management, regardless of the origin.

It is important for the practitioner to recognize the difference between a person with a somatiform disorder and a ***malingerer.*** Faking the symptoms of a disease to avoid work or to benefit from insurance settlements, malingerers tend to be defensive, evasive, and suspicious. They are reluctant to be examined or to discuss their symptoms, lest the pretense be discovered.

In contrast to the malingerer, who has conscious motivations for faking a disease, is the patient suffering from a complicated psychologic picture called ***Munchausen's syndrome*** (factitious disorder). This individual self-induces physical or psychologic symptoms for the sole purpose of assuming a patient role. An example is a nondiabetic person who purposely injects insulin and presents with hypoglycemic crisis in the emergency room. There may be a history of medical problems in childhood that required extensive treatment or hospitalization. These patients are frequently health care workers or persons who have had a significant association with a physician. This background provides them with the knowledge to present a convincing history and complaints. They have dependent, exploitive, or masochistic personality traits. Treatment is difficult and requires intervention by a specialist.

Whether or not stress leads to secondary problems depends in part on its magnitude. The classic proof of this statement was provided by the Holmes-Rahe scale, developed in the 1940s, in which life events (divorce, pregnancy, buying a house, starting a new job) were rated in terms of the amount of social readjustment they imposed (Table 13.16). On one end of the scale was the death of a spouse (100 units), and on the other end, minor violations of the law (11 units). Any person who experienced changes over a year's time that added up to more than 300 points was found to be at risk for the development of a serious physical or mental illness. Although the Holmes-Rahe scale still applies, many psychologists now feel that everyday annoyances contribute more to stress-related problems than do major life events. They contend that most persons have a remarkable capacity to withstand a tragedy but are ill equipped to handle the smaller chronic strains of life. Those who adjust best have a sense of being in control of their lives. Perhaps even more importantly, they have a strong network of friends and family to provide social support. The notion that isolation is the fastest route to mental and physical breakdown has long been used by penal systems and prisoner-of-war camps. It is also suggested by the high rate of suicide and depression among older persons who have been retired from jobs, set apart from their families, and faced with the death of friends. While no one can completely avoid stress, ▶ ***stress reduction*** can be accomplished by learning to recognize and avoid stressful stimuli and by employing carefully selected relaxation techniques.

FAMILY SYSTEMS

Theorists such as Bowen, Manuchin, and Toman view the total family as being greater than the sum of its members. They describe closed family systems (those whose members have very little involvement with outside persons or activities) and open family systems (those whose members accept and welcome change). Family balance is more likely to occur in open systems. It also depends on the maturity rating of individual members. At the top of the rating scale are principal-oriented persons who have a solid self-image and very distinct views ("I" stands) and who take an intellectual approach to decision making. At the bottom of the scale are relationship-oriented persons who act to gain increased attention, who are concerned about "what people think," and who have an emotional approach to decision making.

TABLE 13.16 SOCIAL READJUSTMENT RATING SCALE (SRRS)

Event	Scale of Impact
Death of spouse	100
Divorce	73
Marital separation	65
Jail term	63
Death of close family member	63
Personal injury or illness	53
Marriage	50
Fired from job	47
Marital reconciliation	45
Retirement	45
Change in health of family member	44
Pregnancy	40
Difficulty with sex life	39
Gain of new family member	39
Business readjustment	39
Change in financial status	38
Death of close friend	37
Change in line of work	36
Change in number of marital arguments	35
Mortgage or loan above $10,000	31
Foreclosure of mortgage or loan	30
Change in work responsibilities	29
Child leaving home	29
Trouble with in-laws	29
Outstanding personal achievement	28
Change in working status of wife	26
Beginning or ending of school session	26
Change in living conditions	25
Change of personal habits	24
Trouble with boss	23
Change in work hours or conditions	20
Change of residence	20
Change of school	20
Change in recreation habits	19
Change in church activities	19
Change in social activities	18
Mortgage or loan less than $10,000	17
Change in sleeping habits	16
Change in number of family get-togethers	15
Change in eating habits	15
Vacation	13
Christmas	12
Minor violations of the law	11

Source: Developed by Holmes and colleagues, 1967, 1970.

Persons with similar maturity levels tend to marry. Thus, maturity levels tend to pass from one generation to the next.

Family function is best understood from circular responses (triangling or feedback loops), which can have healthy or unhealthy outcomes. Projection of uncontrolled anger, for example, has been identified as the basic maladaptation in most instances of ***domestic violence,*** a problem of increasing concern. Today Americans are more likely to be injured by the aggressive behavior of a family member than by a stranger on the street. Nearly one-third of all homicides occur in the home, and nearly one-third of the policemen killed in the line of duty die while responding to family disturbances. Bodily injury is only one manifestation of the problem. Other forms include forced sexual activity, destruction of property, cruelty to pets, withholding food or medications, and neglect. Persons who are threatened with future harm, kept in forced isolation, and/or deliberately humiliated may be considered psychologically battered.

Research has only recently shed some light on the etiology of domestic violence. One study compared satisfied, discordant (but nonabusive), and abusive couples. Abusive individuals were significantly different in terms of assertiveness, marital adjustment, alcoholism, and sex role attitudes from those in the happily married group. However, similar results were obtained from wives in discordant and abused relationships. This suggests that discord per se is not the cause of abuse. Instead, it appears to be directly related to some distinguishing characteristics of abusive husbands. These men were found to be considerably less assertive than normal with their wives in day-to-day living. They had generally poor communication skills and tended to turn all feelings into anger, the only emotion they were comfortable expressing. Also, abusive husbands had a higher than normal incidence of alcoholism. Many had been abused themselves or had witnessed abusive behavior as children.

It has been proposed that battering occurs in three distinct phases. Phase I involves tension buildup and is characterized by minor incidents such as throwing things, pushing, shoving, or shaking. The woman usually responds by becoming compliant, passive, or withdrawn. She may use denial and rationalization to regain psychologic equilibrium. Fearing that the aggression may spill over to outsiders, the woman isolates herself and her spouse from supportive persons, thus increasing the opportunity for violence against herself. Each minor battering adds to mounting residual tension and phase II erupts in volatile, uncontrolled violence by the man which can last for periods ranging from 2 to 24 hours. During the attack, most women concentrate on protecting themselves as well as they can. Afterward they experience depression, malaise, withdrawal, and helplessness. Medical treatment may be delayed because of embarrassment or lack of transportation or because the partner will not allow it. Phase III is marked by a period of tenderness and contrition. The man pleads for forgiveness, apologizes, lavishes gifts, and tells the woman that he will never behave that way again. He believes he will live up to this promise. One damaging misconception is that women remain in abusive relationships because they deserve beatings or are masochistic. Women may give many rationalizations, but fear seems to be the major reason that so many stay.

Because so many battered women are afraid to speak out or ask for help, they frequently hide the real cause of their injuries and invent explanations. Therefore, providers need to be aware of certain signs and symptoms that are characteristic of abuse (Table 13.17). It may be several days before help is sought for acute injuries. The battered woman may be pregnant; in fact, the first pregnancy often marks the beginning of the abuse. It is also common for the woman to be accompanied by the batterer. He may be adamantly opposed to leaving her alone for an interview or exam. If abusive behavior is suspected, providers can ask, "How do people in your family express anger?" Such a direct question cuts through denial and gives the patient permission to talk about family discord. Answers may reveal important information about levels of impulse control and about the frequency and severity of violent behavior.

By law, health care providers must report suspected cases of child abuse to the appropriate state agency. In cases of adult battering, it is inappropriate to initiate legal proceedings against the patient's will unless a gunshot wound is present. Victims are usually the best judge of a batterer's response, and if they insist that they are safe and want to return home, they must be allowed to do so. Any other

TABLE 13.17 INDICATIONS OF DOMESTIC ABUSE OR NEGLECT

Sign	Discussion
In general	Signs of physical beatings may recur regularly, particularly after the abuser has been away from or confined to home for any length of time (e.g., after business trips, weekends at home, or family vacations). Poor or conflicting explanations may be given about the injury by both the victim and the abuser. In addition, victims seen for medical care often display blunted affect, extreme dependency or apprehension, unusual aggressiveness, depression, or paranoia. They may seem wary of adult contacts or afraid to go home.
Beatings	Fractures, particularly of the skull, nose, and facial structures. Bruises, welts, lacerations, or abrasions that usually involve the face, torso, buttocks, and/or thighs. Lesions often found in clusters, in patterns that reflect the weapon used (e.g., electric cord, belt buckle), and in various stages of healing.
Burns	Usually inflicted on soles, palms, back, or buttocks. Wounds made by lighted cigars or cigarettes, by irons, or by immersing body parts in scalding water, fires, or burners (e.g., sock-like or glove-like lesions involving the extremities, doughnut-shaped lesions of the genitalia and buttocks).
Restraint	Rope burns on arms, legs, or buttocks.
Neglect	Victims have poor hygiene or are inappropriately dressed. Due to starvation, they may be constantly hungry, underweight, and malnourished. There may be unattended physical and medical needs and accidents related to lack of needed supervision. Begging, stealing, and other unlawful practices are not uncommon.

course of action may place a battered person in greater danger. Information about ▶ ***organizations for abused adults*** should be offered. Many of these organizations offer temporary housing, legal aid, counseling, and group support. Even if the woman does not act on the information at the time, she may use the knowledge in the future. It is not helpful to push the woman to leave her home, since she often loves the man and wants to believe in him. Depending and relying on each other, many couples will reject intervention that focuses on separation. A more realistic goal is to decrease the frequency and intensity of the batterings. This strategy appears to be successful if the man and woman become involved in separate treatment. Marital counseling is not recommended as an initial intervention, since it may imply that the battered partner is at least partially responsible for being beaten. In fact, an important part of treatment is to place the sole responsibility for violent behavior on the batterer. Both individuals must realize that while their relationship is dysfunctional, it is not to blame for acts of battering.

Another channel for family dysfunction is incest. Recent statistics indicate that about 20 million women in the United States may have been childhood victims of ***incest or sexual abuse.*** The acute problems associated with this situation tend to reside in the province of pediatric primary care, but occasionally the adult primary care provider will encounter the issue as a retrospective report during a routine physical exam (e.g., during a family planning visit) or while taking a detailed history. If the volunteered information seems to cause sudden distress for the patient, further discussion is indicated in order to provide support and an opportunity to vent feelings about the situation, and to consider the possibility of referral for individual or group therapy. There are a number of ▶ ***organizations for victims of childhood sexual abuse.*** This is important since victims of sexual abuse often have a number of residual sexual and interpersonal problems, including decreased sexual desire, sexual performance problems, guilt, and low self-esteem. In addition, persons

TABLE 13.18 DEVELOPMENTAL TASKS

Age and Task	Socialization	Cognitive Growth	Body Image	Signs of Failure
Infancy (0–18 months) Trust versus mistrust; resultant strength—hope; resultant problem—withdrawal	Sole relationships with nurturing figures. Oral activity predominant. Stranger anxiety at 7 months. Begins to accept discipline at 12 months. Begins play at 15 months.	Learns through positive feedback from sensory gratification. Rudimentary verbal communication.	Can separate self from surroundings by age 12 months.	Excessive crying. Failure to gain weight. Lack of smiling.
Toddler (18–36 months) Autonomy versus doubt and shame; resultant strength—will; resultant problem—compulsion	Main relationships with family figures. Predominant activity is play, including parallel play. Coordination improves. Begins to respond to discipline based on reward or punishment.	Rapid speech development. Uses full sentences with pronouns to communicate. Preoperational thinking.	Recognizes urine and stool as part of self. Explores body. Begins to gain self-image from praise.	Failure to toilet train or develop speech. Does not conform to any discipline. Excessive tantrums.
Preschool (3–6 years) Initiative versus guilt; resultant strength—purpose; resultant problem—inhibition	Relationships still with family figures. Symbolic group play rich in fantasy. Uses play to express feelings. Few feelings for others. Interested in gender. Learns to cooperate. Tentative independence in leaving home.	Competent use of language. Needs and enjoys books, stories, and other learning routines. Communicates with one person at a time. Uses images for expression.	Concern with body safety. Places importance on appraisals from adults other than parents. Can separate self and objects from environment.	Bedwetting. Temper tantrums. Excessive concern for comfort habits to point of disrupting play. Poor language skills. Lacks responsibility for self.
School age (6–12 years) Industry versus inferiority; resultant strength—competence; resultant problem—inertia	Relationships not only with family but also with peers. Engages in organized games with rigid rules. Ritualistic. Enjoys sports and collecting things.	Uses language to increase knowledge and socialization. Reads for enjoyment. Eager to learn. Concrete thinking.	Self-concept expands through input from peers and teachers. Begins to have concern for others. Still self-involved. Expresses feelings.	Somatasizes. Few friends, but "teacher's pet." Antisocial. Dependent behavior.
Adolescence (12–18 years) Identity versus role confusion; resultant strength—fidelity; resultant problem—repudiation	In early adolescence, relates to peers of same sex; later relates to those of opposite sex. Most activities are outside the home. Enjoys TV, movies, music, and reading.	Ability to acquire and use knowledge at height. Abstract thinking. Deductive reasoning. Highly imaginative.	Distinct and stable self-image. Knows strengths and limitations. Accepts physique and sex role.	Lack of self-control. Running away from home or dropping out of school. Drug or alcohol abuse. Psychosomatic illness. Isolation.
Early adulthood (18–40 years) Intimacy versus isolation; resultant strength—love; resultant problem—exclusivity	Relationships evolve from sexual and competitive interests. Pursues marriage and career. Starts family. Enjoys social and recreational activities.	Continues to add to knowledge base, particularly through life experience. Successfully balances work, family, and recreation. Provides secure upbringing for offspring.	Works toward desired place in society. Secure in sexuality and physical well-being.	Unstable family relationships. Failure to keep jobs. Failure to relax or have fun. Alcoholism.
Middle adulthood (40–60 years) Generativity versus stagnation; resultant strength—care; resultant problem—rejection	Relationships and activities center on spouse, family, friends, and coworkers. Role reversal with own parents.	Has accumulated experience and knowledge. May take up new hobbies and interests.	Notes decline in physical strength and well-being.	Persistent midlife crisis. Depression.
Older adulthood (60–death) Integrity versus despair; resultant strength—wisdom; resultant problem—disdain	Main relationships with family and close friends. Activities remain the same but may be reduced.	Mental capacity remains until organic problems develop.	May be affected by multiple health problems. Becomes dependent on children.	Withdrawal, depression, confusion, failure to thrive.

who were victims of sexual abuse as children may sometimes become abusers as adults. However, if the report emerges as an incidental detail (e.g., as part of a detailed sexual history) without eliciting distress, all that may be called for is a sensitive, nonjudgmental attitude.

DEVELOPMENTAL MILESTONES

Life is marked by physical change—growth, maturity, decline. Psychologic changes also occur. Early theorists (e.g., Freud and Sullivan) contended that along with physical growth, psychologic development was completed by the end of adolescence. More recent theorists (e.g., Erikson and Levinson) proposed that physical and psychologic changes occur in stages right up to the end of life. Each stage is characterized by inherent "tasks," as noted in Table 13.18. With the successful completion of these tasks, the individual reaches a "developmental milestone" and moves on to the next stage. In this way, psychologic growth occurs, its development progressing slowly. Hopefully, the final result is a sense of culmination rather than decline.

The transition from one stage of life to the next may be smooth. Alternatively, it may be accompanied by turmoil, despair, or other unsettling feelings referred to as a ***developmental crisis.*** The feelings can be a healthy response spurring individuals to reassess their present direction, future goals, or past outcomes. By deciding which aspects of life have been successfully completed and hold significance, the individual continues to grow. Thus, ***midlife crisis*** may characterize the passage from middle to later adulthood when physical function begins to decline and the period of major decisions (career, marriage. lifestyle) comes to a close. Crisis is also common among the elderly, who are faced with many changes: death of friends, decreased physical capacity, major health problems, and loss of position in the family, work place, or community. Although a crisis is self-limited and usually resolves within 8 weeks, many patients require intervention (see the discussion of anxiety).

During late adulthood, patients review their lives, searching for meaning and satisfaction in preparation for ***death,*** the final stage of development. Five stages of death have been identified. These stages and their sequence can vary, and are not seen in all dying patients. The initial stage is one of shock and denial. Patients often respond with the belief that "this can't be happening to me" and feel extremely isolated. Denial then gives way to anger and rage. The patient asks, "Why me?" Often this is the most difficult period for the family and the health care provider because anger may be directed toward them. The bargaining stage is a plea for life extension and/or pain relief. Most bargains are made with God and are not verbalized with others. When the bargaining is recognized as futile, the fourth stage, depression, ensues, with a focus on past and impending loss. This grief prepares the individual for the final stage, acceptance. At this point, the inevitability and nearness of death are acknowledged, and it becomes important that patients know that they are not alone. Health care workers and family members may experience these same stages while caring for the dying patient. In terms of understanding these stages, emotional support heads the list of ▶ ***considerations for the dying patient.*** Making arrangements for physical care and pain control is equally important. Religious retreats for the dying, hospices, home health aid, and hospital or nursing home care are some of the possibilities. Wherever possible, patients and loved ones should be helped to put their lives in order as a final consideration.

Details of Management

▸ *Organizations for Mental Illness*

Laboratory Tests: None.

Therapeutic Measures: None.

Patient Education: The National Alliance for the Mentally Ill is an organization whose sole purpose is to act as an advocate for the chronically mentally ill. As part of this effort, they support the education of medical and other care providers about the nature of chronic mental illness (avoiding the typical view of mental illness as primarily a manifestation of social dysfunction that may be readily alleviated by psychotherapy). The organization is made up of families of persons with a chronic mental illness, and as such is uniquely qualified to understand the needs of mentally ill persons and the difficulties confronting them and their families. They are active in educating families about mental illness, facilitating their contacts with the mental health services system (e.g., explaining procedures of hospital admission and release), and in other ways enabling them to provide the type of support that persons suffering from chronic mental illness require. Primary care providers can contact the national organization for addresses and phone numbers of local branches and then pass this information on to the families of their patients suffering from chronic mental illness.

National Alliance for the Mentally Ill
1901 North Fort Myer Drive
Suite 500
Arlington, Virginia 22209
Tel.: (703) 524-7600

The Mental Illness Foundation is primarily involved with research funding. However, it can be contacted for patient education pamphlets and also publishes a quarterly newsletter.

Mental Illness Foundation
1457 Broadway, Suite 514
New York, New York 10036
Tel.: (212) 302-0110

Consult nearby psychiatric hospitals or mental health clinics for other resources and check local listings for mental health services (usually listed by county). Information about local support groups may also be obtained by contacting a local information line of the United Way or the National Self-Help Clearinghouse. The National Self-Help Clearinghouse can also provide phone numbers and addresses of regional self-help clearinghouses that may publish lists of local, state, or regional self-help organizations. Contact:

National Self-Help Clearinghouse
33 West 42nd Street, Room 1227
New York, New York 10036
Tel.: (212) 840-1259

Follow-up: If necessary, assist patients in making contacts with support groups and other organizations.

▸ *Office Management of Alcoholism*

Laboratory Tests: None, except as needed initially to determine the extent of related medical complications (particularly of the liver and nervous system).

Therapeutic Measures: In general, group therapy is more effective for alcohol rehabilitation than individual processes, but getting patients to seek an appropriate treatment program may require considerable effort. Patients must be helped to recognize that many of the problems they previously attempted to deal with by alcohol use were brought about by their own alcohol dependency. They must also be helped to realize that abstinence and the development of more effective coping strategies to deal with everyday problems are apt to be beyond their ability without outside help. Often, however, this realization does not develop until the individual fails to control his own drinking behavior (by relapsing) or until distressing consequences such as marital discord or separation, physical abuse, work absenteeism, a decline in work performance, threatened loss of a job or actual job loss, automobile accidents, arrests, or hospitalizations occur. Even then many patients resist the primary care provider's diagnosis of alcoholism because of the associated social stigma. Thus, it is often helpful to allow the patient to reach that conclusion alone. A prepared alcoholism questionnaire such as the Michigan Alcoholism Screening Test (MAST) or the one available from Alcoholics Anonymous can help simplify the process of self-diagnosis. At all times, a patient, supportive, nonjudgmental approach on the part of the primary care provider is important to help an alcoholic patient reach the point where he or she is able to admit the problem, acknowledge the need for professional intervention, and desire that assistance so that referral to an appropriate treatment facility can be initiated. It is also important to emphasize that success can be achieved through specialized rehabilitation programs available in hospitals and Alcoholics Anonymous. Inpatient admission to a specialized program is invariably more successful than outpatient treatment; the latter should be reserved for stable, healthy, and detoxified patients. Alcoholics Anonymous (AA) groups are available throughout the country, and, according to one report, have about a 35% success rate among new applicants. These groups provide the support and encouragement of others who have the same problem with alcohol (and similar expertise in rationalizing the problem). They also provide socialization in a non-drinking environment, and an opportunity for the patient to help other members and thereby increase personal self-esteem and confidence without having to turn to alcohol. It is particularly helpful if the members of the AA group have more in common than the drinking problem (e.g., there are groups of physicians and dentists).

General or psychiatric hospitalization should be used only for the treatment of medical or psychiatric conditions other than alcoholism that are serious enough to warrant such admission, and specific treatment of the alcoholism should be continued once the acute medical or psychiatric condition has been handled. Criteria for general hospital admission include unconsciousness or head injury, serious hemorrhaging, serious withdrawal syndrome (with impending delirium tremens), fever, convulsions, dehydration or significant malnutrition and vitamin deficiency, disulfiram-alcohol reaction, signs of hepatic disease (e.g., jaundice), or other significant medical conditions warranting hospitalization. As stated above, acute psychiatric hospitalization is indicated only when a severe acute psychiatric condition other than alcoholism is present (e.g., psychosis, depression, or a behavioral disorder) that is itself serious enough to warrant hospitalization. Further, except for the rare instance of short-term management of acute withdrawal symptoms (or for independent medical or psychiatric conditions), there is little justification for pharmacologic management of alcoholism. The exception to this general rule is the use of disulfiram (Antabuse), but there are mixed reports about its success. In general, the best results are obtained with patients who are already highly motivated to continue alcohol abstinence and have a positive, ongoing relationship with the care provider prescribing the drug. The use of disulfiram to prevent drinking in patients who are not motivated to abstain does not seem to have much long-term success. Disulfiram therapy should not exclude participation in a rehabilitation program.

Patient Education: Perhaps the most essential realization that one can help the alcoholic patient to achieve is that he alone is responsible for the consequences of his actions and that his desire for and involvement in his own rehabilitation are vital for its success.

Follow-up: Once a patient has joined a rehabilitation program or an AA group, continue to schedule him (or her) and possibly his spouse for regular, frequent, short office visits (for an appropriate fee) for at least 1–2 years. This will reassure the patient of the care provider's continued interest in his success and will provide opportunities to encourage him to continue his abstinence and regular involvement in an AA group. Initially, visits should be weekly; later, they may be scheduled every 2 weeks and then every month. Whenever possible, enlist the support of a spouse or family and encourage them to join similar support groups such as Al-Anon (for spouses of alcoholics) and Al-Ateen (for children from about 12 to 20 years of age).

▸ *Alcohol Treatment Programs and Support Groups*

Laboratory Tests: None.

Therapeutic Measures: None.

Patient Education: For information about treatment programs for alcoholics, consult local listings for psychiatric hospitals or mental health clinics offering such programs or for private institutions that deal specifically with the treatment of alcoholism. For support groups for alcoholic patients, contact local listings for Alcoholics Anonymous chapters or one of the following:

Alcoholics Anonymous
P.O. Box 459
Grand Central Station
New York, New York 10163
Tel.: (212) 473-6200

Alcoholics Anonymous
World Services Office
468 Park Avenue South
New York, New York 10016
Tel.: (212) 686-1100

For information about Al-Anon (support groups for family members and friends of alcoholics), Al-Ateen (for teenage children of alcoholics), or Adult Children of Alcoholics chapters, consult local listings or contact:

Al-Anon/Al-Ateen Information Center
1 Park Avenue
New York, New York 10016
Tel.: (212) 683-1771 or (212) 254-7230

Further information, patient education pamphlets, and assistance in making referrals to treatment programs and support groups may be obtained by contacting:

National Council on Alcoholism
12 West 21st Street
New York, New York 10010
Tel.: (212) 206-6770

Clearinghouse for Alcohol Information
P.O. Box 2345
Rockville, Maryland 20852
Tel.: (301) 468-2600

National Self-Help Clearing House
Graduate School and University Center
City University of New York
33 West 42nd Street, Room 1227
New York, New York 10036
Tel.: (212) 840-1259

Follow-up: If needed, assist patients in making contacts with support groups.

▸ *Drug Abuse Organizations*

Laboratory Tests: None.

Therapeutic Measures: None.

Patient Education: For information about local treatment programs and support groups for substance abusers, contact:

Pills Anonymous (in some areas called Drugs Anonymous)
P.O. Box 473, Ansonia Station
New York, New York 10023
Tel.: (212) 874-0700

Narcotics Anonymous
25 St. Mark's Place
New York, New York 10003
Tel.: (212) 420-9400 is a 24-hour hotline number (not toll-free)

Information and referrals to other groups may also be obtained from the National Federation of Parents for Drug-Free Youths by calling 1-800-554-5437.

Follow-up: Assist patients in making contacts with support groups as needed.

▸ *Proper Care of the Rape Victim*

Laboratory Tests: After securing written informed consent (see below), the following should be done: Using sterile cotton swabs, collect material from the vaginal walls and cervix to make two air-dried smears on clean glass slides. Obtain similar samples from the mouth (swab around the molars and cheeks) and anus if indicated (by report or other evidence of oral or anal-genital contact) and prepare fixed slides from these samples. Carefully label all slides. Prepare a wet mount from secretions obtained by swabbing the same areas with a premoistened cotton swab, placing the samples at once on a slide with a drop of saline and covering them with a coverslip. Examine the slides for motile or nonmotile spermatozoa under high-dry magnification and record the percentage of motile forms. Culture the vagina, anus, and/or mouth (as indicated) for *Neisseria gonorrhoeae* and *Chlamydia*, and obtain a Papanicolaou smear of the cervix. Perform pregnancy tests to rule out concurrent pregnancy and repeat these tests if the next menses is missed. Draw blood typing and VDRL, and repeat VDRL in 6 weeks. If the patient's history includes forced ingestion or injection of alcohol or drugs, obtain blood (10 mL without anticoagulant) and urine (100 mL) specimens.

All specimens must be carefully and legibly labeled with the patient's name, date, sampling site (i.e., vaginal fornix, vulva, anus), and examiner's name, and accounted for from the time of the initial exam until the time they appear in court. The patient's chart should contain a list of all specimens taken and the sampling sites, the name of the person present with the patient during the exam, and the person to whom the specimens were delivered. Transfer to a pathologist or laboratory technician should be done directly (*not* via messenger) and in the presence of witnesses, and a receipt must be obtained.

Therapeutic Measures: Whenever possible, the exam of a rape victim should take place in an emergency room, but when this is not possible, it is important to provide empathetic support and to explain carefully the nature and purpose of all procedures (history, physical exam, collection of evidence, taking of photographs, medical and preventive treatment, and release of information and evidence to the police) in order to provide the patient with some sense of control during the exam and the collection of evidence. You may wish to begin by first stating to the victim that what has happened is terrible and that you want to help. After explaining the procedures, obtain written informed consent from the patient, keeping in mind at all times that she has the right to refuse any part of the exam as well as to forbid the release of any information or evidence to the legal authorities. Consent forms should be obtained well before the need arises and should be readily available. A bulletin published by the American College of Obstetricians and Gynecologists (ACOG) in 1978 contains a consent form and guidelines (ACOG, 1 Wacker Drive, Chicago, Illinois 60601). This should be signed by the patient in the presence of a witness, and someone besides the person taking the history and examining the patient should remain with her at all times. If the patient wishes, it may be helpful to have someone she knows accompany her (a friend, family member, or roommate), but if no such person is available, it may be some other trained person (e.g., a nurse or a volunteer provided by a rape crisis center) who is sensitive, supportive, and able to listen.

The history, which should be recorded in the patient's own words, should include the following information:

If birth control is used and the type of method.

Date of last normal menstrual period.

Time of most recent coitus prior to the assault.

Gravidity and parity.

Time, location, and other details about the alleged attack.

Number of assailants.

If any injuries were sustained.

The nature of any genital contact (e.g., vaginal penetration, oral-genital contact, anal-genital contact) and whether there was penetration of the vagina by penis, hands or foreign objects.

Whether ejaculation occurred.

Whether a condom was used by the attacker.

If the victim knew the alleged attacker and, if so, the nature of the relationship.

Whether there were physical or verbal threats.

Whether, how, and to what extent the victim resisted.

Whether the victim or attacker had been using alcohol or other drugs.

How the victim has reacted to the attack emotionally and behaviorally. Did she come directly to you? Did she bathe or change her clothing? Is she calm, agitated, or confused? Note the types of coping strategies used by the victim during and after the attack.

Have the patient stand on a white sheet to disrobe. Any hair, leaves, dirt, or other substances found should be placed in separate clean paper bags or envelopes, labeled, and kept as evidence. Also to be collected and appropriately labeled are any hairs obtained by gently but thoroughly combing the patient's vulva, five pubic hairs, and five head hairs of the patient for comparison (these should be pulled, not cut), scrapings from under the patient's fingernails, the patient's underwear, and any torn or stained clothing. All collected evidence should be carefully and legibly labeled and accounted for from the time of the initial exam until the time it appears as evidence in the courtroom.

Examine the patient, noting any external evidence of trauma (bruises, scratches, cuts), and document and/or photograph these findings. Note also the patient's emotional state and vital signs, and examine the scalp, neck, and face for bruises, cuts, or signs of attempted strangulation. Examine the back, breasts, and chest (for bruises and tenderness), abdomen (for masses, tenderness, rebound), pelvic area (look particularly for evidence of trauma), and thighs. Explain to the patient the need to check this particular area of her body, even though she may feel very vulnerable under the circumstances. Check for semen stains (dry yellow-white with some flaking) on the thighs, in the pubic hair, and around the vulva, and use Wood's light to examine the entire body and genitalia for semen, which fluoresces. Swab any positive areas with a premoistened swab for identification of acid phosphatase (from prostatic secretions). Examine the vagina and cervix for blood, fluid, and discharge. Wait until all specimens have been obtained before attempting to wipe the vagina for visualization. Examine any laceration in this region carefully, because what appears to be a small cut may in actuality be a deep stab wound, and save any foreign body (including a tampon) found in the vagina. The pelvic exam should be performed gently, using a narrow speculum that is lubricated only with water (other lubricants may interfere with the chemical test for acid phosphatase). Note the condition of the hymen and write a brief statement about what you find (e.g., "Hymen was recently ruptured" or "Remnants of hymen are visible, with no evidence of trauma"). Obtain all other samples and cultures mentioned in the previous section, and perform a bimanual exam of the uterus and adnexa, searching for evidence of trauma, tenderness, masses, hematoma, or pregnancy. Do a rectal exam and check for blood, stains of semen or lubricant, and evidence of trauma; wait until specimens have been obtained from this area before doing a digital exam (if indicated).

Since about 3–4% of rape victims contract gonorrhea, and because of the possibility of false-negative results on the culture and the potential difficulty of establishing follow-up visits, gonorrhea prophylaxis should be provided at the initial visit (see Chapter 9). However, syphilis develops in only about 0.1% of rape victims, so only the VDRL should be performed and a return visit scheduled to repeat the test (and rule out pregnancy) in 6 weeks. If the syphilis test is positive, treat as indicated (see Chapter 9). If pregnancy is a possibility as a result of the rape, administer high-dose estrogen within 72 hours of the incident or insert an intrauterine device (see Chapter 9) to prevent implantation. Submit all collected evidence (slides, laboratory reports, photographs, clothing, etc.) to the police as evidence and obtain a written receipt at that time.

Patient Education: Discuss the concept of rape trauma syndrome. At some point, victims may be offered information on local support groups. Consult local listings for groups or contact Victims Anonymous, an organization providing information about support groups for victims of sexual assault and abuse, at:

Victims Anonymous
9514-9 Reseda Blvd., # 605
North Ridge, California 91324
Tel.: (818) 993-1139

Also, many states and counties have hotlines for victims of sexual assault (and/or domestic violence) that can provide these persons with immediate telephone access to trained counselors; many are toll-free. These numbers should be obtained well in advance by primary care providers (before being called upon to care for a rape victim) so that they can be readily provided to patients. Other organizations that may provide referral information are the National Organization for Women (NOW) and Planned Parenthood. Contact local chapters of these organizations or:

National NOW
1401 New York Avenue, NW
Suite 800
Washington, D.C. 20005-2102
Tel.: (202) 347-2279

Planned Parenthood Federation
810 7th Avenue
New York, New York 10019
Tel.: (212) 541-7800 or (212) 603-4600

Follow-up: Schedule a return visit in 6 weeks (or earlier if this is considered necessary to ensure continuity of care and provide an opportunity for support and counseling).

▸ Office Management of Depression

Laboratory Tests: As needed to rule out underlying causes of symptoms (e.g., hyperparathyroidism, hypothyroidism, anemia, pancreatic tumor, Cushing's syndrome). Complete blood count, urinalysis, T_4, and VDRL are standard, and electrocardiographic evaluation before and during treatment with tricyclics are indicated for patients with conduction defects and possibly for those receiving high-dose tricyclic therapy. A blood or urine test may be advisable for women who are uncertain about their pregnancy status to avoid inadvertent fetal exposure to medications. A few tests, such as the dexamethasone suppression test (DST), thyroid-releasing hormone (TRH) stimulation test, urinary assay for MHPG, and measurement of cerebrospinal 5-HIAA, are being used to demonstrate physical changes in depression, but none are absolutely effective for screening purposes.

Therapeutic Measures: For conditions in which anxiety (often accompanied by somatic complaints and insomnia) is the predominant feature, an antianxiety drug (e.g., one of the benzodiazepines) may be indicated. However, a tranquilizer will only allay the anxiety, and depression disguised by these symptoms will become more obvious when this type of drug is used. Therefore, benzodiazepines are not recommended for treatment of depression.

The character of any diagnosed depression (e.g., whether it is reactive, endogenous, or part of a bipolar disorder) should be determined in order to choose an appropriate treatment plan. The most common type, reactive depression, accounts for about 70% of the depressions treated in the United States every year. Depressions of this type are precipitated by an identifiable adverse life experience such as the death of a significant person, financial difficulties, marital failure, or some other loss, or may follow physical illness, occur as a side effect of certain medications, or occur secondary to some other psychiatric disorder. Those related to a major loss are termed "grief reactions" and those related to a physical or psychologic condition are called "secondary depressions." Grief reactions often do not require medication, but will respond to such nonspecific treatments as support and concern on the part of the primary care provider, a change in environment, the passage of time, and sometimes professional counseling. In fact, drug treatment of normal grief reactions may actually interfere with the normal process of grieving. However, any depression that is severe (interferes with normal daily functioning) or prolonged (several weeks to months, depending on the severity of the loss) should generally be treated with drugs and possibly psychotherapy. Treatment of a depression secondary to a medical or psychiatric condition should generally be postponed until the underlying disorder is evaluated and treatment begun. Then, if indicated, an antidepressant medication may be used in combination with the treatment of an underlying physical condition. However, depressions secondary to another psychiatric disorder are best managed by a psychiatrist.

Endogenous depression, the second most common type of depression (accounting for about 25% of all depressions), is thought to be based on a genetic-biochemical abnormality that interferes with the individual's coping ability. Characteristically, there are disturbances of vital or "vegetative" functions (e.g., normal rhythms of sleep, appetite, sex, and motor activity), and often there is a diurnal variation in the intensity of symptoms (worse in the morning and improve as the day goes on). If, as in reactive depression, there is an identifiable precipitating factor (e.g., a loss), the response in the endogenous depression is often exaggerated in proportion to the life event, and symptoms tend to persist in spite of improvement in the patient's life circumstances. In this condition, relapses tend to occur.

When medication is indicated for a primary depression, tricyclic antidepressants are usually the drugs of choice (see Table 13.12), but there is evidence that patients with atypical depressive symptoms (e.g., overeating and weight gain, overwhelming anxiety, agitation, phobias, obsessive-compulsive features, hypersomnia, and somatic complaints) may respond better to monoamine oxidase (MAO) inhibitors (see Table 13.12). Agoraphobia (fear of open public places or of situations where crowds might be found) with secondary depression and pain syndromes with depression also seem to be particularly responsive to MAO inhibitors. Of the first-generation tricyclics, imipramine, protriptyline, and desipramine are relatively non-sedating and are thus most effective with patients whose depressions are characterized as withdrawn or retarded, while amitriptyline, nortriptyline, and doxepin are better choices for anxious or agitated, depressed patients since these drugs are more sedating.

Other considerations for choosing an antidepressant include a positive response to a particular drug in the past or a family history of a response to a particular antidepressant, the patient's age, and any concurrent illnesses, particularly diseases of the cardiovascular (acute myocardial infarction is an absolute contraindication to antidepressant therapy), genitourinary, gastrointestinal, or central nervous systems, since these drugs vary somewhat in their hypotensive, cardiotoxic, and anticholinergic effects. For example, trazodone, which ranks low in anticholinergic effects, is the best choice for older men who have prostatic hypertrophy, and doxepin may offer relatively low cardiotoxicity for patients with cardiac disease. The anticholinergic potency of amitriptyline may make it a good choice for patients with concurrent gastrointestinal disorders (except esophageal hiatus hernia). A previous trial with a particular drug should not be considered unsuccessful unless the patient failed to respond to the maximum tolerated dosages given over a period of 4–6 weeks. The most common reasons for unsuccessful treatment with antidepressant medications are poor selection of treatable depressions, failure to warn patients of potential side effects, underdosage (either iatrogenic or due to poor patient compliance), and the typical delay in onset of action (1–4 weeks). Most patients will obtain relief of anxiety and insomnia very early in therapy (within the first few days of treatment), and increased energy and decreased concern with somatic complaints usually occur in the second or third week of therapy. However, relief of the depression is often not evident until the fourth week, and sexual dysfunction may also not be relieved for several weeks. Therefore, it is important to warn the patient of potential side effects and to explain the expected course of therapy at the onset in order to avoid discouragement and noncompliance.

The initial dosage is similar for most of the tricyclic antidepressants (usually 75–150 mg/day in three divided doses), with the exception of protriptyline (15–40 mg/day). Variables such as the severity of the depression, availability of follow-up, and the age and general health of the patient may modify the dosage (e.g., elderly patients generally require much lower dosages than younger adults). Once a medication is begun, the dosage is increased gradually to obtain a maximum response with a minimum number of side effects. Typically, if the initial dosage is well tolerated after 1–7 days, the daily dosage is increased by 25–50 mg one to three times per week until side effects occur, a positive response is obtained, or the standard dosage level of 150 mg/day (less for protriptyline) is reached (this usually occurs during the first week). After side effects are minimized, the total daily amount may be given in a single evening dose, taking advantage of the sedative properties of the medications. For most patients, a daily dosage of 150–200 mg is sufficient to obtain relief of symptoms. However, if a response to standard-dose therapy does not take place after 2 weeks and no side effects have occurred, the dosage can again be increased gradually until side effects, a clinical response, or the maximum dosage range is reached (see Table 13.12). If a response is still not obtained after 1 month of high-dose therapy, blood drug levels should be monitored or a different medication tried. Blood plasma levels can vary considerably (up to 30-fold) among individuals receiving similar dosages, and those that are higher than the recommended range (a plasma steady state of approximately 100 ng/mL is optimum for most of the tricyclics) can be countertherapeutic. Another tricyclic, usually one with an opposite neurotransmitter effect (regarding serotonin-norepinephrine uptake), or an MAO inhibitor may be tried, but if a response has not been obtained after two treatment attempts, a psychiatric consultation should be obtained.

After 3 weeks of treatment with one tricyclic at maximum doses with no significant response, the switch to another one may sometimes be made with full therapeutic doses. For instance, if amitriptyline is often chosen for the first trial, and a switch to desipramine or amoxapine is intended, either one can be substituted for amitriptyline at the same dosage level instead of reinitiating therapy with the second drug in the usual way, since both have less sedative and anticholinergic actions and are therefore generally better tolerated. Once a clinical response is obtained, the drug should be continued at that dosage for several weeks to months and thereafter gradually decreased, monitoring the patient closely for recurrence of symptoms in order to provide the lowest effective dose for the duration of the depression. In most cases, tapering can begin within 3–9 months of therapy, decreasing by 25–50 mg every month or so, until the dosage is about one-half to one-third of that required during the acute illness. The patient should continue this maintenance therapy for a period of time. Then, depending on the clinical response, the drug may again be gradually decreased until the patient requires no medication. However, if there is a history of prior attacks of depression, treatment should be continued for at least 3–6 months after remission (unless the duration of the illness was very brief and was followed by good treatment results), and it may be preferable to continue prolonged maintenance therapy rather than to treat the illness episodically. Maintenance dosages are usually one-third to one-half of the peak amount, but the lowest effective dose for the individual patient is recommended, and periodic attempts to reduce this dose should be made.

MAO inhibitors may be effective for depressions with the specific features mentioned above (e.g., high levels of anxiety, somatic complaints, overeating and weight gain, agitation, phobic and obsessive-compulsive features, hypersomnia) or for patients who have been unresponsive to complete trials of tricyclics (allowing a 1- to 2-week "washout" period after discontinuing the tricyclic before initiating treatment with an MAO inhibitor). The initial dosage of phenelzine is usually 45–60 mg/day and may be increased to 75–90 mg/day if necessary. Tranylcypromine is usually begun at a dosage of about 20 mg/day and isocarboxazid at 10–20 mg/day, and either may be increased to 30 mg/day if needed. Therapeutic levels of MAO inhibitors tend to be more quickly achieved than those of tricyclics, since there is a shorter lag in clinical response and a narrower range of dosages. However, it is vital that patients be instructed to avoid ingestion of tyramine-containing foods and sympathomimetic drugs while taking MAO inhibitors because of the potential for hypertensive crises.

Patients with a primary depression that is bipolar (manic-depressive) should be treated with lithium carbonate (alone or in combination with an antidepressant). The depressive phase of this illness may be indistinguishable from an endogenous depression, but a history of episodes of manic or hypomanic behavior will help identify a bipolar affective disorder. Also, some patients with severe recurrent unipolar depression that tricyclics and MAO inhibitors have not effectively alleviated or prevented may respond to lithium therapy. The decision of a primary care provider to initiate lithium therapy for severe bipolar or unipolar primary depression should be made only after consultation with a psychiatrist because of the extremely narrow therapeutic range and the danger of drug toxicity. Lithium therapy is discussed in more detail elsewhere.

Patient Education: Patients should be encouraged to maintain positive social contacts and a normal, active life but to make changes in counterproductive behaviors (e.g., overworking, inactivity, excessive alcohol use, recreational drug use). Napping should also be avoided, since it may worsen insomnia. Avoidable major life changes such as marriage or divorce, taking a vacation or leave of absence from work, moving, or changing jobs are to be discouraged during depression, since all changes tend to introduce a certain amount of stress into the person's life, and excessive stress can worsen the illness. Other specific measures to reduce stress should be recommended (see "Stress Reduction"), including meditative relaxation techniques, progressive muscle relaxation, biofeedback, regular physical exercise (walking, jogging, biking, swimming, etc.), participation in recreational activities that the patient enjoys, talking out feelings with a family member or close friend, and individual or group psychotherapy. The complicating effects of alcoholism and drug abuse on depression should be discussed and patients with complicating substance abuse problems encouraged to join Alcoholics Anonymous or another substance abuse support group. All patients receiving antidepressant drug therapy should be warned against using alcohol because of its interaction with antidepressants. Women should be advised to avoid becoming pregnant while receiving antidepressant therapy because of the risk of fetal drug exposure.

Patients receiving antidepressants should be warned about the typical delay in onset of action (1–4 weeks) of these drugs and about the need to obtain an optimum dosage gradually. Potential side effects should be discussed and patients urged to bring any side effects to the physician's attention whenever they occur. Most of the side effects of tricyclics are minor and well tolerated, and patients can often be encouraged to continue taking the medication when it is explained that the unpleasant sensations are indications that the drug is beginning to have an effect. The most significant side effects include cardiac and anticholinergic effects. Palpitations, tachycardia, orthostatic hypotension, arrhythmias (at high doses), cardiac conduction prolongations, dry mouth, constipation, urinary retention, blurred vision, loss of libido, decreased orgasm, erectile or ejaculatory difficulties, reduced seizure threshold, photosensitivity (infrequent), oversedation, confusional reactions (usually in patients over age 40), tremor, and agitation have all been know to occur. There is also a wide range of interactions of tricyclics with other drugs (including alcohol) and serious cardiovascular and CNS effects of overdosage (including tachycardia, hypotension, respiratory deficiency, convulsive seizures, heart blocks, arrhythmias, coma with shock, hyperpyrexia, smooth muscle paralysis, and delirium). The effects of tricyclic overdoses are of particular concern, since any patient with a depression serious enough to warrant drug therapy should be considered a potential suicide, and the potential lethal dosage may be only 10 times the therapeutic daily dosage (or even less).

Patients receiving MAO inhibitors should be instructed to avoid ingestion of sympathomimetic amines in the form of sympathomimetic drugs or tyramine- or levodopa-containing foods because these may precipitate a severe hypertensive crisis. The following is a list of foods that the patient should be told to avoid (provide patients with a written list):

Sausage
Bologna
Liver (all types)
Sardines
Anchovies
Pickled herring
Caviar
Chinese pea pods
Broad pod beans
Beer
Ale
Wines (especially red wine and sherry)
Avocados
Raisins

Meat prepared with tenderizer	Canned figs
Aged cheeses	Excessive chocolate
Concentrated yeast extract	Soy sauce
Yogurt	Overripe fruits
Sour cream	

Also to be avoided are reserpine, meperidine, and all stimulants, including excessive caffeine and prescription and over-the-counter cold remedies and diet aids (most contain phenylpropanolamine). There are also a number of drugs that may enhance the action of MAO inhibitors (e.g., thiazide diuretics) and lead to hypotension; patients should be advised to contact the physician if there is any doubt about the compatibility of a particular medication with the MAO inhibitor. Postural hypotension is a common side effect, so patients should be cautioned about sitting or standing suddenly and taking hot baths. Other potential side effects of MAO inhibitor therapy are dizziness, delayed micturition, dry mouth, constipation, tachycardia, sweating, tremor, nausea, drowsiness, insomnia, agitation, and toxic psychosis. A craving for sweets (and resultant weight gain) and anorgasmia may occur with long-term therapy. A hypertensive crisis should be treated by giving phentolamine, 1.2 mg IV every 5 minutes as needed, to lower blood pressure. The need to keep all of these drugs away from children should be emphasized.

Follow-up: Schedule frequent, short (15- to 20-minute) visits on a regular basis for all depressed patients. Initially, the patient should be seen at least two or three times per week; the frequency may be decreased later as the patient improves. Some patients (e.g., irresponsible, substance-abusing, or possibly suicidal patients or those in ill health) require closer observation and more frequent follow-up. It may be helpful to obtain the assistance of family members for such patients. Female patients should be questioned about their menstrual history, and other means of pregnancy detection should be used if necessary to avoid inadvertent fetal exposure to drugs. One should periodically question patients about alcohol or drug abuse, review all prescription and nonprescription medications being taken by the patient, and discontinue all nonvital ones. For medical and legal reasons, the patient's suicide potential should be ascertained at each visit (see "Suicide Prevention"), and drug prescriptions strictly controlled. It is recommended that prescriptions be limited to a total of 1.5 g (i.e., less than a lethal dose), which may be less than a 1- or 2-week supply at moderate dosages. For some patients, it may be simplest to give a new prescription at each visit or to have a responsible family member or other adult dispense the medication. Unlimited refill orders are never justified. Immediate psychiatric consultation is indicated if suicide is considered to be even a remote possibility. One should ask patients direct questions about thoughts of suicide, as well as about other feelings. Feelings of helplessness, hopelessness, lack of plans for life in the future, and a well-thought-out plan for committing suicide ("if he were planning to do so") are all indicators of suicide risk, as is a history of previous suicide attempts. Such patients may be candidates for hospitalization and possibly ECT. When referring such a patient, it is important to discuss one's concerns openly, as well as one's reasons for believing that a specialist would be better able to help the patient. To avoid giving the patient the impression that he is being abandoned because you are tired of him, assure him that you will continue to be his primary care provider, and schedule at least one return visit after the patient has seen the specialist for the first time. Maintain contact with the psychiatrist as well, to avoid prescribing incompatible drugs in your continued medical care of the patient.

▸ *The Patient Taking Lithium*

Laboratory Tests: The decision to initiate lithium therapy should be made by a psychiatrist only after a complete work-up, including a medical history and physical exam, complete blood count, T_4, blood urea nitrogen, creatinine, serum electrolytes, serum calcium and phosphorus (to help rule out hypercalcemia, related renal disease), urinalysis, and electrocardiogram. It is particularly important to obtain a kidney history for familial, primary, and secondary renal disease (e.g., hypertension, diabetes, and other sequelae). Also, many experts recommend a 24-hour creatinine clearance test (as an index of glomerular function), or a urine concentration test (to assess renal tubular function) or both. A urine or blood pregnancy test may be indicated for women who are uncertain of their pregnancy status. Acute renal failure, acute myocardial infarction, first trimester of pregnancy (use during pregnancy carries a serious risk for the fetus, especially of right heart abnormalities), later trimesters of pregnancy (less risk), breast feeding, and myasthenia gravis are generally accepted contraindications to lithium therapy. The feasibility of long-term prophylactic lithium therapy should be discussed with the patient and family, and informed consent obtained and documented.

Often the psychiatrist will opt to initiate therapy but will have the patient return to the primary care provider for periodic blood level determinations and most of the routine follow-up care. The daily dosage necessary to achieve therapeutic blood levels is determined by giving a test dose of 600 mg lithium carbonate and then drawing a blood sample 24 hours later. Thereafter lithium is administered (in two divided doses) according to the total daily amount listed next to the 24-hour lithium level in the following table:

24-hour Lithium Level	Predicted Total Daily Dose
Less than 0.05 mEq/L	3,600 mg
0.05–0.09 mEq/L	2,700 mg
0.10–0.14 mEq/L	1,800 mg
0.15–0.19 mEq/L	1,200 mg
0.20–0.23 mEq/L	900 mg
0.24–0.30 mEq/L	600 mg
More than 0.30 mEq/L	300 mg

Therapeutic Measures: At the start of therapy, weekly blood level determinations should be made (blood for the lithium levels should always be drawn *12 hours after the last dose*) until the lithium level stabilizes within desired therapeutic limits. These range from 1.0 to 1.6 mEq/L for acute manic attacks (there is often a lag of 4 to 10 days to obtain these high serum levels, so a neuroleptic such as haloperidol, 5–30 mg/day orally, may be used and then gradually withdrawn as the therapeutic lithium levels are established) and from 0.4 to 1.0 mEq/L for prophylactic maintenance. Maintenance levels vary from individual to individual, but should be limited to the lowest dose possible in order to protect the kidneys while preventing psychiatric relapse. Until recently, blood levels of 0.6 to 1.2 mEq/L were considered standard, but there is some evidence that many patients may be successfully managed with a plasma level as low as 0.5 to 0.7 mEq/L. The dosage required to achieve therapeutic blood levels also varies considerably from individual to individual, but the usual range for healthy young patients is 900–1,500 mg/day (in two divided doses), and that for healthy elderly patients is 300–900 mg/day (in two divided doses). Dosages for patients in ill health (e.g., with chronic renal failure or hyponatremia) should be individually titrated. Once the patient has been stabilized within the therapeutic range, lithium levels can be checked every few weeks and then monthly. Serum levels for patients who have remained stable (within the therapeutic range) for several months to a year may be checked as often as the provider feels is necessary (usually every 3–4 months). Lithium levels should also be checked whenever there is any condition that may result in altered sodium levels (e.g., diarrhea, excessive perspiration, dehydration, or use of diuretics) or when there are signs or symptoms of lithium toxicity.

Great caution should be exercised in treating elderly patients and those with disorders involving the kidney, thyroid, brain (especially epilepsy), heart, gastrointestinal tract, or electrolyte balance. The incidence of toxicity is higher in elderly patients, so they may need to be maintained on slightly lower serum levels than those used with younger patients. Chronic renal failure and hyponatremia will induce lithium retention and require lower dosages and closer clinical and laboratory monitoring. Dose reductions are required if a low-sodium diet is followed, and similar adjustments may be needed when there are changes in the patient's general health or renal status, or when other medications are used. Patients using a thiazide diuretic have increased lithium reabsorption from the proximal renal tubules, resulting in increased serum lithium levels; the lithium dosage should be reduced by 25–40% when the patient is receiving 50 mg/day of hydrochlorothiazide. Potassium-sparing diuretics (spironolactone, triamterene, amiloride) may cause increased serum lithium levels to a lesser extent, requiring careful monitoring and lithium dosage adjustments. Loop diuretics (furosemide, bumetanide, ethacrynic acid) do not appear to cause lithium retention. Furosemide (Lasix) is thought to be the safest diuretic for use in lithium-treated patients, but it should be coprescribed only when clearly indicated and with appropriate caution and monitoring.

High lithium blood level peaks should always be avoided. Divided dose administration is imperative (two doses/day), and missed doses should never be made up. Mealtime administration is helpful for slowing the absorption rate. Lithium overdosage may occur accidentally or intentionally, or may result from poor monitoring, salt or fluid depletion, or kidney disease. Toxic effects usually begin at blood levels above 1.5 mEq/L, with frank toxicity occurring at levels above 2.0 mEq/L. Signs and symptoms of lithium intoxication include polyuria, polydipsia, anorexia, nausea, vomiting, diarrhea, increasing neurologic dysfunction (e.g., tremors, vertigo, ataxia, confusion, stupor, seizures, marked muscle weakness, hyperreflexia, rigidity, opisthotonos) in the absence of the anticholinergic syndrome, slurred speech, dysarthria, blurred vision, drowsiness, grunting, nystagmus, nephropathy (nephrogenic diabetes insipidus, renal failure), incontinence, anuria, hypotension, arrhythmia, coma, and possibly death at extremely high levels. Treatment includes discontinuation of lithium (and of oral diuretic therapy), monitoring and maintenance of vital functions, induced emesis and gastric lavage (for recent massive ingestions or serum levels above 3 mEq/L), IV administration of fluids and electrolytes, maintenance of adequate hydration and sodium, and monitoring of lithium and electrolyte levels. For significant intoxication with normal renal function, forced diuresis with an osmotic diuretic (e.g., mannitol, urea) and saline to increase renal clearance may be indicated. Acetazolamide (Diamox) is also helpful in decreasing lithium reabsorption in the proximal tubule, as is urinary alkalinization with sodium bicarbonate. For more severe intoxication (extremely ill patients with coma or seizures, or possibly patients with a serum lithium level of 4.0 mEq/L or higher), hemodialysis or peritoneal dialysis may be necessary. A benzodiazepine may be given as needed for agitation and/or reported seizures, or phenytoin may be given for seizures.

Patient Education: Discuss the drug, its side effects, and precautions with the patient and family, and provide them with written instructions about taking the drug, diet, and what to report (e.g., side effects, unusual fluid loss through sweating, etc.). Women should be warned about the risks of fetal exposure to lithium and advised to avoid pregnancy during therapy. Bottle feeding is recommended for mothers and infants, since lithium is excreted in the breast milk (the concentration in breast milk is one-third to one-half that in serum). Have patients take the drug on a divided dose schedule (two doses/day) and with meals to slow absorption. Stress the importance of a stable diet, with fairly uniform salt and fluid intake and avoidance of dehydration. Instruct patients never to "make up" forgotten doses; to report any side effects (polyuria, polydipsia, tremor), concomitant drug use, changes in general health, or episodes of abnormal sweating, vomiting, or diarrhea; and to omit doses if they are actively vomiting or not eating. Emphasize the importance of compliance with therapy regardless of the absence of mood swings (loss of episodes of mania may be undesirable for many patients with bipolar affective disorder, making compliance difficult) and of scheduled follow-up visits.

Follow-up: At each visit, question patients about side effects and discuss compliance with therapy, diet (including fluid and salt intake), and any concerns they may have. Questions about menstrual history and/or other means of pregnancy detection are important for preventing inadvertent fetal exposure to lithium. With all patients who have affective disorders (i.e., involving depression), it is important to ascertain the mental status and suicide risk (discussed in more detail under "Suicide Prevention"). Overtly psychotic, hypomanic, or manic symptoms and the possibility of suicide (or any uncertainty about suicide potential) are indications for referral and possibly hospitalization. The frequency of clinical and laboratory monitoring of lithium and electrolyte levels should be as described above, but more frequent follow-up and monitoring of lithium levels are required for patients who have had unusual sodium and/or fluid losses (following a low-sodium diet, vomiting, diarrhea, excessive perspiration, dehydration, use of diuretics, excessive alcohol or caffeine intake); elderly patients; patients with cardiac, brain, gastrointestinal, electrolyte balance, renal, or thyroid disturbances; and patients exhibiting any of the signs or symptoms suggestive of toxicity. In addition to regular blood level determinations, the general health, thyroid function, and renal status of patients on lithium therapy should be evaluated annually. Apart from the regular questioning about lithium-related conditions, the yearly evaluation should include blood pressure determination, urinalysis, and blood urea nitrogen and serum creatinine determinations. Creatinine clearance and urine concentration tests are also recommended when there are any signs of renal disease. Any indication of renal abnormality calls for a review of the history and repetition of kidney function tests, and possibly more extensive work-up and consultation with a specialist.

▸ *Suicide Prevention*

Laboratory Tests: None.

Therapeutic Measures: Whenever a patient's symptoms or answers to questions suggest a diagnosis of depression, it is extremely important to evaluate during the initial interview and *at each follow-up visit* the potential for suicide. Classically, suicide attempts occur when the patient is going into or coming out of a depression (i.e., when he or she still has some energy to carry out the attempt), which emphasizes the importance of early diagnosis and extensive follow-up of all depressed patients. One of the most important ways of assessing a suicide risk is to discuss the question with the patient. Contrary to the prevailing concern that talking about suicide will "put the idea into the depressed patient's mind," questioning the patient makes the act less likely. It also helps in evaluating the degree of risk as well as identifying the most appropriate method of management. Almost all patients who are depressed have already had at least an occasional thought about suicide, so discussion will not put a new idea into their minds. However, bringing the subject into the open in a sensitive, nonjudgmental way helps to defuse whatever anxiety or guilt the patient may have associated with the idea and make the patient feel more comfortable about discussing "forbidden" thoughts and feelings. Most patients appreciate the concern that prompted the question and feel relieved to realize that they are not unique or "crazy" to have had such ideas. However, the question should be asked in a way that does not make answering "yes" difficult. One possible way to word the question is, "I'm concerned about one thing. Everyone who has this illness [depression] at one time or another begins to think that his family, friends, and everyone else would be much better off without him. I'm sure that has happened to you, hasn't it?" Suggesting that every depressed person has had this thought (instead of blurting out, "You haven't been thinking about suicide, have you?") enables the patient to answer yes with relief instead of guilt or embarrassment. At that point it can be followed up with, "Can you tell me about it?" or "But my most important concern is *how close* you are to actually doing it. Can you tell me about this?" At some point, ask the patient, "Have you ever thought about *how* you would do it?" On the basis of the patient's answers, the decision of whether or not to hospitalize can be discussed. If the patient says that he or she is very close to suicide or is noncommittal, or has a specific, well-thought-out plan for self-destruction, referral and hospitalization are indicated. But if, after the issue has been discussed a little and the stigma removed, the patient can look you in the eye and say that although he or she has considered suicide, there is no thought of following through on it just now, chances are that this answer can be trusted. However, it is important to ask the patient to promise to contact you whenever suicidal impulses become strong and to provide a number(s) where you can be reached. Making this contract is a very important strategy that is commonly used by psychiatrists and other mental health care professionals, since most persons will keep that promise if they believe that they will receive a caring response. (It is useless to ask patients to promise not to commit suicide, since anyone who could confidently make such a promise would not be suicidal.) Any patient who cannot look you in the eye and make such a promise is probably not a good candidate for outpatient management.

A large percentage of low-risk but nevertheless potentially suicidal patients can be safely managed on a closely monitored outpatient basis. If the patient is not at severe risk of suicide (suicidal thoughts are fleeting and indefinite, and the patient does not consider them serious) and is able to care for himself, if he can promise to contact you when things become worse, and if other complicating factors are absent, office management on a primary care basis is feasible. In addition to the usual treatment measures (see "Office Management of Depression"), the following should be kept in mind to lessen the possibility of suicide:

Treat all serious depressions aggressively with appropriate antidepressants, avoiding underdosage, which is a common cause of treatment failure. The risk of a suicide attempt by overdose should be kept in mind and minimized, but that possibility does *not* call for withholding antidepressant medications.

To whatever extent possible, remove potential instruments for suicide from the patient's environment, including firearms and medications such as sedatives and hypnotics. Find out what the patient perceives as an acceptable means of suicide to assist in this step. For instance, some patients will readily consider a drug overdose when they are extremely suicidal but would never contemplate using razor blades. Enlist the support of family members in this endeavor.

Limit antidepressant prescriptions to a total amount that is less than a potentially lethal dose (e.g., 1.5 g for most of the tricyclics) without automatic refills. Use questioning about expected side effects as a gauge of treatment compliance. Larger quantities may be prescribed for economic reasons if another responsible adult is available to hold most of them and provide the patient with only nonlethal quantities or to administer single doses.

Treat every suicide gesture as a serious attempt (and an indication for referral), since there is no sure way to distinguish between a manipulative gesture and a resolute attempt. Remember that any person who makes such an attempt is distressed, and to dismiss any gesture as unimportant may prompt the patient to make a more serious attempt the next time because he feels that no one cares, because he is embarrassed, or because he wishes to "show you." Repeated threats or nonserious gestures may indicate a manipulative or hysterical patient; seek consultation for advice on the management of such a patient if a psychiatrist has determined (usual after a few hospitalizations) that actual suicide is not likely. Avoid simply dismissing the behavior as unimportant and conveying an attitude of noncaring.

Referral to a psychiatrist should be made when there is suicide potential or a depression not responding to treatment. It is also indicated for persons whose illness is long-standing or complex or who lack insight into their difficulties (these may require more intensive therapy than is available on a primary care basis). Prior to the referral, discuss with the patient why you feel that this step is indicated. The referral of a depressed patient must be handled very carefully. It may be helpful to say something like, "I know that you're still feeling awful and by now you may be beginning to feel hopeless, but you must take my word that your situation is *not* hopeless. However, although I still expect you to recover completely, you have not had as quick a response to therapy as I had hoped for." Then explain that you would like the patient to see Dr. X (refer to him or her by name in the initial discussion). Describe Dr. X as a psychiatrist whom you respect and frequently work with, who has had specialized training and more experience in treating this illness. Explaining that the visits with the psychiatrist will be similar to those the patient has had with you, and that you are interested in hearing the psychiatrist's advice, can help to allay fears about what to expect and communicate that you are still interested in the patient. Take time to discuss any questions or concerns that the patient has about the referral and mention that you feel that the delay in response may be due to your not having taken all of the best possible steps in treatment in this particular case (taking the blame off of the patient's shoulders). Using this discussion to communicate your continuing concern for the patient's well-being and your availability for other medical care is critical, since a depressed patient with decreased self-esteem may perceive the referral as a sign that you are tired of him and wish to be rid of him or that you blame him or see him as hopeless and have given up on him. Finally, scheduling at least one more follow-up visit after the patient has seen the psychiatrist for the first time will help to demonstrate the sincerity of your concern.

Whether the patient is referred or managed in the primary care setting, it is important to notify the family or other persons in the patient's support system of your concerns and explain the need for supervision. If possible, discuss this matter with the patient first in order to explain the need for this measure and to decide which family members or other persons are likely to be the most accepting and supportive of the patient at this time. Emphasize to these persons the need for tact, since a perception of being watched may make the patient feel worse and intensify the suicidal tendencies.

A major depression characterized by feelings of despair, hopelessness, helplessness, and unworthiness, and a preconceived, available means for committing suicide, is unquestionably an indication for immediate hospitalization under the care of a psychiatrist. Unless contraindicated, ECT will probably be administered. In addition to the existence of a concrete and feasible plan for self-destruction, other factors to be considered in deciding whether to hospitalize a patient include a complicating substance abuse problem, a family history of suicide, previous attempts at suicide, reports of recent suicide threats to family members or friends (or actual attempts), level of responsibility (a mother of small children or a college president overseeing several employees may be less likely to give up on life than a retired widower who never remarried), and the absence or presence of a support system of reliable, caring, and nurturing persons (family members, co-workers, friends). Threats of suicide may be indirect, such as "I know my family will be better off without me" or "If anything ever happens to me, I know you'll be able to carry on."

Patient Education: This is the same as for depression (see "Office Management of Depression"). In addition to giving patients your telephone number so that you can be contacted when they have strong suicidal tendencies, it is a good idea to provide them with the number of a local suicide hotline where they can obtain immediate telephone contact with trained counselors. Not only is this a good backup in the event that you cannot be reached quickly when the patient needs you most, but it can be presented as a possible source of readily available, trained persons with whom the patient can talk when other persons (i.e., friends, family) are not accessible.

Follow-up: Schedule frequent, brief (15- to 20-minute) visits and evaluate the suicide risk during each contact. (See also "Office Management of Depression.")

▸ *Anxiety Reaction*

Laboratory Tests: As needed to rule out other causes of the physical symptoms (e.g., hyperthyroidism, myocardial infarction, congestive heart failure, anemia, adrenal insufficiency, hypoglycemia, cerebral arteriosclerosis, labyrinthitis, and drug reaction).

Therapeutic Measures: Distinguish an anxiety reaction from transient situational disturbances (stress reaction or adjustment disorder) in which anxiety, depression, and a number of physical symptoms may develop in response to episodic stress. Transient situational disturbances are nonpsychopathologic responses to stress that exceed the adaptive capacity of an individual, and will usually respond to identification of the precipitating stress (e.g., college exams, changes in interpersonal relationships, work deadlines, financial difficulties) and reassurance. Patients in whom anxiety is rooted in a more complex disorder (obsessive-compulsive disorder, somatiform disorder) should be referred for psychiatric evaluation and therapy.

Reduction of the patient's life stresses and augmentation of his or her defensive structuring are the primary concerns in treating anxiety neurosis. Psychotherapy is the treatment of choice, so referral to a professional counselor is important, but some strategies for stress management and suggestions about environmental restructuring can be presented on a primary care basis during regular office visits.

Early recognition and removal of a source of stress before the symptoms become severe is important. This requires careful attention to daily events that evoke an anxiety response, as well as factors that function as alleviators, and may be assisted by having patients keep a daily log of such factors. Specific relaxation techniques may be helpful in reducing anxiety, and some of them may be easily taught during a single office visit (see "Stress Reduction"). Yoga, meditation, progressive relaxation, biofeedback, and regular physical exercise are some of the methods that may be tried; in most cases, a combination of approaches (e.g., meditation plus physical exercise) may be more effective than any one method.

The benzodiazepines are the drugs of choice for most patients with anxiety reaction. They have a high therapeutic-toxic ratio and a low risk of physical dependency compared to other agents (e.g., barbiturates, antipsychotic agents, and other sedative-hypnotics), and are effective in ameliorating anxiety without causing excessive CNS depression. However, they should be reserved for relief of severe, incapacitating symptoms and prescribed only for a limited period of time. Elimination of all anxiety is not desirable, since anxiety may serve a useful function by motivating the patient to work with alternative nondrug therapies. Medications should be an adjunct to the overall treatment plan, which includes psychotherapy, modification of lifestyle, relaxation therapy, and development of alternative coping strategies, and should be limited to the smallest effective dosage and discontinued at the earliest possible time. Factors to be considered in choosing a particular benzodiazepine include the patient's age, concurrent illnesses, liver status, concurrent drug therapy, desirability of sedative effects (i.e., for insomnia), and the risk of drug dependence. In general, longer-acting drugs (prazepam, clorazepate, diazepam, chlordiazepoxide, and halazepam) are preferred, since their prolonged action necessitates less frequent dosing and the withdrawal effects are less severe than those of shorter-acting agents. A long-acting agent is also preferable in dependency-prone individuals (suggested by a history of drug or alcohol abuse, a tendency for the patient to overemphasize the need for drug therapy, reported loss of prescriptions, or requests for prescriptions by telephone). The shorter-acting agents, tempazepam, oxazepam, and lorazepam, do not undergo oxidative metabolism in the liver and are thus preferred for patients with liver disease or those receiving concurrent drug therapy. (Alprazolam also has a short half-life, but does undergo oxidative hepatic metabolism and is therefore not a preferred agent for patients with these factors.) Diazepam (Valium) and chlordiazepoxide (Librium) are the most commonly prescribed benzodiazepines; the recommended dosage for diazepam is 2–5 mg three to four times a day and for chlordiazepoxide it is 5–10 mg three to four times a day, but some patients require much less frequent doses and should be told to resort to the drug only when the need is strong.

In certain patients who exhibit primarily somatic anxiety, often in the cardiovascular system, beta blockers (alprenolol, oxprenolol, practolol, propranolol, sotalol) may be the drugs of choice, since they are helpful in relieving peripheral somatic symptoms. However, merely relieving these symptoms is not helpful when the anxiety is predominantly central or psychic (marked by apprehensive expectation, dread, etc.) and somatic complaints are of secondary importance, as is common in most cases of anxiety reaction. The advantage of beta blockers over benzodiazepines is that they cause a low incidence of drowsiness, tolerance, dependence, and abuse, but benzodiazepines are far superior drugs for the treatment of most forms of anxiety.

Patient Education: Tell the patient at the onset of therapy that the drug will be prescribed for a fixed period of time, and discuss the risks of psychologic or physical dependence. Discuss the actions and other side effects of benzodiazepines, including sedation, disturbed sleep patterns, and depression. Depression as a side effect of benzodiazepine use occurs most frequently when a misdiagnosis is made about an underlying depression that is disguised by symptoms of anxiety. The development of an increasingly depressed mood calls for discontinuation of the antianxiety agent and treatment for depression (e.g., with a tricyclic or MAO inhibitor as indicated). Paradoxical reactions such as agitation and confusion may also arise as side effects, but these occur less frequently with benzodiazepines than with barbiturates. Warn patients not to use alcohol while taking a benzodiazepine, and discuss any other drugs the patient may be taking (prescription and nonprescription) and the potential for adverse drug interactions. Suggest that patients wait to see how they react to the drug before attempting to drive or operate machinery while using an anxiolytic. Advise patients to reduce or eliminate caffeine intake and stress the importance of a healthy, balanced diet and adequate rest. Encourage patients to pursue nondrug approaches to anxiety reduction such as hypnosis, meditation, biofeedback, relaxation, regular physical exercise, and psychotherapy, and provide instructions for simple meditative or progressive relaxation techniques (see "Stress Reduction"). Discuss environmental manipulation as a means of eliminating some of the stresses that may be contributing factors, and offer referral for psychotherapy as an alternative to chronic anxiolytic use.

Follow-up: Schedule frequent, brief (15- to 20-minute) follow-up visits with patients taking anxiolytics, particularly at the onset of therapy. Initially the patient should be seen two or three times weekly, and the presence or absence of a positive response to the drug should be noted after 1 week (relief of symptoms is usually evident within a week and is optimal within 4–6 weeks when a benzodiazepine is clinically effective). Question the patient about any side effects and be alert for depression or other adverse drug reactions (e.g., drowsiness, fatigue, bradycardia, visual disturbances). After the patient begins to experience relief of symptoms, the frequency of visits may be decreased (e.g., to every week or so), but they should continue throughout therapy. It is a good idea to limit the drug prescription to a 2-week supply without refill to facilitate compliance. Limit the dose prescribed to the minimum effective dose and make every effort to minimize the duration of therapy ($\frac{1}{2}$ to 4 weeks); brief, intermittent drug therapy is preferable to long-term therapy. Treatment with 5–10 mg diazepam daily (or the equivalent) for longer than 2 months calls for tapered withdrawal of the medication (reducing the dose by approximately 10% per day). Cross-dependent tolerance may occur in some patients, necessitating higher therapeutic doses, but a daily dosage of 40 mg diazepam (or the equivalent) should be avoided, because such high doses may result in severe withdrawal syndromes. Use follow-up visits to offer support, advice, and hope for improvement by helping the patient to identify and discuss factors contributing to the anxiety state (e.g., feelings of isolation, recent loss, fear of aging or death, a recent move into a nursing home). Involvement of family members or friends may be advisable if they are contributing to or reinforcing the patient's anxiety and diminishing his or her hope for a cure. If therapy is unsuccessful, referral to a specialist is indicated. The reason should be carefully explained to the patient and the possibility of continued primary care follow-up visits offered. It is important that such a patient not receive the impression that he is tiresome and that referral is a way to get rid of him.

▸ *Panic Attack*

Laboratory Tests: As needed to rule out physical causes of symptoms (e.g., cardiac disorders).

Therapeutic Measures: During the acute attack, the patient should be kept in a safe, isolated room so that he cannot harm himself or others. Have someone remain with the patient (at a distance of several feet) to reassure and monitor him. Sedate him with diazepam (Valium, 5–10 mg, IM or IV) or chlordiazepoxide (Librium, 50–100 mg, IM or IV) as soon as possible. If necessary, this may be followed in 3–4 hours by a repeat dose (5–10 mg diazepam or 25–50 mg chlordiazepoxide). Arrange for immediate psychiatric consultation, since the attack may signify the beginning of psychosis. Also, since this disorder tends to be recurrent, maintenance therapy may be required. Tricyclics and tetracyclic antidepressants at near-therapeutic doses (e.g., imipramine, 75–150 mg/day orally) will often provide relief for panic attacks. MAO inhibitors have been shown to be as effective as the tricyclics for this disorder, but have the disadvantage of requiring careful dietary regulation and are therefore not recommended as a first choice. Therapy with one benzodiazepine, alprazolam (Xanax), has also been effective for some patients at high dosage levels (10 mg/day), but the drawbacks of long-term benzodiazepine use must be considered. Beta blockers (e.g., propranolol) are also effective in reducing the peripheral somatic symptoms of panic attacks but are not helpful if the primary feature is psychic anxiety.

Patient Education: Offer support and reassurance, and explain the need for psychiatric consultation. When maintenance therapy with a particular medication is decided upon, discuss the actions, side effects, and drug interactions of that agent. Caution patients against the concomitant use of benzodiazepines and alcohol or other CNS depressant drugs, and explain the dietary restrictions (and provide a written list of foods to be avoided) if a MAO inhibitor is decided upon. Encourage patients to continue in psychotherapy, and discuss stress management and anxiety reduction strategies (see "Stress Reduction").

Follow-up: As needed to monitor the effectiveness of therapy and patient compliance.

▶ *Stress Reduction*

Laboratory Tests: None.

Therapeutic Measures: Instruct the patient in general and specific measures to reduce the amount and negative effects of psychologic stress. General measures include maintenance of a healthy diet (without excessive alcohol or caffeine intake), a regular exercise program, frequent involvement in enjoyable recreation (sports, reading, music, painting, hobbies), and adequate rest. Patients should be encouraged to experience all of their feelings, positive and negative, fully and to talk about negative feelings. Patients who have difficulty handling changes in unacceptable situations may benefit from instruction in problem-solving strategies by a professional counselor. Advise patients to avoid making several changes at once, since any changes, even positive ones, may be stressful if they occur all at the same time. Also, involvement in group activities and maintenance of close social ties are important in resisting the harmful consequences of stress.

Passive or mildly depressed patients seem to benefit most from deep breathing or meditative relaxation, but these techniques may also be used with active patients to supplement an exercise or movement therapy program. Many of these techniques may be taught in 5 to 10 minutes during a single office visit. Breath control is a simple and effective technique for reducing emotional tension based on the fact that in a state of tension, breathing automatically becomes shallow, rapid, and confined to the chest region (using primarily the intercostal muscles), whereas in a state of relaxation, breathing tends to deepen and slow down, and the abdominal muscles become primarily involved. By consciously slowing and deepening breathing, one can induce a state of relaxation that will generalize to the entire body. The steps of the breath control technique are as follows:

1. Sit or lie in a comfortable position with the arms and legs uncrossed and the body in alignment; loosen any restrictive clothing. Close your eyes and consciously surrender the weight of your body, allowing the chair to support you.
2. Take in a slow, deep breath from the diaphragm (to a mental count of 4). Pause, holding the breath (to a mental count of 4), and then exhale slowly and completely (to a mental count of 7 or 8), ending with a slight sigh. As you exhale, allow the muscles of the jaw, shoulders, back, arms, and legs to relax.

3. Repeat for several breaths. (It is preferable not to count the number of breaths, but simply to continue until you feel relaxed or for a period of about 15–20 minutes). Do this twice daily.
4. Supplement these deep-breathing sessions with mini-sessions throughout the day whenever you feel tense, or use an event or activity as a signal to remind you to focus on your breathing. For example, whenever the phone rings at work, take a slow, deep breath and count from 10 to 1 slowly before answering, or put a colored piece of tape on the clock as a reminder to breathe deeply whenever you look at it.

Meditation reduces tension and promotes relaxation by focusing attention away from stressful thoughts. There are a number of variations, but two simple ones are awareness meditation and meditation to a mantra (a soothing word or sound). In Awareness meditation, the meditator is instructed to do the following:

1. Sit in a comfortable and quiet position, with the eyes closed and any restrictive clothing loosened. You may find that moving a couple of inches from side to side two or three times before stopping will help you find a position that feels aligned. Tell yourself that for the next 5 (or 10, 15, or 20) minutes you are going to relax and care for yourself. Begin to breathe slowly, deeply, and regularly from the diaphragm.
2. Do a mental inventory of your body; as you become aware of any part of your body that is tense, purposefully relax it. (It may be easiest to do this with exhalations.) As you become more deeply relaxed, scan your body again, noticing any areas of tension and relaxing them.
3. When you begin to feel a sense of inner calm or balance, simply continue to sit and experience this relaxation for as long as you wish. If distracting or disturbing thoughts arise, note them and allow them to go; do not think of them as good or bad or worry about their interference, but simply be aware of them and notice that they pass as readily as they occurred. At the conclusion, rest for a minute or two before returning to your normal activities.
4. Repeat this once or twice daily.

Another variation, meditation to a mantra, is done as follows:

1. Sit in a comfortable position, with the eyes closed. Begin to breathe slowly, deeply, and regularly.
2. Slowly and silently (mentally) repeat a word, sound, or phrase that you find relaxing or comforting. (A word such as "one," "peace," or "relax" may be suggested if you cannot decide on one at first.) The silent mantra may or may not be coordinated with the breathing. If it is, it may be repeated with each inhalation and exhalation, or it may be repeated only with each exhalation.
3. Some variations of mantra meditation (e.g., transcendental meditation) instruct the meditator to ignore distracting thoughts purposefully and focus on the mantra. Others suggest that the meditator simply notice that a thought has entered the mind and then effortlessly allow the thought to leave as he returns to the focus on his breathing. This "permissiveness" supposedly allows the patient to become desensitized to any distracting or stressful thoughts that may arise during meditation.

4. Repeat for a period of 10–20 minutes once or twice a day. Rest for a minute or two at the conclusion before resuming your normal activities.

Meditation should be used cautiously with hysterical or excessively dependent patients and is not advisable for psychotic ones. It is most helpful for patients with chronic tension, depression, or anxiety states. Imaginative patients who have learned to meditate may also use visualization of peaceful scenes (e.g., a meadow, mountain top, ocean shore) to deepen their feeling of relaxation.

Active patients who find it difficult to relax readily may be taught the simple technique of progressive muscle relaxation, which consists of progressively contracting and then relaxing the major muscle groups. Eventually the patient becomes able to institute deep skeletal muscle relaxation at will, which helps to dissipate emotional tension. Progressive muscle relaxation is particularly helpful for patients with chronic anxiety or psychosomatic disorders, and may be used in conjunction with breath control, meditation, or visualization. The steps of the technique are as follows:

1. Sit or lie in a comfortable position, with the eyes closed. Through the nose, inhale deeply, using the muscles of the abdomen rather than those of the chest. Hold the breath for a few seconds and then exhale sharply through the mouth all at once, dropping and relaxing the shoulders, arms, jaw, and other body parts as you exhale. Repeat this a few times.
2. Inhale and hold the breath, and at the same time tighten the entire right arm by making a fist. Focus on tightening the fist and raise the entire arm about 6 in. off the floor (if you are lying down) or the body (if you are sitting).
3. Release the breath all at once through the mouth and allow the arm to drop to the floor or your side. Roll the arm slightly and note how it feels in comparison to the left arm.
4. Repeat (steps 2 and 3) once more with the right arm.
5. Repeat the entire procedure with the left arm twice.
6. Repeat with the rest of the body, progressing next to the entire right leg, left leg, abdomen, chest, shoulders, back, neck, and face. (Do the procedure twice for each body part.)
7. Conclude by lying (or sitting) relaxed and experiencing how the muscles feel while loose and free of tension. This may be followed by meditation.

Active or restless patients seem to benefit most from physical exercise programs, sometimes supplemented by meditation. Stretching exercises (several books teaching a variety of standing and floor stretching exercises are available) or simple repetitive exercises (e.g., walking, jogging, biking, swimming) are the most helpful, or the patient may prefer to seek instruction in one of the many available movement therapies, such as t'ai chi ch'uan, hatha yoga, or aikido. Patients who suffer from stress-related psychosomatic disorders but who are not tense or anxious are best referred to a professional for biofeedback-assisted relaxation training. Patients who seem to be deriving an important secondary gain (attention, freedom from responsibilities, etc.) should be referred for psychologic counseling. Also, for stress related to thinking patterns (e.g., unrealistic or distorted ideas), some form of cognitive therapy (psychotherapy) aimed at locating and correcting destructive thought patterns is appropriate.

Patient Education: It may be helpful to create a one- to two-page hand-out explaining the elements of a particular technique (meditative relaxation, progressive muscle relaxation) for the patient to refer to later on at home, along with a short list of available books or cassettes tapes on such topics as stress-reduction, meditation, and yoga.

Follow-up: Use follow-up visits to encourage the patient's adherence to a chosen technique or program or to suggest an alternative technique if a particular one is unsuccessful.

▸ *Organizations for Abused Adults and Victims of Childhood Sexual Abuse*

Laboratory Tests: None.

Therapeutic Measures: None.

Patient Education: Let Incest Victims Emerge (LIVE) is a support organization for adult survivors of childhood incest. Contact LIVE at (914) 425-2405 for information about similar local organizations. Other helpful organizations are as follows:

VOICE (Victims of Incest Can Emerge)
P.O. Box 142
Westminster, California 92684

National Coalition Against Domestic Violence
2401 Virginia Avenue
Suite 306
Washington, D.C. 20037
Tel.: (202) 223-2256

Other possible sources of information about support groups include local psychotherapists, mental health clinics, the National Organization for Women (NOW), and Planned Parenthood:

National NOW
1401 New York Avenue, NW
Suite 800
Washington, D.C. 20005-2102
Tel.: (202) 347-2279

Planned Parenthood Federation
810 7th Avenue
New York, New York 10019
Tel.: (212) 541-7800 or (212) 603-4600

Also, check local listings for both of these organizations.

Follow-up: Provide assistance as needed in making contact with support groups.

▸ *Considerations for the Dying Patient*

Laboratory Tests: None.

Therapeutic Measures: The issue of whether or not to tell a patient (or certain family members) if the diagnosis is unfavorable is continually debated. As a general rule, remember that your first responsibility is to the patient, and that he has a right to be told (or not be told) whatever information is available about his condition. By the time the diagnosis has been confirmed, more than one previous visit is likely to have occurred, including one in which the differential diagnosis (which probably included the correct one) was discussed, so the patient may already have communicated a desire to be told everything. In that case, he should be told all that there is to know, but the way he is given the information will depend on a number of variables, including how he responds. During the visit in which a patient with a condition carrying a poor prognosis (e.g., a carcinoma) is first told of the diagnosis, little else that you say is apt to be heard. For this reason, it is important to arrange for several (frequent) follow-up visits in order to discuss the appropriate course of therapy, expected treatment outcome, and other questions or concerns the patient may have. In all instances, it is important to present even the total truth about a condition in such a way that the patient is allowed some (reasonable) measure of hope. This may not necessarily be the hope for recovery, but it should certainly include the hope that the patient will retain some measure of control over his life and circumstances and can expect whatever support and assistance he requires to make the remainder of his life bearable. Under no circumstances should you lie about the chances of a recovery that is nonexistent, but it is important to be sensitive to the times when a patient, no matter how much he has expressed a desire to be told the truth, resists the full impact of that truth, and to not try to force the issue. Whenever possible, you should also present the truth in a way which does not emphasize the negative aspects. For instance, you may initially avoid using the word "cancer" until you see how the patient responds, but if the patient asks, you should be very clear. When a patient asks what his chances are of surviving, it is always truthful to say that you do not really know but that you have some statistics you can share with him. Be very careful in using statistics; try to present them in the best possible way and, if there is no positive way to present them (i.e., if the odds of survival are 1 in 1,000), avoid them altogether. If the patient's family requests that you not tell the patient, consider whether this is due to a valid concern about the patient's ability to handle the news or whether it is their attempt to avoid having to deal with the implications. Once again, while you should be sensitive to the needs of family members, your primary responsibility is to the patient, and if he has said that he wishes to know the truth about his condition, explain this to the family or discuss it with the patient and try to assist him in involving the family in discussions. On the other hand, the wishes of patients who state that they do not wish to know about a bad prognosis or who continually resist attempts to give them information should be respected. They may be coping with the situation in the only way available to them, and have the right to do so. However, you should continue to make more open discussion of the condition or the patient's feelings available to the patient (i.e., by spending time with the patient and communicating your support and willingness to listen), should his desire change, *without* pressing the issue.

It is also not necessary that the primary care provider be the only one the patient talks with about his condition. It is only important that the patient have at least one person with whom he can talk freely if he so desires. It is helpful to ask patients at some point if there is anyone else they would like to talk with, since there may be a particular person (nurse, social worker, member of the clergy) who has established such rapport with them that discussion of feelings is greatly facilitated. The presence of such a person does not, however, negate your responsibility to be available for the same purposes.

Also, the decision to terminate medical treatment (except for palliative efforts) should be made with the full involvement and consent of the patient and family. At that time, the alternatives for management and location of an optimum environment can be discussed, including the possibility of home or hospice care and the possibility of drawing up a living will (in which the patient specifies the types of treatment he wishes to receive or not receive under certain circumstances). Regardless of the nature of these decisions or who else becomes involved in the patient's care, at no time should you withdraw emotionally or otherwise from the patient or family. While it may be important to maintain some emotional distance from the situation in order to avoid becoming unhealthily involved, it is important to confront your own feelings about the patient's condition. Your acceptance of your own mortality is also an important aspect of the relationship with the patient and his family; primary care providers who are unwilling to confront their own mortality may foster shame in a dying patient or find themselves unable to be as compassionate and supportive as the patient deserves. It may be helpful for the provider to discuss these feelings with a friend or colleague, and to ask others how they handle similar situations.

Patient Education: There are a number of local and national resources available for patients and families confronted with a terminal illness. Organizations that deal with cancer include the following:

CanSurmount
777 Third Avenue
New York, New York 10017
Tel.: (212) 371-2900

I Can Cope
(same address and phone number as above)

Other helpful resources include The Concern for Dying, an organization that distributes "The Living Will." Another is The National Hospice Organization, which includes groups and institutions concerned with providing care for terminally ill patients and their families. It provides information about local hospice facilities and ways to incorporate the hospice philosophy in other settings.

The Concern for Dying
250 W. 57th Street
New York, New York 10019
Tel.: (212) 246-6962

The National Hospice Organization
1901 N. Ft. Myer Drive
Arlington, Virginia 22209
Tel.: (703) 243-5900

Follow-up: Maintain close, open contact with patients and family members throughout the course of illness.

BIBLIOGRAPHY

American Psychiatric Association. *Diagnostic and Statistical Manual of Mental Disorders,* 3rd ed. Washington, D.C., 1980.

Anstett RE, Poole SR. Depressive equivalents in adults. *American Family Physician,* 25(3):151–156.

Bassuk EL. The prevention of suicide: Is it possible? *Emergency Decisions,* (Mar.) 1985, 24–35.

Bellak L, Sheehy M. The broad role of ego functions. *American Journal of Psychiatry,* 1976, 133:1259.

Berkow RB (ed.). *The Merck Manual of Diagnosis and Therapy,* 14th ed. Merck Sharp & Dohme Research Laboratories, Rahway, N.J., 1982.

Burgess AW. *Psychiatric Nursing in the Hospital and the Community.* Prentice-Hall, Englewood Cliffs, N.J., 1981.

Cadoret RJ. The family physician and the psychiatrist: A complementary management team. *Family Practice Recertification,* 1982, 4(1):49–54.

Cain R, Cain N. A compendium of psychiatric drugs. In: Backer B, Dubbert P, Eisenman E (eds.): *Psychiatric/Mental Health Nursing: Contemporary Readings.* Van Nostrand, New York, 1978, pp. 313–348.

Carlson JP, Murray CL, Martinson P. The hospice concept: Comfort care for dying patients. *Postgraduate Medicine,* 1985, 77(2):55–66.

Cordoba OA. Antipsychotic medications: Clinical use and effectiveness. *Hospital Practice,* (Dec.) 1981, 99–108.

Davidson J. When and how to use MAO inhibitors. *PA Drug Update,* (Apr.) 1983, 50–63.

DeGennaro M, et al. Antidepressant drug therapy. *American Journal of Nursing,* (July) 1981, 81:1304.

Devaul RA, Jervey FL. Delirium: A neglected medical emergency. *American Family Physician,* (Dec.) 1981, 24(6):152–157.

Dipalma JR. Cocaine abuse and toxicity. *American Family Physician,* (Nov.) 1981, 24(5):236–238.

Donlon PT. Problems in family practice: Primary affective disorders. *Journal of Family Practice,* 1979, 9(4):689–699.

Drake VK. Battered women: A health care problem in disguise. *Image,* (June) 1982, 14:40.

Dunham HW. Schizophrenia: The impact of sociocultural factors. *Hospital Practice,* (Aug.) 1977, 61–668.

Epstein LJ. Clinical management of anxiety: Psychiatric consultation. In: *Diagnosis and Treatment of Anxiety in the Aged,* Part IV: *Clinical Management of Anxiety.* Hoffmann-La Roche, 1979, pp. 23–31.

Erikson E. *The Life Cycle Completed.* Norton, New York, 1982, pp. 32–33.

Fann WE. Pharmacological management of anxiety in the elderly. In: *Diagnosis and Treatment of Anxiety in the Aged,* Part IV: *Clinical Management of Anxiety.* Hoffmann-La Roche, 1979, pp. 43–54.

Feighner J. Pharmacological management of depression. *Family Practice Recertification,* 1982, 4(1):13–22.

Frederick C. The role of the nurse in crisis intervention and suicide prevention. In: Backer B, Dubbert P, Eisenman E (eds.): *Psychiatric/Mental Health Nursing: Contemporary Readings.* Van Nostrand, New York, 1978, pp. 193–203.

Fuller E. Psychiatric emergency!: Caring for the suicidal patient. *Patient Care,* (Nov.) 1980, 101–134.

Garvey MJ, Tollefson G. Suicide. *American Family Physician,* 1982, 25(5):157–159.

Gaylin W. *Feelings.* Harper & Row, New York, 1979.

Geyman JP. Office management of anxiety in older patients. In: *Diagnosis and Treatment of Anxiety in the Aged,* Part IV: *Clinical Management of Anxiety.* Hoffmann-La Roche, 1979, pp. 5–20.

Goldfrank L, Osborn H. Lithium toxicity. (RS Weisman, ed.). *Physician Assistant and Health Practitioner,* (Sept.) 1980, 67–72.

Goldfrank L, et al. Withdrawal? *Physician Assistant and Health Practitioner,* (Sept.) 1982, 13–32.

Gottheil E, Weinstein SP. Cocaine: Today's drug. *Medical Times,* (Oct.) 1983, 33–37.

Graber RF (ed.). The physician as healer: Helping your patient face death. *Patient Care,* 1985, 19(10):40–69.

Harris E. Lithium. *American Journal of Nursing,* (July) 1981, 81:1310.

Hasan MK, Mooney RP. Once-a-day drug regimen for psychiatric patients. *American Family Physician,* (Oct.) 1981, 24(4):123–125.

Hawkins RO Jr, Friedman E. Human sexuality: A content area for continuing medical education. *The PA Journal,* (winter) 1978, 8(4):217–219.

Herzog DB. Anorexia nervosa: A treatment challenge. *Drug Therapy,* (Mar.) 1982, 103–110.

Hoff L, Resing M. Was this suicide preventable? *American Journal of Nursing,* (July) 1982, 82:1106.

Hollister L. Office management of depression: Diagnosis. *Consultant,* (Jan.) 1980, 221–223.

Hollister L. Office management of depression: Treatment. *Consultant,* (Feb.) 1980, 121–127.

Holmes TH, Rahe RH. The social readjustment rating scale. *Journal of Psychosomatic Research,* 1967, 11(2):213–218.

Houghton B. Domestic violence training: Treatment of adult victims of family violence. *Journal of the New York State Nurses Association,* (Dec.) 1981, 12:25.

Imboden JB, Urbaitis JC. Practical psychiatry in medicine, part 15: Schizophrenic disorders. *Journal of Family Practice,* 1979, 9(5):939–970.

Janowsky DS. Management of depression in the elderly. *Family Practice Recertification,* 1982, 4(1):37–47.

Kiev A. *The Courage to Live.* Crowell, New York, 1979.

Koop CE. Statement on marijuana. *Medical Times,* (Oct.) 1983, 70–71.

Kozier B, Erb G. *Fundamentals of Nursing.* Addison-Wesley, Calif., 1979.

Krupp MA, Chatton MJ, Werdegar D (eds.). *Current Medical Diagnosis and Treatment 1985.* Lange, Los Altos, Calif., 1984.

Landers DF. Alcohol withdrawal syndrome. *American Family Physician,* (May) 1983, 27(5):114–118.

Lantner IL, O'Brien JE, Voth HM. Answering questions about marijuana use. *Patient Care,* (May) 1980, 112–148.

Levenson AJ. Clinical manifestations of anxiety: A psychiatrists's viewpoint. In: *Diagnosis and Treatment of Anxiety in the Aged,* Part III: *Clinical Manifestations of Anxiety.* Hoffmann-La Roche, 1979, pp. 15–22.

Lipman AG. What are the pharmacologic effects of marijuana? *Modern Medicine,* (Mar. 15–30) 1979, 105–106.

Lippmann S. Antidepressant pharmacotherapy. *American Family Physician,* 1982, 25(6):145–153.

Lippmann S. Lithium's effects on the kidney. *Postgraduate Medicine,* 1982, 71(3):99–108.

Loebl S, Spratto G. *The Nurse's Drug Handbook* 3rd ed. Wiley, New York, 1986.

Manschreck TC. Drug treatment of schizophrenia: Principles and limitations. *Drug Therapy,* (Sept.) 1983, 185–203.

McCandless H. Managing depression in family practice. *Family Practice Recertification,* 1982, 4(1):25–35.

McLaughlin BE. Recognizing the depressed patient—in time. *Diagnosis,* (May) 1980, 73–81.

Meredith HL. Munchausen syndrome. *Physician Assistant and Health Practitioner,* (Feb.) 1980, 33–38.

Miller MS. *Child Stress.* Doubleday, New York, 1982.

Nadelson CC, Notman MT. Caring for the rape victim: How to conduct the initial examination. *The Female Patient,* 1985, 10(3):84–91.

Nemiah J. The dynamic bases of psychopathology. In: *The Harvard Guide to Modern Psychiatry.* Harvard University Press, Cambridge, Mass., 1978.

Ostchega Y, Jacob JG. Providing "safe conduct": Helping your patient cope with cancer. *Nursing 84,* (Apr.) 1984, 42–47.

Pasguali E, et al. *Mental Health Nursing.* Mosby, St. Louis, 1981.

Peplau H. *Interpersonal Relations in Nursing.* Putnam, New York, 1952.

Pfizer Laboratories Division. Controlled substances: Uses and effects (table). Pfizer, New York, 1982.

Provenzale JM. Anorexia nervosa: Thinness as illness. *Postgraduate Medicine,* (Oct.) 1983, 74(4):83–89.

Richardson JI. The manipulative patient spells trouble. *Nursing 81,* (Jan.) 1981, 11:49.

Rohde J, et al. Diagnosis and treatment of anorexia nervosa. *Journal of Family Practice,* 1980, 10(6):1007–1012.

Salzberger GJ. Tardive dyskinesia: Prevalence and risk factors in long-term neuroleptic therapy. *Medical Times* (Feb.) 1985, 57–60.

Satir V. Conjoint family therapy. *Science and Behavior,* 1967.

Sausser GJ, Fishburne SB Jr, Everett VD. Outpatient detoxification of the alcoholic. *Journal of Family Practice,* 1982, 14(5):863–867.

Skom JH. Combating prescription drug abuse. *Medical Times,* (Oct.) 1983, 43–50.

Sternburg JK, Scheibel W. Terminal care. *Journal of Family Practice,* 1982, 14(6):995–1008.

Stuart G, Sundeen S. *Principles and Practice of Psychiatric Nursing.* Mosby, St. Louis, 1979.

Sutterley D, Donnelly G. *Perspectives in Human Development.* Lippincott, Philadelphia, 1973.

Talley JH. Suicide prevention: On not being part of the problem. *Consultant,* (June) 1983, 33–41.

Tennant FS Jr, Pumphrey EA. Management of opioid-dependent patients. *Medical Times,* (Oct.) 1983, 59–62.

Thompson TL III, Thompson WL. Treating depression: Tricyclics, tetracyclics, and other options. *Modern Medicine,* (Aug.) 1983, 87–109.

Tollefson G, Lesar T, Teubner-Rhodes D. Anxiety states and benzodiazepines. *American Family Physician,* 1983, 27(5):151–158.

Vaillant GE, Milofsky ES. Natural history of male alcoholism, part IV: Paths to recovery. *Archives of General Psychiatry,* (Feb.) 1982, 39:127–133.

Weisman AD. Coping with illness. In: Hackett T, Cassem N (eds.): *Massachusetts General Hospital Handbook of General Hospital Psychiatry.* St. Louis, 1978, pp. 264–75.

Wertheimer AJ. Examination of the rape victim. *Postgraduate Medicine,* 1982, 71(3):173–180.

Widmer RB. Early identification of the depressed patient. *Family Practice Recertification,* 1982, 4(1):7–12.

Wyngaarden JB, Smith LH Jr (eds.). *Cecil Textbook of Medicine,* 16th ed., Vols. 1 and 2. Saunders, Philadelphia, 1982.

Zisook S, Hall RCW, Gammon E. Drug treatment of depression: A classification system for agent selection. *Postgraduate Medicine,* 1980, 67(5):153–161.

Index